SAUNDERS
PHARMACEUTICAL
WORD BOOK

1997

ELLEN DRAKE, CMT
RANDY DRAKE, BS

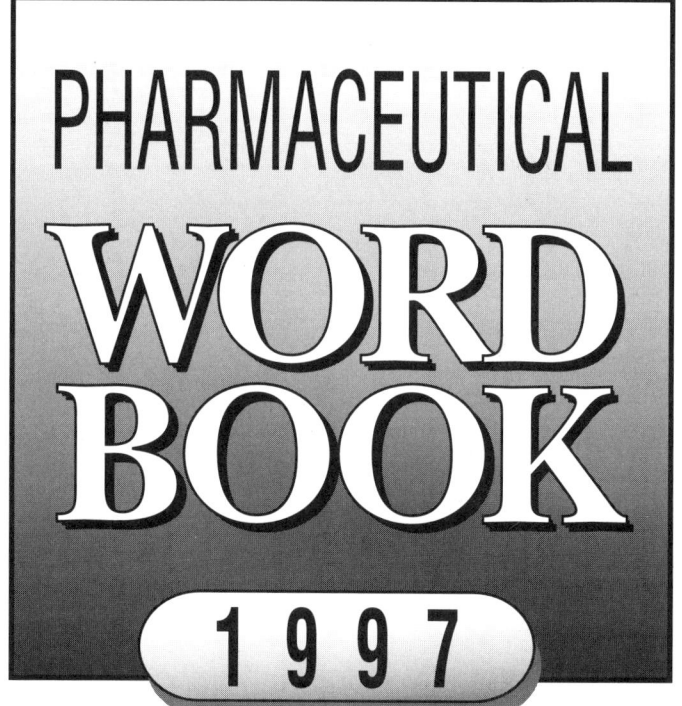

SAUNDERS

PHARMACEUTICAL WORD BOOK

1997

W.B. SAUNDERS COMPANY
A Division of Harcourt Brace & Company
Philadelphia London Toronto Montreal Sidney Tokyo

W.B. SAUNDERS COMPANY
A Division of
Harcourt Brace & Company

The Curtis Center
Independence Square West
Philadelphia, Pennsylvania 19106

SAUNDERS PHARMACEUTICAL WORD BOOK 1997   ISBN 0-7216-7249-3

Copyright © 1997, 1996, 1995, 1994, 1992 by W.B. Saunders Company.

All rights reserved. No part of this publication may be reproduced or transmitted in any form or by any means, electronic or mechanical, including photocopying, recording, or any information storage and retrieval system, without permission in writing from the publisher.

ISSN 1072-7779

Printed in the United States of America.

Last digit is the print number: 9   8   7   6   5   4   3   2   1

To the Lord Jesus

"Hear attentively the thunder of His voice,
    And the rumbling that comes from His mouth.
He sends it forth under the whole heaven,
    His lightning to the ends of the earth.
After it a voice roars;
    He thunders with His majestic voice,
    And He does not restrain them when His voice is heard.
God thunders marvelously with His voice;
    He does great things which we cannot comprehend.
For He says to the snow, 'Fall on the earth';
    Likewise to the gentle rain and the heavy rain of His strength.
He seals the hand of every man,
    That all men may know His work.
The animals enter dens,
    And remain in their lairs.
From the chamber of the south comes the whirlwind,
    And cold from the scattering winds of the north.
By the breath of God ice is given,
    And the broad waters are frozen.
Also with moisture, He saturates the thick clouds;
    He scatters His bright clouds.
And they swirl about, being turned by His guidance,
    That they may do whatever He commands them
    On the face of the whole earth.
He causes it to come,
    Whether for correction,
        Or for His land,
            Or for mercy.

Stand still and consider the wondrous works of God."

— Job 37:2–14

Preface

What an exciting time to be in the healthcare profession! New drugs are being introduced every month, offering newer and more effective treatments. New uses for old drugs are being explored, and entirely new classes of drugs are being discovered. As always, we include this cutting-edge product research within these pages. Investigational and orphan drugs account for some 1676 entries in this edition. Many drugs newly approved for marketing this year have appeared in previous editions as "investigational." With each annual edition, you will keep up-to-date on the latest pharmaceutical research and will truly receive "tomorrow's news today"!

For the first time this year, we have used the Internet as an information source. Many pharmaceutical companies, research hospitals, and government agencies provide the latest information through this medium, and we have taken full advantage of the resources provided. We have also been granted access to online services usually restricted to physicians only. In hundreds of hours of online research, we have found the most useful and reliable sources of drug information.

This 1997 edition includes dosages for generic drugs, completing our goal to include dosages for all products. This information is presented in a slightly different format from dosages for brand name drugs (included last year). We invite you to compare the entry formats on pages xi and xii.

Among the 23,857 entries are over 1200 changes from last year's edition, including over 500 brand new entries! Other interesting statistics appear in the "Notes on Using the Text" at the bottom of page ix.

Appendix E, The Most-Prescribed Drugs, has been a popular "quick reference" for transcriptionists and transcription students alike. The list has been updated for 1997, with changes in prescribing patterns reflected by several additions and deletions to last year's list. This list covers over 50% of prescriptions filled at retail pharmacies (i.e., *not* hospital formularies).

In the main section of the book, drug names, whether trade, generic, or chemical, are in bold print for greater ease of reading. Brand (trade) names appear with appropriate capitalization, with generic and chemical names shown in lower case—the way transcription style guides recommend they be typed.

We think you will find this fifth edition more complete and more valuable than ever; however, no book is ever perfect. We plan to keep our database current by adding new entries as the information becomes available. Although we have diligently tried to be as accurate and comprehensive as possible, we will certainly welcome your comments regarding additions, inconsistencies, or inaccuracies. Please send them to us at W.B. Saunders Company, The Curtis Center, Independence Square West, Philadelphia, PA 19106. We welcome your suggestions.

ELLEN DRAKE, CMT
RANDY DRAKE, BS
Orlando, Florida

Notes on Using the Text

The purpose of the *Saunders Pharmaceutical Word Book* is to provide the medical transcriptionist (as well as medical record administrators and technicians, coders, nurses, ward clerks, court reporters, legal secretaries, medical assistants, allied health students, and even physicians) a quick, easy-to-use reference that gives not only the correct spellings and capitalizations of drugs, but the designated uses of those drugs, the cross-referencing of brand names to generics, and the usual methods of administration (e.g., capsule, IV, cream). The indication of the preferred nonproprietary (generic) names and the agencies adopting these names (e.g., USAN, USP) should be particularly useful to those writing for publication. The reader will also find various trademarked or proprietary names (e.g., Spansule, Dosepak) that are not drugs but are closely associated with the packaging or administration of drugs.

There are four different ways to refer to drugs. One of these ways is not the name of the drug itself but the class to which it belongs—aminoglycosides for example. Inexperienced transcriptionists sometimes confuse these classes with the names of drugs. If you cannot find what you think is a drug in this reference, it may be that you are looking for a class of drugs. Try your dictionary. Every drug, however, has three names. The first is the *chemical name*, which describes its chemical composition and how the molecules are arranged. It is often long and complex, sometimes containing numbers, Greek letters, italicized letters, and hyphens between elements. This name is rarely used in dictation except in research hospitals and sometimes in the laboratory section when the blood or urine is examined for traces of the drug. The second name for a drug is the *nonproprietary* or *generic name*. This is a name chosen by the discovering manufacturer or agency and submitted to a nomenclature committee (the United States Adopted Names Council, for example). The name is simpler than the chemical name but often reflects the chemical entity. It is arrived at by using guidelines provided by the nomenclature committee and must be unique. There is increasing emphasis on the adoption of the same nonproprietary name by various nomenclature committees worldwide. The third name for a drug is the *trade* or *brand name*. There may be several trade names for the same generic drug, each marketed by a different company. These are the ones that are highly advertised, and sometimes have unusual capitalization. An interesting article on the naming of drugs is "Pharmaceutical Nomenclature: The Lawless Language" in *Perspectives on the Medical Transcription Profession.*[1] *Understanding Pharmacology*[2] also discusses the naming of drugs.

Special effort has been made to include experimental and investigational drugs (1033 entries), chemotherapy drugs (761 entries) and drug protocols (521 entries), drugs that have been recently discontinued by the manufacturer or withdrawn from the market by the Food and Drug Administration (1511 entries), and orphan drugs (739 entries). Orphan drugs are those products that have limited commercial appeal and are used for the treatment of relatively rare disease conditions. The government and FDA encourage the marketing of orphan drugs through subsidized research and the streamlining of the approval process. In an effort to provide necessary information without the book becoming too large and unwieldy, any drug withdrawn from the market five years ago or more is not included; therefore, drugs discontinued in 1991 or earlier have been dropped.

We have included many foreign names of drugs for our Canadian friends, and also because we have so many visitors to the United States from other countries (and they get sick, too). The international and British spellings of generic drugs are cross-referenced to the American spellings, and vice versa. Occasionally there will be three different spellings—one American, one international, and another British—which are all cross-referenced to each other. Other special features that may be useful, especially for students, are commonly used prescribing abbreviations and the sound-alike list which are found in the appendices. Another appendix gives the investigational codes (assigned to drugs before they are named), cross-referenced to their subsequent generic names. The Most-Prescribed Drugs and Therapeutic Drug Levels appendices will be useful as well.

This information was compiled using a variety of sources including direct communication with over 500 drug companies. The orphan entries are taken directly from the latest list issued by the FDA. When sources differed, we ranked our sources as to reliability and went with what we thought was the most reliable source. We recognize that there may be several published ways in which to type a single drug, but we have chosen to use only one of those ways. In the instance of internal capitalization (e.g., pHisoHex), it should be recognized that in most instances it is acceptable to type such words with initial capitalization only (Phisohex).

While we have made every attempt to include as much necessary information as possible, we have by no means tried to provide *prescribing information* as defined by the FDA. The given uses/actions for a particular drug are not all-inclusive, and the indications, contraindications, and side effects are not listed. Physicians should consult the *Physicians' Desk Reference*, package insert, or some other acceptable source for prescribing information.

How the Book Is Arranged

All entries are in alphabetical order by word. Initial numbers, chemical prefixes (*N*-, *p*-, *l*-, *d*-, etc.), and punctuation (prime, ampersands, etc.) are ignored. For example, L-dopa would be alphabetized under "dopa," but levodopa under "levo."

We have indicated brand names with initial capital letters unless an unusual combination of capitals and lower case has been designated by the manufacturer (e.g., pHisoHex, ALternaGEL). Generic names are rendered in lower case. Where the same name can be either generic or brand, both have been included.

Notes on Using the Text xi

The general format of a *generic* entry is:

entry council(s) *designated use* [other references] dosages 👂 sound-alike(s)
| #1 | | #2 | | #3 | | #4 | | #5 | | #6 |

1. The name of the drug (in bold).
2. The various agencies that have approved the name, shown in small caps, which may be any or all of the following (listed according to appearance in the book):
   USAN   United States Adopted Name Council
   USP   United States Pharmacopeial Convention
   NF   National Formulary
   FDA   U.S. Food & Drug Administration
   INN   International Nonproprietary Name (a project of the World Health Organization)
   BAN   British Approved Name
   JAN   Japanese Accepted Name
   DCF   Dénomination Commune Française (French)
3. The designated use, sometimes referred to as the drug's "therapeutic action." This is provided only for official FDA-approved names or other names for the same substance (e.g., the British name of an official U.S. generic). This entry is always in italic.
4. The entry in brackets is one of four cross-references:
   see: refers the reader to the "official" name(s).
   now: for an older generic name no longer used, refers reader to the current official name(s).
   also: a substance that has two or more different names, each officially recognized by one of the above groups, will cross-reference the other name(s).
   q.v.   Latin for quod vide; which see. Used exclusively for abbreviations, it invites the reader to turn to the reference in parentheses.
   If there is more than one cross reference, alternate names will follow the order of the above agency list; i.e., U.S. names, then international names, then British, Japanese, and French names. The first cross-reference will always be to the approved U.S. name, unless the entry itself is the U.S. name.
5. Dosage information, including the delivery form(s), is given for medications that may be dispensed generically. No dosage information appears for drugs dispensed only under the brand name, or for those containing multiple ingredients. Some drugs may be available in more than one strength, indicated by a comma in the dosage field:

   phentermine HCl USP *anorexiant; CNS stimulant* 8, 15, 18.75, 30, 37.5 mg oral

   A semicolon in the dosage field separates different delivery forms, such as:
   nitroglycerin USP *coronary vasodilator; antianginal* [also: glyceryl trinitrate] 2.5, 6.5, 9 mg oral; 5 mg/mL injection; 16–187.5 mg transdermal; 2% topical
   (Note that the oral and transdermal forms come in multiple strengths.)
6. Sound-alike drugs follow the "ear" icon.

xii Notes on Using the Text

The general format for a *brand name* entry is:

Entry	form(s)	℞/OTC	*designated use*	[generics]	dosages	👂 sound-alike(s)
#1	#2	#3	#4	#5	#6	#7

1. The drug name (in bold), which almost always starts with a capital letter.
2. The form of administration; e.g., tablets, capsules, syrup. (Sometimes these words are slurred by the dictator causing confusion regarding the name.)
3. The ℞ or OTC status. A few drugs may be either ℞ or OTC depending on strength or various state laws.[3]
4. The designated use in italics as for generics. These are more complete or less complete as supplied by the individual drug companies.
5. The brackets that follow contain the generic names of the active ingredients to which the reader may refer for further information.
6. Dosage information follows the generics. For multi-ingredient drugs, a bullet separates the dosages of each ingredient, listed in the same order as the generics. For example,
    Ser-Ap-Es tablets ℞ *antihypertensive* [hydrochlorothiazide; reserpine; hydralazine HCl] 15•0.1•25 mg
   shows a three-ingredient product containing 15 mg hydrochlorothiazide, 0.1 mg reserpine, and 25 mg hydralazine HCl.

   Some drugs may have more than one strength, indicated by a comma in the dosage field:
   Nitrodisc transdermal patch ℞ *antianginal* [nitroglycerin] 16, 24, 32 mg

   A semicolon in the dosage field separates either different products listed together, such as:
   Pred Mild; Pred Forte eye drop suspension ℞ *ophthalmic topical corticosteroidal anti-inflammatory* [prednisolone acetate] 0.12%; 1%

   Or different delivery forms:
   Phenergan tablets, suppositories, injection ℞ *antihistamine; motion sickness; sleep aid; antiemetic; sedative* [promethazine HCl] 12.5, 25 mg; 12.5, 25, 50 mg; 25, 50 mg/mL
   (Note that all three forms of Phenergan come in multiple strengths.)

   Liquid delivery forms show the strength per usual dose where appropriate. Thus injectables and drops are usually shown per milliliter (mL), with oral liquids and syrups shown per 5 mL or 15 mL.

   The $\triangleq$ symbol indicates that dosage information has not been supplied by the manufacturer for one or more ingredients.

   The $\pm$ symbol is used when a value *cannot* be given because the generic entry refers to multiple ingredients.
7. Sound-alike drugs follow the "ear" icon.

A Brief Note on the Transcription of Drugs

Many references are available describing several acceptable ways to transcribe drug information when dictated. For exhaustive discussions of these methods, the reader is referred to Fordney and Diehl's *Medical Transcription Guide: Do's and Don'ts*,[4] or the American Medical Association *Manual of Style*.[5]

Although some institutions favor capitalizing every drug, others promote not capitalizing any drug, and yet others put drugs in all capital letters, the generally accepted style today for the transcription of medical reports for hospital and doctors' office charts (see the AMA *Manual of Style* for publications) is to capitalize the initial letter of brand name drugs and lower case generic name drugs. The institution may also designate that brand name drugs with unusual capitalization may be typed with initial capital letter only, or typed using the manufacturer's scheme.

In general, commas are omitted between the drug name, the dosage, and the instructions for purposes of simplification. Items in a series may be separated by either commas (if no internal commas are used) or semicolons. A simple series might be typed thus:

Procardia, nitroglycerin sublingual, and Tolinase

or

Procardia 10 mg three times a day, nitroglycerin 1/150 p.r.n., and Tolinase 100 mg twice a day.

or

Procardia 10 mg t.i.d., nitroglycerin 1/150 p.r.n., and Tolinase 100 mg b.i.d.

A more complex or lengthy list of medications, or a list with internal commas, may require the use of semicolons to separate the items in a series. For example,

Procardia 10 mg, one 3 times a day; nitroglycerin 1/150 p.r.n., to take one with onset of pain, a second in five minutes, and a third five minutes later, if no relief to go immediately to the ER; Tolinase 100 mg, one 2 times a day; and Coumadin 2.5 mg on Mondays, Wednesdays, and Fridays, and 5 mg on Tuesdays, Thursdays, and Saturdays...

Note that the "one" following Procardia 10 mg and Tolinase 100 mg is not necessary, but many doctors dictate something like this; when they do, it is acceptable to place a comma after the dosage. In addition, when two numbers are adjacent to each other, write out one number and use a numeral for the other.

The typing of chemicals with superscripts or subscripts, italics, small capitals, and Greek letters often presents a problem to the medical transcriptionist. In general, Greek letters are written out (alpha-, beta-, gamma-, etc.). Italics and small capitals are written as standard letters followed by a hyphen (dl-alpha-tocopherol, L-dopa).

When typing nonproprietary (generic) isotope names, element symbols should be included with the name. It may appear to be redundant, but it is the correct form. Therefore, we would type sodium pertechnetate Tc 99m, iodohippurate sodium I 131, or sodium iodide I 125. Occasionally the physician may simply dictate isotopes such as Tc 99m, iodine 131 or I 131, or sodium iodide I 125, and unless he is indicating a trademarked name, it should be typed with a space, no hyphen, and no superscript. This reference indicates proper capitalization, spacing, and hyphenation of isotope entries.

Other combinations of letters and numbers are usually written without spaces or hyphens (OKT1, OKT3, T101, SC1), but this is a complex subject and is dealt with extensively in the AMA *Manual of Style*.

---

[1] Dirckx, John, M.D.: "Pharmaceutical Nomenclature: The Lawless Language," *Perspectives on the Medical Transcription Profession*, Vol. 1, No. 4. Modesto: Health Professions Institute, 1991, p. 9.

[2] Turley, Susan M., CMT: *Understanding Pharmacology*. Englewood Cliffs: Regents/Prentice Hall, 1991.

[3] Some states are moving toward the creation of a third class of drugs between ℞ and OTC. These medications, while not being readily available on the shelf, could be dispensed by a licensed pharmacist without a doctor's prescription.

[4] Fordney, Marilyn and Diehl, Marcy: *Medical Transcription Guide: Do's and Don'ts*. Philadelphia: W.B. Saunders Co., 1990.

[5] American Medical Association: *Manual of Style*, 8th ed. Baltimore: Williams & Wilkins, 1989.

A (vitamin A) [q.v.]

A and D ointment OTC *moisturizer; emollient* [fish liver oil (vitamins A and D); cholecalciferol; lanolin] ≟

A and D Medicated ointment OTC *topical diaper rash treatment* [zinc oxide; vitamins A and D] ≟

A + D (ara-C, daunorubicin) *chemotherapy protocol*

A-200 shampoo concentrate (discontinued 1995) OTC *pediculicide* [pyrethrins; piperonyl butoxide] 0.33%•4%

A-200 Pyrinate gel (discontinued 1992) OTC *pediculicide* [pyrethrins; piperonyl butoxide technical; petroleum distillate]

AA (ara-C, Adriamycin) *chemotherapy protocol*

AA-HC Otic ear drops ℞ *topical corticosteroidal anti-inflammatory; antibacterial/antifungal* [hydrocortisone; acetic acid] 1%•2%

abamectin USAN, INN *antiparasitic*

abanoquil INN, BAN

Abbokinase IV or intracoronary artery infusion ℞ *thrombolytic* [urokinase] 250,000 IU/vial

Abbokinase Open-Cath liquid for catheter clearance ℞ *thrombolytic* [urokinase] 5000 IU/mL

Abbo-Pac (trademarked packaging form) *unit dose package*

Abbott HIVAB HIV-1 EIA test kit (name changed to HIVAB HIV-1 EIA in 1995)

Abbott HIVAG-1 test kit (name changed to HIVAG-1 in 1995)

Abbott HTLV I EIA test kit (name changed to Human T-Lymphotropic Virus Type I EIA in 1995)

Abbott HTLV III Confirmatory EIA test kit for professional use (discontinued 1995) *in vitro diagnostic aid for HTLV III antibody* [enzyme immunoassay (EIA)]

Abbott TestPack Plus hCG-Urine Plus test kit for professional use *in vitro diagnostic aid for urine pregnancy test* [monoclonal antibody-based enzyme immunoassay]

Abbott TestPack Strep A kit (name changed to Test Pack in 1995)

ABC (Adriamycin, BCNU, cyclophosphamide) *chemotherapy protocol*

ABC to Z tablets OTC *vitamin/mineral/ iron supplement* [multiple vitamins & minerals; ferrous fumarate; folic acid; biotin] ≟•18 mg•0.4 mg•30 μg

abciximab (monoclonal antibody 7E3) USAN, INN *monoclonal antibody; antiplatelet agent for acute arterial occlusive disorders*

ABCM (Adriamycin, bleomycin, cyclophosphamide, mitomycin) *chemotherapy protocol*

ABD (Adriamycin, bleomycin, DTIC) *chemotherapy protocol*

ABDIC (Adriamycin, bleomycin, DIC, [CCNU, prednisone]) *chemotherapy protocol*

ABDV (Adriamycin, bleomycin, DTIC, vinblastine) *chemotherapy protocol*

ABE (antitoxin botulism equine) [see: botulism equine antitoxin, trivalent]

abecarnil INN *investigational anxiolytic*

Abelcet suspension for IV infusion ℞ *systemic antifungal for aspergillosis* [amphotericin B lipid complex (ABLC)] 5 mg/mL

Abitrexate IV or IM injection ℞ *antineoplastic for leukemia; systemic antipsoriatic; antirheumatic* [methotrexate sodium]

ABLC [see: TLC ABLC]

ABLC (amphotericin B lipid complex) [q.v.]

ablukast USAN, INN *antiasthmatic; leukotriene antagonist*

ablukast sodium USAN *antiasthmatic; leukotriene antagonist*

ABP (Adriamycin, bleomycin, prednisone) *chemotherapy protocol*

ABPP (aminobromophenylpyrimidinone) [see: bropirimine]

absorbable cellulose cotton [see: cellulose, oxidized]

absorbable dusting powder [see: dusting powder, absorbable]

absorbable gelatin film [see: gelatin film, absorbable]
absorbable gelatin powder [see: gelatin powder, absorbable]
absorbable gelatin sponge [see: gelatin sponge, absorbable]
absorbable surgical suture [see: suture, absorbable surgical]
Absorbase OTC *ointment base* [water-in-oil emulsion of cholesterolized petrolatum and purified water]
absorbent gauze [see: gauze, absorbent]
Absorbine Antifungal cream, powder OTC *topical antifungal* [tolnaftate] 1%
Absorbine Antifungal Foot aerosol powder OTC *topical antifungal* [miconazole nitrate] 2%
Absorbine Arthritic Pain lotion (discontinued 1994) OTC *counterirritant* [methyl salicylate; camphor; menthol; methyl nicotinate] 10% • 3.25% • 1.25% • 1%
Absorbine Athlete's Foot Care liquid OTC *topical antifungal* [tolnaftate] 1%
Absorbine Jock Itch powder OTC *topical antifungal* [tolnaftate] 1%
Absorbine Jr. liniment OTC *counterirritant* [menthol] 1.27%, 4%
Absorbine Jr. Antifungal spray liquid OTC *topical antifungal* [tolnaftate] 1%
Absorbine Jr. Extra Strength liquid OTC *counterirritant* [menthol] 4%
Absorbine Power gel OTC *counterirritant* [menthol] 4%
abunidazole INN
ABV (actimomycin D, bleomycin, vincristine) *chemotherapy protocol*
ABV (Adriamycin, bleomycin, vinblastine) *chemotherapy protocol*
ABVD (Adriamycin, bleomycin, vinblastine, dacarbazine) *chemotherapy protocol*
ABVD/MOPP (alternating cycles of ABVD and MOPP) *chemotherapy protocol*
AC (Adriamycin, carmustine) *chemotherapy protocol*
AC (Adriamycin, CCNU) *chemotherapy protocol*
AC (Adriamycin, cisplatin) *chemotherapy protocol*

AC; A-C (Adriamycin, cyclophosphamide) *chemotherapy protocol*
AC 137 *investigational antidiabetic*
AC625 *investigational amylin blocker antihypertensive for overweight patients*
ACA-147 *investigational AcylCoA cholesterol acyltransferase inhibitor for reducing serum cholesterol*
acacia NF, JAN *suspending agent; emollient; demulcent*
Acacia senegal [see: acacia]
acadesine USAN, INN, BAN *platelet aggregation inhibitor*
A-Caine Rectal ointment (discontinued 1995) OTC *topical anesthetic; vasoconstrictor; astringent* [diperodon HCl; pyrilamine maleate; phenylephrine HCl; bismuth subcarbonate; zinc oxide] 0.25% • 0.1% • 0.25% • 0.2% • 5% ⑨ Anocaine
acamprosate 6473 INN
acamylophenine [see: camylofin]
acaprazine INN
acarbose USAN, INN, BAN α-*glucosidase inhibitor; antidiabetic agent*
ACAT (AcylCoA transferase) inhibitor *investigational agent to lower serum cholesterol levels*
Accolate ℞ *investigational leukotriene receptor antagonist for asthma* [zafirlukast]
Accu-Chek Advantage reagent strips for home use OTC *in vitro diagnostic aid for blood glucose*
Accu-Pak (trademarked packaging form) *unit dose blister pack*
Accupep HPF powder OTC *enteral nutritional therapy for GI impairment*
Accupril film-coated tablets ℞ *antihypertensive; angiotensin-converting enzyme (ACE) inhibitor* [quinapril HCl] 5, 10, 20, 40 mg
Accurbron syrup ℞ *antiasthmatic* [theophylline; alcohol 7.5%] 150 mg/15 mL ⑨ Accutane
Accusens T multi-sample kit (discontinued 1995) *in vitro diagnostic aid for taste dysfunction*
AccuSite injection ℞ *investigational agent for genital warts*

Accutane capsules ℞ *internal keratolytic for severe cystic acne* [isotretinoin] 10, 20, 40 mg ⓓ Accurbron

ACD solution (acid citrate dextrose; anticoagulant citrate dextrose) [see: anticoagulant citrate dextrose solution]

ACD whole blood [see: blood, whole]

ACe (Adriamycin, cyclophosphamide) *chemotherapy protocol*

ACE (Adriamycin, cyclophosphamide, etoposide) *chemotherapy protocol* [also: CAE]

acebrochol INN, DCF

aceburic acid INN, DCF

acebutolol USAN, INN, BAN *antihypertensive; antiarrhythmic; antiadrenergic (β-receptor)* [also: acebutolol HCl]

acebutolol HCl JAN *antihypertensive; antiarrhythmic; antiadrenergic (β-receptor)* [also: acebutolol] 200, 400 mg oral

acecainide INN *antiarrhythmic* [also: acecainide HCl]

acecainide HCl USAN *antiarrhythmic* [also: acecainide]

acecarbromal INN *CNS depressant; sedative; hypnotic*

aceclidine USAN, INN *cholinergic*

aceclofenac INN, BAN

acedapsone USAN, INN, BAN *antimalarial; antibacterial; leprostatic*

acediasulfone sodium INN, DCF

acedoben INN

acefluranol INN, BAN

acefurtiamine INN

acefylline clofibrol INN

acefylline piperazine INN, DCF [also: acepifylline]

aceglaton JAN [also: aceglatone]

aceglatone INN [also: aceglaton]

aceglutamide INN *antiulcerative* [also: aceglutamide aluminum]

aceglutamide aluminum USAN, JAN *antiulcerative* [also: aceglutamide]

Acel-Imune IM injection ℞ *immunization against diphtheria, tetanus and pertussis* [diphtheria & tetanus toxoids & acellular pertussis vaccine (DTaP)] 7.5 LfU•5 LfU•300 HAU per 0.5 mL

acemannan USAN, INN *antiviral; immunomodulator; investigational (Phase I) for AIDS*

acemetacin INN, BAN, JAN

acemethadone [see: methadyl acetate]

aceneuramic acid INN

acenocoumarin [see: acenocoumarol]

acenocoumarol NF, INN [also: nicoumalone]

Aceon tablets (discontinued 1994) ℞ *antihypertensive; ACE inhibitor* [perindopril erbumine] 2, 4, 8 mg

aceperone INN

Acephen suppositories OTC *analgesic; antipyretic* [acetaminophen] 120, 320, 650 mg

acephenazine dimaleate [see: acetophenazine maleate]

acepifylline BAN [also: acefylline piperazine]

acepromazine INN, BAN *veterinary sedative* [also: acepromazine maleate]

acepromazine maleate USAN *veterinary sedative* [also: acepromazine]

aceprometazine INN, DCF

acequinoline INN, DCF

ACES soft capsules OTC *vitamin supplement* [vitamins A, C, and E; selenium methionine]

acesulfame INN, BAN

Aceta tablets, elixir OTC *analgesic; antipyretic* [acetaminophen] 325, 500 mg; 160 mg/5 mL

Aceta with Codeine tablets ℞ *narcotic analgesic* [codeine phosphate; acetaminophen] 30•300 mg

Aceta-Gesic tablets OTC *antihistamine; analgesic* [phenyltoloxamine citrate; acetaminophen] 30•325 mg

***p*-acetamidobenzoic acid** [see: acedoben]

6-acetamidohexanoic acid [see: acexamic acid]

4-acetamidophenyl acetate [see: diacetamate]

acetaminocaproic acid [see: acexamic acid]

acetaminophen USP *analgesic; antipyretic* [also: paracetamol] 80, 325, 500, 650 mg oral; 120, 130, 160 mg/5 mL oral; 120, 300, 325, 650 mg suppositories

acetaminophenol [see: acetaminophen]
acetaminosalol INN, DCF
acetanilid (or acetanilide) NF
acetannin [see: acetyltannic acid]
acetarsol INN, BAN, DCF [also: acetarsone]
acetarsone NF [also: acetarsol]
acetarsone salt of arecoline [see: drocarbil]
Acetasol ear drops ℞ *antibacterial/antifungal* [acetic acid] 2%
Acetasol HC ear drops ℞ *topical corticosteroidal anti-inflammatory; antibacterial/antifungal* [hydrocortisone; acetic acid] 1%•2%
acetazolamide USP, INN, BAN, JAN *carbonic anhydrase inhibitor; anticonvulsant* 125, 250 mg oral; 500 mg injection
acetazolamide sodium USP, JAN *carbonic anhydrase inhibitor*
acetcarbromal [see: acecarbromal]
acet-dia-mer-sulfonamide (sulfacetamide, sulfadiazine & sulfamerazine) [q.v.]
acetergamine INN
Acetest reagent tablets for professional use *in vitro diagnostic aid for acetone (ketones) in the urine or blood*
acetiamine INN
acetic acid NF, JAN *acidifying agent* 0.25%
acetic acid, aluminum salt [see: aluminum acetate]
acetic acid, calcium salt [see: calcium acetate]
acetic acid, diluted NF *bladder irrigant*
acetic acid, ethyl ester [see: ethyl acetate]
acetic acid, glacial USP, INN *acidifying agent*
acetic acid, potassium salt [see: potassium acetate]
acetic acid, sodium salt trihydrate [see: sodium acetate]
acetic acid, zinc salt dihydrate [see: zinc acetate]
acetic acid 5-nitrofurfurylidenehydrazide [see: nihydrazone]
aceticyl [see: aspirin]
acetilum acidulatum [see: aspirin]
acetiromate INN

acetohexamide USAN, USP, INN, BAN, JAN *sulfonylurea-type antidiabetic* 250, 500 mg oral
acetohydroxamic acid (AHA) USAN, USP, INN *urease enzyme inhibitor*
acetol [see: aspirin]
acetomenaphthone BAN
acetomeroctol
acetone NF *solvent; antiseptic*
acetophen [see: aspirin]
acetophenazine INN *antipsychotic* [also: acetophenazine maleate]
acetophenazine maleate USAN, USP *antipsychotic* [also: acetophenazine]
***p*-acetophenetidide** (*withdrawn from market*) [see: phenacetin]
acetophenetidin (*withdrawn from market*) [now: phenacetin]
acetorphine INN, BAN *enkephalinase inhibitor for acute diarrhea; investigational for opioid withdrawal and GERD*
acetosal [see: aspirin]
acetosalic acid [see: aspirin]
acetosalin [see: aspirin]
acetosulfone sodium USAN *antibacterial; leprostatic* [also: sulfadiasulfone sodium]
acetoxyphenylmercury [see: phenylmercuric acetate]
acetoxythymoxamine [see: moxisylyte]
acetphenarsine [see: acetarsone]
acetphenetidin (*withdrawn from market*) [now: phenacetin]
acetphenolisatin [see: oxyphenisatin acetate]
acetrizoate sodium USP [also: sodium acetrizoate]
acetrizoic acid USP
acetryptine INN
acetsalicylamide [see: salacetamide]
acet-theocin sodium [see: theophylline sodium acetate]
aceturate USAN, INN *combining name for radicals or groups*
acetyl adalin [see: acetylcarbromal]
acetyl L-carnitine [see: levacecarnine]
acetyl sulfisoxazole [see: sulfisoxazole acetyl]
***l*-acetyl-α-methadol (LAAM)** [see: levomethadyl acetate]

p-acetylaminobenzaldehyde thiosemicarbazone [see: thioacetazone; thiacetazone]
acetylaminobenzene [see: acetanilid]
N-acetyl-*p*-aminophenol (APAP; NAPA) [see: acetaminophen]
acetylaniline [see: acetanilid]
acetylated polyvinyl alcohol *viscosity-increasing agent*
acetyl-bromo-diethylacetylcarbamide [see: acecarbromal]
acetylcarbromal [see: acecarbromal]
acetylcholine chloride USP, INN, BAN, JAN *cardiac depressant; cholinergic; miotic; peripheral vasodilator*
acetylcysteine (N-acetylcysteine) USAN, USP, INN, BAN *mucolytic inhaler; investigational immunomodulator for AIDS; (orphan: severe acetaminophen overdose)* [also: N-acetyl-L-cysteine]
acetylcysteine sodium *mucolytic* 10%, 20% inhalation
acetyldigitoxin (α-acetyldigitoxin) NF, INN
acetyldihydrocodeinone [see: thebacon]
N-acetyl-DL-leucine [see: acetylleucine]
acetylin [see: aspirin]
acetylkitasamycin JAN *antibacterial* [also: kitasamycin; kitasamycin tartrate]
acetyl-L-carnitine (ALCAR) *investigational cognition enhancer for Alzheimer's disease*
N-acetyl-L-cysteine JAN *mucolytic inhaler; investigational immunomodulator for AIDS; (orphan: severe acetaminophen overdose)* [also: acetylcysteine]
N-acetyl-L-cysteine salicylate [see: salnacedin]
acetylleucine (N-acetyl-DL-leucine) INN
acetylmethadol INN, DCF *narcotic analgesic* [also: methadyl acetate]
acetyloleandomycin [see: troleandomycin]
2-acetyloxybenzoic acid [see: aspirin]
acetylpheneturide JAN [also: pheneturide]
acetylphenylisatin [see: oxyphenisatin acetate]
N-acetylprocainamide (NAPA) *(orphan status withdrawn 1996)*
acetylpropylorvinol [see: acetorphine]
acetylresorcinol [see: resorcinol monoacetate]
acetylsal [see: aspirin]
N-acetylsalicylamide [see: salacetamide]
acetylsalicylate aluminum [see: aspirin aluminum]
acetylsalicylic acid (ASA) [now: aspirin]
acetylsalicylic acid, phenacetin & caffeine [see: APC]
acetylspiramycin JAN *antibacterial* [also: spiramycin]
acetylsulfamethoxazole JAN *broad-spectrum bacteriostatic* [also: sulfamethoxazole; sulphamethoxazole; sulfamethoxazole sodium]
N^1-acetylsulfanilamide [see: sulfacetamide]
acetyltannic acid USP
acetyltannin [see: acetyltannic acid]
acevaltrate INN
acexamic acid INN, DCF
ACFUCY (actinomycin D, fluorouracil, cyclophosphamide) *chemotherapy protocol*
Aches-N-Pain tablets (discontinued 1996) OTC *nonsteroidal anti-inflammatory drug (NSAID); antiarthritic; analgesic* [ibuprofen] 200 mg
Achromycin eye drop suspension, ophthalmic ointment (discontinued 1995) ℞ *ophthalmic antibiotic* [tetracycline HCl] 10 mg/mL; 10 mg/g ② actinomycin; Aureomycin
Achromycin IV or IM injection (discontinued 1992) ℞ *broad-spectrum antibiotic* [tetracycline HCl] 100, 250, 500 mg
Achromycin topical ointment (discontinued 1995) OTC *broad-spectrum antibacterial* [tetracycline HCl] 3%
Achromycin V capsules, oral suspension ℞ *broad-spectrum antibiotic* [tetracycline HCl] 250, 500 mg; 125 mg/5 mL
aciclovir INN, JAN *antiviral* [also: acyclovir]
acid acriflavine [see: acriflavine HCl]

acid citrate dextrose (ACD) [see: anticoagulant citrate dextrose solution]

acid histamine phosphate [see: histamine phosphate]

Acid Mantle OTC *cream base*

acid trypaflavine [see: acriflavine HCl]

acidogen [see: glutamic acid HCl]

acidol HCl [see: betaine HCl]

acidophilus [see: *Lactobacillus acidophilus*]

acidulated phosphate fluoride (sodium fluoride & hydrofluoric acid) *dental caries prophylactic*

Acidulin Pulvules (capsules) (discontinued 1992) OTC *gastric acidifier* [glutamic acid HCl]

acidum acetylsalicylicum [see: aspirin]

acifran USAN, INN *antihyperlipoproteinemic*

aciglumin [see: glutamic acid HCl]

Aci-jel vaginal jelly OTC *acidity modifier* [acetic acid; oxyquinolone sulfate] 0.921%•0.025%

acinitrazole BAN *veterinary antibacterial* [also: nithiamide; aminitrozole]

acipimox INN, BAN

acistrate INN *combining name for radicals or groups*

acitemate INN

acitretin USAN, INN, BAN *antipsoriatic*

acivicin USAN, INN *antineoplastic*

Aclacin ℞ *investigational antibiotic antineoplastic for acute nonlymphocytic leukemia* [aclarubicin HCl]

aclacinomycin A [now: aclarubicin]

aclantate INN

aclarubicin USAN, INN, BAN *antibiotic antineoplastic* [also: aclarubicin HCl]

aclarubicin HCl JAN *antibiotic antineoplastic* [also: aclarubicin]

aclatonium napadisilate INN, BAN, JAN

Aclophen long-acting tablets ℞ *decongestant; antihistamine; analgesic* [phenylephrine HCl; chlorpheniramine maleate; acetaminophen] 40•8•500 mg

Aclovate ointment, cream ℞ *topical corticosteroidal anti-inflammatory* [alclometasone dipropionate] 0.05%

ACM (Adriamycin, cyclophosphamide, methotrexate) *chemotherapy protocol*

A.C.N. tablets OTC *vitamin supplement* [vitamins A, B₃, and C] 25,000 IU•25 mg•250 mg

Acne Lotion 10 OTC *antibacterial and exfoliant for acne* [colloidal sulfur] 10%

Acne-5 lotion, mask OTC *topical keratolytic for acne* [benzoyl peroxide] 5%

Acne-10 lotion OTC *topical keratolytic for acne* [benzoyl peroxide] 10%

Acne-Aid cleansing bar (discontinued 1994) OTC *medicated cleanser for acne* [surfactant blend] 6.3%

Acne-Aid cream (discontinued 1994) OTC *keratolytic for acne* [benzoyl peroxide] 10%

Acnederm lotion (discontinued 1993) OTC *topical acne treatment* [sulfur; zinc sulfate; zinc oxide; isopropyl alcohol] 5%•1%•10%•21%

Acno lotion OTC *topical acne treatment* [sulfur] 3%

Acno Cleanser liquid OTC *topical cleanser for acne* [isopropyl alcohol] 60%

Acnomel cream OTC *topical acne treatment* [sulfur; resorcinol; alcohol] 8%•2%•11%

Acnophill ointment (discontinued 1992) OTC *topical acne treatment* [precipitated sulfur; zinc oxide] 5%•10%

Acnotex lotion OTC *topical acne treatment* [sulfur; resorcinol; isopropyl alcohol] 8%•2%•20%

acodazole INN *antineoplastic* [also: acodazole HCl]

acodazole HCl USAN *antineoplastic* [also: acodazole]

aconiazide INN *(orphan: tuberculosis)*

aconitine USP

ACOP (Adriamycin, cyclophosphamide, Oncovin, prednisone) *chemotherapy protocol*

ACOPP; A-COPP (Adriamycin, cyclophosphamide, Oncovin, procarbazine, prednisone) *chemotherapy protocol*

acortan [see: corticotropin]

acoxatrine INN

9-acridinamine monohydrochloride [see: aminacrine HCl]

acridinyl anisidide [see: amsacrine]

acridinylamine methanesulfon anisidide (AMSA) [see: amsacrine]
acridorex INN
acriflavine NF
acriflavine HCl NF [also: acriflavinium chloride]
acriflavinium chloride INN [also: acriflavine HCl]
acrihellin INN
acrinol JAN [also: ethacridine lactate; ethacridine]
acrisorcin USAN, USP, INN *antifungal*
acrivastine USAN, INN, BAN *antihistamine*
acrocinonide INN, DCF
acronine USAN, INN *antineoplastic*
acrosoxacin BAN *antibacterial* [also: rosoxacin]
ACT oral rinse OTC *topical dental caries preventative* [sodium fluoride; alcohol 7%] 0.05%
actagardin INN
Actagen tablets, syrup OTC *decongestant; antihistamine* [pseudoephedrine HCl; triprolidine HCl] 60•2.5 mg; 30•1.25 mg/5 mL
Actagen-C Cough syrup ℞ *narcotic antitussive; decongestant; antihistamine* [codeine phosphate; pseudoephedrine HCl; triprolidine HCl] 10•30•2 mg/5 mL
Actamin; Actamin Extra tablets OTC *analgesic; antipyretic* [acetaminophen]
Actamin Super tablets OTC *analgesic; antipyretic* [acetaminophen; caffeine] ≟
actaplanin USAN, INN, BAN *veterinary growth stimulant*
actarit INN
ACTH powder for IM or subcu injection ℞ *steroid* [corticotropin] 40 U/vial
ACTH (adrenocorticotropic hormone) [see: corticotropin]
ACTH-40 subcu or IM injection (discontinued 1994) ℞ *steroid* [corticotropin repository] 40 U/mL
ACTH-80 subcu or IM injection ℞ *steroid* [corticotropin repository] 80 U/mL
Acthar powder for IM or subcu injection ℞ *steroid* [corticotropin] 25, 40 U/vial
Acthar Gel [see: H.P. Acthar Gel]

ActHIB powder for injection ℞ *pediatric vaccine for meningitis caused by Haemophilus influenzae type b (HIB) virus* [Hemophilus b conjugate vaccine; tetanus toxoid] 10•24 μg/0.5 mL
ActHIB/acellular DTP ℞ *investigational pediatric vaccine for children younger than 5 months old* [Hemophilus b conjugate vaccine; acellular diphtheria & tetanus toxoids & pertussis vaccine]
ActHIB/DTacP ℞ *investigational pediatric vaccine for children younger than 5 months old* [Hemophilus b conjugate vaccine; diphtheria & tetanus toxoids & acellular pertussis vaccine]
ActHIB/DTP IM injection ℞ *pediatric vaccine for diphtheria, tetanus, pertussis, and Haemophilus influenzae type b (HIB)* [Hemophilus b conjugate vaccine; diphtheria & tetanus toxoids & pertussis vaccine (DTP)] 20 μg/mL
Acthrel ℞ *(orphan: diagnostic aid for adrenocorticotropic hormone-dependent Cushing syndrome)* [corticorelin ovine triflutate]
ActiBath effervescent tablets OTC *moisturizer; emollient* [colloidal oatmeal] 20%
Acticel ℞ *investigational treatment for Parkinson's disease, stroke, burns, and venous ulcers* [fibroblast growth factor]
Acticort 100 lotion ℞ *topical corticosteroid* [hydrocortisone] 1%
Actidil syrup OTC *antihistamine* [triprolidine HCl; alcohol 4%] 1.25 mg/5 mL ▣ Actifed
Actidil tablets (discontinued 1993) OTC *antihistamine* [triprolidine HCl] 2.5 mg
Actidose with Sorbitol oral suspension OTC *adsorbent antidote for poisoning; reduces intestinal transit time* [activated charcoal; sorbitol] 25•≟ g/120 mL; 50•≟ g/240 mL
Actidose-Aqua oral suspension OTC *adsorbent antidote for poisoning* [activated charcoal] 25 g/120 mL, 50 g/240 mL
Actifed capsules (discontinued 1993) OTC *decongestant; antihistamine* [pseudoephedrine HCl; triprolidine HCl] ▣ Actidil

Actifed syrup (discontinued 1995) OTC *decongestant; antihistamine* [pseudoephedrine HCl; triprolidine HCl] 30•1.25 mg/5 mL

Actifed tablets OTC *decongestant; antihistamine* [pseudoephedrine HCl; triprolidine HCl] 60•2.5 mg

Actifed 12-Hour sustained-release capsules (discontinued 1993) OTC *decongestant; antihistamine* [pseudoephedrine HCl; triprolidine HCl]

Actifed Allergy daytime caplets + nighttime caplets OTC *decongestant; (antihistamine/sleep aid added at night)* [pseudoephedrine HCl; (diphenhydramine HCl added at night)] 30 mg; 30•25 mg

Actifed Plus caplets, tablets OTC *decongestant; antihistamine; analgesic* [pseudoephedrine HCl; triprolidine HCl; acetaminophen] 30•1.25•500 mg

Actifed Sinus daytime caplets + nighttime caplets OTC *decongestant; analgesic; (antihistamine/sleep aid added at night)* [pseudoephedrine HCl; acetaminophen; (diphenhydramine HCl added at night)] 30•325 mg; 30•500•25 mg

Actifed with Codeine Cough syrup ℞ *narcotic antitussive; decongestant; antihistamine* [codeine phosphate; pseudoephedrine HCl; triprolidine HCl; alcohol 4.3%] 10•30•1.25 mg/5 mL

Actigall capsules ℞ *gallstone dissolving agent; (orphan: primary biliary cirrhosis)* [ursodiol] 300 mg

Actimmune subcu injection ℞ *biologic response modifier; for chronic granulomatous disease (orphan)* [interferon gamma-1b] 100 μg (3 million U)

Actinex cream ℞ *antineoplastic for actinic keratoses (AK)* [masoprocol] 10%

actinium *element (Ac)*

actinomycin C BAN *antibiotic antineoplastic* [also: cactinomycin] ⑨ Achromycin; Aureomycin

actinomycin D JAN *antibiotic antineoplastic* [also: dactinomycin] ⑨ Achromycin; Aureomycin

actinoquinol INN *ultraviolet screen* [also: actinoquinol sodium]

actinoquinol sodium USAN *ultraviolet screen* [also: actinoquinol]

actinospectocin [see: spectinomycin]

Actisite periodontal fiber ℞ *oral antibiotic for periodontitis* [tetracycline] 12.7 mg/23 cm

actisomide USAN, INN *antiarrhythmic*

Activase IV infusion ℞ *tissue plasminogen activator for acute MI, pulmonary embolism, and stroke* [alteplase] 20, 50, 100 mg/vial (11.6, 29, 58 million IU/vial)

activated attapulgite [see: attapulgite, activated]

activated carbon

activated charcoal [see: charcoal, activated]

activated 7-dehydrocholesterol [see: cholecalciferol]

activated ergosterol [see: ergocalciferol]

activated prothrombin complex BAN

actodigin USAN, INN *cardiotonic*

Act-O-Vial (trademarked packaging form) *vial system*

Actron tablets OTC *nonsteroidal anti-inflammatory drug (NSAID); analgesic; antiarthritic* [ketoprofen] 12.5 mg

ACU-dyne ointment, perineal wash concentrate, prep solution, skin cleanser, prep swabs, swabsticks OTC *broad-spectrum antimicrobial* [povidone-iodine]

ACU-dyne Douche concentrate OTC *antiseptic/germicidal; vaginal cleanser and deodorizer* [povidone-iodine]

Acular eye drops ℞ *ocular nonsteroidal anti-inflammatory drug (NSAID); antipruritic for allergic conjunctivitis* [ketorolac tromethamine] 0.5%

Acupaque ℞ *investigational broad-spectrum contrast agent for x-ray and CT scans* [iodixanol]

Acutrim 16 Hour; Acutrim Late Day; Acutrim II precision-release tablets OTC *diet aid* [phenylpropanolamine HCl] 75 mg

acycloguanosine [see: acyclovir]

acyclovir USAN, USP, BAN *antiviral* [also: aciclovir]

acyclovir redox [see: redox-acyclovir]

acyclovir sodium USAN *antiviral*

acylpyrin [see: aspirin]

AD-439 *investigational (Phase II) antiviral for HIV and AIDS*

AD-519 *investigational (Phase II) antiviral for HIV and AIDS*

adafenoxate INN

Adagen IM injection ℞ *enzyme replacement; (orphan: severe combined immunodeficiency disease)* [pegademase bovine] 250 U/mL

Adalat capsules ℞ *antianginal* [nifedipine] 10, 20 mg

Adalat CC; Adalat Oros sustained-release tablets ℞ *antianginal; antihypertensive* [nifedipine] 30, 60, 90 mg

adamantanamine [see: amantadine]

adamantanamine HCl [see: amantadine HCl]

adamexine INN

adapalene USAN, INN, BAN *investigational synthetic retinoid analog for acne*

Adapettes solution OTC *rewetting solution for hard contact lenses*

Adapettes Especially for Sensitive Eyes solution OTC *rewetting solution for soft contact lenses*

Adapin capsules ℞ *anxiolytic; antidepressant* [doxepin HCl] 10, 25, 50, 75, 100, 150 mg ② Atabrine; Ativan; Betapen

adaprolol maleate USAN *ophthalmic antihypertensive (β-blocker)*

Adapt solution (discontinued 1995) OTC *wetting/rewetting solution for hard contact lenses*

adatanserin INN *anxiolytic; antidepressant* [also: adatanserin HCl]

adatanserin HCl USAN *anxiolytic; antidepressant* [also: adatanserin]

AdatoSil 5000 intraocular injection ℞ *retinal tamponade for retinal detachment* [polydimethylsiloxane] 10, 15 mL

Adavite tablets OTC *vitamin supplement* [multiple vitamins; folic acid; biotin] ±•400•35 μg

Adavite-M tablets OTC *vitamin/mineral/iron supplement* [multiple vitamins & minerals; iron; folic acid; biotin] ±•27 mg•0.4 mg•30 μg

ADBC (Adriamycin, DTIC, bleomycin, CCNU) *chemotherapy protocol*

ADC with Fluoride drops ℞ *pediatric vitamin supplement and dental caries preventative* [vitamins A, C, and D; fluoride] 1500 IU•35 mg•400 IU•0.5 mg per mL

Adcon-L gel ℞ *investigational agent to inhibit excess scar formation following back surgery*

Adderall tablets ℞ *CNS stimulant for attention deficit hyperactivity disorder (ADHD), narcolepsy, and obesity* [dextroamphetamine sulfate; dextroamphetamine saccharate; amphetamine aspartate; amphetamine sulfate] 2.5•2.5•2.5•2.5, 5•5•5•5 mg

ADD-Vantage (trademarked delivery system) *intravenous drug admixture system*

ADE cream, ointment OTC *topical antioxidant* [vitamins A, D, and E]

ADE (ara-C, daunorubicin, etoposide) *chemotherapy protocol*

Adeflor chewable tablets, drops (discontinued 1992) ℞ *pediatric vitamin supplement and dental caries preventative* [multiple vitamins; fluoride]

Adeflor M tablets ℞ *pediatric vitamin deficiency and dental caries prevention* [multiple vitamins; fluoride; calcium; iron] ±•1•250•30 mg

ADEKs chewable tablets OTC *vitamin/mineral supplement* [multiple vitamins & minerals; folic acid; biotin] ±•200•50 μg

ADEKs pediatric drops OTC *vitamin/mineral supplement* [multiple vitamins & minerals; biotin] ±•15 μg

adelmidrol INN

ademetionine INN

Adenazole ℞ *investigational antineoplastic* [8-chlorocamp]

Adenic injection ℞ *nutrient* [adenosine phosphate]

adenine USP, JAN *amino acid*

adenine arabinoside (ara-A) [see: vidarabine]

Adenocard IV injection ℞ *antiarrhythmic* [adenosine] 3 mg/mL

Adenoscan IV infusion ℞ *cardiac diagnostic aid; cardiac stressor; adjunct to thallium 201 myocardial perfusion scintigraphy* [adenosine] 3 mg/mL

adenosine USAN, BAN *antiarrhythmic for paroxysmal supraventricular tachycardia; diagnostic aid; (orphan: brain tumors)*

adenosine monophosphate (AMP) [see: adenosine phosphate]

adenosine phosphate USAN, INN, BAN *nutrient; treatment for varicose veins and herpes infections* 25 mg/mL IM injection

adenosine triphosphate (ATP) disodium JAN

5′-adenylic acid [see: adenosine phosphate]

adepsine oil [see: mineral oil]

Adequate M Improved tablets (discontinued 1992) ℞ *vitamin/mineral/iron supplement* [multiple vitamins & minerals; iron; folic acid]

adhesive bandage [see: bandage, adhesive]

adhesive tape [see: tape, adhesive]

adibendan INN

A-DIC (Adriamycin, dacarbazine) *chemotherapy protocol*

adicillin INN, BAN

adimolol INN

adinazolam USAN, INN, BAN *antidepressant; sedative*

adinazolam mesylate USAN *antidepressant*

Adipex-P tablets ℞ *anorexiant* [phentermine HCl] 37.5 mg

adiphenine INN *smooth muscle relaxant* [also: adiphenine HCl]

adiphenine HCl USAN *smooth muscle relaxant* [also: adiphenine]

adipiodone INN, JAN [also: iodipamide]

adipiodone meglumine JAN *radiopaque medium* [also: iodipamide meglumine]

Adipost slow-release capsules ℞ *anorexiant* [phendimetrazine tartrate] 105 mg

aditeren INN

aditoprim INN

Adlone injection ℞ *glucocorticoids* [methylprednisolone acetate] 40, 80 mg/mL

adnephrine [see: epinephrine]

ADOAP (Adriamycin, Oncovin, ara-C, prednisone) *chemotherapy protocol*

Adolph's Salt Substitute; Adolph's Seasoned Salt Substitute OTC *salt substitute* [potassium chloride] 64 mEq/5 g; 35 mEq/5 g

ADOP (Adriamycin, Oncovin, prednisone) *chemotherapy protocol*

Adosar ℞ *investigational antineoplastic for solid tumors and leukemia* [adozelesin]

adosopine

adozelesin USAN, INN *antineoplastic*

Adprin-B coated tablets OTC *analgesic; antipyretic; anti-inflammatory; antirheumatic* [aspirin, buffered with calcium carbonate, magnesium oxide, and magnesium carbonate] 325, 500 mg

ADR (Adriamycin) [see: doxorubicin HCl]

adrafinil INN

adrenal [see: epinephrine]

Adrenalin Chloride eye drops ℞ *antiglaucoma agent* [epinephrine HCl]

Adrenalin Chloride nose drops OTC *nasal decongestant* [epinephrine HCl] 0.1%

Adrenalin Chloride solution for inhalation OTC *bronchodilator for bronchial asthma* [epinephrine HCl] 1:100

Adrenalin Chloride subcu, IV, IM or intracardiac injection ℞ *bronchodilator for bronchial asthma, bronchospasm and COPD; vasopressor for shock* [epinephrine HCl] 1:1000 (1 mg/mL)

adrenaline BAN *vasoconstrictor; bronchodilator; topical antiglaucoma agent; vasopressor for shock* [also: epinephrine] ⓘ adrenalone

adrenaline bitartrate [see: epinephrine bitartrate]

adrenaline HCl [see: epinephrine HCl]

adrenalone USAN, INN *ophthalmic adrenergic* ⓘ adrenaline

adrenamine [see: epinephrine]

adrenine [see: epinephrine]

adrenochromazone [see: carbazochrome salicylate]

adrenochrome [see: carbazochrome salicylate]

adrenochrome guanylhydrazone mesilate JAN

adrenochrome monoaminoguanidine sodium methylsulfonate

[see: adrenochrome guanylhydrazone mesilate]
adrenochrome monosemicarbazone sodium salicylate [see: carbazochrome salicylate]
adrenocorticotrophin [see: corticotropin]
adrenocorticotropic hormone (ACTH) [see: corticotropin]
adrenone [see: adrenalone]
Adria + BCNU (Adriamycin, BCNU) *chemotherapy protocol*
Adria-L-PAM (Adriamycin, L-phenylalanine mustard) *chemotherapy protocol*
Adriamycin PFS (preservative-free solution) IV injection ℞ *antibiotic antineoplastic* [doxorubicin HCl] 2 mg/mL
Adriamycin RDF (rapid dissolution formula) IV injection ℞ *antibiotic antineoplastic* [doxorubicin HCl] 10, 20, 50, 150 mg/vial
Adria-Oncoline Chemo-Pin (trademarked delivery system)
Adrin tablets (discontinued 1993) ℞ *peripheral vasodilator* [nylidrin HCl] 6, 12 mg
Adrotest SL sublingual tablets ℞ *investigational treatment for hypogonadism* [testosterone]
Adrucil IV injection ℞ *antimetabolic antineoplastic; (orphan: adjuvant to colorectal and esophageal cancer)* [fluorouracil] 50 mg/mL
ADS (azodisal sodium) [now: olsalazine sodium]
adsorbed diphtheria toxoid [see: diphtheria toxoid, adsorbed]
Adsorbocarpine eye drops ℞ *antiglaucoma agent; direct-acting miotic* [pilocarpine HCl] 1%, 2%, 4%
Adsorbonac eye drops OTC *corneal edema-reducing agent* [hypertonic saline solution] 2%, 5%
Adsorbotear eye drops OTC *ocular moisturizer/lubricant* [hydroxyethylcellulose] 0.4%
ADT (trademarked dosage form) *alternate-day therapy*
Advance liquid (discontinued 1993) OTC *total or supplementary infant feeding* 390 mL concentrate, 1 qt. ready-to-use
Advance test stick for home use OTC *in vitro diagnostic aid for urine pregnancy test*
Advanced Care Cholesterol Test kit for home use OTC *in vitro diagnostic aid for cholesterol in the blood*
"Advanced Formula" products [see under product name]
Advantage 24 vaginal gel OTC *spermicidal contraceptive (for use with a diaphragm)* [nonoxynol 9] 3.5%
Advera liquid OTC *enteral nutritional therapy for HIV and AIDS patients* [lactose-free formula] 240 mL
Advil tablets, caplets OTC *nonsteroidal anti-inflammatory drug (NSAID); antiarthritic; analgesic* [ibuprofen] 200 mg ② Avail
Advil, Children's oral suspension OTC *nonsteroidal anti-inflammatory drug (NSAID); antiarthritic; analgesic* [ibuprofen] 100 mg/5 mL
Advil Cold & Sinus caplets OTC *decongestant; analgesic* [pseudoephedrine HCl; ibuprofen] 30•200 mg
AE-0047 *investigational calcium antagonist for hypertension and to improve cerebral blood flow*
A-E-R pads OTC *astringent* [hamamelis water] 50%
Aeroaid spray OTC *antiseptic; antibacterial; antifungal* [thimerosal; alcohol 72%] 1:1000
AeroBid; AeroBid-M oral inhalation aerosol ℞ *corticosteroid for bronchial asthma* [flunisolide] 200 μg/dose
AeroCaine aerosol solution OTC *topical local anesthetic* [benzocaine; benzethonium chloride] 13.6%•0.5%
AeroChamber (trademarked form) *aerosol holding chamber*
Aerodine aerosol OTC *broad-spectrum antimicrobial* [povidone-iodine]
Aerofreeze spray OTC *topical vapocoolant anesthetic* [trichloromonofluoromethane; dichlorodifluoromethane] ?•?
Aerolate oral solution (discontinued 1993) ℞ *bronchodilator* [theophylline] 150 mg/15 mL

Aerolate Sr.; Aerolate Jr.; Aerolate III timed-action capsules ℞ *bronchodilator* [theophylline] 260 mg; 130 mg; 65 mg

Aeropin ℞ *(orphan: cystic fibrosis)* [heparin, 2-0-desulfated]

Aeroseb-Dex aerosol spray ℞ *topical corticosteroid* [dexamethasone] 0.01%

Aeroseb-HC aerosol spray ℞ *topical corticosteroid; antiseborrheic* [hydrocortisone] 0.5%

aerosol OT [see: docusate sodium]

aerosolized pooled immune globulin [see: globulin, aerosolized pooled immune]

Aerosporin powder for IV, IM or intrathecal injection ℞ *bactericidal antibiotic* [polymyxin B sulfate] 500,000 U

AeroTherm aerosol solution OTC *topical local anesthetic* [benzocaine; benzethonium chloride] 13.6%•0.5%

Aerotrol (trademarked form) *inhalation aerosol*

AeroZoin spray OTC *skin protectant* [benzoin; isopropyl alcohol 44.8%] 30%

AErrane ℞ *investigational anesthetic* [isoflurane]

aethylis chloridum [see: ethyl chloride]

AF102B *investigational M-1 agonist for Alzheimer's disease*

afalanine INN

Affirm DP kit ℞ *investigational microbial identification test system for periodontal disease*

afloqualone INN, JAN

AFM (Adriamycin, fluorouracil, methotrexate [with leucovorin rescue]) *chemotherapy protocol*

afovirsen INN

Afrin extended-release tablets OTC *nasal decongestant* [pseudoephedrine sulfate] 120 mg ⓓ Afrinol; aspirin

Afrin nasal spray, nose drops OTC *nasal decongestant* [oxymetazoline HCl] 0.05%

Afrin Children's Nose Drops OTC *nasal decongestant* [oxymetazoline HCl] 0.025%

Afrin Moisturizing Saline Mist solution OTC *nasal moisturizer* [sodium chloride (saline)] 0.64%

Afrin Saline Mist solution (name changed to Afrin Moisturizing Saline Mist in 1996)

Afrin Sinus nasal spray OTC *nasal decongestant* [oxymetazoline HCl] 0.05%

Afrinol (name changed to Afrin in 1993) ⓓ Afrin

Aftate for Athlete's Foot gel, powder, spray powder, spray liquid OTC *topical antifungal* [tolnaftate] 1%

Aftate for Jock Itch gel, powder, spray powder OTC *topical antifungal* [tolnaftate] 1%

afurolol INN

A/G Pro tablets OTC *dietary supplement* [protein hydrolysate; multiple vitamins, minerals, and amino acids] 542•≛ mg

AG-337 *investigational antineoplastic*

aganodine INN

agar NF, JAN *suspending agent*

agar-agar [see: agar]

aggregated albumin [see: albumin, aggregated]

aggregated radio-iodinated I 131 serum albumin [see: albumin, aggregated iodinated I 131 serum]

aglepristone INN

agofollin [see: estradiol]

Agoral emulsion OTC *laxative* [mineral oil; phenolphthalein] 4.2•0.2 g/15 mL ⓓ Argyrol

Agoral Plain emulsion OTC *emollient laxative* [mineral oil] 1.4 g/5 mL

Agrelin ℞ *investigational antineoplastic* [anagrelide]

agurin [see: theobromine sodium acetate]

AHA (acetohydroxamic acid) [q.v.]

AHA (alpha hydroxy acids) [see: glycolic acid]

AH-chew chewable tablets ℞ *decongestant; antihistamine; anticholinergic* [phenylephrine HCl; chlorpheniramine maleate; methscopolamine nitrate] 10•2•1.25 mg

AH-chew D chewable tablets ℞ *decongestant* [phenylephrine HCl] 10 mg

AHF (antihemophilic factor) [q.v.]

AHG (antihemophilic globulin) [see: antihemophilic factor]

A-Hydrocort IV or IM injection ℞ *glucocorticoids* [hydrocortisone sodium succinate] 100, 250, 500, 1000 mg/vial

AI204 *investigational T-cell receptor peptide vaccine for rheumatoid arthritis*

AIDS vaccine (several different compounds are included in this general category; e.g., gp120, rgp160, rgp160 MN, rp24) *investigational (Phase I to III) antiviral for AIDS/HIV*

air, compressed [see: air, medical]

air, medical USP *medicinal gas*

Airet solution for inhalation ℞ *bronchodilator* [albuterol sulfate] 0.083%z

Airomir metered dose inhaler *investigational CFC-free aerosol propellant to replace CFC-based propellants in other inhalers*

AI-RSA (*orphan: autoimmune uveitis*)

ajmaline JAN

Akarpine eye drops ℞ *antiglaucoma agent; direct-acting miotic* [pilocarpine HCl] 1%, 2%, 4%

AKBeta eye drops ℞ *topical antiglaucoma agent (β-blocker)* [levobunolol HCl] 0.25%, 0.5%

AK-Biocholine tablets OTC *vitamin supplement* [choline bitartrate; citrus bioflavonoids]

AK-Chlor eye drops, ophthalmic ointment ℞ *ophthalmic antibiotic* [chloramphenicol] 5 mg/mL; 10 mg/g

AK-Cide eye drop suspension, ophthalmic ointment ℞ *ophthalmic topical corticosteroidal anti-inflammatory; bacteriostatic* [prednisolone acetate; sulfacetamide sodium] 0.5%•10%

AK-Con eye drops ℞ *topical ocular decongestant/vasoconstrictor* [naphazoline HCl] 0.1%

AK-Con-A eye drops (discontinued 1995) ℞ *topical ocular decongestant and antihistamine* [naphazoline HCl; pheniramine maleate] 0.025%•0.3%

AK-Dex eye drops, ophthalmic ointment ℞ *ophthalmic topical corticosteroidal anti-inflammatory* [dexamethasone sodium phosphate] 0.1%; 0.05%

AK-Dilate eye drops ℞ *ocular decongestant/vasoconstrictor; mydriatic* [phenylephrine HCl] 2.5%, 10%

AK-Fluor IV injection ℞ *corneal disclosing agent* [fluorescein] 10%, 25%

AK-Homatropine eye drops ℞ *mydriatic; cycloplegic* [homatropine hydrobromide] 5%

Akineton IV or IM injection ℞ *anticholinergic; antiparkinsonian agent* [biperiden lactate] 5 mg/mL

Akineton tablets ℞ *anticholinergic; antiparkinsonian agent* [biperiden HCl] 2 mg

aklomide USAN, INN, BAN *coccidiostat for poultry*

AK-Mycin ophthalmic ointment (discontinued 1995) ℞ *ophthalmic antibiotic* [erythromycin] 5 mg/g ② Akne-Mycin

AK-NaCl eye drops, ophthalmic ointment OTC *corneal edema-reducing agent* [hypertonic saline solution] 5%

AK-Nefrin eye drops OTC *topical ocular decongestant* [phenylephrine HCl] 0.12%

Akne-mycin ointment, topical solution ℞ *topical antibiotic for acne* [erythromycin] 2% ② Ak-Mycin

AK-Neo-Cort eye drop suspension (discontinued 1992) ℞ *topical ophthalmic corticosteroidal anti-inflammatory; antibiotic* [hydrocortisone acetate; neomycin sulfate]

AK-Neo-Dex eye drops ℞ *topical ophthalmic corticosteroidal anti-inflammatory; antibiotic* [dexamethasone sodium phosphate; neomycin sulfate] 0.1%•0.35%

Akoline C.B. capsules, caplets (discontinued 1995) OTC *dietary lipotropic with vitamin supplementation* [choline; inositol; methionine; multiple B vitamins; vitamin C; lemon bioflavonoids] 111•111•28•±•100•100 mg

Akoline CB with Zinc caplets OTC *dietary lipotropic with vitamin and zinc supplementation* [choline; inositol; methionine; multiple B vitamins; vitamin C; bioflavonoid; zinc amino acid chelate]

AK-Pentolate eye drops ℞ *mydriatic; cycloplegic* [cyclopentolate HCl] 1%

AK-Poly-Bac ophthalmic ointment ℞ *ophthalmic antibiotic* [polymyxin B sulfate; bacitracin zinc] 10,000•500 U/g

AK-Pred eye drops ℞ *ophthalmic topical corticosteroidal anti-inflammatory* [prednisolone sodium phosphate] 0.125%, 1%

AKPro eye drops ℞ *antiglaucoma agent* [dipivefrin HCl] 0.1%

AK-Rinse ophthalmic solution OTC *extraocular irrigating solution* [sterile isotonic solution]

AK-Spore eye drops ℞ *ophthalmic antibiotic* [polymyxin B sulfate; neomycin sulfate; gramicidin] 10,000 U•1.75 mg•0.025 mg per mL

AK-Spore ophthalmic ointment ℞ *ophthalmic antibiotic* [polymyxin B sulfate; neomycin sulfate; bacitracin zinc] 10,000 U•3.5 mg•400 U per g

AK-Spore H.C. ear drops, otic suspension ℞ *topical corticosteroidal anti-inflammatory; antibiotic* [hydrocortisone; neomycin sulfate; polymyxin B sulfate] 1%•5 mg•10,000 U per mL

AK-Spore H.C. eye drop suspension ℞ *topical ophthalmic corticosteroidal anti-inflammatory; antibiotic* [hydrocortisone; neomycin sulfate; polymyxin B sulfate] 1%•0.35%•10,000 U per mL

AK-Spore H.C. ointment ℞ *topical ophthalmic corticosteroidal anti-inflammatory; antibiotic* [hydrocortisone; neomycin sulfate; bacitracin zinc; polymyxin B sulfate] 1%•0.35%•400 U/g•10,000 U/g

AK-Sulf eye drops, ophthalmic ointment ℞ *ophthalmic bacteriostatic* [sulfacetamide sodium] 10%

AK-Taine eye drops (discontinued 1995) ℞ *topical ophthalmic anesthetic* [proparacaine HCl] 0.5%

AKTob eye drops ℞ *ophthalmic antibiotic* [tobramycin] 0.3%

AK-Tracin ophthalmic ointment ℞ *ophthalmic antibiotic* [bacitracin] 500 U/g

AK-Trol eye drop suspension, ophthalmic ointment ℞ *topical ophthalmic corticosteroidal anti-inflammatory; antibiotic* [dexamethasone; neomycin sulfate; polymyxin B sulfate] 0.1%•0.35%•10,000 U/mL; 0.1%•0.35%•10,000 U/g

Akwa Tears eye drops OTC *ocular moisturizer/lubricant* [polyvinyl alcohol] 1.4%

Akwa Tears ophthalmic ointment OTC *ocular moisturizer/lubricant* [white petrolatum; mineral oil]

AK-Zol tablets (discontinued 1993) ℞ *antiglaucoma; anticonvulsant; diuretic* [acetazolamide] 250 mg

AL-721 investigational (Phase I/II) *antiviral for AIDS*

ALA Photodynamic Therapy ℞ *investigational treatment for psoriasis and actinic keratoses*

alacepril INN, JAN

Ala-Cort cream, lotion ℞ *topical corticosteroid* [hydrocortisone] 1%

alafosfalin INN, BAN

Alamag oral suspension OTC *antacid* [aluminum hydroxide; magnesium hydroxide] 225•200 mg/5 mL ⓘ Alma-Mag

Alamag Plus oral suspension OTC *antacid; antiflatulent* [aluminum hydroxide; magnesium hydroxide; simethicone] 225•200•25 mg/5 mL

alamecin USAN *antibacterial*

alanine (L-alanine) USAN, USP, INN *nonessential amino acid; symbols: Ala, A*

alanine nitrogen mustard [see: melphalan]

alanosine INN

alaproclate USAN, INN *antidepressant*

Ala-Quin cream ℞ *topical corticosteroid; antifungal; antibacterial* [hydrocortisone; clioquinol] 0.5%•3%

Ala-Scalp lotion ℞ *topical corticosteroid* [hydrocortisone] 2%

AlaSTAT lab test for professional use ℞ *test for allergic reaction to latex*

Alasulf vaginal cream ℞ *bacteriostatic antibiotic; antiseptic; vulnerary* [sulfanilamide; aminacrine HCl; allantoin] 15%•0.2%•2%

Ala-Tet capsules (discontinued 1992) ℞ *broad-spectrum antibiotic* [tetracycline HCl] 250, 500 mg

Alatone tablets (discontinued 1993) ℞ *potassium-sparing diuretic* [spironolactone]

alazanine triclofenate INN

Alazide tablets (discontinued 1993) ℞ *diuretic* [spironolactone; hydrochlorothiazide]

Alazine tablets (discontinued 1993) ℞ *antihypertensive; vasodilator* [hydralazine HCl]

Albalon eye drops ℞ *topical ocular decongestant/vasoconstrictor* [naphazoline HCl] 0.1%

Albalon-A Liquifilm eye drops (discontinued 1993) ℞ *topical ocular decongestant and antihistamine* [naphazoline HCl; antazoline phosphate]

Albamycin capsules ℞ *bacteriostatic antibiotic* [novobiocin sodium] 250 mg

Albay subcu or IM injection ℞ *venom sensitivity testing (subcu); venom desensitization therapy (IM)* [extract of honeybee, yellow jacket, yellow hornet, white-faced hornet, wasp, and mixed vespid]

albendazole USAN, INN, BAN *anthelmintic; investigational (Phase III) for AIDS-related microsporidiosis*

albendazole oxide INN, BAN

Albenza tablets ℞ *investigational anthelmintic for hydatid cyst disease due to tapeworm larvae infestation* [albendazole]

Albright solution (sodium citrate and citric acid) *urine alkalizer; compounding agent*

albucid [see: sulfacetamide]

albumin, aggregated USAN *lung imaging aid (with technetium Tc 99m)*

albumin, aggregated iodinated I 131 serum USAN, USP *radioactive agent*

albumin, chromated Cr 51 serum USAN *radioactive agent*

albumin, human USP *blood volume supporter* 5%, 25% injection

albumin, iodinated (^{125}I) human serum INN *radioactive agent; blood volume test* [also: albumin, iodinated I 125 serum]

albumin, iodinated (^{131}I) human serum INN, JAN *radioactive agent; intrathecal imaging agent; blood volume test* [also: albumin, iodinated I 131 serum]

albumin, iodinated I 125 USP *radioactive agent; blood volume test*

albumin, iodinated I 125 serum USAN, USP *radioactive agent; blood volume test* [also: iodinated (^{125}I) human serum albumin]

albumin, iodinated I 131 USP *radioactive agent; intrathecal imaging agent; blood volume test*

albumin, iodinated I 131 serum USAN, USP *radioactive agent; intrathecal imaging agent; blood volume test* [also: iodinated (^{131}I) human serum albumin]

albumin, normal human serum [now: albumin, human]

Albuminar-5; Albuminar-25 IV infusion ℞ *blood volume expander for shock, burns, and hypoproteinemia* [human albumin] 5%; 25%

Albunex injection ℞ *ultrasound heart imaging agent* [albumin, human (sonicated)] 5%

Albustix reagent strips for professional use *in vitro diagnostic aid for albumin (protein) in the urine*

Albutein 5%; Albutein 25% IV infusion ℞ *blood volume expander for shock, burns, and hypoproteinemia* [human albumin] 5%; 25%

albuterol USAN, USP *bronchodilator* [also: salbutamol]

albuterol sulfate USAN, USP *bronchodilator* [also: salbutamol sulfate] 2, 4 mg oral; 2 mg/5 mL oral; 0.083%, 0.5% inhalation; 90 μg aerosol

albutoin USAN, INN *anticonvulsant*

Alcaine Drop-Tainers (eye drops) ℞ *topical ophthalmic anesthetic* [proparacaine HCl] 0.5%

Alcar ℞ *investigational treatment for Alzheimer's disease* [levacecarnine]

ALCAR (acetyl-L-carnitine) [q.v.]

Alcare foam OTC *topical antiseptic* [ethyl alcohol] 62%

alclofenac USAN, INN, BAN, JAN *anti-inflammatory*

alclometasone INN, BAN *topical corticosteroidal anti-inflammatory* [also: alclometasone dipropionate]

alclometasone dipropionate USAN, USP, JAN *topical corticosteroidal anti-inflammatory* [also: alclometasone]

alcloxa USAN, INN *astringent; keratolytic* [also: aluminum chlorohydroxy allantoinate]

Alco-Gel OTC *topical antiseptic for instant sanitation of hands* [ethyl alcohol] 60% ☒ aloe gel

alcohol USP *topical anti-infective/antiseptic; astringent; solvent* [also: ethanol]

alcohol, dehydrated USP *antidote* [also: ethanol, dehydrated]

alcohol, diluted NF *solvent*

alcohol, rubbing USP, INN *rubefacient*

5% Alcohol and 5% Dextrose in Water; 10% Alcohol and 5% Dextrose in Water IV infusion ℞ *for caloric replacement and rehydration* [alcohol; dextrose] 5%•5%; 10%•5%

Alcon Saline Especially for Sensitive Eyes solution OTC *rinsing/storage solution for soft contact lenses* [preserved saline solution]

Alconefrin nose drops, nasal spray OTC *nasal decongestant* [phenylephrine HCl] 0.25%, 0.5%

Alconefrin 12 nose drops OTC *nasal decongestant* [phenylephrine HCl] 0.16%

alcuronium chloride USAN, INN, BAN, JAN *skeletal muscle relaxant*

Aldactazide tablets ℞ *diuretic; antihypertensive* [spironolactone; hydrochlorothiazide] 25•25, 50•50 mg ☒ Aldactone

Aldactone tablets ℞ *potassium-sparing diuretic* [spironolactone] 25, 50, 100 mg ☒ Aldactazide

alderlin [see: pronethalol]

aldesleukin USAN, INN, BAN *antineoplastic; biologic response modifier; immunostimulant; (orphan: immunodeficiency diseases)*

aldesulfone sodium INN, DCF *antibacterial; leprostatic* [also: sulfoxone sodium]

aldioxa USAN, INN, JAN *astringent; keratolytic*

Aldoclor-150; Aldoclor-250 film-coated tablets ℞ *antihypertensive* [chlorothiazide; methyldopa] 150•250 mg; 250•250 mg

aldocorten [see: aldosterone]

Aldomet IV injection ℞ *antihypertensive* [methyldopate HCl] 250 mg/5 mL ☒ Aldoril

Aldomet tablets, oral suspension ℞ *antihypertensive* [methyldopa] 125, 250, 500 mg; 250 mg/5 mL

Aldoril 15; Aldoril 25; Aldoril D30; Aldoril D50 film-coated tablets ℞ *antihypertensive* [hydrochlorothiazide; methyldopa] 15•250 mg; 25•250 mg; 30•500 mg; 50•500 mg ☒ Aldomet; Elavil

aldosterone INN, BAN, DCF

Alec ℞ *(orphan: neonatal respiratory distress syndrome)* [dipalmitoylphosphatidylcholine; phosphatidylglycerol]

alendronate sodium USAN *bone resorption inhibitor; biphosphonate*

alendronic acid INN, BAN

Alenic Alka chewable tablets OTC *antacid* [aluminum hydroxide; magnesium trisilicate] 80•20 mg

Alenic Alka liquid OTC *antacid* [aluminum hydroxide; magnesium carbonate] 31.7•137.3 mg/5 mL

Alenic Alka, Extra Strength chewable tablets OTC *antacid* [aluminum hydroxide; magnesium carbonate] 160•105 mg

alentemol INN *antipsychotic; dopamine agonist* [also: alentemol hydrobromide]

alentemol hydrobromide USAN *antipsychotic; dopamine agonist* [also: alentemol]

alepride INN

Aler C 500 capsules OTC *vitamin supplement* [vitamin C]

Aler-Key capsules OTC *dietary supplement* [multiple vitamins; bioflavonoids; bovine adrenal concentrate]

Alersule sustained-release capsules (discontinued 1995) ℞ *decongestant; antihistamine* [phenylephrine HCl; chlorpheniramine maleate] 20•8 mg

Alersule Forte sustained-release capsules (discontinued 1992) ℞ *decongestant; antihistamine; anticholinergic* [phenylephrine HCl; chlorpheniramine maleate; methscopolamine nitrate]

alestramustine INN

aletamine HCl USAN *antidepressant* [also: alfetamine]

Aleve tablets OTC *nonsteroidal anti-inflammatory drug (NSAID); antiarthritic; analgesic* [naproxen (from naproxen sodium)] 200 (220) mg

alexidine USAN, INN *antibacterial*

alexitol sodium INN, BAN

alfacalcidol INN, BAN, JAN

alfadex INN

alfadolone INN, DCF [also: alphadolone]

alfaprostol USAN, INN, BAN *veterinary prostaglandin*

alfaxalone INN, JAN, DCF [also: alphaxalone]

Alfenta IV or IM injection ℞ *narcotic analgesic; anesthetic* [alfentanil HCl] 500 μg/mL

alfentanil INN, BAN *narcotic analgesic* [also: alfentanil HCl]

alfentanil HCl USAN *narcotic analgesic* [also: alfentanil]

Alferon LDO (low dose oral) ℞ *investigational (Phase I/II) cytokine for AIDS and ARC* [interferon alfa-n3]

Alferon N intralesional injection ℞ *antineoplastic for condylomata acuminata; investigational (Phase I/II) cytokine for AIDS and ARC* [interferon alfa-n3] 5 mIU

alfetamine INN *antidepressant* [also: aletamine HCl]

alfetamine HCl [see: aletamine HCl]

alfuzosin INN, BAN *antihypertensive (α-blocker); investigational treatment for urinary incontinence* [also: alfuzosin HCl]

alfuzosin HCl USAN *antihypertensive (α-blocker); investigational treatment for urinary incontinence* [also: alfuzosin]

algeldrate USAN, INN *antacid*

Algenic Alka liquid OTC *antacid* [aluminum hydroxide; magnesium carbonate; EDTA]

Algenic Alka Improved chewable tablets OTC *antacid* [aluminum hydroxide; sodium bicarbonate; magnesium trisilicate]

algestone INN *anti-inflammatory* [also: algestone acetonide]

algestone acetonide USAN, BAN *anti-inflammatory* [also: algestone]

algestone acetophenide USAN *progestin*

Algicon chewable tablets (discontinued 1992) OTC *antacid* [aluminum hydroxide; magnesium carbonate]

algin [see: sodium alginate]

alginic acid NF, BAN *tablet binder and emulsifying agent*

alginic acid, sodium salt [see: sodium alginate]

alglucerase USAN, INN, BAN *glucocerebrosidase enzyme replenisher; for Gaucher's disease (orphan)*

alibendol INN, DCF

aliconazole INN

alidine dihydrochloride [see: anileridine]

alidine phosphate [see: anileridine]

alifedrine INN

aliflurane USAN, INN *inhalation anesthetic*

alimadol INN

alimemazine INN *antipruritic; antihistamine* [also: trimeprazine tartrate; trimeprazine; alimemazine tartrate]

alimemazine tartrate JAN *antipruritic; antihistamine* [also: trimeprazine tartrate; alimemazine; trimeprazine]

Alimentum ready-to-use liquid OTC *hypoallergenic infant food* [casein protein formula]

alinidine INN, BAN

alipamide USAN, INN, BAN *diuretic; antihypertensive*

aliphatic alcohol compound *investigational treatment for herpes simplex*

alisactide [see: alsactide]

alisobumal [see: butalbital]

alitame USAN *sweetener*

alizapride INN

Alkaban-AQ IV injection (discontinued 1995) ℞ *antineoplastic* [vinblastine sulfate] 1 mg/mL

Alka-Mints chewable tablets OTC *antacid* [calcium carbonate] 850 mg

Alka-Seltzer effervescent tablets OTC *antacid; analgesic* [sodium bicarbonate; citric acid; aspirin; phenylalanine] 1700•1000•325•9 mg

Alka-Seltzer, Extra Strength effervescent tablets OTC *antacid; analgesic* [sodium bicarbonate; citric acid; aspirin] 1985•1000•500 mg

Alka-Seltzer, Gold effervescent tablets OTC *antacid* [sodium bicarbonate; citric acid; potassium bicarbonate] 958•832•312 mg

Alka-Seltzer, Original effervescent tablets OTC *antacid; analgesic* [sodium bicarbonate; citric acid; aspirin] 1916•1000•325 mg

Alka-Seltzer Advanced Formula effervescent tablets (discontinued 1994) OTC *antacid; analgesic* [sodium bicarbonate; calcium carbonate; acetaminophen; citric acid; potassium bicarbonate] 465•280•325•900•300 mg

Alka-Seltzer Plus Allergy Liqui-Gels; Alka-Seltzer Plus Cold Liqui-Gels (capsules) OTC *decongestant; antihistamine; analgesic* [pseudoephedrine HCl; chlorpheniramine maleate; acetaminophen] 30•2•250 mg

Alka-Seltzer Plus Cold & Cough tablets OTC *antitussive; decongestant; antihistamine; analgesic; antipyretic* [dextromethorphan hydrobromide; phenylpropanolamine bitartrate; chlorpheniramine maleate; aspirin] 10•20•2•325 mg

Alka-Seltzer Plus Cold & Cough Liqui-Gels (capsules) OTC *antitussive; decongestant; antihistamine; analgesic* [dextromethorphan hydrobromide; pseudoephedrine HCl; chlorpheniramine maleate; acetaminophen] 10•30•2•250 mg

Alka-Seltzer Plus Cold Medicine; Alka-Seltzer Plus Cold Tablets for oral solution OTC *decongestant; antihistamine; analgesic; antipyretic* [phenylpropanolamine bitartrate; brompheniramine maleate; aspirin] 20•2•325 mg; 24.08•2•325 mg

Alka-Seltzer Plus Flu & Body Aches Non-Drowsy Liqui-Gels (capsules) OTC *antitussive; decongestant; analgesic* [dextromethorphan hydrobromide; pseudoephedrine HCl; acetaminophen] 10•30•250 mg

Alka-Seltzer Plus Night-Time Cold tablets OTC *antitussive; decongestant; antihistamine; analgesic; antipyretic* [dextromethorphan hydrobromide; phenylpropanolamine bitartrate; doxylamine succinate; aspirin] 10•20•6.25•500 mg

Alka-Seltzer Plus Night-Time Cold Liqui-Gels (capsules) OTC *antitussive; decongestant; antihistamine; analgesic* [dextromethorphan hydrobromide; pseudoephedrine HCl; doxylamine succinate; acetaminophen] 10•30•6.25•250 mg

Alka-Seltzer Plus Sinus tablets OTC *decongestant; analgesic; antipyretic* [phenylpropanolamine bitartrate; aspirin] 20•325 mg

Alka-Seltzer Plus Sinus Allergy tablets (discontinued 1995) OTC *decongestant; antihistamine; analgesic; antipyretic* [phenylpropanolamine bitartrate; brompheniramine maleate; aspirin] 24.08•2•500 mg

Alka-Seltzer with Aspirin effervescent tablets OTC *antacid; analgesic* [sodium bicarbonate; citric acid; aspirin] 1900•1000•325, 1900•1000•500 mg

alkavervir (Veratrum viride alkaloids)

Alkeran tablets, powder for IV infusion ℞ *antineoplastic for ovarian, testicular, and breast cancers, lymphomas; multiple myeloma (orphan)* [melphalan] 2 mg; 50 mg

Alkets chewable tablets OTC *antacid* [calcium carbonate] 500, 750 mg

alkyl aryl sulfonate *surfactant/wetting agent*

alkylbenzyldimethylammonium chloride [see: benzalkonium chloride]

alkyldimethylbenzylammonium chloride [see: benzalkonium chloride]

alkylpolyaminoethylglycine JAN

alkylpolyaminoethylglycine HCl JAN

allantoin USAN, BAN *topical vulnerary*

Allbee C-800 film-coated tablets OTC *vitamin supplement* [multiple B vitamins; vitamins C and E] ±•800•45 mg

Allbee C-800 plus Iron film-coated tablets OTC *vitamin/iron supplement* [ferrous fumarate; multiple B vitamins; vitamins C and E; folic acid] 27 mg•±•800 mg•45 IU•0.4 mg

Allbee with C caplets OTC *vitamin supplement* [multiple B vitamins; vitamin C] ±•300 mg

Allbee-T tablets OTC *vitamin supplement* [multiple B vitamins; vitamin C] ±•500 mg

Allegra capsules ℞ *nonsedating antihistamine* [fexofenadine HCl] 60 mg

allegron [see: nortriptyline]

Allent sustained-release capsules ℞ *decongestant; antihistamine* [pseudoephedrine HCl; brompheniramine maleate] 120•12 mg

Aller-Chlor tablets, syrup OTC *antihistamine* [chlorpheniramine maleate] 4 mg; 2 mg/5 mL

Allercon tablets OTC *decongestant; antihistamine* [pseudoephedrine HCl; triprolidine HCl] 60•2.5 mg

Allercreme Skin lotion OTC *moisturizer; emollient*

Allercreme Ultra Emollient cream OTC *moisturizer; emollient*

Allerest eye drops OTC *topical ocular decongestant/vasoconstrictor* [naphazoline HCl] 0.012%

Allerest tablets OTC *decongestant; antihistamine* [pseudoephedrine HCl; chlorpheniramine maleate] 30•2 mg

Allerest, Children's chewable tablets OTC *pediatric decongestant and antihistamine* [phenylpropanolamine HCl; chlorpheniramine maleate] 9.4•1 mg

Allerest 12 Hour nasal spray OTC *nasal decongestant* [oxymetazoline HCl] 0.05%

Allerest 12 Hour sustained-release caplets OTC *decongestant; antihistamine* [phenylpropanolamine HCl; chlorpheniramine maleate] 75•12 mg

Allerest Headache; Allerest Sinus Pain Formula tablets OTC *decongestant; antihistamine; analgesic* [pseudoephedrine HCl; chlorpheniramine maleate; acetaminophen] 30•2•325 mg; 30•2•500 mg

Allerest No Drowsiness tablets OTC *decongestant; analgesic* [pseudoephedrine HCl; acetaminophen] 30•325 mg

Allerfrim tablets, syrup OTC *decongestant; antihistamine* [pseudoephedrine HCl; triprolidine HCl] 60•2.5 mg; 30•1.25 mg/5 mL

Allerfrin with Codeine syrup ℞ *narcotic antitussive; decongestant; antihistamine* [codeine phosphate; pseudoephedrine HCl; triprolidine HCl] 10•30•1.25 mg/5 mL

Allergan Enzymatic tablets OTC *enzymatic cleaner for soft contact lenses* [papain] ⑫ allergen; Auralgan

Allergan Hydrocare [see: Hydrocare]

Allergan Sorbi-Care Saline solution (discontinued 1992) OTC *rinsing/storage solution for soft contact lenses* [preserved saline solution]

Allergen Ear Drops ℞ *topical local anesthetic; analgesic* [benzocaine; antipyrine] 1.4%•5.4%

allergenic extracts (aqueous, glycerinated, or alum-precipitated) *over 900 allergens available for diagnosis of and desensitization to specific allergies*

Allergy tablets OTC *antihistamine* [chlorpheniramine maleate] 4 mg

Allergy Cold tablets (discontinued 1995) OTC *decongestant; antihistamine* [pseudoephedrine HCl; triprolidine HCl] 60•2.5 mg

Allergy Drops eye drops OTC *topical ocular decongestant/vasoconstrictor* [naphazoline HCl] 0.012%; 0.03%

Allergy Relief Medicine tablets (discontinued 1995) OTC *decongestant; antihistamine* [phenylpropanolamine HCl; chlorpheniramine maleate] 25•4 mg

AlleRid capsules OTC *decongestant* [pseudoephedrine HCl]

AllerMax caplets, oral liquid OTC *antihistamine* [diphenhydramine HCl] 25, 50 mg; 12.5 mg/5 mL

Allermed capsules OTC *nasal decongestant* [pseudoephedrine HCl] 60 mg

Allerphed syrup OTC *decongestant; antihistamine* [pseudoephedrine HCl; triprolidine HCl] 30•1.25 mg/5 mL

Allersone ointment (discontinued 1992) ℞ *topical corticosteroid; anesthetic; astringent* [hydrocortisone; diperodon HCl; zinc oxide]

Allersule Forte sustained-release capsules (discontinued 1992) ℞ *decongestant; antihistamine; anticholinergic* [phenylephrine HCl; chlorpheniramine maleate; methscopolamine nitrate]

Allervax ℞ *investigational antiallergic*

alletorphine BAN, INN

All-Nite Cold Formula liquid OTC *antitussive; decongestant; antihistamine; analgesic* [dextromethorphan hydrobromide; pseudoephedrine HCl; doxylamine succinate; acetaminophen; alcohol 25%] 5•10•1.25•167 mg/5 mL

allobarbital USAN, INN *hypnotic*

allobarbitone [see: allobarbital]

alloclamide INN, DCF

allocupreide sodium INN, DCF

Alloderm *investigational skin graft for third-degree burns and plastic surgery* [processed human donor skin]

allomethadione INN, DCF [also: aloxidone]

allopurinol USAN, USP, INN, BAN, JAN *xanthine oxidase inhibitor for gout; (orphan: kidney transplants)* 100, 300 mg oral

allopurinol riboside *(orphan: leishmaniasis; Chagas disease)*

allopurinol sodium *(orphan: leukemia, lymphoma, and solid tumor malignancies)*

Allpyral subcu or IM injection ℞ *allergenic sensitivity testing (subcu); allergenic desensitization therapy (IM)* [allergenic extracts, alum-precipitated]

all-*trans*-retinoic acid [see: tretinoin]

allyl isothiocyanate USAN

allylbarbituric acid [now: butalbital]

allylestrenol INN, JAN [also: allyloestrenol]

allyl-isobutylbarbituric acid [see: butalbital]

allylisopropylmalonylurea [see: aprobarbital]

4-allyl-2-methoxyphenol [see: eugenol]

N-allylnoretorphine [see: alletorphine]

N-allylnoroxymorphone HCl [see: naloxone HCl]

allyloestrenol BAN [also: allylestrenol]

allyprodine INN, BAN, DCF

5-allyl-5-*sec*-butylbarbituric acid [see: talbutal]

allylthiourea INN

allypropymal [see: aprobarbital]

Almacone chewable tablets, liquid OTC *antacid; antiflatulent* [aluminum hydroxide; magnesium hydroxide; simethicone] 200•200•20 mg; 200•200•20 mg/5 mL

Almacone II liquid OTC *antacid; antiflatulent* [aluminum hydroxide; magnesium hydroxide; simethicone] 400•400•40 mg/5 mL

almadrate sulfate USAN, INN *antacid*

almagate USAN, INN *antacid*

almagodrate INN

Alma-Mag oral suspension (discontinued 1994) OTC *antacid* [aluminum hydroxide; magnesium hydroxide] ⊇ Alamag

Alma-Mag, Improved liquid (discontinued 1994) OTC *antacid; antiflatulent* [aluminum hydroxide; magnesium hydroxide; simethicone] 40•40•5 mg/mL

Alma-Mag #4 Improved chewable tablets (discontinued 1994) OTC *antacid; antiflatulent* [aluminum hydroxide; magnesium hydroxide; simethicone] 200•200•25 mg

almasilate INN, BAN

Almebex Plus B₁₂ liquid OTC *vitamin supplement* [multiple B vitamins] ≜

almecillin INN

almestrone INN

alminoprofen INN, JAN

almitrine INN, BAN

almokalant INN *investigational antiarrhythmic*

almond oil NF *emollient and perfume; oleaginous vehicle*

Almora tablets OTC *magnesium supplement* [magnesium gluconate] 500 mg

almoxatone INN

alnespirone INN

Alodopa-15; Alodopa-25 tablets ℞ *antihypertensive* [hydrochlorothiazide; methyldopa]

aloe USP ▣ Alco-Gel

Aloe Grande lotion OTC *moisturizer; emollient; skin protectant* [vitamins A and E; aloe] 3333.3•50•≟ U/g

Aloe Vesta Perineal solution OTC *emollient/protectant* [propylene glycol; aloe vera gel]

alofilcon A USAN *hydrophilic contact lens material*

aloin BAN

ALOMAD (Adriamycin, Leukeran, Oncovin, methotrexate, actinomycin D, dacarbazine) *chemotherapy protocol* ▣ Alomide

Alomide Drop-Tainers (eye drops) ℞ *antiallergic agent for vernal keratoconjunctivitis (orphan)* [lodoxamide tromethamine] 0.1% ▣ ALOMAD

alonacic INN

alonimid USAN, INN *sedative; hypnotic*

Alophen Pills tablets OTC *laxative* [phenolphthalein] 60 mg

Alophen Pills No. 973 tablets (name changed to Alophen Pills in 1995)

aloracetam INN

alosetron INN, BAN *antiemetic* [also: alosetron HCl]

alosetron HCl USAN *antiemetic; investigational antipsychotic for schizophrenia (clinical trials discontinued 1994)* [also: alosetron]

alovudine USAN, INN *antiviral*

aloxidone BAN [also: allomethadione]

aloxiprin INN, BAN, DCF

aloxistatin INN

alozafone INN

alpertine USAN, INN *antipsychotic*

alpha amylase (α-amylase) USAN *anti-inflammatory*

alpha hydroxy acids (AHA) [see: glycolic acid]

alpha interferon-2A [see: interferon alfa-2A]

alpha interferon-2B [see: interferon alfa-2B]

alpha interferon-N1 [see: interferon alfa-N1]

alpha interferon-N3 [see: interferon alfa-N3]

Alpha Keri Moisturizing Soap bar OTC *therapeutic skin cleanser*

Alpha Keri Spray; Alpha Keri Therapeutic Bath Oil OTC *bath emollient*

***d*-alpha tocopherol** [see: vitamin E]

***dl*-alpha tocopherol** [see: vitamin E]

***d*-alpha tocopheryl acetate** [see: vitamin E]

***dl*-alpha tocopheryl acetate** [see: vitamin E]

***d*-alpha tocopheryl acid succinate** [see: vitamin E]

***dl*-alpha tocopheryl acid succinate** [see: vitamin E]

Alpha Zeta tablets (discontinued 1994) OTC *vitamin/mineral/iron supplement* [ferrous fumarate; multiple vitamins & minerals; folic acid; biotin] 27 mg•≟•0.4 mg•45 µg

alpha$_1$ PI (alpha$_1$-proteinase inhibitor) [q.v.]

alpha$_1$-antitrypsin, recombinant *(orphan: alpha$_1$-antitrypsin deficiency)* [see: alpha$_1$-proteinase inhibitor]

alpha$_1$-proteinase inhibitor (alpha$_1$ PI) *investigational (Phase II) antiviral for HIV; congenital alpha$_1$ PI deficiency (orphan)*

***l*-alpha-acetyl-methadol (LAAM)** *(orphan: heroin addiction)*

alphacemethadone [see: alphacetylmethadol]

alphacetylmethadol BAN, INN, DCF

alpha-chymotrypsin [see: chymotrypsin]

alpha-cypermethrin BAN

Alphaderm cream (discontinued 1992) ℞ *topical corticosteroid* [hydrocortisone]

alpha-D-galactosidase *digestive enzyme*

alphadolone BAN [also: alfadolone]

alpha-estradiol [see: estradiol]

alpha-estradiol benzoate [see: estradiol benzoate]

alpha-galactosidase A *(orphan: Fabry's disease)*

1-alpha-hydroxy vitamin D$_2$ *investigational osteoporosis treatment*

alpha-hypophamine [see: oxytocin]

alphameprodine INN, BAN, DCF

alphamethadol INN, BAN, DCF

alpha-methyldopa [now: methyldopa]

Alphamin IM injection (discontinued 1994) ℞ *antianemic; vitamin B_{12} supplement* [hydroxocobalamin] 1000 μg/mL

Alphamul emulsion (discontinued 1994) OTC *stimulant laxative* [castor oil] 60%

Alphanate powder for IV injection ℞ *antihemophilic* [antihemophilic factor VIII:C, solvent/detergent treated] ≟

AlphaNine IV injection ℞ *hemostatic; for factor IX deficiency; coagulant for hemophilia B (orphan)* [coagulation factor IX (human)] ≟

AlphaNine SD IV injection ℞ *antihemophilic for factor IX deficiency; coagulant for hemophilia B (orphan)* [coagulation factor IX (human), solvent/detergent treated] ≟

alpha-phenoxyethyl penicillin, potassium [see: phenethicillin potassium]

alphaprodine INN, BAN [also: alphaprodine HCl]

alphaprodine HCl USP [also: alphaprodine]

alphasone acetophenide [now: algestone acetonide]

Alphatrex cream, ointment, lotion ℞ *topical corticosteroid* [betamethasone dipropionate] 0.05%

alphaxalone BAN [also: alfaxalone]

Alphosyl cream (discontinued 1992) OTC *topical antipsoriatic; antiseborrheic; vulnerary* [coal tar extract; allantoin]

Alphosyl lotion OTC *topical antipsoriatic; antiseborrheic; vulnerary* [coal tar extract; allantoin]

alpidem USAN, INN, BAN *anxiolytic*

alpiropride INN

alprafenone INN

alprazolam USAN, USP, INN, BAN, JAN *anxiolytic; sedative; treatment of panic disorders and agoraphobia* 0.25, 0.5, 1, 2 mg, 0.5 mg/5 mL, 1 mg/mL oral

alprenolol INN, BAN *antiadrenergic (β-receptor)* [also: alprenolol HCl]

alprenolol HCl USAN, JAN *antiadrenergic (β-receptor)* [also: alprenolol]

alprenoxime HCl USAN *antiglaucoma agent*

alprostadil USAN, USP, INN, BAN, JAN *vasodilator; platelet aggregation inhibitor; treatment for erectile dysfunction*

alprostadil alfadex BAN

Alramucil effervescent powder OTC *bulk laxative* [psyllium hydrophilic mucilloid] 3.6 g/packet

Alredase ℞ *investigational aldose reductase inhibitor for diabetic neuropathy* [tolrestat]

alrestatin INN *aldose reductase enzyme inhibitor* [also: alrestatin sodium]

alrestatin sodium USAN *aldose reductase enzyme inhibitor* [also: alrestatin]

alsactide INN

alseroxylon JAN *antihypertensive; rauwolfia derivative*

ALT (autolymphocyte therapy) [q.v.]

Altace capsules ℞ *antihypertensive; angiotensin-converting enzyme (ACE) inhibitor* [ramipril] 1.25, 2.5, 5, 10 mg

altanserin INN *serotonin antagonist* [also: altanserin tartrate]

altanserin tartrate USAN *serotonin antagonist* [also: altanserin]

altapizone INN

alteconazole INN

alteplase USAN, INN, BAN, JAN *tissue plasminogen activator (tPA); investigational treatment for stroke*

ALternaGEL liquid OTC *antacid* [aluminum hydroxide gel] 600 mg/5 mL

althiazide USAN *antihypertensive* [also: altizide]

altizide INN, DCF *antihypertensive* [also: althiazide]

altoqualine INN

Altracin (*orphan: pseudomembranous enterocolitis*) [bacitracin]

altrenogest USAN, INN, BAN *veterinary progestin*

altretamine USAN, INN, BAN *antineoplastic; for ovarian adenocarcinoma (orphan)*

altumomab USAN, INN *radiodiagnostic monoclonal antibody; anticarcinoembryonic antigen (anti-CEA)* [also: indium In 111 altumomab pentetate]

altumomab pentetate USAN *monoclonal antibody conjugate* [also: indium In 111 altumomab pentetate]

Alu-Cap capsules OTC *antacid* [aluminum hydroxide gel] 400 mg

Aludrox oral suspension OTC *antacid; antiflatulent* [aluminum hydroxide; magnesium hydroxide; simethicone] 307•103•<u>?</u> mg/5 mL

alukalin [see: kaolin]

alum, ammonium USP *topical astringent*

alum, potassium USP *topical astringent* [also: aluminum potassium sulfate]

Alumadrine tablets ℞ *decongestant; antihistamine; analgesic* [phenylpropanolamine HCl; chlorpheniramine maleate; acetaminophen] 25•4•500 mg

alumina & magnesia USP *antacid*

aluminopara-aminosalicylate calcium (alumino *p*-aminosalicylate calcium) JAN

aluminosilicic acid, magnesium salt hydrate [see: silodrate]

aluminum *element (Al)*

aluminum, micronized *astringent*

aluminum acetate USP *topical astringent; Burow solution*

aluminum aminoacetate [see: dihydroxyaluminum aminoacetate]

aluminum ammonium sulfate dodecahydrate [see: alum, ammonium]

aluminum bismuth oxide [see: bismuth aluminate]

aluminum carbonate, basic USAN, USP *antacid*

aluminum chlorhydroxide [now: aluminum chlorohydrate]

aluminum chlorhydroxide alcohol soluble complex [now: aluminum chlorohydrex]

aluminum chloride USP *topical astringent for hyperhidrosis*

aluminum chloride, basic [see: aluminum sesquichlorohydrate]

aluminum chloride hexahydrate [see: aluminum chloride]

aluminum chloride hydroxide hydrate [see: aluminum chlorohydrate]

aluminum chlorohydrate USAN *anhidrotic*

aluminum chlorohydrex USAN *topical astringent*

aluminum chlorohydrol propylene glycol complex [now: aluminum chlorohydrex]

aluminum chlorohydroxy allantoinate JAN *astringent; keratolytic* [also: alcloxa]

aluminum clofibrate INN, BAN, JAN

aluminum dihydroxyaminoacetate [see: dihydroxyaluminum aminoacetate]

aluminum flufenamate JAN

aluminum glycinate, basic [see: dihydroxyaluminum aminoacetate]

aluminum hydroxide gel USP *antacid* 320, 450, 600 mg/5 mL oral

aluminum hydroxide gel, dried USP, JAN *antacid*

aluminum hydroxide glycine [see: dihydroxyaluminum aminoacetate]

aluminum hydroxide hydrate [see: algeldrate]

aluminum hydroxychloride [now: aluminum chlorohydrate]

aluminum magnesium carbonate hydroxide dihydrate [see: almagate]

aluminum magnesium hydroxide carbonate hydrate [see: hydrotalcite]

aluminum magnesium hydroxide oxide sulfate [see: almadrate sulfate]

aluminum magnesium hydroxide oxide sulfate hydrate [see: almadrate sulfate]

aluminum magnesium hydroxide sulfate [see: magaldrate]

aluminum magnesium hydroxide sulfate hydrate [see: magaldrate]

aluminum monostearate NF, JAN

aluminum oxide

Aluminum Paste ointment OTC *occlusive skin protectant* [metallic aluminum] 10%

aluminum phosphate gel USP *antacid (disapproved for use as an antacid in 1989)*

aluminum potassium sulfate JAN *topical astringent* [also: alum, potassium]

aluminum potassium sulfate dodecahydrate [see: alum, potassium]

aluminum sesquichlorohydrate USAN *anhidrotic*

aluminum silicate, natural JAN

aluminum silicate, synthetic JAN

aluminum sodium carbonate hydroxide [see: dihydroxyaluminum sodium carbonate]

aluminum subacetate USP *topical astringent*

aluminum sulfate USP

aluminum sulfate hydrate [see: aluminum sulfate]

aluminum zirconium glycine tetrachloro hydrate complex [see: aluminum zirconium tetrachlorohydrex gly]

aluminum zirconium glycine trichloro hydrate complex [see: aluminum zirconium trichlorohydrex gly]

aluminum zirconium octachlorohydrate USP *anhidrotic*

aluminum zirconium octachlorohydrex gly USP *anhidrotic*

aluminum zirconium pentachlorohydrate USP *anhidrotic*

aluminum zirconium pentachlorohydrex gly USP *anhidrotic*

aluminum zirconium tetrachlorohydrate USP *anhidrotic*

aluminum zirconium tetrachlorohydrex gly USAN, USP *anhidrotic*

aluminum zirconium trichlorohydrate USP *anhidrotic*

aluminum zirconium trichlorohydrex gly USAN, USP *anhidrotic*

Alupent tablets, syrup, inhalation aerosol powder, solution for inhalation ℞ *bronchodilator* [metaproterenol sulfate] 10, 20 mg; 10 mg/5 mL; 0.65 mg/dose; 0.4%, 0.6%, 5%

Alurate elixir ℞ *sedative; hypnotic* [aprobarbital] 40 mg/5 mL

alusulf INN

Alu-Tab film-coated tablets OTC *antacid* [aluminum hydroxide gel] 500 mg

ALVAC-120TMG *investigational (Phase I) vaccine for HIV*

ALVAC-HIV 1 *investigational (Phase I) vaccine for HIV*

alverine INN, BAN *anticholinergic* [also: alverine citrate]

alverine citrate USAN, NF *anticholinergic* [also: alverine]

alvircept sudotox USAN, INN *antiviral; investigational for AIDS*

Al-Vite tablets (discontinued 1993) ℞ *vitamin supplement* [multiple vitamins]

Alzene ℞ *investigational treatment for Alzheimer's disease and epilepsy*

amabevan [see: carbarsone]

amacetam HCl [now: pramiracetam HCl]

amacetam sulfate [now: pramiracetam sulfate]

Amacodone tablets (discontinued 1995) ℞ *narcotic analgesic* [hydrocodone bitartrate; acetaminophen] 5•500 mg

amadinone INN *progestin* [also: amadinone acetate]

amadinone acetate USAN *progestin* [also: amadinone]

amafolone INN, BAN

amalgucin

amanozine INN

amantadine INN, BAN *antiviral; antiparkinsonian* [also: amantadine HCl]

amantadine HCl USAN, USP, JAN *antiviral; antiparkinsonian* [also: amantadine] 100 mg oral; 50 mg/5 mL oral

amantanium bromide INN

amantocillin INN

Amaphen capsules ℞ *analgesic; antipyretic; sedative* [acetaminophen; caffeine; butalbital] 325•40•50 mg

Amaphen with Codeine #3 capsules (discontinued 1995) ℞ *narcotic analgesic; sedative* [codeine phosphate; acetaminophen; caffeine; butalbital] 30•325•40•50 mg

amaranth (FD&C Red No. 2) USP

amarsan [see: acetarsone]

Amaryl tablets ℞ *once-daily sulfonylurea-type antidiabetic* [glimepiride] 1, 2, 4 mg

Amatine ℞ *investigational hypotension treatment* [midodrine]

ambamustine INN

ambasilide INN *investigational antiarrhythmic*

ambazone INN, BAN, DCF

ambenonium chloride USP, INN, BAN, JAN *anticholinesterase muscle stimulant*

ambenoxan INN, BAN

Ambenyl Cough syrup ℞ *narcotic antitussive; antihistamine* [codeine phosphate; bromodiphenhydramine

HCl; alcohol 5%] 10•12.5 mg/5 mL
℞ Aventyl

Ambenyl-D liquid OTC *antitussive; decongestant; expectorant* [dextromethorphan hydrobromide; pseudoephedrine HCl; guaifenesin; alcohol 9.5%] 10•30•100 mg/5 mL

Ambi 10 bar OTC *therapeutic skin cleanser*

Ambi 10 cream OTC *topical keratolytic for acne* [benzoyl peroxide] 10%

Ambi Skin Tone cream OTC *hyperpigmentation bleaching agent; sunscreen* [hydroquinone; padimate O]

ambicromil INN, BAN *prophylactic antiallergic* [also: probicromil calcium]

ambicromil calcium [see: probicromil calcium]

Ambien film-coated tablets ℞ *imidazopyridine-type sedative/hypnotic* [zolpidem tartrate] 5, 10 mg

AmBisome ℞ *investigational antifungal for immunocompromised patients* [liposomal formulation of amphotericin B]

ambomycin USAN, INN *antineoplastic*

ambroxol INN [also: ambroxol HCl]

ambroxol HCl JAN [also: ambroxol]

ambruticin USAN, INN *antifungal*

ambucaine INN, DCF

ambucetamide INN, BAN

ambuphylline USAN *diuretic; smooth muscle relaxant* [also: bufylline]

ambuside USAN, INN, BAN *diuretic*

ambuterol [see: mabuterol]

ambutonium bromide BAN

ambutoxate [see: ambucaine]

amcinafal USAN, INN *anti-inflammatory*

amcinafide USAN, INN *anti-inflammatory*

amcinonide USAN, USP, INN, BAN, JAN *topical corticosteroid*

Amcort IM injection ℞ *glucocorticoid* [triamcinolone diacetate] 40 mg/mL

amdinocillin USAN, USP *antibacterial* [also: mecillinam]

amdinocillin pivoxil USAN *antibacterial* [also: pivmecillinam; pivmecillinam HCl]

ameban [see: carbarsone]

amebarsone [see: carbarsone]

amebucort INN

amechol [see: methacholine chloride]

amedalin INN *antidepressant* [also: amedalin HCl]

amedalin HCl USAN *antidepressant* [also: amedalin]

ameltolide USAN, INN, BAN *anticonvulsant*

Amen tablets ℞ *progestin for secondary amenorrhea or abnormal uterine bleeding* [medroxyprogesterone acetate] 10 mg

amenozine [see: amanozine]

Americaine ointment, anorectal ointment, aerosol spray OTC *topical local anesthetic* [benzocaine] 20%

Americaine Anesthetic Lubricant gel ℞ *anesthetic lubricant for upper GI procedures* [benzocaine] 20%

Americaine First Aid ointment OTC *topical local anesthetic* [benzocaine] 20%

Americaine Otic ear drops ℞ *topical local anesthetic* [benzocaine] 20%

americium *element* (Am)

Amesec capsules (discontinued 1993) OTC *antiasthmatic; bronchodilator; decongestant* [aminophylline; ephedrine HCl]

amesergide USAN, INN *serotonin antagonist; investigational antidepressant*

ametantrone INN *antineoplastic* [also: ametantrone acetate]

ametantrone acetate USAN *antineoplastic* [also: ametantrone]

ametazole BAN [also: betazole HCl; betazole]

A-Methapred powder for injection ℞ *glucocorticoid; anti-inflammatory; immunosuppressant* [methylprednisolone sodium succinate] 40, 125, 500, 1000 mg/vial

amethocaine BAN *topical anesthetic* [also: tetracaine]

amethocaine HCl BAN *local anesthetic* [also: tetracaine HCl]

amethopterin [now: methotrexate]

amezepine INN

amezinium metilsulfate INN, JAN

amfebutamone INN *aminoketone antidepressant* [also: bupropion HCl; bupropion]

amfebutamone HCl [see: bupropion HCl]

amfecloral INN, BAN *anorectic* [also: amphecloral]
amfenac INN, BAN *anti-inflammatory* [also: amfenac sodium]
amfenac sodium USAN, JAN *anti-inflammatory* [also: amfenac]
amfepentorex INN, DCF
amfepramone INN, DCF *anorexiant* [also: diethylpropion HCl; diethylpropion]
amfepramone HCl *anorexiant* [see: diethylpropion HCl]
amfetamine INN *CNS stimulant* [also: amphetamine sulfate; amphetamine]
amfetaminil INN
amfilcon A USAN *hydrophilic contact lens material*
amflutizole USAN, INN *gout suppressant*
amfodyne [see: imidecyl iodine]
amfomycin INN, DCF *antibacterial* [also: amphomycin]
amfonelic acid USAN, INN, BAN *CNS stimulant*
Amgenal Cough syrup ℞ *narcotic antitussive; antihistamine* [codeine phosphate; bromodiphenhydramine HCl] 10•12.5 mg/5 mL
AMI-227 *investigational contrast agent for magnetic imaging of the heart, brain, and lymphatic system*
amibiarson [see: carbarsone]
Amicar tablets, syrup, IV infusion ℞ *systemic hemostatic to control excessive bleeding* [aminocaproic acid] 500 mg; 250 mg/mL; 250 mg/mL ⓥ Amikin
amicarbalide INN, BAN
amicibone INN
amicloral USAN *veterinary food additive*
amicycline USAN, INN *antibacterial*
amidantel INN, BAN
amidapsone USAN, INN *antiviral for poultry*
Amidate IV ℞ *general anesthetic* [etomidate] 2 mg/mL
amidefrine mesilate INN *adrenergic* [also: amidephrine mesylate; amidephrine]
amidephrine BAN *adrenergic* [also: amidephrine mesylate; amidefrine mesilate]
amidephrine mesylate USAN *adrenergic* [also: amidefrine mesilate; amidephrine]

amidofebrin [see: aminopyrine]
amidol [see: dimepheptanol]
amidone HCl [see: methadone HCl]
amidopyrazoline [see: aminopyrine]
amidopyrine [now: aminopyrine]
amidotrizoate sodium [see: diatrizoate sodium]
amidotrizoic acid JAN *radiopaque medium* [also: diatrizoic acid]
Ami-Drix sustained-release tablets (discontinued 1995) ℞ *decongestant; antihistamine* [pseudoephedrine sulfate; dexbrompheniramine maleate] 120•6 mg
amiflamine INN
amifloverine INN, DCF
amifloxacin USAN, INN, BAN *broad-spectrum fluoroquinolone-type antibiotic*
amifloxacin mesylate USAN *antibacterial*
amifostine USAN, INN, BAN *topical radioprotectant; systemic chemoprotective agent for cisplatin and paclitaxel (orphan)* [USAN previously used: ethiofos]
Amigesic film-coated tablets, film-coated caplets, capsules ℞ *analgesic; antipyretic; anti-inflammatory; antirheumatic* [salsalate] 500 mg; 750 mg; 500 mg
AMI-HS *investigational contrast agent for magnetic imaging of the liver*
amikacin USP, INN, BAN *antibacterial*
amikacin sulfate USAN, USP, JAN *aminoglycoside bactericidal antibiotic* 50, 250 mg/mL injection
amikhelline INN
Amikin IV or IM injection, pediatric injection ℞ *aminoglycoside-type antibiotic* [amikacin sulfate] 250 mg/mL; 50 mg/mL ⓥ Amicar
amilomer INN
amiloride INN, BAN *potassium-sparing diuretic* [also: amiloride HCl]
amiloride HCl USAN, USP *potassium-sparing diuretic; (orphan: cystic fibrosis)* [also: amiloride]
Amina-21 capsules OTC *dietary supplement* [multiple amino acids]
aminacrine BAN *topical anti-infective/ antiseptic* [also: aminacrine HCl; aminoacridine]

aminacrine HCl USAN *topical anti-infective/antiseptic* [also: aminoacridine; aminacrine]

Amin-Aid Instant Drink powder OTC *enteral nutritional therapy for acute or chronic renal failure* [essential amino acids]

aminarsone [see: carbarsone]

amindocate INN

amine resin [see: polyamine-methylene resin]

amineptine INN

Aminess 5.2% IV infusion ℞ *nutritional therapy for renal failure* [multiple essential amino acids]

aminicotin [see: niacinamide]

aminitrozole INN *veterinary antibacterial* [also: nithiamide; acinitrazole]

Amino LIV powder OTC *dietary supplement* [multiple amino acids]

Amino VIL powder OTC *dietary supplement* [multiple amino acids]

aminoacetic acid JAN *nonessential amino acid; urologic irrigant; symbols:* Gly, G [also: glycine]

aminoacridine INN *topical anti-infective/antiseptic* [also: aminacrine HCl; aminacrine]

aminoacridine HCl [see: aminacrine HCl]

9-aminoacridine monohydrochloride [see: aminacrine HCl]

***p*-aminobenzenearsonic acid** [see: arsanilic acid]

***p*-aminobenzenesulfonamide** [see: sulfanilamide]

***p*-aminobenzene-sulfonylacetylimide** [see: sulfacetamide]

aminobenzoate potassium USP *analgesic; "possibly effective" for scleroderma and other skin diseases*

aminobenzoate sodium USP *analgesic*

***p*-aminobenzoic acid** [see: aminobenzoic acid]

aminobenzoic acid (4-aminobenzoic acid) USP *ultraviolet screen*

aminobenzylpenicillin [see: ampicillin]

γ-amino-β-hydroxybutyric acid JAN

aminobromophenylpyrimidinone (ABPP) [see: bropirimine]

γ-aminobutyric acid JAN

aminocaproic acid USAN, USP, INN, BAN *systemic hemostatic* [also: ε-aminocaproic acid] 250 mg/mL injection

JAN *systemic hemostatic* [also: aminocaproic acid]

aminocardol [see: aminophylline]

Amino-Cerv pH 5.5 vaginal cream ℞ *emollient; antifungal; anti-inflammatory* [urea; sodium propionate; methionine; cystine; inositol] 8.34%•0.5%•0.83%•0.35%•0.83%

aminodeoxykanamycin [see: bekanamycin]

2-aminoethanethiol [see: cysteamine]

2-aminoethanethiol HCl [see: cysteamine HCl]

2-aminoethanol [see: monoethanolamine]

aminoethyl nitrate (2-aminoethyl nitrate) INN, DCF

amino-ethyl-propanol [see: ambuphylline]

aminoethylsulfonic acid JAN [also: taurine]

aminoform [see: methenamine]

aminoglutethimide USP, INN, BAN *adrenocortical suppressant; antineoplastic*

aminoguanidine monohydrochloride [see: pimagedine HCl]

6-aminohexanoic acid [see: aminocaproic acid]

aminohippurate sodium USP *renal function test* [also: *p*-aminohippurate sodium] 20% injection

***p*-aminohippurate sodium** JAN *renal function test* [also: aminohippurate sodium]

aminohippuric acid (*p*-aminohippuric acid) USP

aminohydroxypropylidene diphosphonate (APD) [see: pamidronate disodium]

aminoisobutanol [see: ambuphylline]

aminoisometradine [see: methionine]

aminometradine INN, BAN

Amino-Min-D capsules OTC *dietary supplement* [calcium carbonate; multiple minerals; vitamin D] 250 mg•±•100 IU

aminonat [see: protein hydrolysate]

Amino-Opti-C sustained-release tablets OTC *dietary supplement* [vitamin

C; lemon & rose hips bioflavonoids; rutin; hesperidin] 1000•250•<u>2</u>•<u>2</u> mg

Amino-Opti-E capsules OTC *dietary supplement* [vitamin E] 165 mg

aminopentamide sulfate [see: dimevamide]

aminophenazone INN [also: aminopyrine]

aminophenazone cyclamate INN

***p*-aminophenylarsonic acid** [see: arsanilic acid]

aminophylline USP, INN, BAN, JAN *smooth muscle relaxant; bronchodilator* 100, 200 mg oral; 105 mg/5 mL oral; 250 mg/10 mL injection; 250, 500 suppositories

Aminoprel capsules (discontinued 1992) OTC *dietary supplement* [multiple amino acids & minerals; vitamins B_6 and C]

aminopromazine INN, DCF [also: proquamezine]

aminopterin sodium INN, BAN, DCF *investigational antineoplastic for breast and ovarian cancer*

4-aminopyridine [see: fampridine]

aminopyrine NF, JAN [also: aminophenazone]

aminoquin naphthoate [see: pamaquine naphthoate]

aminoquinol INN

aminoquinoline [see: aminoquinol]

4-aminoquinoline [see: chloroquine phosphate]

8-aminoquinoline [see: primaquine phosphate]

aminoquinuride INN

aminorex USAN, INN, BAN *anorectic*

aminosalicylate calcium USP [also: calcium para-aminosalicylate]

aminosalicylate potassium USP

aminosalicylate sodium (*p*-aminosalicylate sodium) USP *bacteriostatic; tuberculosis retreatment* (*orphan: Crohn's disease*)

aminosalicylic acid (**4-aminosalicylic acid**) USP *antibacterial; tuberculostatic;* (*orphan: ulcerative colitis; tuberculosis*)

5-aminosalicylic acid (**5-ASA**) [see: mesalamine]

aminosalyle sodium [see: aminosalicylate sodium]

aminosidine (*orphan: Mycobacterium avium complex; visceral leishmaniasis*)

aminosidine sulfate [see: paromomycin sulfate]

aminosuccinic acid [see: aspartic acid]

Aminosyn (pH6) 8.5% IV infusion (discontinued 1992) ℞ *total parenteral nutrition; peripheral parenteral nutrition* [multiple essential and nonessential amino acids]

Aminosyn 3.5% (5%, 7%, 8.5%, 10%); Aminosyn (pH6) 10%; Aminosyn II 3.5% (5%, 7%, 8.5%, 10%, 15%); Aminosyn-PF 7% (10%) IV infusion ℞ *total parenteral nutrition (except 3.5%); peripheral parenteral nutrition (all)* [multiple essential and nonessential amino acids]

Aminosyn 3.5% M; Aminosyn II 3.5% M IV infusion ℞ *peripheral parenteral nutrition* [multiple essential and nonessential amino acids; electrolytes]

Aminosyn 7% (8.5%) with Electrolytes; Aminosyn II 7% (8.5%, 10%) with Electrolytes IV infusion ℞ *total parenteral nutrition; peripheral parenteral nutrition* [multiple essential and nonessential amino acids; electrolytes]

Aminosyn II 3.5% in 5% (25%) Dextrose; Aminosyn II 4.25% in 10% (20%, 25%) Dextrose; Aminosyn II 5% in 25% Dextrose IV infusion ℞ *total parenteral nutrition (except 3.5% in 5%); peripheral parenteral nutrition (not 20% and 25%)* [multiple essential and nonessential amino acids; dextrose]

Aminosyn II 3.5% M in 5% Dextrose; Aminosyn II 4.25% M in 10% Dextrose IV infusion ℞ *total parenteral nutrition (4.25% in 10% only); peripheral parenteral nutrition (both)* [multiple essential and nonessential amino acids & electrolytes; dextrose]

Aminosyn-HBC 7% IV infusion ℞ *nutritional therapy for high metabolic stress* [multiple branched-chain essential and nonessential amino acids; electrolytes]

Aminosyn-RF 5.2% IV infusion ℞ *nutritional therapy for renal failure* [multiple essential amino acids]

aminothiazole INN

aminotrate phosphate [see: trolnitrate phosphate]

aminoxaphen [see: aminorex]

aminoxytriphene INN

aminoxytropine tropate HCl [see: atropine oxide HCl]

Amio-Aqueous ℞ *antiarrhythmic for acute ventricular tachycardia and fibrillation (orphan)* [amiodarone HCl]

amiodarone USAN, INN, BAN *ventricular antiarrhythmic; for acute ventricular tachycardia and fibrillation (orphan)*

amiodarone HCl *antiarrhythmic (orphan: acute ventricular tachycardia and fibrillation)*

Amipaque powder for injection ℞ *parenteral radiopaque agent* [metrizamide] 13.5%, 18.75%

amiperone INN

amiphenazole INN, BAN

amipizone INN

amipramidine [see: amiloride HCl]

amiprilose INN *anti-inflammatory* [also: amiprilose HCl]

amiprilose HCl USAN *anti-inflammatory* [also: amiprilose]

amiquinsin INN *antihypertensive* [also: amiquinsin HCl]

amiquinsin HCl USAN *antihypertensive* [also: amiquinsin]

amisometradine NF, INN, BAN

amisulpride INN

amiterol INN

Ami-Tex LA long-acting tablets ℞ *decongestant; expectorant* [phenylpropanolamine HCl; guaifenesin] 75•400 mg

amithiozone [see: thioacetazone; thiacetazone]

amitivir INN *investigational influenza vaccine*

Amitone chewable tablets OTC *antacid* [calcium carbonate] 350 mg

amitraz USAN, INN, BAN *scabicide*

amitriptyline INN, BAN *antidepressant* [also: amitriptyline HCl] ② nortriptyline

amitriptyline HCl USP, JAN *tricyclic antidepressant* [also: amitriptyline] 10, 25, 50, 75, 100, 150 mg oral; 10 mg/mL injection

amitriptylinoxide INN

amixetrine INN, DCF

amlexanox USAN, INN, JAN *antiallergic*

amlodipine INN, BAN *antianginal; antihypertensive; calcium channel blocker* [also: amlodipine besylate]

amlodipine besylate USAN *antianginal; antihypertensive; calcium channel blocker* [also: amlodipine]

amlodipine maleate USAN *antianginal; antihypertensive*

ammoidin [see: methoxsalen]

[^{13}N]ammonia [see: ammonia N 13]

ammonia [see: ammonia spirit, aromatic]

ammonia N 13 USAN, USP *radioactive diagnostic aid for cardiac and liver imaging*

ammonia solution, strong NF *solvent; source of ammonia* [also: ammonia water]

ammonia spirit, aromatic USP *respiratory stimulant*

ammonia water JAN *solvent; source of ammonia* [also: ammonia solution, strong]

ammoniated mercury [see: mercury, ammoniated]

ammonio methacrylate copolymer NF *coating agent*

ammonium alum [see: alum, ammonium]

ammonium benzoate USP

ammonium biphosphate *urinary acidifier*

ammonium carbonate NF *source of ammonia*

ammonium chloride USP, JAN *acidifier; nonprescription diuretic* 500 mg oral; 5 mEq/mL (26.75%) injection

ammonium 2-hydroxypropanoate [see: ammonium lactate]

ammonium ichthosulfonate [see: ichthammol]

ammonium lactate (lactic acid neutralized with ammonium hydroxide) USAN *antipruritic; emollient for xerosis*
ammonium mandelate USP
ammonium molybdate USP *dietary molybdenum supplement* 25 µg/mL injection
ammonium molybdate tetrahydrate [see: ammonium molybdate]
ammonium phosphate NF *pharmaceutic aid*
ammonium salicylate NF
ammonium tetrathiomolybdate (*orphan: Wilson's disease*)
ammonium valerate NF
ammophyllin [see: aminophylline]
AMO Endosol; AMO Endosol Extra ophthalmic solution ℞ *intraocular irrigating solution* [balanced saline solution]
AMO Vitrax intraocular injection ℞ *viscoelastic agent for ophthalmic surgery* [hyaluronate sodium] 30 mg/mL
amobarbital USP, INN, JAN *sedative; hypnotic; anticonvulsant* [also: amylobarbitone]
amobarbital sodium USP, JAN *hypnotic; sedative; anticonvulsant*
amocaine chloride [see: amolanone HCl]
amocarzine INN
amodiaquine USP, INN, BAN *antiprotozoal*
amodiaquine HCl USP *antimalarial*
Amodopa tablets ℞ *antihypertensive* [methyldopa] 125, 250, 500 mg
amogastrin INN, JAN
amolanone INN
amolanone HCl [see: amolanone]
amonafide INN *investigational antineoplastic*
Amonidrin tablets (discontinued 1994) OTC *expectorant* [guaifenesin] 200 mg
Amoni-Opti-E capsules OTC *vitamin supplement* [vitamin E]
amoproxan INN, DCF
amopyroquine INN
amorolfine USAN, INN, BAN *antimycotic*
Amosan powder OTC *oral antibacterial* [sodium peroxyborate monohydrate]
amoscanate INN

amosulalol INN [also: amosulalol HCl]
amosulalol HCl JAN [also: amosulalol]
amotriphene [see: aminoxytriphene]
amoxapine USAN, USP, INN, BAN, JAN *tricyclic antidepressant* 25, 50, 100, 150 mg oral ⓦ amoxicillin; Amoxil
amoxecaine INN
amoxicillin USAN, USP, JAN *bactericidal antibiotic* [also: amoxicilline; amoxycillin] 250 mg oral ⓦ amoxapine
amoxicillin trihydrate *bactericidal antibiotic* 250, 500 mg oral; 125, 250 mg/5 mL oral; 50 mg/mL oral
amoxicilline INN *bactericidal antibiotic* [also: amoxicillin; amoxycillin]
Amoxil capsules, powder for oral suspension, chewable tablets, pediatric drops ℞ *penicillin-type antibiotic* [amoxicillin trihydrate] 250, 500 mg; 125, 250 mg/5 mL; 125, 250 mg; 50 mg/mL ⓦ amoxapine
amoxycillin BAN *bactericidal antibiotic* [also: amoxicillin; amoxicilline]
amoxydramine camsilate INN [also: amoxydramine camsylate]
amoxydramine camsylate DCF [also: amoxydramine camsilate]
AMP; A$_5$MP (adenosine monophosphate) [see: adenosine phosphate]
amperozide INN, BAN *investigational antipsychotic for schizophrenia*
amphecloral USAN *anorectic* [also: amfecloral]
amphenidone INN
amphetamine BAN *CNS stimulant* [also: amphetamine sulfate; amfetamine]
***d*-amphetamine** [see: dextroamphetamine]
(+)-amphetamine [see: dextroamphetamine]
***l*-amphetamine** [see: levamphetamine]
(−)-amphetamine [see: levamphetamine]
amphetamine aspartate *CNS stimulant*
amphetamine complex (resin complex of amphetamine & dextroamphetamine) [q.v.]
amphetamine phosphate, dextro [see: dextroamphetamine phosphate]
amphetamine succinate, levo [see: levamphetamine succinate]

amphetamine sulfate USP *CNS stimulant* [also: amfetamine; amphetamine] 5, 10 mg oral

amphetamine sulfate, dextro [see: dextroamphetamine sulfate]

Amphocil ℞ *investigational antifungal for immunocompromised patients* [lipid-complex formulation of amphotericin B]

amphocortrin [see: amphomycin]

Amphojel tablets, oral suspension OTC *antacid* [aluminum hydroxide gel] 300, 600 mg; 320 mg/5 mL

amphomycin USAN, BAN *antibacterial* [also: amfomycin]

amphotalide INN, DCF

Amphotec injection ℞ *investigational antifungal for immunocompromised patients* [amphotericin B colloidal dispersion]

amphotericin B USP, INN, BAN, JAN *antifungal* 50 mg/vial injection

amphotericin B lipid complex (ABLC) *systemic antifungal (orphan: cryptococcal meningitis)*

ampicillin USAN, USP, INN, BAN, JAN *bactericidal antibiotic*

ampicillin sodium USAN, USP, JAN *bactericidal antibiotic* 125, 250, 500, 1000, 2000, 10,000 g/vial injection

ampicillin trihydrate *bactericidal antibiotic* 250, 500 mg oral; 125, 250, 500 mg/5 mL oral; 100 mg/mL oral

ampiroxicam INN, BAN

Amplicor Chlamydia test kit for professional use *in vitro diagnostic aid for Chlamydia trachomatis* [DNA amplification test]

Amplicor HIV Monitor test kit for professional use *in vitro diagnostic aid for HIV in blood* [polymerase chain reaction (PCR) test]

Ampligen ℞ *investigational antiviral/immunomodulator (orphan: AIDS; renal carcinoma; melanoma; chronic fatigue)* [poly I: poly C12U]

amprocidum [see: amprolium]

amprolium USP, INN, BAN *coccidiostat for poultry*

amprotropine phosphate

ampyrimine INN

ampyzine INN *CNS stimulant* [also: ampyzine sulfate]

ampyzine sulfate USAN *CNS stimulant* [also: ampyzine]

amquinate USAN, INN *antimalarial*

amrinone USAN, INN, BAN *cardiotonic*

amrinone lactate *vasodilator for congestive heart failure*

amrubicin INN

AMSA; m-AMSA (acridinylamine methanesulfon anisidide) [see: amsacrine]

amsacrine USAN, INN, BAN *investigational antineoplastic; for acute adult leukemia (orphan)*

Amsidyl ℞ *investigational antineoplastic; for acute adult leukemia (orphan)* [amsacrine]

amsonate INN, BAN *combining name for radicals or groups*

amtolmetin guacil INN

Amvisc; Amvisc Plus intraocular injection ℞ *viscoelastic agent for ophthalmic surgery* [hyaluronate sodium] 12 mg/mL; 16 mg/mL

amyl alcohol, tertiary [see: amylene hydrate]

amyl nitrite USP, JAN *vasodilator; antianginal* 0.3 mL inhalant

amylase [see: alpha amylase]

amylene hydrate NF *solvent*

amylmetacresol INN, BAN

amylobarbitone BAN *sedative; hypnotic; anticonvulsant* [also: amobarbital]

amylocaine BAN

amylopectin sulfate, sodium salt [see: sodium amylosulfate]

amylosulfate sodium [see: sodium amylosulfate]

Amytal Sodium powder for injection ℞ *sedative; hypnotic; anxiolytic; anticonvulsant* [amobarbital sodium]

Amytal Sodium Pulvules (capsules) (discontinued 1992) ℞ *sedative; hypnotic; anxiolytic; anticonvulsant* [amobarbital sodium]

ANA-756 *investigational once-daily vasodilator for hypertension*

Anacin caplets, tablets OTC *analgesic; antipyretic; anti-inflammatory* [aspirin; caffeine] 400•32 mg; 400•32, 500•32 mg

Anacin, Aspirin Free caplets, gel caplets, tablets OTC *analgesic; antipyretic* [acetaminophen] 500 mg

Anacin P.M., Aspirin Free film-coated caplets OTC *antihistaminic sleep aid; analgesic* [diphenhydramine HCl; acetaminophen] 25•500 mg

Anacin-3 caplets, tablets (name changed to Aspirin Free Anacin in 1992)

Anacin-3, Children's chewable tablets, liquid (discontinued 1993) OTC *analgesic; antipyretic* [acetaminophen] 80 mg; 160 mg/5 mL

Anacin-3, Infants' drops (discontinued 1993) OTC *analgesic; antipyretic* [acetaminophen] 100 mg/mL

Anadrol-50 tablets ℞ *anabolic steroid for anemias* [oxymetholone] 50 mg

anafebrina [see: aminopyrine]

Anafranil capsules ℞ *treatment of obsessive-compulsive disorders* [clomipramine HCl] 25, 50, 75 mg ⓓ enalapril

anagestone INN *progestin* [also: anagestone acetate]

anagestone acetate USAN *progestin* [also: anagestone]

anagrelide INN *antithrombotic; (orphan: polycythemia vera; essential thrombocythemia; thrombocytosis)* [also: anagrelide HCl]

anagrelide HCl USAN *antithrombotic* [also: anagrelide]

Ana-Guard Epinephrine injection ℞ *emergency treatment of anaphylaxis* [epinephrine] 1:1000

Anaids tablets (discontinued 1994) ℞ *antacid; sedative* [calcium carbonate; phenobarbital sodium]

anakinra USAN *nonsteroidal anti-inflammatory drug (NSAID); inflammatory bowel disease suppressant*

Ana-Kit ℞ *emergency treatment of anaphylaxis* [epinephrine; chlorpheniramine maleate; alcohol pads; tourniquet] 1:100,000•2 mg

Analbalm emulsion (discontinued 1994) OTC *counterirritant* [methyl salicylate; camphor; menthol] 10%•3%•1.25% ⓓ Analpram

Analgesia Creme OTC *topical analgesic* [trolamine salicylate] 10%

Analgesic Balm OTC *counterirritant* [methyl salicylate; menthol]

analgesine [see: antipyrine]

Analpram-HC anorectal cream ℞ *topical corticosteroidal anti-inflammatory; local anesthetic* [hydrocortisone acetate; pramoxine] 1%•1%, 2.5%•1% ⓓ Analbalm

Anamine syrup ℞ *decongestant; antihistamine* [pseudoephedrine HCl; chlorpheniramine maleate] 30•2 mg/5 mL

Anamine T.D. sustained-release capsules ℞ *decongestant; antihistamine* [pseudoephedrine HCl; chlorpheniramine maleate] 120•8 mg

ananain (orphan: *enzymatic debridement of severe burns*)

Anandron (foreign name for U.S. investigational product Nilandron)

Anaplex liquid ℞ *decongestant; antihistamine* [pseudoephedrine HCl; chlorpheniramine maleate] 30•2 mg/5 mL

Anaplex HD syrup ℞ *narcotic antitussive; decongestant; antihistamine* [hydrocodone bitartrate; phenylephrine HCl; chlorpheniramine maleate] 1.7•5•2 mg/5 mL

Anaplex SR sustained-release capsules (discontinued 1995) ℞ *decongestant; antihistamine* [pseudoephedrine HCl; chlorpheniramine maleate] 120•8 mg

Anaprox; Anaprox DS film-coated tablets ℞ *nonsteroidal anti-inflammatory drug (NSAID); antiarthritic; analgesic* [naproxen (from naproxen sodium)] 250 (275) mg; 500 (550) mg

anarel [see: guanadrel sulfate]

anaritide INN, BAN *antihypertensive; diuretic* [also: anaritide acetate]

anaritide acetate USAN *antihypertensive; diuretic* (orphan: *renal failure; adjunct to renal transplant*) [also: anaritide]

Anaspaz tablets ℞ *anticholinergic; antispasmodic* [hyoscyamine sulfate] 0.125 mg

anastrozole USAN, INN, BAN *antineoplastic; aromatase inhibitor for advanced breast cancer*

Anatrast paste ℞ *GI contrast radiopaque agent* [barium sulfate] 100%

Anatuss film-coated tablets ℞ *antitussive; decongestant; expectorant; analgesic* [dextromethorphan hydrobromide; phenylpropanolamine HCl; guaifenesin; acetaminophen] 15•25•100•325 mg

Anatuss syrup OTC *antitussive; decongestant; expectorant* [dextromethorphan hydrobromide; phenylpropanolamine HCl; guaifenesin] 15•25•100 mg/5 mL

Anatuss DM tablets, syrup OTC *antitussive; decongestant; expectorant* [dextromethorphan hydrobromide; pseudoephedrine HCl; guaifenesin] 20•60•400 mg; 10•30•100 mg/5 mL

Anatuss LA long-acting tablets ℞ *decongestant; expectorant* [pseudoephedrine HCl; guaifenesin] 120•400 mg

anaxirone INN

anayodin [see: chiniofon]

anazocine INN

anazolene sodium USAN, INN *blood volume and cardiac output test* [also: sodium anoxynaphthonate]

Anbesol liquid, gel OTC *topical oral anesthetic; antipruritic/counterirritant; antiseptic* [benzocaine; phenol; alcohol 70%] 6.3%•0.5%

Anbesol, Baby gel OTC *topical oral anesthetic* [benzocaine] 7.5%

Anbesol, Maximum Strength liquid, gel OTC *mucous membrane anesthetic* [benzocaine; alcohol 60%] 20%

ancarolol INN

Ancef powder for IV or IM injection ℞ *cephalosporin-type antibiotic* [cefazolin sodium] 0.25, 0.5, 1, 5, 10 g

Ancet liquid OTC *soap-free therapeutic skin cleanser*

ancitabine INN [also: ancitabine HCl]

ancitabine HCl JAN [also: ancitabine]

Ancobon capsules ℞ *antifungal* [flucytosine] 250, 500 mg ② Oncovin

ancrod USAN, INN, BAN *anticoagulant; (orphan: thrombocytopenia or thrombosis)*

andolast INN

Andozac ℞ *investigational treatment for benign prostatic hyperplasia*

Andro 100 IM injection (discontinued 1994) ℞ *androgen replacement for delayed puberty or breast cancer* [testosterone] 100 mg/mL

Andro 100; Andro 200 [see: depAndro 100; depAndro 200]

Andro L.A. 200 IM injection ℞ *androgen replacement for delayed puberty or breast cancer* [testosterone enanthate] 200 mg/mL

Androcur *(orphan: severe hirsutism)* [cyproterone acetate]

Andro-Cyp 100; Andro-Cyp 200 IM injection (discontinued 1994) ℞ *androgen replacement for delayed puberty or breast cancer* [testosterone cypionate] 100 mg/mL; 200 mg/mL

Androderm transdermal patch (for nonscrotal area) ℞ *hormone replacement therapy for hypogonadism* [testosterone] 2.5 mg/day (12.2 mg)

Andro/Fem IM injection (discontinued 1995) ℞ *estrogen/androgen for menopausal vasomotor symptoms* [estradiol cypionate; testosterone cypionate] 2•50 mg/mL

Androgyn [see: depAndrogyn]

Androgyn L.A. IM injection (discontinued 1994) ℞ *estrogen/androgen for menopausal vasomotor symptoms* [estradiol valerate; testosterone enanthate] 4•90 mg/mL

Android-10; Android-25 tablets ℞ *androgen for male hypogonadism, cryptorchidism, impotence, and female breast cancer* [methyltestosterone] 10 mg; 25 mg

Androlone-D 200 IM injection ℞ *anabolic steroid for anemia of renal insufficiency* [nandrolone decanoate] 200 mg/mL

Andronate 100; Andronate 200 IM injection (discontinued 1994) ℞ *androgen replacement for delayed puberty or breast cancer* [testosterone cypionate] 100 mg/mL; 200 mg/mL

Andropository-200 IM injection ℞ *androgen replacement for delayed puberty or breast cancer* [testosterone enanthate] 200 mg/mL

androstanazole [now: stanozolol]
androstane [see: androstanolone; stanolone]
androstanolone INN [also: stanolone]
androtest P [see: testosterone propionate]
Androvite tablets OTC *vitamin/mineral/iron supplement* [multiple vitamins & minerals; iron; folic acid; biotin] ≟•3•0.06•≟ mg
Anectine IV or IM injection, Flo-Pack (powder for injection) ℞ *neuromuscular blocker* [succinylcholine chloride] 20 mg/mL; 500, 1000 mg
Anergan 25 injection (discontinued 1995) ℞ *antihistamine; motion sickness; sleep aid; antiemetic; sedative* [promethazine HCl] 25 mg/mL
Anergan 50 injection ℞ *antihistamine; motion sickness; sleep aid; antiemetic; sedative* [promethazine HCl] 50 mg/mL
anertan [see: testosterone propionate]
Anestacon jelly ℞ *mucous membrane anesthetic* [lidocaine HCl] 2%
anesthesin [see: benzocaine]
anesthrone [see: benzocaine]
anethaine [see: tetracaine HCl]
anethole NF *flavoring agent*
anetholtrithion JAN
aneurine HCl [see: thiamine HCl]
Anexsia 5/500; Anexsia 7.5/650 tablets ℞ *narcotic analgesic* [hydrocodone bitartrate; acetaminophen] 5•500 mg; 7.5•650 mg
Angio-Conray injection ℞ *parenteral angiography radiopaque agent* [iothalamate sodium] 80%
angiotensin II INN
angiotensin II receptor antagonist *investigational treatment for hypertension and congestive heart failure*
angiotensin II receptor blocker *investigational treatment for hypertension*
angiotensin amide USAN, NF, BAN *vasoconstrictor* [also: angiotensinamide]
angiotensinamide INN *vasoconstrictor* [also: angiotensin amide]
Angiovist 282 injection ℞ *parenteral radiopaque agent* [diatrizoate meglumine] 60%

Angiovist 292; Angiovist 370 injection ℞ *parenteral radiopaque agent* [diatrizoate meglumine; diatrizoate sodium] 52%•8%; 66%•10%
anhydrohydroxyprogesterone [now: ethisterone]
anhydrous lanolin [see: lanolin, anhydrous]
anidoxime USAN, INN, BAN *analgesic*
anilamate INN
anileridine USP, INN, BAN *narcotic analgesic*
anileridine HCl USP *narcotic analgesic*
anilopam INN *analgesic* [also: anilopam HCl]
anilopam HCl USAN *analgesic* [also: anilopam]
Animal Shapes chewable tablets OTC *vitamin supplement* [multiple vitamins; folic acid] ≟•0.3 mg
Animal Shapes + Iron chewable tablets OTC *vitamin/iron supplement* [multiple vitamins; iron; folic acid] ≟•15•0.3 mg
anion exchange resin [see: polyamine-methylene resin]
anipamil INN
aniracetam USAN, INN *mental performance enhancer*
anirolac USAN, INN *anti-inflammatory; analgesic*
anisacril INN
anise oil NF
anisindione NF, INN, BAN *anticoagulant*
anisopirol INN
anisopyradamine [see: pyrilamine maleate]
anisotropine methylbromide USAN, JAN *anticholinergic; peptic ulcer adjunct* [also: octatropine methylbromide] 50 mg oral
anisoylated plasminogen streptokinase activator complex (APSAC) [see: anistreplase]
anistreplase USAN, INN, BAN *fibrinolytic; thrombolytic enzyme*
anitrazafen USAN, INN *topical anti-inflammatory*
Anocaine Hemorrhoidal suppositories (discontinued 1992) OTC *topical local anesthetic; astringent* [benzo-

caine; zinc oxide; bismuth subgallate; balsam Peru] ② A-Caine

anodynine [see: antipyrine]

anodynon [see: ethyl chloride]

Anodynos tablets (discontinued 1995) OTC *analgesic; antipyretic; anti-inflammatory* [aspirin; salicylamide; caffeine] 420.6•34.4•34.4 mg

Anodynos DHC tablets (discontinued 1994) ℞ *narcotic analgesic* [hydrocodone bitartrate; acetaminophen]

Anodynos Forte tablets OTC *antihistamine; decongestant; analgesic; antipyretic* [chlorpheniramine maleate; phenylephrine HCl; acetaminophen; salicylamide; caffeine]

Anoquan capsules ℞ *analgesic; antipyretic; sedative* [acetaminophen; caffeine; butalbital] 325•40•50 mg

Anorex capsules (discontinued 1996) ℞ *anorexiant* [phendimetrazine tartrate] 35 mg

anovlar [see: norethindrone & ethinyl estradiol]

anoxomer USAN *antioxidant; food additive*

anoxynaphthonate sodium [see: anazolene sodium]

anpirtoline INN

Ansaid tablets ℞ *nonsteroidal anti-inflammatory drug (NSAID); antiarthritic* [flurbiprofen] 50, 100 mg

ansamycin [see: rifabutin]

ansoxetine INN

Answer; Answer 2; Answer Plus 2 test kit for home use (discontinued 1995) OTC *in vitro diagnostic aid for urine pregnancy test*

Answer Ovulation test kit for home use OTC *in vitro diagnostic aid to predict ovulation time*

Answer Plus; Answer Quick & Simple test kit for home use OTC *in vitro diagnostic aid for urine pregnancy test*

Antabuse tablets ℞ *deterrent to alcohol consumption* [disulfiram] 250, 500 mg

Antacid chewable tablets OTC *antacid* [calcium carbonate] 500, 750 mg

Antacid oral suspension OTC *antacid* [aluminum hydroxide; magnesium hydroxide] 225•200 mg/5 mL

antafenite INN

Anta-Gel; Anta-Gel II oral suspension (discontinued 1994) OTC *antacid; antiflatulent* [aluminum hydroxide; magnesium hydroxide; simethicone] 40•40•4 mg/mL; 80•80•6 mg/mL

antastan [see: antazoline HCl]

antazoline INN, BAN [also: antazoline HCl]

antazoline HCl USP [also: antazoline]

antazoline phosphate USP *antihistamine*

Antazoline-V eye drops (discontinued 1995) ℞ *topical ocular decongestant and antihistamine* [naphazoline HCl; antazoline phosphate] 0.05%•0.5%

antazonite INN

antelmycin INN *anthelmintic* [also: anthelmycin]

anterior pituitary

anthelmycin USAN *anthelmintic* [also: antelmycin]

anthiolimine INN

Anthra-Derm ointment ℞ *topical antipsoriatic* [anthralin] 0.1%, 0.25%, 0.5%, 1%

anthralin USP *antipsoriatic* [also: dithranol]

anthramycin USAN *antineoplastic* [also: antramycin]

anthraquinone of cascara [see: cascara sagrada]

anti pan T lymphocyte monoclonal antibody (orphan: bone marrow transplants; graft vs. host disease) [also: anti-T lymphocyte immunotoxin XMMLY-H65-RTA]

anti-A blood grouping serum USP *in vitro blood testing*

antib [see: thioacetazone; thiacetazone]

anti-B blood grouping serum USP *in vitro blood testing*

anti-B4-blocked ricin [see: ricin (blocked) ...]

antibason [see: methylthiouracil]

AntibiŌtic ear drops, otic suspension ℞ *topical corticosteroidal anti-inflammatory; antibiotic* [hydrocortisone; neomycin sulfate; polymyxin B sulfate] 1%•5 mg•10,000 U per mL

Antibiotic Ear Solution ℞ *topical corticosteroidal anti-inflammatory; antibiotic* [hydrocortisone; neomycin sulfate; polymyxin B sulfate] 1%•5 mg•10,000 U per mL

Antibiotic Ear Suspension ℞ *topical corticosteroidal anti-inflammatory; antibiotic* [hydrocortisone; neomycin sulfate; polymyxin B sulfate] 1%•5 mg•10,000 U per mL

anti-C blood grouping serum [see: blood grouping serum, anti-C]

anti-c blood grouping serum [see: blood grouping serum, anti-c]

anti-CD3 [see: muromonab-CD3]

anti-CD5 monoclonal antibodies *investigational treatment for graft vs. host disease, rheumatoid arthritis, and type I diabetes*

anticoagulant citrate dextrose (ACD) solution USP *anticoagulant for storage of whole blood and during cardiac surgery*

anticoagulant citrate phosphate dextrose adenine solution USP *anticoagulant for storage of whole blood*

anticoagulant citrate phosphate dextrose solution USP *anticoagulant for storage of whole blood*

anticoagulant heparin solution USP *anticoagulant for storage of whole blood*

anticoagulant sodium citrate solution USP *anticoagulant for plasma and for blood for fractionation*

anticytomegalovirus monoclonal antibodies (*orphan status withdrawn 1994*)

anti-D antibodies [see: Rh$_0$(D) immune globulin]

Antide ℞ *investigational LHRH antagonist for hormone-dependent cancers and gynecologic disorders*

anti-E blood grouping serum [see: blood grouping serum, anti-E]

anti-e blood grouping serum [see: blood grouping serum, anti-e]

antienite INN

antiepilepsirine [now: ilepcimide]

antiestrogen [see: tamoxifen citrate]

antifebrin [see: acetanilide]

antifolic acid [see: methotrexate]

antiformin, dental JAN [also: sodium hypochlorite, diluted]

antihemophilic factor (AHF) USP *antihemophilic*

Antihemophilic Factor (Porcine) Hyate:C powder for IV injection ℞ *antihemophilic to correct coagulation deficiency* [antihemophilic factor VIII:C] 400–700 porcine units/vial

antihemophilic factor, human [now: antihemophilic factor]

antihemophilic factor, recombinant (rFVIII) *for hemophilia A* (*orphan*)

antihemophilic factor A [see: antihemophilic factor]

antihemophilic factor B [see: factor IX complex]

antihemophilic globulin (AHG) [see: antihemophilic factor]

antihemophilic human plasma [now: plasma, antihemophilic human]

antihemophilic plasma, human [now: plasma, antihemophilic human]

antiheparin [see: protamine sulfate]

Antihist-1 tablets OTC *antihistamine* [clemastine fumarate] 1.34 mg

anti-HIV T-cell *investigational (Phase I/II) gene therapy for HIV*

anti-idiotypic antibody vaccine *investigational treatment for small cell lung cancer*

anti-IgE humanized monoclonal antibody *investigational treatment for allergic rhinitis and asthma*

anti-inhibitor coagulant complex *antihemophilic*

anti-J5MAB (*orphan status withdrawn 1993*)

Antilirium IV or IM injection ℞ *cholinergic to reverse anticholinergic overdose;* (*orphan: Friedreich's and other ataxias*) [physostigmine salicylate] 1 mg/mL

antilymphocyte immunoglobulin BAN

antimelanoma antibody XMMME-001-DTPA 111 indium (*orphan: diagnostic imaging for metastatic melanoma*)

antimelanoma antibody XMMME-001-RTA (*orphan: stage III melanoma*)

Antiminth oral suspension OTC *anthelmintic* [pyrantel pamoate] 50 mg/mL

antimony *element* (Sb)

antimony potassium tartrate USP *antischistosomal*

antimony sodium tartrate USP, JAN *antischistosomal*
antimony sodium thioglycollate USP
antimony sulfide [see: antimony trisulfide colloid]
antimony trisulfide colloid USAN *pharmaceutic aid*
antimonyl potassium tartrate [see: antimony potassium tartrate]
anti-MY9-blocked ricin [see: ricin (blocked) ...]
Antinea cream (discontinued 1992) OTC *topical antifungal; keratolytic* [benzoic acid; salicylic acid] 6%•3%
Antiox capsules OTC *vitamin supplement* [vitamins C and E; beta carotene] 120 mg•100 IU•25 mg
anti-pellagra vitamin [see: niacin]
anti-pernicious anemia principle [see: cyanocobalamin]
antipyrine USP, JAN *analgesic;* (*orphan: tests hepatic drug-metabolizing capacity*) [also: phenazone]
N-antipyrinylnicotinamide [see: nifenazone]
antirabies serum (ARS) USP *passive immunizing agent*
anti-Rh antibodies [see: $Rh_0(D)$ immune globulin]
anti-Rh typing serums [now: blood grouping serums]
antiscorbutic vitamin [see: ascorbic acid]
Antispas IM injection ℞ *gastrointestinal antispasmodic* [dicyclomine HCl] 10 mg/mL
Antispasmodic elixir ℞ *GI anticholinergic; sedative* [atropine sulfate; scopolamine hydrobromide; hyoscyamine sulfate; phenobarbital] 0.0194•0.0065•0.1037•16.2 mg/5 mL
antisterility vitamin [see: vitamin E]
anti-T lymphocyte immunotoxin XMMLY-H65-RTA (*orphan: bone marrow transplants; graft vs. host disease*) [also: anti pan T lymphocyte monoclonal antibody]
anti-tac, humanized (*orphan: prevent renal allograft rejection and graft vs. host disease*)
anti-TAP-72 immunotoxin (*orphan: metastatic colorectal adenocarcinoma*)

antithrombin III (AT-III) INN, BAN *for thrombosis and pulmonary emboli of congenital AT-III deficiency* (*orphan*)
antithrombin III, human [see: antithrombin III]
antithrombin III concentrate IV [see: antithrombin III]
antithymocyte globulin [see: lymphocyte immune globulin, antithymocyte]
antithymocyte serum (*orphan: prevent allograft rejection*) [see: lymphocyte immune globulin, antithymocyte]
anti-TNF (tumor necrosis factor) monoclonal antibody *investigational treatment for septic shock and rheumatoid arthritis*
antitoxin botulism equine (ABE) [see: botulism equine antitoxin, trivalent]
α_1-**antitrypsin** [see: alpha$_1$-antitrypsin]
Anti-Tuss syrup OTC *expectorant* [guaifenesin; alcohol 3.5%] 100 mg/5 mL
antivenin (Crotalidae) polyvalent USP *passive immunizing agent for pit viper (rattlesnake, copperhead, and cottonmouth moccasin) bites*
antivenin (Crotalidae) polyvalent (ovine) Fab (*orphan: Crotalidae snake bite*)
antivenin (Crotalidae) purified (avian) (*orphan: Crotalidae snake bite*)
antivenin (Latrodectus mactans) USP *passive immunizing agent for black widow spider bites* 6000 U/vial
antivenin (Micrurus fulvius) USP *passive immunizing agent for coral snake bites*
Antivert; Antivert/25; Antivert/50 tablets ℞ *anticholinergic; antihistamine; antivertigo agent; motion sickness preventative* [meclizine HCl] 12.5 mg; 25 mg; 50 mg
Antivert/25 chewable tablets (discontinued 1995) ℞ *anticholinergic; antihistamine; antivertigo agent; motion sickness preventative* [meclizine HCl] 25 mg
antixerophthalmic vitamin [see: vitamin A]
antrafenine INN
antramycin INN *antineoplastic* [also: anthramycin]

Antril ℞ *(orphan: sepsis; rheumatoid arthritis; graft vs. host disease; leukemia)* [anakinra]

Antrizine tablets ℞ *anticholinergic; antihistamine; antivertigo agent; motion sickness preventative* [meclizine HCl] 12.5, 25, 50 mg

Antrocol capsules, tablets (discontinued 1995) ℞ *GI anticholinergic; sedative* [atropine sulfate; phenobarbital] 0.195•16 mg

Antrocol elixir ℞ *GI anticholinergic; sedative* [atropine sulfate; phenobarbital] 0.195•16 mg/5 mL

Antrypol (available only from the Centers for Disease Control) ℞ *investigational anti-infective for trypanosomiasis and onchocerciasis* [suramin sodium]

antrypol [see: suramin sodium]

Anturane tablets, capsules ℞ *uricosuric for gout* [sulfinpyrazone] 100 mg; 200 mg ⑨ Artane

Anucort HC rectal suppositories ℞ *topical corticosteroidal anti-inflammatory* [hydrocortisone acetate] 25 mg

Anumed rectal suppositories OTC *temporary relief of hemorrhoidal symptoms* [bismuth subgallate; bismuth resorcin compound; benzyl benzoate; zinc oxide; peruvian balsam] 2.25%•1.75%•1.2%•11%•1.8%

Anumed HC rectal suppositories ℞ *topical corticosteroidal anti-inflammatory* [hydrocortisone acetate] 10 mg

Anuprep HC rectal suppositories (discontinued 1995) ℞ *topical corticosteroidal anti-inflammatory; antipruritic* [hydrocortisone acetate] 25 mg

Anuprep Hemorrhoidal rectal suppositories (discontinued 1995) OTC *temporary relief of hemorrhoidal symptoms* [bismuth subgallate; bismuth resorcin compound; benzyl benzoate; peruvian balsam; zinc oxide] 2.25%•1.75%•1.2%•1.8%•11%

Anusol anorectal ointment OTC *topical local anesthetic; astringent* [pramoxine HCl; zinc oxide] 1%•12.5% ⑨ Aplisol

Anusol rectal suppositories OTC *emollient* [topical starch] 51%

Anusol-HC anorectal cream ℞ *topical corticosteroidal anti-inflammatory* [hydrocortisone] 2.5%

Anusol-HC rectal suppositories ℞ *topical corticosteroidal anti-inflammatory* [hydrocortisone acetate] 25 mg

Anusol-HC 1 ointment (discontinued 1995) ℞ *topical corticosteroid* [hydrocortisone acetate] 1%

Anxanil film-coated tablets ℞ *anxiolytic* [hydroxyzine HCl] 25 mg

Anzemet ℞ *investigational antiemetic for nausea following chemotherapy, radiation therapy, or operations* [dolasetron]

AOPA (ara-C, Oncovin, prednisone, asparaginase) *chemotherapy protocol*

AOPE (Adriamycin, Oncovin, prednisone, etoposide) *chemotherapy protocol*

Aosept solution + Aodisc (tablet) OTC *two-step chemical disinfecting system for soft contact lenses* [hydrogen peroxide based] 3%

AP injection ℞ *diagnosis and treatment of allergies* [epidermal/environmental allergenic extracts]

AP (Adriamycin, Platinol) *chemotherapy protocol*

Apacet chewable tablets OTC *analgesic; antipyretic* [acetaminophen] 80 mg

apafant INN

apalcillin sodium USAN, INN *antibacterial*

APAP drops, elixir, tablets, chewable tablets, caplets, suppositories OTC *analgesic; antipyretic* [acetaminophen]

APAP (N-acetyl-p-aminophenol) [see: acetaminophen]

Apatate chewable tablets, liquid OTC *vitamin supplement* [vitamins B_1, B_6, and B_{12}] 15•0.5•0.025 mg; 15•0.5•0.025 mg/5 mL

Apatate with Fluoride liquid ℞ *pediatric vitamin supplement and dental caries preventative* [vitamins B_1, B_6, and B_{12}; fluoride] 15•0.5•0.025•0.5 mg/5 mL

apaxifylline USAN, INN *selective adenosine A_1 antagonist for cognitive deficits*

apazone USAN *anti-inflammatory* [also: azapropazone]

APC (AMSA, prednisone, chlorambucil) *chemotherapy protocol*

APC (aspirin, phenacetin & caffeine) [q.v.]

APD (aminohydroxypropylidene diphosphonate) [see: pamidronate disodium]

APE (Adriamycin, Platinol, etoposide) *chemotherapy protocol*

APE (ara-C, Platinol, etoposide) *chemotherapy protocol*

Apetil liquid OTC *vitamin/mineral supplement* [multiple B vitamins; multiple minerals] ≛•≛

Aphrodyne tablets ℞ *no approved uses; sympatholytic; mydriatic; aphrodisiac* [yohimbine HCl] 5.4 mg

apicillin [see: ampicillin]

apicycline INN

apiquel fumarate [see: aminorex]

A.P.L. powder for IM injection ℞ *hormone for prepubertal cryptorchidism and hypogonadism; ovulation stimulant* [chorionic gonadotropin] 500, 1000, 2000 U/mL

Aplisol intradermal injection ℞ *tuberculosis skin test* [tuberculin purified protein derivative] 5 U/0.1 mL ⌽ Anusol; Apresoline

Aplitest single-use intradermal puncture test device ℞ *tuberculosis skin test* [tuberculin purified protein derivative] 5 U

aplonidine HCl [see: apraclonidine HCl]

APO (Adriamycin, prednisone, Oncovin) *chemotherapy protocol*

apodol [see: anileridine HCl]

Apo-Ipravent solution for inhalation (available only in Canada) ℞ *bronchodilator* [ipratropium bromide] 250 μg/mL

apomorphine BAN *emetic* [also: apomorphine HCl]

apomorphine HCl USP *emetic (orphan: late-stage Parkinson's disease)* [also: apomorphine]

apovincamine INN

Appedrine tablets OTC *nonprescription diet aid; vitamin/mineral supplement* [phenylpropanolamine HCl; multiple vitamins and minerals; folic acid] 25•≛•0.4 mg ⌽ aprindine; ephedrine

APPG (aqueous penicillin G procaine) [see: penicillin G procaine]

Appli-Kit (trademarked form) *ointment and adhesive dosage covers*

Appli-Ruler (trademarked name) OTC *dose-determining pads*

Appli-Tape (trademarked name) OTC *dosage covers*

apraclonidine INN, BAN *topical adrenergic for glaucoma* [also: apraclonidine HCl]

apraclonidine HCl USAN *topical adrenergic for glaucoma* [also: apraclonidine]

apramycin USAN, INN, BAN *antibacterial*

Aprazone capsules ℞ *uricosuric for gout* [sulfinpyrazone]

Apresazide 25/25; Apresazide 50/50; Apresazide 100/50 capsules ℞ *antihypertensive* [hydralazine HCl; hydrochlorothiazide] 25•25 mg; 50•50 mg; 100•50 mg

Apresoline IV or IM injection (discontinued 1993) ℞ *antihypertensive; vasodilator* [hydralazine HCl] 20 mg/mL ⌽ Aplisol; Priscoline

Apresoline tablets ℞ *antihypertensive; vasodilator* [hydralazine HCl] 10, 25, 50, 100 mg

Apresoline-Esidrix tablets (discontinued 1992) ℞ *antihypertensive; diuretic* [hydralazine HCl; hydrochlorothiazide]

apricot kernel water JAN

aprikalim INN *investigational antianginal*

Aprim ℞ *investigational potassium channel opener for angina* [aprikalim]

aprindine USAN, INN, BAN *antiarrhythmic* ⌽ Appedrine; ephedrine

aprindine HCl USAN, JAN *antiarrhythmic*

aprobarbital NF, INN, DCF *sedative*

Aprodine tablets, syrup OTC *decongestant; antihistamine* [pseudoephedrine HCl; triprolidine HCl] 60•2.5 mg; 30•1.25 mg/5 mL

Aprodine with Codeine syrup ℞ *narcotic antitussive; decongestant; antihistamine* [codeine phosphate; pseudoephedrine HCl; triprolidine HCl] 10•30•1.25 mg/5 mL

aprofene INN

aprosulate sodium INN

aprotinin USAN, INN, BAN, JAN *systemic hemostatic to reduce blood loss in coronary surgery (orphan); protease inhibitor*

Aprozide 25/25; Aprozide 50/50; Aprozide 100/50 capsules ℞ *antihypertensive* [hydrochlorothiazide; hydralazine HCl]

A.P.S. (aspirin, phenacetin & salicylamide) [q.v.]

APSAC (anisoylated plasminogen streptokinase activator complex) [see: anistreplase]

aptazapine INN *antidepressant* [also: aptazapine maleate]

aptazapine maleate USAN *antidepressant* [also: aptazapine]

aptocaine INN, BAN, DCF

apyron [see: magnesium salicylate]

Aqua Gem-E soft capsules OTC *vitamin supplement* [vitamin E]

Aqua-Ban enteric-coated tablets OTC *diuretic* [ammonium chloride; caffeine] 325•100 mg

Aqua-Ban, Maximum Strength tablets OTC *diuretic* [pamabrom] 50 mg

Aqua-Ban Plus enteric-coated tablets OTC *diuretic* [ammonium chloride; caffeine; ferrous sulfate] 650•200•6 mg

Aquabase OTC *ointment base*

Aquacare cream, lotion OTC *moisturizer; emollient; keratolytic* [urea] 10%

Aquachloral Supprettes (suppositories) ℞ *sedative; hypnotic* [chloral hydrate] 324, 648 mg

aquaday [see: menadione]

aquakay [see: menadione]

AquaMEPHYTON IM or subcu injection ℞ *coagulant; correct anticoagulant-induced prothrombin deficiency; vitamin K supplement* [phytonadione] 2, 10 mg/mL

Aquanil lotion OTC *moisturizer; emollient*

Aquanil Cleanser lotion OTC *soap-free therapeutic skin cleanser*

Aquaphilic OTC *ointment base*

Aquaphilic with Carbamide OTC *ointment base* [urea] 10%, 20%

Aquaphor OTC *ointment base*

Aquaphor Antibiotic ointment (discontinued 1994) OTC *topical antibiotic* [polymyxin B sulfate; bacitracin zinc] 10,000•500 U/g

Aquaphyllin syrup ℞ *bronchodilator* [theophylline] 80 mg/15 mL

AquaSite eye drops OTC *ocular moisturizer/lubricant* [polyethylene glycol 400] 0.2%

Aquasol A capsules, IM injection ℞ *vitamin deficiency therapy* [vitamin A] 25,000, 50,000 IU; 50,000 IU/mL

Aquasol A drops OTC *vitamin supplement* [vitamin A] 5000 IU/0.1 mL

Aquasol E capsules, drops OTC *vitamin supplement* [vitamin E] 73.5 mg, 400 IU; 50 mg/mL

AquaTar gel OTC *topical antipsoriatic; antiseborrheic* [coal tar extract] 2.5%

Aquatensen tablets ℞ *diuretic; antihypertensive* [methyclothiazide] 5 mg

aqueous penicillin G procaine (APPG) [see: penicillin G procaine]

Aquest IM injection ℞ *estrogen replacement therapy; antineoplastic for prostatic and breast cancer* [estrone] 2 mg/mL

aquinone [see: menadione]

AR-121 *investigational (Phase I/II) antiviral for AIDS*

AR-177 *investigational (Phase I) antiviral oligonucleotide for AIDS*

AR-623 *investigational antineoplastic for leukemia and Kaposi sarcoma (orphan)*

ara-A (adenine arabinoside) [see: vidarabine]

ara-AC (azacytosine arabinoside) [see: fazarabine]

arabinofuranosylcytosine [see: cytarabine]

arabinoluranosylcytosine HCl [see: cytarabine HCl]

arabinosyl cytosine [see: cytarabine]

ara-C (cytosine arabinoside) [see: cytarabine] ⑨ ERYC

ara-C, DepoFoam encapsulated *investigational (Phase II) antineoplastic for leptomeningeal leukemia, lymphoma, and solid tumors*

ara-C + 6-TG (ara-C, thioguanine) *chemotherapy protocol*

ara-C + ADR (ara-C, Adriamycin) *chemotherapy protocol*

ara-C + DNR + PRED + MP (ara-C, daunorubicin, prednisolone, mercaptopurine) *chemotherapy protocol*

arachis oil [see: peanut oil]

ara-C-HU (ara-C, hydroxyurea) *chemotherapy protocol*

ara-cytidine [see: cytarabine]

Aralen HCl IM injection ℞ *antimalarial; amebicide* [chloroquine HCl] 50 mg/mL ⧈ Arlidin

Aralen Phosphate film-coated tablets, injection ℞ *antimalarial; amebicide* [chloroquine phosphate] 500 mg; 5 mg

Aralen Phosphate with Primaquine Phosphate tablets (discontinued 1996) ℞ *malaria prophylaxis* [chloroquine phosphate; primaquine phosphate] 500•79 mg

Aramine IV, subcu or IM injection ℞ *vasopressor for acute hypotensive shock, anaphylaxis, or traumatic shock* [metaraminol bitartrate] 10 mg/mL

aranidipine INN

aranotin USAN, INN *antiviral*

araprofen INN

arbaprostil USAN, INN *gastric antisecretory*

arbekacin INN

Arbon tablets (discontinued 1994) OTC *vitamin/mineral/iron supplement* [multiple vitamins & minerals; ferrous fumarate; folic acid] ≛•18•0.4 mg

Arbon Plus tablets (discontinued 1994) OTC *vitamin/mineral/iron supplement* [multiple vitamins & minerals; ferrous fumarate; folic acid; biotin] ≛•27 mg•0.4 mg•150 μg

arbutamine INN, BAN *cardiac stimulant* [also: arbutamine HCl]

arbutamine HCl USAN *cardiac stimulant* [also: arbutamine]

Arcet tablets (discontinued 1995) ℞ *sedative; analgesic; antipyretic* [butalbital; acetaminophen; caffeine] 50•325•40 mg

arcitumomab *investigational imaging agent for detection of recurrent or metastatic colorectal cancer*

arclofenin USAN, INN *hepatic function test*

Arcobee with C caplets OTC *vitamin supplement* [multiple B vitamins; vitamin C] ≛•300 mg

Arco-Lase chewable tablets OTC *digestive enzymes* [amylase; protease; lipase; cellulase] 30•6•25•2 mg

Arco-Lase Plus tablets ℞ *digestive enzymes; antispasmodic; sedative* [amylase; protease; lipase; cellulase; hyoscyamine sulfate; atropine sulfate; phenobarbital] 30•6•25•2•0.1•0.02•7.5 mg

Arcotinic liquid (discontinued 1992) OTC *hematinic* [iron; liver fraction 1; multiple B vitamins; alcohol 3%] 64.8•180•≛ mg/15 mL

Arcotinic tablets (discontinued 1995) OTC *hematinic* [ferrous fumarate & ferrous sulfate; desiccated liver; ascorbic acid] 102.5•200•250 mg

ardacin INN

ardeparin sodium USAN, INN *anticoagulant*

Arduan powder for IV injection ℞ *nondepolarizing neuromuscular blocker; adjunct to anesthesia* [pipecuronium bromide] 10 mg/vial

arecoline acetarsone salt [see: drocarbil]

arecoline hydrobromide NF

Aredia powder for IV infusion ℞ *bone resorption suppressant for Paget's disease, hypercalcemia, and multiple myeloma* [pamidronate disodium] 30, 60, 90 mg

arfalasin INN

arfendazam INN

Arfonad IV infusion (discontinued 1995) ℞ *antihypertensive for hypertensive emergencies* [trimethaphan camsylate] 50 mg/mL

argatroban INN, JAN

Argesic cream OTC *topical analgesic; counterirritant* [methyl salicylate; trolamine]

Argesic-SA tablets ℞ *analgesic; antiinflammatory* [salsalate] 500 mg

argimesna INN

arginine (L-arginine) USP, INN *nonessential amino acid; ammonia detoxi-*

cant; pituitary function diagnostic aid; symbols: Arg, R
arginine butyrate *(orphan: beta-hemoglobinopathies and beta-thalassemia; sickle cell disease)*
arginine glutamate (**L-arginine L-glutamate**) USAN, BAN, JAN *ammonia detoxicant*
arginine HCl USAN, USP, JAN *ammonia detoxicant; pituitary (growth hormone) function diagnostic aid*
L-arginine monohydrochloride [see: arginine HCl]
8-L-arginine vasopressin [see: vasopressin]
8-arginineoxytocin [see: argiprestocin]
8-L-argininevasopressin tannate [see: argipressin tannate]
argipressin INN, BAN *antidiuretic* [also: argipressin tannate]
argipressin tannate USAN *antidiuretic* [also: argipressin]
argiprestocin INN
argon *element* (Ar)
argyn [see: silver protein, mild]
Argyrol S.S. 10% eye drops (discontinued 1994) OTC *ophthalmic antiseptic* [silver protein, mild] 10% ② Agoral
Argyrol S.S. 20% eye drops (discontinued 1995) ℞ *ophthalmic mucus staining and coagulating agent; topical antiseptic* [silver protein, mild] 20%
ARI-509 *investigational aldose reductase inhibitor for the secondary complications of long-term diabetes*
arildone USAN, INN *antiviral*
Arimidex film-coated tablets ℞ *nonsteroidal aromatase inhibitor for advanced breast cancer* [anastrozole] 1 mg
Aristocort ointment, cream ℞ *topical corticosteroid* [triamcinolone acetonide] 0.1%, 0.5%; 0.025%, 0.1%, 0.5%
Aristocort tablets ℞ *glucocorticoid* [triamcinolone] 1, 2, 4, 8 mg
Aristocort A ointment, cream ℞ *topical corticosteroid* [triamcinolone acetonide in a water-washable base] 0.1%; 0.025%, 0.1%, 0.5%
Aristocort Forte IM injection ℞ *glucocorticoid* [triamcinolone diacetate] 40 mg/mL

Aristocort Intralesional injection ℞ *glucocorticoid* [triamcinolone diacetate] 25 mg/mL
Aristospan Intra-articular injection ℞ *glucocorticoid* [triamcinolone hexacetonide] 20 mg/mL
Aristospan Intralesional injection ℞ *glucocorticoid* [triamcinolone hexacetonide] 5 mg/mL
Arkin Z (commercially available in Japan) ℞ *investigational treatment for congestive heart failure* [vesnarinone]
Arlidin tablets (discontinued 1993) ℞ *vasodilator* [nylidrin HCl] 6, 12 mg ② Aralen
A.R.M. (Allergy Relief Medicine) caplets OTC *decongestant; antihistamine* [phenylpropanolamine HCl; chlorpheniramine maleate] 25•4 mg
Arm-A-Med (trademarked packaging form) *single-dose plastic vial*
Arm-A-Vial (trademarked packaging form) *single-dose plastic vial*
Armour Thyroid tablets ℞ *hypothyroidism; thyroid cancer* [thyroid, desiccated] 15, 30, 60, 90, 120, 180, 240, 300 mg
arnica *claimed to relieve sprains and bruises (of dubious value)*
arnolol INN
aromatic ammonia spirit [see: ammonia spirit, aromatic]
aromatic cascara fluidextract [see: cascara fluidextract, aromatic]
aromatic cascara sagrada [see: cascara fluidextract, aromatic]
aromatic elixir NF *flavored and sweetened vehicle*
aronixil INN
Aropax (name changed to Paxil in 1992)
arotinolol INN [also: arotinolol HCl]
arotinolol HCl JAN [also: arotinolol]
arprinocid USAN, INN, BAN *coccidiostat*
arpromidine INN
Arrestin IM injection ℞ *anticholinergic; antiemetic* [trimethobenzamide HCl] 100 mg/mL
ARS (antirabies serum) [q.v.]
arsambide [see: carbarsone]

arsanilic acid INN, BAN *investigational (Phase I/II) immunomodulator for AIDS (orphan)*

arseclor [see: dichlorophenarsine HCl]

arsenic *element (As)*

arsenic acid, sodium salt [see: sodium arsenate]

arsenic trioxide JAN

arsenobenzene [see: arsphenamine]

arsenobenzol [see: arsphenamine]

arsenphenolamine [see: arsphenamine]

Arsobal (available only from the Centers for Disease Control) ℞ *investigational anti-infective for trypanosomiasis* [melarsoprol]

arsphenamine USP

arsthinenol DCF [also: arsthinol]

arsthinol INN [also: arsthinenol]

Artane tablets, elixir, Sequels (sustained-release capsules) ℞ *anticholinergic; antiparkinsonian agent* [trihexyphenidyl HCl] 2, 5 mg; 2 mg/5 mL; 5 mg ② Anturane

arteflene USAN, INN *antimalarial*

artegraft USAN *arterial prosthetic aid*

artemether INN

artemisinin INN

arterenol [see: norepinephrine bitartrate]

artesunate INN

Artha-G tablets OTC *analgesic; anti-inflammatory* [salsalate] 750 mg

ArthriCare, Double Ice gel OTC *counterirritant* [menthol; camphor] 4%•3.1%

ArthriCare, Odor Free rub OTC *counterirritant* [menthol; methyl nicotinate; capsaicin] 1.25%•0.25%•0.025%

ArthriCare Daytime Formula (name changed to Odor Free ArthriCare in 1992)

ArthriCare Triple Medicated gel OTC *counterirritant* [methyl salicylate; menthol; methyl nicotinate] 30%•1.5%•0.7%

Arthriten tablets OTC *analgesic; antipyretic* [acetaminophen; magnesium salicylate; caffeine (buffered with magnesium carbonate, magnesium oxide, and calcium carbonate)] 250•250•32.5 mg

Arthritis Foundation Ibuprofen tablets OTC *nonsteroidal anti-inflammatory drug (NSAID); antiarthritic; analgesic* [ibuprofen] 200 mg

Arthritis Foundation Nighttime caplets OTC *antihistaminic sleep aid; analgesic* [diphenhydramine citrate; acetaminophen] 25•500 mg

Arthritis Foundation Pain Reliever tablets OTC *analgesic; antipyretic; anti-inflammatory; antirheumatic* [aspirin] 500 mg

Arthritis Foundation Pain Reliever, Aspirin Free caplets OTC *analgesic; antipyretic* [acetaminophen] 500 mg

Arthritis Hot Creme OTC *counterirritant* [methyl salicylate; menthol] 15%•10%

Arthritis Pain Formula caplets OTC *analgesic; antipyretic; anti-inflammatory; antirheumatic* [aspirin, buffered with magnesium hydroxide and aluminum hydroxide] 500 mg

Arthritis Pain Formula Aspirin-Free tablets OTC *analgesic; antipyretic* [acetaminophen] 500 mg

"Arthritis Strength" products [see under product name]

Arthropan IM injection ℞ *analgesic; antipyretic; anti-inflammatory; antirheumatic* [choline salicylate] 870 mg/5 mL

Arthrotec ℞ *investigational antiarthritic* [diclofenac sodium; misoprostol]

articaine INN [also: carticaine]

Articulose L.A. IM injection ℞ *glucocorticoids* [triamcinolone diacetate] 40 mg/mL

Articulose-50 IM injection ℞ *glucocorticoids* [prednisolone acetate] 50 mg/mL

Artificial Tears eye drops OTC *ocular moisturizer/lubricant*

Artificial Tears ophthalmic ointment OTC *ocular moisturizer/lubricant* [white petrolatum; mineral oil; lanolin]

Artificial Tears Plus eye drops OTC *ocular moisturizer/lubricant* [polyvinyl alcohol] 1.4%

artilide INN *antiarrhythmic* [also: artilide fumarate]

artilide fumarate USAN *antiarrhythmic* [also: artilide]

Arvin *investigational treatment for stroke; (orphan: thrombocytopenia or thrombosis)* [ancrod]

AS-013 *investigational prostaglandin for peripheral arterial occlusive disease*

⁷⁴As [see: sodium arsenate As 74]

A.S.A. Enseals (enteric-release tablets), suppositories OTC *analgesic; antipyretic; anti-inflammatory* [aspirin]

5-ASA (5-aminosalicylic acid) [see: mesalamine]

ASA (acetylsalicylic acid) [see: aspirin]

Asacol delayed-release tablets ℞ *treatment of active ulcerative colitis, proctosigmoiditis and proctitis* [mesalamine] 400 mg

Asbron-G Inlay-Tabs (tablets), elixir (discontinued 1996) ℞ *antiasthmatic; bronchodilator; expectorant* [theophylline; guaifenesin] 150•100 mg; 150•100 mg/15 mL

ascorbic acid (L-ascorbic acid) USP, INN, BAN, JAN *vitamin C; antiscorbutic; urinary acidifier* 25, 50, 100, 250, 500, 1000, 1500 oral; 500 mg/5 mL oral; 250, 500 mg/mL injection

L-ascorbic acid, monosodium salt [see: sodium ascorbate]

L-ascorbic acid 6-palmitate [see: ascorbyl palmitate]

Ascorbicap timed-release capsules OTC *vitamin supplement* [ascorbic acid] 500 mg

ascorbyl palmitate NF *antioxidant*

Ascriptin; Ascriptin A/D coated tablets OTC *analgesic; antipyretic; anti-inflammatory; antirheumatic* [aspirin, buffered with magnesium hydroxide, aluminum hydroxide, and calcium carbonate] 325, 500 mg; 325 mg

Asendin tablets ℞ *tricyclic antidepressant* [amoxapine] 25, 50, 100, 150 mg

aseptichrome [see: merbromin]

ASHAP; A-SHAP (Adriamycin, Solu-Medrol, high-dose ara-C, Platinol) *chemotherapy protocol*

Asmalix elixir ℞ *bronchodilator* [theophylline] 80 mg/15 mL

asobamast INN, BAN

asocainol INN

asparaginase (L-asparaginase) USAN, JAN *antineoplastic for acute lymphocytic leukemia* [also: colaspase]

asparagine (L-asparagine) *nonessential amino acid; symbols: Asn, N*

L-asparagine amidohydrolase [see: asparaginase]

aspartame USAN, NF, INN, BAN *sweetener*

L-aspartate potassium JAN

aspartic acid (L-aspartic acid) USAN, INN *nonessential amino acid; symbols: Asp, D*

aspartocin USAN, INN *antibacterial*

A-Spas S/L sublingual tablets ℞ *anticholinergic; antispasmodic* [hyoscyamine sulfate] 0.125 mg

Aspegic ℞ *(orphan: sickle cell crisis)* [lysine acetylsalicylate]

Aspercin; Aspercin Extra tablets OTC *analgesic; anti-inflammatory; antipyretic* [aspirin]

Aspercreme cream OTC *topical analgesic* [trolamine salicylate] 10%

Aspercreme Rub lotion OTC *topical analgesic* [trolamine salicylate] 10%

Aspergillus oryase **proteinase** [see: asperkinase]

Aspergum chewing gum tablets OTC *analgesic; antipyretic; anti-inflammatory; antirheumatic* [aspirin] 227.5 mg

asperkinase

asperlin USAN *antibacterial; antineoplastic*

Aspermin; Aspermin Extra tablets OTC *analgesic; anti-inflammatory; antipyretic* [aspirin]

aspidosperma USP

aspirin USP, BAN, JAN *analgesic; antipyretic; anti-inflammatory; antirheumatic* 325, 500, 650, 975 mg oral; 120, 200, 300, 600 mg suppositories ② Afrin

aspirin, buffered USP *analgesic; antipyretic; anti-inflammatory; antirheumatic* 325 mg oral

aspirin aluminum NF, JAN

aspirin DL-lysine JAN

Aspirin EC enteric-coated tablets OTC *analgesic; antipyretic; anti-inflammatory* [aspirin]

Aspirin Lite Coat tablets OTC *analgesic; antipyretic; anti-inflammatory* [aspirin]

Aspirin with Codeine No. 2, No. 3, and No. 4 tablets ℞ *narcotic analgesic* [codeine phosphate; aspirin] 15•325 mg; 30•325 mg; 60•325 mg

Aspirin-Free Pain Relief tablets OTC *analgesic; antipyretic* [acetaminophen] 325, 500 mg

Aspirol (trademarked delivery form) *crushable ampule for inhalation*

aspogen [see: dihydroxyaluminum aminoacetate]

aspoxicillin INN, JAN

Asprimox; Asprimox Extra Protection for Arthritis Pain caplets OTC *analgesic; antipyretic; anti-inflammatory; antirheumatic* [aspirin, buffered] 325 mg

aspro [see: aspirin]

Asproject IM injection (discontinued 1992) ℞ *analgesic; antipyretic; anti-inflammatory; antirheumatic* [sodium thiosalicylate] 50 mg/mL

astatine *element (At)*

Astelin ℞ *investigational antiasthmatic* [azelastine]

astemizole USAN, INN, BAN *antiallergic; antihistamine*

Astenose ℞ *investigational anticoagulant to block vascular restenosis following cardiac surgery*

AsthmaHaler inhalation aerosol OTC *bronchodilator for bronchial asthma* [epinephrine bitartrate] 0.3 mg/dose

AsthmaNefrin solution for inhalation OTC *bronchodilator for bronchial asthma* [racepinephrine] 2.25%

astifilcon A USAN *hydrophilic contact lens material*

Astramorph PF IV, subcu or IM injection ℞ *narcotic analgesic; preoperative sedative and anxiolytic* [morphine sulfate] 0.5, 1 mg/mL

Astroglide vaginal gel OTC *lubricant* [glycerin; propylene glycol]

astromicin INN *antibacterial* [also: astromicin sulfate]

astromicin sulfate USAN, JAN *antibacterial* [also: astromicin]

AT-III (antithrombin III) [q.v.]

Atabrine HCl tablets (discontinued 1993) ℞ *antimalarial; anthelmintic for giardiasis and cestodiasis* [quinacrine HCl] 100 mg ☒ Adapin

atamestane INN *investigational aromatase inhibitor for cancer*

ataprost INN

Atarax tablets, syrup ℞ *anxiolytic* [hydroxyzine HCl] 10, 25, 50 mg; 10 mg/5 mL ☒ Marax

Atarax 100 tablets ℞ *anxiolytic* [hydroxyzine HCl] 100 mg

atarvet [see: acepromazine]

atenolol USAN, INN, BAN, JAN *antiadrenergic (β-receptor)* 25, 50, 100 mg oral ☒ timolol

atevirdine INN *antiviral* [also: atevirdine mesylate]

atevirdine mesylate USAN *antiviral; investigational (Phase II) for HIV and AIDS* [also: atevirdine]

Atgam IV infusion ℞ *immunizing agent for allograft rejection* [lymphocyte immune globulin, antithymocyte globulin (equine)] 50 mg/mL

athyromazole [see: carbimazole]

atipamezole USAN, INN, BAN α_2-receptor antagonist

atiprosin INN *antihypertensive* [also: atiprosin maleate]

atiprosin maleate USAN *antihypertensive* [also: atiprosin]

Ativan tablets, IV or IM injection ℞ *anxiolytic* [lorazepam] 0.5, 1, 2 mg; 2, 4 mg/mL ☒ Adapin; Avitene

atlafilcon A USAN *hydrophilic contact lens material*

ATnativ powder for IV infusion ℞ *congenital antithrombin III deficiency (orphan)* [antithrombin III, human] 500 IU

atolide USAN, INN *anticonvulsant*

Atolone tablets ℞ *glucocorticoid* [triamcinolone] 4 mg

atorvastatin calcium USAN *antihyperlipidemic*

atosiban USAN, INN *oxytocin antagonist*

atovaquone USAN, INN, BAN *antipneumocystic; antiprotozoal; for Pneumocystis carinii pneumonia (orphan)*

ATP (adenosine triphosphate) [see: adenosine triphosphate disodium]

atracurium besilate INN *skeletal muscle relaxant; nondepolarizing neuro-*

muscular blocker; adjunct to anesthesia [also: atracurium besylate]

atracurium besylate USAN, BAN *skeletal muscle relaxant; nondepolarizing neuromuscular blocker; adjunct to anesthesia* [also: atracurium besilate]

Atretol tablets ℞ *anticonvulsant* [carbamazepine] 200 mg

Atrigel (trademarked delivery system) *sustained-release delivery*

atrimustine INN

atrinositol INN

Atrocholin tablets (discontinued 1992) OTC *laxative; hydrocholeretic* [dehydrocholic acid]

Atrofed tablets (discontinued 1993) OTC *decongestant; antihistamine* [pseudoephedrine HCl; triprolidine HCl]

Atrohist L.A. sustained-release tablets (discontinued 1993) ℞ *antihistamine; decongestant; anticholinergic* [brompheniramine maleate; phenyltoloxamine citrate; pseudoephedrine HCl; atropine sulfate]

Atrohist Pediatric oral suspension ℞ *pediatric decongestant and antihistamine* [phenylephrine tannate; chlorpheniramine tannate; pyrilamine tannate] 5•2•12.5 mg/5 mL

Atrohist Pediatric sustained-release capsules ℞ *pediatric decongestant and antihistamine* [pseudoephedrine HCl; chlorpheniramine maleate] 60•4 mg

Atrohist Plus sustained-release tablets ℞ *decongestant; antihistamine; anticholinergic* [phenylpropanolamine HCl; phenylephrine HCl; chlorpheniramine maleate; hyoscyamine sulfate; atropine sulfate; scopolamine hydrobromide] 50•25•8•0.19•0.04•0.01 mg

Atrohist Sprinkle sustained-release capsules (name changed to Atrohist Pediatric in 1995)

atromepine INN, DCF

Atromid-S capsules ℞ *antihyperlipidemic (cholesterol-lowering)* [clofibrate] 500 mg

AtroPen auto-injector (automatic IM injection device) ℞ *antidote for organophosphorous or carbamate insecticides* [atropine sulfate] 2

atropine USP, BAN *anticholinergic*

Atropine Care eye drops ℞ *mydriatic; cycloplegic* [atropine sulfate] 1%

Atropine Care ophthalmic ointment (discontinued 1993) ℞ *mydriatic; cycloplegic* [atropine sulfate]

atropine methonitrate INN, BAN *anticholinergic* [also: methylatropine nitrate]

atropine methylnitrate [see: methylatropine nitrate]

atropine oxide INN *anticholinergic* [also: atropine oxide HCl]

atropine oxide HCl USAN *anticholinergic* [also: atropine oxide]

atropine propionate [see: prampine]

atropine sulfate USP, JAN *GI antispasmodic; bronchodilator; cycloplegic; mydriatic* [also: atropine sulphate] 0.4, 0.6 mg oral; 1%, 2% eye drops; 0.05, 0.1, 0.3, 0.4, 0.5, 0.8, 1 mg/mL injection

atropine sulphate BAN *GI antispasmodic; bronchodilator; cycloplegic; mydriatic* [also: atropine sulfate]

Atropine-1 eye drops ℞ *mydriatic; cycloplegic* [atropine sulfate] 1%

Atropisol Dropperettes (eye drops) ℞ *cycloplegic; mydriatic* [atropine sulfate] 1%

Atrosept sugar-coated tablets ℞ *urinary anti-infective; analgesic; antispasmodic; acidifier* [methenamine; phenyl salicylate; atropine sulfate; methylene blue; hyoscyamine sulfate; benzoic acid] 40.8•18.1•0.03•5.4•0.03•4.5 mg

Atrovent nasal spray, solution for inhalation, inhalation aerosol ℞ *bronchodilator* [ipratropium bromide] 0.03%, 0.06%; 0.02%; 18 μg/dose

A/T/S topical solution, gel ℞ *topical antibiotic for acne* [erythromycin] 2%

Attain liquid OTC *enteral nutritional therapy* [lactose-free formula]

attapulgite, activated USP *suspending agent; GI adsorbent*

Attenuvax powder for subcu injection ℞ *measles vaccine* [measles virus vaccine, live attenuated] 0.5 mL

Atuss HD liquid ℞ *narcotic antitussive; decongestant; antihistamine*

[hydrocodone bitartrate; phenylephrine HCl; chlorpheniramine maleate] 2.5•5•2 mg/5 mL

[198]Au [see: gold Au 198]

augmented betamethasone dipropionate *topical corticosteroid*

Augmentin film-coated tablets, chewable tablets, powder for oral suspension ℞ *penicillin-type antibiotic* [amoxicillin trihydrate; clavulanate potassium] 250•125, 500•125, 875•125 mg; 125•31.25, 250•62.5 mg; 125•31.25, 250•62.5 mg/5 mL

Auralgan Otic ear drops ℞ *topical local anesthetic; analgesic* [benzocaine; antipyrine] 1.4%•5.4% ⓡ Allergan; allergen

auranofin USAN, INN, BAN, JAN *antirheumatic (29% gold)*

Aureomycin ointment (discontinued 1996) OTC *topical antibiotic* [chlortetracycline HCl] 3% ⓡ Achromycin; actinomycin

Aureomycin ophthalmic ointment (discontinued 1995) ℞ *ophthalmic antibiotic and antiprotozoal* [chlortetracycline HCl] 10 mg/g

aureoquin [now: quinetolate]

Auriculin *investigational treatment for acute kidney failure; (orphan: adjunct to renal transplant)* [anaritide acetate]

Aurinol Ear Drops (discontinued 1992) OTC *antibacterial/antifungal* [chloroxylenol; acetic acid; benzalkonium chloride]

Auro Ear Drops OTC *agent to emulsify and disperse ear wax* [carbamide peroxide] 6.5%

Aurocaine ear drops (discontinued 1992) OTC *agent to emulsify and disperse ear wax* [carbamide]

Aurocaine 2 ear drops (discontinued 1992) OTC *antibacterial/antifungal* [boric acid]

Auro-Dri ear drops OTC *antibacterial/antifungal* [boric acid] 2.75%

Aurolate IM injection ℞ *antirheumatic* [gold sodium thiomalate] 50 mg/mL

aurolin [see: gold sodium thiosulfate]

auropin [see: gold sodium thiosulfate]

Aurorix (commercially available overseas) ℞ *investigational antidepressant* [moclobemide]

aurosan [see: gold sodium thiosulfate]

aurothioglucose USP *antirheumatic (50% gold)*

aurothioglycanide INN, DCF

aurothiomalate disodium [see: gold sodium thiomalate]

aurothiomalate sodium [see: gold sodium thiomalate]

Auroto Otic ear drops ℞ *topical local anesthetic; analgesic* [antipyrine; benzocaine] 1.4%•5.4%

Autohaler (delivery form) *breath-activated metered-dose inhaler*

auto-injector (delivery device) *automatic IM injection device*

autolymphocyte therapy (ALT) *(orphan: renal cancer)*

Autoplex T IV injection or drip ℞ *antihemophilic to correct factor VIII deficiency and coagulation deficiency* [anti-inhibitor coagulant complex, heat treated] ‽

autoprothrombin I [see: factor VII]

autoprothrombin II [see: factor IX]

AV (Adriamycin, vincristine) *chemotherapy protocol*

Avail tablets OTC *vitamin/mineral/iron supplement* [multiple vitamins & minerals; iron; folic acid] ≛•18•0.4 mg ⓡ Advil

Avalgesic lotion (discontinued 1994) OTC *counterirritant* [methyl salicylate; menthol; camphor; methyl nicotinate; capsicum oleoresin]

Avan ℞ *investigational treatment for Alzheimer's disease* [idebenone]

AVC vaginal cream, vaginal suppositories ℞ *broad-spectrum bacteriostatic* [sulfanilamide] 15%; 1.05 g

Aveeno lotion OTC *moisturizer; emollient* [colloidal oatmeal] 1%

Aveeno Anti-Itch cream, lotion OTC *topical poison ivy treatment* [calamine; pramoxine HCl; camphor] 3%•1%•0.3%

Aveeno Cleansing bar OTC *soap-free therapeutic skin cleanser* [colloidal oatmeal] 51%

Aveeno Cleansing for Acne-Prone Skin bar OTC *medicated cleanser for acne* [salicylic acid; colloidal oatmeal]

Aveeno Moisturizing cream OTC *moisturizer; emollient* [colloidal oatmeal] 1%

Aveeno Oilated Bath packets OTC *bath emollient* [colloidal oatmeal; mineral oil] 43%•⚠

Aveeno Regular Bath packets OTC *bath emollient* [colloidal oatmeal] 100%

Aveeno Shave gel OTC *moisturizer; emollient* [oatmeal flour] ⚠

Aveeno Shower & Bath oil OTC *bath emollient* [colloidal oatmeal] 5%

Aventyl solution ℞ *tricyclic antidepressant* [nortriptyline HCl] 10 mg/5 mL ⚠ Ambenyl; Bentyl

Aventyl HCl Pulvules (capsules) ℞ *tricyclic antidepressant* [nortriptyline HCl] 10, 25 mg

avertin [see: tribromoethanol]

avicatonin INN

avilamycin USAN, INN, BAN *antibacterial*

avinar [see: uredepa]

Avitene Hemostat fiber (discontinued 1996) ℞ *topical hemostatic aid for surgery* [microfibrillar collagen hemostat] ⚠ Ativan

Avitene Hemostat nonwoven web ℞ *topical hemostatic aid in surgery* [microfibrillar collagen hemostat] ⚠ Ativan

Aviva ℞ *investigational treatment for Alzheimer's disease (clinical trials discontinued 1994)* [linopirdine]

avizafone INN, BAN

avobenzone USAN, INN *sunscreen*

Avonex powder for IM injection ℞ *immunomodulator for multiple sclerosis* [interferon beta-1a] 33 μg (6.6 million IU)/vial

avoparcin USAN, INN, BAN *glycopeptide antibiotic*

AVP (actinomycin D, vincristine, Platinol) *chemotherapy protocol*

avridine USAN, INN *antiviral*

axamozide INN

axerophthol [see: vitamin A]

axetil USAN, INN *combining name for radicals or groups*

Axid Pulvules (capsules) ℞ *histamine H_2 antagonist for treatment of gastric and duodenal ulcers* [nizatidine] 150, 300 mg

Axid AR tablets OTC *histamine H_2 antagonist for gastric and duodenal ulcers* [nizatidine] 75 mg

Axocet capsules ℞ *analgesic; antipyretic; sedative* [acetaminophen; butalbital] 650•50 mg

Axotal tablets ℞ *analgesic; antipyretic; anti-inflammatory; sedative* [aspirin; butalbital] 650•50 mg

Axsain (name changed to Zostrix-HP in 1992)

Aygestin tablets ℞ *progestin for amenorrhea, abnormal uterine bleeding, or endometriosis* [norethindrone acetate] 5 mg

Ayr Saline nasal mist, nose drops, nasal gel OTC *nasal moisturizer* [sodium chloride (saline)] 0.65%

5-AZA (5-azacitidine) [see: azacitidine]

azabon USAN, INN *CNS stimulant*

azabuperone INN

azacitidine (5-AZA; 5-AZC) USAN, INN *antineoplastic*

azaclorzine INN *coronary vasodilator* [also: azaclorzine HCl]

azaclorzine HCl USAN *coronary vasodilator* [also: azaclorzine]

azaconazole USAN, INN *antifungal*

azacosterol INN *avian chemosterilant* [also: azacosterol HCl]

azacosterol HCl USAN *avian chemosterilant* [also: azacosterol]

AZA-CR [see: azacitidine]

Azactam powder for IV or IM injection ℞ *monobactam-type bactericidal antibiotic* [aztreonam] 0.5, 1, 2 g

azacyclonol INN, BAN [also: azacyclonol HCl]

azacyclonol HCl NF [also: azacyclonol]

5-azacytosine arabinoside (ara-AC) [see: fazarabine]

5-AZA-2'-deoxycytidine (orphan: *acute leukemia*)

azaftozine INN

azalanstat dihydrochloride USAN *hypolipidemic*

azalomycin INN, BAN

azaloxan INN *antidepressant* [also: azaloxan fumarate]

azaloxan fumarate USAN *antidepressant* [also: azaloxan]

azamethiphos BAN

azamethonium bromide INN, BAN

azamulin INN

azanator INN *bronchodilator* [also: azanator maleate]

azanator maleate USAN *bronchodilator* [also: azanator]

azanidazole USAN, INN, BAN *antiprotozoal*

azaperone USAN, INN, BAN *antipsychotic*

azapetine BAN

azapetine phosphate [see: azapetine]

azaprocin INN

azapropazone INN, BAN, DCF *antiinflammatory* [also: apazone]

azaquinzole INN

azaribine USAN, INN, BAN *antipsoriatic*

azarole USAN *immunoregulator*

azaserine USAN, INN *antifungal*

azasetron INN

azaspirium chloride INN

azastene

azatadine INN, BAN *antihistamine* [also: azatadine maleate]

azatadine maleate USAN, USP *antihistamine* [also: azatadine]

azatepa INN *antineoplastic* [also: azetepa]

azathioprine USAN, USP, INN, BAN, JAN *immunosuppressant*

azathioprine sodium USP *immunosuppressant* 100 mg injection

5-AZC (5-azacitidine) [see: azacitidine]

Azdone tablets ℞ *narcotic analgesic* [hydrocodone bitartrate; aspirin] 5•500 mg

azdU (azidouridine) [q.v.]

azelaic acid INN *topical antimicrobial and keratolytic*

azelastine INN, BAN *antiallergic; antiasthmatic* [also: azelastine HCl]

azelastine HCl USAN, JAN *antiallergic; antiasthmatic* [also: azelastine]

Azelex cream ℞ *antimicrobial and keratolytic for inflammatory acne vulgaris* [azelaic acid] 20%

azelnidipine INN

azepexole INN, BAN

azephine [see: azapetine phosphate]

azepinamide [see: glypinamide]

azepindole USAN, INN *antidepressant*

azetepa USAN, BAN *antineoplastic* [also: azatepa]

azetirelin INN

azidamfenicol INN, BAN, DCF

azidoamphenicol [see: azidamfenicol]

azidocillin INN, BAN

3′-azido-2′,3′dideoxyuridine (orphan: AIDS)

azidothymidine (AZT) [now: zidovudine]

azidouridine (azdU) *investigational (Phase I) antiviral for AIDS/ARC/HIV*

azimexon INN

azimilide dihydrochloride USAN *antiarrhythmic; antifibrillatory*

azintamide INN

azinthiamide [see: azintamide]

azipramine INN *antidepressant* [also: azipramine HCl]

azipramine HCl USAN *antidepressant* [also: azipramine]

aziridinyl benzoquinone [see: diaziquone]

azithromycin USAN, USP, INN, BAN *macrolide antibacterial antibiotic*

azithromycin dihydrate *macrolide antibiotic*

azlocillin USAN, INN, BAN *antibacterial*

azlocillin sodium USP *antibacterial*

Azmacort oral inhalation aerosol ℞ *corticosteroid for bronchial asthma* [triamcinolone acetonide] 100 μg/dose

Azo Gantanol film-coated tablets (discontinued 1995) ℞ *urinary antiinfective; urinary analgesic* [sulfamethoxazole; phenazopyridine HCl] 500•100 mg

Azo Gantrisin film-coated tablets (discontinued 1995) ℞ *urinary anti-infective; urinary analgesic* [sulfisoxazole; phenazopyridine HCl] 500•50 mg

azoconazole [now: azaconazole]

azodisal sodium (ADS) [now: olsalazine sodium]

azolimine USAN, INN *diuretic* ② Azulfidine

azosemide USAN, INN, JAN *diuretic*

Azo-Standard tablets OTC *urinary analgesic* [phenazopyridine HCl] 95 mg

Azostix reagent strips for professional use *in vitro diagnostic aid to estimate the amount of BUN in whole blood*

Azo-Sulfisoxazole tablets ℞ *urinary anti-infective; urinary analgesic* [sulfisoxazole; phenazopyridine HCl] 500•50 mg

azotomycin USAN, INN *antibiotic antineoplastic*

azovan blue BAN *blood volume test* [also: Evans blue]

azovan sodium [see: Evans blue]

AZT (azidothymidine) [now: zidovudine]

Aztec ℞ *investigational (Phase III) controlled-release formulation for early HIV and AIDS* [zidovudine]

AZT-P-ddI *investigational (Phase I) antiviral for AIDS*

aztreonam USAN, USP, INN, BAN, JAN *monobactam-type bactericidal antibiotic*

azulene sulfonate sodium JAN [also: sodium gualenate]

Azulfidine oral suspension (discontinued 1995) ℞ *broad-spectrum bacteriostatic; anti-inflammatory for ulcerative colitis* [sulfasalazine] 250 mg/5 mL ②

azolimine

Azulfidine tablets ℞ *broad-spectrum bacteriostatic; anti-inflammatory for ulcerative colitis* [sulfasalazine] 500 mg

Azulfidine EN-tabs enteric-coated tablets ℞ *broad-spectrum bacteriostatic; anti-inflammatory for ulcerative colitis* [sulfasalazine] 500 mg

azumolene INN *skeletal muscle relaxant* [also: azumolene sodium]

azumolene sodium USAN *skeletal muscle relaxant* [also: azumolene]

azure A carbacrylic resin [see: azuresin]

azuresin NF, BAN

B

B Complex + C timed-release tablets OTC *vitamin supplement* [multiple B vitamins; vitamin C] ≛•500 mg

B Complex with C and B-12 injection ℞ *parenteral vitamin supplement* [multiple vitamins] ≛

B Complex-50 sustained-release tablets OTC *vitamin supplement* [multiple B vitamins; folic acid; biotin] ≛•400•50 µg

B Complex-150 sustained-release tablets OTC *vitamin supplement* [multiple B vitamins; folic acid; biotin] ≛•400•150 µg

B & O Supprettes No. 15A; B & O Supprettes No. 16A suppositories ℞ *narcotic analgesic* [belladonna extract; opium] 16.2•30 mg; 16.2•60 mg

B vitamins [see: vitamin B]

B_1 (vitamin B_1) [see: thiamine HCl]

B_2 (vitamin B_2) [see: riboflavin]

B_3 (vitamin B_3) [see: niacin; niacinamide]

B_5 (vitamin B_5) [see: calcium pantothenate]

B_6 (vitamin B_6) [see: pyridoxine HCl]

B_8 (vitamin B_8) [see: adenosine phosphate]

B_{12} (vitamin B_{12}) [see: cyanocobalamin]

B_{12a} (vitamin B_{12a}) [see: hydroxocobalamin]

B_{12b} (vitamin B_{12b}) [see: hydroxocobalamin]

B-50 tablets OTC *vitamin supplement* [multiple B vitamins; folic acid; biotin] ≛•100•50 µg

B-50 timed-release tablets (discontinued 1995) OTC *vitamin supplement* [multiple B vitamins; folic acid; biotin] ≛•100•50 µg

B-100 tablets, timed-release tablets OTC *vitamin supplement* [multiple B vitamins; folic acid; biotin] ≛•100•100 µg; ≛•400•50 µg

B-125; B-150 tablets (discontinued 1992) OTC *vitamin supplement* [multiple B vitamins; folic acid; biotin]

B_c (vitamin B_c) [see: folic acid]

B_t (vitamin B_t) [see: carnitine]

Babee Teething lotion OTC *topical oral anesthetic; antiseptic* [benzocaine; cetalkonium chloride] 2.5%•0.02%

Baby Vitamin drops OTC *vitamin supplement* [multiple vitamins] ≛

Baby Vitamin with Iron drops OTC *vitamin/iron supplement* [multiple vitamins; iron] ≛•10 mg/mL

Babylax [see: Fleet Babylax]

B-A-C tablets (discontinued 1992) ℞ *analgesic; antipyretic; anti-inflammatory; sedative* [aspirin; caffeine; butalbital] 650•40•50 mg

BAC (BCNU, ara-C, cyclophosphamide) *chemotherapy protocol*

BAC (benzalkonium chloride) [q.v.]

bacampicillin INN, BAN *bactericidal antibiotic* [also: bacampicillin HCl]

bacampicillin HCl USAN, USP, JAN *bactericidal antibiotic* [also: bacampicillin]

BACI ℞ *investigational anti-infective for AIDS-related cryptosporidiosis* [cryptosporidium hyperimmune bovine colostrum IgG concentrate]

Bacid capsules OTC *dietary supplement; fever blister treatment; not generally regarded as safe and effective as an antidiarrheal* [*Lactobacillus acidophilus*] 500 million cultures ⍾ Banacid

Baciguent ointment OTC *topical antibiotic* [bacitracin] 500 U/g

Baci-IM powder for IM injection ℞ *bactericidal antibiotic* [bacitracin] 50,000 U

bacillus Calmette-Guérin (BCG) vaccine [see: BCG vaccine]

bacitracin USP, INN, BAN, JAN *bactericidal antibiotic; (orphan: pseudomembranous enterocolitis)* 500 U/g topical; 50,000 U/vial injection ⍾ Bacitrin; Bactrim

bacitracin zinc USP, BAN *bactericidal antibiotic*

bacitracins zinc complex [see: bacitracin zinc]

Bacitrin ointment OTC *topical antibiotic* [bacitracin] ⍾ bacitracin

Backache Maximum Strength Relief film-coated caplets OTC *analgesic; antirheumatic* [magnesium salicylate] 467 mg

Back-Pack (trademarked packaging form) *unit-of-use package*

baclofen (L-baclofen) USAN, USP, INN, BAN, JAN *muscle relaxant; intractable spasticity (orphan); (orphan: trigeminal neuralgia)* 10, 20 mg oral; 10 mg/20 mL injection; 10 mg/5 mL injection

bacmecillinam INN

Bacmin tablets ℞ *vitamin/mineral/iron supplement* [multiple vitamins & minerals; iron; folic acid; biotin] ≛•27•0.8•0.15 mg

BACOD (bleomycin, Adriamycin, CCNU, Oncovin, dexamethasone) *chemotherapy protocol*

BACON (bleomycin, Adriamycin, CCNU, Oncovin, nitrogen mustard) *chemotherapy protocol*

BACOP (bleomycin, Adriamycin, cyclophosphamide, Oncovin, prednisone) *chemotherapy protocol*

BACT (BCNU, ara-C, cyclophosphamide, thioguanine) *chemotherapy protocol*

Bactal Soap liquid (discontinued 1992) OTC *disinfectant/antiseptic* [triclosan]

bactericidal and permeability-increasing (BPI) protein *investigational treatment for gram-negative sepsis*

bacteriostatic sodium chloride [see: sodium chloride]

Bacteriostatic Sodium Chloride Injection ℞ *IV diluent* [sodium chloride (saline)] 0.9% (normal)

Bacti-Cleanse liquid OTC *soap-free therapeutic skin cleanser* [benzalkonium chloride] ≛

Bacticort eye drop suspension (discontinued 1995) ℞ *topical ophthalmic corticosteroidal anti-inflammatory; antibiotic* [hydrocortisone; neomycin sulfate; polymyxin B sulfate] 1%•0.35%•10,000 U/mL

Bactigen B Streptococcus-CS slide test for professional use *in vitro diagnostic aid for Group B streptococcal antigens in vaginal and cervical swabs*

Bactigen Meningitis Panel slide test for professional use *in vitro diagnostic aid for H influenzae, N meningitidis,* *and S pneumoniae in various fluids* [latex agglutination test]

Bactigen N meningitidis slide test for professional use ℞ *in vitro diagnostic aid for Neisseria meningitidis* [latex agglutination test]

Bactigen S Pneumonia test kit for professional use (discontinued 1996) *in vitro diagnostic aid for Streptococcus pneumoniae antigens in various fluids*

Bactigen Salmonella-Shigella slide test for professional use *in vitro diagnostic aid for salmonella and shigella* [latex agglutination test]

Bactigen Strep B slide test for professional use (discontinued 1996) *in vitro diagnostic aid for Group B streptococcal antigens in various fluids*

Bactine Antiseptic Anesthetic aerosol (discontinued 1995) OTC *topical local anesthetic; antiseptic* [lidocaine HCl; benzalkonium chloride] 2.5%•0.13%

Bactine Antiseptic Anesthetic liquid, spray OTC *topical local anesthetic; antiseptic* [lidocaine HCl; benzalkonium chloride] 2.5%•0.13%

Bactine First Aid Antibiotic ointment OTC *topical antibiotic* [polymyxin B sulfate; neomycin sulfate; bacitracin]

Bactine First Aid Antibiotic Plus Anesthetic ointment OTC *topical antibiotic; topical local anesthetic* [polymyxin B sulfate; neomycin sulfate; bacitracin; diperodon HCl] 5000 U•3.5 mg•400 U•10 mg per g

Bactine Hydrocortisone; Maximum Strength Bactine cream OTC *topical corticosteroid* [hydrocortisone] 0.5%; 1%

Bactocill capsules, powder for IV or IM injection ℞ *bactericidal antibiotic (penicillinase-resistant penicillin)* [oxacillin sodium] 250, 500 mg; 0.25, 0.5, 1, 2, 4, 10 g ② Pathocil

BactoShield aerosol foam, solution OTC *broad-spectrum antimicrobial; germicidal* [chlorhexidine gluconate; alcohol 4%] 4%

BactoShield 2 solution OTC *broad-spectrum antimicrobial; germicidal* [chlorhexidine gluconate; alcohol 4%] 2%

Bactrim; Bactrim DS tablets ℞ *anti-infective; antibacterial* [trimethoprim; sulfamethoxazole] 80•400 mg; 160•800 mg ② bacitracin

Bactrim IV infusion ℞ *anti-infective; antibacterial* [trimethoprim; sulfamethoxazole] 80•400 mg/5 mL

Bactrim Pediatric oral suspension ℞ *anti-infective; antibacterial* [trimethoprim; sulfamethoxazole] 40•200 mg/5 mL

Bactroban ointment ℞ *topical antibiotic for impetigo* [mupirocin] 2%

Bactroban Nasal ointment in single-use tubes ℞ *antibiotic for iatrogenic methicillin-resistant Staphylococcus aureus (MRSA) infections* [mupirocin calcium] 2%

bakeprofen INN

baker's yeast *natural source of protein and B-complex vitamins*

BAL (British antilewisite) [now: dimercaprol]

BAL in Oil deep IM injection ℞ *antidote for arsenic, gold, and mercury poisoning; lead poisoning adjunct* [dimercaprol in peanut oil] 100 mg/mL

balafilcon A USAN *hydrophilic contact lens material*

Balanced B-100 tablets (discontinued 1992) OTC *vitamin B supplement* [multiple B vitamins; folic acid; biotin; inositol]

Baldex eye drops, ophthalmic ointment (discontinued 1993) ℞ *ophthalmic topical corticosteroidal anti-inflammatory* [dexamethasone sodium phosphate]

balipramine BAN [also: depramine]

Balmex ointment OTC *moisturizer; emollient; astringent; antiseptic* [peruvian balsam; zinc oxide; bismuth subnitrate]

Balmex Baby powder OTC *topical diaper rash treatment* [zinc oxide; balsam Peru; corn starch]

Balmex Emollient lotion OTC *moisturizer; emollient*

Balneol Perianal Cleansing lotion OTC *emollient/protectant* [mineral oil; lanolin]

Balnetar bath oil OTC *antipsoriatic; antiseborrheic; antipruritic; emollient* [coal tar] 2.5%
balsalazide INN, BAN
balsalazide disodium USAN *gastrointestinal anti-inflammatory*
balsalazide sodium [see: balsalazide disodium]
balsalazine [see: balsalazide]
balsam Peru [see: peruvian balsam]
balsan [see: peruvian balsam]
bamaluzole INN
bambermycin INN, BAN *antibacterial antibiotic* [also: bambermycins]
bambermycins USAN *antibacterial antibiotic* [also: bambermycin]
bambuterol INN, BAN
bamethan INN, BAN *vasodilator* [also: bamethan sulfate]
bamethan sulfate USAN, JAN *vasodilator* [also: bamethan]
bamifylline INN, BAN *bronchodilator* [also: bamifylline HCl]
bamifylline HCl USAN *bronchodilator* [also: bamifylline]
bamipine INN, BAN, DCF
bamnidazole USAN, INN *antiprotozoal* (*Trichomonas*)
BAMON (bleomycin, Adriamycin, methotrexate, Oncovin, nitrogen mustard) *chemotherapy protocol*
Banacid tablets OTC *antacid* [magnesium hydroxide; aluminum hydroxide; magnesium trisilicate] ② Bacid
Banadyne-3 solution OTC *topical oral anesthetic; antipruritic/counterirritant; antiseptic* [lidocaine; menthol; alcohol 45%] 4%•1%
Banalg lotion OTC *counterirritant* [methyl salicylate; camphor; menthol] 4.9%•2%•1%
Banalg Hospital Strength lotion OTC *counterirritant* [methyl salicylate; menthol] 14%•3%
Bancap capsules (discontinued 1994) ℞ *analgesic; antipyretic; sedative* [acetaminophen; butalbital] 325•50 mg
Bancap HC capsules ℞ *narcotic analgesic* [hydrocodone bitartrate; acetaminophen] 5•500 mg
bandage, adhesive USP *surgical aid*
bandage, gauze USP *surgical aid*

Banesin tablets (discontinued 1994) OTC *analgesic; antipyretic* [acetaminophen] 500 mg
Banex liquid ℞ *decongestant; antihistamine; expectorant* [phenylpropanolamine HCl; phenylephrine HCl; guaifenesin]
Banflex IV or IM injection ℞ *skeletal muscle relaxant* [orphenadrine citrate] 30 mg/mL
Bangesic liniment (discontinued 1994) OTC *counterirritant* [menthol; camphor; methyl salicylate; eucalyptus oil]
banocide [see: diethylcarbamazine citrate]
Banophen elixir OTC *antihistamine* [diphenhydramine HCl] 12.5 mg/5 mL
Banophen Decongestant capsules OTC *decongestant; antihistamine* [pseudoephedrine HCl; diphenhydramine HCl] 60•25 mg ② Barophen
BanSmoke gum (discontinued 1995) OTC *smoking deterrent* [benzocaine] 6 mg
Banthīne tablets ℞ *anticholinergic; peptic ulcer treatment adjunct* [methantheline bromide] 50 mg ② Brethine
Bantron tablets OTC *smoking deterrent* [lobeline sulfate alkaloids; tribasic calcium phosphate; magnesium carbonate] 2•130•130 mg
baquiloprim INN, BAN
Barbased tablets, elixir (discontinued 1992) ℞ *sedative; hypnotic* [butabarbital sodium]
barbenyl [see: phenobarbital]
barbexaclone INN
Barbidonna elixir (discontinued 1995) ℞ *anticholinergic; sedative* [atropine sulfate; scopolamine hydrobromide; hyoscyamine hydrobromide; phenobarbital] 0.034•0.01•0.174•21.6 mg/5 mL
Barbidonna; Barbidonna No. 2 tablets ℞ *GI anticholinergic; sedative* [atropine sulfate; scopolamine hydrobromide; hyoscyamine hydrobromide; phenobarbital] 0.025•

0.0074•0.1286•16 mg; 0.025•0.0074•0.1286•32 mg

barbiphenyl [see: phenobarbital]

Barbita sugar-coated tablets (discontinued 1993) ℞ *long-acting barbiturate sedative, hypnotic and anticonvulsant* [phenobarbital]

barbital NF, INN, JAN [also: barbitone]

barbital, soluble [now: barbital sodium]

barbital sodium NF, INN [also: barbitone sodium]

barbitone BAN [also: barbital]

barbitone sodium BAN [also: barbital sodium]

Barc liquid OTC *pediculicide* [pyrethrins; piperonyl butoxide; petroleum distillate] 0.18%•2.2%•5.52%

Baricon powder for suspension ℞ *GI contrast radiopaque agent* [barium sulfate] 98%

Baridium tablets OTC *urinary analgesic* [phenazopyridine HCl] 100 mg

barium *element (Ba)*

barium hydroxide lime USP *carbon dioxide absorbent*

barium sulfate USP, JAN *GI radiopaque medium*

barmastine USAN, INN *antihistamine*

BarnesHind Saline for Sensitive Eyes solution OTC *rinsing/storage solution for soft contact lenses* [preserved saline solution]

barnidipine INN

Barobag suspension (discontinued 1993) ℞ *GI contrast radiopaque agent* [barium sulfate] 97%

Baro-cat suspension ℞ *GI contrast radiopaque agent* [barium sulfate] 1.5%

Baroflave powder ℞ *GI contrast radiopaque agent* [barium sulfate]

Barophen elixir (discontinued 1995) ℞ *GI anticholinergic; sedative* [atropine sulfate; scopolamine hydrobromide; hyoscyamine sulfate; phenobarbital] 0.0194•0.0065•0.1037•16.2 mg/5 mL ② Banophen

Baros effervescent granules ℞ *GI contrast radiopaque agent* [sodium bicarbonate; tartaric acid; simethicone] 460•420•≛ mg/g

barosmin [see: diosmin]

Barosperse powder for suspension ℞ *GI contrast radiopaque agent* [barium sulfate] 95%

Barosperse, Liquid suspension ℞ *GI contrast radiopaque agent* [barium sulfate] 60%

Barotrast oral suspension ℞ *GI contrast medium* [barium sulfate]

Barriere cream *investigational protective hand cream*

barucainide INN

BAS (benzyl analogue of serotonin) [see: benanserin HCl]

Basaljel tablets, capsules, suspension OTC *antacid* [aluminum carbonate gel, basic] 500 mg; 500 mg; 400 mg/5 mL

basic aluminum acetate [see: aluminum subacetate]

basic aluminum aminoacetate [see: dihydroxyaluminum aminoacetate]

basic aluminum carbonate [see: aluminum carbonate, basic]

basic aluminum chloride [see: aluminum sesquichlorohydrate]

basic aluminum glycinate [see: dihydroxyaluminum aminoacetate]

basic bismuth carbonate [see: bismuth subcarbonate]

basic bismuth gallate [see: bismuth subgallate]

basic bismuth nitrate [see: bismuth subnitrate]

basic bismuth potassium bismuthotartrate [see: bismuth potassium tartrate]

basic bismuth salicylate [see: bismuth subsalicylate]

basic fibroblast growth factor (bFGF) [see: ersofermin]

basic fuchsin [see: fuchsin, basic]

basic zinc acetate [see: zinc acetate, basic]

basifungin USAN, INN *antifungal*

Basis Glycerin Soap; Basis Superfatted Soap bar (discontinued 1992) OTC *therapeutic skin cleanser*

batanopride INN *antiemetic* [also: batanopride HCl]

batanopride HCl USAN *antiemetic* [also: batanopride]

batebulast INN

batelapine INN *antipsychotic* [also: batelapine HCl]
batelapine maleate USAN *antipsychotic* [also: batelapine]
batilol INN
batimastat USAN, INN *antineoplastic; matrix metalloproteinase inhibitor*
batoprazine INN
batroxobin INN, JAN
batyl alcohol [see: batilol]
batylol [see: batilol]
Baumodyne ointment, gel (discontinued 1992) OTC *counterirritant* [methyl salicylate; menthol; eucalyptus oil; methylparaben; butylparaben]
BAVIP (bleomycin, Adriamycin, vinblastine, imidazole carboxamide, prednisone) *chemotherapy protocol*
baxitozine INN
Bayer, Therapy caplets (name changed to Bayer Enteric Coated in 1994)
Bayer Arthritis Regimen delayed-release enteric-coated tablets OTC *analgesic; antipyretic; anti-inflammatory; antirheumatic* [aspirin] 500 mg
Bayer Aspirin, Genuine; Maximum Bayer Aspirin film-coated tablets, film-coated caplets OTC *analgesic; antipyretic; anti-inflammatory; antirheumatic* [aspirin] 325 mg; 500 mg
Bayer Aspirin Regimen delayed-release enteric-coated tablets and caplets OTC *analgesic; antipyretic; anti-inflammatory; antirheumatic* [aspirin] 81, 325 mg
Bayer Buffered tablets (discontinued 1995) OTC *analgesic; antipyretic; anti-inflammatory; antirheumatic* [aspirin, buffered] 325 mg
Bayer Children's Aspirin chewable tablets OTC *analgesic; antipyretic; anti-inflammatory; antirheumatic* [aspirin] 81 mg
Bayer Enteric 500 delayed-release enteric-coated caplets (name changed to Bayer Arthritis Regimen in 1995)
Bayer Enteric Coated delayed-release enteric-coated caplets (name changed to Bayer Aspirin Regimen in 1995)
Bayer Low Adult Strength delayed-release enteric-coated tablets (name changed to Bayer Aspirin Regimen in 1995)
Bayer Plus caplets OTC *analgesic; antipyretic; anti-inflammatory; antirheumatic* [aspirin, buffered with calcium carbonate, magnesium carbonate and magnesium oxide] 500 mg
Bayer Select Allergy Sinus, Aspirin-Free caplets OTC *decongestant; antihistamine; analgesic* [pseudoephedrine HCl; chlorpheniramine maleate; acetaminophen] 30•2•500 mg
Bayer Select Backache caplets OTC *analgesic; antipyretic; anti-inflammatory; antirheumatic* [magnesium salicylate] 580 mg
Bayer Select Chest Cold caplets OTC *antitussive; analgesic* [dextromethorphan hydrobromide; acetaminophen] 15•500 mg
Bayer Select Flu Relief caplets OTC *antitussive; decongestant; antihistamine; analgesic* [dextromethorphan hydrobromide; pseudoephedrine HCl; chlorpheniramine maleate; acetaminophen] 15•30•2•500 mg
Bayer Select Head & Chest Cold, Aspirin-Free caplets OTC *antitussive; decongestant; expectorant; analgesic* [dextromethorphan hydrobromide; pseudoephedrine HCl; guaifenesin; acetaminophen] 10•30•100•325 mg
Bayer Select Head Cold; Bayer Select Sinus Pain Relief caplets OTC *decongestant; analgesic; antipyretic* [pseudoephedrine HCl; acetaminophen] 30•500 mg
Bayer Select Headache caplets OTC *analgesic; antipyretic* [acetaminophen; caffeine] 500•65 mg
Bayer Select Menstrual caplets OTC *analgesic; antipyretic; diuretic* [acetaminophen; pamabrom] 500•25 mg
Bayer Select Night Time Cold caplets OTC *antitussive; decongestant; antihistamine; analgesic* [dextromethorphan hydrobromide; pseudoephedrine HCl; triprolidine HCl; acetaminophen] 15•30•1.25•500 mg

Bayer Select Night Time Pain Relief caplets OTC *antihistaminic sleep aid; analgesic* [diphenhydramine HCl; acetaminophen] 25•500 mg

Bayer Select Pain Relief Formula caplets OTC *nonsteroidal anti-inflammatory drug (NSAID); analgesic* [ibuprofen] 200 mg

Bayer Timed Release, 8-Hour caplets OTC *analgesic; antipyretic; anti-inflammatory; antirheumatic* [aspirin] 650 mg

Baylocaine 2% Viscous; Baylocaine 4% solution ℞ *topical anesthetic for mouth and pharynx* [lidocaine HCl]

Baypress ℞ *investigational antihypertensive; calcium channel blocker* [nitrendipine]

bazinaprine INN

B-Between capsules OTC *vitamin supplement* [multiple B vitamins]

BBVP-M (BCNU, bleomycin, VePesid, prednisone, methotrexate) *chemotherapy protocol*

BC tablets, powder OTC *analgesic; antipyretic; anti-inflammatory* [aspirin; salicylamide; caffeine] 325•95•16 mg; 650•145•32 mg/packet

B$_c$ (vitamin B$_c$) [see: folic acid]

BC Arthritis Strength powder OTC *analgesic; antipyretic; anti-inflammatory* [aspirin; salicylamide; caffeine] 742•222•36 mg

BC Cold Powder Non-Drowsy Formula packets (name changed to BC Cold-Sinus Powder in 1995)

BC Cold-Sinus Powder packets OTC *decongestant; analgesic; antipyretic* [phenylpropanolamine HCl; aspirin] 25•650 mg

BC Cold-Sinus-Allergy Powder packets OTC *decongestant; antihistamine; analgesic; antipyretic* [phenylpropanolamine HCl; chlorpheniramine maleate; aspirin] 25•4•650 mg

BC Multi Symptom Cold Powder packets (name changed to BC Cold-Sinus-Allergy Powder in 1995)

B-C with Folic Acid tablets ℞ *vitamin supplement* [multiple B vitamins; vitamin C; folic acid] ±•500•0.5 mg

B-C with Folic Acid Plus tablets ℞ *vitamin/mineral/iron supplement* [multiple vitamins & minerals; ferrous fumarate; folic acid; biotin] ±•27•0.8•0.15 mg

BCAA (branched-chain amino acids) *(orphan: amyotrophic lateral sclerosis)* [see: isoleucine; leucine; valine]

BCAP (BCNU, cyclophosphamide, Adriamycin, prednisone) *chemotherapy protocol*

BCAVe; B-CAVe (bleomycin, CCNU, Adriamycin, Velban) *chemotherapy protocol*

B-C-Bid caplets OTC *vitamin supplement* [multiple B vitamins; vitamin C] ±•300 mg

BCD (bleomycin, cyclophosphamide, dactinomycin) *chemotherapy protocol*

B-C-E & Zinc tablets (discontinued 1993) OTC *vitamin/zinc supplement* [vitamin E; vitamin C; multiple B vitamins; zinc]

BCG vaccine (bacillus Calmette-Guérin) USP *active bacterin for tuberculosis*

B-CHOP (bleomycin, Cytoxin, hydroxydaunomycin, Oncovin, prednisone) *chemotherapy protocol*

BCMF (bleomycin, cyclophosphamide, methotrexate, fluorouracil) *chemotherapy protocol*

BCNU (bis-chloroethyl-nitrosourea) [see: carmustine]

B-Compleet tablets OTC *vitamin supplement* [multiple B vitamins; vitamin C]

B-Compleet-50; B-Compleet-100 cellulose-coated caplet OTC *vitamin supplement* [multiple B vitamins]

B-Complex elixir OTC *vitamin supplement* [multiple B vitamins] ±

B-Complex "50"; B-Complex "100" tablets (discontinued 1992) OTC *vitamin B supplement* [multiple B vitamins; folic acid; inositol; biotin; choline bitartrate]

B-Complex and B-12 tablets OTC *vitamin supplement* [multiple B vitamins; protease] ±•10 mg

B-Complex with B-12 tablets OTC *vitamin supplement* [multiple B vitamins] ±

B-Complex/Vitamin C caplets OTC *vitamin supplement* [multiple B vitamins; vitamin C] ± •300 mg

BCOP (BCNU, cyclophosphamide, Oncovin, prednisone) *chemotherapy protocol*

BCP (BCNU, cyclophosphamide, prednisone) *chemotherapy protocol*

BC-Vite tablets OTC *vitamin supplement* [multiple B vitamins; vitamin C]

BCVP (BCNU, cyclophosphamide, vincristine, prednisone) *chemotherapy protocol*

BCVPP (BCNU, cyclophosphamide, vinblastine, procarbazine, prednisone) *chemotherapy protocol*

BCX-34 *investigational agent for psoriasis and cutaneous T-cell lymphoma*

B-D glucose chewable tablets OTC *glucose elevating agent* [glucose] 5 g

bDNA (branched DNA) assay *investigational in vitro diagnostic aid for HIV in the blood*

B-DOPA (bleomycin, DTIC, Oncovin, prednisone, Adriamycin) *chemotherapy protocol*

BEAC (BCNU, etoposide, ara-C, cyclophosphamide) *chemotherapy protocol*

BEAM (BCNU, etoposide, ara-C, melphalan) *chemotherapy protocol*

Beano liquid, tablets OTC *digestive aid* [alpha-D-galactosidase enzyme]

Bebulin VH ℞ *investigational coagulant for hemophilia B* [factor IX complex]

BE-C 800 with Iron tablets OTC *vitamin/iron supplement* [vitamin E; vitamin C; multiple B vitamins; iron]

becanthone HCl USAN *antischistosomal* [also: becantone]

becantone INN *antischistosomal* [also: becanthone HCl]

becanthone HCl [see: becanthone HCl]

becaplermin USAN *recombinant platelet-derived growth factor B for chronic dermal ulcers*

Because vaginal foam OTC *spermicidal contraceptive* [nonoxynol 9] 8%

beciparcil INN

beclamide INN, BAN, DCF

becliconazole INN

beclobrate INN, BAN

beclometasone INN *corticosteroidal inhalant for asthma; intranasal steroid* [also: beclomethasone dipropionate; beclomethasone; beclomethasone dipropionate]

beclometasone dipropionate JAN *corticosteroidal inhalant for asthma; intranasal steroid* [also: beclomethasone dipropionate; beclomethasone; beclomethasone]

beclomethasone BAN *corticosteroidal inhalant for asthma; intranasal steroid* [also: beclomethasone dipropionate; beclomethasone; beclomethasone dipropionate]

beclomethasone dipropionate USAN, USP *corticosteroidal inhalant for asthma; intranasal steroid* [also: beclomethasone; beclomethasone; beclomethasone dipropionate]

beclotiamine INN

Beclovent oral inhalation aerosol ℞ *corticosteroid for bronchial asthma* [beclomethasone dipropionate] 42 μg/dose

Becomject-100 injection (discontinued 1996) ℞ *parenteral vitamin therapy* [multiple B vitamins] ±

Beconase nasal inhalation aerosol ℞ *intranasal steroidal anti-inflammatory* [beclomethasone dipropionate] 42 μg/dose

Beconase AQ nasal spray ℞ *intranasal steroidal anti-inflammatory* [beclomethasone dipropionate] 0.042%

beechwood creosote [see: creosote carbonate]

beef tallow JAN

Beelith tablets OTC *dietary supplement* [vitamin B_6; magnesium oxide] 20• 362 mg

Beepen-VK tablets, powder for oral solution ℞ *bactericidal antibiotic* [penicillin V potassium] 250, 500 mg; 125, 250 mg/5 mL

Beesix IM or IV injection (discontinued 1994) ℞ *vitamin deficiency therapy; antidote to isoniazid poisoning* [pyridoxine HCl] 100 mg/mL

beeswax, white JAN [also: wax, white]

beeswax, yellow JAN [also: wax, yellow]
Bee-T-Vites film-coated tablets (discontinued 1995) OTC *vitamin supplement* [multiple B vitamins; vitamin C] ± •300 mg
Bee-Zee tablets OTC *vitamin/zinc supplement* [multiple vitamins; zinc] ± •22.5 mg
befiperide INN
befloxatone INN
befunolol INN [also: befunolol HCl]
befunolol HCl JAN [also: befunolol]
befuraline INN
behepan [see: cyanocobalamin]
bekanamycin INN *antibiotic* [also: bekanamycin sulfate]
bekanamycin sulfate JAN *antibiotic* [also: bekanamycin]
belarizine INN
belfosdil USAN, INN *antihypertensive; calcium channel blocker*
Belganyl (available only from the Centers for Disease Control) ℞ *investigational anti-infective for trypanosomiasis and onchocerciasis* [suramin sodium]
Belix elixir OTC *antihistamine* [diphenhydramine HCl] 12.5 mg/5 mL
Bellacane elixir ℞ *GI anticholinergic; sedative* [atropine sulfate; scopolamine hydrobromide; hyoscyamine sulfate; phenobarbital] 0.0194•0.0065•0.1037•16.2 mg/5 mL
Bellacane tablets ℞ *GI anticholinergic; sedative* [hyoscyamine sulfate; phenobarbital] 0.125•15 mg
Bellacane SR sustained-release tablets ℞ *GI anticholinergic; sedative; analgesic* [belladonna alkaloids; phenobarbital; ergotamine tartrate] 0.2•40•0.6 mg
belladonna extract USP *GI/GU anticholinergic/antispasmodic; antiparkinsonian* 27–33 mg/100 mL oral
Bellafoline tablets ℞ *GI anticholinergic; antispasmodic; antiparkinsonian agent* [belladonna extract] 0.25 mg
Bell/ans tablets OTC *antacid* [sodium bicarbonate] 520 mg
Bellatal tablets ℞ *long-acting barbiturate sedative, hypnotic, and anticonvulsant* [phenobarbital] 16.2 mg

Bellergal-S tablets ℞ *GI anticholinergic; sedative; analgesic* [belladonna extract; phenobarbital; ergotamine tartrate] 0.2•40•0.6 mg
beloxamide USAN, INN *antihyperlipoproteinemic*
Bel-Phen-Ergot SR sustained-release tablets ℞ *GI anticholinergic; sedative; analgesic* [belladonna alkaloids; phenobarbital; ergotamine tartrate] 0.2•40•0.6 mg
bemarinone INN *cardiotonic; positive inotropic; vasodilator* [also: bemarinone HCl]
bemarinone HCl USAN *cardiotonic; positive inotropic; vasodilator* [also: bemarinone]
bemegride USP, INN, BAN, JAN
bemesetron USAN, INN *antiemetic*
bemetizide INN, BAN
Beminal 500 tablets OTC *vitamin supplement* [multiple B vitamins; vitamin C] ± •500 mg ⑨ Benemid
bemitradine USAN, INN *antihypertensive; diuretic*
bemoradan USAN, INN *cardiotonic*
BEMP (bleomycin, Eldisine, mitomycin, Platinol) *chemotherapy protocol*
benactyzine INN, BAN
benactyzine HCl *mild antidepressant; anticholinergic*
Bena-D 10; Bena-D 50 injection (discontinued 1996) ℞ *antihistamine; motion sickness preventative; sleep aid; antiparkinsonian* [diphenhydramine HCl] 10 mg/mL; 50 mg/mL
Benadryl elixir (name changed to Benadryl Allergy in 1995) ⑨ Bentyl; Benylin; Caladryl
Benadryl tablets, capsules, Kapseals (capsules), injection OTC *antihistamine; motion sickness preventative; sleep aid; antiparkinsonian* [diphenhydramine HCl] 25 mg; 25 mg; 50 mg; 10, 50 mg/mL ⑨ Bentyl; Benylin; Caladryl
Benadryl; Benadryl 2% cream, spray OTC *topical antihistamine* [diphenhydramine HCl] 1%; 2% ⑨ Bentyl; Benylin; Caladryl

Benadryl Allergy Kapseals (sealed capsules), tablets, chewable tablets, liquid OTC *antihistamine; motion sickness preventative; sleep aid; antiparkinsonian* [diphenhydramine HCl] 25 mg; 25 mg; 12.5 mg; 12.5 mg/5 mL ▣ Bentyl; Benylin; Caladryl

Benadryl Allergy Decongestant liquid OTC *pediatric decongestant and antihistamine* [pseudoephedrine HCl; diphenhydramine HCl] 30•12.5 mg/5 mL ▣ Bentyl; Benylin; Caladryl

Benadryl Allergy/Sinus Headache caplets OTC *decongestant; antihistamine; analgesic* [pseudoephedrine HCl; diphenhydramine HCl; acetaminophen] 30•12.5•500 mg ▣ Bentyl; Benylin; Caladryl

Benadryl Cold Nighttime Formula liquid (discontinued 1995) OTC *decongestant; antihistamine; analgesic* [pseudoephedrine HCl; diphenhydramine HCl; acetaminophen; alcohol 10%] 10•8.3•167 mg/5 mL ▣ Bentyl; Benylin; Caladryl

Benadryl Cold/Flu tablets (discontinued 1996) OTC *decongestant; antihistamine; analgesic* [pseudoephedrine HCl; diphenhydramine HCl; acetaminophen] 30•12.5•500 mg ▣ Bentyl; Benylin; Caladryl

Benadryl Decongestant elixir (name changed to Benadryl Allergy Decongestant in 1995) ▣ Bentyl; Benylin; Caladryl

Benadryl Decongestant Kapseals (capsules) (discontinued 1993) OTC *decongestant; antihistamine* [pseudoephedrine HCl; diphenhydramine HCl] ▣ Bentyl; Benylin; Caladryl

Benadryl Decongestant Allergy film-coated tablets OTC *decongestant; antihistamine* [pseudoephedrine HCl; diphenhydramine HCl] 60•25 mg ▣ Bentyl; Benylin; Caladryl

Benadryl Dye-Free liquid OTC *antihistamine* [diphenhydramine HCl] 6.25 mg/5 mL ▣ Bentyl; Benylin; Caladryl

Benadryl Dye-Free Allergy Liqui Gels OTC *antihistamine* [diphenhydramine HCl] 25 mg ▣ Bentyl; Benylin; Caladryl

Benadryl Itch Relief spray, cream, stick OTC *topical antihistamine; astringent* [diphenhydramine HCl; zinc acetate] 2%•0.1% ▣ Bentyl; Benylin; Caladryl

Benadryl Itch Relief, Children's spray, cream OTC *topical antihistamine; astringent* [diphenhydramine HCl; zinc acetate] 1%•0.1% ▣ Bentyl; Benylin; Caladryl

Benadryl Itch Stopping Gel; Benadryl Itch Stopping Gel Children's Formula OTC *topical antihistamine; astringent* [diphenhydramine HCl; zinc acetate] 2%•1%; 1%•1% ▣ Bentyl; Benylin; Caladryl

Benadryl Plus Night-Time (name changed to Benadryl Cold in 1992) ▣ Bentyl; Benylin; Caladryl

benafentrine INN

Benahist 10; Benahist 50 injection (discontinued 1996) ℞ *antihistamine; motion sickness preventative; sleep aid; antiparkinsonian* [diphenhydramine HCl] 10 mg/mL; 50 mg/mL

Ben-Allergin-50 injection ℞ *antihistamine; motion sickness preventative; sleep aid; antiparkinsonian* [diphenhydramine HCl] 50 mg/mL

benanserin HCl

benapen [see: benethamine penicillin]

benaprizine INN *anticholinergic* [also: benapryzine HCl; benapryzine]

benapryzine BAN *anticholinergic* [also: benapryzine HCl; benaprizine]

benapryzine HCl USAN *anticholinergic* [also: benaprizine; benapryzine]

Ben-Aqua 5; Ben-Aqua 10 gel OTC *topical keratolytic for acne* [benzoyl peroxide] 5%; 10%

Ben-Aqua 5; Ben-Aqua 10 lotion (discontinued 1994) OTC *topical keratolytic for acne* [benzoyl peroxide]

Benatol ℞ *investigational beta blocker for hypertension* [bevantolol]

benaxibine INN

benazepril INN, BAN *antihypertensive; angiotensin-converting enzyme (ACE) inhibitor* [also: benazepril HCl]

benazepril HCl USAN *antihypertensive; angiotensin-converting enzyme (ACE) inhibitor* [also: benazepril]
benazeprilat USAN, INN *angiotensin-converting enzyme inhibitor*
bencianol INN
bencisteine INN, DCF
benclonidine INN
bencyclane INN [also: bencyclane fumarate]
bencyclane fumarate JAN [also: bencyclane]
bendacalol mesylate USAN *antihypertensive*
bendamustine INN
bendazac USAN, INN, BAN, JAN *antiinflammatory*
bendazol INN, DCF
benderizine INN
bendrofluazide BAN *diuretic; antihypertensive* [also: bendroflumethiazide]
bendroflumethiazide USP, INN *diuretic; antihypertensive* [also: bendrofluazide]
Benegyn vaginal cream (discontinued 1993) ℞ *bacteriostatic antibiotic; antiseptic; vulnerary* [sulfanilamide; aminacrine HCl; allantoin] 15%•0.2%•2%
Benemid film-coated tablets (discontinued 1996) ℞ *uricosuric for gout* [probenecid] 500 mg ② Beminal
benethamine penicillin INN, BAN
benexate INN
benexate HCl JAN
benfluorex INN, DCF
benfosformin INN, DCF
benfotiamine INN, JAN, DCF
benfurodil hemisuccinate INN, DCF
bengal gelatin [see: agar]
Ben-Gay gel, lotion (discontinued 1992) OTC *counterirritant* [methyl salicylate; menthol]
Ben-Gay Original ointment OTC *counterirritant* [methyl salicylate; menthol] 18.3%•16%
Ben-Gay Regular Strength; Ben-Gay Extra Strength cream OTC *counterirritant* [methyl salicylate; menthol] 15%•10%; 30%•8%
Ben-Gay Ultra Strength cream OTC *counterirritant* [methyl salicylate; menthol; camphor] 30%•10%•4%

Ben-Gay Vanishing Scent gel OTC *counterirritant* [menthol; camphor] 3%•?
benhepazone INN
benidipine INN
benmoxin INN, DCF
Benoject-10; Benoject-50 injection (discontinued 1996) ℞ *antihistamine; motion sickness preventative; sleep aid; antiparkinsonian* [diphenhydramine HCl] 10 mg/mL; 50 mg/mL
benolizime INN
Benoquin cream ℞ *depigmenting agent for vitiligo* [monobenzone] 20%
benorilate INN, DCF [also: benorylate]
benorterone USAN, INN *antiandrogen*
benorylate BAN [also: benorilate]
benoxafos INN
benoxaprofen USAN, INN, BAN *antiinflammatory; analgesic*
benoxinate HCl USP *topical anesthetic* [also: oxybuprocaine; oxybuprocaine HCl]
Benoxyl #5 lotion, mask OTC *topical keratolytic for acne* [benzoyl peroxide] 5% ② PanOxyl
Benoxyl 10 lotion OTC *topical keratolytic for acne* [benzoyl peroxide] 10%
benpenolisin INN
benperidol USAN, INN, BAN *antipsychotic*
benproperine INN [also: benproperine phosphate]
benproperine phosphate JAN [also: benproperine]
benrixate INN, DCF
bensalan USAN, INN *disinfectant*
benserazide USAN, INN, BAN *decarboxylase inhibitor* [also: benserazide HCl]
benserazide HCl JAN *decarboxylase inhibitor* [also: benserazide]
bensuldazic acid INN, BAN
Bensulfoid cream OTC *topical acne treatment* [colloidal sulfur; resorcinol; alcohol] 8%•2%•12%
Bensulfoid tablets (discontinued 1994) ℞ *antibacterial and exfoliant for acne* [sulfur] 130 mg
bensylyte HCl [see: phenoxybenzamine HCl]
bentazepam USAN, INN *sedative*
bentemazole INN
bentiamine INN

bentipimine INN
bentiromide USAN, INN, BAN, JAN *pancreas function test*
bentonite NF, JAN *suspending agent*
Bentyl capsules, tablets, IM injection, syrup ℞ *gastrointestinal antispasmodic* [dicyclomine HCl] 10 mg; 20 mg; 10 mg/mL; 10 mg/5 mL ② Aventyl; Benadryl; Bontril
benurestat USAN, INN *urease enzyme inhibitor*
Benylin Adult oral liquid OTC *antitussive* [dextromethorphan hydrobromide; alcohol 5%] 15 mg/5 mL ② Benadryl
Benylin Cough syrup (name changed to Benylin Adult in 1995) ② Benadryl
Benylin Decongestant liquid (discontinued 1995) OTC *decongestant; antihistamine* [pseudoephedrine HCl; diphenhydramine HCl; alcohol 5%] 30•12.5 mg/5 mL ② Benadryl
Benylin DM syrup OTC *antitussive* [dextromethorphan hydrobromide] 10 mg/5 mL ② Benadryl
Benylin DM-D; Children's Benylin DM-D syrup (available only in Canada) OTC *antitussive; decongestant* [dextromethorphan hydrobromide; pseudoephedrine HCl] 15•30 mg/5 mL; 7.5•15 mg/5 mL ② Benadryl
Benylin DM-D-E syrup (available only in Canada) OTC *antitussive; decongestant; expectorant* [dextromethorphan hydrobromide; pseudoephedrine HCl; guaifenesin; alcohol 5%] 15•30•100, 15•30•200 mg/5 mL ② Benadryl
Benylin DM-E syrup (available only in Canada) OTC *antitussive; expectorant* [dextromethorphan hydrobromide; guaifenesin; alcohol 5%] 15•100 mg/5 mL ② Benadryl
Benylin Expectorant liquid OTC *antitussive; expectorant* [dextromethorphan hydrobromide; guaifenesin] 5•100 mg/5 mL ② Benadryl
Benylin Multi-Symptom liquid OTC *antitussive; decongestant; expectorant* [dextromethorphan hydrobromide; pseudoephedrine HCl; guaifenesin] 5•15•100 mg/5 mL ② Benadryl
Benylin Pediatric oral liquid OTC *antitussive* [dextromethorphan hydrobromide] 7.5 mg/5 mL ② Benadryl
Benza solution OTC *topical antiseptic* [benzalkonium chloride] 1:750
Benzac AC 2½; Benzac W 2½; Benzac 5; Benzac AC 5; Benzac W 5; Benzac 10; Benzac AC 10; Benzac W 10 gel ℞ *topical keratolytic for acne* [benzoyl peroxide] 2.5%; 2.5%; 5%; 5%; 5%; 10%; 10%; 10%
Benzac AC Wash 2½; Benzac AC Wash 5; Benzac W Wash 5; Benzac AC Wash 10; Benzac W Wash 10 liquid ℞ *topical keratolytic for acne* [benzoyl peroxide] 2.5%; 5%; 5%; 10%; 10%
5 Benzagel; 10 Benzagel gel ℞ *topical keratolytic for acne* [benzoyl peroxide] 5%; 10%
benzaldehyde NF *flavoring agent*
benzalkonium chloride (BAC) NF, INN, BAN, JAN *preservative; bacteriostatic antiseptic; surfactant/wetting agent* 17% topical
Benzamycin gel ℞ *topical antibiotic and keratolytic for acne* [erythromycin; benzoyl peroxide] 30•50 mg/mL
benzaprinoxide INN
benzarone INN, DCF
Benzashave shaving cream ℞ *topical keratolytic for acne* [benzoyl peroxide] 5%, 10%
benzathine benzylpenicillin INN *bactericidal antibiotic* [also: penicillin G benzathine; benzathine penicillin; benzylpenicillin benzathine]
benzathine penicillin BAN *bactericidal antibiotic* [also: penicillin G benzathine; benzathine benzylpenicillin; benzylpenicillin benzathine]
benzathine penicillin G [see: penicillin G benzathine]
benzatropine INN *antiparkinsonian; anticholinergic* [also: benztropine mesylate; benztropine]
benzazoline HCl [see: tolazoline HCl]

benzbromaron JAN *uricosuric* [also: benzbromarone]
benzbromarone USAN, INN, BAN *uricosuric* [also: benzbromaron]
benzchinamide [see: benzquinamide]
benzchlorpropamide [see: beclamide]
Benzedrex inhaler ℞ *nasal decongestant* [propylhexedrine] 250 mg
benzene ethanol [see: phenylethyl alcohol]
benzene hexachloride, gamma [now: lindane]
benzeneacetic acid, sodium salt [see: sodium phenylacetate]
benzenebutanoic acid, sodium salt [see: sodium phenylbutyrate]
1,3-benzenediol [see: resorcinol]
benzenemethanol [see: benzyl alcohol]
benzestrofol [see: estradiol benzoate]
benzestrol USP, INN, BAN
benzethacil [see: penicillin G benzathine]
benzethidine INN, BAN, DCF
benzethonium chloride USP, INN, BAN, JAN *topical anti-infective; preservative*
benzetimide INN *anticholinergic* [also: benzetimide HCl]
benzetimide HCl USAN *anticholinergic* [also: benzetimide]
benzfetamine INN *anorexiant; CNS stimulant* [also: benzphetamine HCl; benzphetamine]
benzhexol BAN *anticholinergic; antiparkinsonian* [also: trihexyphenidyl HCl; trihexyphenidyl]
N-benzhydryl-N-methylpiperazine [see: cyclizine HCl]
benzilone bromide [see: benzilonium bromide]
benzilonium bromide USAN, INN, BAN *anticholinergic*
2-benzimidazolepropionic acid [see: procodazole]
benzin, petroleum JAN
benzindamine HCl [see: benzydamine HCl]
benzindopyrine INN *antipsychotic* [also: benzindopyrine HCl]
benzindopyrine HCl USAN *antipsychotic* [also: benzindopyrine]
benzinoform [see: carbon tetrachloride]
benziodarone INN, BAN, DCF
benzmalecene INN
benzmethoxazone [see: chlorthenoxazine]
benznidazole INN
benzoaric acid [see: ellagic acid]
benzoate & phenylacetate (sodium benzoate & sodium phenylacetate) *to prevent or treat hyperammonemia in urea cycle enzymopathy* (orphan)
benzobarbital INN
benzocaine USP, INN, BAN *topical anesthetic; nonprescription diet aid* [also: ethyl aminobenzoate] 5% topical
benzoclidine INN
Benzocol cream (discontinued 1995) OTC *topical local anesthetic* [benzocaine] 5%
benzoctamine INN, BAN *sedative; muscle relaxant* [also: benzoctamine HCl]
benzoctamine HCl USAN, INN *sedative; muscle relaxant* [also: benzoctamine]
Benzodent ointment OTC *topical oral anesthetic* [benzocaine] 20%
benzodepa USAN, INN *antineoplastic*
benzodiazepine HCl [see: medazepam HCl]
benzododecinium chloride INN
Benzodyne ear drops (discontinued 1992) OTC *antibacterial/antifungal* [chloroxylenol; acetic acid; benzalkonium chloride]
benzogynestryl [see: estradiol benzoate]
benzoic acid USP, JAN *antifungal; urinary acidifier*
benzoic acid, phenylmethyl ester [see: benzyl benzoate]
benzoic acid, potassium salt [see: potassium benzoate]
benzoic acid, sodium salt [see: sodium benzoate]
benzoin USP, JAN *topical protectant*
Benzoin Compound tincture OTC *skin protectant* [benzoin; aloe; alcohol 74–80%]
benzol [see: benzene ...]
benzonatate USP, INN, BAN *antitussive* 100 mg oral
benzophenone
benzopyrrolate [see: benzopyrronium]
benzopyrronium bromide INN

benzoquinone amidoinohydrazone thiosemicarbazone hydrate [see: ambazone]
benzoquinonium chloride
benzorphanol [see: levophenacylmorphan]
benzosulfinide [see: saccharin]
benzosulphinide sodium [see: saccharin sodium]
benzothiozon [see: thioacetazone; thiacetazone]
benzotript INN
Benzox-10 gel ℞ *topical keratolytic for acne* [benzoyl peroxide] 10%
benzoxiquine USAN, INN *antiseptic/disinfectant*
benzoxonium chloride INN
benzoyl *p*-aminosalicylate (B-PAS) [see: benzoylpas calcium]
benzoyl peroxide USAN, USP *keratolytic* 5%, 10% topical
***m*-benzoylhydratropic acid** [see: ketoprofen]
benzoylmethylecgonine [see: cocaine]
benzoylpas calcium USAN, USP *antibacterial; tuberculostatic* [also: calcium benzamidosalicylate]
benzoylsulfanilamide [see: sulfabenzamide]
benzoylthiamindisulfide [see: bisbentiamine]
benzoylthiaminmonophosphate [see: benfotiamine]
benzphetamine BAN *anorexiant; CNS stimulant* [also: benzphetamine HCl; benzfetamine]
benzphetamine chloride [see: benzphetamine HCl]
benzphetamine HCl NF *anorexiant; CNS stimulant* [also: benzfetamine; benzphetamine]
benzpiperylon [see: benzpiperylone]
benzpiperylone INN
benzpyrinium bromide NF, INN
benzquercin INN
benzquinamide USAN, INN, BAN *postanesthesia antinauseant and antiemetic*
benzthiazide USP, INN, BAN *diuretic; antihypertensive*

benztropine BAN *antiparkinsonian; anticholinergic* [also: benztropine mesylate; benzatropine]
benztropine mesylate USP *antiparkinsonian; anticholinergic* [also: benzatropine; benztropine] 0.5, 1, 2 mg oral
benztropine methanesulfonate [see: benztropine mesylate]
benzydamine INN, BAN *analgesic; antipyretic; anti-inflammatory* [also: benzydamine HCl]
benzydamine HCl USAN, JAN *analgesic; antipyretic; anti-inflammatory* [also: benzydamine]
benzydroflumethiazide [see: bendroflumethiazide]
benzyl alcohol NF, INN, JAN *antimicrobial agent; antiseptic; local anesthetic*
benzyl analogue of serotonin (BAS) [see: benanserin HCl]
benzyl antiserotonin [see: benanserin HCl]
benzyl benzoate USP, JAN
benzyl carbinol [see: phenylethyl alcohol]
S-benzyl thiobenzoate [see: tibenzate]
benzylamide [see: beclamide]
N-benzylanilinoacetamidoxime [see: cetoxime]
2-benzylbenzimidazole [see: bendazol]
benzyldimethyltetradecylammonium chloride [see: miristalkonium chloride]
benzyldodecyldimethylammonium chloride [see: benzododecinium chloride]
benzylhexadecyldimethylammonium [see: cetalkonium]
benzylhexadecyldimethylammonium chloride [see: cetalkonium chloride]
benzylhydrochlorothiazide JAN
***p*-benzyloxyphenol** [see: monobenzone]
benzylpenicillin INN, BAN *(orphan: penicillin hypersensitivity assessment)*
benzylpenicillin benzathine JAN *bactericidal antibiotic* [also: penicillin G benzathine; benzathine benzylpenicillin; benzathine penicillin]

benzylpenicillin potassium BAN, JAN *antibacterial* [also: penicillin G potassium]

benzylpenicillin procaine [see: penicillin G procaine]

benzylpenicillin sodium BAN *antibacterial* [also: penicillin G sodium]

benzylpenicilloic acid [see: benzylpenicillin]

benzylpenicilloyl polylysine USP *penicillin sensitivity test*

benzylpenilloic acid [see: benzylpenicillin]

benzylsulfamide INN, DCF

benzylsulfanilamide [see: benzylsulfamide]

BEP (bleomycin, etoposide, Platinol) *chemotherapy protocol*

bepafant INN

bepanthen [see: panthenol]

beperidium iodide INN

bephene oxinaphthoate [see: bephenium hydroxynaphthoate]

bephenium embonate [see: bephenium hydroxynaphthoate]

bephenium hydroxynaphthoate USP, INN, BAN

bepiastine INN, DCF

bepridil INN, BAN *vasodilator; antianginal; calcium channel blocker* [also: bepridil HCl]

bepridil HCl USAN *vasodilator; antianginal; calcium channel blocker* [also: bepridil]

beractant USAN *pulmonary surfactant; for neonatal respiratory distress syndrome (orphan)*

beraprost USAN, INN *platelet aggregation inhibitor*

beraprost sodium USAN *platelet aggregation inhibitor*

berberine chloride JAN

berberine sulfate JAN

berberine tannate JAN

berculon A [see: thioacetazone; thiacetazone]

berefrine USAN, INN *mydriatic*

bergenin JAN

berkelium *element (Bk)*

berlafenone INN

bermastine [see: barmastine]

bermoprofen INN

Berocca tablets ℞ *vitamin supplement* [multiple B vitamins; vitamin C; folic acid] ±•500•0.5 mg

Berocca Parenteral Nutrition injection ℞ *parenteral vitamin supplement* [multiple vitamins; folic acid; biotin] ±•400•60 μg/mL

Berocca Plus tablets ℞ *vitamin/mineral/iron supplement* [multiple vitamins & minerals; ferrous fumarate; folic acid; biotin] ±•27•0.8•0.15 mg

Berotec ℞ *investigational bronchodilator; antiasthmatic* [fenoterol hydrobromide]

Berplex tablets ℞ *vitamin supplement* [multiple vitamins]

Berplex Plus tablets ℞ *vitamin/mineral/iron supplement* [multiple vitamins & minerals; ferrous fumarate; folic acid; biotin] ±•27•0.8•0.15 mg

bertosamil INN

beryllium *element (Be)*

berythromycin USAN, INN *antiamebic; antibacterial*

besigomsin INN

besilate INN *combining name for radicals or groups* [also: besylate]

besipirdine INN *investigational cognition enhancer for Alzheimer's disease*

besipirdine HCl USAN *investigational cognition enhancer for Alzheimer's disease*

Besta capsules (discontinued 1993) OTC *vitamin/mineral supplement* [multiple vitamins & minerals]

besulpamide INN

besunide INN

besylate USAN *combining name for radicals or groups* [also: besilate]

beta carotene USAN, USP *ultraviolet screen; vitamin A precursor* [also: betacarotene]

beta cyclodextrin NF *sequestering agent* [also: betadex]

Beta-2 solution for inhalation ℞ *bronchodilator* [isoetharine HCl] 1%

betacarotene INN *ultraviolet screen; vitamin A precursor* [also: beta carotene]

betacetylmethadol INN, BAN

Betachron E-R extended-release capsules ℞ *antianginal; antihypertensive; migraine preventative* [propranolol HCl] 60, 80, 120, 160 mg

betadex INN *sequestering agent* [also: beta cyclodextrin]

beta-D-galactosidase *digestive enzyme* [see: tilactase]

Betadine aerosol, gauze pads, lubricating gel, cream, mouthwash, ointment, perineal wash, skin cleanser, foam, solution, swab, swabsticks, surgical scrub OTC *broad-spectrum antimicrobial* [povidone-iodine] 5%; 10%; 5%; 5%; 0.5%; 10%; 10%; 7.5%; 7.5%; 10%; 10%; 10%; 7.5%

Betadine shampoo OTC *broad-spectrum antimicrobial for dandruff* [povidone-iodine] 7.5%

Betadine 5% Sterile Ophthalmic Prep solution ℞ *broad-spectrum antimicrobial for eye surgery* [povidone-iodine] 5%

Betadine First Aid Antibiotics + Moisturizer ointment OTC *topical antibiotic* [polymyxin B sulfate; bacitracin zinc] 10,000•500 IU/g

Betadine Medicated vaginal suppositories, vaginal gel OTC *broad-spectrum antimicrobial* [povidone-iodine] 10%

Betadine Medicated Douche; Betadine Medicated Disposable Douche; Betadine Premixed Medicated Disposable Douche solution OTC *broad-spectrum antimicrobial* [povidone-iodine] 10%

beta-estradiol [see: estradiol]

beta-estradiol benzoate [see: estradiol benzoate]

betaeucaine HCl [now: eucaine HCl]

Betafectan ℞ *investigational agent to prevent postsurgical infections* [PCAG glucan]

Betagan Liquifilm eye drops ℞ *topical antiglaucoma agent (β-blocker)* [levobunolol HCl] 0.25%, 0.5% ② Betagen

Betagen ointment, solution, surgical scrub OTC *broad-spectrum antimicrobial* [povidone-iodine] 1%; 10%; 7.5% ② Betagan

beta-glucocerebrosidase [see: alglucerase]

betahistine INN, BAN *vasodilator* [also: betahistine HCl; betahistine mesilate]

betahistine HCl USAN *vasodilator* [also: betahistine; betahistine mesilate]

betahistine mesilate JAN *vasodilator* [also: betahistine HCl; betahistine]

beta-hypophamine [see: vasopressin]

betaine HCl USP *electrolyte replenisher (orphan: homocystinuria)*

BetaKine ℞ *investigational connective tissue growth stimulator for chronic ulcers and macular holes* [transforming growth factor beta]

beta-lactone [see: propiolactone]

betameprodine INN, BAN, DCF

betamethadol INN, BAN, DCF

betamethasone USAN, USP, INN, BAN, JAN *corticosteroid*

betamethasone acetate USP, JAN *corticosteroid*

betamethasone acibutate INN, BAN *corticosteroid*

betamethasone benzoate USAN, USP, BAN *corticosteroid*

betamethasone dipropionate USAN, USP, BAN, JAN *corticosteroid* 0.05% topical

betamethasone dipropionate, augmented *corticosteroid*

betamethasone sodium phosphate USP, BAN, JAN *corticosteroid* 4 mg/mL injection

betamethasone valerate USAN, USP, BAN, JAN *corticosteroid* 0.1% topical

betamicin INN *antibacterial* [also: betamicin sulfate]

betamicin sulfate USAN *antibacterial* [also: betamicin]

betamipron INN

betanaphthol NF

betanidine INN *antihypertensive* [also: bethanidine sulfate; bethanidine; betanidine sulfate]

betanidine sulfate JAN *antihypertensive* [also: bethanidine sulfate; betanidine; bethanidine]

Betapace tablets ℞ *antiarrhythmic; for life-threatening ventricular arrhythmias (orphan); β-blocker* [sotalol HCl] 80, 120, 160, 240 mg

Betapen-VK film-coated tablets, powder for oral solution ℞ *bactericidal antibiotic* [penicillin V potassium] 250, 500 mg; 125, 250 mg/5 mL ② Adapin; Phenaphen

betaprodine INN, BAN, DCF

beta-propiolactone [see: propiolactone]
beta-pyridylcarbinol [see: nicotinyl alcohol]
Betasept liquid OTC *broad-spectrum antimicrobial; germicidal* [chlorhexidine gluconate; alcohol 4%] 4%
Betaseron powder for subcu injection ℞ *immunomodulator for multiple sclerosis; (orphan: non-A, non-B hepatitis; multiple carcinomas; AIDS)* [interferon beta-1b] 0.3 mg (9.6 mIU)/vial
Beta-Tim eye drops (available only in Canada) ℞ *antiglaucoma agent (β-blocker)* [timolol maleate] 0.25%, 0.5%
Betatrex cream, ointment, lotion ℞ *topical corticosteroid* [betamethasone valerate] 0.1%
Beta-Val cream, lotion ℞ *topical corticosteroid* [betamethasone valerate] 0.1%
Beta-Val ointment (discontinued 1994) ℞ *topical corticosteroid* [betamethasone valerate] 0.1%
betaxolol INN, BAN *antianginal; antihypertensive; topical antiglaucoma agent (β-blocker)* [also: betaxolol HCl]
betaxolol HCl USAN, USP *antianginal; antihypertensive; topical antiglaucoma agent (β-blocker)* [also: betaxolol]
betazole INN [also: betazole HCl; ametazole]
betazole HCl USP [also: betazole; ametazole]
betazolium chloride [see: betazole HCl]
bethanechol chloride USP, BAN, JAN *cholinergic urinary stimulant* 5, 10, 25, 50 mg oral
bethanidine BAN *antihypertensive* [also: bethanidine sulfate; betanidine; betanidine sulfate]
bethanidine sulfate USAN *antihypertensive (orphan: primary ventricular fibrillation)* [also: betanidine; bethanidine; betanidine sulfate]
betiatide USAN, INN, BAN *pharmaceutic aid*
Betimol eye drops ℞ *ocular antihypertensive; antiglaucoma agent (β-blocker)* [timolol hemihydrate] 0.25%, 0.5%

Betnesol ℞ *investigational topical steroidal anti-inflammatory*
Betoptic; Betoptic S Drop-Tainer (eye drops) ℞ *topical antiglaucoma agent (β-blocker)* [betaxolol HCl] 0.5% (5.6 mg/mL); 0.25% (2.8 mg/mL)
betoxycaine INN
betoxycaine HCl [see: betoxycaine]
betula oil [see: methyl salicylate]
Betuline lotion OTC *counterirritant* [methyl salicylate; camphor; menthol; peppermint oil]
bevantolol INN, BAN *antianginal; antihypertensive; antiarrhythmic* [also: bevantolol HCl]
bevantolol HCl USAN *antianginal; antihypertensive; antiarrhythmic* [also: bevantolol]
bevonium methylsulphate BAN [also: bevonium metilsulfate]
bevonium metilsulfate INN [also: bevonium methylsulphate]
bezafibrate USAN, INN, BAN, JAN *antihyperlipoproteinemic*
bezitramide INN, BAN, DCF
bezomil INN *combining name for radicals or groups*
bFGF (basic fibroblast growth factor) [see: ersofermin]
B.F.I. Antiseptic powder OTC *topical antiseptic* [bismuth-formic-iodide] 16%
BHA (butylated hydroxyanisole) [q.v.]
BHAPs (bisheteroarylpiperazines) *a class of antiviral drugs*
BHD (BCNU, hydroxyurea, dacarbazine) *chemotherapy protocol*
BHDV; BHD-V (BCNU, hydroxyurea, dacarbazine, vincristine) *chemotherapy protocol*
BHT (butylated hydroxytoluene) [q.v.]
bialamicol INN, BAN *antiamebic* [also: bialamicol HCl]
bialamicol HCl USAN *antiamebic* [also: bialamicol]
biallylamicol [see: bialamicol]
biantrazole [now: losoxantrone HCl]
biapenem USAN, INN *antibacterial*
Biavax II powder for subcu injection ℞ *rubella and mumps vaccine* [rubella

& mumps virus vaccine, live] 1000•20,000 U/0.5 mL

Biaxin Filmtabs (film-coated tablets), granules for oral suspension ℞ *macrolide antibacterial antibiotic* [clarithromycin] 250, 500 mg; 125, 250 mg/5 mL

bibenzonium bromide INN, BAN

bibrocathin [see: bibrocathol]

bibrocathol INN, DCF

Bicalma chewable tablets (discontinued 1994) OTC *antacid* [calcium carbonate; magnesium trisilicate]

bicalutamide USAN, INN, BAN *antiandrogen for prostatic cancer*

Bichloracetic Acid liquid ℞ *cauterant; keratolytic* [dichloroacetic acid] 10 mL ⑫ dichloroacetic acid

bicifadine INN *analgesic* [also: bicifadine HCl]

bicifadine HCl USAN *analgesic* [also: bicifadine]

Bicillin C-R; Bicillin C-R 900/300 IM injection, Tubex (cartridge-needle unit) ℞ *bactericidal antibiotic* [penicillin G benzathine; penicillin G procaine] 150,000•150,000 U/mL; 900,000•300,000 U ⑫ V-Cillin; Wycillin

Bicillin L-A IM injection, Tubex (cartridge-needle units) ℞ *bactericidal antibiotic* [penicillin G benzathine] 300,000 U/mL; 600,000 U/mL

biciromab USAN, INN, BAN *antifibrin monoclonal antibody*

Bicitra solution ℞ *urinary alkalinizing agent* [sodium citrate; citric acid] 500•334 mg/5 mL

biclodil INN *antihypertensive; vasodilator* [also: biclodil HCl]

biclodil HCl USAN *antihypertensive; vasodilator* [also: biclodil]

biclofibrate INN, DCF

biclotymol INN, DCF

BiCNU powder for IV injection ℞ *antineoplastic for brain, colon, and stomach tumors, melanomas, lymphomas and multiple myeloma* [carmustine] 100 mg

bicozamycin INN

Bicozene cream OTC *topical local anesthetic; antifungal* [benzocaine; resorcinol] 6%•1.67%

bicyclomycin [see: bicozamycin]

bidCAP (trademarked dosage form) *twice-daily capsule*

Bidil ℞ *investigational vasodilator for congestive heart failure* [hydralazine; isosorbide]

bidimazium iodide INN, BAN

bidisomide USAN, INN *antiarrhythmic*

Biebrich scarlet red [see: scarlet red]

Biebrich scarlet-picroaniline blue

bietamiverine INN

bietamiverine HCl [see: bietamiverine]

bietaserpine INN, DCF

bifemelane INN [also: bifemelane HCl]

bifemelane HCl JAN [also: bifemelane]

bifepramide INN

bifeprofen INN

bifluranol INN, BAN

bifonazole USAN, INN, BAN, JAN *antifungal*

bile acids, oxidized [see: dehydrocholic acid]

bile salts BAN *laxative*

Bilezyme tablets (discontinued 1995) ℞ *digestive enzymes* [amylase; protease; dehydrocholic acid; desoxycholic acid] 30•6•200•50 mg

Bili-Labstix reagent strips *in vitro diagnostic aid for multiple urine products*

Bilivist capsules ℞ *oral cholecystographic radiopaque agent* [ipodate sodium] 500 mg

Bilopaque capsules ℞ *oral cholecystographic radiopaque agent* [tyropanoate sodium] 750 mg

Bilron Pulvules (capsules) (discontinued 1992) OTC *choleretic; fat digestive aid* [bile salts]

Biltricide tablets ℞ *anthelmintic* [praziquantel] 600 mg

bimakalim INN

bimazol [see: carbimazole]

bimethadol [see: dimepheptanol]

bimethoxycaine lactate

bindarit USAN, INN *antirheumatic*

bindazac [see: bendazac]

binedaline INN

binfloxacin USAN, INN *veterinary antibacterial*

binifibrate INN

biniramycin USAN, INN *antibacterial antibiotic*

binizolast INN

binodaline [see: binedaline]

binospirone INN *anxiolytic* [also: binospirone mesylate]

binospirone mesylate USAN *anxiolytic* [also: binospirone]

Bio-Acerola C Complex wafers OTC *dietary supplement* [vitamin C; citrus bioflavonoids; rutin] 500•10•5 mg

bioallethrin BAN

Biocef capsules, powder for oral suspension ℞ *cephalosporin-type antibiotic* [cephalexin monohydrate] 500 mg; 125, 250 mg/5 mL

Bioclate powder for IV injection ℞ *antihemophilic to correct coagulation deficiency* [antihemophilic factor VIII, recombinant] 250, 500, 1000 IU

BioCox intradermal injection ℞ *diagnostic aid for coccidioidomycosis* [coccidioidin] 1:100, 1:10

Biocult-GC culture paddles for professional use *in vitro diagnostic aid for Neisseria gonorrhoeae*

Bioday with Iron tablets OTC *vitamin/iron supplement* [multiple vitamins; iron; folic acid]

Biodel Implant/BCNU biodegradable polymer implant ℞ *(orphan: recurrent malignant glioma)* [carmustine]

Biodine Topical solution OTC *broad-spectrum antimicrobial* [povidone-iodine] 1%

Bioferon (working name during investigational testing; name changed to Avonex upon product launch in 1996)

bioflavonoids *vitamin P*

biogastrone [see: carbenoxolone]

Biohist-LA timed-release tablets ℞ *decongestant; antihistamine* [pseudoephedrine HCl; carbinoxamine maleate] 120•8 mg

biological indicator for dry-heat sterilization USP *sterilization indicator*

biological indicator for ethylene oxide sterilization USP *sterilization indicator*

biological indicator for steam sterilization USP *sterilization indicator*

Biomox capsules, powder for oral suspension ℞ *penicillin-type antibiotic* [amoxicillin trihydrate] 250, 500 mg; 250 mg/5 mL

Bion Tears eye drops OTC *ocular moisturizer/lubricant* [hydroxypropyl methylcellulose] 0.3%

bioral [see: carbenoxolone]

Bio-Rescue ℞ *(orphan: acute iron poisoning)* [dextran; deferoxamine]

bioresmethrin INN

bios I [see: inositol]

bios II [see: biotin]

Biosynject ℞ *(orphan: newborn hemolytic disease; ABO blood incompatibility of organ or bone marrow transplants)* [trisaccharides A and B]

Bio-Tab film-coated tablets ℞ *tetracycline-type antibiotic* [doxycycline hyclate] 100 mg

Biotab tablets OTC *decongestant; antihistamine; analgesic* [phenylpropanolamine HCl; phenyltoloxamine citrate; acetaminophen]

Biotel diabetes test kit (discontinued 1995) *in vitro diagnostic aid for urine glucose*

Biotel kidney reagent strips *in vitro diagnostic aid for urine hemoglobin, RBCs, and albumin (predictor of kidney diseases)*

Biotel u.t.i. test kit for home use (discontinued 1995) *in vitro diagnostic aid for urine nitrite (predictor of urinary tract infections)*

biotexin [see: novobiocin]

biotin USP, INN, JAN *B complex vitamin; vitamin H*

Biotin Forte tablets OTC *vitamin supplement* [multiple B vitamins; vitamin C; folic acid; biotin] ±•200 mg•800 μg•3 mg, ±•100 mg•800 μg•5 mg

BioTropin ℞ *investigational drug for AIDS (orphan: Turner syndrome; growth delay; severe burns; anovulation)* [somatropin]

BIP (bleomycin, ifosfamide [with mesna rescue], Platinol) *chemotherapy protocol*
bipenamol INN *antidepressant* [also: bipenamol HCl]
bipenamol HCl USAN *antidepressant* [also: bipenamol]
biperiden USP, INN, BAN, JAN *anticholinergic; antiparkinsonian*
biperiden HCl USP, BAN, JAN *anticholinergic; antiparkinsonian*
biperiden lactate USP, BAN, JAN *anticholinergic; antiparkinsonian*
biphasic insulin [see: insulin, biphasic]
biphenamine HCl USAN *topical anesthetic; antibacterial; antifungal* [also: xenysalate]
Biphetamine 12½; Biphetamine 20 capsules (discontinued 1993) ℞ *CNS stimulant; amphetamine* [dextroamphetamine; amphetamine] 6.25•6.25 mg; 10•10 mg
biprofenide [see: bifepramide]
birch oil, sweet [see: methyl salicylate]
biriperone INN
bisacodyl USP, INN, BAN, JAN *stimulant laxative* 5 mg oral; 10 mg suppositories
bisacodyl tannex USAN *laxative*
bisantrene INN *antineoplastic* [also: bisantrene HCl]
bisantrene HCl USAN *antineoplastic* [also: bisantrene]
bisaramil INN
bisatin [see: oxyphenisatin acetate]
bisbendazole INN
bisbentiamine INN, JAN
bisbutiamine [see: bisbutitiamine]
bisbutitiamine JAN
bis-chloroethyl-nitrosourea (BCNU) [see: carmustine]
Bisco-Lax suppositories OTC *stimulant laxative* [bisacodyl] 10 mg
bisdequalinium diacetate JAN
bisfenazone INN, DCF
bisfentidine INN
bisheteroarylpiperazines (BHAPs) *a class of antiviral drugs*
bishydroxycoumarin [now: dicumarol]
bisibutiamine JAN [also: sulbutiamine]
Bismatrol chewable tablets, liquid OTC *antidiarrheal; antinauseant* [bismuth subsalicylate] 262 mg; 524 mg/5 mL

bismucatebrol [see: bibrocathol]
bismuth *element (Bi)*
bismuth, milk of USP *antacid; astringent*
bismuth aluminate USAN
bismuth betanaphthol USP
bismuth carbonate USAN
bismuth carbonate, basic [see: bismuth subcarbonate]
bismuth citrate USP
bismuth cream [see: bismuth, milk of]
bismuth gallate, basic [see: bismuth subgallate]
bismuth glycollylarsanilate BAN [also: glycobiarsol]
bismuth hydroxide [see: bismuth, milk of]
bismuth hydroxide nitrate oxide [see: bismuth subnitrate]
bismuth magma [now: bismuth, milk of]
bismuth magnesium aluminosilicate JAN
bismuth oxycarbonate [see: bismuth subcarbonate]
bismuth potassium tartrate NF
bismuth sodium triglycollamate USP
bismuth subcarbonate USAN, JAN *antacid; GI adsorbent*
bismuth subgallate USAN, USP *antacid; GI adsorbent*
bismuth subnitrate USP, JAN *skin protectant*
bismuth subsalicylate (BSS) USAN, JAN *antiperistaltic; antacid; GI adsorbent*
bisnafide dimesylate USAN *antineoplastic; DNA and RNA synthesis inhibitor*
bisobrin INN *fibrinolytic* [also: bisobrin lactate]
bisobrin lactate USAN *fibrinolytic* [also: bisobrin]
Bisodol chewable tablets (discontinued 1994) OTC *antacid* [magnesium hydroxide; calcium carbonate]
Bisodol powder (discontinued 1994) OTC *antacid* [sodium bicarbonate; magnesium carbonate]
bisoprolol USAN, INN, BAN *antihypertensive (β-blocker)*
bisoprolol fumarate USAN, JAN *antihypertensive (β-blocker)*
bisorcic INN

bisoxatin INN, BAN *laxative* [also: bisoxatin acetate]

bisoxatin acetate USAN *laxative* [also: bisoxatin]

bispecific antibody 520C9x22 (*orphan: ovarian cancer*)

bispyrithione magsulfex USAN *antibacterial; antidandruff; antifungal*

bis-tropamide [now: tropicamide]

bithionol NF, INN, BAN, JAN *investigational anti-infective for paragonimiasis and fascioliasis*

bithionolate sodium USAN *topical anti-infective* [also: sodium bitionolate]

bithionoloxide INN

Bitin (available only from the Centers for Disease Control) ℞ *investigational anti-infective for paragonimiasis and fascioliasis* [bithionol]

bitipazone INN

bitolterol INN, BAN *bronchodilator* [also: bitolterol mesylate; bitolterol mesilate]

bitolterol mesilate JAN *bronchodilator* [also: bitolterol mesylate; bitolterol]

bitolterol mesylate USAN *bronchodilator* [also: bitolterol; bitolterol mesilate]

bitoscanate INN

bivalirudin USAN *antithrombotic; anticoagulant*

bizelesin USAN, INN *antineoplastic*

B-Ject-100 injection ℞ *parenteral vitamin therapy* [multiple B vitamins] ≟

black widow spider antivenin [see: antivenin (Latrodectus mactans)]

Black-Draught syrup OTC *laxative* [casanthranol; senna extract] 90•≟ mg/15 mL

Black-Draught tablets, granules OTC *laxative* [senna concentrate] 600 mg; 1.65 g per ½ tsp.

Blairex Hard Contact Lens Cleaner solution (discontinued 1993) OTC *cleaning solution for hard contact lenses*

Blairex Lens Lubricant solution OTC *rewetting solution for soft contact lenses*

Blairex Sterile Saline aerosol solution OTC *rinsing/storage solution for soft contact lenses* [preservative-free saline solution]

blastomycin NF

Blem-Derm cream OTC *acne* [benzoyl peroxide]

BlemErase lotion OTC *topical keratolytic for acne* [benzoyl peroxide] 10%

Blenoxane powder for IM, IV or subcu injection ℞ *antibiotic antineoplastic for lymphoma, squamous cell and testicular cancers, and pleural effusion* [bleomycin sulfate] 15 U

BLEO-COMF (bleomycin, cyclophosphamide, Oncovin, methotrexate, fluorouracil) *chemotherapy protocol*

bleomycin (BLM) INN, BAN *glycopeptide antibiotic antineoplastic* [also: bleomycin sulfate; bleomycin HCl] ⑤ Cleocin

bleomycin HCl JAN *glycopeptide antibiotic antineoplastic* [also: bleomycin sulfate; bleomycin]

bleomycin sulfate USAN, USP, JAN *glycopeptide antibiotic antineoplastic; malignant pleural effusion (orphan)* [also: bleomycin; bleomycin HCl]

Bleph-10 eye drops, ophthalmic ointment ℞ *ophthalmic bacteriostatic* [sulfacetamide sodium] 10%

Blephamide eye drop suspension, ophthalmic ointment ℞ *ophthalmic topical corticosteroidal anti-inflammatory; bacteriostatic* [prednisolone acetate; sulfacetamide sodium] 0.2%•10%

Blink-N-Clean solution (discontinued 1992) OTC *rewetting solution for hard contact lenses*

Blinx ophthalmic solution OTC *extraocular irrigating solution* [sterile isotonic solution]

BlisterGard liquid OTC *skin protectant*

Blistex ointment OTC *topical antipruritic/counterirritant; mild local anesthetic; vulnerary* [camphor; phenol; allantoin] 0.5%•0.5%•1%

Blistik lip balm OTC *antipruritic/counterirritant; mild local anesthetic; skin protectant; sunscreen (SPF 10)* [camphor; phenol; allantoin; dimethicone; padimate O; oxybenzone] 0.5%•0.5%•1%•2%•6.6%•2.5%

Blis-To-Sol liquid OTC *topical antifungal; keratolytic* [tolnaftate] 1%

Blis-To-Sol powder OTC *topical antifungal* [zinc undecylenate] 12%

BLM (bleomycin) [q.v.]

Blocadren tablets ℞ *antihypertensive; migraine preventative; β-blocker* [timolol maleate] 5, 10, 20 mg

blocked ricin conjugated murine monoclonal antibody [see: ricin (blocked) conjugated murine MCA]

blood, whole USP *blood replenisher*

blood, whole human [now: blood, whole]

blood cell growth factor *investigational antineoplastic*

blood cells, human red [now: blood cells, red]

blood cells, red USP *blood replenisher*

blood group specific substances A, B & AB USP *blood neutralizer*

blood grouping serum, anti-A [see: anti-A blood grouping serum]

blood grouping serum, anti-B [see: anti-B blood grouping serum]

blood grouping serum, anti-C USP *for in vitro blood testing*

blood grouping serum, anti-c USP *for in vitro blood testing*

blood grouping serum, anti-D USP *for in vitro blood testing*

blood grouping serum, anti-E USP *for in vitro blood testing*

blood grouping serum, anti-e USP *for in vitro blood testing*

Blood Nutrients capsule OTC *vitamin/mineral supplement* [multiple vitamins & minerals]

Bluboro powder packets OTC *astringent wet dressing (modified Burow solution)* [aluminum sulfate; calcium acetate]

Blue Gel OTC *pediculicide* [pyrethrins; piperonyl butoxide; petroleum distillate] 0.3%•3%•1.2%

Blue Gel Muscular Pain Reliever gel OTC *counterirritant* [menthol] 2

bluensomycin INN *antibiotic*

BM 14802 *investigational antipsychotic for schizophrenia (clinical trials discontinued 1994)*

B-MOPP (bleomycin, nitrogen mustard, Oncovin, procarbazine, prednisone) *chemotherapy protocol*

BMP (BCNU, methotrexate, procarbazine) *chemotherapy protocol*

BMP-1 to BMP-8 (bone morphogenetic proteins) [q.v.]

BMS 180048 *investigational antimigraine agent*

BMS 181101 *investigational antidepressant*

BMY 14802 *investigational antipsychotic for schizophrenia*

BMY-45622 *(orphan status withdrawn 1994)*

B-Nutron tablets (discontinued 1992) OTC *vitamin/mineral supplement* [multiple vitamins & minerals]

BOAP (bleomycin, Oncovin, Adriamycin, prednisone) *chemotherapy protocol*

Bo-Cal tablets OTC *dietary supplement* [calcium; vitamin D; magnesium] 250 mg•100 IU•125 mg

boforsin [see: colforsin]

bofumustine INN

Boil n Soak solution (discontinued 1992) OTC *rinsing/storage solution for soft contact lenses* [preserved saline solution]

Boil-Ease ointment OTC *topical local anesthetic* [benzocaine] 20%

bolandiol INN *anabolic* [also: bolandiol dipropionate]

bolandiol dipropionate USAN, JAN *anabolic* [also: bolandiol]

bolasterone USAN, INN *anabolic*

bolazine INN

BOLD (bleomycin, Oncovin, lomustine, dacarbazine) *chemotherapy protocol*

boldenone INN, BAN *anabolic* [also: boldenone undecylenate]

boldenone undecylenate USAN *anabolic* [also: boldenone]

bolenol USAN, INN *anabolic*

bolmantalate USAN, INN, BAN *anabolic*

bolus alba [see: kaolin]

Bolvidon ℞ *investigational antidepressant* [mianserin]

bometolol INN

BOMP (bleomycin, Oncovin, Matulane, prednisone) *chemotherapy protocol*

BOMP (bleomycin, Oncovin, mitomycin, Platinol) *chemotherapy protocol*

Bonamil Infant Formula with Iron powder, oral liquid OTC *total or supplementary infant feeding* 453 g; 384, 946 mL

bone ash [see: calcium phosphate, tribasic]

Bone Meal tablets OTC *dietary supplement* [calcium; phosphorus] 236•118 mg

bone morphogenetic protein-2 (BMP-2) *investigational bone growth stimulant*

bone morphogenetic proteins (BMPs) *class of factors that regulate bone formation, growth, and development (investigational)*

bone powder, purified [see: calcium phosphate, tribasic]

Bonefos ℞ *(orphan: increased bone resorption due to malignancy)* [disodium clodronate tetrahydrate]

Bonine chewable tablets OTC *anticholinergic; antihistamine; antivertigo agent; motion sickness preventative* [meclizine HCl] 25 mg

Bontril slow-release capsules ℞ *anorexiant* [phendimetrazine tartrate] 105 mg ⊘ Bentyl; Vontrol

Bontril PDM tablets ℞ *anorexiant* [phendimetrazine tartrate] 35 mg

Boost liquid OTC *enteral nutritional therapy* [milk-based formula] 237 mL

BOP (BCNU, Oncovin, prednisone) *chemotherapy protocol*

BOPAM (bleomycin, Oncovin, prednisone, Adriamycin, mechlorethamine, methotrexate) *chemotherapy protocol*

bopindolol INN

BOPP (BCNU, Oncovin, procarbazine, prednisone) *chemotherapy protocol*

boracic acid [see: boric acid]

borax [see: sodium borate]

boric acid NF, JAN *acidifying agent; ocular emollient; antiseptic; astringent* 10% topical

2-bornanone [see: camphor]

bornaprine INN, BAN

bornaprolol INN

bornelone USAN, INN *ultraviolet screen*

bornyl acetate USAN

borocaptate sodium B 10 USAN *antineoplastic; radioactive agent* [also: sodium borocaptate (^{10}B)]

Borocell ℞ *(orphan: boron neutron capture therapy for glioblastoma multiforme)* [monomercaptoundecahydro-closo-DO decaborate sodium]

Borofair Otic ear drops ℞ *antibacterial/antifungal; astringent* [acetic acid; aluminum acetate] 2%•?

Borofax Skin Protectant ointment OTC *astringent* [zinc oxide] 15%

boroglycerin NF

boron *element (B)*

Boropak powder packets OTC *astringent wet dressing (modified Burrow solution)* [aluminum sulfate; calcium acetate]

bosentan USAN, INN *endothelin receptor antagonist for vasospastic diseases*

Boston Advance Cleaner; Boston Cleaner solution OTC *cleaning solution for rigid gas permeable contact lenses*

Boston Advance Comfort Formula solution OTC *disinfecting/wetting/soaking solution for rigid gas permeable contact lenses*

Boston Advance Conditioning Solution (name changed to Boston Advance Comfort Formula in 1995)

Boston Advance Rewetting Drops (name changed to Boston Rewetting Drops in 1995)

Boston Conditioning Solution OTC *disinfecting/wetting/soaking solution for rigid gas permeable contact lenses*

Boston Reconditioning Drops (discontinued 1993) OTC *cleaning/soaking solution for hard contact lenses*

Boston Rewetting Drops OTC *rewetting solution for rigid gas permeable contact lenses*

botiacrine INN

Botox powder for extraocular muscle injection ℞ *blepharospasm and strabismus of dystonia; (orphan: pediatric cerebral palsy)* [botulinum toxin, type A] 100 U

BottomBetter ointment OTC *topical diaper rash treatment*

botulinum toxin, type A *blepharospasm and strabismus of dystonia; (orphan: pediatric cerebral palsy)*

botulinum toxin, type B *(orphan: cervical dystonia)*

botulinum toxin, type F *(orphan: spasmodic torticollis; cervical dystonia; essential blepharospasm)*

botulinum toxoid, pentavalent (ABCDE) *investigational vaccine (available only from the Centers for Disease Control)*

botulism antitoxin USP *passive immunizing agent*

botulism equine antitoxin, trivalent *passive immunizing agent*

botulism immune globulin *(orphan: infant botulism)*

Bounty Bears chewable tablets OTC *vitamin supplement* [multiple vitamins; folic acid] ±•0.3 mg

Bounty Bears Plus Iron chewable tablets OTC *vitamin/iron supplement* [multiple vitamins; iron; folic acid] ±•15•0.3 mg

bourbonal [see: ethyl vanillin]

bovactant BAN

bovine colostrum *(orphan: AIDS-related diarrhea)*

bovine fibrin BAN

bovine immunoglobulin concentrate, Cryptosporidium parvum *(orphan: treatment of cryptosporidiosis in immunocompromised patients)*

bovine superoxide dismutase (bSOD) [see: orgotein]

bovine whey protein concentrate *(orphan: treatment of cryptosporidiosis in immunocompromised patients)*

boxidine USAN, INN *antihyperlipoproteinemic*

Boyol salve OTC *topical anti-infective; anesthetic* [ichthammol; benzocaine] 10%•?•🅑 *boil*

B.P. 5%; B.P. 10% lotion OTC *keratolytic for acne* [benzoyl peroxide]

B.P. Gel 5%; B.P. Gel 10% OTC *keratolytic for acne* [benzoyl peroxide]

B-PAS (benzoyl para-aminosalicylate) [see: benzoylpas calcium]

BPI (bactericidal and permeability-increasing) protein [q.v.]

B-Plex tablets ℞ *vitamin supplement* [multiple B vitamins; vitamin C; folic acid] ±•500•0.5 mg

BQ tablets (discontinued 1993) OTC *decongestant; antihistamine; analgesic* [phenylpropanolamine HCl; chlorpheniramine maleate; acetaminophen]

BR-96 *investigational antineoplastic* [doxorubicin monoclonal antibody immunoconjugate]

Bradycor ℞ *investigational analgesic for systemic inflammatory response syndrome and sepsis*

brain-derived neurotrophic factor *investigational agent for brain and nerve degenerative diseases*

brallobarbital INN

BranchAmin 4% IV infusion ℞ *nutritional therapy for high metabolic stress* [multiple branched-chain essential amino acids]

branched DNA (bDNA) assay *investigational in vitro diagnostic aid for HIV in the blood*

branched-chain amino acids (BCAA) *(orphan: amyotrophic lateral sclerosis)* [see: isoleucine; leucine; valine]

Brasivol cream OTC *abrasive cleanser for acne* [aluminum oxide]

Brasivol Base (discontinued 1994) OTC *topical acne cleanser* [surfactant cleansing base with neutral soaps]

Bravavir ℞ *investigational (awaiting approval) antiviral for varicella zoster and herpes zoster in AIDS* [sorivudine]

brazergoline INN

Breathe Free nasal spray OTC *nasal moisturizer* [sodium chloride (saline)] 0.65%

Breezee Mist Aerosol powder OTC *topical antifungal; anhidrotic* [undecylenic acid; menthol; aluminum chlorhydrate]

Breezee Mist Antifungal powder OTC *topical antifungal* [tolnaftate] 1%

brefonalol INN

bremazocine INN

Breonesin capsules OTC *expectorant* [guaifenesin] 200 mg
brequinar INN *antineoplastic* [also: brequinar sodium]
brequinar sodium USAN *antineoplastic* [also: brequinar]
bretazenil USAN, INN *anxiolytic*
Brethaire oral inhalation aerosol ℞ *bronchodilator* [terbutaline sulfate] 0.2 mg/dose
Brethine tablets, IV or subcu injection ℞ *bronchodilator* [terbutaline sulfate] 2.5, 5 mg; 1 mg/mL ⓓ Banthine
bretylium tosilate INN *antiadrenergic; antiarrhythmic* [also: bretylium tosylate]
bretylium tosylate USAN, BAN *antiadrenergic; antiarrhythmic* [also: bretylium tosilate] 500, 1000 mg/vial injection
Bretylol IV or IM injection ℞ *antiarrhythmic* [bretylium tosylate] 50 mg/mL ⓓ Brevital
Brevibloc IV infusion ℞ *β-blocker for supraventricular tachycardia* [esmolol HCl] 10, 250 mg/mL
Brevicon tablets ℞ *monophasic oral contraceptive* [norethindrone; ethinyl estradiol] 0.5 mg•35 μg
Brevital Sodium powder for IV injection ℞ *general anesthetic* [methohexital sodium] 0.5, 2.5, 5 g ⓓ Bretylol
Brevoxyl gel ℞ *keratolytic for acne* [benzoyl peroxide] 4%
brewer's yeast *natural source of protein and B-complex vitamins*
Brexin-L.A. sustained-release capsules ℞ *decongestant; antihistamine* [pseudoephedrine HCl; chlorpheniramine maleate] 120•8 mg
Bricanyl tablets, IV or subcu injection ℞ *bronchodilator* [terbutaline sulfate] 2.5, 5 mg; 1 mg/mL
brifentanil INN *narcotic analgesic* [also: brifentanil HCl]
brifentanil HCl USAN *narcotic analgesic* [also: brifentanil]
Brik-Paks (trademarked delivery form) *ready-to-use liquid containers*
brimonidine INN *ophthalmic adrenergic* [also: brimonidine tartrate]
brimonidine tartrate USAN *ophthalmic adrenergic* [also: brimonidine]

brinaldix [see: clopamide]
brinase INN [also: brinolase]
brinazarone INN
brindoxime INN
brinolase USAN *fibrinolytic enzyme* [also: brinase]
Bristoject (trademarked delivery form) *prefilled disposable syringe*
British antilewisite (BAL) [now: dimercaprol]
brivudine INN
BRL 46470 *investigational antipsychotic for schizophrenia (clinical trials discontinued 1994)*
BRL55834 *investigational antiasthmatic*
brobactam INN
brobenzoxaldine [see: broxaldine]
broclepride INN
brocresine USAN, INN, BAN *histidine decarboxylase inhibitor*
brocrinat USAN, INN *diuretic*
brodimoprim INN
brofaromine INN *investigational reversible/selective MAO inhibitor*
Brofed elixir ℞ *decongestant; antihistamine* [pseudoephedrine HCl; brompheniramine maleate] 30•4 mg/5 mL
brofezil INN, BAN
brofoxine USAN, INN *antipsychotic*
brolaconazole INN
brolamfetamine INN
Brolene ℞ *(orphan: Acanthamoeba keratitis)* [propamidine isethionate] 0.1%
bromacrylide INN
bromadel [see: carbromal]
bromadoline INN *analgesic* [also: bromadoline maleate]
bromadoline maleate USAN *analgesic* [also: bromadoline]
Bromaline elixir OTC *decongestant; antihistamine* [phenylpropanolamine HCl; brompheniramine maleate] 12.5•2 mg/5 mL
Bromaline Plus captabs (discontinued 1995) OTC *decongestant; antihistamine; analgesic* [phenylpropanolamine HCl; brompheniramine maleate; acetaminophen] 12.5•2•500 mg
bromamid INN
Bromanate elixir OTC *decongestant; antihistamine* [phenylpropanolamine

HCl; brompheniramine maleate] 12.5•2 mg/5 mL

Bromanate DC Cough syrup ℞ *narcotic antitussive; decongestant; antihistamine* [codeine phosphate; phenylpropanolamine HCl; brompheniramine maleate; alcohol] 10•12.5•2 mg/5 mL

Bromanyl syrup ℞ *narcotic antitussive; antihistamine* [codeine phosphate; bromodiphenhydramine HCl] 10•12.5 mg/5 mL

bromanylpromide [see: bromamid]

Bromarest DX Cough syrup ℞ *antitussive; decongestant; antihistamine* [dextromethorphan hydrobromide; pseudoephedrine HCl; brompheniramine maleate; alcohol 0.95%] 10•30•2 mg/5 mL

Bromatane elixir OTC *antihistamine* [brompheniramine maleate]

Bromatane DX Cough syrup ℞ *antitussive; decongestant; antihistamine* [dextromethorphan hydrobromide; pseudoephedrine HCl; brompheniramine maleate] 10•30•2 mg/5 mL

Bromatapp elixir (name changed to Cold & Allergy in 1995)

Bromatapp extended-release tablets OTC *decongestant; antihistamine* [phenylpropanolamine HCl; brompheniramine maleate] 75•12 mg

Bromatapp Extended timed-release tablets (discontinued 1993) ℞ *decongestant; antihistamine* [phenylpropanolamine HCl; phenylephrine HCl; brompheniramine maleate]

Bromatol elixir OTC *decongestant; antihistamine* [brompheniramine maleate; phenylpropanolamine HCl]

bromauric acid NF

bromazepam USAN, INN, BAN, JAN *minor tranquilizer*

bromazine INN, DCF *antihistamine* [also: bromodiphenhydramine HCl; bromodiphenhydramine]

bromazine HCl [see: bromodiphenhydramine HCl]

brombenzonium [see: bromhexine HCl]

bromchlorenone USAN, INN *topical anti-infective*

bromebric acid INN, BAN

bromelain JAN *anti-inflammatory; proteolytic enzymes* [also: bromelains]

bromelains USAN, INN, BAN *anti-inflammatory; proteolytic enzymes* [also: bromelain]

bromelin [see: bromelains]

bromerguride INN

brometenamine INN, DCF

bromethol [see: tribromoethanol]

Bromfed syrup OTC *decongestant; antihistamine* [pseudoephedrine HCl; brompheniramine maleate] 30•2 mg/5 mL ⑫ Bromphen

Bromfed tablets, timed-release capsules ℞ *decongestant; antihistamine* [pseudoephedrine HCl; brompheniramine maleate] 60•4 mg; 120•12 mg

Bromfed-DM Cough syrup ℞ *antitussive; decongestant; antihistamine* [dextromethorphan hydrobromide; pseudoephedrine HCl; brompheniramine maleate] 10•30•2 mg/5 mL

Bromfed-PD timed-release capsules ℞ *pediatric decongestant and antihistamine* [pseudoephedrine HCl; brompheniramine maleate] 60•6 mg

bromfenac INN *long-acting analgesic* [also: bromfenac sodium]

bromfenac sodium USAN *long-acting analgesic* [also: bromfenac]

Bromfenex extended-release capsules ℞ *decongestant; antihistamine* [pseudoephedrine HCl; brompheniramine maleate] 120•12 mg

Bromfenex PD extended-release capsules ℞ *pediatric decongestant and antihistamine* [pseudoephedrine HCl; brompheniramine maleate] 60•6 mg

bromhexine INN, BAN *expectorant; mucolytic; (orphan: keratoconjunctivitis sicca of Sjögren syndrome)* [also: bromhexine HCl]

bromhexine HCl USAN, JAN *expectorant; mucolytic* [also: bromhexine]

bromindione USAN, INN, BAN *anticoagulant*

bromine *element (Br)*

bromisoval INN [also: bromisovalum; bromvalerylurea; bromovaluree]

bromisovalum NF [also: bromisoval; bromvalerylurea; bromovaluree]

2-bromo-α-ergocryptine [see: bromocriptine]
bromocamphor [see: camphor, monobromated]
bromociclen INN [also: bromocyclen]
bromocriptine USAN, INN, BAN *prolactin enzyme inhibitor*
bromocriptine mesilate JAN *prolactin enzyme inhibitor; antiparkinsonian* [also: bromocriptine mesylate]
bromocriptine mesylate USAN, USP *prolactin enzyme inhibitor; antiparkinsonian* [also: bromocriptine mesilate]
bromocyclen BAN [also: bromociclen]
bromodiethylacetylurea [see: carbromal]
bromodiphenhydramine BAN *antihistamine* [also: bromodiphenhydramine HCl; bromazine]
bromodiphenhydramine HCl USP *antihistamine* [also: bromazine; bromodiphenhydramine]
bromofenofos INN
bromoform USP
bromofos INN
1-bromoheptadecafluorooctane [see: perflubron]
bromoisovaleryl urea (BVU) [see: bromisovalum]
Bromophen T.D. sustained-release tablets ℞ *decongestant; antihistamine* [phenylpropanolamine HCl; phenylephrine HCl; brompheniramine maleate] 15•15•12 mg ② Bromphen
bromophenol blue
bromophin [see: apomorphine HCl]
bromophos [see: bromofos]
bromopride INN, DCF
Bromo-Seltzer effervescent granules OTC *antacid; analgesic; antipyretic* [sodium bicarbonate; citric acid; acetaminophen] 2781•2224•325 mg/dose
bromotheophyllinate aminoisobutanol [see: pamabrom]
bromotheophyllinate pyranisamine [see: pyrabrom]
bromotheophyllinate pyrilamine [see: pyrabrom]
8-bromotheophylline [see: pamabrom]
Bromotuss with Codeine syrup ℞ *narcotic antitussive; antihistamine* [codeine phosphate; bromodiphenhydramine HCl] 10•12.5 mg/5 mL
bromovaluree DCF [also: bromisovalum; bromisoval; bromvalerylurea]
11-bromovincamine [see: brovincamine]
bromovinyl arabinosyluracil (BV-araU) [see: sorivudine]
bromoxanide USAN, INN *anthelmintic*
bromperidol USAN, INN, BAN, JAN *antipsychotic*
bromperidol decanoate USAN, BAN *antipsychotic*
Bromphen elixir OTC *antihistamine* [brompheniramine maleate] 2 mg/5 mL ② Bromfed; Bromophen
Bromphen sustained-release tablets, elixir (discontinued 1995) OTC *decongestant; antihistamine* [phenylpropanolamine HCl; brompheniramine maleate] 75•12 mg; 12.5•2 mg/5 mL ② Bromfed; Bromophen
Bromphen DC with Codeine Cough syrup ℞ *narcotic antitussive; decongestant; antihistamine* [codeine phosphate; phenylpropanolamine HCl; brompheniramine maleate] 10•12.5•2 mg/5 mL
Bromphen DX Cough syrup ℞ *antitussive; decongestant; antihistamine* [dextromethorphan hydrobromide; pseudoephedrine HCl; brompheniramine maleate; alcohol 0.95%] 10•30•2 mg/5 mL
brompheniramine INN, BAN *antihistamine* [also: brompheniramine maleate]
Brompheniramine Cough syrup OTC *antitussive; decongestant; antihistamine* [dextromethorphan hydrobromide; pseudoephedrine HCl; brompheniramine maleate; alcohol 0.95%] 10•30•2 mg/5 mL
Brompheniramine DC Cough syrup ℞ *narcotic antitussive; decongestant; antihistamine* [codeine phosphate; phenylpropanolamine HCl; brompheniramine maleate; alcohol 1.15%] 10•12.5•2 mg/5 mL
brompheniramine maleate USP *antihistamine* [also: brompheniramine] 4, 8, 12 mg oral; 2 mg/5 mL oral

Brompton's Cocktail; Brompton's Mixture (refers to any oral narcotic/alcoholic solution containing morphine and either cocaine or a phenothiazine derivative) *prophylaxis for chronic, severe pain*

Bromtapp elixir OTC *antihistamine* [brompheniramine maleate]

bromvalerylurea JAN [also: bromisovalum; bromisoval; bromovaluree]

Bronchial capsules ℞ *antiasthmatic; bronchodilator; expectorant* [theophylline; guaifenesin] 150•90 mg

Broncho Saline solution OTC *diluent for inhalation bronchodilators; solution for tracheal lavage* [saline solution] 0.9%

Broncholate softgels, syrup ℞ *decongestant; expectorant* [ephedrine HCl; guaifenesin] 12.5•200 mg; 6.25•100 mg/5 mL ② Brondelate

Broncholate CS liquid (discontinued 1994) ℞ *narcotic antitussive; decongestant; expectorant* [codeine phosphate; ephedrine HCl; guaifenesin]

Brondecon tablets, elixir (discontinued 1993) ℞ *antiasthmatic; bronchodilator; expectorant* [oxtriphylline; guaifenesin] ② Bronitin

Brondelate elixir ℞ *antiasthmatic; bronchodilator; expectorant* [theophylline; guaifenesin] 192•150 mg/15 mL ② Broncholate

Bronitin tablets (discontinued 1993) OTC *antiasthmatic; bronchodilator; decongestant; antihistamine* [theophylline; ephedrine HCl; guaifenesin; pyrilamine maleate] ② Brondecon

Bronitin Mist inhalation aerosol OTC *bronchodilator for bronchial asthma* [epinephrine bitartrate] 0.3 mg/dose

Bronkaid tablets (discontinued 1995) OTC *antiasthmatic; bronchodilator; expectorant* [theophylline; ephedrine sulfate; guaifenesin] 100•24•100 mg

Bronkaid Dual Action caplets OTC *decongestant; expectorant* [ephedrine sulfate; guaifenesin] 25•400 mg

Bronkaid Mist inhalation aerosol OTC *bronchodilator for bronchial asthma* [epinephrine nitrate & epinephrine HCl] 0.5%

Bronkephrine subcu or IM injection (discontinued 1996) ℞ *bronchodilator* [ethylnorepinephrine HCl] 2 mg/mL

Bronkodyl capsules ℞ *bronchodilator* [theophylline] 100, 200 mg

Bronkolixir elixir (discontinued 1995) OTC *antiasthmatic; bronchodilator; decongestant; expectorant; sedative* [theophylline; ephedrine sulfate; guaifenesin; phenobarbital] 3•2.4•10•0.8 mg/mL

Bronkometer inhalation aerosol ℞ *bronchodilator* [isoetharine mesylate] 0.61% (340 μg/dose)

Bronkosol solution for inhalation ℞ *bronchodilator* [isoetharine HCl] 1%

Bronkotabs tablets (discontinued 1995) OTC *antiasthmatic; bronchodilator; decongestant; expectorant; sedative* [theophylline; ephedrine sulfate; guaifenesin; phenobarbital] 100•24•100•8 mg

Bronkotuss Expectorant liquid ℞ *decongestant; antihistamine; expectorant* [ephedrine sulfate; chlorpheniramine maleate; guaifenesin; hydriodic acid; alcohol 5%] 8.2•4•100•1.67 mg/5 mL

bronopol INN, BAN, JAN

Brontex tablets, liquid ℞ *narcotic antitussive; expectorant* [codeine phosphate; guaifenesin] 10•300 mg; 2.5•75 mg/5 mL

broparestrol INN, DCF

broperamole USAN, INN *anti-inflammatory*

bropirimine USAN, INN *antineoplastic; antiviral; investigational (Phase II) immunomodulator for AIDS (Kaposi sarcoma)*

broquinaldol INN

brosotamide INN, DCF

brosuximide INN

Brotane tablets, elixir OTC *antihistamine* [brompheniramine maleate]

Brotane DX Cough syrup ℞ *antihistamine; antitussive* [pseudoephedrine HCl; brompheniramine maleate; dextromethorphan hydrobromide]

brotianide INN, BAN

brotizolam USAN, INN, BAN, JAN *hypnotic*
brovanexine INN
brovavir [see: sorivudine]
brovincamine INN [also: brovincamine fumarate]
brovincamine fumarate JAN [also: brovincamine]
broxaldine INN, DCF
broxaterol INN
broxitalamic acid INN
broxuridine INN
broxyquinoline INN, DCF
brucine sulfate NF
B-Salt Forte ophthalmic solution ℞ *intraocular irrigating solution* [balanced saline solution]
bSOD (bovine superoxide dismutase) [see: orgotein]
BSS (bismuth subsalicylate) [q.v.]
BSS; BSS Plus ophthalmic solution ℞ *intraocular irrigating solution* [balanced saline solution]
BTS67,583 *investigational antidiabetic*
bucainide INN *antiarrhythmic* [also: bucainide maleate]
bucainide maleate USAN *antiarrhythmic* [also: bucainide]
Bucast ℞ *investigational (Phase II) antiviral glucosidase inhibitor for HIV* [MDL 28,574 (code name—generic name not yet approved)]
Bucet capsules ℞ *sedative; analgesic* [butalbital; acetaminophen] 50•650 mg
bucetin INN, BAN, JAN
buchu [see: diosmin]
buciclovir INN
bucillamine INN, JAN
bucindolol INN, BAN *antihypertensive; investigational treatment for congestive heart failure* [also: bucindolol HCl]
bucindolol HCl USAN *antihypertensive; investigational treatment for congestive heart failure* [also: bucindolol]
bucladesine INN [also: bucladesine sodium]
bucladesine sodium JAN [also: bucladesine]
Bucladin-S Softabs (discontinued 1994) ℞ *anticholinergic; antiemetic; motion sickness preventative* [buclizine HCl] 50 mg
buclizine INN, BAN *antinauseant; antiemetic; anticholinergic; motion sickness relief* [also: buclizine HCl]
buclizine HCl USAN *antinauseant; antiemetic; anticholinergic; motion sickness relief* [also: buclizine]
buclosamide INN, BAN, DCF
bucloxic acid INN, DCF
bucolome INN, JAN
bucricaine INN
bucrilate INN *tissue adhesive* [also: bucrylate]
bucromarone USAN, INN *antiarrhythmic*
bucrylate USAN *tissue adhesive* [also: bucrilate]
bucumolol INN [also: bucumolol HCl]
bucumolol HCl JAN [also: bucumolol]
budesonide USAN, INN, BAN, JAN *anti-inflammatory*
budipine INN
budotitane INN
budralazine INN, JAN
Buf-Bar (discontinued 1994) OTC *medicated cleanser for acne* [sulfur] 3%
bufenadine [see: bufenadrine]
bufenadrine INN
bufeniode INN, DCF
bufetolol INN [also: bufetolol HCl]
bufetolol HCl JAN [also: bufetolol]
bufexamac INN, BAN, JAN, DCF
bufezolac INN
Buffaprin; Buffaprin Extra tablets (discontinued 1992) OTC *analgesic; anti-inflammatory; antipyretic* [buffered aspirin]
buffered aspirin [see: aspirin, buffered]
Bufferin coated tablets, coated caplets OTC *analgesic; antipyretic; anti-inflammatory; antirheumatic* [aspirin, buffered with calcium carbonate, magnesium oxide, and magnesium carbonate] 325, 500 mg
Bufferin, Arthritis Strength; Bufferin Extra Strength tablets (discontinued 1993) OTC *analgesic; antipyretic; anti-inflammatory; antirheumatic* [aspirin, buffered with magnesium carbonate and aluminum glycinate]

Bufferin, Tri-Buffered caplets (discontinued 1993) OTC *analgesic; antipyretic; anti-inflammatory; antirheumatic* [aspirin, buffered with calcium carbonate, magnesium oxide, and magnesium carbonate]

Bufferin, Tri-Buffered tablets (discontinued 1993) OTC *analgesic; antipyretic; anti-inflammatory; antirheumatic* [aspirin, buffered with calcium carbonate, magnesium oxide, and magnesium carbonate] 325 mg

Bufferin AF Nite Time tablets OTC *antihistaminic sleep aid; analgesic* [diphenhydramine HCl; acetaminophen] 30•500 mg

Buffets II tablets OTC *analgesic; antipyretic; anti-inflammatory; antacid* [acetaminophen; aspirin; caffeine; aluminum hydroxide] 162•227•32.4•50 mg

Buffex tablets OTC *analgesic; antipyretic; anti-inflammatory; antirheumatic* [aspirin, buffered with aluminum glycinate and magnesium carbonate] 325 mg

Buffinol; Buffinol Extra tablets (discontinued 1992) OTC *analgesic; anti-inflammatory; antipyretic* [buffered aspirin]

bufilcon A USAN *hydrophilic contact lens material*

buflomedil INN, BAN, DCF

bufogenin INN

buformin USAN, INN *antidiabetic*

Buf-Puf Acne Cleansing bar OTC *medicated cleanser for acne* [salicylic acid; vitamin E] 2%•≟

Buf-Puf Medicated pads OTC *medicated cleansing pad for acne* [salicylic acid; alcohol]

bufrolin INN, BAN

bufuralol INN, BAN

bufylline BAN *diuretic; smooth muscle relaxant* [also: ambuphylline]

Bugs Bunny Children's chewable tablets (discontinued 1994) OTC *vitamin supplement* [multiple vitamins; folic acid] ≟•0.3 mg

Bugs Bunny Complete chewable tablets OTC *vitamin/mineral/calcium/iron supplement* [multiple vitamins & minerals; calcium; iron; folic acid; biotin] ≟•100•18•0.4•0.04 mg

Bugs Bunny Plus Iron chewable tablets OTC *vitamin/iron supplement* [multiple vitamins; iron; folic acid] ≟•15•0.3 mg

Bugs Bunny Vitamins and Minerals (name changed to Bugs Bunny Complete in 1993)

Bugs Bunny with Extra C Children's chewable tablets OTC *vitamin supplement* [multiple vitamins; folic acid] ≟•0.3 mg

bumadizone INN, DCF

bumecaine INN

bumepidil INN

bumetanide USAN, USP, INN, BAN, JAN *loop diuretic* 0.25 mg/mL injection

bumetrizole USAN, INN *ultraviolet screen*

Bumex tablets, IV or IM injection ℞ *loop diuretic* [bumetanide] 0.5, 1, 2 mg; 0.25 mg/mL

Buminate 5%; Buminate 25% IV infusion ℞ *blood volume expander for shock, burns, and hypoproteinemia* [human albumin] 5%; 25%

bunaftine INN

bunamidine INN, BAN *anthelmintic* [also: bunamidine HCl]

bunamidine HCl USAN *anthelmintic* [also: bunamidine]

bunamiodyl INN [also: buniodyl]

bunamiodyl sodium [see: bunamiodyl; buniodyl]

bunaprolast USAN, INN *antiasthmatic; 5-lipoxygenase inhibitor*

bunapsilate INN *combining name for radicals or groups*

bunazosin INN [also: bunazosin HCl]

bunazosin HCl JAN [also: bunazosin]

bundlin [now: sedecamycin]

buniodyl BAN [also: bunamiodyl]

bunitrolol INN [also: bunitrolol HCl]

bunitrolol HCl JAN [also: bunitrolol]

bunolol INN *antiadrenergic (β-receptor)* [also: bunolol HCl]

bunolol HCl USAN *antiadrenergic (β-receptor)* [also: bunolol]

buparvaquone INN, BAN

buphenine INN, BAN *peripheral vasodilator* [also: nylidrin HCl]

Buphenyl tablets, powder for oral solution ℞ *antihyperammonemic for urea cycle disorders* [sodium phenylbutyrate] 500 mg; 3 g/tsp, 8.6 g/tbsp

bupicomide USAN, INN *antihypertensive*

bupivacaine INN, BAN *injectable local anesthetic* [also: bupivacaine HCl]

bupivacaine HCl USAN, USP, JAN *injectable local anesthetic* [also: bupivacaine] 0.25%, 0.5%, 0.75%

bupranol [see: bupranolol]

bupranolol INN, DCF [also: bupranolol HCl]

bupranolol HCl JAN [also: bupranolol]

Buprenex IV or IM injection ℞ *narcotic agonist-antagonist analgesic* [buprenorphine HCl] 0.324 mg/mL

buprenorphine INN, BAN *narcotic agonist-antagonist analgesic* [also: buprenorphine HCl]

buprenorphine HCl USAN, JAN *narcotic agonist-antagonist analgesic* [also: buprenorphine]

buprenorphine & naloxone (*orphan: opiate withdrawal*)

bupropion BAN *aminoketone antidepressant* [also: bupropion HCl; amfebutamone]

bupropion HCl USAN *aminoketone antidepressant* [also: amfebutamone; bupropion]

buquineran INN, BAN

buquinolate USAN, INN *coccidiostat for poultry*

buquiterine INN

buramate USAN, INN *anticonvulsant; antipsychotic*

burefrine [now: berefrine]

Burntame topical spray (discontinued 1992) OTC *antiseptic; topical anesthetic* [8-hydroxyquinoline; benzocaine]

burodiline INN

Buro-Sol solution OTC *astringent wet dressing (Burow solution)* [aluminum sulfate] 0.23%

Burow solution [see: aluminum acetate]

buserelin INN, BAN *gonad-stimulating principle; antineoplastic* [also: buserelin acetate]

buserelin acetate USAN, JAN *gonad-stimulating principle; antineoplastic* [also: buserelin]

BuSpar tablets ℞ *azapirone anxiolytic* [buspirone HCl] 5, 10, 15 mg

BuSpar ER ℞ *investigational once-daily anxiolytic* [buspirone HCl]

buspirone INN, BAN *azapirone anxiolytic; minor tranquilizer* [also: buspirone HCl]

buspirone HCl USAN *azapirone anxiolytic; minor tranquilizer* [also: buspirone]

busulfan USP, INN, JAN *alkylating antineoplastic* (*orphan: bone marrow transplants*) [also: busulphan]

busulphan BAN *alkylating antineoplastic* [also: busulfan]

butabarbital USP *sedative; hypnotic* [also: secbutobarbitone] ⓦ butalbital

butabarbital sodium USP *sedative; hypnotic* [also: secbutabarbital sodium] 15, 30 mg oral; 30 mg/5 mL oral

butacaine INN, BAN [also: butacaine sulfate]

butacaine sulfate USP [also: butacaine]

Butace capsules (discontinued 1994) ℞ *analgesic; antipyretic; sedative* [acetaminophen; caffeine; butalbital] 325•40•50 mg

butacetin USAN

butacetoluide [se

butaclamol INN
butaclamol HC

butaclamol HCl
[also: butaclam

butadiazamide

butafosfan INN

butalamine IN

Butalan elixir (
sedative; hypr

butalbital USA
butabarbita

Butalbital Compound tablets, capsules ℞ *analgesic; antipyretic; antiinflammatory; sedative* [aspirin; caffeine; butalbital] 325•40•50 mg

butalgin [see: methadone HCl]

butallylonal NF

butamben USAN, USP *topical anesthetic*

butamben picrate USAN *topical local anesthetic* 1% topical

butamirate INN *antitussive* [also: butamirate citrate; butamyrate]

butamirate citrate USAN *antitussive* [also: butamirate; butamyrate]

butamisole INN *veterinary anthelmintic* [also: butamisole HCl]

butamisole HCl USAN *veterinary anthelmintic* [also: butamisole]

butamiverine [see: butaverine]

butamoxane INN

butamyrate BAN *antitussive* [also: butamirate citrate; butamirate]

butane (n-butane) NF *aerosol propellant*

butanilicaine INN, BAN

butanixin INN

butanserin INN

butantrone INN

butaperazine USAN, INN *antipsychotic*

butaperazine maleate USAN *antipsychotic*

butaprost USAN, INN, BAN *bronchodilator*

butaverine INN, DCF

butaxamine INN *antidiabetic; antihyperlipoproteinemic* [also: butoxamine HCl; butoxamine]

Butazolidin tablets, capsules (discontinued 1992) ℞ *antirheumatic* [phenylbutazone] 100 mg ⓓ Butisol

butedronate tetrasodium USAN *bone imaging aid*

butedronic acid INN

butelline [see: butacaine sulfate]

butenafine INN

butenemal [see: vinbarbital]

buteprate USAN, INN *combining name for radicals or groups*

buterizine USAN, INN *peripheral vasodilator*

Butesin Picrate ointment OTC *topical local anesthetic* [butamben picrate] 1%

butetamate INN [also: butethamate]

butethal NF [also: butobarbitone]

butethamate BAN [also: butetamate]

butethamine HCl NF

butethanol [see: tetracaine]

buthalital sodium INN [also: buthalitone sodium]

buthalitone sodium BAN [also: buthalital sodium]

buthiazide USAN *diuretic; antihypertensive* [also: butizide]

Butibel tablets, elixir ℞ *GI anticholinergic; sedative* [belladonna extract; butabarbital sodium] 15•15 mg; 15•15 mg/5 mL ⓓ butalbital

butibufen INN

butidrine INN, DCF

butikacin USAN, INN, BAN *antibacterial*

butilfenin USAN, INN *hepatic function test*

butinazocine INN

butinoline INN

butirosin INN *antibacterial antibiotic* [also: butirosin sulfate; butirosin sulphate]

butirosin sulfate USAN *antibacterial antibiotic* [also: butirosin; butirosin sulphate]

butirosin sulphate BAN *antibacterial antibiotic* [also: butirosin sulfate; butirosin]

Butisol Sodium tablets, elixir ℞ *sedative; hypnotic* [butabarbital sodium] 15, 30, 50, 100 mg; 30 mg/5 mL ⓓ Butazolidin

butixirate USAN, INN *analgesic; antirheumatic*

butixocort INN

butizide INN *diuretic; antihypertensive* [also: buthiazide]

butobarbitone BAN [also: butethal]

butobendine INN

butoconazole INN, BAN *antifungal* [also: butoconazole nitrate]

butoconazole nitrate USAN, USP *antifungal* [also: butoconazole]

butocrolol INN

butoctamide INN [also: butoctamide semisuccinate]

butoctamide semisuccinate JAN [also: butoctamide]

butofilolol INN

butonate USAN, INN *anthelmintic*

butopamine USAN, INN *cardiotonic*

butopiprine INN, DCF

butoprozine INN *antiarrhythmic; antianginal* [also: butoprozine HCl]

butoprozine HCl USAN *antiarrhythmic; antianginal* [also: butoprozine]

butopyrammonium iodide INN

butopyronoxyl USP

butorphanol USAN, INN, BAN *analgesic; antitussive*

butorphanol tartrate USAN, USP, BAN, JAN *narcotic agonist-antagonist analgesic; antitussive*
butoxamine BAN *antidiabetic; antihyperlipoproteinemic* [also: butoxamine HCl; butaxamine]
butoxamine HCl USAN *antidiabetic; antihyperlipoproteinemic* [also: butaxamine; butoxamine]
2-butoxyethyl nicotinate [see: nicoboxil]
butoxylate INN
butoxyphenylacethydroxamic acid [see: bufexamac]
butriptyline INN, BAN *antidepressant* [also: butriptyline HCl]
butriptyline HCl USAN *antidepressant* [also: butriptyline]
butropium bromide INN, JAN
butydrine [see: butidrine]
butyl alcohol NF *solvent*
butyl aminobenzoate (butyl *p*-aminobenzoate) [now: butamben]
butyl *p*-aminobenzoate picrate [see: butamben picrate]
butyl chloride NF
butyl 2-cyanoacrylate [see: enbucrilate]
butyl DNJ (deoxynojirimycin) [see: deoxynojirimycin]
butyl *p*-hydroxybenzoate [see: butylparaben]
butyl methoxydibenzoylmethane [see: avobenzone]
butyl parahydroxybenzoate JAN *antifungal agent* [also: butylparaben]
***p*-butylaminobenzoyldiethylaminoethyl HCl** JAN
butylated hydroxyanisole (BHA) NF, BAN *antioxidant*
butylated hydroxytoluene (BHT) NF, BAN *antioxidant*
α-butylbenzyl alcohol [see: fenipentol]
1-butylbiguanide [see: buformin]
N-butyl-deoxynojirimycin [see: deoxynojirimycin]
butylmesityl oxide [see: butopyronoxyl]
butylparaben NF *antifungal agent* [also: butyl parahydroxybenzoate]
butylphenamide
butylphenylsalicylamide [see: butylphenamide]
butylscopolamine bromide JAN
butynamine INN
butyrylcholesterinase (*orphan: reduction and clearance of serum cocaine levels; postsurgical apnea*)
butyrylperazine [see: butaperazine]
O-butyrylthiamine disulfide [see: bisbutitiamine]
butyvinyl [see: vinylbital]
buzepide metiodide INN, DCF
BVAP (BCNU, vincristine, Adriamycin, prednisone) *chemotherapy protocol*
BV-araU (bromovinyl arabinosyluracil) [see: sorivudine]
BVCPP (BCNU, vinblastine, cyclophosphamide, procarbazine, prednisone) *chemotherapy protocol*
BVDS (bleomycin, Velban, doxorubicin, streptozocin) *chemotherapy protocol*
BVPP (BCNU, vincristine, procarbazine, prednisone) *chemotherapy protocol*
BVU (bromoisovaleryl urea) [see: bromisovalum]
BW 12C (*orphan: sickle cell disease*)
BW B759U (DHPG) (*orphan status withdrawn 1993*)
Byclomine capsules, tablets ℞ *gastrointestinal antispasmodic* [dicyclomine HCl] 10 mg; 20 mg ② Hycomine
Bydramine Cough Syrup OTC *antihistamine; antitussive* [diphenhydramine HCl; alcohol 5%] 12.5 mg/5 mL ② Hydramine

C (vitamin C) [see: ascorbic acid]
C & E softgels OTC *vitamin supplement* [vitamins C and E] 500•400 mg
C Factors "1000" Plus tablets OTC *dietary supplement* [vitamin C; citrus & rose hips bioflavonoids; rutin; hesperidin complex] 1000•250•50•25 mg
C Speridin sustained-release tablets OTC *dietary supplement* [ascorbic acid; hesperidin; lemon bioflavonoids] 500•100•100
C vitamin [see: ascorbic acid]
C1-esterase-inhibitor, human, pasteurized *(orphan: acute angioedema)*
C1-inhibitor *(orphan: acute angioedema)*
CA (cyclophosphamide, Adriamycin) *chemotherapy protocol*
⁴⁵Ca [see: calcium chloride Ca 45]
⁴⁷Ca [see: calcium chloride Ca 47]
cabastine INN
cabergoline INN *investigational dopamine agonist for Parkinson's disease and gynecologic disorders*
cabis bromatum [see: bibrocathol]
CABOP; CA-BOP (Cytoxin, Adriamycin, bleomycin, Oncovin, prednisone) *chemotherapy protocol*
CABS (CCNU, Adriamycin bleomycin, streptozocin) *chemotherapy protocol*
cabufocon A USAN *hydrophobic contact lens material*
cabufocon B USAN *hydrophobic contact lens material*
CAC (cisplatin, ara-C, caffeine) *chemotherapy protocol*
cacao butter JAN
Cachexon ℞ *(orphan: cachexia of AIDS)* [L-glutathione, reduced]
cactinomycin USAN, INN *antibiotic antineoplastic* [also: actinomycin C]
CAD (cyclophosphamide, Adriamycin, dacarbazine) *chemotherapy protocol*
CAD (cytarabine [and] daunorubicin) *chemotherapy protocol*
cade oil [see: juniper tar]
cadexomer INN
cadexomer iodine USAN, INN, BAN *antiseptic; antiulcerative*

cadmium *element (Cd)*
cadralazine INN, BAN, JAN
CAE (cyclophosphamide, Adriamycin, etoposide) *chemotherapy protocol* also: ACE
CAF (cyclophosphamide, Adriamycin, fluorouracil) *chemotherapy protocol*
cafaminol INN
Cafatine suppositories ℞ *migraine-specific vasoconstrictor* [ergotamine tartrate; caffeine] 2•200 mg
Cafatine-PB tablets ℞ *migraine treatment; vasoconstrictor; anticholinergic; sedative* [ergotamine tartrate; caffeine; sodium pentobarbital; belladonna extract] 1•100•30•0.125 mg
cafedrine INN, BAN
Cafergot tablets, suppositories ℞ *migraine treatment; vasoconstrictor* [ergotamine tartrate; caffeine] 1•100 mg; 2•100 mg
Cafetrate suppositories ℞ *migraine-specific vasoconstrictor* [ergotamine tartrate; caffeine] 2•100 mg
Caffedrine timed-release tablets, timed-release capsules OTC *CNS stimulant; analeptic* [caffeine] 200 mg
caffeine USP, BAN, JAN *CNS stimulant; diuretic; (orphan: apnea of prematurity)*
caffeine, citrated NF
caffeine monohydrate [see: caffeine, citrated]
CAFP (cyclophosphamide, Adriamycin, fluorouracil, prednisone) *chemotherapy protocol*
CAFTH (cyclophosphamide, Adriamycin, fluorouracil, tamoxifen, Halotestin) *chemotherapy protocol*
CAFVP (cyclophosphamide, Adriamycin, fluorouracil, vincristine, prednisone) *chemotherapy protocol*
Cal Carb-HD powder OTC *calcium supplement* [calcium carbonate] 2.5 g/packet
Caladryl cream OTC *topical antihistamine; astringent; antipruritic/anesthetic* [diphenhydramine HCl; calamine] 1%•8% ⓘ Benadryl

Caladryl lotion OTC *topical poison ivy treatment* [calamine; pramoxine HCl; alcohol 2.2%] 8%•1%

Caladryl spray (discontinued 1994) OTC *topical antihistamine; astringent; antipruritic/anesthetic* [diphenhydramine HCl; calamine; alcohol 10%] 1%•8%

Caladryl Clear lotion OTC *topical poison ivy treatment* [pramoxine HCl; zinc acetate; camphor; alcohol 2%] 1%•0.1%• ≟ •2%

Caladryl for Kids cream OTC *topical poison ivy treatment* [calamine; pramoxine HCl; camphor] 8%•1%• ≟

Cala-gen lotion OTC *topical antihistamine; antipruritic/anesthetic* [diphenhydramine HCl; alcohol 2%] 1%

Calamatum spray OTC *topical poison ivy treatment* [calamine; zinc oxide; menthol; camphor; benzocaine]

calamine USP, JAN *topical protectant; astringent*

Calamox ointment OTC *topical poison ivy treatment* [calamine] 17 g/100 g ⓓ Camalox

Calamycin lotion OTC *topical antihistamine; astringent; anesthetic* [pyrilamine maleate; zinc oxide; calamine; benzocaine; chloroxylenol; alcohol 2%]

Calan film-coated tablets ℞ *antianginal; antiarrhythmic; antihypertensive; calcium channel blocker* [verapamil HCl] 40, 80, 120 mg

Calan SR film-coated sustained-release tablets ℞ *antihypertensive; calcium channel blocker* [verapamil HCl] 120, 180, 240 mg

Cal-Bid tablets (discontinued 1992) OTC *dietary supplement* [calcium; vitamins C and D]

Calbonate chewable tablets OTC *antacid* [calcium carbonate]

Calcet tablets OTC *dietary supplement* [calcium; vitamin D] 152.8 mg•100 IU

Calcet Plus tablets OTC *vitamin/calcium/iron supplement* [multiple vitamins; calcium; iron; folic acid] ≟ • 152.8•18•0.8 mg

Calcibind powder ℞ *to reduce hypercalciuria and prevent stone formation* [cellulose sodium phosphate] 2.5 g/packet

CalciCaps tablets OTC *dietary supplement* [dibasic calcium phosphate; calcium gluconate; calcium carbonate; vitamin D] 125 mg (Ca)•60 mg (P)•67 IU

CalciCaps with Iron tablets OTC *dietary supplement* [dibasic calcium phosphate; calcium gluconate; calcium carbonate; vitamin D; ferrous gluconate] 125 mg (Ca)•60 mg (P)•67 IU•7 mg

Calci-Chew chewable tablets OTC *calcium supplement* [calcium carbonate] 1.25 g

Calciday-667 tablets OTC *calcium supplement* [calcium carbonate] 667 mg

calcidiol [see: calcifediol]

Calcidrine syrup ℞ *narcotic antitussive; expectorant* [codeine; calcium iodide; alcohol 6%] 8.4•152 mg/5 mL

calcifediol USAN, USP, INN *calcium regulator*

calciferol [now: ergocalciferol]

Calciferol tablets, IM injection ℞ *vitamin deficiency therapy* [ergocalciferol (vitamin D_2)] 50,000 IU; 500,000 IU/mL

Calciferol Drops OTC *vitamin supplement* [ergocalciferol] 8000 IU/mL

Calcijex injection ℞ *treatment of hypocalcemia in dialysis patients; decreases severity of psoriatic lesions* [calcitriol] 1, 2 µg/mL

Calcilac tablets (discontinued 1994) OTC *antacid* [calcium carbonate; glycine]

Calcimar intranasal spray (commercially available in Italy, Belgium, and Spain) ℞ *investigational treatment for postmenopausal osteoporosis* [calcitonin (salmon)]

Calcimar subcu or IM injection ℞ *calcium regulator for hypercalcemia, Paget's disease, and postmenopausal osteoporosis* [calcitonin (salmon)] 200 IU/mL

Calci-Mix capsules OTC *calcium supplement* [calcium carbonate] 1250 mg

Calciparine IV or deep subcu injection (discontinued 1995) ℞ *anticoagulant* [heparin calcium] 5000 U/dose

calcipotriene USAN *antipsoriatic* [also: calcipotriol]

calcipotriol INN, BAN *antipsoriatic* [also: calcipotriene]

calcitonin (human) USAN, INN, BAN, JAN *calcium regulator; for Paget's disease (osteitis deformans) of bone (orphan)* ② calcitriol

calcitonin (salmon) USAN, INN, BAN *calcium regulator for hypercalcemia, postmenopausal osteoporosis, and Paget's disease*

calcitonin salmon (synthesis) JAN *synthetic analog of calcitonin (salmon); calcium regulator* [also: salcatonin]

calcitriol USAN, INN, BAN, JAN *calcium regulator* ② calcitonin

Calcitrol ℞ *investigational antipsoriatic*

calcium *element (Ca)*

calcium, oyster shell [see: calcium carbonate]

Calcium 600 tablets OTC *dietary supplement* [calcium carbonate] 600 mg

Calcium 600 + D tablets OTC *dietary supplement* [calcium; vitamin D] 600 mg•125 IU

Calcium 600 with Vitamin D tablets OTC *dietary supplement* [calcium; vitamin D] 600 mg•100 IU

calcium acetate USP, JAN *buffering agent; for hyperphosphatemia of end-stage renal failure (orphan)*

calcium aminacyl B-PAS (benzoyl para-aminosalicylate) [see: benzoylpas calcium]

calcium 4-aminosalicylate trihydrate [see: aminosalicylate calcium]

calcium amphomycin [see: amphomycin]

calcium ascorbate USP *vitamin C; antiscorbutic* 500 mg oral; 1652 mg/½ tsp. oral

calcium benzamidosalicylate INN, BAN *antibacterial; tuberculostatic* [also: benzoylpas calcium]

calcium benzoyl *p*-aminosalicylate (B-PAS) [see: benzoylpas calcium]

calcium benzoylpas [see: benzoylpas calcium]

calcium bis-dioctyl sulfosuccinate [see: docusate calcium]

calcium bromide JAN

calcium carbimide INN [also: cyanamide]

calcium carbonate USP *antacid; calcium replenisher (orphan: hyperphosphatemia of end-stage renal disease)* [also: precipitated calcium carbonate] 500, 600, 650, 1250 mg oral; 1250 mg/5 mL oral

calcium carbonate, precipitated [now: calcium carbonate]

calcium carbophil *bulk laxative*

calcium caseinate *dietary supplement; infant formula modifier*

calcium chloride USP, JAN *calcium replenisher*

calcium chloride Ca 45 USAN *radioactive agent*

calcium chloride Ca 47 USAN *radioactive agent*

calcium chloride dihydrate [see: calcium chloride]

calcium citrate USP *calcium supplement*

calcium citrate tetrahydrate [see: calcium citrate]

calcium clofibrate INN

calcium cyanamide [see: calcium carbimide]

calcium D-glucarate tetrahydrate [see: calcium saccharate]

calcium D-gluconate lactobionate monohydrate [see: calcium glubionate]

calcium dioctyl sulfosuccinate [see: docusate calcium]

calcium disodium edathamil [see: edetate calcium disodium]

calcium disodium edetate JAN *heavy metal chelating agent* [also: edetate calcium disodium; sodium calcium edetate; sodium calciumedetate]

Calcium Disodium Versenate IM, IV, or subcu injection ℞ *lead chelation therapy; antidote to lead poisoning and lead encephalopathy* [edetate calcium disodium] 200 mg/mL

calcium dobesilate INN

calcium doxybensylate [see: calcium dobesilate]

calcium edetate sodium [see: edetate calcium disodium]

calcium EDTA (ethylene diamine tetraacetic acid) [see: edetate calcium disodium]

calcium folinate INN, BAN, JAN *antianemic; folate replenisher; antidote to folic acid antagonist* [also: leucovorin calcium]

calcium glubionate USAN, INN *calcium replenisher*

calcium gluceptate USP *calcium replenisher* [also: calcium glucoheptonate] 1100 mg/5 mL injection

calcium glucoheptonate INN, DCF *calcium replenisher* [also: calcium gluceptate]

calcium gluconate (calcium D-gluconate) USP *calcium replenisher; (orphan: hydrofluoric acid burns)* 500, 650, 975, 1000 mg oral; 10% injection

calcium glycerinophosphate [see: calcium glycerophosphate]

calcium glycerophosphate NF, JAN

calcium hopantenate JAN

calcium hydroxide USP *astringent*

calcium hydroxide phosphate [see: calcium phosphate, tribasic]

calcium hypophosphite NF

calcium iodide

calcium iododocosanoate [see: iodobehenate calcium]

calcium lactate USP, JAN *calcium replenisher* 325, 650 mg oral

calcium lactate hydrate [see: calcium lactate]

calcium lactate pentahydrate [see: calcium lactate]

calcium lactobionate USP *calcium supplement*

calcium lactobionate dihydrate [see: calcium lactobionate]

calcium lactophosphate NF

calcium L-aspartate JAN

calcium levofolinate [see: levoleucovorin calcium]

calcium levulate [see: calcium levulinate]

calcium levulinate USP *calcium replenisher*

calcium levulinate dihydrate [see: calcium levulinate]

calcium mandelate USP

calcium oxide [see: lime]

Calcium Oyster Shell tablets (discontinued 1993) OTC *dietary supplement* [calcium carbonate]

calcium pantothenate (calcium D-pantothenate) USP, INN, JAN *vitamin B_5; enzyme cofactor* [also: pantothenic acid] 25, 100, 218, 250, 500, 545 mg oral

calcium pantothenate, racemic (calcium DL-pantothenate) USP *vitamin; enzyme cofactor*

calcium para-aminosalicylate JAN [also: aminosalicylate calcium]

calcium phosphate, dibasic USP, JAN *calcium replenisher; tablet base*

calcium phosphate, monocalcium [see: calcium phosphate, dibasic]

calcium phosphate, tribasic NF *calcium replenisher* [also: durapatite; hydroxyapatite]

calcium polycarbophil USAN, USP *bulk laxative*

calcium polystyrene sulfonate JAN

calcium polysulfide & calcium thiosulfate [see: lime, sulfurated]

calcium saccharate USP, INN *stabilizer*

calcium silicate NF *tablet excipient*

calcium sodium ferriclate INN *hematinic* [also: ferriclate calcium sodium]

calcium stearate NF, JAN *tablet and capsule lubricant*

calcium sulfate NF *tablet and capsule diluent*

calcium tetracemine disodium [see: edetate calcium disodium]

calcium trisodium pentetate INN, BAN *plutonium chelating agent* [also: pentetate calcium trisodium]

calcium 10-undecenoate [see: calcium undecylenate]

calcium undecylenate USAN *antifungal*

calciumedetate sodium [see: edetate calcium disodium]

Calcort (commercially available in Germany) ℞ *investigational antiinflammatory for rheumatoid arthritis and asthma* [deflazacort]

CaldeCort aerosol spray OTC *topical corticosteroid* [hydrocortisone] 0.5%

CaldeCort; CaldeCort Light with Aloe cream OTC *topical corticosteroid* [hydrocortisone acetate] 0.5%

Calderol capsules R *increase serum calcium levels* [calcifediol] 20, 50 μg

Caldesene ointment OTC *moisturizer; emollient; astringent; antiseptic* [cod liver oil (vitamins A and D); zinc oxide; lanolin]

Caldesene powder OTC *topical antifungal* [calcium undecylenate] 10%

caldiamide INN *pharmaceutic aid* [also: caldiamide sodium]

caldiamide sodium USAN, BAN *pharmaceutic aid* [also: caldiamide]

Calel D tablets OTC *dietary supplement* [calcium carbonate; cholecalciferol] 500 mg•200 IU

CALF (cyclophosphamide, Adriamycin, leucovorin [rescue], fluorouracil) *chemotherapy protocol*

CALF-E (cyclophosphamide, Adriamycin, leucovorin [rescue], fluorouracil, ethinyl estradiol) *chemotherapy protocol*

Calfer-Vite tablets (discontinued 1992) OTC *antianemic* [ferrous fumarate; vitamins A and D; multiple B vitamins; sodium ascorbate]

Calglycine chewable tablets OTC *antacid* [calcium carbonate; glycine] 420•150 mg

Cal-Guard softgels OTC *calcium supplement* [calcium carbonate] 50 mg

Calicylic Creme (discontinued 1994) OTC *topical keratolytic; topical analgesic* [salicylic acid; trolamine] 10%• ?

californium *element (Cf)*

calioben [see: calcium iodobehenate]

Calmol 4 rectal suppositories OTC *emollient; astringent* [cocoa butter; zinc oxide] 80%•10%

Calm-X tablets OTC *anticholinergic; antiemetic; antivertigo agent; motion sickness preventative* [dimenhydrinate] 50 mg

Calmylin oral solution (available only in Canada) OTC *antitussive; decongestant; expectorant* [dextromethorphan hydrobromide; pseudoephedrine HCl; guaifenesin] 3•6•20 mg/mL

Calmylin #1 syrup (available only in Canada) OTC *antihistamine* [dextromethorphan hydrobromide] 3 mg/mL

Calmylin #2 oral solution (available only in Canada) OTC *antitussive; decongestant* [dextromethorphan hydrobromide; pseudoephedrine HCl] 3•6 mg/mL

Calmylin #4 oral solution (available only in Canada) OTC *antitussive; antihistamine; expectorant* [dextromethorphan hydrobromide; diphenhydramine HCl; ammonium chloride] 2.5•3•25 mg/mL

Calmylin Codeine oral solution (available only in Canada) R *narcotic antitussive; decongestant; expectorant* [codeine phosphate; pseudoephedrine HCl; guaifenesin] 0.66•6•20 mg/mL

Calmylin Cough & Cold oral solution (available only in Canada) OTC *antitussive; decongestant; expectorant; analgesic* [dextromethorphan hydrobromide; pseudoephedrine HCl; guaifenesin; acetaminophen] 1•2•6.67•21.67 mg/mL

Calmylin Expectorant syrup (available only in Canada) OTC *expectorant* [guaifenesin] 20 mg/mL

Calmylin Pediatric syrup (available only in Canada) OTC *pediatric antitussive and decongestant* [dextromethorphan hydrobromide; pseudoephedrine HCl] 1.5•3 mg/mL

Cal-Nor injection (discontinued 1992) R *calcium replacement* [calcium glycerophosphate; calcium levulinate]

Calohist lotion OTC *astringent; topical antihistamine; antipruritic* [calamine; diphenhydramine HCl; camphor]

calomel NF

Calphosan IV injection R *calcium replacement* [calcium glycerophosphate; calcium lactate] 50•50 mg/10 mL (0.08 mEq/mL)

Calphron tablets R *buffering agent; for hyperphosphatemia in end-stage renal failure (orphan)* [calcium acetate] 667 mg

Cal-Plus tablets OTC *calcium supplement* [calcium carbonate] 1.5 g

calteridol INN *pharmaceutic aid* [also: calteridol calcium]

calteridol calcium USAN, BAN *pharmaceutic aid* [also: calteridol]

Caltrate 600 film-coated tablets OTC *calcium supplement* [calcium carbonate] 1.5 g

Caltrate 600 + D tablets OTC *dietary supplement* [calcium carbonate; vitamin D] 600 mg•200 IU

Caltrate 600 + Iron/Vitamin D film-coated tablets OTC *dietary supplement* [calcium carbonate; ferrous fumarate; vitamin D] 600 mg•18 mg•125 IU

Caltrate Jr. chewable tablets OTC *calcium supplement* [calcium carbonate] 750 mg

Caltrate Plus tablets OTC *dietary supplement* [calcium carbonate; vitamin D; various minerals] 600 mg•200 IU• ≛

Caltro tablets OTC *dietary supplement* [calcium, vitamin D] 250 mg•125 IU

calusterone USAN, INN *antineoplastic*

CAM (cyclophosphamide, Adriamycin, methotrexate) *chemotherapy protocol*

Cama Arthritis Pain Reliever tablets OTC *analgesic; antipyretic; antiinflammatory; antirheumatic* [aspirin, buffered with magnesium oxide and aluminum hydroxide] 500 mg

Camalox chewable tablets (discontinued 1992) OTC *antacid* [magnesium hydroxide; aluminum hydroxide; calcium carbonate] ② Calamox

Camalox oral suspension (discontinued 1994) OTC *antacid* [aluminum hydroxide; magnesium hydroxide; calcium carbonate] 45•40•50 mg/mL

Cam-Ap-Es tablets (discontinued 1995) ℞ *antihypertensive* [hydrochlorothiazide; reserpine; hydralazine HCl] 15•0.1•25 mg

camazepam INN

CAMB (Cytoxin, Adriamycin, methotrexate, bleomycin) *chemotherapy protocol*

cambendazole USAN, INN, BAN *anthelmintic*

CAMELEON (cytosine arabinoside, methotrexate, Leukovorin, Oncovin) *chemotherapy protocol*

camellia oil JAN

CAMEO (cyclophosphamide, Adriamycin, methotrexate, etoposide, Oncovin) *chemotherapy protocol*

Cameo Oil OTC *bath emollient*

CAMF (cyclophosphamide, Adriamycin, methotrexate, folinic acid) *chemotherapy protocol*

camiglibose USAN, INN *antidiabetic*

camiverine INN

camonagrel INN

camostat INN [also: camostat mesilate]

camostat mesilate JAN [also: camostat]

CAMP (cyclophosphamide, Adriamycin, methotrexate, procarbazine HCl) *chemotherapy protocol*

Campath 1H ℞ *investigational treatment for non-Hodgkin's lymphoma and rheumatoid arthritis*

camphetamide [see: camphotamide]

Campho-Phenique liquid, gel OTC *mild anesthetic; anti-infective; counterirritant* [camphor; phenol; eucalyptus oil] 10.8%•4.7%• ≛

Campho-Phenique Antibiotic Plus Pain Reliever ointment OTC *topical antibiotic; local anesthetic* [polymyxin B sulfate; neomycin sulfate; bacitracin zinc; lidocaine] 5000 U•3.5 mg•500 U•40 mg per g

camphor (d-camphor; dl-camphor) USP, JAN *topical antipruritic; mild local anesthetic; counterirritant* [also: trans-π-oxocamphor]

camphor, monobromated USP

camphorated opium tincture [now: paregoric]

camphorated parachlorophenol [see: parachlorophenol, camphorated]

camphoric acid USP

camphotamide INN, DCF

Camptosar IV infusion ℞ *I inhibitor; antineoplastic for metastatic cervical, colon, and rectal cancers* [irinotecan HCl]

camptothecin-11 (CPT-11) [see: irinotecan]

camsilate INN *combining name for radicals or groups* [also: camsylate]

camsylate USAN, BAN *combining name for radicals or groups* [also: camsilate]
camylofin INN, DCF
canbisol INN
candicidin USAN, USP, INN, BAN *antifungal*
Candida albicans skin test antigen *diagnostic aid for diminished cellular immunity; test for HIV patients to assess TB antigen response*
CandidaSure reagent slides for professional use *in vitro diagnostic aid for Candida albicans in the vagina*
Candin intradermal injection ℞ *diagnostic aid for diminished cellular immunity; test for HIV patients to assess TB antigen response* [Candida albicans skin test antigen] 0.1 mL
candocuronium iodide INN
candoxatril USAN, INN, BAN *antihypertensive; investigational treatment for congestive heart failure*
candoxatrilat USAN, INN, BAN *antihypertensive*
Cankaid oral solution (discontinued 1992) OTC *topical oral anti-inflammatory/anti-infective* [carbamide peroxide] 10%
cannabinol INN, BAN *antiemetic; antinauseant*
canrenoate potassium USAN *aldosterone antagonist* [also: canrenoic acid; potassium canrenoate]
canrenoic acid INN, BAN *aldosterone antagonist* [also: canrenoate potassium; potassium canrenoate]
canrenone USAN, INN *aldosterone antagonist*
cantharides JAN
cantharidin *topical keratolytic*
Cantharone liquid (discontinued 1994) ℞ *topical keratolytic* [cantharidin] 0.7%
Cantharone Plus liquid (discontinued 1994) ℞ *topical keratolytic* [salicylic acid; podophyllum; cantharidin] 30%•2%•1%
Cantil tablets ℞ *treatment for peptic ulcer* [mepenzolate bromide] 25 mg
Cantri vaginal cream (discontinued 1992) ℞ *bacteriostatic; antiseptic; vulnerary* [sulfisoxazole; aminacrine HCl; allantoin] 10%•0.2%•2%
CAO (cyclophosphamide, Adriamycin, Oncovin) *chemotherapy protocol*
CAP (cellulose acetate phthalate) [q.v.]
CAP (cyclophosphamide, Adriamycin, prednisone) *chemotherapy protocol*
CAP; CAP-I (cyclophosphamide, Adriamycin, Platinol) *chemotherapy protocol*
CAP-II (cyclophosphamide, Adriamycin, high-dose Platinol) *chemotherapy protocol*
Capastat Sulfate powder for IM injection ℞ *tuberculostatic* [capreomycin sulfate] 1 g/10 mL ② Cepastat
CAP-BOP (cyclophosphamide, Adriamycin, procarbazine, bleomycin, Oncovin, prednisone) *chemotherapy protocol*
capecitabine USAN, INN *antineoplastic*
Capiscint ℞ *investigational imaging agent for atherosclerotic plaque* [monoclonal antibodies]
Capital with Codeine oral suspension ℞ *narcotic analgesic* [codeine phosphate; acetaminophen] 12•120 mg/5 mL
Capitrol shampoo ℞ *antiseborrheic; antibacterial; antifungal* [chloroxine] 2% ② captopril
caplet (dosage form) *capsule-shaped tablet*
capmul 8210 [see: monoctanoin]
capobenate sodium USAN *antiarrhythmic*
capobenic acid USAN, INN *antiarrhythmic*
Capoten tablets ℞ *antihypertensive; angiotensin-converting enzyme (ACE) inhibitor* [captopril] 12.5, 25, 50, 100 mg
Capozide 25/15; Capozide 25/25; Capozide 50/15; Capozide 50/25 tablets ℞ *antihypertensive* [captopril; hydrochlorothiazide] 25•15 mg; 25•25 mg; 50•15 mg; 50•25 mg
CAPPr (cyclophosphamide, Adriamycin, Platinol, prednisone) *chemotherapy protocol*

capreomycin INN, BAN *bactericidal antibiotic; tuberculostatic* [also: capreomycin sulfate]

capreomycin sulfate USAN, USP, JAN *bactericidal antibiotic; tuberculostatic* [also: capreomycin]

capromab INN *monoclonal antibody for diagnosis of prostate cancer* [also: capromab pendetide]

capromab pendetide USAN *monoclonal antibody for diagnosis of prostate cancer* [also: capromab]

Capros ℞ *investigational oral timed-release analgesic for severe pain*

caproxamine INN, BAN

capsaicin *topical analgesic; counterirritant*

capsicum JAN

capsicum oleoresin *topical analgesic; counterirritant*

Capsin lotion OTC *topical analgesic* [capsaicin] 0.025%, 0.075%

Capsulets (trademarked form) *sustained-release caplet*

captab (dosage form) *capsule-shaped tablet*

captamine INN *depigmentor* [also: captamine HCl]

captamine HCl USAN *depigmentor* [also: captamine]

captodiame INN, BAN

captodiame HCl [see: captodiame]

captodiamine HCl [see: captodiame]

captopril USAN, USP, INN, BAN, JAN *antihypertensive; angiotensin-converting enzyme (ACE) inhibitor* 12.5, 25, 50, 100 mg oral ▼ Capitrol

Captrix cream OTC *topical analgesic* [capsaicin]

capuride USAN, INN *hypnotic*

Capzasin-P cream OTC *topical analgesic* [capsaicin] 0.025%

caracemide USAN, INN *antineoplastic*

Carafate tablets, oral suspension ℞ *treatment for duodenal ulcer* [sucralfate] 1 g; 1 g/10 mL

caramel NF *coloring agent*

caramiphen INN, BAN

caramiphen edisylate

caramiphen HCl [see: caramiphen]

caraway NF

caraway oil NF

carazolol INN, BAN

carbachol USP, INN, BAN, JAN *ophthalmic cholinergic; miotic for surgery; antiglaucoma agent* [also: carbacholine chloride]

carbacholine chloride DCF *ophthalmic cholinergic; miotic for surgery; antiglaucoma agent* [also: carbachol]

carbacrylamine resins

carbadipimidine HCl [see: carpipramine dihydrochloride]

carbadox USAN, INN, BAN *antibacterial*

carbaldrate INN

carbamate choline chloride [see: carbachol]

carbamazepine USAN, USP, INN, BAN, JAN *analgesic; anticonvulsant* 100, 200 mg oral

carbamide [see: urea]

carbamide peroxide USP *topical dental anti-infective*

N-carbamoylarsanilic acid [see: carbarsone]

carbamoylcholine chloride [see: carbachol]

O-carbamoylsalicylic acid lactam [see: carsalam]

carbamylcholine chloride [see: carbachol]

carbamylmethylcholine chloride [see: bethanechol chloride]

carbantel INN *anthelmintic* [also: carbantel lauryl sulfate]

carbantel lauryl sulfate USAN *anthelmintic* [also: carbantel]

carbaril INN [also: carbaryl]

carbarsone USP, INN

carbaryl BAN [also: carbaril]

carbasalate calcium INN *analgesic* [also: carbaspirin calcium]

carbaspirin calcium USAN *analgesic* [also: carbasalate calcium]

Carbastat solution ℞ *direct-acting miotic for ophthalmic surgery* [carbachol] 0.01%

carbazeran USAN, INN *cardiotonic*

carbazochrome INN, JAN

carbazochrome salicylate INN

carbazochrome sodium sulfonate INN

carbazocine INN

carbenicillin INN, BAN *antibacterial* [also: carbenicillin disodium; carbenicillin sodium]

carbenicillin disodium USAN, USP *antibacterial* [also: carbenicillin; carbenicillin sodium]

carbenicillin indanyl sodium USAN, USP *bactericidal antibiotic* [also: carindacillin]

carbenicillin phenyl sodium USAN *antibacterial* [also: carfecillin]

carbenicillin potassium USAN *antibacterial*

carbenicillin sodium JAN *antibacterial* [also: carbenicillin disodium; carbenicillin]

carbenoxolone INN, BAN *glucocorticoid* [also: carbenoxolone sodium]

carbenoxolone sodium USAN *glucocorticoid* [also: carbenoxolone]

carbenzide INN

carbesilate INN *combining name for radicals or groups*

carbetapentane citrate NF [also: pentoxyverine]

carbetapentane tannate

carbetimer USAN, INN *antineoplastic*

carbetocin INN, BAN

Carbex tablets ℞ *antiparkinsonian* [selegiline HCl] 5 mg

carbidopa USAN, USP, INN, BAN, JAN *decarboxylase inhibitor; antiparkinsonian (when used with levodopa)*

carbifene INN *analgesic* [also: carbiphene HCl; carbiphene]

carbimazole INN, BAN

carbinoxamine INN, BAN *antihistamine* [also: carbinoxamine maleate]

Carbinoxamine Compound syrup, pediatric drops ℞ *antitussive; decongestant; antihistamine* [dextromethorphan hydrobromide; pseudoephedrine HCl; carbinoxamine maleate] 15•60•4 mg/5 mL; 4•25•2 mg/mL

carbinoxamine maleate USP *antihistamine* [also: carbinoxamine]

carbiphene BAN *analgesic* [also: carbiphene HCl; carbifene]

carbiphene HCl USAN *analgesic* [also: carbifene; carbiphene]

Carbiset tablets ℞ *decongestant; antihistamine* [pseudoephedrine HCl; carbinoxamine maleate] 60•4 mg

Carbiset-TR timed-release tablets ℞ *decongestant; antihistamine* [pseudoephedrine HCl; carbinoxamine maleate] 120•8 mg

Carbocaine injection ℞ *injectable local anesthetic* [mepivacaine HCl] 1%, 1.5%, 2%, 3%

Carbocaine with Neo-Cobefrin injection ℞ *injectable local anesthetic* [mepivacaine HCl; levonordefrin] 2%•1:20,000

carbocisteine INN, BAN *mucolytic* [also: carbocysteine]

carbocloral USAN, INN, BAN *hypnotic*

carbocromen INN *coronary vasodilator* [also: chromonar HCl]

carbocysteine USAN *mucolytic* [also: carbocisteine]

Carbodec tablets, syrup ℞ *decongestant; antihistamine* [pseudoephedrine HCl; carbinoxamine maleate] 60•4 mg; 60•4 mg/5 mL

Carbodec DM syrup, pediatric drops ℞ *antitussive; decongestant; antihistamine* [dextromethorphan hydrobromide; pseudoephedrine HCl; carbinoxamine maleate] 15•60•4 mg/5 mL; 4•25•2 mg/mL

Carbodec TR timed-release tablets ℞ *decongestant; antihistamine* [pseudoephedrine HCl; carbinoxamine maleate] 120•8 mg

carbodimid calcium [see: calcium carbimide]

carbofenotion INN [also: carbophenothion]

carbol-fuchsin solution (or paint) USP *antifungal*

carbolic acid [see: phenol]

carbolin [see: carbachol]

carbolonium bromide BAN [also: hexcarbacholine bromide]

carbomer INN, BAN *emulsifying and suspending agent* [also: carbomer 910]

carbomer 1342 NF *emulsifying and suspending agent*

carbomer 910 USAN, NF *emulsifying and suspending agent* [also: carbomer]

carbomer 934 USAN, NF *emulsifying and suspending agent*
carbomer 934P USAN, NF *emulsifying and suspending agent*
carbomer 940 USAN, NF *emulsifying and suspending agent*
carbomer 941 USAN, NF *emulsifying and suspending agent*
carbomycin INN
carbon *element* (C)
carbon, activated
carbon dioxide (CO_2) USP *respiratory stimulant*
carbon tetrachloride NF *solvent*
carbonic acid, calcium salt [see: calcium carbonate]
carbonic acid, dilithium salt [see: lithium carbonate]
carbonic acid, dipotassium salt [see: potassium carbonate]
carbonic acid, disodium salt [see: sodium carbonate]
carbonic acid, magnesium salt [see: magnesium carbonate]
carbonic acid, monoammonium salt [see: ammonium carbonate]
carbonic acid, monopotassium salt [see: potassium bicarbonate]
carbonic acid, monosodium salt [see: sodium bicarbonate]
carbonis detergens, liquor (LCD) [see: coal tar]
carbophenothion BAN [also: carbofenotion]
carboplatin USAN, INN, BAN *alkylating antineoplastic*
carboprost USAN, INN, BAN *oxytocic*
carboprost methyl USAN *oxytocic*
carboprost trometanol BAN *oxytocic; prostaglandin-type abortifacient* [also: carboprost tromethamine]
carboprost tromethamine USAN, USP *oxytocic; prostaglandin-type abortifacient* [also: carboprost trometanol]
Carboptic Drop-Tainers (eye drops) ℞ *antiglaucoma agent; direct-acting miotic* [carbachol] 3%
carboquone INN
carbose D [see: carboxymethylcellulose sodium]
carbovir (*orphan: AIDS*)
carboxyimamidate [see: carbetimer]

carboxymethylcellulose calcium NF *tablet disintegrant*
carboxymethylcellulose sodium USP *suspending and viscosity-increasing agent; tablet excipient* [also: carmellose; carmellose sodium]
carboxymethylcellulose sodium 12 NF *suspending and viscosity-increasing agent*
carbromal NF, INN
carbubarb INN
carbubarbital [see: carbubarb]
carburazepam INN
carbutamide INN, BAN
carbuterol INN, BAN *bronchodilator* [also: carbuterol HCl]
carbuterol HCl USAN *bronchodilator* [also: carbuterol]
carcainium chloride INN
carcinoembryonic antigen (CEA)
cardamom seed NF
Cardec-DM syrup, pediatric syrup, pediatric drops ℞ *antitussive; decongestant; antihistamine* [dextromethorphan hydrobromide; pseudoephedrine HCl; carbinoxamine maleate] 15•60•4 mg/5 mL; 15•60•4 mg/5 mL; 4•25•2 mg/mL
Cardec-S syrup ℞ *decongestant; antihistamine* [pseudoephedrine HCl; carbinoxamine maleate] 60•4 mg/5 mL
Cardene capsules ℞ *antianginal; antihypertensive* [nicardipine HCl] 20, 30 mg
Cardene I.V. injection ℞ *antihypertensive* [nicardipine HCl] 2.5 mg/mL
Cardene QD ℞ *investigational once-daily antihypertensive* [nicardipine HCl]
Cardene SR sustained-release capsules ℞ *antihypertensive* [nicardipine HCl] 30, 45, 60 mg
Cardenz tablets OTC *vitamin/mineral supplement* [multiple vitamins & minerals]
Cardiac T test ℞ *in vitro test for troponin T (indicator of cardiac damage) in whole blood*
cardiamid [see: nikethamide]
Cardilate oral or sublingual tablets (discontinued 1995) ℞ *antianginal* [erythrityl tetranitrate] 10 mg
Cardio-Green (CG) powder for IV injection ℞ *in vivo diagnostic aid for*

cardiac output, hepatic function, or ophthalmic angiography [indocyanine green] 25, 50 mg

Cardiolite injection ℞ *myocardial perfusion agent for cardiac SPECT imaging* [technetium Tc 99m sestamibi] 5 mL

Cardi-Omega 3 capsules OTC *dietary supplement* [omega-3 fatty acids; multiple vitamins & minerals] 1000•≛ mg

cardioplegic solution (calcium chloride, magnesium chloride, potassium chloride, sodium chloride) [q.v.]

Cardioquin tablets ℞ *antiarrhythmic* [quinidine polygalacturonate] 275 mg

Cardioxane ℞ *investigational adjunct to chemotherapy*

Cardizem IV injection, Lyo-Ject (prefilled syringe) ℞ *calcium channel blocker for atrial fibrillation or paroxysmal supraventricular tachycardia (PSVT)* [diltiazem HCl] 5 mg/mL

Cardizem tablets ℞ *antianginal; calcium channel blocker* [diltiazem HCl] 30, 60, 90, 120 mg

Cardizem SR; Cardizem CD sustained-release capsules ℞ *antihypertensive; antianginal; calcium channel blocker* [diltiazem HCl] 60, 90, 120 mg; 120, 180, 240, 300 mg

cardophyllin [see: aminophylline]

Cardura tablets ℞ *antihypertensive; antiadrenergic; treatment for benign prostatic hyperplasia* [doxazosin mesylate] 1, 2, 4, 8 mg

carebastine INN

carena [see: aminophylline]

carfecillin INN, BAN *antibacterial* [also: carbenicillin phenyl sodium]

carfenazine INN *antipsychotic* [also: carphenazine maleate; carphenazine]

carfentanil INN *narcotic analgesic* [also: carfentanil citrate]

carfentanil citrate USAN *narcotic analgesic* [also: carfentanil]

carfimate INN

Carfin tablets ℞ *anticoagulant* [warfarin sodium]

cargentos [see: silver protein]

cargutocin INN

carindacillin INN, BAN *antibacterial* [also: carbenicillin indanyl sodium]

carisoprodol USP, INN, BAN *skeletal muscle relaxant* 350 mg oral

Cari-Tab chewable tablets (discontinued 1992) ℞ *pediatric vitamin deficiency and dental caries prevention* [vitamins A, C, and D; fluoride]

carmantadine USAN, INN *antiparkinsonian*

carmellose INN *suspending agent; tablet excipient* [also: carboxymethylcellulose sodium; carmellose sodium]

carmellose sodium BAN *suspending agent; tablet excipient* [also: carboxymethylcellulose sodium; carmellose]

carmetizide INN

carminomycin HCl [now: carubicin HCl]

carmofur INN

Carmol 10 lotion OTC *moisturizer; emollient; keratolytic* [urea] 10%

Carmol 20 cream OTC *moisturizer; emollient; keratolytic* [urea] 20%

Carmol HC cream ℞ *topical corticosteroid; moisturizer; emollient* [hydrocortisone acetate; urea] 1%•10%

carmoxirole INN

carmustine USAN, INN, BAN *alkylating antineoplastic; (orphan: polymer implant for recurrent malignant glioma)*

Carnation Follow-Up; Carnation GoodStart liquid, powder OTC *total or supplementary infant feeding*

carnauba wax [see: wax, carnauba]

carnidazole USAN, INN, BAN *antiprotozoal*

carnitine INN *vitamin* B_t

L-carnitine [see: levocarnitine]

Carnitor tablets, oral solution, IV injection or infusion ℞ *carnitine replenisher for deficiency of genetic origin or end-stage renal disease (orphan)* [levocarnitine] 330 mg; 100 mg/mL; 500 mg/2.5 mL, 1 g/5 mL

carocainide INN

β-carotene [see: beta carotene]

caroverine INN

caroxazone USAN, INN *antidepressant*

Carozyme capsules OTC *dietary supplement* [multiple enzymes]

carperidine INN, BAN
carperone INN
carphenazine BAN *antipsychotic* [also: carphenazine maleate; carfenazine]
carphenazine maleate USAN, USP *antipsychotic* [also: carfenazine; carphenazine]
carpindolol INN
carpipramine INN
carpipramine dihydrochloride [see: carpipramine]
carpolene [now: carbomer 934P]
carprazidil INN
carprofen USAN, INN, BAN *nonsteroidal anti-inflammatory drug (NSAID); analgesic; antipyretic*
carpronium chloride INN
Carpuject (trademarked delivery system) *prefilled cartridge-needle unit*
Carpuject Smartpak (trademarked delivery system) *prefilled cartridge-needle unit package*
carrageenan NF *suspending and viscosity-increasing agent*
Carrisyn ℞ *investigational (Phase I) antiviral/immunomodulator for AIDS/ARC* [acemannan]
carsalam INN, BAN
carsatrin INN *cardiotonic* [also: carsatrin succinate]
carsatrin succinate USAN *cardiotonic* [also: carsatrin]
cartazolate USAN, INN *antidepressant*
carteolol INN, BAN *antiadrenergic; topical antiglaucoma agent (β-blocker)* [also: carteolol HCl]
carteolol HCl USAN *antiadrenergic; topical antiglaucoma agent (β-blocker)* [also: carteolol]
carticaine BAN [also: articaine]
Cartrix (delivery system) *prefilled syringes*
Cartrol Filmtabs (film-coated tablets) OTC *antihypertensive; β-blocker* [carteolol HCl] 2.5, 5 mg
carubicin INN *antineoplastic* [also: carubicin HCl]
carubicin HCl USAN *antineoplastic* [also: carubicin]
carumonam INN, BAN *antibacterial* [also: carumonam sodium]

carumonam sodium USAN *antibacterial* [also: carumonam]
carvedilol USAN, INN, BAN *antianginal; antihypertensive; α- and β-blocker*
carvotroline HCl USAN *antipsychotic*
Carwin ℞ *investigational treatment for hypertension and congestive heart failure* [xamoterol]
carzelesin USAN *antineoplastic*
carzenide INN
casanthranol USAN, USP *laxative*
cascara fluidextract, aromatic USP *laxative*
cascara sagrada USP *stimulant laxative* 325 mg oral
cascara sagrada fluid extract (*orphan: oral drug overdose*)
cascarin [see: casanthranol]
Casec powder OTC *protein supplement* [calcium caseinate]
Casodex film-coated tablets ℞ *antiandrogen for prostatic cancer* [bicalutamide] 50 mg
cassia oil [see: cinnamon oil]
CAST (Color Allergy Screening Test) reagent sticks for professional use *in vitro diagnostic aid for immunoglobulin E in serum*
Castaderm liquid OTC *topical antifungal; astringent; antiseptic* [resorcinol; boric acid; acetone; basic fuchsin; phenol; alcohol 9%]
Castel Minus; Castel Plus liquid OTC *topical antifungal* [resorcinol; acetone; basic fuchsin; alcohol 11.5%]
Castellani Paint solution (name changed to Castellani Paint Modified in 1996)
Castellani Paint Modified solution ℞ *topical antifungal; antibacterial* [basic fuchsin; phenol; resorcinol]
Castellani's paint [see: carbol-fuchsin solution]
Castile soap
castor oil USP *stimulant laxative*
CAT (cytarabine, Adriamycin, thioguanine) *chemotherapy protocol*
Cataflam tablets ℞ *nonsteroidal anti-inflammatory drug (NSAID); antiarthritic; analgesic for primary dysmenorrhea* [diclofenac potassium] 50 mg

catalase *catalytic neutralizing agent and rinse for contact lenses*

Catapres tablets ℞ *antihypertensive* [clonidine HCl] 0.1, 0.2, 0.3 mg ▢ Catarase; Combipres; Ser-Ap-Es

Catapres-TTS-1; Catapres-TTS-2; Catapres-TTS-3 transdermal patch ℞ *antihypertensive* [clonidine] 2.5 mg; 5 mg; 7.5 mg

Catarase 1:5,000 ophthalmic solution ℞ *enzymatic zonulolytic for intracapsular lens extraction* [chymotrypsin] 300 U ▢ Catapres

Catarase 1:10,000 ophthalmic solution (discontinued 1993) ℞ *enzymatic zonulolytic for intracapsular lens extraction* [chymotrypsin] 150 U ▢ Catapres

Catatrol ℞ *investigational bicyclic antidepressant; (orphan: cataplexy; narcolepsy)* [viloxazine]

catgut suture [see: absorbable surgical suture]

cathine INN

cathinone INN

cathomycin sodium [see: novobiocin sodium]

Catrix ℞ *investigational antineoplastic for breast, cervical, ovarian, uterine, and endometrial cancer*

Catrix Correction cream OTC *moisturizer; emollient*

CatVax ℞ *investigational allergic desensitization to cats*

CAV (cyclophosphamide, Adriamycin, vinblastine) *chemotherapy protocol*

CAV (cyclophosphamide, Adriamycin, vincristine) *chemotherapy protocol* also: VAC

CAVe; CA-Ve (CCNU, Adriamycin, vinblastine) *chemotherapy protocol*

CAVE (cyclophosphamide, Adriamycin, vincristine, etoposide) *chemotherapy protocol*

Caverject powder for intracavernosal injection ℞ *vasodilator for erectile dysfunction* [alprostadil] 10, 20 μg/mL

CAVP16 (cyclophosphamide, Adriamycin, VP-16) *chemotherapy protocol*

C-B Time liquid (discontinued 1992) OTC *vitamin supplement* [multiple B vitamins; vitamin C]

C-B Time; C-B Time 500 timed-release tablets (discontinued 1995) OTC *vitamin supplement* [multiple B vitamins; vitamin C] ± •200 mg; ± •500 mg

CBV (cyclophosphamide, BCNU, VePesid) *chemotherapy protocol*

CBV (cyclophosphamide, BCNU, VP-16-213) *chemotherapy protocol*

CC (carboplatin, cyclophosphamide) *chemotherapy protocol*

CCD 1042 *(orphan: infantile spasms)*

CC-Galactosidase *(orphan: Fabry's disease)* [alpha-galactosidase A]

CCM (cyclophosphamide, CCNU, methotrexate) *chemotherapy protocol*

CCNU (chloroethyl-cyclohexyl-nitrosourea) [see: lomustine]

C-Crystals crystals OTC *vitamin supplement* [vitamin C]

CCV-AV (CCNU, cyclophosphamide, vincristine [alternates with] Adriamycin, vincristine) *chemotherapy protocol*

CCVPP (CCNU, cyclophosphamide, Velban, procarbazine, prednisone) *chemotherapy protocol*

CD (cytarabine, daunorubicin) *chemotherapy protocol*

CD4, human truncated 369 AA polypeptide *(orphan: AIDS)*

CD4, recombinant soluble human (rCD4) *investigational (Phase I) antiviral for AIDS/ARC (orphan)*

CD4 immunoadhesin [see: CD4 immunoglobulin G, recombinant human]

CD4 immunoglobulin G, recombinant human *investigational (Phase I) antiviral for maternal/fetal transfer of HIV (orphan)*

CD4-IgG [see: CD4 immunoglobulin G, recombinant human]

CD4-PE40 [see: alvircept sudotox]

CD5-T lymphocyte immunotoxin *(orphan: graft vs. host disease or graft rejection in bone marrow transplants)*

CD6-blocked ricin *investigational treatment for cutaneous T-cell lymphoma*

CD-18 *investigational treatment for inflammatory disorders*

CD19 [see: anti-B4-blocked ricin]

CD-33 [see: ricin (blocked) conjugated murine MCA myeloid cells]

CD-40 ligand *investigational cytokine for rheumatoid arthritis, AIDS, and hyperimmunoglobulin M (HIM) syndrome*

CD-45 monoclonal antibodies *(orphan: organ transplant rejection)*

CdA (2-chloro-2′-deoxyadenosine) [see: cladribine]

CDC (carboplatin, doxorubicin, cyclophosphamide) *chemotherapy protocol*

CDDP; C-DDP (cis-diamminedichloroplatinum) [see: cisplatin]

CDDP/VP (CDDP, VePesid) *chemotherapy protocol*

CDE (cyclophosphamide, doxorubicin, etoposide) *chemotherapy protocol*

CDP-cholin [see: citicoline]

CEA (carcinoembryonic antigen)

CEAker ℞ *(orphan: detection of tumor foci in colorectal carcinoma)* [indium In 111 murine anti-CEA monoclonal anitbody, type ZCE 025]

CEA-Scan ℞ *investigational imaging agent for detection of recurrent or metastatic colorectal cancer* [arcitumomab]

CEB (carboplatin, etoposide, bleomycin) *chemotherapy protocol*

Cebid Timecelles (sustained-release capsules) OTC *vitamin supplement* [ascorbic acid] 500 mg

CECA (cisplatin, etoposide, cyclophosphamide, Adriamycin) *chemotherapy protocol*

Ceclor Pulvules (capsules), powder for oral suspension ℞ *cephalosporin-type antibiotic* [cefaclor] 250, 500 mg; 125, 187, 250, 375 mg/5 mL

Ceclor CD; Ceclor SR ℞ *investigational twice-daily cephalosporin-type antibiotic* [cefaclor]

Cecon solution OTC *vitamin supplement* [vitamin C] 100 mg/mL

Cedax capsules, oral suspension ℞ *cephalosporin-type antibiotic for respiratory infections* [ceftibuten] 400 mg; 90, 180 mg/mL

cedefingol USAN *antipsoriatic; antineoplastic adjunct*

Cedilanid-D IV or IM injection (discontinued 1993) ℞ *cardiac glycoside to increase cardiac output; antiarrhythmic* [deslanoside] 0.2 mg/mL

CeeNu capsules, dose pack (two 100 mg + two 40 mg + two 10 mg capsules) ℞ *antineoplastic for brain, colon, lung, and renal tumors, lymphomas, melanomas, and multiple myeloma* [lomustine] 10, 40, 100 mg;

CEF (cyclophosphamide, epirubicin, fluorouracil) *chemotherapy protocol*

cefacetrile INN *antibacterial* [also: cephacetrile sodium]

cefacetrile sodium [see: cephacetrile sodium]

cefaclor USAN, USP, INN, BAN, JAN *bactericidal antibiotic* 250, 500 mg oral; 125, 187, 250, 375 mg/5 mL oral suspension

cefadroxil USAN, USP, INN, BAN *bactericidal antibiotic* 125, 250, 500 mg/5 mL oral suspension

cefadroxil monohydrate *bactericidal antibiotic* 500, 1000 mg

Cefadyl powder for IV or IM injection ℞ *cephalosporin-type antibiotic* [cephapirin sodium] 0.5, 1, 2, 4, 20 g

cefalexin INN, JAN *bactericidal antibiotic* [also: cephalexin]

cefaloglycin INN *antibacterial* [also: cephaloglycin]

cefalonium INN [also: cephalonium]

cefaloram INN [also: cephaloram]

cefaloridine INN *antibacterial* [also: cephaloridine]

cefalotin INN *bactericidal antibiotic* [also: cephalothin sodium; cephalothin]

cefalotin sodium [see: cephalothin sodium]

cefamandole USAN, INN *antibacterial* [also: cephamandole]

cefamandole nafate USAN, USP *bactericidal antibiotic* [also: cephamandole nafate]

cefamandole sodium USP *antibacterial*

Cefanex capsules (discontinued 1995) ℞ *cephalosporin-type antibiotic* [cephalexin monohydrate] 250, 500 mg

cefaparole USAN, INN *antibacterial*
cefapirin INN, BAN *antibacterial* [also: cephapirin sodium]
cefapirin sodium [see: cephapirin sodium]
cefatrizine USAN, INN, BAN *antibacterial*
cefazaflur INN *antibacterial* [also: cefazaflur sodium]
cefazaflur sodium USAN *antibacterial* [also: cefazaflur]
cefazedone INN, BAN
cefazolin USP, INN *systemic antibacterial* [also: cephazolin] ② cephalexin; cephalothin
cefazolin sodium USAN, USP *bactericidal antibiotic* [also: cephazolin sodium] 0.25, 0.5, 1, 5, 10, 20 g injection
cefbuperazone USAN, INN *antibacterial*
cefcanel INN
cefcanel daloxate INN
cefdinir USAN, INN *antibacterial*
cefedrolor INN
cefempidone INN, BAN
cefepime USAN, INN *antibacterial*
cefepime HCl USAN *cephalosporin-type antibiotic*
cefetamet USAN, INN *veterinary antibacterial*
cefetecol USAN, INN, BAN *antibacterial*
cefetrizole INN
cefivitril INN
cefixime USAN, USP, INN, BAN *bactericidal antibiotic*
Cefizox powder for IV or IM injection ℞ *cephalosporin-type antibiotic* [ceftizoxime sodium] 0.5, 1, 2, 10 g
cefmenoxime INN *antibacterial* [also: cefmenoxime HCl]
cefmenoxime HCl USAN, USP *antibacterial* [also: cefmenoxime]
cefmepidium chloride INN
cefmetazole USAN, INN *antibacterial*
cefmetazole sodium USAN, USP, JAN *bactericidal antibiotic*
cefminox INN
Cefobid powder for IV or IM injection ℞ *cephalosporin-type antibiotic* [cefoperazone sodium] 1, 2 g
cefodizime INN *investigational antibiotic*

Cefol Filmtabs (film-coated tablets) ℞ *vitamin supplement* [multiple vitamins; folic acid] ≛•0.5 mg
cefonicid INN, BAN *antibacterial* [also: cefonicid monosodium]
cefonicid monosodium USAN *antibacterial* [also: cefonicid]
cefonicid sodium USAN, USP *bactericidal antibiotic*
cefoperazone INN, BAN *antibacterial* [also: cefoperazone sodium]
cefoperazone sodium USAN, USP *bactericidal antibiotic* [also: cefoperazone]
ceforanide USAN, USP, INN, BAN *bactericidal antibiotic*
Cefotan powder for IV or IM injection ℞ *cephalosporin-type antibiotic* [cefotetan disodium] 1, 2, 10 g
cefotaxime INN, BAN *antibacterial* [also: cefotaxime sodium] ② cefoxitin
cefotaxime sodium USAN, USP *bactericidal antibiotic* [also: cefotaxime]
cefotetan USAN, INN, BAN *antibacterial*
cefotetan disodium USAN, USP *bactericidal antibiotic*
cefotiam INN, BAN *antibacterial* [also: cefotiam HCl]
cefotiam HCl USAN *antibacterial* [also: cefotiam]
cefoxazole INN [also: cephoxazole]
cefoxitin USAN, INN, BAN *cephalosporin-type antibiotic* ② cefotaxime
cefoxitin sodium USAN, USP, BAN *cephalosporin-type antibiotic*
cefpimizole USAN, INN *antibacterial*
cefpimizole sodium USAN, JAN *antibacterial*
cefpiramide USAN, USP, INN *antibacterial*
cefpiramide sodium USAN, JAN *antibacterial*
cefpirome INN, BAN *antibacterial* [also: cefpirome sulfate]
cefpirome sulfate USAN, JAN *antibacterial* [also: cefpirome]
cefpodoxime INN, BAN *bactericidal antibiotic* [also: cefpodoxime proxetil]
cefpodoxime proxetil USAN, JAN *bactericidal antibiotic* [also: cefpodoxime]
cefprozil USAN, INN *bactericidal antibiotic*
cefprozil monohydrate
cefquinome INN, BAN *veterinary antibacterial*

cefquinome sulfate USAN *veterinary antibacterial*
cefradine INN *bactericidal antibiotic* [also: cephradine]
Cefrom ℞ *investigational cephalosporin antibiotic* [cefpirome]
cefrotil INN
cefroxadine USAN, INN *antibacterial*
cefsulodin INN, BAN *antibacterial* [also: cefsulodin sodium]
cefsulodin sodium USAN *antibacterial* [also: cefsulodin]
cefsumide INN
ceftazidime USAN, USP, INN, BAN, JAN *bactericidal antibiotic*
cefteram INN
ceftezole INN
ceftibuten USAN, INN, BAN *antibacterial antibiotic*
Ceftin film-coated tablets, oral suspension ℞ *cephalosporin-type antibiotic* [cefuroxime axetil] 125, 250, 500 mg; 125 mg/5 mL
ceftiofur INN, BAN *veterinary antibacterial* [also: ceftiofur HCl]
ceftiofur HCl USAN *veterinary antibacterial* [also: ceftiofur]
ceftiofur sodium USAN *veterinary antibacterial*
ceftiolene INN
ceftioxide INN
ceftizoxime INN, BAN *bactericidal antibiotic* [also: ceftizoxime sodium] ② cefuroxime
ceftizoxime sodium USAN, USP *bactericidal antibiotic* [also: ceftizoxime]
ceftriaxone INN, BAN *bactericidal antibiotic* [also: ceftriaxone sodium]
ceftriaxone sodium USAN, USP *bactericidal antibiotic* [also: ceftriaxone]
cefuracetime INN, BAN
cefuroxime USAN, INN, BAN *cephalosporin-type antibiotic* ② ceftizoxime
cefuroxime axetil USAN, USP, BAN *cephalosporin-type antibiotic*
cefuroxime pivoxetil USAN *cephalosporin-type antibiotic*
cefuroxime sodium USP, BAN *cephalosporin-type antibiotic* 0.75, 1.5, 7.5 g injection
cefuzonam INN

Cefzil film-coated tablets, powder for oral suspension ℞ *cephalosporin-type antibiotic* [cefprozil] 250, 500 mg; 125, 250 mg/5 mL ② Kefzol
Cefzon (foreign name for U.S. product Omnicef)
Celestone tablets, syrup *glucocorticoids* [tamethasone] 0.6 mg; 0.6 mg/5 mL
Celestone Phosphate IV, IM injection ℞ *glucocorticoids* [betamethasone sodium phosphate] 4 mg/mL
Celestone Soluspan intrabursal, intra-articular, intralesional injection ℞ *glucocorticoids* [betamethasone sodium phosphate; betamethasone acetate] 3•3 mg/mL
celiprolol INN, BAN *antiadrenergic (β-receptor)* [also: celiprolol HCl]
celiprolol HCl USAN *antiadrenergic (β-receptor)* [also: celiprolol]
cellacefate INN *tablet-coating agent* [also: cellulose acetate phthalate; cellacephate]
cellacephate BAN *tablet-coating agent* [also: cellulose acetate phthalate; cellacefate]
CellCept capsules ℞ *immunosuppressant for renal transplants* [mycophenolate mofetil] 250 mg
Cellufresh eye drops OTC *ocular moisturizer/lubricant* [carboxymethylcellulose] 0.5%
cellulase USAN *digestive enzyme*
cellulolytic enzyme [see: cellulase]
cellulose, absorbable [see: cellulose, oxidized]
cellulose, ethyl ester [see: ethylcellulose]
cellulose, hydroxypropyl methyl ether [see: hydroxypropyl methylcellulose]
cellulose, microcrystalline NF *tablet and capsule diluent* [also: dispersible cellulose]
cellulose, oxidized USP *topical local hemostatic*
cellulose, oxidized regenerated USP *local hemostatic*
cellulose, sodium carboxymethyl [see: carboxymethylcellulose sodium]
cellulose acetate NF *tablet-coating agent; insoluble polymer membrane*

cellulose acetate butyrate [see: cabufocon A; cabufocon B]
cellulose acetate dibutyrate [see: porofocon A; porofocon B]
cellulose acetate phthalate (CAP) NF *tablet-coating agent* [also: cellacefate; cellacephate]
cellulose carboxymethyl ether, sodium salt [see: carboxymethylcellulose sodium]
cellulose diacetate [see: cellulose acetate]
cellulose dihydrogen phosphate, disodium salt [see: cellulose sodium phosphate]
cellulose disodium phosphate [see: cellulose sodium phosphate]
cellulose ethyl ether [see: ethylcellulose]
cellulose gum, modified [now: croscarmellose sodium]
cellulose methyl ether [see: methylcellulose]
cellulose nitrate [see: pyroxylin]
cellulose sodium phosphate (CSP) USAN, USP *antiurolithic*
cellulosic acid [see: cellulose, oxidized]
Celluvisc solution OTC *ocular moisturizer/lubricant* [carboxymethylcellulose] 1%
celmoleukin INN *immunostimulant*
Celontin Kapseals (capsules) ℞ *anticonvulsant* [methsuximide] 150, 300 mg
celucloral INN, BAN
Cel-U-Jec IV, IM injection ℞ *glucocorticoids* [betamethasone sodium phosphate] 4 mg/mL
CEM (cytosine arabinoside, etoposide, methotrexate) *chemotherapy protocol*
Cemill 500; Cemill 1000 sustained-release tablets OTC *vitamin supplement* [ascorbic acid]
Cemill plus Bioflavonoids tablets OTC *vitamin supplement* [ascorbic acid; bioflavonoids; rutin]
Cenafed syrup OTC *nasal decongestant* [pseudoephedrine HCl] 30 mg/5 mL
Cenafed tablets (discontinued 1993) OTC *nasal decongestant* [pseudoephedrine HCl] 60 mg

Cenafed Plus tablets OTC *decongestant; antihistamine* [pseudoephedrine HCl; tripolidine HCl] 60•2.5 mg
Cena-K liquid ℞ *potassium supplement* [potassium chloride] 20, 40 mEq/15 mL
Cenocort A-40 injection (discontinued 1994) ℞ *corticosteroid* [triamcinolone acetonide] 40 mg/mL
Cenocort Forte injection (discontinued 1994) ℞ *corticosteroid* [triamcinolone diacetate] 40 mg/mL
Cenolate IV, IM, or subcu injection ℞ *antiscorbutic* [sodium ascorbate] 562.5 mg/mL
Centara ℞ *investigational treatment for arthritis and multiple sclerosis; transplant rejection preventative* [chimeric monoclonal antibody anti-CD4]
Center-Al subcu or IM injection ℞ *allergenic sensitivity testing (subcu); allergenic desensitization therapy (IM)* [allergenic extracts, alum-precipitated]
CenTNF ℞ *investigational treatment for sepsis, rheumatoid arthritis & Crohn's disease* [anti-TNF (tumor necrosis factor)]
CentoRx (name changed to ReoPro upon its release in 1995)
Centovir (orphan status withdrawn 1994) [human IgM monoclonal antibody (C-58) to cytomegalovirus (CMV)]
Centoxin ℞ *(orphan: gram-negative bacteremia in endotoxin shock)* [nebacumab]
Centrafree tablets OTC *antianemic* [ferrous fumarate; multiple vitamins]
Centrax capsules, tablets (discontinued 1995) ℞ *anxiolytic* [prazepam] 5, 10, 20 mg; 10 mg
centrazene [see: simtrazene]
centrophenoxine [see: meclofenoxate]
Centrovite Advanced Formula tablets (name changed to Cerovite Advanced Formula in 1995)
Centrovite Jr. tablets (name changed to Cerovite Jr. in 1995)
Centrum tablets OTC *antianemic* [ferrous fumarate; multiple vitamins]
Centrum, Advanced Formula liquid OTC *vitamin/mineral/iron supplement* [multiple vitamins & minerals; fer-

rous fumarate; biotin; alcohol 6.7%]
≐•9•0.3 mg/15 mL

Centrum, Advanced Formula tablets OTC *vitamin/mineral/iron supplement* [multiple vitamins & minerals; ferrous fumarate; folic acid; biotin] ≐•18 mg•0.4 mg•30 μg

Centrum Jr. + Extra C; Centrum Jr. + Extra Calcium chewable tablets OTC *vitamin/mineral/calcium/iron supplement* [multiple vitamins & minerals; calcium; iron; folic acid; biotin] ≐•108•18•0.4•0.045 mg; ≐•160•18•0.4•0.045 mg

Centrum Jr. with Iron tablets OTC *vitamin/mineral/iron supplement* [multiple vitamins & minerals; iron; folic acid; biotin] ≐•18 mg•0.4 mg•45 μg

Centrum Silver tablets OTC *geriatric vitamin/mineral supplement* [multiple vitamins & minerals; folic acid; biotin] ≐•400•30 μg

Centura ℞ *investigational treatment for multiple sclerosis* [monoclonal antibody IgG]

Centurion A-Z tablets (name changed to Multi-Vitamin Mineral with Beta-Carotene in 1995)

Ceo-Two suppository OTC *laxative* [sodium bicarbonate; potassium bitartrate]

CEP (CCNU, etoposide, prednimustine) *chemotherapy protocol*

Cēpacol mouthwash/gargle OTC *oral antiseptic* [cetylpyridinium chloride] 0.05%

Cēpacol Anesthetic troches OTC *topical oral anesthetic; antiseptic* [benzocaine; cetylpyridinium chloride] 10 mg•0.07%

Cēpacol Throat lozenges OTC *oral antiseptic* [cetylpyridinium chloride] 0.07%

Cēpastat Sore Throat lozenges OTC *topical antipruritic/counterirritant; mild local anesthetic* [phenol] 14.5, 29 mg ② Capastat

cephacetrile sodium USAN, USP *antibacterial* [also: cefacetrile]

cephalexin USAN, USP, BAN *bactericidal antibiotic* [also: cefalexin] ② cefazolin; cephalothin

cephalexin HCl USAN, USP *bactericidal antibiotic*

cephalexin HCl monohydrate *bactericidal antibiotic*

cephalexin monohydrate *bactericidal antibiotic* 250, 500, 1000 mg oral; 125, 250 mg/5 mL oral suspension

cephaloglycin USAN, USP, BAN *antibacterial* [also: cefaloglycin]

cephalonium BAN [also: cefalonium]

cephaloram BAN [also: cefaloram]

cephaloridine USAN, USP, BAN *antibacterial* [also: cefaloridine]

cephalosporin N [see: adicillin]

cephalothin BAN *bactericidal antibiotic* [also: cephalothin sodium; cefalotin] ② cefazolin; cephalexin

cephalothin sodium USAN, USP *bactericidal antibiotic* [also: cefalotin; cephalothin] 1, 2 g/vial injection

cephamandole BAN *antibacterial* [also: cefamandole]

cephamandole nafate BAN *antibacterial* [also: cefamandole nafate]

cephapirin sodium USAN, USP *bactericidal antibiotic* [also: cefapirin] 0.5, 1, 2, 4, 20 g/vial injection ② cephradine

cephazolin BAN *systemic antibacterial* [also: cefazolin]

cephazolin sodium BAN *systemic antibacterial* [also: cefazolin sodium]

cephoxazole BAN [also: cefoxazole]

cephradine USAN, USP, BAN *bactericidal antibiotic* [also: cefradine] 250, 500 mg oral; 125, 250 mg/5 mL oral ② cephapirin

Cephulac syrup ℞ *prevent and treat portal-systemic encephalopathy* [lactulose] 10 g/15 mL

Cepralan ℞ *investigational antiarrhythmic* [cifenline]

Ceprate SC ℞ *investigational stem cell concentration system for bone marrow transplants for breast cancer* [monoclonal antibodies]

Ceptaz powder for IV or IM injection ℞ *cephalosporin-type antibiotic* [ceftazidime pentahydrate] 1, 2, 10 g

ceramide trihexosidase (CTH) *(orphan: enzyme-replacement therapy for Fabry's disease)*

ceramide trihexosidase & alpha-galactosidase A *(orphan: Fabry's disease)*

ceranapril *investigational once-daily ACE inhibitor for hypertension; investigational treatment for dementia*

Cerebyx IV or IM injection ℞ *hydantoin-type anticonvulsant* [fosphenytoin sodium (phenytoin sodium equivalent)] 150 (100), 750 (500) mg/vial

CereCRIB ℞ *investigational analgesic* [cellular implants]

Ceredase IV infusion ℞ *enzyme replacement in Gaucher's disease (orphan)* [alglucerase] 10, 80 U/mL

cerelose [see: glucose]

Cerespan timed-release capsules (discontinued 1996) ℞ *peripheral vasodilator* [papaverine HCl] 150 mg

Cerestat ℞ *investigational treatment for stroke* [CNS 1102 (code name—generic name not yet approved)]

Cerezyme powder for IV infusion ℞ *enzyme replacement therapy for Gaucher's disease* [imiglucerase] 40 U/mL

cerium *element (Ce)*

cerium oxalate USP

ceronapril USAN, INN *antihypertensive*

Cerose-DM liquid OTC *antitussive; decongestant; antihistamine* [dextromethorphan hydrobromide; phenylephrine HCl; chlorpheniramine maleate; alcohol 2.4%] 15•10•4 mg/5 mL

Cerovite; Cerovite Advanced Formula tablets OTC *vitamin/mineral/iron supplement* [multiple vitamins & minerals; ferrous fumarate; folic acid; biotin] $\pm$ •18 mg•0.4 mg•30 μg

Cerovite Jr. tablets OTC *vitamin/mineral/iron supplement* [multiple vitamins & minerals; ferrous fumarate; folic acid; biotin] $\pm$ •18 mg•0.4 mg•45 μg

Cerovite Senior tablets OTC *geriatric vitamin/mineral supplement* [multiple vitamins and minerals; folic acid; biotin] $\pm$ •200•30 μg

Certagen film-coated tablets OTC *vitamin/mineral/iron supplement* [multiple vitamins & minerals; ferrous fumarate; folic acid; biotin] $\pm$ •18 mg•0.4 mg•30 μg

Certagen liquid OTC *vitamin/mineral/iron supplement* [multiple vitamins & minerals; iron; biotin; alcohol 6.6%] $\pm$ •9•0.3 mg

Certagen Senior tablets OTC *geriatric vitamin/mineral supplement* [multiple vitamins & minerals; folic acid; biotin] $\pm$ •200•30 μg

CertaVite tablets OTC *vitamin/mineral/iron supplement* [multiple vitamins & minerals; ferrous fumarate; folic acid; biotin] $\pm$ •18 mg•0.4 mg•30 μg

Certa-Vite Golden tablets OTC *geriatric vitamin/mineral supplement* [multiple vitamins & minerals; biotin] $\pm$ •30 μg

Cerubidine powder for IV injection (discontinued 1996) ℞ *antibiotic antineoplastic for multiple nonlymphocytic leukemias* [daunorubicin HCl] 20 mg

ceruletide USAN, INN, BAN *gastric secretory stimulant*

ceruletide diethylamine USAN *gastric secretory stimulant*

Cerumenex ear drops ℞ *agent to emulsify and disperse ear wax* [trolamine polypeptide oleate-condensate] 10%

Cervene injection ℞ *investigational treatment for stroke, benzodiazepine-induced hypotension, and opiate reversal* [nalmefene]

Cervidil vaginal insert ℞ *prostaglandin for cervical ripening at term* [dinoprostone] 10 mg

cesium *element (Cs)*

cesium (^{131}Cs) chloride INN *radioactive agent* [also: cesium chloride Cs 131]

cesium chloride Cs 131 USAN *radioactive agent* [also: cesium (^{131}Cs) chloride]

Ceta liquid OTC *soap-free therapeutic skin cleanser*

Ceta Plus capsules ℞ *narcotic analgesic* [hydrocodone bitartrate; acetaminophen] 5•500 mg

cetaben INN *antihyperlipoproteinemic* [also: cetaben sodium]

cetaben sodium USAN *antihyperlipoproteinemic* [also: cetaben]

Cetacaine gel, liquid, ointment, aerosol ℞ *topical local anesthetic; antiseptic* [benzocaine; tetracaine HCl; butamben] 14%•2%•2%

Cetacort lotion ℞ *topical corticosteroid* [hydrocortisone] 0.25%, 0.5%, 1%

cetalkonium *antiseptic*

cetalkonium chloride USAN, INN, BAN *topical anti-infective*

Cetamide ophthalmic ointment ℞ *ophthalmic bacteriostatic* [sulfacetamide sodium] 10%

cetamolol INN *antiadrenergic (β-receptor)* [also: cetamolol HCl]

cetamolol HCl USAN *antiadrenergic (β-receptor)* [also: cetamolol]

Cetane timed-release capsules (discontinued 1992) OTC *vitamin supplement* [ascorbic acid] 500 mg

Cetaphil cream, lotion OTC *soap-free therapeutic skin cleanser*

Cetapred ophthalmic ointment ℞ *ophthalmic topical corticosteroidal antiinflammatory; bacteriostatic* [prednisolone acetate; sulfacetamide sodium] 0.25%•10%

cethexonium chloride INN

cetiedil INN *peripheral vasodilator* [also: cetiedil citrate]

cetiedil citrate USAN *peripheral vasodilator; (orphan status withdrawn 1993)* [also: cetiedil]

cetirizine INN, BAN *antihistamine* [also: cetirizine HCl]

cetirizine HCl USAN *antihistamine* [also: cetirizine]

cetobemidone [see: ketobemidone]

cetocycline INN *antibacterial* [also: cetocycline HCl]

cetocycline HCl USAN *antibacterial* [also: cetocycline]

cetofenicol INN *antibacterial* [also: cetophenicol]

cetohexazine INN

cetomacrogol 1000 INN, BAN

cetophenicol USAN *antibacterial* [also: cetofenicol]

cetophenylbutazone [see: kebuzone]

cetostearyl alcohol NF *emulsifying agent*

cetotetrine HCl [now: cetocycline HCl]

cetotiamine INN

cetoxime INN, BAN

cetoxime HCl [see: cetoxime]

cetraxate INN *GI antiulcerative* [also: cetraxate HCl]

cetraxate HCl USAN *GI antiulcerative* [also: cetraxate]

cetrimide INN, BAN

cetrimonium bromide INN *topical antiseptic* [also: cetrimonium chloride]

cetrimonium chloride BAN *topical antiseptic* [also: cetrimonium bromide]

cetyl alcohol NF *emulsifying and stiffening agent*

cetyl esters wax NF *stiffening agent*

cetyldimethylbenzyl ammonium chloride [see: cetalkonium chloride]

cetylpyridinium chloride USP, INN, BAN *topical antiseptic; preservative*

cetyltrimethyl ammonium bromide

CEV (cyclophosphamide, etoposide, vincristine) *chemotherapy protocol*

Cevalin IV, IM, or subcu injection ℞ *antiscorbutic* [ascorbic acid] 500 mg/mL

Cevi-Bid timed-release capsules OTC *vitamin supplement* [ascorbic acid] 500 mg

Cevi-Fer timed-release capsules ℞ *hematinic* [ferrous fumarate; ascorbic acid; folic acid] 20•300•1 mg

Ce-Vi-Sol drops OTC *vitamin supplement* [ascorbic acid; alcohol 5%] 35 mg/0.6 mL

cevitamic acid [see: ascorbic acid]

cevitan [see: ascorbic acid]

ceylon gelatin [see: agar]

Cezin capsules OTC *vitamin/mineral supplement* [multiple vitamins & minerals]

Cezin-S capsules ℞ *geriatric vitamin/mineral supplement* [multiple vitamins & minerals; folic acid] ± •0.5 mg

CF (carboplatin, fluorouracil) *chemotherapy protocol*

CF (cisplatin, fluorouracil) *chemotherapy protocol*

CFL (cisplatin, fluorouracil, leucovorin [rescue]) *chemotherapy protocol*

CFM (cyclophosphamide, fluorouracil, mitoxantrone) *chemotherapy protocol* [also: CNF; FNC]

CFP (cyclophosphamide, fluorouracil, prednisone) *chemotherapy protocol*

CFPT (cyclophosphamide, fluorouracil, prednisone, tamoxifen) *chemotherapy protocol*

CFTR (cystic fibrosis transmembrane conductance regulator) [q.v.]
CG (Cardio-Green) [q.v.]
CG (chorionic gonadotropin) [see: gonadotropin, chorionic]
C-Gel soft capsules OTC *vitamin supplement* [vitamin C]
CGF (Control Gel Formula) dressing [see: DuoDERM CGF]
CGP 57701 ℞ *investigational penem antibiotic*
CH1VPP; Ch1VPP (chlorambucil, vinblastine, procarbazine, prednisone) *chemotherapy protocol*
CHAD (cyclophosphamide, hexamethylmelamine, Adriamycin, DDP) *chemotherapy protocol*
chalk, precipitated [see: calcium carbonate, precipitated]
CHAMOCA (Cytoxan, hydroxyurea, actinomycin D, methotrexate, Oncovin, calcium folinate, Adriamycin) *chemotherapy protocol*
CHAP (cyclophosphamide, Hexalen, Adriamycin, Platinol) *chemotherapy protocol*
CHAP (cyclophosphamide, hexamethylmelamine, Adriamycin, Platinol) *chemotherapy protocol*
Chap Stick Medicated Lip Balm stick, jar, squeezable tube OTC *counterirritant; moisturizer; protectant; emollient* [camphor; menthol; phenol] 1%•0.6%•0.5%
CharcoAid oral suspension OTC *adsorbent antidote for poisoning* [activated charcoal] 15 g/120 mL, 30 g/150 mL
CharcoAid 2000 oral liquid, granules OTC *adsorbent antidote for poisoning* [activated charcoal] 15 g/120 mL, 50 g/240 mL; 15 g
charcoal *gastric adsorbent/detoxicant; antiflatulent* 260 mg oral
charcoal, activated USP *general purpose antidote/adsorbent* 15, 30, 40, 120, 240 g, 208 mg/mL oral
Charcoal Plus enteric-coated tablets OTC *adsorbent; detoxicant; antiflatulent* [activated charcoal; simethicone] 200•40 mg

CharcoCaps capsules OTC *adsorbent; detoxicant; antiflatulent* [charcoal] 260 mg
Chardonna-2 tablets ℞ *GI anticholinergic; sedative* [belladonna extract; phenobarbital] 15•15 mg
chaulmosulfone INN
Chealamide IV infusion ℞ *calcium-lowering agent; antiarrhythmic for digitalis toxicity* [edetate disodium] 150 mg/mL
Checkmate gel (discontinued 1992) ℞ *topical dental caries preventative* [acidulated phosphate fluoride]
chelafrin [see: epinephrine]
Chelated Magnesium tablets OTC *magnesium supplement* [magnesium amino acid chelate] 500 mg
Chelated Manganese tablets OTC *manganese supplement* [manganese] 20, 50 mg
chelen [see: ethyl chloride]
Chemet capsules ℞ *heavy metal chelating agent; (orphan: cystine kidney stones; lead and mercury poisoning)* [succimer] 100 mg
Chemo-Pin (trademarked form) *chemical-dispensing pin*
Chemstrip 2 GP; Chemstrip 2 LN; Chemstrip 4 the OB; Chemstrip 6; Chemstrip 7; Chemstrip 8; Chemstrip 9; Chemstrip 10 with SG; Chemstrip uGK reagent strips *in vitro diagnostic aid for multiple urine products*
Chemstrip bG reagent strips for home use OTC *in vitro diagnostic aid for blood glucose*
Chemstrip K reagent strips for professional use *in vitro diagnostic aid for acetone (ketones) in the urine*
Chemstrip Micral reagent strips for professional use *in vitro diagnostic aid for albumin (protein) in the urine*
Chemstrip uG reagent strips for home use OTC *in vitro diagnostic aid for urine glucose*
Chenatal tablets OTC *prenatal vitamin/mineral supplement* [multiple vitamins & minerals]
chenic acid [now: chenodiol]

Chenix tablets (discontinued 1994) ℞ *anticholelithogenic; for radiolucent gallstones (orphan)* [chenodiol] 250 mg

chenodeoxycholic acid INN, BAN *anticholelithogenic* [also: chenodiol]

chenodiol USAN *anticholelithogenic; for radiolucent gallstones (orphan)* [also: chenodeoxycholic acid]

Cheracol Cough syrup ℞ *narcotic antitussive; expectorant* [codeine phosphate; guaifenesin; alcohol 1.75%] 10•100 mg/5 mL

Cheracol D Cough liquid OTC *antitussive; expectorant* [dextromethorphan hydrobromide; guaifenesin; alcohol 4.75%] 10•100 mg/5 mL

Cheracol Nasal spray OTC *nasal decongestant* [oxymetazoline HCl] 0.05%

Cheracol Plus liquid OTC *antitussive; decongestant; antihistamine* [dextromethorphan hydrobromide; phenylpropanolamine HCl; chlorpheniramine maleate; alcohol 8%] 6.7•8.3•1.3 mg/5 mL

Cheracol Sinus sustained-action tablets (discontinued 1995) OTC *decongestant; antihistamine* [pseudoephedrine sulfate; dexbrompheniramine maleate] 120•6 mg

Cheracol Sore Throat spray OTC *topical antipruritic/counterirritant; mild local anesthetic* [phenol] 1.4%

Cheralin Expectorant liquid (discontinued 1994) OTC *expectorant* [potassium guaiacolsulfonate; ammonium chloride; antimony potassium tartrate; alcohol]

Cheralin with Codeine liquid (discontinued 1994) ℞ *narcotic antitussive; expectorant* [codeine phosphate; potassium guaiacolsulfonate; ammonium chloride; antimony potassium tartrate]

Cherapas tablets (discontinued 1993) ℞ *antihypertensive* [hydrochlorothiazide; reserpine; hydralazine HCl]

cherry juice NF

Chewable C chewable tablets OTC *vitamin supplement* [sodium ascorbate & ascorbic acid] 100, 250, 300, 500 mg

Chewable Multivitamins with Fluoride tablets ℞ *pediatric vitamin supplement and dental caries preventative* [multiple vitamins; fluoride; folic acid] ≟•1•0.3 mg

Chewable Triple Vitamins with Fluoride tablets ℞ *pediatric vitamin supplement and dental caries preventative* [vitamins A, C, and D; fluoride] 2500 IU•60 mg•400 IU•1 mg

Chew-C chewable tablets OTC *vitamin supplement* [sodium ascorbate; ascorbic acid]

Chew-Vites chewable tablets OTC *vitamin supplement* [multiple vitamins; folic acid]

ChexUP; Chex-Up; CHEX-UP (cyclophosphamide, hexamethylmelamine, fluorouracil, Platinol) *chemotherapy protocol*

CHF (cyclophosphamide, hexamethylmelamine, fluorouracil) *chemotherapy protocol*

Chibroxin Ocumeter (eye drops) ℞ *ophthalmic antibiotic* [norfloxacin] 3 mg/mL

Chiggerex ointment OTC *topical local anesthetic; counterirritant* [benzocaine; camphor; menthol] ≟

Chigger-Tox liquid OTC *topical local anesthetic* [benzocaine] ≟

Children's Formula Cough syrup OTC *pediatric antitussive and expectorant* [dextromethorphan hydrobromide; guaifenesin] 5•50 mg/5 mL

chillifolinum [see: quillifoline]

chimeric (murine variable, human constant) MAb to CD20 (*orphan: non-Hodgkin's B-cell lymphoma*)

chimeric L6 monoclonal antibodies *investigational chemotherapy rescue agent*

chimeric M-T412 (human-murine) IgG monoclonal anti-CD4 (*orphan: multiple sclerosis*)

Chinese gelatin [see: agar]

Chinese isinglass [see: chiniofon]

chinethazone [see: quinethazone]

chiniofon NF, INN

chitosan [see: poliglusam]

CHL + PRED (chlorambucil, prednisone) *chemotherapy protocol*

Chlamydiazyme reagent kit for professional use *in vitro diagnostic aid for*

Chlamydia trachomatis [solid phase enzyme immunoassay]

Chlo-Amine chewable tablets ℞ *antihistamine* [chlorpheniramine maleate] 2 mg

chlophedianol BAN *antitussive* [also: chlophedianol HCl; clofedanol]

chlophedianol HCl USAN *antitussive* [also: clofedanol; chlophedianol]

chlophenadione [see: clorindione]

chloquinate [see: cloquinate]

Chlor-100 injection ℞ *antihistamine; anaphylaxis* [chlorpheniramine maleate] 100 mg/mL

chloracyzine INN

Chlorafed liquid OTC *decongestant; antihistamine* [pseudoephedrine HCl; chlorpheniramine maleate] 30•2 mg/5 mL

Chlorafed; Chlorafed HS Timecelles (sustained-release capsules) ℞ *decongestant; antihistamine* [pseudoephedrine HCl; chlorpheniramine maleate] 120•8 mg; 60•4 mg

chloral betaine USAN, NF, BAN *sedative* [also: cloral betaine]

chloral hydrate USP, BAN *hypnotic; sedative* 500 mg oral; 250, 500 mg/5 mL oral

chloral hydrate betaine [see: chloral betaine]

chloralformamide USP

chloralodol INN [also: chlorhexadol]

chloralose (α-chloralose) INN

chloralurethane [see: carbocloral]

chlorambucil USP, INN, BAN *alkylating antineoplastic*

chloramidobenzol [see: clofenamide]

chloramine [now: chloramine-T]

chloramine-T NF [also: tosylchloramide sodium]

chloramiphene [see: clomiphene citrate]

chloramphenicol USP, INN, BAN, JAN *bacteriostatic antibiotic; antirickettsial* 250 mg oral; 5 mg/mL eye drops; 10 mg/g topical

chloramphenicol palmitate USP, JAN *antibacterial; antirickettsial* 150 mg/5 mL oral

chloramphenicol pantothenate complex USAN *antibacterial; antirickettsial* [also: cloramfenicol pantotenate complex]

chloramphenicol sodium succinate USP, JAN *antibacterial; antirickettsial* 100 mg/mL injection

chloranautine [see: dimenhydrinate]

chlorarsen [see: dichlorophenarsine HCl]

Chloraseptic lozenges, throat spray (discontinued 1994) OTC *topical antipruritic/counterirritant; mild local anesthetic* [phenol] 32.5 mg; 1.4%

Chloraseptic mouthwash/gargle OTC *topical antipruritic/counterirritant; mild local anesthetic* [phenol] 1.4%

Chloraseptic, Children's lozenges OTC *topical oral anesthetic* [benzocaine] 5 mg

Chloraseptic, Children's throat spray OTC *topical antipruritic/counterirritant; mild local anesthetic* [phenol] 0.5%

Chloraseptic Sore Throat lozenges OTC *topical oral anesthetic; antipruritic/counterirritant* [benzocaine; menthol] 6•10 mg

Chlorate tablets OTC *antihistamine* [chlorpheniramine maleate] 4 mg

chlorazanil INN

chlorazanil HCl [see: chlorazanil]

chlorazodin INN [also: chloroazodin]

chlorazone [see: chloramine-T]

chlorbenzoxamine INN

chlorbenzoxamine HCl [see: chlorbenzoxamine]

chlorbetamide INN, BAN

chlorbutanol [see: chlorobutanol]

chlorbutin [see: chlorambucil]

chlorbutol BAN *antimicrobial agent* [also: chlorobutanol]

chlorcinnazine [see: clocinizine]

chlorcyclizine INN, BAN *antihistamine* [also: chlorcyclizine HCl]

chlorcyclizine HCl USP *antihistamine* [also: chlorcyclizine]

chlordantoin USAN, BAN *antifungal* [also: clodantoin]

chlordiazepoxide USP, INN, BAN *anxiolytic; minor tranquilizer; alcohol withdrawal therapy*

chlordiazepoxide HCl USAN, USP, BAN *sedative* 5, 10, 25 mg oral

chlordimorine INN

Chlordrine S.R. sustained-release capsules ℞ *decongestant; antihistamine* [pseudoephedrine HCl; chlorpheniramine maleate] 120•8 mg

Chloresium ointment, solution OTC *vulnerary and deodorant for wounds, burns, and ulcers* [chlorophyllin copper complex] 0.5%; 0.2%

Chloresium tablets OTC *systemic deodorant for ostomy, breath, and body odors* [chlorophyllin copper complex] 14 mg

chlorethate [see: clorethate]

chlorethyl [see: ethyl chloride]

chlorfenisate [see: clofibrate]

chlorfenvinphos BAN [also: clofenvinfos]

Chlorgest-HD liquid ℞ *narcotic antitussive; decongestant; antihistamine* [hydrocodone bitartrate; phenylephrine HCl; chlorpheniramine maleate] 1.67•5•4 mg/5 mL

chlorguanide HCl [see: chloroguanide HCl]

chlorhexadol BAN [also: chloralodol]

chlorhexidine INN, BAN *antimicrobial* [also: chlorhexidine gluconate]

chlorhexidine gluconate USAN *antimicrobial; (orphan: oral mucositis)* [also: chlorhexidine]

chlorhexidine HCl USAN, BAN *topical anti-infective*

chlorhexidine phosphanilate USAN *antibacterial*

chlorimiphenin [see: imiclopazine]

chlorimpiphenine [see: imiclopazine]

chlorinated & iodized peanut oil [see: chloriodized oil]

chlorindanol USAN *spermaticide* [also: clorindanol]

chlorine *element (Cl)*

chloriodized oil USP

chlorisondamine chloride INN, BAN

chlorisondamone chloride [see: chlorisondamine chloride]

chlormadinone INN, BAN *progestin* [also: chlormadinone acetate]

chlormadinone acetate USAN, NF *progestin* [also: chlormadinone]

chlormerodrin NF, INN, BAN

chlormerodrin (^{197}Hg) INN *renal function test; radioactive agent* [also: chlormerodrin Hg 197]

chlormerodrin Hg 197 USAN, USP *renal function test; radioactive agent* [also: chlormerodrin (^{197}Hg)]

chlormerodrin Hg 203 USAN, USP *renal function test; radioactive agent*

chlormeroprin [see: chlormerodrin]

chlormethazanone [see: chlormezanone]

chlormethiazole BAN [also: clomethiazole]

chlormethine INN *alkylating antineoplastic* [also: mechlorethamine HCl; mustine; nitrogen mustard N-oxide HCl]

chlormethylencycline [see: clomocycline]

chlormezanone INN, BAN *mild anxiolytic*

chlormidazole INN, BAN

chlornaphazine INN

chloroacetic acid [see: monochloroacetic, dichloroacetic, or trichloroacetic acid]

chloroazodin USP [also: chlorazodin]

5-chlorobenzoxazolinone [see: chlorzoxazone]

chlorobutanol NF, INN *antimicrobial agent; preservative* [also: chlorbutol]

8-chlorocamp *investigational antineoplastic*

chlorochine [see: chloroquine]

chlorocresol USAN, NF, INN *antiseptic; disinfectant*

2-chloro-2'-deoxyadenosine (CdA) [now: cladribine]

chlorodeoxylincomycin [see: clindamycin]

chloroethane [see: ethyl chloride]

chloroform NF *solvent*

chloroguanide HCl USP [also: proguanil]

chloroguanide triazine pamoate [see: cycloguanil pamoate]

chloro-iodohydroxyquinoline [see: clioquinol]

chlorolincomycin [see: clindamycin]

chloromethapyrilene citrate [see: chlorothen citrate]

Chloromycetin cream (discontinued 1994) ℞ *broad-spectrum topical antibiotic* [chloramphenicol] 1%

Chloromycetin Kapseals (capsules) (discontinued 1996) ℞ *broad-spectrum bacteriostatic antibiotic* [chloramphenicol] 250 mg

Chloromycetin powder for eye drops, ophthalmic ointment ℞ *ophthalmic antibiotic* [chloramphenicol] 25 mg/15 mL; 10 mg/g

Chloromycetin Hydrocortisone powder for eye drops ℞ *ophthalmic topical corticosteroidal anti-inflammatory; broad-spectrum antibiotic* [hydrocortisone acetate; chloramphenicol] 0.5%•0.25%

Chloromycetin Otic ear drops ℞ *broad-spectrum antibiotic* [chloramphenicol] 0.5%

Chloromycetin Palmitate oral suspension (discontinued 1994) ℞ *broad-spectrum bacteriostatic antibiotic* [chloramphenicol palmitate] 150 mg/5 mL

Chloromycetin Sodium Succinate powder for IV injection ℞ *broad-spectrum bacteriostatic antibiotic* [chloramphenicol sodium succinate] 100 mg/mL

p-**chlorophenol** [see: parachlorophenol]

chlorophenothane NF [also: clofenotane; dicophane]

chlorophenoxamide [see: clefamide]

chlorophenylmercury [see: phenylmercuric chloride]

chlorophyll, water soluble [see: chlorophyllin]

chlorophyllin *vulnerary; deodorant for wounds and ulcers (topical); for ostomy, breath, and body odors (oral)* 20 mg oral

chlorophyllin copper complex USAN *deodorant for wounds and ulcers (topical); for ostomy, breath, and body odors (oral)*

chloroprednisone INN

chloroprednisone acetate [see: chloroprednisone]

chloroprocaine INN *local anesthetic* [also: chloroprocaine HCl]

chloroprocaine HCl USP *injectable local anesthetic* [also: chloroprocaine]

Chloroptic eye drops ℞ *ophthalmic antibiotic* [chloramphenicol] 5 mg/mL

Chloroptic S.O.P. ophthalmic ointment ℞ *ophthalmic antibiotic* [chloramphenicol] 10 mg/g

chloropyramine INN [also: halopyramine]

chloropyrilene INN, BAN [also: chlorothen citrate]

chloroquine USP, INN, BAN *antiamebic; antimalarial*

chloroquine diphosphate [see: chloroquine phosphate]

chloroquine HCl USP *amebicide; antimalarial* [also: chloroquine]

chloroquine phosphate USP, BAN *antimalarial; amebicide; lupus erythematosus suppressant* 250 mg oral

chloroserpidine INN

Chloroserpine tablets (discontinued 1995) ℞ *antihypertensive* [chlorothiazide; reserpine] 250•0.125 mg

N-**chlorosuccinimide** [see: succinchlorimide]

chlorothen citrate NF [also: chloropyrilene]

chlorothenium citrate [see: chlorothen citrate]

chlorothenylpyramine [see: chlorothen]

chlorothiazide USP, INN, BAN *diuretic; antihypertensive* 250, 500 mg oral

chlorothiazide sodium USAN, USP *diuretic; antihypertensive*

chlorothymol NF

chlorotrianisene USP, INN, BAN *estrogen for hormone replacement therapy or inoperable prostatic cancer*

chloroxine USAN *antiseborrheic*

chloroxylenol USP, INN, BAN *bacteriostatic*

chlorozone [see: chloramine-T]

chlorpenthixol [see: clopenthixol]

Chlorphed-LA nasal spray OTC *nasal decongestant* [oxymetazoline HCl] 0.05%

Chlorphedrine SR sustained-release capsules ℞ *decongestant; antihistamine* [pseudoephedrine HCl; chlorpheniramine maleate] 120•8 mg

chlorphenamine INN *antihistamine* [also: chlorpheniramine maleate; chlorpheniramine]

chlorphenamine maleate [see: chlorpheniramine maleate]

chlorphenecyclane [see: clofenciclan]

chlorphenesin INN, BAN *skeletal muscle relaxant* [also: chlorphenesin carbamate]

chlorphenesin carbamate USAN, JAN *skeletal muscle relaxant* [also: chlorphenesin]

chlorphenindione [see: clorindione]

chlorpheniramine BAN *antihistamine* [also: chlorpheniramine maleate; chlorphenamine] ⑦ chlorphentermine

chlorpheniramine maleate USP *antihistamine* [also: chlorphenamine; chlorpheniramine] 4, 8, 12 mg oral; 2 mg/5 mL oral; 100 mg/mL injection

chlorpheniramine polistirex USAN *antihistamine*

chlorpheniramine tannate

chlorphenoctium amsonate INN, BAN

chlorphenotane [see: chlorophenothane]

chlorphenoxamine INN, BAN [also: chlorphenoxamine HCl]

chlorphenoxamine HCl USP [also: chlorphenoxamine]

chlorphentermine INN, BAN *anorectic* [also: chlorphentermine HCl] ⑦ chlorpheniramine

chlorphentermine HCl USAN *anorectic* [also: chlorphentermine]

chlorphenylindandione [see: clorindione]

chlorphthalidone [see: chlorthalidone]

Chlor-Pro injection ℞ *antihistamine* [chlorpheniramine maleate] 10, 100 mg/mL

chlorprocaine chloride [see: chloroprocaine HCl]

chlorproethazine INN [also: chlorproethazine HCl]

chlorproethazine HCl [also: chlorproethazine]

chlorproguanil INN, BAN

chlorproguanil HCl [see: chlorproguanil]

chlorpromazine USP, INN, BAN *antiemetic; antipsychotic; antidopaminergic; intractable hiccough relief*

chlorpromazine HCl USP, BAN *antiemetic; antipsychotic; intractable hiccough relief* 10, 25, 50, 100, 200 mg oral; 10 mg/5 mL oral; 30, 100 mg/mL oral; 25 mg/mL injection

chlorpropamide USP, INN, BAN *sulfonylurea-type antidiabetic* 100, 250 mg oral

chlorprophenpyridamine maleate [see: chlorpheniramine maleate]

chlorprothixene USAN, USP, INN, BAN *antipsychotic*

chlorprothixene HCl *antipsychotic*

chlorprothixene lactate *antipsychotic*

chlorpyrifos BAN

chlorquinaldol INN, BAN

Chlor-Rest tablets OTC *decongestant; antihistamine* [phenylpropanolamine HCl; chlorpheniramine maleate] 18.7•2 mg

Chlorspan-12 timed-release capsules ℞ *antihistamine* [chlorpheniramine maleate] 12 mg

Chlortab-4 tablets (discontinued 1996) ℞ *antihistamine* [chlorpheniramine maleate] 4 mg

Chlortab-8 timed-release tablets (discontinued 1996) ℞ *antihistamine* [chlorpheniramine maleate] 8 mg

chlortalidone INN *diuretic* [also: chlorthalidone]

Chlor-Tel Slocaps (sustained-release capsules) ℞ *antihistamine* [chlorpheniramine maleate]

chlortetracycline INN, BAN *antibacterial antibiotic; antiprotozoal* [also: chlortetracycline bisulfate]

chlortetracycline bisulfate USP *antibacterial; antiprotozoal* [also: chlortetracycline]

chlortetracycline calcium

chlortetracycline HCl USP, BAN *antibacterial antibiotic; antiprotozoal*

chlorthalidone USAN, USP, BAN *diuretic; antihypertensive* [also: chlortalidone] 25, 50, 100 mg oral

chlorthenoxazin BAN [also: chlorthenoxazine]

chlorthenoxazine INN [also: chlorthenoxazin]

chlorthiazide [see: chlorothiazide]

chlortrianisestrol [see: chlorotrianisene]

Chlor-Trimeton Repetabs (repeat-action tablets) (name changed to

Chlor-Trimeton 12 Hour Allergy in 1993)

Chlor-Trimeton tablets, syrup, injection OTC *antihistamine; anaphylaxis (IV only)* [chlorpheniramine maleate] 4 mg; 2 mg/5 mL; 10 mg/mL

Chlor-Trimeton 4 Hour Relief tablets OTC *decongestant; antihistamine* [pseudoephedrine sulfate; chlorpheniramine maleate] 60•4 mg

Chlor-Trimeton 8 Hour Allergy; Chlor-Trimeton 12 Hour Allergy timed-release tablets OTC *antihistamine* [chlorpheniramine maleate] 8 mg; 12 mg

Chlor-Trimeton 12 Hour Relief sustained-release tablets OTC *decongestant; antihistamine* [pseudoephedrine sulfate; chlorpheniramine maleate] 120•8 mg

Chlor-Trimeton Allergy tablets OTC *antihistamine* [chlorpheniramine maleate] 4 mg

Chlor-Trimeton Allergy-Sinus caplets OTC *decongestant; antihistamine; analgesic* [phenylpropanolamine HCl; chlorpheniramine maleate; acetaminophen] 12.5•2•500 mg

Chlor-Trimeton Decongestant (name changed to Chlor-Trimeton 4 Hour Relief & 12 Hour Relief in 1992)

Chlor-Trimeton Sinus caplets (name changed to Chlor-Trimeton Allergy-Sinus in 1993)

chlorzoxazone USP, INN, BAN, JAN *skeletal muscle relaxant* 250, 500 mg oral

chlosudimeprimylum [see: clopamide]

ChlVPP (chlorambucil, vinblastine, procarbazine, prednisone) *chemotherapy protocol*

ChlVPP/EVA (chlorambucil, vinblastine, procarbazine, prednisone, etoposide, vincristine, Adriamycin) *chemotherapy protocol*

CHO (cyclophosphamide, hydroxydaunomycin, Oncovin) *chemotherapy protocol*

CHO cells, recombinant [see: CD4, human truncated]

CHOB (cyclophosphamide, hydroxydaunomycin, Oncovin, bleomycin) *chemotherapy protocol*

CHOD (cyclophosphamide, hydroxydaunomycin, Oncovin, dexamethasone) *chemotherapy protocol*

Choice dm oral liquid OTC *enteral nutritional therapy for abnormal glucose tolerance* [lactose-free formula] 240 mL

Cholac syrup ℞ *prevent and treat portal-systemic encephalopathy* [lactulose] 10 g/15 mL

cholalic acid [see: dehydrocholic acid]

Cholan-DH tablets (discontinued 1992) OTC *laxative; hydrocholeretic* [dehydrocholic acid]

Cholan-HMB tablets OTC *laxative; hydrocholeretic* [dehydrocholic acid] 250 mg

Cholebrine tablets ℞ *oral cholecystographic radiopaque agent* [iocetamic acid] 750 mg

cholecalciferol USP, BAN, JAN *vitamin D_3; antirachitic* [also: colecalciferol] 1000 IU oral

Choledyl tablets, pediatric syrup, elixir (discontinued 1996) ℞ *bronchodilator* [oxtriphylline] 100, 200 mg; 50 mg/5 mL; 100 mg/5 mL

Choledyl SA sustained-action tablets ℞ *bronchodilator* [oxtriphylline] 400, 600 mg

cholera vaccine USP *active bacterin for cholera (Vibrio cholerae)* 16 U/mL SC or IM injection

cholesterin [see: cholesterol]

cholesterol NF *emulsifying agent*

cholestrin [see: cholesterol]

cholestyramine BAN *bile salts ion-exchange resin; antihyperlipoproteinemic* [also: cholestyramine resin; colestyramine]

cholestyramine resin USP *bile salts ion-exchange resin; antihyperlipoproteinemic* [also: colestyramine; cholestyramine]

cholic acid [see: dehydrocholic acid]

Cholidase tablets OTC *dietary lipotropic with vitamin supplementation* [choline; inositol; vitamins B_6, B_{12}, and E] 185•150•2.5•0.005•7.5 mg

choline *dietary lipotropic supplement* 250, 300, 500, 650 mg oral
choline alfoscerate INN
choline bitartrate NF 250 mg oral
choline bromide hexamethylenedicarbamate [see: hexacarbacholine bromide]
choline chloride INN *(orphan: choline deficiency of long-term parenteral nutrition)*
choline chloride acetate [see: acetylcholine chloride]
choline chloride carbamate [see: carbachol]
choline chloride succinate [see: succinylcholine chloride]
choline dihydrogen citrate NF 650 mg oral
choline gluconate INN
choline glycerophosphate [see: choline alfoscerate]
choline magnesium trisalicylate (choline salicylate + magnesium salicylate) [q.v.] 500, 750, 1000 mg (293•362, 440•544, 587•725 mg) oral
choline perchlorate, nitrate ester [see: nitricholine perchlorate]
choline salicylate USAN, INN, BAN *analgesic; antipyretic; anti-inflammatory; antirheumatic*
choline theophyllinate INN, BAN *bronchodilator* [also: oxtriphylline]
Cholinoid capsules OTC *dietary lipotropic with vitamin supplementation* [choline; inositol; multiple B vitamins; vitamin C; lemon bioflavonoids] 111•111• ± •100•100 mg
Cholografin Meglumine injection ℞ *parenteral cholecystographic and cholangiographic radiopaque agent* [iodipamide meglumine] 10.3%, 52%
Choloxin tablets ℞ *antihyperlipidemic (cholesterol-lowering)* [dextrothyroxine sodium] 2, 4, 6 mg
Cholybar resin bar (discontinued 1994) ℞ *cholesterol-lowering antihyperlipidemic* [cholestyramine resin] 4 g
chondodendron tomentosum [see: tubocurarine chloride]
chondroitin 4-sulfate [see: danaparoid sodium]

chondroitin 6-sulfate [see: danaparoid sodium]
chondroitin sulfate sodium JAN
Chooz chewable tablets OTC *antacid* [calcium carbonate] 500 mg
CHOP (cyclophosphamide, hydroxydaunomycin, Oncovin, prednisone) *chemotherapy protocol*
CHOP-BLEO (cyclophosphamide, hydroxydaunomycin, Oncovin, prednisone, bleomycin) *chemotherapy protocol*
CHOPE (cyclophosphamide, hydroxydaunomycin, Oncovin, prednisone, etoposide) *chemotherapy protocol*
CHOR (cyclophosphamide, hydroxydaunomycin, Oncovin, radiation therapy) *chemotherapy protocol*
Chorex-5; Chorex-10 powder for IM injection ℞ *hormone for prepubertal cryptorchidism and hypogonadism; ovulation stimulant* [chorionic gonadotropin] 500 U/mL; 1000 U/mL
Chorigon powder for injection (discontinued 1995) ℞ *hormone for prepubertal cryptorchidism and hypogonadism* [chorionic gonadotropin] 1000 U/mL
chorionic gonadotrophin [see: gonadotropin, chorionic]
chorionic gonadotropin (CG) [see: gonadotropin, chorionic]
Choron-10 powder for IM injection ℞ *hormone for prepubertal cryptorchidism and hypogonadism; ovulation stimulant* [chorionic gonadotropin] 1000 U/mL
CHP (chlorhexidine phosphanilate) [q.v.]
Christmas factor [see: factor IX complex]
Chromagen capsules ℞ *hematinic* [ferrous fumarate; cyanocobalamin; ascorbic acid; intrinsic factor concentrate] 66 mg•10 µg•250 mg•100 mg
Chromagen OB capsules (discontinued 1992) OTC *vitamin/mineral/iron supplement* [multiple vitamins & minerals; iron; folic acid]

Chroma-Pak IV injection ℞ *intravenous nutritional therapy* [chromic chloride hexahydrate] 20.5, 102.5 μg/mL

chromargyre [see: merbromin]

chromated albumin [see: albumin, chromated Cr 51 serum]

Chromelin Complexion Blender OTC *skin darkening agent for vitiligo and hypopigmented areas* [dihydroxyacetone] 5%

chromic acid, disodium salt [see: sodium chromate Cr 51]

chromic chloride USP *dietary chromium supplement* 4, 20 μg/mL injection

chromic chloride Cr 51 USAN *radioactive agent*

chromic chloride hexahydrate [see: chromic chloride]

chromic phosphate Cr 51 USAN *radioactive agent*

chromic phosphate P 32 USAN, USP *antineoplastic; radioactive agent*

chromium *element (Cr)*

Chromium Chloride IV injection ℞ *intravenous nutritional therapy* [chromic chloride hexahydrate] 4 μg/mL

chromium chloride [see: chromic chloride Cr 51]

chromium chloride hexahydrate [see: chromic chloride]

chromocarb INN

chromonar HCl USAN *coronary vasodilator* [also: carbocromen]

Chronosule (trademarked dosage form) *sustained-action capsule*

Chronotab (trademarked dosage form) *sustained-action tablet*

Chronulac syrup ℞ *laxative* [lactulose] 10 g/15 mL

chrysazin (*withdrawn from market by FDA*) [see: danthron]

CHVP (cyclophosphamide, hydroxydaunomycin, VM-26, prednisone) *chemotherapy protocol*

Chymex solution ℞ *in vivo pancreatic function test* [bentiromide] 500 mg/7.5 mL

Chymodiactin powder for intradiscal injection ℞ *enzyme for herniated nucleus pulposus* [chymopapain] 4 nKat

chymopapain USAN, INN, BAN *proteolytic enzyme for herniated lumbar discs*

chymotrypsin USP, INN, BAN *proteolytic enzyme; zonulolytic for intracapsular lens extraction*

C.I. acid orange 24 monosodium salt (color index) [see: resorcin brown]

C.I. basic violet 3 (color index) [see: gentian violet]

C.I. basic violet 14 monohydrochloride (color index) [see: fuchsin, basic]

C.I. direct blue 53 tetrasodium salt (color index) [see: Evans blue]

C.I. mordant yellow 5, disodium salt (color index) [see: olsalazine sodium]

CI-979 *investigational selective muscarinic agonist for Alzheimer's disease*

CI-980 *investigational antineoplastic mitotic inhibitor*

CI-988 *investigational cholecystokinin-B receptor antagonist for obsessive-compulsive disorders (OCD)*

ciadox INN

ciamexon INN, BAN

cianergoline INN

cianidanol INN

cianidol [see: cianidanol]

cianopramine INN

ciapilome INN

Ciba Vision Cleaner for Sensitive Eyes solution OTC *surfactant cleaning solution for soft contact lenses*

Ciba Vision Saline aerosol solution OTC *rinsing/storage solution for soft contact lenses* [preservative-free saline solution]

Cibacalcin subcu or IM injection (discontinued 1996) ℞ *calcium regulator for Paget's disease (osteitis deformans) of bone (orphan)* [calcitonin (human)] 0.5 mg/vial

Cibadrex ℞ *investigational antihypertensive*

Cibalith-S syrup (discontinued 1994) ℞ *antipsychotic/antimanic* [lithium citrate] 8 mEq/5 mL

cibenzoline INN, BAN *antiarrhythmic* [also: cifenline]

cibenzoline succinate JAN *antiarrhythmic* [also: cifenline succinate]

cicaprost INN

cicaprost clathrate *investigational prostacyclin analog for metastatic tumors and cardiovascular disease*
cicarperone INN
ciclacillin INN, BAN *antibacterial* [also: cyclacillin]
ciclactate INN
ciclafrine INN *antihypotensive* [also: ciclafrine HCl]
ciclafrine HCl USAN *antihypotensive* [also: ciclafrine]
ciclazindol USAN, INN, BAN *antidepressant*
cicletanine USAN, INN, BAN *antihypertensive*
ciclindole INN *antidepressant* [also: cyclindole]
cicliomenol INN
ciclobendazole INN, BAN *anthelmintic* [also: cyclobendazole]
ciclofenazine INN *antipsychotic* [also: cyclophenazine HCl]
ciclofenazine HCl [see: cyclophenazine HCl]
cicloheximide INN *antipsoriatic* [also: cycloheximide]
ciclonicate INN
ciclonium bromide INN
ciclopirox USAN, INN, BAN *antifungal*
ciclopirox olamine USAN, USP, JAN *antifungal*
ciclopramine INN
cicloprofen USAN, INN, BAN *antiinflammatory*
cicloprolol INN *antiadrenergic (β-receptor)* [also: cicloprolol HCl; cycloprolol]
cicloprolol HCl USAN *antiadrenergic (β-receptor)* [also: cicloprolol; cycloprolol]
ciclosidomine INN, BAN
ciclosporin INN *immunosuppressive* [also: cyclosporine; cyclosporin]
ciclotate INN *combining name for radicals or groups*
ciclotizolam INN, BAN
ciclotropium bromide INN
cicloxilic acid INN
cicloxolone INN, BAN
cicortonide INN
cicrotoic acid INN
cideferron INN

Cidex; Cidex-7; Cidex Plus 28 *solution* OTC *broad-spectrum antimicrobial* [glutaral] 2%; 2%; 3.2%
cidofovir USAN, INN *antiviral for AIDS-related cytomegalovirus retinitis, genital warts, and herpes simplex*
cidoxepin INN *antidepressant* [also: cidoxepin HCl]
cidoxepin HCl USAN *antidepressant* [also: cidoxepin]
cifenline USAN *antiarrhythmic* [also: cibenzoline]
cifenline succinate USAN *antiarrhythmic* [also: cibenzoline succinate]
cifostodine INN
ciglitazone USAN, INN *antidiabetic*
cignolin [see: anthralin]
ciheptolane INN
ciladopa INN, BAN *antiparkinsonian; dopaminergic agent* [also: ciladopa HCl]
ciladopa HCl USAN *antiparkinsonian; dopaminergic agent* [also: ciladopa]
cilansetron INN *investigational treatment for irritable bowel syndrome*
cilastatin INN, BAN *enzyme inhibitor* [also: cilastatin sodium]
cilastatin sodium USAN, JAN *enzyme inhibitor* [also: cilastatin]
cilazapril USAN, INN, BAN, JAN *antihypertensive; ACE inhibitor*
cilazaprilat INN, BAN
cilexetil USAN *combining name for radicals or groups*
ciliary neurotrophic factor *(orphan: amyotrophic lateral sclerosis)*
ciliary neurotrophic factor, recombinant human *(orphan: spinal and progressive muscular atrophies; amyotrophic and primary lateral scleroses)*
cilobamine INN *antidepressant* [also: cilobamine mesylate]
cilobamine mesylate USAN *antidepressant* [also: cilobamine]
cilofungin USAN, INN *antifungal*
ciloprost [see: iloprost]
cilostamide INN
cilostazol INN
Ciloxan Drop-Tainers (eye drops) ℞ *ophthalmic antibiotic* [ciprofloxacin HCl] 3.5 mg/mL
ciltoprazine INN
cilutazoline INN

cimaterol USAN, INN *repartitioning agent*
cimemoxin INN
cimepanol INN
cimetidine USAN, USP, INN, BAN, JAN *treatment of GI ulcers; histamine H_2 antagonist* 200, 300, 400, 800 mg oral ② dimethicone
cimetidine HCl USAN *antagonist to histamine H_2 receptors* 300 mg/5 mL oral; 300 mg/2 mL injection
cimetropium bromide INN
cimoxatone INN
cinalukast USAN, INN *antiasthmatic*
cinametic acid INN
cinamolol INN
cinanserin INN *serotonin inhibitor* [also: cinanserin HCl]
cinanserin HCl USAN *serotonin inhibitor* [also: cinanserin]
cinaproxen INN
cincaine chloride [see: dibucaine HCl]
cinchocaine INN, BAN *local anesthetic* [also: dibucaine]
cinchocaine HCl BAN *local anesthetic* [also: dibucaine HCl]
cinchonidine sulfate NF
cinchonine sulfate NF
cinchophen NF, INN, BAN
cinecromen INN
cinepaxadil INN
cinepazet INN, BAN *antianginal* [also: cinepazet maleate]
cinepazet maleate USAN *antianginal* [also: cinepazet]
cinepazic acid INN
cinepazide INN, BAN
cinfenine INN
cinfenoac INN, BAN
cinflumide USAN, INN *muscle relaxant*
cingestol USAN, INN *progestin*
cinitapride INN
cinmetacin INN
cinnamaldehyde NF
cinnamaverine INN
cinnamedrine USAN, INN *smooth muscle relaxant*
cinnamedrine HCl *smooth muscle relaxant*
cinnamic aldehyde [now: cinnamaldehyde]
cinnamon NF
cinnamon oil NF

cinnarizine USAN, INN, BAN *antihistamine*
cinnarizine clofibrate INN
cinnofuradione INN
cinnofuron [see: cinnofuradione]
cinnopentazone INN *anti-inflammatory* [also: cintazone]
cinnopropazone [see: apazone]
Cinobac capsules ℞ *urinary antibacterial* [cinoxacin] 250, 500 mg
cinoctramide INN
cinodine HCl USAN *veterinary antibacterial*
cinolazepam INN
cinoquidox INN
cinoxacin USAN, USP, INN, BAN *urinary antibacterial* 250, 500 mg oral
cinoxate USAN, USP, INN *ultraviolet screen*
cinoxolone INN, BAN
cinoxopazide INN
cinperene USAN, INN *antipsychotic*
cinprazole INN
cinpropazide INN
Cin-Quin tablets, capsules (discontinued 1992) ℞ *antiarrhythmic* [quinidine sulfate]
cinromide USAN, INN *anticonvulsant*
cintazone USAN *anti-inflammatory* [also: cinnopentazone]
cintramide INN *antipsychotic* [also: cintriamide]
cintriamide USAN *antipsychotic* [also: cintramide]
cinuperone INN
cioteronel USAN, INN *antiandrogen*
cipamfylline USAN *antiviral agent; tumor necrosis factor alpha inhibitor*
cipionate INN *combining name for radicals or groups* [also: cypionate]
ciprafamide INN
Cipralan ℞ *investigational antiarrhythmic* [cifenline succinate]
Cipramil ℞ *investigational treatment for depression and Alzheimer's disease* [citalopram]
ciprazafone INN
ciprefadol INN *analgesic* [also: ciprefadol succinate]
ciprefadol succinate USAN *analgesic* [also: ciprefadol]

Cipro film-coated tablets, Cystitis Pack (6 tablets), IV infusion ℞ *broad-spectrum fluoroquinolone-type antibiotic; investigational treatment for cystic fibrosis* [ciprofloxacin] 100, 250, 500, 750 mg; 100 mg; 200, 400 mg

ciprocinonide USAN, INN *adrenocortical steroid*

ciprofibrate USAN, INN, BAN *antihyperlipoproteinemic*

ciprofloxacin USAN, INN, BAN *broad-spectrum bactericidal antibiotic; investigational treatment for cystic fibrosis*

ciprofloxacin HCl USAN, USP, JAN *broad-spectrum bactericidal antibiotic*

cipropride INN

ciproquazone INN

ciproquinate INN *coccidiostat for poultry* [also: cyproquinate]

ciprostene INN *platelet antiaggregatory agent* [also: ciprostene calcium]

ciprostene calcium USAN *platelet antiaggregatory agent* [also: ciprostene]

ciproximide INN *antipsychotic; antidepressant* [also: cyproximide]

ciramadol USAN, INN *analgesic*

ciramadol HCl USAN *analgesic*

cirazoline INN

Circavite-T tablets OTC *vitamin/mineral/iron supplement* [multiple vitamins & minerals; iron] ± • 12 mg

cirolemycin USAN, INN *antineoplastic; antibacterial*

cisapride USAN, INN, BAN, JAN *peristaltic stimulant; treatment for nocturnal heartburn due to gastroesophageal reflux disease*

cisatracurium besylate USAN *nondepolarizing neuromuscular blocker*

CISCA; CisCA (cisplatin, cyclophosphamide, Adriamycin) *chemotherapy protocol*

CISCA$_{II}$/VB$_{IV}$ (cisplatin, cyclophosphamide, Adriamycin, vinblastine, bleomycin) *chemotherapy protocol*

cisclomiphene [now: enclomiphene]

cisconazole USAN, INN *antifungal*

cis-**DDP (diamminedichloroplatinum)** [see: cisplatin]

cis-**diamminedichloroplatinum (DDP)** [see: cisplatin]

cismadinone INN

cisplatin USAN, USP, INN, BAN *alkylating antineoplastic*

cis-**platinum** [now: cisplatin]

cis-**platinum II** [now: cisplatin]

9-*cis*-**retinoic acid** *investigational (Phase I/III) for AIDS-related Kaposi sarcoma (orphan: acute promyelocytic leukemia)*

13-*cis*-**retinoic acid** [see: isotretinoin]

cistinexine INN

citalopram INN, BAN *investigational treatment for depression and Alzheimer's disease*

Citanest Forte injection ℞ *injectable local anesthetic for dental procedures* [prilocaine HCl; epinephrine] 4% • 1:200,000

Citanest Plain injection ℞ *injectable local anesthetic for dental procedures* [prilocaine HCl] 4%

citatepine INN

citenamide USAN, INN *anticonvulsant*

citenazone INN

citicoline INN *investigational treatment for ischemic stroke*

citicoline sodium USAN *treatment for stroke and head trauma*

citidoline [see: citicoline]

citiolone INN

Citra pH oral solution OTC *antacid* [sodium citrate] 450 mg/5 mL

Citracal tablets OTC *calcium supplement* [calcium citrate] 900 mg

Citracal 1500+D tablets (discontinued 1993) OTC *dietary supplement* [calcium citrate; vitamin D]

Citracal Caplets + D OTC *dietary supplement* [calcium citrate; vitamin D] 315 mg • 200 IU

Citracal Liquitab effervescent tablets OTC *calcium supplement* [calcium citrate] 23.76 mg

Citralax effervescent granules OTC *laxative* [magnesium citrate; magnesium sulfate]

citrate dextrose [see: ACD solution]

citrate of magnesia [see: magnesium citrate]

citrate phosphate dextrose [see: anticoagulant citrate phosphate dextrose solution]

citrate phosphate dextrose adenine [see: anticoagulant citrate phosphate dextrose adenine solution]
citrated caffeine [see: caffeine, citrated]
citric acid USP *pH adjusting agent*
citric acid, glucono-delta-lactone & magnesium carbonate *for renal and bladder apatite calculi (orphan)*
citric acid, magnesium oxide & sodium carbonate [see: Suby solution G]
citrin [see: bioflavonoids]
Citrocarbonate effervescent granules OTC *antacid* [sodium bicarbonate; sodium citrate] 780•1820 mg/dose
Citro-Flav 200 capsules OTC *dietary supplement* [citrus bioflavonoids complex] 200 mg
Citrolith tablets ℞ *urinary alkalinizing agent* [potassium citrate; sodium citrate] 50•950 mg
Citro-Nesia solution (discontinued 1993) OTC *laxative* [magnesium citrate]
Citrotein powder, liquid OTC *enteral nutritional therapy* [lactose-free formula]
citrovorum factor [see: leucovorin calcium]
Citrucel powder OTC *bulk laxative* [methylcellulose] 2 g/tbsp.
Citrucel Sugar Free powder OTC *bulk laxative* [methylcellulose; phenylalanine] 2 g•52 mg per tbsp.
citrus bioflavonoids [see: bioflavonoids]
Citrus-flav C 500 tablets OTC *dietary supplement* [vitamin C; citrus & acerola bioflavonoids; hesperidin; rutin] 200•250•40•10 mg
CIVPP (chlorambucil, vinblastine, procarbazine, prednisone) *chemotherapy protocol*
cladribine *antineoplastic; (orphan: hairy cell and chronic lymphocytic leukemias; chronic multiple sclerosis)*
Claforan powder for IV or IM injection ℞ *cephalosporin-type antibiotic* [cefotaxime sodium] 0.5, 1, 2, 10 g
clamidoxic acid INN, BAN
clamoxyquin BAN *antiamebic* [also: clamoxyquin HCl; clamoxyquine]
clamoxyquin HCl USAN *antiamebic* [also: clamoxyquine; clamoxyquin]

clamoxyquine INN *antiamebic* [also: clamoxyquin HCl; clamoxyquin]
clanfenur INN
clanobutin INN
clantifen INN
claretin-12 [see: cyanocobalamin] ⑫ Claritin; Clarityne
clarithromycin USAN, INN, BAN, JAN *macrolide antibacterial antibiotic*
Claritin tablets ℞ *nonsedating antihistamine; treatment for chronic urticaria* [loratadine] 10 mg ⑫ claretin; Clarityne
Claritin-D; Claritin-D 24 Hour extended-release tablets ℞ *decongestant; nonsedating antihistamine* [pseudoephedrine sulfate; loratadine] 120•5 mg; 240•10 mg
Clarityne (Mexican name for U.S. product Claritin) ⑫ claretin; Claritin
clavulanate potassium USAN, USP *β-lactamase inhibitor*
clavulanate potassium & amoxicillin [see: amoxicillin]
clavulanate potassium & ticarcillin [see: ticarcillin disodium]
clavulanic acid INN, BAN
clavulanic acid & amoxicillin [see: amoxicillin]
clavulanic acid & ticarcillin [see: ticarcillin disodium]
clazolam USAN, INN *minor tranquilizer*
clazolimine USAN, INN *diuretic*
clazuril USAN, INN, BAN *coccidiostat for pigeons*
Clean-N-Soak solution OTC *cleaning/soaking solution for hard contact lenses*
Clear Away; Clear Away Plantar (name changed to Dr. Scholl's Clear Away in 1994)
Clear By Design gel OTC *topical keratolytic for acne* [benzoyl peroxide] 2.5%
Clear Eyes eye drops OTC *topical ocular decongestant/vasoconstrictor* [naphazoline HCl] 0.012%
Clear Eyes ACR eye drops OTC *topical ocular decongestant; astringent* [naphazoline HCl; zinc sulfate] 0.012%•0.25%
Clear Total Lice Elimination System kit (shampoo + egg remover enzymes + nit comb) OTC *pediculicide*

[pyrethrins; piperonyl butoxide] 0.3%•3%

Clear Tussin 30 liquid OTC *antitussive; expectorant* [dextromethorphan hydrobromide; guaifenesin] 15•100 mg/5 mL

Clearasil cream, lotion OTC *topical keratolytic for acne* [benzoyl peroxide] 10%

Clearasil Adult Care cream OTC *topical acne treatment* [sulfur; resorcinol; alcohol 10%]

Clearasil Adult Care Medicated Blemish Stick (discontinued 1994) OTC *topical acne treatment* [sulfur; resorcinol; bentonite] 8%•1%•4%

Clearasil Antibacterial Soap bar OTC *medicated cleanser for acne* [triclosan]

Clearasil Clearstick liquid OTC *topical keratolytic for acne* [salicylic acid; alcohol 39%] 1.25%, 2%

Clearasil Daily Face Wash liquid OTC *antiseptic; disinfectant* [triclosan] 0.3%

Clearasil Double Clear; Clearasil Double Textured medicated pads OTC *topical keratolytic for acne* [salicylic acid; alcohol 40%] 1.25%, 2%; 2%

Clearasil Medicated Astringent liquid (name changed to Clearasil Medicated Deep Cleanser in 1994)

Clearasil Medicated Deep Cleanser liquid OTC *topical keratolytic cleanser for acne* [salicylic acid; alcohol 42%] 0.5%

Clearblue test kit for home use (discontinued 1995) OTC *in vitro diagnostic aid for urine pregnancy test*

Clearblue Easy test stick for home use OTC *in vitro diagnostic aid for urine pregnancy test*

Clearly Cala-gel OTC *topical antihistamine* [diphenhydramine HCl] ?

Clearplan Easy test kit for home use OTC *in vitro diagnostic aid to predict ovulation time*

Clearview Chlamydia test for professional use *in vitro diagnostic aid for Chlamydia trachomatis* [color-label immunoassay]

Clearview hCG test kit for professional use (discontinued 1996) *in vitro diagnostic aid for urine pregnancy test*

clebopride USAN, INN *antiemetic*
clefamide INN, BAN

clemastine USAN, BAN *antihistamine*
clemastine fumarate USAN, USP, BAN *antihistamine* 1.34, 2.68 mg; 0.5 mg/5 mL oral
clemeprol INN, BAN
clemizole INN, BAN
clemizole penicillin INN, BAN
clenbuterol INN, BAN
clenpirin INN [also: clenpyrin]
clenpyrin BAN [also: clenpirin]
Clens solution (discontinued 1995) OTC *cleaning solution for hard contact lenses*
clentiazem INN *calcium channel antagonist* [also: clentiazem maleate]
clentiazem maleate USAN *calcium channel antagonist* [also: clentiazem]
Cleocin capsules R *lincosamide-type antibiotic; (orphan: AIDS-related Pneumocystis carinii pneumonia)* [clindamycin HCl] 75, 100, 300 mg ⑨ bleomycin; Lincocin
Cleocin vaginal cream R *antibacterial* [clindamycin phosphate] 2%
Cleocin Pediatric granules for oral solution R *lincosamide-type antibiotic* [clindamycin palmitate HCl] 75 mg/5 mL
Cleocin Phosphate IV infusion, IM injection R *lincosamide-type antibiotic* [clindamycin phosphate] 150 mg/mL
Cleocin T gel, topical solution, lotion, pads R *topical antibiotic for acne* [clindamycin phosphate] 10 mg/mL
Clerz 2 solution OTC *rewetting solution for hard or soft contact lenses*
Clerz Drops solution (discontinued 1993) OTC *rewetting solution for hard contact lenses*
cletoquine INN, BAN
Clexane (European name for U.S. product Lovenox)
clibucaine INN
clidafidine INN
clidanac INN
clidinium bromide USAN, USP, INN, BAN *peptic ulcer adjunct*
Climara transdermal patch R *estrogen replacement therapy for postmenopausal disorders* [estradiol] 50, 100 μg/day
climazolam INN
climbazole INN, BAN
climiqualine INN

clinafloxacin HCl USAN *quinolone antibacterial*

Clinda-Derm topical solution ℞ *topical antibiotic for acne* [clindamycin phosphate] 10 mg/mL

clindamycin USAN, INN, BAN *lincosamide bactericidal antibiotic (orphan: AIDS-related Pneumocystis carinii pneumonia)*

clindamycin HCl USP, BAN *lincosamide bactericidal antibiotic* 75, 150 mg oral

clindamycin palmitate HCl USAN, USP *lincosamide bactericidal antibiotic*

clindamycin phosphate USAN, USP *lincosamide bactericidal antibiotic* 10 mg/mL topical; 150 mg/mL injection

Clindex capsules ℞ *GI anticholinergic; anxiolytic* [clidinium bromide; chlordiazepoxide HCl] 2.5•5 mg

Clinipak (trademarked packaging form) *unit dose package*

Clinistix reagent strips for home use OTC *in vitro diagnostic aid for urine glucose*

Clinitest reagent tablets for home use OTC *in vitro diagnostic aid for urine glucose*

clinocaine HCl [see: procaine HCl]

clinofibrate INN

clinolamide INN

Clinoril tablets ℞ *nonsteroidal anti-inflammatory drug (NSAID); antiarthritic; analgesic* [sulindac] 150, 200 mg

Clinoxide capsules (discontinued 1995) ℞ *GI anticholinergic; anxiolytic* [clidinium bromide; chlordiazepoxide HCl] 2.5•5 mg ⚠ clioxanide; Clipoxide

clioquinol USP, INN, BAN *topical antibacterial; antifungal*

clioxanide USAN, INN, BAN *anthelmintic* ⚠ Clinoxide

clipoxamine [see: cliropamine]

Clipoxide capsules (discontinued 1995) ℞ *GI anticholinergic; anxiolytic* [clidinium bromide; chlordiazepoxide HCl] 2.5•5 mg ⚠ Clinoxide

cliprofen USAN, INN *anti-inflammatory*

cliropamine INN

clobamine mesylate [now: cilobamine mesylate]

clobazam USAN, INN, BAN *minor tranquilizer*

clobedolum [see: clonitazene]

clobenoside INN

clobenzepam INN

clobenzorex INN

clobenztropine INN

clobetasol INN, BAN *topical corticosteroidal anti-inflammatory* [also: clobetasol propionate]

clobetasol propionate USAN *topical corticosteroidal anti-inflammatory* [also: clobetasol] 0.05% topical

clobetasone INN, BAN *anti-inflammatory* [also: clobetasone butyrate]

clobetasone butyrate USAN *anti-inflammatory* [also: clobetasone]

clobutinol INN

clobuzarit INN, BAN

clocanfamide INN

clocapramine INN

clociguanil INN, BAN

clocinizine INN

clocortolone INN *topical corticosteroid* [also: clocortolone acetate]

clocortolone acetate USAN *topical corticosteroid* [also: clocortolone]

clocortolone pivalate USAN, USP *topical corticosteroid*

clocoumarol INN

Clocream cream OTC *moisturizer; emollient* [cod liver oil (vitamins A and E); cholecalciferol; vitamin A palmitate]

clodacaine INN

clodanolene USAN, INN *skeletal muscle relaxant*

clodantoin INN *antifungal* [also: chlordantoin]

clodazon INN *antidepressant* [also: clodazon HCl]

clodazon HCl USAN *antidepressant* [also: clodazon]

Cloderm cream ℞ *topical corticosteroid* [clocortolone pivalate] 0.1%

clodoxopone INN

clodronic acid USAN, INN, BAN *calcium regulator*

clofazimine USAN, INN, BAN *bactericidal; tuberculostatic; leprostatic (orphan)*

clofedanol INN *antitussive* [also: chlophedianol HCl; chlophedianol]

clofedanol HCl [see: chlophedianol HCl]
clofenamic acid INN
clofenamide INN
clofenciclan INN
clofenetamine INN
clofenetamine HCl [see: clofenetamine]
clofenotane INN [also: chlorophenothane; dicophane]
clofenoxyde INN
clofenpyride [see: nicofibrate]
clofenvinfos INN [also: chlorfenvinphos]
clofeverine INN
clofexamide INN
clofezone INN
clofibrate USAN, USP, INN, BAN *antihyperlipoproteinemic* 500 mg oral
clofibric acid INN
clofibride INN
clofilium phosphate USAN, INN *antiarrhythmic*
clofinol [see: nicofibrate]
cloflucarban USAN *disinfectant* [also: halocarban]
clofluperol INN, BAN *antipsychotic* [also: seperidol HCl]
clofluperol HCl [see: seperidol HCl]
clofoctol INN
cloforex INN
clofurac INN
clogestone INN, BAN *progestin* [also: clogestone acetate]
clogestone acetate USAN *progestin* [also: clogestone]
cloguanamil INN, BAN [also: cloguanamile]
cloguanamile BAN [also: cloguanamil]
clomacran INN, BAN *antipsychotic* [also: clomacran phosphate]
clomacran phosphate USAN *antipsychotic* [also: clomacran]
clomegestone INN *progestin* [also: clomegestone acetate]
clomegestone acetate USAN *progestin* [also: clomegestone]
clometacin INN
clometerone INN *antiestrogen* [also: clometherone]
clometherone USAN *antiestrogen* [also: clometerone]

clomethiazole INN [also: chlormethiazole]
clometocillin INN
Clomid tablets ℞ *ovulation stimulant* [clomiphene citrate] 50 mg
clomide [see: aklomide]
clomifene INN *gonad-stimulating principle; ovulation stimulant* [also: clomiphene citrate; clomiphene]
clomifenoxide INN
clominorex USAN, INN *anorectic*
clomiphene BAN *gonad-stimulating principle; ovulation stimulant* [also: clomiphene citrate; clomifene] ⚠ clonidine
clomiphene citrate USAN, USP *gonad-stimulating principle; ovulation stimulant* [also: clomifene; clomiphene] 50 mg oral
clomipramine INN, BAN *tricyclic antidepressant* [also: clomipramine HCl]
clomipramine HCl USAN *tricyclic antidepressant; used for obsessive-compulsive disorders* [also: clomipramine]
clomocycline INN, BAN
clomoxir INN
Clomycin ointment OTC *topical antibiotic; anesthetic* [polymyxin B sulfate; bacitracin; neomycin sulfate; lidocaine] 5000 U•500 U•3.5 mg•40 mg per g
clonazepam USAN, USP, INN, BAN *anticonvulsant (orphan: hyperexplexia)*
clonazoline INN
clonidine USAN, INN, BAN *antihypertensive; investigational analgesic for severe cancer pain* ⚠ clomiphene; Klonopin; quinidine
clonidine HCl USAN, USP, BAN *antihypertensive; (orphan: epidural analgesia in cancer treatment)* 0.1, 0.2, 0.3 mg oral
clonitazene INN, BAN
clonitrate USAN, INN *coronary vasodilator*
clonixeril USAN, INN *analgesic*
clonixin USAN, INN *analgesic*
clopamide USAN, INN, BAN *antihypertensive; diuretic*
clopenthixol USAN, INN, BAN *antipsychotic*
cloperastine INN
cloperidone INN *sedative* [also: cloperidone HCl]

cloperidone HCl USAN *sedative* [also: cloperidone]
clophenoxate [see: meclofenoxate]
clopidogrel INN *investigational preventative for stroke, myocardial ischemia, and peripheral artery disease*
clopidol USAN, INN, BAN *coccidiostat for poultry*
clopimozide USAN, INN *antipsychotic*
clopipazan INN *antipsychotic* [also: clopipazan mesylate]
clopipazan mesylate USAN *antipsychotic* [also: clopipazan]
clopirac USAN, INN, BAN *anti-inflammatory*
cloponone INN, BAN
clopoxide [see: chlordiazepoxide]
clopoxide chloride [see: chlordiazepoxide HCl]
Clopra tablets ℞ *antidopaminergic; antiemetic for chemotherapy; peristaltic* [metoclopramide monohydrochloride monohydrate] 10 mg
cloprednol USAN, INN, BAN *glucocorticoid*
cloprostenol INN, BAN *prostaglandin* [also: cloprostenol sodium]
cloprostenol sodium USAN *prostaglandin* [also: cloprostenol]
cloprothiazole INN
cloquinate INN, BAN
cloquinozine INN
cloracetadol INN
cloral betaine INN *sedative* [also: chloral betaine]
cloramfenicol pantotenate complex INN *antibacterial; antirickettsial* [also: chloramphenicol pantothenate complex]
cloranolol INN
clorarsen [see: dichlorophenarsine HCl]
clorazepate dipotassium USAN, USP *anxiolytic; minor tranquilizer; alcohol withdrawal relief* [also: dipotassium clorazepate] 3.75, 7.5, 15 mg oral
clorazepate monopotassium USAN *minor tranquilizer*
clorazepic acid BAN
cloretate INN *sedative; hypnotic* [also: clorethate]
clorethate USAN *sedative; hypnotic* [also: cloretate]

clorexolone USAN, INN, BAN *diuretic*
clorgiline INN [also: clorgyline]
clorgyline BAN [also: clorgiline]
cloricromen INN
clorridarol INN
clorindanic acid INN
clorindanol INN *spermaticide* [also: chlorindanol]
clorindione INN, BAN
clormecaine INN
clorofene INN *disinfectant* [also: clorophene]
cloroperone INN *antipsychotic* [also: cloroperone HCl]
cloroperone HCl USAN *antipsychotic* [also: cloroperone]
clorophene USAN *disinfectant* [also: clorofene]
cloroqualone INN
clorotepine INN
Clorpactin WCS-90 powder for solution OTC *topical antimicrobial* [oxychlorosene sodium] 2 g
Clorpactin XCB powder for solution (discontinued 1994) OTC *topical antimicrobial* [oxychlorosene] 5 g
clorprenaline INN, BAN *adrenergic; bronchodilator* [also: clorprenaline HCl]
clorprenaline HCl USAN *adrenergic; bronchodilator* [also: clorprenaline]
clorquinaldol [see: chlorquinaldol]
clorsulon USAN, INN *antiparasitic; fasciolicide*
clortermine INN *anorectic* [also: clortermine HCl]
clortermine HCl USAN *anorectic* [also: clortermine]
closantel USAN, INN, BAN *anthelmintic*
closilate INN *combining name for radicals or groups* [also: closylate]
closiramine INN *antihistamine* [also: closiramine aceturate]
closiramine aceturate USAN *antihistamine* [also: closiramine]
clostebol INN [also: clostebol acetate]
clostebol acetate BAN [also: clostebol]
Clostridium botulinum toxin [see: botulinum toxin]
Clostridium botulinum toxin, type A *(orphan: essential blepharospasm)*
closylate USAN, BAN *combining name for radicals or groups* [also: closilate]

clothiapine USAN, BAN *antipsychotic* [also: clotiapine]

clothixamide maleate USAN *antipsychotic* [also: clotixamide]

clotiapine INN *antipsychotic* [also: clothiapine]

clotiazepam INN

cloticasone INN, BAN *anti-inflammatory* [also: cloticasone propionate]

cloticasone propionate USAN *anti-inflammatory* [also: cloticasone]

clotioxone INN

clotixamide INN *antipsychotic* [also: clothixamide maleate]

clotixamide maleate [see: clothixamide maleate]

clotrimazole USAN, USP, INN, BAN, JAN *broad-spectrum antifungal* 1% topical; 100 mg vaginal ② co-trimoxazole

clove oil NF

clovoxamine INN

cloxacepride INN

cloxacillin INN, BAN *antibacterial* [also: cloxacillin benzathine]

cloxacillin benzathine USP *antibacterial* [also: cloxacillin]

cloxacillin sodium USAN, USP *bactericidal antibiotic* 250, 500 mg oral; 125 mg/5 mL oral

Cloxapen capsules ℞ *bactericidal antibiotic (penicillinase-resistant penicillin)* [cloxacillin sodium] 250, 500 mg

cloxazolam INN

cloxestradiol INN

cloxifenol [see: triclosan]

cloximate INN

cloxiquine INN *antibacterial* [also: cloxyquin]

cloxotestosterone INN

cloxphendyl [see: cloxypendyl]

cloxypendyl INN

cloxyquin USAN *antibacterial* [also: cloxiquine]

clozapine USAN, INN, BAN *sedative; antipsychotic for severe schizophrenia*

Clozaril tablets ℞ *antipsychotic* [clozapine] 25, 100 mg

Clusivol syrup (discontinued 1992) OTC *vitamin/mineral supplement* [multiple vitamins & minerals]

Clysodrast powder for oral solution ℞ *laxative for pre-procedure bowel prep* [bisacodyl tannex] 2.5 g/packet

C-Max gradual-release tablets OTC *vitamin/mineral supplement* [various minerals; vitamin C] ≛•1 g

CMC (carboxymethylcellulose) gum [see: carboxymethylcellulose sodium]

CMC (cyclophosphamide, methotrexate, CCNU) *chemotherapy protocol*

CMC-VAP (cyclophosphamide, methotrexate, CCNU, vincristine, Adriamycin, procarbazine) *chemotherapy protocol*

CMF (cyclophosphamide, methotrexate, fluorouracil) *chemotherapy protocol*

CMF/AV (cyclophosphamide, methotrexate, fluorouracil, Adriamycin, Oncovin) *chemotherapy protocol*

CMFAVP (cyclophosphamide, methotrexate, fluorouracil, Adriamycin, vincristine, prednisone) *chemotherapy protocol*

CMFP; CMF-P (cyclophosphamide, methotrexate, fluorouracil, prednisone) *chemotherapy protocol*

CMFPT (cyclophosphamide, methotrexate, fluorouracil, prednisone, tamoxifen) *chemotherapy protocol*

CMFPTH (cyclophosphamide, methotrexate, fluorouracil, prednisone, tamoxifen, Halotestin) *chemotherapy protocol*

CMFT (cyclophosphamide, methotrexate, fluorouracil, tamoxifen) *chemotherapy protocol*

CMFVAT (cyclophosphamide, methotrexate, fluorouracil, vincristine, Adriamycin, testosterone) *chemotherapy protocol*

CMFVP (cyclophosphamide, methotrexate, fluorouracil, vincristine, prednisone) *chemotherapy protocol* [two dosing protocols: Cooper's protocol and SWOG protocol]

CMH (cyclophosphamide, m-AMSA, hydroxyurea) *chemotherapy protocol*

C-MOPP (cyclophosphamide, mechlorethamine, Oncovin, procarbazine, prednisone) *chemotherapy protocol*

CMT tablets ℞ *antiarthritic* [choline magnesium trisalicylate]

CMV (cisplatin, methotrexate, vinblastine) *chemotherapy protocol*

CMV MAb (cytomegalovirus monoclonal antibody) [q.v.]

CMV-IGIV (cytomegalovirus immune globulin intravenous) [see: globulin, immune]

CN2 HCl [see: mechlorethamine HCl]

CNF (cyclophosphamide, Novantrone, fluorouracil) *chemotherapy protocol* [also: CFM; FNC]

CNOP (cyclophosphamide, Novantrone, Oncovin, prednisone) *chemotherapy protocol*

CNS 1102 *investigational treatment for stroke*

Co I (coenzyme I) [see: nadide]

Co Tinic IM injection ℞ *antianemic* [ferrous gluconate; multiple B vitamins; procaine]

CO_2 (carbon dioxide) [q.v.]

^{57}Co [see: cobaltous chloride Co 57]

^{57}Co [see: cyanocobalamin Co 57]

^{58}Co [see: cyanocobalamin (^{58}Co)]

^{60}Co [see: cobaltous chloride Co 60]

^{60}Co [see: cyanocobalamin Co 60]

CoAdvil (name changed to Advil Cold & Sinus in 1992)

coagulation factor IX (human) [see: factor IX complex]

coal tar USP *topical antieczematic; antiseborrheic*

COAP (cyclophosphamide, Oncovin, ara-C, prednisone) *chemotherapy protocol*

Co-Apap tablets OTC *antitussive; decongestant; antihistamine; analgesic* [dextromethorphan hydrobromide; pseudoephedrine HCl; chlorpheniramine maleate; acetaminophen] 15•30•2•325 mg

COAP-BLEO (cyclophosphamide, Oncovin, ara-C, prednisone, bleomycin) *chemotherapy protocol*

COB (cisplatin, Oncovin, bleomycin) *chemotherapy protocol*

cobalamin concentrate USP *vitamin B_{12}; hematopoietic*

cobalt *element (Co)*

cobalt-labeled vitamin B_{12} [see: cyanocobalamin Co 57 & Co 60]

cobaltous chloride Co 57 USAN *radioactive agent*

cobaltous chloride Co 60 USAN *radioactive agent*

cobamamide INN

Cobex IM or subcu injection (discontinued 1994) ℞ *antianemic; vitamin B_{12} supplement* [cyanocobalamin] 100, 1000 μg/mL

cocaine USP, BAN *topical anesthetic for mucous membranes* 4%, 10% topical

cocaine HCl USP *topical anesthetic for mucous membranes* 135 mg oral; 4%, 10% topical

Cocaine Viscous topical solution ℞ *topical mucosal anesthesia* [cocaine] 4%, 10%

cocarboxylase INN [also: co-carboxylase]

co-carboxylase BAN [also: cocarboxylase]

coccidioidin USP *dermal coccidioidomycosis test*

cocculin [see: picrotoxin]

cocoa NF

cocoa butter NF *suppository base; emollient/protectant*

cod liver oil USP, BAN *vitamins A and D source; emollient/protectant*

cod liver oil, nondestearinated NF

codactide INN, BAN

Codafed Expectorant liquid (discontinued 1994) ℞ *narcotic antitussive; decongestant; expectorant* [codeine phosphate; pseudoephedrine HCl; guaifenesin; alcohol] ② Codaphen

Codalan No. 1, No. 2 & No. 3 tablets (discontinued 1992) ℞ *narcotic analgesic* [codeine phosphate; acetaminophen; aspirin; caffeine]

Codamine syrup, pediatric syrup ℞ *narcotic antitussive; decongestant* [hydrocodone bitartrate; phenylpropanolamine HCl] 5•25 mg/5 mL; 2.5•12.5 mg/5 mL

Codaphen tablets (discontinued 1993) ℞ *analgesic* [acetaminophen; codeine phosphate] ⓘ Codafed

CODE (cisplatin, Oncovin, doxorubicin, etoposide) *chemotherapy protocol*

Codegest Expectorant liquid ℞ *narcotic antitussive; decongestant; expectorant* [codeine phosphate; phenylpropanolamine HCl; guaifenesin] 10•12.5•100 mg/5 mL ⓘ Codehist

Codehist DH elixir ℞ *narcotic antitussive; decongestant; antihistamine* [codeine phosphate; pseudoephedrine HCl; chlorpheniramine maleate; alcohol 5.7%] 10•30•2 mg/5 mL ⓘ Codegest

codehydrogenase I [see: nadide]

codeine USP, BAN *antitussive; narcotic analgesic* ⓘ Kaodene

codeine phosphate USP, BAN *antitussive; narcotic analgesic*

codeine polistirex USAN *antitussive*

codeine sulfate USP *narcotic analgesic; antitussive* 15, 30, 60 mg oral; 30, 60 mg/mL injection

codelcortone [see: prednisolone]

co-dergocrine mesylate BAN *cognition adjuvant* [also: ergoloid mesylates]

Codiclear DH syrup ℞ *narcotic antitussive; expectorant* [hydrocodone bitartrate; guaifenesin] 5•100 mg/5 mL

Codimal capsules, film-coated tablets OTC *decongestant; antihistamine; analgesic* [pseudoephedrine HCl; chlorpheniramine maleate; acetaminophen] 30•2•325 mg

Codimal A injection (discontinued 1994) ℞ *antihistamine* [brompheniramine maleate] 10 mg/mL

Codimal DH syrup ℞ *narcotic antitussive; decongestant; antihistamine* [hydrocodone bitartrate; phenylephrine HCl; pyrilamine maleate] 1.66•5•8.33 mg/5 mL

Codimal DM syrup OTC *antitussive; decongestant; antihistamine* [dextromethorphan hydrobromide; phenylephrine HCl; pyrilamine maleate] 10•5•8.33 mg/5 mL

Codimal Expectorant liquid (discontinued 1994) OTC *decongestant; expectorant* [phenylpropanolamine HCl; guaifenesin] 25•100 mg/5 mL

Codimal PH syrup OTC *narcotic antitussive; decongestant; antihistamine* [codeine phosphate; phenylephrine HCl; pyrilamine maleate] 10•5•8.33 mg/5 mL

Codimal-L.A.; Codimal-L.A. Half extended-release capsules ℞ *decongestant; antihistamine* [pseudoephedrine HCl; chlorpheniramine maleate] 120•8 mg; 60•4 mg

codorphone [now: conorphone HCl]

codoxime USAN, INN *antitussive*

Codroxomin IM injection (discontinued 1992) ℞ *antianemic; vitamin B_{12} supplement* [hydroxocobalamin] 1000 μg/mL

coenzyme Q10 *investigational immune stimulant for AIDS; antioxidant; cardiac protectant*

COF/COM (cyclophosphamide, Oncovin, fluorouracil + cyclophosphamide, Oncovin, methotrexate) *chemotherapy protocol*

Coffee Break timed-release caplets (discontinued 1992) OTC *CNS stimulant; analeptic* [caffeine] 200 mg

coffeine [see: caffeine]

cofisatin INN

cofisatine [see: cofisatin]

cogazocine INN

Cogentin tablets, IV or IM injection ℞ *anticholinergic; antiparkinsonian* [benztropine mesylate] 0.5, 1, 2 mg; 1 mg/mL

Co-Gesic tablets ℞ *narcotic analgesic* [hydrocodone bitartrate; acetaminophen] 5•500 mg

Cognex capsules ℞ *cognition adjuvant for Alzheimer's dementia* [tacrine HCl] 10, 20, 30, 40 mg

Co-Hist tablets OTC *decongestant; antihistamine; analgesic* [pseudoephedrine HCl; chlorpheniramine maleate; acetaminophen] 30•2•325 mg

Colabid tablets ℞ *uricosuric for gout* [probenecid; colchicine]

Colace capsules, syrup, drops OTC *stool softener* [docusate sodium] 50, 100 mg; 60 mg/15 mL; 150 mg/15 mL

colaspase BAN *antineoplastic for acute lymphocytic leukemia (ALL)* [also: asparaginase]

Co-Lav powder for oral solution ℞ *pre-procedure bowel evacuant* [polyethylene glycol-electrolyte solution] 60 g/L

Colax tablets OTC *laxative; stool softener* [phenolphthalein; docusate sodium] 65•100 mg

Colazide ℞ *investigational gastrointestinal anti-inflammatory* [balsalazide disodium]

ColBenemid tablets ℞ *uricosuric for gout* [probenecid; colchicine] 500•0.5 mg

colchamine [see: demecolcine]

colchicine USP, JAN *gout suppressant; (orphan: multiple sclerosis)* 0.5, 0.6 mg oral; 1 mg injection

Cold & Allergy elixir OTC *decongestant; antihistamine* [phenylpropanolamine HCl; brompheniramine maleate] 12.5•2 mg/5 mL

cold cream USP

Cold Relief tablets OTC *antitussive; decongestant; antihistamine; analgesic* [dextromethorphan hydrobromide; phenylpropanolamine HCl; chlorpheniramine maleate; acetaminophen] 10•12.5•2•325 mg

Cold Symptoms Relief tablets OTC *antitussive; decongestant; antihistamine; analgesic* [dextromethorphan hydrobromide; pseudoephedrine HCl; chlorpheniramine maleate; acetaminophen] 10•30•2•325 mg

Cold-Gest sustained-release capsules OTC *decongestant; antihistamine* [phenylpropanolamine HCl; chlorpheniramine maleate] 75•8 mg

Coldloc liquid ℞ *decongestant; expectorant* [phenylpropanolamine HCl; phenylephrine HCl; guaifenesin] 20•5•100 mg/5 mL

Coldloc-LA sustained-release caplets ℞ *decongestant; expectorant* [phenylpropanolamine HCl; guaifenesin] 75•600 mg

Coldrine tablets OTC *decongestant; analgesic* [pseudoephedrine HCl; acetaminophen] 30•325 mg

colecalciferol INN *vitamin D_3; antirachitic* [also: cholecalciferol]

Colestid granules ℞ *cholesterol-lowering antihyperlipidemic* [colestipol HCl] 5 g/dose ⓓ colistin

Colestid tablets ℞ *cholesterol-lowering antihyperlipidemic* [colestipol HCl] 1 g

colestipol INN, BAN *antihyperlipoproteinemic; bile acid sequestrant* [also: colestipol HCl] ⓓ colistin

colestipol HCl USAN, USP *antihyperlipoproteinemic; bile acid sequestrant* [also: colestipol]

colestolone USAN, INN *hypolipidemic*

colestyramine INN *bile salts ion-exchange resin; antihyperlipoproteinemic* [also: cholestyramine resin; cholestyramine]

colestyramine resin [see: cholestyramine resin]

colextran INN

Colfed-A sustained-release capsules ℞ *decongestant; antihistamine* [pseudoephedrine HCl; chlorpheniramine maleate] 120•8 mg

colfenamate INN

colforsin USAN, INN *antiglaucoma agent*

colfosceril palmitate USAN, INN, BAN *pulmonary surfactant; for hyaline membrane disease and respiratory distress syndrome (orphan)*

colimecycline INN

colistimethate sodium USAN, USP, INN *bactericidal antibiotic* [also: colistin sulphomethate]

colistin INN, BAN *bactericidal antibiotic* [also: colistin sulfate] ⓓ Colestid; colestipol

colistin methanesulfonate [see: colistimethate sodium]

colistin sulfate USP *bactericidal antibiotic* [also: colistin]

colistin sulphomethate BAN *bactericidal antibiotic* [also: colistimethate sodium]

collagen *ophthalmic implant to block puncta and retain moisture*

collagenase *topical proteolytic enzymes for necrotic tissue debridement*

Collastin Oil Free Moisturizer lotion OTC *moisturizer; emollient* [collagen] ≛

collodion USP *topical protectant*

colloidal aluminum hydroxide [see: aluminum hydroxide gel]

colloidal oatmeal *demulcent*

colloidal silicon dioxide [see: silicon dioxide, colloidal]

Collyrium for Fresh Eyes ophthalmic solution OTC *extraocular irrigating solution* [sterile isotonic solution]

Collyrium Fresh eye drops OTC *topical ocular decongestant/vasoconstrictor* [tetrahydrozoline HCl] 0.05%

ColoCare test kit for home use OTC *in vitro diagnostic aid for fecal occult blood*

Color Allergy Screening Test (CAST) reagent assay tubes ℞ *in vitro diagnostic aid for immunoglobulin E in serum*

Color Ovulation Test kit for home use OTC *in vitro diagnostic aid to predict ovulation time*

ColoScreen slide test for professional use *in vitro diagnostic aid for fecal occult blood*

Colovage powder for oral solution ℞ *pre-procedure bowel evacuant* [polyethylene glycol-electrolyte solution]

Col-Probenecid tablets ℞ *uricosuric for gout* [probenecid; colchicine] 500•0.5 mg

Coltab Children's tablets (discontinued 1993) OTC *pediatric decongestant and antihistamine* [phenylephrine HCl; chlorpheniramine maleate]

colterol INN *bronchodilator* [also: colterol mesylate]

colterol mesylate USAN *bronchodilator* [also: colterol]

Coly-Mycin M powder for IV or IM injection ℞ *bactericidal antibiotic* [colistimethate sodium] 150 mg

Coly-Mycin S powder for oral suspension (discontinued 1996) ℞ *bactericidal antibiotic* [colistin sulfate] 25 mg/5 mL

Coly-Mycin S Otic suspension ℞ *topical corticosteroidal anti-inflammatory; antibiotic* [hydrocortisone acetate; neomycin sulfate; colistin sulfate] 1%•4.71 mg•3 mg per mL

Colyte powder for oral solution ℞ *pre-procedure bowel evacuant* [polyethylene glycol-electrolyte solution]

COM (cyclophosphamide, Oncovin, MeCCNU) *chemotherapy protocol*

COM (cyclophosphamide, Oncovin, methotrexate) *chemotherapy protocol*

COMA-A (cyclophosphamide, Oncovin, methotrexate/citrovorum factor, Adriamycin, ara-C) *chemotherapy protocol*

COMB (cyclophosphamide, Oncovin, MeCCNU, bleomycin) *chemotherapy protocol*

COMB (Cytoxin, Oncovin, methotrexate, bleomycin) *chemotherapy protocol*

Combi-patch ℞ *investigational transdermal patch for hormone replacement therapy* [estrogen; progestin]

Combipres 0.1; Combipres 0.2; Combipres 0.3 tablets ℞ *antihypertensive* [clonidine HCl; chlorthalidone] 0.1•15 mg; 0.2•15 mg; 0.3•15 mg ⑨ Catapres

Combistix reagent strips *in vitro diagnostic aid for multiple urine products*

COMe (Cytoxin, Oncovin, methotrexate) *chemotherapy protocol*

COMF (cyclophosphamide, Oncovin, methotrexate, fluorouracil) *chemotherapy protocol*

Comfort eye drops OTC *topical ocular decongestant/vasoconstrictor* [naphazoline HCl] 0.03%

Comfort Tears eye drops OTC *ocular moisturizer/lubricant* [hydroxyethylcellulose]

ComfortCare GP Wetting & Soaking solution OTC *disinfecting/wetting/soaking solution for rigid gas permeable contact lenses*

Comfortine ointment OTC *moisturizer; emollient; astringent; antiseptic* [vitamins A and D; lanolin; zinc oxide]

Comhist tablets ℞ *decongestant; antihistamine* [phenylephrine HCl; chlorpheniramine maleate; phenyltoloxamine citrate] 10•2•25 mg

Comhist LA long-acting capsules ℞ *decongestant; antihistamine* [phenylephrine HCl; chlorpheniramine maleate; phenyltoloxamine citrate] 20•4•50 mg

COMLA (cyclophosphamide, Oncovin, methotrexate, leucovorin [rescue], ara-C) *chemotherapy protocol*

comosain *(orphan: enzymatic debridement of severe burns)*

COMP (CCNU, Oncovin, methotrexate, procarbazine) *chemotherapy protocol*

COMP (cyclophosphamide, Oncovin, methotrexate, prednisone) *chemotherapy protocol*

Compazine tablets, Spansules (capsules), IV or IM injection, suppositories, syrup ℞ *antiemetic; tranquilizer* [prochlorperazine maleate] 5, 10, 25 mg; 10, 15, 30 mg; 5 mg/mL; 2.5, 5, 25 mg; 5 mg/5 mL

Compete tablets OTC *vitamin/iron supplement* [multiple vitamins; ferrous gluconate; folic acid] ±•27•0.4 mg

Compleat Modified Formula closed system containers OTC *enteral nutritional therapy* [lactose-free formula]

Compleat Modified Formula ready-to-use liquid OTC *enteral nutritional therapy* [lactose-free formula]

Compleat Regular Formula ready-to-use liquid OTC *enteral nutritional therapy* [milk-based formula]

Complere tablets OTC *vitamin/mineral supplement* [multiple vitamins, minerals, and amino acids]

Complete solution OTC *rewetting solution for soft contact lenses*

Complete All-in-One solution OTC *cleaning/disinfecting/rinsing/storage solution for soft contact lenses*

Complete Multi-Purpose solution (name changed to Complete All-In-One in 1995)

Complete Weekly Enzymatic Cleaner effervescent tablets OTC *enzymatic cleaner for soft contact lenses* [subtilisin A]

Complex 15 Face cream OTC *moisturizer; emollient*

Complex 15 Hand & Body cream, lotion OTC *moisturizer; emollient*

Comply liquid OTC *enteral nutritional therapy* [lactose-free formula]

compound 42 [see: warfarin]

compound CB3025 [see: melphalan]
compound E [see: cortisone acetate]
compound F [see: hydrocortisone]
compound insulin zinc suspension INN *antidiabetic* [also: insulin zinc]
compound orange spirit [see: orange spirit, compound]
compound Q [see: trichosanthin]
compound S [see: zidovudine]
compound solution of sodium chloride INN *fluid and electrolyte replenisher* [also: Ringer's injection]
compound solution of sodium lactate INN *electrolyte and fluid replenisher; systemic alkalizer* [also: Ringer's injection, lactated]
Compound W liquid, gel OTC *topical keratolytic* [salicylic acid in collodion] 17%
Compoz gel caps OTC *antihistaminic sleep aid* [diphenhydramine HCl] 25 mg
Compoz Nighttime Sleep Aid tablets OTC *antihistaminic sleep aid* [diphenhydramine HCl] 50 mg
compressible sugar [see: sugar, compressible]
Comtrex caplets, tablets (name changed to Comtrex Multi-Symptom Cold & Flu Relief in 1995)
Comtrex liquid OTC *antitussive; decongestant; antihistamine; analgesic* [dextromethorphan hydrobromide; pseudoephedrine HCl; chlorpheniramine maleate; acetaminophen] 3.3•10•0.67•108.3 mg/5 mL
Comtrex, Cough Formula liquid OTC *antitussive; decongestant; expectorant; analgesic* [dextromethorphan hydrobromide; pseudoephedrine HCl; guaifenesin; acetaminophen; alcohol 20%] 7.5•15•50•125 mg/5 mL
Comtrex, Day & Night daytime caplets + nighttime tablets (discontinued 1995) OTC *antitussive; decongestant; analgesic; (antihistamine added nighttime)* [dextromethorphan hydrobromide; pseudoephedrine HCl; acetaminophen; (chlorpheniramine maleate added nighttime)] 15•30•500 mg daytime; 15•30•500•2 mg nighttime

Comtrex Allergy-Sinus caplets, tablets OTC *decongestant; antihistamine; analgesic* [pseudoephedrine HCl; chlorpheniramine maleate; acetaminophen] 30•2•500 mg

Comtrex Hot Flu Relief powder (discontinued 1995) OTC *antitussive; decongestant; antihistamine; analgesic* [dextromethorphan hydrobromide; pseudoephedrine HCl; chlorpheniramine maleate; acetaminophen] 20•60•4•500 mg/packet

Comtrex Liqui-Gels (liquid-filled capsules) OTC *antitussive; decongestant; antihistamine; analgesic* [dextromethorphan hydrobromide; phenylpropanolamine HCl; chlorpheniramine maleate; acetaminophen] 10•12.5•2•325, 15•12.5•2•500 mg

Comtrex Multi-Symptom, Day & Night daytime caplets + nighttime tablets (discontinued 1995) OTC *antitussive; decongestant; analgesic; (antihistamine added nighttime)* [dextromethorphan hydrobromide; pseudoephedrine HCl; acetaminophen; (chlorpheniramine maleate added nighttime)] 10•30•325 mg daytime; 10•30•325•2 mg nighttime

Comtrex Multi-Symptom Cold & Flu Relief tablets, caplets OTC *antitussive; decongestant; antihistamine; analgesic* [dextromethorphan hydrobromide; pseudoephedrine HCl; chlorpheniramine maleate; acetaminophen] 15•30•2•500 mg

Comtrex Multi-Symptom Cold & Flu Relief Liqui-Gels (capsules) OTC *antitussive; decongestant; antihistamine; analgesic* [dextromethorphan hydrobromide; phenylpropanolamine HCl; chlorpheniramine maleate; acetaminophen] 15•12.5•2•500 mg

Comtrex Non-Drowsy caplets OTC *antitussive; decongestant; analgesic* [dextromethorphan hydrobromide; pseudoephedrine HCl; acetaminophen] 15•30•500 mg

Conceive Ovulation Predictor 5-day test kit for professional use *in vitro diagnostic aid to predict ovulation time*

Conceive Pregnancy test kit for home use OTC *in vitro diagnostic aid for urine pregnancy test*

Concentraid nasal spray, intranasal pipets (discontinued 1994) ℞ *diabetes insipidus; hemophilia A; von Willebrand's disease* [desmopressin acetate]

Concentrated Cleaner solution OTC *cleaning solution for rigid gas permeable contact lenses*

Conceptrol Contraceptive Inserts vaginal suppositories OTC *spermicidal contraceptive* [nonoxynol 9] 150 mg

Conceptrol Disposable Contraceptive vaginal gel OTC *spermicidal contraceptive* [nonoxynol 9] 4%

Condrin-LA sustained-release capsules (discontinued 1995) ℞ *decongestant; antihistamine* [phenylpropanolamine HCl; chlorpheniramine maleate] 75•12 mg

Condylox solution ℞ *topical keratolytic for external genital warts* [podofilox; alcohol 95%] 0.5%

conessine INN

conessine hydrobromide [see: conessine]

Conex lozenges (discontinued 1994) OTC *topical oral anesthetic; antiseptic* [benzocaine; cetylpyridinium chloride] 5•0.5 mg

Conex syrup OTC *decongestant; expectorant* [phenylpropanolamine HCl; guaifenesin] 12.5•100 mg/5 mL

Conex D.A. tablets (discontinued 1993) OTC *decongestant; antihistamine* [phenylpropanolamine HCl; chlorpheniramine maleate]

Conex Plus tablets (discontinued 1993) OTC *decongestant; antihistamine; analgesic* [phenylpropanolamine HCl; chlorpheniramine maleate; acetaminophen]

Conex with Codeine syrup ℞ *narcotic antitussive; decongestant; expectorant* [codeine phosphate; phenylpropanolamine HCl; guaifenesin] 10•12.5•100 mg/5 mL

confectioner's sugar [see: sugar, confectioner's]

Confide test kit for home use OTC *in vitro diagnostic aid for HIV in the blood*

congazone sodium [see: Congo red]

Congespirin for Children chewable tablets (discontinued 1995) OTC *decongestant; analgesic* [phenylephrine HCl; acetaminophen] 1.25•81 mg

Congess JR capsules ℞ *decongestant; expectorant* [pseudoephedrine HCl; guaifenesin] 60•125 mg

Congess SR sustained-release capsules ℞ *decongestant; expectorant* [pseudoephedrine HCl; guaifenesin] 120•250 mg

Congestac caplets OTC *decongestant; expectorant* [pseudoephedrine HCl; guaifenesin] 60•400 mg

Congestant tablets (name changed to Improved Congestant in 1995)

Congestant D tablets OTC *decongestant; antihistamine; analgesic* [phenylpropanolamine HCl; chlorpheniramine maleate; acetaminophen] 12.5•2•325 mg

Congestion Relief tablets OTC *nasal decongestant* [pseudoephedrine HCl] 30, 60 mg

Congestion Relief, Children's liquid OTC *nasal decongestant* [pseudoephedrine HCl] 30 mg/5 mL

Congo red USP

conjugated estrogens [see: estrogens, conjugated]

conorfone INN *analgesic* [also: conorphone HCl]

conorfone HCl [see: conorphone HCl]

conorphone HCl USAN *analgesic* [also: conorfone]

CONPADRI; CONPADRI-I (cyclophosphamide, Oncovin, L-phenylalanine mustard, Adriamycin) *chemotherapy protocol*

Conray; Conray 30; Conray 43 injection ℞ *parenteral radiopaque agent* [iothalamate meglumine] 60%; 30%; 43%

Conray 325; Conray 400 injection ℞ *parenteral radiopaque agent* [iothalamate sodium] 54.3%; 66.8%

consensus interferon *investigational antiviral for hepatitis C and antineoplastic*

Consonar ℞ *investigational reversible/selective MAO inhibitor, type A* [brofaromine]

Constant-T sustained-action tablets (discontinued 1994) ℞ *bronchodilator* [theophylline] 200, 300 mg

Constene ℞ *investigational treatment for constipation* [naloxone]

Constilac syrup ℞ *laxative* [lactulose] 10 g/15 mL

Constulose syrup ℞ *laxative* [lactulose] 10 g/15 mL

Contac 12 Hour sustained-release capsules, sustained-release caplets OTC *decongestant; antihistamine* [phenylpropanolamine HCl; chlorpheniramine maleate] 75•8 mg; 75•12 mg

Contac Cough & Chest Cold liquid OTC *antitussive; decongestant; expectorant; analgesic* [dextromethorphan hydrobromide; pseudoephedrine HCl; guaifenesin; acetaminophen; alcohol 10%] 5•15•50•125 mg/5 mL

Contac Cough Formula liquid (discontinued 1994) OTC *antitussive; expectorant* [dextromethorphan hydrobromide; guaifenesin]

Contac Cough & Sore Throat liquid OTC *antitussive; analgesic* [dextromethorphan hydrobromide; acetaminophen; alcohol 10%] 5•125 mg/5 mL

Contac Day & Night Allergy/Sinus daytime caplets + nighttime caplets OTC *decongestant; analgesic; (antihistamine/sleep aid added nighttime)* [pseudoephedrine HCl; acetaminophen; (diphenhydramine HCl added nighttime)] 60•650 mg daytime; 60•650•50 mg nighttime

Contac Day & Night Cold & Flu daytime caplets + nighttime caplets OTC *decongestant; analgesic; (antitussive added daytime; antihistamine/sleep aid added nighttime)* [pseudoephedrine HCl; acetaminophen; (dextromethorphan hydrobromide added daytime; diphenhydramine HCl added nighttime)] 60•650•30 mg daytime; 60•650•50 mg nighttime

Contac Jr. Non-Drowsy Cold liquid (discontinued 1994) OTC *pediatric antitussive, decongestant, and analgesic* [dextromethorphan hydrobromide; pseudoephedrine HCl; acetaminophen]

Contac Nighttime Cold Medicine liquid (discontinued 1992) OTC *decongestant; antihistamine; antitussive; analgesic* [pseudoephedrine HCl; doxylamine succinate; dextromethorphan hydrobromide; acetaminophen; alcohol]

Contac Non-Drowsy Formula Sinus tablets, caplets (discontinued 1995) OTC *decongestant; analgesic; antipyretic* [pseudoephedrine HCl; acetaminophen] 30•500 mg

Contac Severe Cold & Flu Formula caplets (discontinued 1995) OTC *antitussive; decongestant; antihistamine; analgesic* [dextromethorphan hydrobromide; phenylpropanolamine HCl; chlorpheniramine maleate; acetaminophen] 15•12.5•2•500 mg

Contac Severe Cold & Flu Hot Medicine powder (discontinued 1995) OTC *antitussive; decongestant; antihistamine; analgesic* [dextromethorphan hydrobromide; pseudoephedrine HCl; chlorpheniramine maleate; acetaminophen] 20•60•4•650 mg/packet

Contac Severe Cold & Flu Nighttime liquid OTC *antitussive; decongestant; antihistamine; analgesic* [dextromethorphan hydrobromide; pseudoephedrine HCl; chlorpheniramine maleate; acetaminophen; alcohol 18.5%] 5•10•0.67•167 mg/5 mL

Contac-C Cold Care Formula caplets (Canadian name for U.S. product Contac Severe Cold & Flu Formula)

conteben [see: thioacetazone; thiacetazone]

ConTE-Pak-4 IV injection ℞ *intravenous nutritional therapy* [multiple trace elements (metals)] ±

Contigen urethral injection ℞ *treatment for stress urinary incontinence* [purified collagen implant]

Contrin capsules ℞ *hematinic* [ferrous fumarate; cyanocobalamin; ascorbic acid; intrinsic factor concentrate; folic acid] 110 mg•15 μg•75 mg•240 mg•0.5 mg

Control timed-release capsules OTC *diet aid* [phenylpropanolamine HCl] 75 mg

Control-L liquid (discontinued 1993) OTC *lice treatment* [pyrethrins; piperonyl butoxide; petroleum distillate] 0.3%•3%• ?

ControlPak (trademarked packaging form) *tamper-resistant unit-dose package*

Contuss liquid ℞ *decongestant; expectorant* [phenylpropanolamine HCl; phenylephrine HCl; guaifenesin; alcohol 5%] 20•5•100 mg/5 mL

Cooper's regimen *chemotherapy protocol* [see: CMFVP]

COP [see: creatinolfosfate]

COP (cyclophosphamide, Oncovin, prednisone) *chemotherapy protocol*

COP 1 (copolymer 1) [q.v.]

COPA (Cytoxin, Oncovin, prednisone, Adriamycin) *chemotherapy protocol*

COPA-BLEO (cyclophosphamide, Oncovin, prednisone, Adriamycin, bleomycin) *chemotherapy protocol*

COPAC (CCNU, Oncovin, prednisone, Adriamycin, cyclophosphamide) *chemotherapy protocol*

Copaxone ℞ *investigational treatment for relapsing-remitting multiple sclerosis* [copolymer 1]

COPB (cyclophosphamide, Oncovin, prednisone, bleomycin) *chemotherapy protocol*

COP-BLAM (cyclophosphamide, Oncovin, prednisone, bleomycin, Adriamycin, Matulane) *chemotherapy protocol*

COP-BLEO (cyclophosphamide, Oncovin, prednisone, bleomycin) *chemotherapy protocol*

Cope tablets OTC *analgesic; antipyretic; anti-inflammatory; antacid* [aspirin; caffeine; magnesium hydroxide; aluminum hydroxide] 421•32•50•25 mg

COPE (cyclophosphamide, Oncovin, Platinol, etoposide) *chemotherapy protocol*

Cophene No. 2 sustained-release capsules ℞ *decongestant; antihistamine* [pseudoephedrine HCl; chlorpheniramine maleate] 120•12 mg

Cophene XP liquid ℞ *narcotic antitussive; decongestant; expectorant* [hydrocodone bitartrate; pseudoephedrine HCl; guaifenesin; alcohol 12.5%] 5•60•200 mg/5 mL

Cophene-B subcu or IM injection ℞ *antihistamine; anaphylaxis* [brompheniramine maleate] 10 mg/mL

Cophene-X capsules ℞ *antitussive; decongestant; expectorant* [carbetapentane citrate; phenylephrine HCl; phenylpropanolamine HCl; potassium guaiacolsulfonate] 20•10•10•45 mg

copolymer 1 (COP 1) *(orphan: multiple sclerosis)*

copovithane BAN

COPP (CCNU, Oncovin, procarbazine, prednisone) *chemotherapy protocol*

COPP (cyclophosphamide, Oncovin, procarbazine, prednisone) *chemotherapy protocol*

copper *element (Cu)*

copper chloride dihydrate [see: cupric chloride]

copper gluconate (copper D-gluconate) USP *trace mineral supplement*

copper sulfate pentahydrate [see: cupric sulfate]

copper 10-undecenoate [see: copper undecylenate]

copper undecylenate USAN

copperhead snake antivenin [see: antivenin (Crotalidae) polyvalent]

Co-Pyronil 2 Pulvules (capsules) OTC *decongestant; antihistamine* [pseudoephedrine HCl; chlorpheniramine maleate] 60•4 mg

CoQ10 [see: coenzyme Q10]

Co-Q$_{10}$ soft capsules OTC *dietary supplement* [coenzyme Q$_{10}$]

Coracin ophthalmic ointment (discontinued 1995) ℞ *topical ophthalmic corticosteroidal anti-inflammatory; antibiotic* [hydrocortisone acetate; neomycin sulfate; bacitracin zinc; polymyxin B sulfate] 1%•0.5%•400 U/g•10,000 U/g

coral snake antivenin [see: antivenin (Micrurus fulvius)]

corbadrine INN *adrenergic; vasoconstrictor* [also: levonordefrin]

Cordarone IV infusion ℞ *antiarrhythmic for acute ventricular tachycardia and fibrillation* [amiodarone HCl] 50 mg/mL

Cordarone tablets ℞ *antiarrhythmic for acute ventricular tachycardia and fibrillation (orphan)* [amiodarone HCl] 200 mg

Cordran ointment, lotion, tape ℞ *topical corticosteroid* [flurandrenolide] 0.025%, 0.05%; 0.05%; 4 µg/cm^2

Cordran SP cream ℞ *topical corticosteroid* [flurandrenolide] 0.025%, 0.05%

Cordran-N cream, ointment (discontinued 1993) ℞ *topical corticosteroid; antibiotic* [flurandrenolide; neomycin sulfate]

Coreg film-coated tablets ℞ *antihypertensive; α- and β-blocker* [carvedilol] 6.25, 12.5, 25 mg

Corgard tablets ℞ *antihypertensive; antianginal; β-blocker* [nadolol] 20, 40, 80, 120, 160 mg

coriander oil NF

Coricidin Demilets (chewable tablets) (discontinued 1993) OTC *pediatric decongestant, antihistamine and analgesic* [phenylpropanolamine HCl; chlorpheniramine maleate; acetaminophen]

Coricidin tablets OTC *antihistamine; analgesic* [chlorpheniramine maleate; acetaminophen] 2•325 mg

Coricidin D; Coricidin Sinus Headache tablets OTC *decongestant; antihistamine; analgesic* [phenylpropanolamine HCl; chlorpheniramine maleate; acetaminophen] 12.5•2•325 mg; 12.5•2•500 mg

Coridicin Nasal Mist spray (discontinued 1992) OTC *nasal decongestant* [oxymetazoline HCl]

Corlopam (commercially available overseas) ℞ *investigational vasodilator for severe hypertension and chronic renal failure* [fenoldopam]

cormed [see: nikethamide]

cormetasone INN *topical anti-inflammatory* [also: cormethasone acetate]

cormetasone acetate [see: cormethasone acetate]

cormethasone acetate USAN *topical anti-inflammatory* [also: cormetasone]

Corn Huskers lotion OTC *moisturizer; emollient*

corn oil NF *solvent; caloric replacement*

corpus luteum extract [see: progesterone]

Corque cream ℞ *topical corticosteroid; antifungal; antibacterial* [hydrocortisone; clioquinol] 1%•3%

Correctol tablets (discontinued 1996) OTC *laxative; stool softener* [yellow phenolphthalein; docusate sodium] 65•100 mg

Correctol Extra Gentle soft gel capsules OTC *stool softener* [docusate sodium] 100 mg

Corsevin M ℞ *investigational agent for coagulation disorders and unstable angina* [monoclonal antibodies]

CortaGel OTC *topical corticosteroid* [hydrocortisone] 0.5%, 1%

Cortaid cream, lotion OTC *topical corticosteroid* [hydrocortisone acetate] 1%

Cortaid ointment (discontinued 1993) OTC *topical corticosteroid* [hydrocortisone acetate] 1%

Cortaid pump spray OTC *topical corticosteroid* [hydrocortisone] 0.5%, 1%

Cortaid Faststick roll-on stick OTC *topical corticosteroid* [hydrocortisone acetate; alcohol 55%] 1%

Cortaid with Aloe cream, ointment OTC *topical corticosteroid* [hydrocortisone acetate] 0.5%

Cortatrigen Modified ear drops, otic suspension ℞ *topical corticosteroidal anti-inflammatory; antibiotic* [hydrocortisone; neomycin sulfate; polymyxin B sulfate] 1%•5 mg•10,000 U per mL

Cort-Dome cream ℞ *topical corticosteroid* [hydrocortisone] 0.5%, 1% ⓘ Cortone

Cort-Dome lotion (discontinued 1993) ℞ *topical corticosteroid* [hydrocortisone]

Cort-Dome High Potency rectal suppositories ℞ *topical corticosteroidal anti-inflammatory* [hydrocortisone acetate] 25 mg

Cortef tablets, oral suspension ℞ *glucocorticoids* [hydrocortisone] 5, 10, 20 mg; 10 mg/5 mL

Cortef Feminine Itch cream OTC *topical corticosteroid* [hydrocortisone acetate] 0.5%

Cortenema retention enema ℞ *ulcerative colitis* [hydrocortisone] 100 mg/60 mL ⓘ quart enema

cortenil [see: desoxycorticosterone acetate]

cortexolone [see: cortodoxone]

Cortic ear drops ℞ *topical corticosteroidal anti-inflammatory; topical anesthetic; bacteriostatic* [hydrocortisone; pramoxine HCl; chloroxylenol] 10•10•1 mg/mL

Corticaine anorectal cream (discontinued 1995) OTC *topical corticosteroidal anti-inflammatory; local anesthetic* [hydrocortisone acetate; dibucaine] 0.5%•0.5%

Corticaine cream OTC *topical corticosteroid* [hydrocortisone acetate] 0.5%, 1%

corticorelin ovine triflutate USAN, INN *corticotropin-releasing hormone; diagnostic aid for Cushing syndrome & adrenocortical insufficiency*

corticotrophin INN, BAN *adrenocorticotropic hormone; glucocorticoid; diagnostic aid* [also: corticotropin]

corticotrophin-zinc hydroxide INN *adrenocorticotropic hormone; glucocorticoid; diagnostic aid* [also: corticotropin zinc hydroxide]

corticotropin USP *adrenocorticotropic hormone; glucocorticoid; diagnostic aid* [also: corticotrophin] 40 U/vial injection

corticotropin, repository USP *adrenocorticotropic hormone; glucocorticoid; diagnostic aid*

corticotropin tetracosapeptide [see: cosyntropin]

corticotropin zinc hydroxide USP *adrenocorticotropic hormone; glucocorticoid; diagnostic aid* [also: corticotrophin-zinc hydroxide]

Cortifoam intrarectal foam aerosol ℞ *ulcerative proctitis* [hydrocortisone acetate] 90 mg/dose

Cortin cream ℞ *topical corticosteroid; antifungal; antibacterial* [hydrocortisone; clioquinol] ⓘ Cotrim

cortisol [see: hydrocortisone]
cortisol 21-acetate [see: hydrocortisone acetate]
cortisol 21-butyrate [see: hydrocortisone butyrate]
cortisol 21-cyclopentanepropionate [see: hydrocortisone cypionate]
cortisol cyclopentylpropionate [see: hydrocortisone cypionate]
cortisol 21-valerate [see: hydrocortisone valerate]
cortisone INN, BAN *glucocorticoid* [also: cortisone acetate] ⑫ Cortizone
cortisone acetate USP *glucocorticoid* [also: cortisone] 5, 10, 25 mg oral
Cortisporin cream ℞ *topical corticosteroid; antibiotic* [hydrocortisone acetate; neomycin sulfate; polymyxin B sulfate] 0.5%•0.5%•10,000 U per g
Cortisporin eye drop suspension ℞ *topical ophthalmic corticosteroidal anti-inflammatory; antibiotic* [hydrocortisone; neomycin sulfate; polymyxin B sulfate] 1%•0.35%•10,000 U per mL
Cortisporin ointment ℞ *topical corticosteroid; antibiotic* [hydrocortisone; neomycin sulfate; bacitracin zinc; polymyxin B sulfate] 1%•0.5%•400 U•5,000 U per g
Cortisporin ophthalmic ointment ℞ *topical ophthalmic corticosteroidal anti-inflammatory; antibiotic* [hydrocortisone; neomycin sulfate; bacitracin zinc; polymyxin B sulfate] 1%•0.35%•400 U/g•10,000 U/g
Cortisporin Otic ear drops, otic suspension ℞ *topical corticosteroidal anti-inflammatory; antibiotic* [hydrocortisone; neomycin sulfate; polymyxin B sulfate] 1%•5 mg•10,000 U per mL
cortisuzol INN
cortivazol USAN, INN *glucocorticoid*
Cortizone-5 ointment, cream OTC *topical corticosteroid* [hydrocortisone] 0.5%; 1% ⑫ cortisone
Cortizone-10 ointment OTC *topical corticosteroid* [hydrocortisone] 1%
cortodoxone USAN, INN, BAN *anti-inflammatory*
Cortone Acetate tablets, intra-articular or intralesional injection ℞ *glucocorticoids* [cortisone acetate] 25 mg; 50 mg/mL ⑫ Cort-Dome
Cortril ointment (discontinued 1993) ℞ *topical corticosteroid* [hydrocortisone]
Cortrosyn powder for injection ℞ *multiple sclerosis; infantile spasms; diagnostic purposes* [cosyntropin] 0.25 mg
Corvert IV infusion ℞ *antiarrhythmic for atrial fibrillation/flutter* [ibutilide fumarate] 0.1 mg/mL
Corzide 40/5; Corzide 80/5 tablets ℞ *antihypertensive* [nadolol; bendroflumethiazide] 40•5 mg; 80•5 mg
Cosmegen powder for IV injection ℞ *antibiotic antineoplastic for melanomas, sarcomas, testicular and trophoblastic tumors* [dactinomycin] 0.5 mg
cosmoline [see: petrolatum]
cosyntropin USAN *adrenocorticotropic hormone* [also: tetracosactide; tetracosactrin]
cotarnine chloride NF
cotarnine HCl [see: cotarnine chloride]
Cotazym capsules ℞ *digestive enzymes; antacid* [lipase; protease; amylase; calcium carbonate] 8000 U•30,000 U•30,000 U•25 mg
Cotazym-S capsules containing enteric-coated spheres ℞ *digestive enzymes* [lipase; protease; amylase] 5000•20,000•20,000 U
cotinine INN *antidepressant* [also: cotinine fumarate]
cotinine fumarate USAN *antidepressant* [also: cotinine]
Cotridin syrup (available only in Canada) ℞ *narcotic antitussive; decongestant; antihistamine* [codeine phosphate; pseudoephedrine HCl; triprolidine HCl] 2•6•0.4 mg/mL
Cotridin Expectorant oral solution (available only in Canada) ℞ *narcotic antitussive; decongestant; antihistamine* [codeine phosphate; pseudoephedrine HCl; triprolidine HCl; guaifenesin] 2•6•0.4•20 mg/mL
Cotrim; Cotrim D.S. tablets ℞ *anti-infective; antibacterial* [trimethoprim; sulfamethoxazole] 80•400 mg; 160•800 mg ⑫ Cortin
Cotrim IV infusion (discontinued 1994) ℞ *anti-infective; antibacterial*

[trimethoprim; sulfamethoxazole] 16•80 mg/mL
Cotrim Pediatric oral suspension ℞ *anti-infective; antibacterial* [trimethoprim; sulfamethoxazole] 40•200 mg/5 mL
co-trimoxazole BAN [also: trimethoprim + sulfamethoxazole] ⊡ clotrimazole
cotriptyline INN
cotton, purified USP *surgical aid*
cottonseed oil NF *solvent*
Co-Tuss V liquid ℞ *narcotic antitussive; expectorant* [hydrocodone bitartrate; guaifenesin] 5•100 mg
Cough syrup OTC *antitussive; decongestant; expectorant* [dextromethorphan hydrobromide; phenylephrine HCl; guaifenesin] 10•5•100 mg/5 mL
Cough Formula liquid OTC *antitussive; antihistamine* [dextromethorphan hydrobromide; chlorpheniramine maleate; alcohol 10%] 15•2 mg/5 mL
Cough Formula with Decongestant liquid OTC *antitussive; decongestant* [dextromethorphan hydrobromide; pseudoephedrine HCl; alcohol 10%] 10•20 mg/5 mL
Cough-X lozenges OTC *antitussive; topical oral anesthetic* [dextromethorphan hydrobromide; benzocaine] 5•2 mg
Coulter HIV-1 p24 Antigen Assay test for professional use *in vitro diagnostic aid for HIV in the blood*
Coumadin tablets, powder for injection ℞ *anticoagulant* [warfarin sodium] 1, 2, 2.5, 4, 5, 7.5, 10 mg; 2 mg/mL ⊡ Kemadrin
coumafos INN [also: coumaphos]
coumamycin INN *antibacterial* [also: coumermycin]
coumaphos BAN [also: coumafos]
coumarin NF *anticoagulant (orphan: renal cell carcinoma)*
coumazoline INN
coumermycin USAN *antibacterial* [also: coumamycin]
coumermycin sodium USAN *antibacterial*
coumetarol INN [also: cumetharol]
Counterpain Rub (discontinued 1992) OTC *counterirritant; antiseptic* [methyl salicylate; menthol; eugenol]
Covangesic tablets OTC *decongestant; antihistamine; analgesic* [phenylpropanolamine HCl; phenylephrine HCl; chlorpheniramine maleate; pyrilamine maleate; acetaminophen] 12.5•7.5•2•12.5•275 mg
covatin HCl [see: captodiame HCl]
Covera-HS film-coated, extended-release tablets ℞ *antihypertensive; antianginal; calcium channel blocker* [verapamil HCl] 180, 240 mg
Cozaar film-coated tablets ℞ *antihypertensive; angiotensin II blocker* [losartan potassium] 25, 50 mg
CP (chlorambucil, prednisone) *chemotherapy protocol*
CP (cyclophosphamide, Platinol) *chemotherapy protocol*
CP (cyclophosphamide, prednisone) *chemotherapy protocol*
CPA TR extended-release capsules (discontinued 1993) ℞ *decongestant; antihistamine* [phenylpropanolamine HCl; chlorpheniramine maleate]
CPB (cyclophosphamide, Platinol, BCNU) *chemotherapy protocol*
CPC (cyclophosphamide, Platinol, carboplatin) *chemotherapy protocol*
CPI rectal suppositories (discontinued 1992) OTC *temporary relief of hemorrhoidal symptoms* [bismuth subgallate; bismuth resorcin compound; benzyl benzoate; zinc oxide; balsam Peru] 2.25%•1.75%•1.2%•11%•1.8%
CPM (CCNU, procarbazine, methotrexate) *chemotherapy protocol*
CPOB (cyclophosphamide, prednisone, Oncovin, bleomycin) *chemotherapy protocol*
CPT-11 (camptothecin-11) [see: irinotecan]
^{51}**Cr** [see: albumin, chromated Cr 51 serum]
^{51}**Cr** [see: chromic chloride Cr 51]
^{51}**Cr** [see: chromic phosphate Cr 51]
^{51}**Cr** [see: sodium chromate Cr 51]
CRDS (curdlan sulfate) [q.v.]
Creamy Tar shampoo OTC *antiseborrheic; antipsoriatic; antipruritic; antibacterial* [coal tar] 7.32%

creatinolfosfate INN
Creon capsules containing enteric-coated microspheres ℞ *digestive enzymes* [pancreatin; lipase; protease; amylase] 300 mg•8000 U•13,000 U•30,000 U
Creon 10; Creon 20 capsules containing enteric-coated microspheres ℞ *digestive enzymes* [lipase; amylase; protease] 10,000•33,200•37,500 U; 20,000•66,400•75,000 U
Creon 25 capsules containing enteric-coated microspheres (discontinued 1994) ℞ *digestive enzymes* [lipase; amylase; protease; pancreatin] 25,000 U•74,700 U•62,500 U•300 mg
creosote carbonate USP
Creo-Terpin liquid OTC *antitussive* [dextromethorphan hydrobromide; alcohol 25%] 10 mg/15 mL
cresol NF *disinfectant*
cresotamide INN
cresoxydiol [see: mephenesin]
crestomycin sulfate [see: paromomycin sulfate]
Cresylate ear drops ℞ *antibacterial/antifungal* [m-cresyl acetate; alcohol; chlorobutanol] 25%•25%•1%
cresylic acid [see: cresol]
crilanomer INN
crilvastatin USAN, INN *antihyperlipidemic*
crisnatol INN *antineoplastic* [also: crisnatol mesylate]
crisnatol mesylate USAN *antineoplastic* [also: crisnatol]
Criticare HN ready-to-use liquid OTC *enteral nutritional therapy* [lactose-free formula]
Crixivan capsules ℞ *antiviral protease inhibitor for HIV* [indinavir sulfate] 200, 400 mg
crobefate INN *combining name for radicals or groups*
croconazole INN
crofilcon A USAN *hydrophilic contact lens material*
Crolom eye drops ℞ *mast cell stabilizer; ocular antiallergic/antiviral for vernal keratoconjunctivitis (orphan)* [cromolyn sodium] 4%
cromacate INN *combining name for radicals or groups*
cromakalim INN, BAN
Cro-Man-Zin tablets OTC *mineral supplement* [chromium; manganese; zinc] 0.2•5•25 mg
cromesilate INN *combining name for radicals or groups*
cromitrile INN *antiasthmatic* [also: cromitrile sodium]
cromitrile sodium USAN *antiasthmatic* [also: cromitrile]
cromoglicic acid INN *prophylactic antiasthmatic* [also: cromolyn sodium; cromoglycic acid]
cromoglycic acid BAN *prophylactic antiasthmatic* [also: cromolyn sodium; cromoglicic acid]
cromolyn sodium USAN, USP *prophylactic antiasthmatic; (orphan: mastocytosis; vernal keratoconjunctivitis)* [also: cromoglicic acid; cromoglycic acid] 20 mg/2 mL inhalation
Cronassial ℞ *(orphan: retinitis pigmentosa)* [gangliosides, sodium salts]
cronetal [see: disulfiram]
cronidipine INN
cropropamide INN, BAN
croscarmellose INN *tablet disintegrant* [also: croscarmellose sodium]
croscarmellose sodium USAN, NF *tablet disintegrant* [also: croscarmellose]
crospovidone NF *tablet excipient*
cross-linked carboxymethylcellulose sodium [now: croscarmellose sodium]
cross-linked carmellose sodium [see: croscarmellose sodium]
Crotab ℞ *treatment of Crotalidae snake bites (orphan)* [antivenin (Crotalidae) polyvalent (ovine) Fab]
crotaline antivenin [see: antivenin (Crotalidae) polyvalent]
crotamiton USP, INN, BAN *scabicide*
crotetamide INN [also: crotethamide]
crotethamide BAN [also: crotetamide]
crotoniazide INN
crotonylidenisoniazid [see: crotoniazide]
crotoxyfos BAN
crude tuberculin [see: tuberculin, old]
Cruex cream, aerosol powder OTC *topical antifungal* [undecylenic acid; zinc undecylenate] 20% total; 19% total

Cruex powder OTC *topical antifungal* [calcium undecylenate] 10%

crufomate USAN, INN, BAN *veterinary anthelmintic*

cryofluorane INN *aerosol propellant* [also: dichlorotetrafluoroethane]

cryptenamine acetates

CryptoGAM ℞ *investigational treatment for cryptosporidiosis in immunocompromised patients*

Crypto-LA slide test for professional use *in vitro diagnostic aid for Cryptococcus neoformans antigens*

cryptosporidium hyperimmune bovine colostrum IgG concentrate (*orphan: cryptosporidium-induced diarrhea in AIDS*)

Cryptosporidium parvum **bovine immunoglobulin concentrate** [see: bovine immunoglobulin concentrate]

crystal violet [see: gentian violet]

crystallized trypsin [see: trypsin, crystallized]

Crystamine IM or subcu injection ℞ *antianemic; vitamin B_{12} supplement* [cyanocobalamin] 1000 µg/mL

Crysti 12 IM or subcu injection (discontinued 1994) ℞ *antianemic; vitamin B_{12} supplement* [cyanocobalamin] 1000 µg/mL

Crysti 1000 IM or subcu injection ℞ *antianemic; vitamin B_{12} supplement* [cyanocobalamin] 1000 µg/mL

Crysticillin 300 A.S.; Crysticillin 600 A.S. IM injection ℞ *bactericidal antibiotic* [penicillin G procaine] 300,000 U/mL; 600,000 U/mL

Crysti-Liver IM injection (discontinued 1994) ℞ *antianemic; vitamin supplement* [liver extracts; vitamin B_{12}; folic acid]

Crystodigin tablets ℞ *cardiac glycoside to increase cardiac output; antiarrhythmic* [digitoxin] 0.05, 0.1 mg

crystografin [see: meglumine diatriazole]

^{131}**Cs** [see: cesium chloride Cs 131]

C-Solve OTC *lotion base*

C-Solve 2 topical solution (discontinued 1994) ℞ *topical antibiotic for acne* [erythromycin] 2%

CSP (cellulose sodium phosphate) [q.v.]

CS-T test kit for home use (discontinued 1992) OTC *in vitro diagnostic aid for fecal occult blood*

CT (cisplatin, Taxol) *chemotherapy protocol*

CT (cytarabine, thioguanine) *chemotherapy protocol*

CTAB (cetyltrimethyl ammonium bromide)

CTCb (cyclophosphamide, thiotepa, carboplatin) *chemotherapy protocol*

CTH (ceramide trihexosidase) [q.v.]

C/T/S topical solution ℞ *topical antibiotic for acne* [clindamycin phosphate] 10 mg/mL

C-Tussin Expectorant liquid (discontinued 1992) ℞ *narcotic antitussive; decongestant; expectorant* [codeine phosphate; pseudoephedrine HCl; guaifenesin; alcohol]

Ctx-Plat (cyclophosphamide, Platinol) *chemotherapy protocol*

^{64}**Cu** [see: cupric acetate Cu 64]

Culturette 10 Minute Group A Strep ID slide test for professional use *in vitro diagnostic test for Group A streptococcal antigens in throat swabs* [latex agglutination test]

cumetharol BAN [also: coumetarol]

cupric acetate Cu 64 USAN *radioactive agent*

cupric chloride USP *dietary copper supplement*

cupric sulfate USP *antidote to phosphorus; dietary copper supplement* 0.4, 2 mg/mL injection

Cuprimine capsules ℞ *metal chelating agent for rheumatoid arthritis, Wilson's disease and cystinuria* [penicillamine] 125, 250 mg

cuprimyxin USAN, INN *veterinary antibacterial; antifungal*

Cupri-Pak IV injection (discontinued 1992) ℞ *intravenous nutritional therapy* [cupric sulfate]

cuproxoline INN, BAN

curare [see: tubocurarine chloride]

curdlan sulfate (CRDS) *investigational (Phase I/II) antiviral for HIV*

Curel Moisturizing cream, lotion (discontinued 1993) OTC *moisturizer; emollient*

curium *element (Cm)*

Curosurf ℞ *(orphan: infant respiratory distress syndrome of prematurity)* [pulmonary surfactant replacement (porcine)]

curral [see: diallybarbituric acid]

Curretab tablets ℞ *progestin for secondary amenorrhea or abnormal uterine bleeding* [medroxyprogesterone acetate] 10 mg

Cūtar Bath Oil Emulsion OTC *antipsoriatic; antiseborrheic; antipruritic; emollient* [coal tar] 7.5%

Cūtemol cream OTC *moisturizer; emollient* [allantoin]

Cuticura ointment (discontinued 1995) OTC *topical acne treatment* [sulfur; phenol; oxyquinoline] 0.5%•0.1%•0.05%

Cuticura Acne cream (discontinued 1994) OTC *topical keratolytic for acne* [benzoyl peroxide] 5%

Cuticura Medicated Soap bar OTC *therapeutic skin cleanser* [triclocarban] 1%

Cutivate cream, ointment ℞ *topical corticosteroidal anti-inflammatory* [fluticasone propionate] 0.05%; 0.005%

CV (cisplatin, VePesid) *chemotherapy protocol*

CV Nutrients soft capsules OTC *dietary supplement* [vitamin C; vitamin E; multiple minerals; coenzyme Q_{10}; omega-3 fish oils; garlic]

CVA (cyclophosphamide, vincristine, Adriamycin) *chemotherapy protocol*

CVA-BMP; CVA + BMP (cyclophosphamide, vincristine, Adriamycin, BCNU, methotrexate, procarbazine) *chemotherapy protocol*

CVAD; C-VAD (cyclophosphamide, vincristine, Adriamycin, dexamethasone) *chemotherapy protocol*

CVB (CCNU, vinblastine, bleomycin) *chemotherapy protocol*

CVBD (CCNU, bleomycin, vinblastine, dexamethasone) *chemotherapy protocol*

CVD (cisplatin, vinblastine, dacarbazine) *chemotherapy protocol*

CVEB (cisplatin, vinblastine, etoposide, bleomycin) *chemotherapy protocol*

CVI (carboplatin, VePesid, ifosfamide [with mesna rescue]) *chemotherapy protocol* [also: VIC]

CVM (cyclophosphamide, vincristine, methotrexate) *chemotherapy protocol*

CVP (cyclophosphamide, vincristine, prednisone) *chemotherapy protocol*

CVPP (CCNU, vinblastine, procarbazine, prednisone) *chemotherapy protocol*

CVPP (cyclophosphamide, Velban, procarbazine, prednisone) *chemotherapy protocol*

CVPP-CCNU (cyclophosphamide, vinblastine, procarbazine, prednisone, CCNU) *chemotherapy protocol*

CY-1503 *(orphan: post-ischemic pulmonary reperfusion edema)*

CY-1787 *investigational E-selectin blocker for sepsis*

CY-1899 *(orphan: chronic active hepatitis B)*

cyacetacide INN [also: cyacetazide]

cyacetazide BAN [also: cyacetacide]

CyADIC (cyclophosphamide, Adriamycin, DIC) *chemotherapy protocol*

cyamemazine INN

cyamepromazine [see: cyamemazine]

cyanamide JAN [also: calcium carbimide]

Cyanide Antidote Package ℞ *emergency treatment of cyanide poisoning* [sodium nitrite; sodium thiosulfate; amyl nitrite inhalant] 300 mg•12.5 g•0.3 mL

cyanoacetohydrazide [see: cyacetazide]

cyanocobalamin USP, INN, BAN, JAN *vitamin B_{12}; hematopoietic* 25, 50, 100, 250, 500, 1000 μg oral; 100, 1000 μg/mL injection

cyanocobalamin (^{57}Co) INN *pernicious anemia test; radioactive agent* [also: cyanocobalamin Co 57]

cyanocobalamin (^{58}Co) INN

cyanocobalamin (^{60}Co) INN *pernicious anemia test; radioactive agent* [also: cyanocobalamin Co 60]

cyanocobalamin Co 57 USAN, USP *pernicious anemia test; radioactive agent* [also: cyanocobalamin (^{57}Co)]

cyanocobalamin Co 60 USAN, USP *pernicious anemia test; radioactive agent* [also: cyanocobalamin (^{60}Co)]

Cyanoject IM or subcu injection ℞ *antianemic; vitamin B_{12} supplement* [cyanocobalamin] 1000 μg/mL

cyclacillin USAN, USP *antibacterial* [also: ciclacillin]

cyclamate calcium NF

cyclamic acid USAN, BAN *non-nutritive sweetener (banned in USA)*

cyclamide [see: glycyclamide]

Cyclan capsules ℞ *peripheral vasodilator* [cyclandelate] 200, 400 mg

cyclandelate INN, BAN *peripheral vasodilator* 200, 400 mg oral

cyclarbamate INN, BAN

cyclazocine USAN, INN *analgesic*

cyclazodone INN

cyclexanone INN

cyclic propylene carbonate [see: propylene carbonate]

cyclindole USAN *antidepressant* [also: ciclindole]

Cyclinex-1 powder OTC *formula for infants with urea cycle disorders or gyrate atrophy*

Cyclinex-2 powder OTC *enteral nutritional therapy for urea cycle disorders or gyrate atrophy* [essential amino acids]

cycliramine INN *antihistamine* [also: cycliramine maleate]

cycliramine maleate USAN *antihistamine* [also: cycliramine]

cyclizine USP, INN, BAN *antihistamine; antiemetic; anticholinergic; motion sickness relief*

cyclizine HCl USP, BAN *antiemetic*

cyclizine lactate USP, BAN *antinauseant*

cyclobarbital NF, INN [also: cyclobarbitone]

cyclobarbital calcium NF

cyclobarbitone BAN [also: cyclobarbital]

cyclobendazole USAN *anthelmintic* [also: ciclobendazole]

cyclobenzaprine INN *skeletal muscle relaxant* [also: cyclobenzaprine HCl]

cyclobenzaprine HCl USAN, USP *skeletal muscle relaxant* [also: cyclobenzaprine] 10 mg oral

cyclobutoic acid INN

cyclobutyrol INN

cyclocarbothiamine [see: cycotiamine]

Cyclocort ointment, cream, lotion ℞ *topical corticosteroid* [amcinonide] 0.1%

cyclocoumarol BAN

cyclocumarol [see: cyclocoumarol]

α-cyclodextrin [see: alfadex]

cyclofenil INN, BAN

cyclofilcon A USAN *hydrophilic contact lens material*

cycloguanil embonate INN, BAN *antimalarial* [also: cycloguanil pamoate]

cycloguanil pamoate USAN *antimalarial* [also: cycloguanil embonate]

Cyclogyl Drop-Tainers (eye drops) ℞ *cycloplegic; mydriatic* [cyclopentolate HCl] 0.5%, 1%, 2%

cyclohexanehexol [see: inositol]

cyclohexanesulfamate dihydrate [see: sodium cyclamate]

cyclohexanesulfamic acid *(banned in the USA)* [see: cyclamic acid]

cycloheximide USAN *antipsoriatic* [also: cicloheximide]

p-cyclohexylhydratropic acid [see: hexaprofen]

N-cyclohexyllinoleamide [see: clinolamide]

4-cyclohexyloxybenzoate [see: cyclomethycaine]

1-cyclohexylpropyl carbamate [see: procymate]

N-cyclohexylsulfamic acid *(banned in the USA)* [see: cyclamic acid]

cyclomenol INN

cyclomethicone NF *wetting agent*

cyclomethycaine INN, BAN *local anesthetic* [also: cyclomethycaine sulfate]

cyclomethycaine sulfate USP *local anesthetic* [also: cyclomethycaine]

Cyclomydril Drop-Tainers (eye drops) ℞ *cycloplegic; mydriatic* [cyclopentolate HCl; phenylephrine HCl] 0.2%•1%

cyclonium iodide [see: oxapium iodide]

cyclopentamine INN, BAN [also: cyclopentamine HCl]
cyclopentamine HCl USP [also: cyclopentamine]
cyclopentaphene [see: cyclarbamate]
cyclopenthiazide USAN, INN, BAN *antihypertensive*
cyclopentolate INN, BAN *ophthalmic anticholinergic* [also: cyclopentolate HCl]
cyclopentolate HCl USP *ophthalmic anticholinergic; mydriatic; cycloplegic* [also: cyclopentolate] 1% eye drops
cyclophenazine HCl USAN *antipsychotic* [also: ciclofenazine]
cyclophosphamide USP, INN, BAN *alkylating antineoplastic; immunosuppressive*
cyclopolydimethylsiloxane [see: cyclomethicone]
cyclopregnol INN
cycloprolol BAN *antiadrenergic (β-receptor)* [also: ciclprolol HCl; cicloprolol]
cyclopropane USP, INN *inhalation general anesthetic*
Cyclo-Prostin ℞ *(orphan: primary pulmonary hypertension; heparin replacement for hemodialysis)* [epoprostenol]
cyclopyrronium bromide INN
cycloserine USP, INN, BAN *bacteriostatic; tuberculosis retreatment; investigational treatment for Alzheimer's disease*
L-cycloserine *(orphan: Gaucher's disease)*
Cyclospasmol capsules ℞ *peripheral vasodilator* [cyclandelate] 200, 400 mg
cyclosporin BAN *immunosuppressive* [also: cyclosporine; ciclosporin]
cyclosporin A [now: cyclosporine]
cyclosporine USAN, USP *immunosuppressive for transplants; (orphan: keratoconjunctivitis sicca; corneal melting syndrome)* [also: ciclosporin; cyclosporin]
cyclothiazide USAN, USP, INN, BAN *diuretic; antihypertensive*
cyclovalone INN
cycobemin [see: cyanocobalamin]
cycotiamine INN
cycrimine INN, BAN [also: cycrimine HCl]
cycrimine HCl USP [also: cycrimine]

Cycrin tablets ℞ *progestin for secondary amenorrhea or abnormal uterine bleeding* [medroxyprogesterone acetate] 2.5, 5, 10 mg
cyfluthrin BAN
cyhalothrin BAN
cyheptamide USAN, INN *anticonvulsant*
cyheptropine INN
CyHOP (cyclophosphamide, Halotestin, Oncovin, prednisone) *chemotherapy protocol*
Cyklokapron tablets, IV injection ℞ *systemic hemostatic; (orphan: angioneurotic edema; congenital coagulopathy)* [tranexamic acid] 500 mg; 100 mg/mL
Cylert tablets, chewable tablets ℞ *CNS stimulant for attention deficit hyperactive disorders (ADHD)* [pemoline] 18.75, 37.5, 75 mg; 37.5 mg
Cylex; Cylex Sugar-Free throat lozenges OTC *topical oral anesthetic; antiseptic* [benzocaine; cetylpyridinium chloride] 15•5 mg
cymemoxine [see: cimemoxin]
cynarine INN
Cyomin IM or subcu injection ℞ *antianemic; vitamin B$_{12}$ supplement* [cyanocobalamin] 1000 µg/mL
cypenamine INN, BAN *antidepressant* [also: cypenamine HCl]
cypenamine HCl USAN *antidepressant* [also: cypenamine]
cypionate USAN, BAN *combining name for radicals or groups* [also: cipionate]
cypothrin USAN *veterinary insecticide*
cyprazepam USAN, INN *sedative*
cyprenorphine INN, BAN
cyprenorphine HCl [see: cyprenorphine]
cyprodemanol [see: cyprodenate]
cyprodenate INN
cyproheptadine INN, BAN *antihistamine; antipruritic* [also: cyproheptadine HCl]
cyproheptadine HCl USP, JAN *antihistamine; antipruritic* [also: cyproheptadine] 4 mg oral; 2 mg/5 mL oral
cyprolidol INN *antidepressant* [also: cyprolidol HCl]
cyprolidol HCl USAN *antidepressant* [also: cyprolidol]

cyproquinate USAN *coccidiostat for poultry* [also: ciproquinate]

cyproterone INN, BAN *antiandrogen* [also: cyproterone acetate]

cyproterone acetate USAN *antiandrogen; (orphan: severe hirsutism)* [also: cyproterone]

cyproximide USAN *antipsychotic; antidepressant* [also: ciproximide]

cyren A [see: diethylstilbestrol]

cyren B [see: diethylstilbestrol dipropionate]

cyromazine INN, BAN

Cystagon capsules ℞ *antiurolithic for nephropathic cystinosis (orphan)* [cysteamine bitartrate] 50, 150 mg

cystamin [see: methenamine]

cysteamine USAN, BAN *antiurolithic; (orphan: nephropathic cystinosis)* [also: mercaptamine]

cysteamine bitartrate *antiurolithic for nephropathic cystinosis (orphan)*

cysteamine HCl USAN *antiurolithic*

cysteine (L-cysteine) INN *nonessential amino acid; (orphan: erythropoietic protoporphyria photosensitivity); symbols: Cys, C* [also: cysteine HCl]

cysteine HCl (L-cysteine HCl) USP *nonessential amino acid* [also: cysteine] 50 mg/mL injection

L-cysteine HCl monohydrate [see: cysteine HCl]

Cystex tablets ℞ *urinary anti-infective; analgesic; acidifier* [methenamine; sodium salicylate; benzoic acid] 162•162.5•32 mg

cystic fibrosis gene therapy *(orphan: cystic fibrosis)*

cystic fibrosis transmembrane conductance regulator (CFTR) *(orphan: cystic fibrosis)*

Cysticide ℞ *(orphan: neurocysticercosis)* [praziquantel]

cystine (L-cystine) USAN *amino acid*

Cysto-Conray; Cysto-Conray II intracavitary instillation ℞ *radiopaque agent* [iothalamate meglumine] 43%; 17.2%

cystogen [see: methenamine]

Cystografin; Cystografin Dilute intracavitary instillation ℞ *cholecystographic radiopaque agent* [diatrizoate meglumine] 30%; 18%

Cystospaz tablets ℞ *GI anticholinergic; antispasmodic* [hyoscyamine sulfate] 0.15 mg

Cystospaz-M timed-release capsules ℞ *GI anticholinergic; antispasmodic* [hyoscyamine sulfate] 0.375 mg

CYT-103-Y-90 *investigational antineoplastic for gastrointestinal, ovarian, and colorectal cancer*

CYT-356-In-111 *investigational imaging aid for prostatic cancer detection and staging*

CYT-356-Y-90 *investigational antineoplastic for prostatic cancer*

CYT-372-In-111 *investigational imaging aid for colorectal cancer detection and staging*

CYTABOM (cytarabine, bleomycin, Oncovin, mechlorethamine) *chemotherapy protocol*

Cytadren tablets ℞ *adrenal steroid inhibitor; antisteroidal antineoplastic for corticotropin-producing tumors* [aminoglutethimide] 250 mg

cytarabine USAN, USP, INN, BAN *antimetabolic antineoplastic; antiviral* 100, 500, 1000 mg injection ⑨ vidarabine

cytarabine, depofoam encapsulated *(orphan: neoplastic meningitis)*

cytarabine HCl USAN *antiviral*

CytoGam IV infusion ℞ *adjunct to kidney transplants from CMV seropositive donor to CMV seronegative recipient* [cytomegalovirus immune globulin, solvent/detergent treated] 50 mg/mL

cytomegalovirus immune globulin, human *(orphan: primary cytomegalovirus of organ and bone marrow transplants)*

cytomegalovirus immune globulin intravenous (CMV-IGIV) [see: globulin, immune]

cytomegalovirus immune globulin intravenous (CMV-IGIV) & ganciclovir sodium *(orphan: cytomegalovirus pneumonia in bone marrow transplant patients)*

cytomegalovirus monoclonal antibody (CMV MAb) *investigational antiviral for AIDS*

Cytomel tablets ℞ *thyroid hormone* [liothyronine sodium] 5, 25, 50 μg

Cytosar-U powder for subcu, intrathecal or IV injection ℞ *antimetabolic antineoplastic for multiple leukemias* [cytarabine] 100, 500, 1000, 2000 mg

cytosine arabinoside (ara-C) [see: cytarabine]

cytosine arabinoside HCl [now: cytarabine HCl]

Cytosol liquid ℞ *sterile irrigant* [physiological irrigating solution]

Cytotec tablets ℞ *prevention of NSAID-induced gastric ulcers* [misoprostol] 100, 200 μg

cytotoxic lymphocyte maturation factor [see: interleukin-12]

Cytovene capsules ℞ *antiviral for treatment of cytomegalovirus (CMV); CMV prevention in HIV (orphan)* [ganciclovir] 250 mg

Cytovene powder for IV infusion ℞ *antiviral for cytomegalovirus; CMV retinitis in AIDS (orphan)* [ganciclovir sodium] 500 mg/vial

Cytoxan tablets, powder for IV injection ℞ *alkylating antineoplastic for multiple leukemias, lymphomas, blastomas, sarcomas, and organ cancers* [cyclophosphamide] 25, 50 mg; 100, 200, 500, 1000, 2000 mg

Cytoxan Lyophilized powder for IV injection ℞ *alkylating antineoplastic for multiple leukemias, lymphomas, blastomas, sarcomas, and organ cancers* [cyclophosphamide] 100, 200, 500, 1000, 2000 mg

CY-VA-DACT (Cytoxin, vincristine, Adriamycin, dactinomycin) *chemotherapy protocol*

CYVADIC; CY-VA-DIC; CyVADIC (cyclophosphamide, vincristine, Adriamycin, DIC) *chemotherapy protocol*

CYVMAD (cyclophosphamide, vincristine, methotrexate, Adriamycin, DTIC) *chemotherapy protocol*

D

D (vitamin D) [q.v.]

D-2.5-W; D-5-W; D-10-W; D-20-W; D-25-W; D-30-W; D-40-W; D-50-W; D-60-W; D-70-W ℞ *intravenous nutritional therapy* [dextrose in water]

D$_2$ (vitamin D$_2$) [see: ergocalciferol]

D$_3$ (vitamin D$_3$) [see: cholecalciferol]

D-38.5-W (discontinued 1992) ℞ *intravenous nutritional therapy* [dextrose in water]

d4T [see: stavudine]

D.A. chewable tablets ℞ *decongestant; antihistamine; anticholinergic* [phenylephrine HCl; chlorpheniramine maleate; methscopolamine nitrate] 10•2•1.25 mg

DA (daunorubicin, ara-C) *chemotherapy protocol*

D.A. II tablets ℞ *decongestant; antihistamine; anticholinergic* [phenylephrine HCl; chlorpheniramine maleate; methscopolamine nitrate] 10•4•1.25 mg

D.A. #34 enteric-coated tablets OTC *digestive aid* [pancreatin concentrate; pepsin; ox bile]

DAA (dihydroxyaluminum aminoacetate) [q.v.]

DAB$_{389}$ IL-2 fusion toxin *investigational (Phase I/II) cytokine for HIV*

dacarbazine USAN, USP, INN, BAN *alkylating antineoplastic for metastatic malignant melanoma and Hodgkin's disease* ☒ Dicarbosil; procarbazine

dacemazine INN

dacisteine INN

dacliximab USAN, INN *immunosuppressant monoclonal antibody*

Dacriose ophthalmic solution OTC *extraocular irrigating solution* [sterile isotonic solution]

dactinomycin USAN, USP, BAN *antibiotic antineoplastic* [also: actinomycin D]

dacuronium bromide INN, BAN

DADDS (diacetyl diaminodiphenylsulfone) [see: acedapsone]

dagapamil INN

Daily Care ointment OTC *topical diaper rash treatment* [zinc oxide] 10%

Daily Cleaner solution (discontinued 1993) OTC *surfactant cleaning solution for soft contact lenses*

Daily Vitamins liquid OTC *vitamin supplement* [multiple vitamins] ≟

Daily-Key cellulose-coated caplets OTC *vitamin/mineral supplement* [multiple vitamins & minerals; betaine HCl]

Daily-Vite with Iron & Minerals tablets OTC *vitamin/mineral/iron supplement* [multiple vitamins & minerals; iron; folic acid; biotin] ≟•18•0.4•≟ mg

Dairy Ease chewable tablets OTC *digestive aid for lactose intolerance* [lactase enzyme] 3300 U

Daisy 2 test kit for home use (discontinued 1995) OTC *in vitro diagnostic aid for urine pregnancy test*

Dakin solution [see: sodium hypochlorite]

Dakrina eye drops OTC *ocular moisturizer/lubricant* [vitamin A palmitate; polyvinyl alcohol] 350 IU•0.6%

DAL (daunorubicin, ara-C, L-asparaginase) *chemotherapy protocol*

Dalacin T ℞ *investigational topical anti-acne agent*

Dalalone intra-articular, intralesional, soft tissue, or IM injection ℞ *glucocorticoids* [dexamethasone sodium phosphate] 4 mg/mL

Dalalone D.P. intra-articular, soft tissue, or IM injection ℞ *glucocorticoids* [dexamethasone acetate] 16 mg/mL

Dalalone L.A. intralesional, intra-articular, soft tissue, or IM injection ℞ *glucocorticoids* [dexamethasone acetate] 8 mg/mL

dalanated insulin [see: insulin, dalanated]

dalbraminol INN

Dalcaine injection (discontinued 1994) ℞ *injectable local anesthetic* [lidocaine HCl] 2%

daledalin INN *antidepressant* [also: daledalin tosylate]

daledalin tosylate USAN *antidepressant* [also: daledalin]

dalfopristin USAN, INN *antibacterial*

Dalgan IV, subcu or IM injection ℞ *narcotic agonist-antagonist analgesic* [dezocine] 5, 10, 15 mg/mL

Dallergy sustained-release capsules (discontinued 1994) ℞ *decongestant; antihistamine; anticholinergic* [phenylephrine HCl; chlorpheniramine maleate; methscopolamine nitrate] 20•8•2.5 mg

Dallergy tablets, sustained-release caplets, syrup ℞ *decongestant; antihistamine; anticholinergic* [phenylephrine HCl; chlorpheniramine maleate; methscopolamine nitrate] 10•4•1.25 mg; 20•8•2.5 mg; 10•2•0.625 mg/5 mL

Dallergy-D sustained-release capsules (discontinued 1994) OTC *decongestant; antihistamine* [pseudoephedrine HCl; chlorpheniramine maleate] 120•12 mg

Dallergy-D syrup OTC *decongestant; antihistamine* [phenylephrine HCl; chlorpheniramine maleate] 5•2 mg/5 mL

Dallergy-JR sustained-release capsules ℞ *pediatric decongestant and antihistamine* [pseudoephedrine HCl; brompheniramine maleate] 60•6 mg

Dalmane capsules ℞ *sedative; hypnotic* [flurazepam HCl] 15, 30 mg ② Dialume

d-Alpha Gems soft capsules OTC *vitamin supplement* [vitamin E]

dalteparin sodium USAN, INN, BAN *anticoagulant; antithrombotic; low molecular weight heparin*

daltroban USAN, INN *immunosuppressive*

Damason-P tablets ℞ *narcotic analgesic* [hydrocodone bitartrate; aspirin] 5•500 mg

dambose [see: inositol]

dametralast INN

damotepine INN

D-Amp capsules ℞ *penicillin-type antibiotic* [ampicillin trihydrate] 500 mg

danaparoid sodium USAN, BAN *antithrombotic*

danazol USAN, USP, INN, BAN *anterior pituitary suppressant* 200 mg oral

Danazol-NP ℞ *investigational agent for endometriosis, menorrhagia and fibrocystic breast disease* [danazol nanoparticles]

Danex shampoo (discontinued 1994) OTC *antiseborrheic; antibacterial; antifungal* [pyrithione zinc] 1%

daniquidone BAN

danitamon [see: menadione]

danitracen INN

Danocrine capsules ℞ *androgen for endometriosis, fibrocystic breast disease, and hereditary angioedema* [danazol] 50, 100, 200 mg

danofloxacin INN *veterinary antibacterial* [also: danofloxacin mesylate]

danofloxacin mesylate USAN *veterinary antibacterial* [also: danofloxacin]

danosteine INN

danthron USP, BAN *(withdrawn from market by FDA)* [also: dantron] ⊚ Dantrium

Dantrium capsules, powder for IV injection ℞ *skeletal muscle relaxant (orphan: neuroleptic malignant syndrome)* [dantrolene sodium] 25, 50, 100 mg; 20 mg/vial (0.32 mg/mL) ⊚ danthron

dantrolene USAN, INN, BAN *skeletal muscle relaxant*

dantrolene sodium USAN, BAN *skeletal muscle relaxant (orphan: neuroleptic malignant syndrome)*

dantron INN *(withdrawn from market by FDA)* [also: danthron]

Dapa tablets, capsules OTC *analgesic; antipyretic* [acetaminophen] 325 mg; 500 mg

Dapacin Cold capsules OTC *decongestant; antihistamine; analgesic* [phenylpropanolamine HCl; chlorpheniramine maleate; acetaminophen] 12.5•2•325 mg

Dapex-37.5 capsules (discontinued 1992) ℞ *anorexiant* [phentermine HCl] 37.5 mg

dapiprazole INN α-*adrenergic blocker; antiglaucoma agent; neuroleptic* [also: dapiprazole HCl]

dapiprazole HCl USAN α-*adrenergic blocker; miotic; neuroleptic* [also: dapiprazole]

dapsone USAN, USP, BAN *bactericidal; leprostatic; herpetiform dermatitis suppressant; (orphan: Pneumocystis carinii)*

dapsone & trimethoprim *(orphan: Pneumocystis carinii)*

daptazole [see: amiphenazole]

daptomycin USAN, INN, BAN *antibacterial*

Daranide tablets ℞ *carbonic anhydrase inhibitor; diuretic* [dichlorphenamide] 50 mg ⊚ Daraprim

Daraprim tablets ℞ *antimalarial; toxoplasmosis treatment adjunct* [pyrimethamine] 25 mg ⊚ Daranide

Darbid tablets (discontinued 1994) ℞ *anticholinergic; peptic ulcer treatment adjunct* [isopropamide iodide] 5 mg

darenzepine INN

darglitazone sodium USAN *oral hypoglycemic*

Daricon tablets ℞ *adjunctive therapy for peptic ulcer* [oxyphencyclimine HCl] 10 mg ⊚ Darvon

darodipine USAN, INN *antihypertensive; bronchodilator; vasodilator*

Darvocet-N 50; Darvocet-N 100 tablets ℞ *narcotic analgesic* [propoxyphene napsylate; acetaminophen] 50•325 mg; 100•650 mg ⊚ Darvon-N

Darvon Pulvules (capsules) ℞ *narcotic analgesic* [propoxyphene HCl] 65 mg ⊚ Daricon

Darvon Compound-65 Pulvules (capsules) ℞ *narcotic analgesic* [propoxyphene HCl; aspirin; caffeine] 65•389•32.4 mg

Darvon-N suspension (discontinued 1994) ℞ *narcotic analgesic* [propoxyphene napsylate] 10 mg/mL ⊚ Darvocet-N

Darvon-N tablets ℞ *narcotic analgesic* [propoxyphene napsylate] 100 mg

Dasin capsules (discontinued 1995) OTC *analgesic; antipyretic; anti-inflammatory; bronchodilator; emetic* [aspirin; caffeine; atropine sulfate; ipecac] 130•8•0.13•3 mg

DAT (daunorubicin, ara-C, thioguanine) *chemotherapy protocol* [also: DCT; TAD]

Datelliptium ℞ *investigational antineoplastic for breast cancer* [ellipticine]

datelliptium chloride INN

Datril tablets (discontinued 1993) OTC *analgesic; antipyretic* [acetaminophen] 500 mg

daturine hydrobromide [see: hyoscyamine hydrobromide]

DATVP (daunorubicin, ara-C, thioguanine, vincristine, prednisone) *chemotherapy protocol*

daunomycin [see: daunorubicin HCl]

daunorubicin (DNR) INN, BAN *antibiotic antineoplastic* [also: daunorubicin HCl] ▣ doxorubicin

daunorubicin citrate, liposomal *antibiotic antineoplastic*

daunorubicin HCl USAN, USP, JAN *antibiotic antineoplastic* [also: daunorubicin] ▣ doxorubicin

DaunoXome IV infusion ℞ *antibiotic antineoplastic for advanced AIDS-related Kaposi sarcoma* [daunorubicin citrate, liposomal] 2 mg/mL

DAV (daunorubicin, ara-C, VePesid) *chemotherapy protocol*

DAVA (desacetyl vinblastine amide) [see: vindesine]

DAVH (dibromodulcitol, Adriamycin, vincristine, Halotestin) *chemotherapy protocol*

davitamon [see: menadione]

Dayalets Filmtabs (film-coated tablets) OTC *vitamin supplement* [multiple vitamins; folic acid] ≛•0.4 mg

Dayalets + Iron Filmtabs (film-coated tablets) OTC *vitamin/iron supplement* [multiple vitamins; ferrous sulfate; folic acid] ≛•18•0.4 mg

DayCare caplets, liquid (name changed to DayQuil in 1992)

Daypro film-coated caplets ℞ *nonsteroidal anti-inflammatory drug (NSAID); antiarthritic* [oxaprozin] 600 mg

DayQuil LiquiCaps (soft gel capsules), liquid OTC *antitussive; decongestant; expectorant; analgesic* [dextromethorphan hydrobromide; pseudoephedrine HCl; guaifenesin; acetaminophen] 10•30•100•250 mg; 3.3•10•33.3•108.3 mg/5 mL

DayQuil Allergy Relief 4 Hour tablets OTC *decongestant; antihistamine* [phenylpropanolamine HCl; brompheniramine maleate] 25•4 mg

DayQuil Allergy Relief 12 Hour extended-release tablets OTC *decongestant; antihistamine* [phenylpropanolamine HCl; brompheniramine maleate] 75•12 mg

DayQuil Sinus Pressure & Congestion Relief caplets OTC *decongestant* [phenylpropanolamine HCl; guaifenesin] 25•200 mg

DayQuil Sinus Pressure & Pain Relief caplets OTC *decongestant; analgesic; antipyretic* [pseudoephedrine HCl; acetaminophen] 30•500 mg

Dayto Himbin tablets ℞ *no approved uses; sympatholytic; mydriatic; aphrodisiac* [yohimbine HCl] 5.4 mg

Dayto Sulf vaginal cream ℞ *broad-spectrum bacteriostatic* [sulfathiazole; sulfacetamide; sulfabenzamide] 3.42%•2.86%•3.7%

Dayto-Anase tablets (discontinued 1994) OTC *anti-inflammatory* [bromelains]

Day-Vite tablets (discontinued 1993) OTC *vitamin supplement* [multiple vitamins]

dazadrol INN *antidepressant* [also: dazadrol maleate]

dazadrol maleate USAN *antidepressant* [also: dazadrol]

Dazamide tablets ℞ *anticonvulsant; diuretic* [acetazolamide] 250 mg

dazepinil INN *antidepressant* [also: dazepinil HCl]

dazepinil HCl USAN *antidepressant* [also: dazepinil]

dazidamine INN

dazmegrel USAN, INN, BAN *thromboxane synthetase inhibitor*

dazolicine INN

dazopride INN *peristaltic stimulant* [also: dazopride fumarate]

dazopride fumarate USAN *peristaltic stimulant* [also: dazopride]

dazoquinast INN

dazoxiben INN, BAN *antithrombotic* [also: dazoxiben HCl]
dazoxiben HCl USAN *antithrombotic* [also: dazoxiben]
DBED (dibenzylethylenediamine dipenicillin G) [see: penicillin G benzathine]
DBM (dibromomannitol) [see: mitobronitol]
DC softgels OTC *stool softener* [docusate calcium] 240 mg
DC (daunorubicin, cytarabine) *chemotherapy protocol*
D&C Brown No. 1 (drugs & cosmetics) [see: resorcin brown]
DCA (desoxycorticosterone acetate) [q.v.]
DCF (2'-deoxycoformycin) [see: pentostatin]
DCL Hb (diaspirin crosslinked hemoglobin) [q.v.]
DCMP (daunorubicin, cytarabine, mercaptopurine, prednisone) *chemotherapy protocol*
D-Congest M liquid OTC *antitussive; decongestant; expectorant; analgesic; antipyretic* [dextromethorphan hydrobromide; pseudoephedrine HCl; guaifenesin; acetaminophen]
DCPM (daunorubicin, cytarabine, prednisone, mercaptopurine) *chemotherapy protocol*
DCT (daunorubicin, cytarabine, thioguanine) *chemotherapy protocol* [also: DAT; TAD]
DCV (DTIC, CCNU, vincristine) *chemotherapy protocol*
DDAVP tablets, nasal spray, rhinal tube, subcu or IV injection ℞ *pituitary antidiuretic hormone for hemophilia A and von Willebrand's disease (orphan)* [desmopressin acetate] 0.1, 0.2 mg; 10 μg/dose; 0.1 mg/mL; 4 μg/mL
DDAVP (deamino-D-arginine-vasopressin) [see: desmopressin acetate]
DDAVP High Concentration nasal spray ℞ *(orphan: hemophilia A; von Willebrand's disease)* [desmopressin acetate] 1.5 mg/mL
DDC; ddC (dideoxycytidine) [see: zalcitabine]
o,p'-DDD [now: mitotane]

DDI; ddI (dideoxyinosine) [see: didanosine]
DDP; cis-DDP (diamminedichloroplatinum) [see: cisplatin]
DDS (diaminodiphenylsulfone) [now: dapsone]
DDT (dichlorodiphenyltrichloroethane) [see: chlorophenothane]
DDVP (dichlorovinyl dimethyl phosphate) [see: dichlorvos]
DEA (diethanolamine) [q.v.]
deacetyllanatoside C [see: deslanoside]
deadly nightshade leaf [see: belladonna extract]
deamino-D-arginine-vasopressin (DDAVP) [see: desmopressin acetate]
deanil INN *combining name for radicals or groups*
deanol BAN [also: deanol aceglumate]
deanol aceglumate INN [also: deanol]
deanol acetamidobenzoate
3-deazaguanine *investigational antineoplastic*
deba [see: barbital]
deboxamet INN
Debrisan beads, paste ℞ *debrider and cleanser for wet wounds* [dextranomer]
debrisoquin sulfate USAN *antihypertensive* [also: debrisoquine]
debrisoquine INN, BAN *antihypertensive* [also: debrisoquin sulfate]
Debrox ear drops OTC *agent to emulsify and disperse ear wax* [carbamide peroxide] 6.5%
Decabid extended-release tablets (approved by the FDA in 1989, but never released by the manufacturer) ℞ *antiarrhythmic* [indecainide HCl]
Decaderm gel (discontinued 1993) ℞ *topical corticosteroid* [dexamethasone] ⓘ Decadron
Decadron tablets, elixir ℞ *glucocorticoids* [dexamethasone] 0.5, 0.75, 1.5, 4 mg; 0.5 mg/5 mL ⓘ Decaderm; Percodan
Decadron Phosphate cream ℞ *topical corticosteroid* [dexamethasone sodium phosphate] 0.1%
Decadron Phosphate intra-articular, intralesional, soft tissue or IM injection ℞ *glucocorticoids* [dexamethasone sodium phosphate] 4 mg/mL

Decadron Phosphate IV injection ℞ *glucocorticoids* [dexamethasone sodium phosphate] 24 mg/mL

Decadron Phosphate Ocumeter (eye drops), ophthalmic ointment ℞ *ophthalmic topical corticosteroidal anti-inflammatory* [dexamethasone sodium phosphate] 0.1%; 0.05%

Decadron Phosphate Respihaler, Turbinaire (name changed to Dexacort Phosphate in 1994)

Decadron with Xylocaine soft tissue injection ℞ *glucocorticoids* [dexamethasone sodium phosphate; lidocaine HCl] 4•10 mg/mL

Decadron-LA intralesional, intra-articular, soft tissue, or IM injection ℞ *glucocorticoids* [dexamethasone acetate] 8 mg/mL

Deca-Durabolin IM injection ℞ *anabolic steroid for anemia of renal insufficiency* [nandrolone decanoate] 50, 100, 200 mg/mL

Decagen tablets OTC *vitamin/mineral/iron supplement* [multiple vitamins & minerals; iron; folic acid; biotin] ±•18 mg•0.4 mg•30 μg

Decaject intra-articular, intralesional, soft tissue, or IM injection ℞ *glucocorticoids* [dexamethasone sodium phosphate] 4 mg/mL

Decaject-L.A. intralesional, intra-articular, soft tissue, or IM injection ℞ *glucocorticoids* [dexamethasone acetate] 8 mg/mL

DECAL (dexamethasone, etoposide, cisplatin, ara-C, L-asparaginase) *chemotherapy protocol*

decamethonium bromide USP, INN [also: decamethonium iodide]

decamethonium iodide BAN [also: decamethonium bromide]

Decapeptyl injection ℞ *(orphan: ovarian carcinoma of epithelial origin)* [triptorelin pamoate]

decapinol [see: delmopinol]

Decaspray aerosol (discontinued 1996) ℞ *topical corticosteroid* [dexamethasone] 0.04%

decavitamin USP

Decholin tablets OTC *laxative; hydrocholeretic* [dehydrocholic acid] 250 mg

decicain [see: tetracaine HCl]

decil INN *combining name for radicals or groups*

decimemide INN

decitabine USAN, INN, BAN *antineoplastic*

decitropine INN

declaben [now: Iodelaben]

declenperone USAN, INN *veterinary sedative*

Declomycin capsules, film-coated tablets ℞ *broad-spectrum antibiotic* [demeclocycline HCl] 150 mg; 150, 300 mg

decloxizine INN

Decofed syrup OTC *nasal decongestant* [pseudoephedrine HCl] 30 mg/5 mL

Decohistine elixir (discontinued 1993) OTC *decongestant; antihistamine* [phenylephrine HCl; chlorpheniramine maleate]

Decohistine DH liquid ℞ *narcotic antitussive; decongestant; antihistamine* [codeine phosphate; pseudoephedrine HCl; chlorpheniramine maleate; alcohol 5.8%] 10•30•2 mg/5 mL

decominol INN

Deconal syrup OTC *decongestant; antihistamine* [phenylpropanolamine HCl; phenylephrine HCl; phenyltoloxamine citrate; chlorpheniramine maleate] ② Deconsal

Deconamine tablets, syrup ℞ *decongestant; antihistamine* [pseudoephedrine HCl; chlorpheniramine maleate] 60•4 mg; 30•2 mg/5 mL

Deconamine CX tablets, liquid ℞ *narcotic antitussive; decongestant; expectorant* [hydrocodone bitartrate; pseudoephedrine HCl; guaifenesin] 5•30•300 mg; 5•60•200 mg/5 mL

Deconamine SR sustained-release capsules ℞ *decongestant; antihistamine* [pseudoephedrine HCl; chlorpheniramine maleate] 120•8 mg

Decongestabs sustained-release tablets ℞ *decongestant; antihistamine* [phenylpropanolamine HCl; phenylephrine HCl; chlorpheniramine maleate; phenyltoloxamine citrate] 40•10•5•15 mg

Decongestant sustained-release tablets ℞ *decongestant; antihistamine* [phenylpropanolamine HCl; phenylephrine HCl; chlorpheniramine maleate; phenyltoloxamine citrate] 40•10•5•15 mg

Decongestant tablets OTC *decongestant; antihistamine; analgesic* [phenylephrine HCl; chlorpheniramine maleate; acetaminophen] 5•2•325 mg

Decongestant Expectorant liquid ℞ *narcotic antitussive; decongestant; expectorant* [codeine phosphate; pseudoephedrine HCl; guaifenesin; alcohol 7.5%] 10•30•100 mg/5 mL

Decongestant S.R. sustained-release tablets (discontinued 1995) ℞ *decongestant; antihistamine* [phenylpropanolamine HCl; phenylephrine HCl; chlorpheniramine maleate; phenyltoloxamine citrate] 40•10•5•15 mg

Deconomed SR sustained-release capsules ℞ *decongestant; antihistamine* [pseudoephedrine HCl; chlorpheniramine maleate] 120•8 mg

Deconsal II sustained-release tablets ℞ *decongestant; expectorant* [pseudoephedrine HCl; guaifenesin] 60•600 mg ② Deconal

Deconsal Pediatric syrup ℞ *narcotic antitussive; decongestant; expectorant* [codeine phosphate; pseudoephedrine HCl; guaifenesin; alcohol 6%] 10•30•100 mg ② Deconal

Deconsal Sprinkle sustained-release capsules ℞ *decongestant; expectorant* [phenylephrine HCl; guaifenesin] 10•300 mg ② Deconal

decoquinate USAN, INN, BAN *coccidiostat for poultry*

Decotan caplets (discontinued 1993) ℞ *decongestant; antihistamine* [phenylephrine tannate; chlorpheniramine tannate; pyrilamine tannate]

dectaflur USAN, INN *dental caries prophylactic*

Decubitex ointment, powder (discontinued 1992) ℞ *decubitus ulcer treatment* [Biebrich scarlet red sulfonated; zinc oxide]

Declyenes ointment OTC *topical antifungal* [undecylenic acid; zinc undecylenate]

deditonium bromide INN

Deep-Down Rub OTC *counterirritant* [methyl salicylate; menthol; camphor] 15%•5%•0.5%

DEET (diethyltoluamide) [q.v.]

DeFed-60 tablets OTC *nasal decongestant* [pseudoephedrine HCl] 60 mg

defenfluramine *investigational obesity treatment*

Defen-LA sustained-release tablets ℞ *decongestant; expectorant* [pseudoephedrine HCl; guaifenesin] 60•600 mg

deferoxamine USAN, INN *iron-chelating agent* [also: desferrioxamine]

deferoxamine HCl USAN

deferoxamine mesylate USAN, USP *antidote to iron poisoning; iron-chelating agent* [also: desferrioxamine mesylate]

defibrotide INN, BAN (*orphan: thrombotic thrombocytopenic purpura*)

deflazacort USAN, INN, BAN *antiinflammatory; investigational treatment for rheumatoid arthritis and asthma*

defosfamide INN

defungit sodium salt [see: bensuldazic acid]

Defy eye drops ℞ *ophthalmic antibiotic* [tobramycin] 0.3%

Degas chewable tablets OTC *antiflatulent* [simethicone] 80 mg

Degest 2 eye drops OTC *topical ocular decongestant/vasoconstrictor* [naphazoline HCl] 0.012%

Dehist subcu or IM injection ℞ *antihistamine; anaphylaxis* [brompheniramine maleate] 10 mg/mL

Dehist sustained-release capsules (discontinued 1994) OTC *decongestant; antihistamine* [phenylpropanolamine HCl; chlorpheniramine maleate] 75•8 mg

dehydrated alcohol [see: alcohol, dehydrated]

dehydrex (*orphan: recurrent corneal erosion*)

dehydroacetic acid NF *preservative*

dehydroandrosterone [see: prasterone]

dehydrocholate sodium USP [also: sodium dehydrocholate]

7-dehydrocholesterol, activated [now: cholecalciferol]

dehydrocholic acid USP, INN, BAN, JAN *choleretic; laxative* 250 mg oral

dehydrocholin [see: dehydrocholic acid]

dehydroemetine INN, BAN, DCF *investigational anti-infective for amebiasis and amebic dysentery*

dehydroepiandrosterone (DHEA) *investigational (Phase I/II) immunomodulator for AIDS (orphan: systemic lupus erythematosus)*

Del Aqua-5; Del Aqua-10 gel ℞ *topical keratolytic for acne* [benzoyl peroxide] 5%; 10%

Delacort lotion (discontinued 1993) OTC *topical corticosteroid* [hydrocortisone] ② Delcort

Deladiol-40 IM injection (discontinued 1996) ℞ *estrogen replacement therapy for postmenopausal disorders; antineoplastic for prostatic cancer* [estradiol valerate in oil] 40 mg/mL

Deladumone IM injection (discontinued 1995) ℞ *estrogen/androgen for menopausal vasomotor symptoms* [estradiol valerate; testosterone enanthate] 4•90 mg/mL

delanterone INN

Delaprem (commercially available in several foreign countries) ℞ *investigational tocolytic and bronchodilator* [hexoprenaline sulfate]

delapril INN *antihypertensive; angiotensin-converting enzyme inhibitor* [also: delapril HCl]

delapril HCl USAN *antihypertensive; angiotensin-converting enzyme inhibitor* [also: delapril]

Delatest IM injection (discontinued 1994) ℞ *androgen replacement for delayed puberty or breast cancer* [testosterone enanthate] 100 mg/mL

Delatestryl IM injection ℞ *androgen replacement for delayed puberty or breast cancer* [testosterone enanthate] 200 mg/mL

delavirdine mesylate USAN *antiviral; reverse transcriptase inhibitor; investigational (Phase III) for AIDS/HIV*

delayed-release aspirin [see: aspirin]

Delcap (trademarked dosage form) *unit dispensing cap*

Delcort cream OTC *topical corticosteroid* [hydrocortisone] 0.5%, 1% ② Delacort

delequamine HCl USAN α_2 *adrenoreceptor antagonist for sexual dysfunction*

delergotrile INN

Delestrogen IM injection ℞ *estrogen replacement therapy for postmenopausal disorders; antineoplastic for prostatic cancer* [estradiol valerate in oil] 10, 20, 40 mg/mL

delfantrine INN

delfaprazine INN

Delfen Contraceptive vaginal foam OTC *spermicidal contraceptive* [nonoxynol 9] 12.5%

delmadinone INN, BAN *progestin; antiandrogen; antiestrogen* [also: delmadinone acetate]

delmadinone acetate USAN *progestin; antiandrogen; antiestrogen* [also: delmadinone]

delmetacin INN

delmopinol INN

Del-Mycin topical solution ℞ *topical antibiotic for acne* [erythromycin] 2%

delnav [see: dioxathion]

delorazepam INN

deloxolone INN

***m*-delphene** [see: diethyltoluamide]

delprostenate INN, BAN

Delsym sustained-action liquid OTC *antitussive* [dextromethorphan polistirex] 30 mg/5 mL

Delta-Cortef tablets ℞ *glucocorticoids* [prednisolone] 5 mg

deltacortone [see: prednisone]

Delta-D tablets OTC *vitamin supplement* [cholecalciferol] 400 IU

deltafilcon A USAN *hydrophilic contact lens material*

deltafilcon B USAN *hydrophilic contact lens material*

delta-1-hydrocortisone [see: prednisolone]

Deltalin Gelseals (filled elastic capsules) (discontinued 1993) ℞ *vitamin deficiency therapy* [ergocalciferol] 50,000 IU

Deltasone tablets ℞ *glucocorticoids* [prednisone] 2.5, 5, 10, 20, 50 mg

delta-9-tetrahydrocannabinol (THC) [see: dronabinol]

delta-9-THC (tetrahydrocannabinol) [see: dronabinol]

Delta-Tritex cream, ointment ℞ *topical corticosteroid* [triamcinolone acetonide] 0.1%

Deltavac vaginal cream ℞ *bacteriostatic antibiotic; antiseptic; vulnerary* [sulfanilamide; aminacrine HCl; allantoin] 15%•0.2%•2%

deltra-stab [see: prednisolone]

delvaridine mesylate *investigational (Phase III) reverse transcriptase inhibitor for HIV*

Del-Vi-A capsules ℞ *vitamin deficiency therapy* [vitamin A] 50,000 IU

Demadex tablets, IV injection ℞ *loop diuretic* [torsemide] 5, 10, 20, 100 mg; 10 mg/mL

Demazin Repetabs (repeat-action tablets), syrup OTC *decongestant; antihistamine* [phenylpropanolamine HCl; chlorpheniramine maleate] 25•4 mg; 12.5•2 mg/5 mL

dembrexine INN, BAN

dembroxol [see: dembrexine]

demecarium bromide USP, INN, BAN *antiglaucoma agent; reversible cholinesterase inhibitor miotic*

demeclocycline USP, BAN *antibacterial*

demeclocycline HCl USP, BAN *gram-negative and gram-positive bacteriostatic; antirickettsial*

demecolcine INN, BAN

demecycline USAN, INN *antibacterial*

demegestone INN

demekastigmine bromide [see: demecarium bromide]

demelverine INN

Demerol APAP tablets (discontinued 1992) ℞ *narcotic analgesic* [meperidine HCl; acetaminophen] ⓘ Demulen; dicumarol; Dymelor; Temaril

Demerol HCl tablets, syrup, IV or IM injection ℞ *narcotic analgesic* [meperidine HCl] 50, 100 mg; 50 mg/5 mL; 50, 100 mg/mL

demetacin [see: delmetacin]

11-demethoxyreserpine [see: deserpidine]

demethylchlortetracycline (DMCT) [now: demeclocycline]

demethylchlortetracycline HCl [see: demeclocycline HCl]

N-demethylcodeine [see: norcodeine]

demexiptiline INN

Demi-Regroton tablets ℞ *antihypertensive* [chlorthalidone; reserpine] 25•0.125 mg

democonazole INN

Demolin liniment OTC *topical analgesic* [methyl salicylate; camphor; racemic menthol; mustard oil] ⓘ Demulen

demoxepam USAN, INN *minor tranquilizer*

demoxytocin INN

Demser capsules ℞ *antihypertensive for pheochromocytoma* [metyrosine] 250 mg

Demulen 1/35; Demulen 1/50 tablets ℞ *monophasic oral contraceptive* [ethynodiol diacetate; ethinyl estradiol] 1 mg•35 μg; 1 mg•50 μg ⓘ Demerol; Demolin

denatonium benzoate USAN, NF, INN, BAN *alcohol denaturant; flavoring agent*

denaverine INN

denbufylline INN, BAN

denipride INN

denofungin USAN *antifungal; antibacterial*

denopamine INN

Denorex shampoo OTC *antiseborrheic; antipsoriatic; antipruritic; antibacterial* [coal tar; menthol; alcohol] 9%•1.5•7.5%; 12.5%•1.5%•10.4%

Denov extended-release capsules ℞ *antihistamine; decongestant* [chlorpheniramine maleate; pseudoephedrine HCl]

denpidazone INN

Denquel toothpaste OTC *tooth desensitizer* [potassium nitrate] 5%

dental antiformin [see: antiformin, dental]

dental-type silica [see: silica, dental-type]

Dent's Lotion-Jel lotion/gel OTC *topical oral anesthetic* [benzocaine]

Dent's Toothache Gum; Dent's Toothache Drops OTC *topical oral anesthetic* [benzocaine]

denyl sodium [see: phenytoin sodium]

denzimol INN

2'-deoxycoformycin (DCF) [see: pentostatin]
deoxycorticosterone acetate [see: desoxycorticosterone acetate]
deoxycorticosterone pivalate [see: desoxycorticosterone pivalate]
deoxycortolone pivalate BAN *salt-regulating adrenocortical steroid* [also: desoxycorticosterone pivalate]
deoxycortone BAN *salt-regulating adrenocortical steroid* [also: desoxycorticosterone acetate; desoxycortone]
deoxyephedrine HCl [see: methamphetamine HCl]
12-deoxyerythromycin [see: berythromycin]
3'-deoxy-3-fluorodeoxythymidine *investigational antiviral for AIDS (clinical trials discontinued 1994)*
deoxynojirimycin (DNJ) *investigational (Phase II) antiviral for AIDS/ARC*
deoxyribonuclease, recombinant human (rhDNase) [see: dornase alfa]
deoxyribonucleic acid (DNA)
15-deoxyspergualin trihydrochloride [now: gusperimus trihydrochloride]
Depacin Cold Capsules OTC *decongestant; antihistamine; analgesic* [phenylpropanolamine HCl; chlorpheniramine maleate; acetaminophen]
Depakene capsules ℞ *anticonvulsant* [valproic acid] 250 mg
Depakene syrup ℞ *anticonvulsant* [valproate sodium] 250 mg/5 mL
Depakote delayed-release tablets, sprinkle capsules ℞ *anticonvulsant; antipsychotic for manic episodes; migraine preventative (delayed-release form only)* [divalproex sodium] 125, 250, 500 mg; 125 mg
depAndro 100; depAndro 200 IM injection ℞ *androgen replacement for delayed puberty or breast cancer* [testosterone cypionate] 100 mg/mL; 200 mg/mL
depAndrogyn IM injection ℞ *estrogen/androgen for menopausal vasomotor symptoms* [estradiol cypionate; testosterone cypionate] 2•50 mg/mL
Depen titratable tablets ℞ *metal chelating agent for rheumatoid arthritis, Wilson's disease, and cystinuria* [penicillamine] 250 mg
depepsen [see: sodium amylosulfate]
depGynogen IM injection ℞ *hormone replacement therapy for postmenopausal disorders* [estradiol cypionate in oil] 5 mg/mL
Depitol tablets ℞ *anticonvulsant* [carbamazepine] 200 mg
depMedalone 40; depMedalone 80 intralesional, soft tissue, and IM injection ℞ *glucocorticoid; anti-inflammatory; immunosuppressant* [methylprednisolone acetate] 40 mg/mL; 80 mg/mL
Depo-Estradiol Cypionate IM injection ℞ *hormone replacement therapy for postmenopausal disorders* [estradiol cypionate in oil] 5 mg/mL
DepoGen IM injection ℞ *hormone replacement therapy for postmenopausal disorders* [estradiol cypionate in oil] 5 mg/mL
Depoject intralesional, soft tissue, and IM injection ℞ *glucocorticoid; anti-inflammatory; immunosuppressant* [methylprednisolone acetate] 40, 80 mg/mL
Depo-Medrol intralesional, soft tissue, and IM injection ℞ *glucocorticoid; anti-inflammatory; immunosuppressant* [methylprednisolone acetate] 20, 40, 80 mg/mL
Deponit transdermal patch ℞ *antianginal* [nitroglycerin] 16, 32 mg
Depopred-40; Depopred-80 intralesional, soft tissue, and IM injection ℞ *glucocorticoid; anti-inflammatory; immunosuppressant* [methylprednisolone acetate] 40 mg/mL; 80 mg/mL
Depo-Provera IM injection ℞ *hormonal adjunct for metastatic endometrial and renal carcinoma; long-term injectable contraceptive* [medroxyprogesterone acetate] 150, 400 mg/mL
Depotest 100; Depotest 200 IM injection ℞ *androgen replacement for delayed puberty or breast cancer* [testosterone cypionate] 100 mg/mL; 200 mg/mL
Depo-Testadiol IM injection ℞ *estrogen/androgen for menopausal vasomo-*

tor symptoms [estradiol cypionate; testosterone cypionate] 2•50 mg/mL

Depotestogen IM injection ℞ *estrogen/androgen for menopausal vasomotor symptoms* [estradiol cypionate; testosterone cypionate] 2•50 mg/mL

Depo-Testosterone IM injection ℞ *androgen replacement for delayed puberty or breast cancer* [testosterone cypionate] 100, 200 mg/mL

depramine INN [also: balipramine]

Depranol ℞ *(orphan: sickle cell disease)* [OM 401 (code name—generic name not yet approved)]

deprenyl (L-deprenyl) [see: selegiline HCl]

deprodone INN, BAN

Deproist Expectorant with Codeine liquid ℞ *narcotic antitussive; decongestant; expectorant* [codeine phosphate; pseudoephedrine HCl; guaifenesin; alcohol 8.2%] 10•30•100 mg/5 mL

Deprol tablets (discontinued 1995) ℞ *psychotherapeutic agent* [meprobamate; benactyzine HCl] 400•1 mg

deprostil USAN, INN *gastric antisecretory*

deptropine INN, BAN

deptropine citrate [see: deptropine]

Dequadin lozenges *investigational sore throat emollient*

dequalinium chloride INN, BAN

Dequasine tablets OTC *dietary supplement* [multiple minerals & amino acids; vitamin C] ⁑•200 mg

Deracyn SR tablets ℞ *investigational antidepressant for panic disorder and anxiety* [adinazolam mesylate]

Derifil tablets OTC *systemic deodorant for ostomy, breath, and body odors* [chlorophyllin] 100 mg

Derma Comb cream ℞ *topical corticosteroid; antifungal* [triamcinolone acetonide; nystatin]

Derma Viva lotion OTC *moisturizer; emollient*

Dermabase OTC *cream base*

Dermabet cream ℞ *topical corticosteroid* [betamethasone valerate]

Dermacoat aerosol OTC *topical local anesthetic* [benzocaine] 4.5%

Dermacort cream, lotion ℞ *topical corticosteroid* [hydrocortisone] 1% ② DermiCort

DermaFlex gel OTC *topical local anesthetic* [lidocaine] 2.5%

Dermagraft ℞ *investigational skin substitute*

Dermal-Rub balm OTC *counterirritant* [methyl salicylate; camphor; racemic manthol; cajuput oil]

Dermamycin cream OTC *topical antihistamine* [diphenhydramine HCl] 2%

Derma-Pax lotion OTC *topical antihistamine; antiseptic; antipruritic* [pyrilamine maleate; chlorpheniramine maleate; alcohol 35%] 0.44%•0.06%

Dermarest gel OTC *topical antihistamine; antifungal* [diphenhydramine HCl; resorcinol] 2%•2%

Dermarest Dricort Creme OTC *topical corticosteroid* [hydrocortisone acetate] 1%

Dermarest Plus gel, spray OTC *topical antihistamine; counterirritant* [diphenhydramine HCl; menthol] 2%•1%

Dermasept Antifungal liquid spray OTC *antifungal; antiseptic; anesthetic; astringent* [tolnaftate; tannic acid; zinc chloride; benzocaine; methylbenzethonium HCl; undecylenic acid; alcohol 58.539%] 1.017%•6.098%•5.081%•2.032%•3.049%•5.081%

Dermasil lotion OTC *bath emollient*

Derma-Smoothe/FS oil ℞ *topical corticosteroid; emollient* [fluocinolone acetonide] 0.01%

Dermassage lotion (discontinued 1992) OTC *moisturizer; emollient*

dermatan sulfate [see: danaparoid sodium]

dermatol [see: bismuth subgallate]

Dermatol 10 lotion *moisturizer* [urea]

Dermatop cream ℞ *topical corticosteroid* [prednicarbate] 0.1%

Dermatophytin shallow subcu or intradermal injection (discontinued 1996) ℞ *diagnosis and treatment of Trichophyton-induced skin infections* [Trichophyton extract] 5 mL (undiluted or 1:30)

Dermatophytin "O" shallow subcu or intradermal injection (discontinued 1996) ℞ *diagnosis and treatment of oidiomycin (Candida)-induced infections* [Candida albicans extract] 5 mL (undiluted or 1:100)

Derm-Cleanse liquid OTC *soap-free therapeutic skin cleanser*

DermeD cream (discontinued 1992) OTC *moisturizer; emollient* [vitamins A and D]

DermiCort cream, lotion OTC *topical corticosteroid* [hydrocortisone] ② Dermacort

Dermidon cream (discontinued 1992) OTC *topical antihistamine; antibacterial; antipruritic; anesthetic* [pyrilamine maleate; phenyltoloxamine citrate; diperodon HCl; benzalkonium chloride; menthol; camphor]

Dermol HC anorectal cream, anorectal ointment ℞ *topical corticosteroidal anti-inflammatory* [hydrocortisone] 1%, 2.5%; 1%

Dermolate Anti-Itch cream OTC *topical corticosteroid* [hydrocortisone] 0.5%

Dermolin liniment OTC *counterirritant; topical antiseptic* [methyl salicylate; camphor; racemic menthol; mustard oil; alcohol 8%]

Dermoplast aerosol spray, lotion OTC *topical local anesthetic* [benzocaine; menthol] 20%•0.5%; 8%•0.5%

Dermovan OTC *cream base*

Dermoxyl gel (discontinued 1995) OTC *topical keratolytic for acne* [benzoyl peroxide] 2.5%, 5%, 10%

Dermprotective Factor (DPF) (trademarked ingredient) *aromatic syrup* [eriodictyon]

Dermtex HC with Aloe cream OTC *topical corticosteroid* [hydrocortisone] 0.5%

Dermuspray aerosol spray ℞ *topical enzyme for wound debridement* [trypsin; balsam Peru] 0.1•72.5 mg/0.82 mL

derpanicate INN

DES (diethylstilbestrol) [q.v.]

desacetyl vinblastine amide (DAVA) [see: vindesine]

desacetyl-lanatoside C [see: deslanoside]

desaglybuzole [see: glybuzole]

desamino-oxytocin [see: demoxytocin]

desaspidin INN

desciclovir USAN, INN *antiviral*

descinolone INN *glucocorticoid* [also: descinolone acetonide]

descinolone acetonide USAN *glucocorticoid* [also: descinolone]

Desenex foam, soap OTC *topical antifungal* [undecylenic acid] 10%

Desenex powder, aerosol powder, ointment, cream OTC *topical antifungal* [undecylenic acid; zinc undecylenate] 25% total

Desenex spray liquid OTC *topical antifungal* [tolnaftate] 1%

Desenex, Prescription Strength cream OTC *topical antifungal* [clotrimazole] 1%

Desenex, Prescription Strength spray liquid, spray powder OTC *topical antifungal* [miconazole nitrate] 2%

Desenex Antifungal cream OTC *topical antifungal* [miconazole nitrate] 2%

deserpidine INN, BAN *antihypertensive; peripheral antiadrenergic; rauwolfia derivative* ② desipramine

Desert Pure Calcium film-coated tablets OTC *calcium supplement* [calcium carbonate; vitamin D] 500 mg•125 IU

Desferal powder for IM, IV, or subcu injection ℞ *adjunct treatment for iron intoxication or overload* [deferoxamine mesylate] 500 mg ② Disophrol

desferrioxamine BAN *iron-chelating agent* [also: deferoxamine]

desferrioxamine mesylate BAN *antidote to iron poisoning; iron-chelating agent* [also: deferoxamine mesylate]

desflurane USAN, INN *inhalation general anesthetic*

desglugastrin INN

desipramine INN, BAN *tricyclic antidepressant* [also: desipramine HCl] ② deserpidine

desipramine HCl USAN, USP *tricyclic antidepressant* [also: desipramine] 10, 25, 50, 75, 100, 150 mg oral

desirudin USAN *anticoagulant; thrombin inhibitor*

Desitin ointment OTC *moisturizer; emollient; astringent; antiseptic* [cod liver oil; zinc oxide]

Desitin with Zinc Oxide powder OTC *topical diaper rash treatment* [zinc oxide; corn starch] 10%•88.2%

deslanoside USP, INN, BAN *cardiotonic; cardiac glycoside*

deslorelin USAN, INN *LHRH agonist; (orphan: central precocious puberty)*

desmethylmoramide INN

desmophosphamide [see: defosfamide]

desmopressin INN, BAN *posterior pituitary antidiuretic hormone* [also: desmopressin acetate]

desmopressin acetate USAN *posterior pituitary antidiuretic hormone for hemophilia A and von Willebrand's disease (orphan)* [also: desmopressin]

desocriptine INN

Desogen tablets ℞ *monophasic oral contraceptive* [desogestrel; ethinyl estradiol] 0.15 mg•30 μg

desogestrel USAN, INN, BAN *progestin*

desolone [see: deprodone]

desomorphine INN, BAN

desonide USAN, INN, BAN *topical corticosteroidal anti-inflammatory* 0.05% topical

DesOwen ointment, cream, lotion ℞ *topical corticosteroidal anti-inflammatory* [desonide] 0.05%

desoximetasone USAN, USP, INN *topical corticosteroidal anti-inflammatory* [also: desoxymethasone] 0.05%, 0.25% topical ② dexamethasone

desoxycorticosterone acetate (DCA; DOCA) USP *salt-regulating adrenocortical steroid* [also: desoxycortone; deoxycortone]

desoxycorticosterone pivalate USP *salt-regulating adrenocortical steroid* [also: deoxycortolone pivalate]

desoxycorticosterone trimethylacetate USP

desoxycortone INN *salt-regulating adrenocortical steroid* [also: desoxycorticosterone acetate; deoxycortone]

l-desoxyephedrine *nasal decongestant*

desoxyephedrine HCl [see: methamphetamine HCl]

desoxymethasone BAN *topical corticosteroidal anti-inflammatory* [also: desoximetasone]

Desoxyn Gradumets (sustained-release tablets), tablets ℞ *CNS stimulant* [methamphetamine HCl] 5, 10, 15 mg; 5 mg ② digitoxin; digoxin

desoxyribonuclease [see: fibrinolysin & desoxyribonuclease]

Despec controlled-release capsules (discontinued 1994) ℞ *decongestant; expectorant* [guaifenesin; phenylpropanolamine HCl]

Despec liquid ℞ *decongestant; expectorant* [phenylephrine HCl; phenylpropanolamine HCl; guaifenesin] 20•5•100 mg/5 mL

Desquam-E; Desquam-E 5; Desquam-E 10 gel ℞ *topical keratolytic for acne* [benzoyl peroxide] 2.5%; 5%; 10%

Desquam-X 2.5 gel (discontinued 1995) ℞ *topical keratolytic for acne* [benzoyl peroxide] 2.5%

Desquam-X 5; Desquam-X 10 gel ℞ *topical keratolytic for acne* [benzoyl peroxide] 5%; 10%

Desquam-X 5 Wash; Desquam-X 10 Wash liquid ℞ *topical keratolytic for acne* [benzoyl peroxide] 5%; 10%

de-Stat solution (discontinued 1995) OTC *cleaning/soaking solution for hard contact lenses*

de-Stat 3; de-Stat 4 solution OTC *cleaning/disinfecting/soaking solution for rigid gas permeable contact lenses*

destradiol [see: estradiol]

63-desulfohirudin [see: desirudin]

Desyrel film-coated tablets, Dividose (multiple-scored tablets) ℞ *antidepressant* [trazodone HCl] 50, 100 mg; 150, 300 mg

DET (diethyltryptamine)

detajmium bitartrate INN

Detane gel OTC *topical local anesthetic* [benzocaine] 7.5%

detanosal INN

Detect-A-Strep slide tests for professional use *in vitro diagnostic aid for streptococcal antigens in throat swabs*

Detecto-Seal (trademarked packaging form) *tamper-resistant parenteral package*

deterenol INN *ophthalmic adrenergic* [also: deterenol HCl]

deterenol HCl USAN *ophthalmic adrenergic* [also: deterenol]

detigon HCl [see: chlophedianol HCl]

detirelix INN *luteinizing hormone-releasing hormone (LHRH) antagonist* [also: detirelix acetate]

detirelix acetate USAN *luteinizing hormone-releasing hormone (LHRH) antagonist* [also: detirelix]

detomidine INN, BAN *veterinary analgesic; sedative* [also: detomidine HCl]

detomidine HCl USAN *veterinary analgesic; sedative* [also: detomidine]

detorubicin INN

detralfate INN

detrothyronine INN

Detussin liquid ℞ *narcotic antitussive; decongestant* [hydrocodone bitartrate; pseudoephedrine HCl; alcohol 5%] 5•60 mg/5 mL

Detussin Expectorant liquid ℞ *narcotic antitussive; decongestant; expectorant* [hydrocodone bitartrate; pseudoephedrine HCl; guaifenesin; alcohol] 5•60•200 mg/5 mL

deuterium oxide USAN *radioactive agent*

devapamil INN

devazepide USAN *cholecystokinin antagonist*

Devrom chewable tablets OTC *systemic deodorizer for ostomy and incontinence odors* [bismuth subgallate] 200 mg

Dex4 Glucose tablets OTC *glucose elevating agent* [glucose] ?

Dexacen LA-8 injection (discontinued 1994) ℞ *corticosteroid* [dexamethasone acetate] 8 mg/mL

Dexacen-4 injection (discontinued 1994) ℞ *corticosteroid* [dexamethasone sodium phosphate]

Dexacidin eye drop suspension, ophthalmic ointment ℞ *topical ophthalmic corticosteroidal anti-inflammatory; antibiotic* [dexamethasone; neomycin sulfate; polymyxin B sulfate] 0.1%• 0.35%•10,000 U/mL; 0.1%• 0.35%•10,000 U/g

Dexacort Phosphate Respihaler (oral inhalation aerosol) ℞ *corticosteroid for bronchial asthma* [dexamethasone sodium phosphate] 84 µg/dose

Dexacort Phosphate Turbinaire (nasal inhalation aerosol) ℞ *intranasal steroidal anti-inflammatory* [dexamethasone sodium phosphate; alcohol 2%] 84 µg/dose

Dex-A-Diet timed-release capsules, timed-release caplets (discontinued 1992) OTC *diet aid* [phenylpropanolamine HCl] 75 mg

Dex-A-Diet plus Vitamin C timed-release capsules (discontinued 1992) OTC *diet aid* [phenylpropanolamine HCl; vitamin C] 75•200 mg

Dexafed Cough syrup OTC *antitussive; decongestant; expectorant* [dextromethorphan hydrobromide; phenylephrine HCl; guaifenesin] 10•5• 100 mg/5 mL

Dexameth tablets ℞ *glucocorticoids* [dexamethasone] 0.5, 0.75, 1.5, 4 mg

dexamethasone USP, INN, BAN *corticosteroid* 0.25, 0.5, 0.75, 1, 1.5, 2, 4, 6 mg oral; 0.5 mg/5 mL oral; 0.5 mg/0.5 mL oral ? desoximetasone

dexamethasone acefurate USAN, INN *corticosteroid*

dexamethasone acetate USAN, USP, BAN *corticosteroid* 8 mg/mL injection

dexamethasone dipropionate USAN *corticosteroid*

dexamethasone sodium phosphate USP, BAN *corticosteroid* 0.05%, 0.1% eye drops; 4, 10 mg/mL injection

dexamfetamine INN *CNS stimulant* [also: dextroamphetamine; dexamphetamine]

dexamisole USAN, INN *antidepressant*

dexamphetamine BAN *CNS stimulant* [also: dextroamphetamine; dexamfetamine]

Dexamycin ophthalmic ointment ℞ *topical corticosteroid; antibiotic* [dexamethasone; neomycin sulfate; polymyxin B sulfate]

Dexaphen S.A. sustained-release tablets ℞ *decongestant; antihistamine* [pseudoephedrine sulfate; dexbrompheniramine maleate] 120•6 mg

Dexasone intra-articular, intralesional, soft tissue, or IM injection ℞ *glucocorticoids* [dexamethasone sodium phosphate] 4 mg/mL

Dexasone L.A. intralesional, intra-articular, soft tissue, or IM injection ℞ *glucocorticoids* [dexamethasone acetate] 8 mg/mL

Dexasporin eye drop suspension (discontinued 1995) ℞ *topical ophthalmic corticosteroidal anti-inflammatory; antibiotic* [dexamethasone; neomycin sulfate; polymyxin B sulfate] 0.1% • 0.35% • 10,000 U/mL

Dexasporin ophthalmic ointment ℞ *topical ophthalmic corticosteroidal anti-inflammatory; antibiotic* [dexamethasone; neomycin sulfate; polymyxin B sulfate] 0.1% • 0.35% • 10,000 U/g

Dexatrim extended-release tablets, timed-release capsules OTC *diet aid* [phenylpropanolamine HCl] 75 mg

Dexatrim plus Vitamin C timed-release capsules OTC *diet aid* [phenylpropanolamine HCl; vitamin C] 75 • 180 mg

Dexatrim Plus Vitamins timed-release caplets (diet aid) + caplets (vitamins) OTC *diet aid + vitamin/mineral/iron supplement* [(phenylpropanolamine HCl; vitamin C) + (multiple vitamins/minerals; iron; folic acid; biotin)] (75 • 60 mg) + (± • 18 • 0.4 • 0.03 mg)

Dexatrim Pre-Meal timed-release capsules OTC *diet aid* [phenylpropanolamine HCl] 25 mg

Dexatuss sugar-free syrup OTC *antitussive; expectorant* [dextromethorphan hydrobromide; guaifenesin]

dexbrompheniramine INN, BAN *antihistamine* [also: dexbrompheniramine maleate]

dexbrompheniramine maleate USP *antihistamine* [also: dexbrompheniramine]

Dexchlor extended-release tablets ℞ *antihistamine* [dexchlorpheniramine maleate] 4, 6 mg

dexchlorpheniramine INN *antihistamine* [also: dexchlorpheniramine maleate]

dexchlorpheniramine maleate USP *antihistamine* [also: dexchlorpheniramine] 4, 6 mg oral

dexclamol INN *sedative* [also: dexclamol HCl]

dexclamol HCl USAN *sedative* [also: dexclamol]

Dexedrine Spansules (sustained-release capsules), tablets ℞ *amphetamine; CNS stimulant* [dextroamphetamine sulfate] 5, 10, 15 mg; 5 mg ⓘ dextran

dexetimide USAN, INN, BAN *anticholinergic*

dexetozoline INN

dexfenfluramine INN, BAN *anorexiant; appetite suppressant; serotonin reuptake inhibitor* [also: dexfenfluramine HCl]

dexfenfluramine HCl USAN *anorexiant; appetite suppressant; serotonin reuptake inhibitor* [also: dexfenfluramine]

dexibuprofen INN *analgesic; cyclooxygenase inhibitor; anti-inflammatory* [also: dexibuprofen lysine]

dexibuprofen lysine USAN *analgesic; cyclooxygenase inhibitor; anti-inflammatory* [also: dexibuprofen]

deximafen USAN, INN *antidepressant*

dexindoprofen INN

Dexitac timed-release capsules (discontinued 1992) OTC *CNS stimulant; analeptic* [caffeine]

dexivacaine USAN, INN *anesthetic*

dexlofexidine INN

dexmedetomidine USAN, INN, BAN *tranquilizer*

dexnorgestrel acetime [now: norgestimate]

Dexone intra-articular, intralesional, soft tissue, or IM injection ℞ *glucocorticoids* [dexamethasone sodium phosphate] 4 mg/mL

Dexone tablets ℞ *glucocorticoids* [dexamethasone] 0.5, 0.75, 1.5, 4 mg

Dexone LA intralesional, intra-articular, soft tissue, or IM injection ℞ *glucocorticoids* [dexamethasone acetate] 8 mg/mL

dexormaplatin USAN, INN *antineoplastic*

DexOtic eye drops (discontinued 1992) ℞ *ophthalmic topical corticosteroidal anti-inflammatory* [dexamethasone sodium phosphate]

dexoxadrol INN *CNS stimulant; analgesic* [also: dexoxadrol HCl]

dexoxadrol HCl USAN *CNS stimulant; analgesic* [also: dexoxadrol]
dexpanthenol USAN, USP, INN, BAN *cholinergic; antipruritic; postoperative prophylaxis for paralytic ileus 250 mg/mL injection*
dexpemedolac USAN *analgesic*
dexpropranolol HCl USAN *antiarrhythmic; antiadrenergic (β-receptor)* [also: dexpropranolol]
dexproxibutene INN
dexrazoxane USAN, INN, BAN *cardioprotectant for doxorubicin-induced cardiomyopathy (orphan); chelates intracellular iron*
dexsecoverine INN
dexsotalol HCl USAN *class III antiarrhythmic*
dextilidine INN
dextran INN, BAN *blood flow adjuvant; plasma volume extender* [also: dextran 40] ② Dexedrine; dextrin
dextran, high molecular weight [see: dextran 70]
dextran, low molecular weight [see: dextran 40]
dextran 1 *monovalent hapten for prevention of dextran-induced anaphylactic reactions*
dextran 40 USAN *blood flow adjuvant; plasma volume extender* [also: dextran] *10% injection*
dextran 70 USAN *plasma volume extender; viscosity-increasing agent 6% injection*
dextran 75 USAN *plasma volume extender; viscosity-increasing agent 6% injection*
dextran & deferoxamine (*orphan: acute iron poisoning*)
dextran sulfate *investigational (Phase II) antiviral for AIDS/ARC/HIV;* (*orphan: cystic fibrosis*)
dextran sulfate, sodium salt, aluminum complex [see: detralfate]
dextran sulfate sodium (*orphan: AIDS*)
dextranomer INN, BAN *wound debrider/cleanser*
dextrates USAN, NF *tablet binder and diluent*
dextriferron NF, INN, BAN

dextrin NF, BAN *suspending agent; tablet binder and diluent* ② dextran
dextroamphetamine USAN *CNS stimulant* [also: dexamfetamine; dexamphetamine]
dextroamphetamine phosphate USP
dextroamphetamine saccharate *CNS stimulant*
dextroamphetamine sulfate USP *CNS stimulant 5, 10, 15 mg oral*
dextrobrompheniramine maleate [see: dexbrompheniramine maleate]
dextrochlorpheniramine maleate [see: dexchlorpheniramine maleate]
dextrofemine INN
dextromethorphan USP, INN, BAN *antitussive*
dextromethorphan hydrobromide USP, BAN *antitussive 10 mg/5 mL oral*
dextromethorphan polistirex USAN *antitussive*
dextromoramide INN, BAN
dextromoramide tartrate [see: dextromoramide]
dextro-pantothenyl alcohol [see: dexpanthenol]
dextropropoxyphene chloride [see: propoxyphene HCl]
dextropropoxyphene INN, BAN *narcotic analgesic* [also: propoxyphene HCl]
dextropropoxyphene HCl BAN [also: propoxyphene HCl]
dextrorphan INN, BAN *investigational glutamate receptor antagonist for neurodegenerative disorders*
dextrorphan HCl *treatment of cerebral ischemia*
dextrose USP *fluid and nutrient replenisher; parenteral antihypoglycemic*
5% Dextrose and Electrolyte #48; 5% Dextrose and Electrolyte #75; 10% Dextrose and Electrolyte #48 IV infusion ℞ *intravenous nutritional/electrolyte therapy* [combined electrolyte solution; dextrose]
dextrose excipient NF *tablet excipient*
50% Dextrose with Electrolyte Pattern A (or N) IV infusion ℞ *intravenous nutritional/electrolyte therapy* [combined electrolyte solution; dextrose]
50% Dextrose with Electrolyte Pattern B IV infusion (discontinued

1994) ℞ *intravenous nutritional/electrolyte therapy* [combined electrolyte solution; dextrose]

Dextrostat tablets ℞ *amphetamine; CNS stimulant* [dextroamphetamine sulfate] 5 mg

Dextrostix reagent strips for home use OTC *in vitro diagnostic aid for blood glucose*

dextrothyronine [see: detrothyronine]

dextrothyroxine BAN *antihyperlipoproteinemic* [also: dextrothyroxine sodium]

dextrothyroxine sodium USAN, USP, INN *antihyperlipoproteinemic* [also: dextrothyroxine]

dexverapamil INN *investigational adjunct to chemotherapy*

Dey-Dose (delivery system) *nebulizer*

Dey-Lube ophthalmic ointment (discontinued 1992) ℞ *ocular moisturizer/lubricant*

Dey-Lute (delivery system) *nebulizer*

Dey-Pak Sodium Chloride 0.45% & 0.9% solution OTC *for respiratory therapy and tracheal lavage* [sodium chloride] 0.45%; 0.9%

Dey-Pak Sodium Chloride 3% & 10% solution ℞ *for inducing sputum production for specimen collection* [sodium chloride] 3%; 10%

Dey-Vial Sodium Chloride 0.9% solution OTC *for respiratory therapy and tracheal lavage* [sodium chloride] 0.9%

dezaguanine USAN, INN *antineoplastic*

dezaguanine mesylate USAN *antineoplastic*

dezinamide *investigational antiepileptic*

dezocine USAN, INN *narcotic analgesic*

d-Film gel (discontinued 1993) OTC *cleaning gel for hard contact lenses*

DFMO (difluoromethylornithine) [see: eflornithine]

DFMO (difluoromethylornithine) HCl [see: eflornithine HCl]

DFMO-MGBG (eflornithine, mitoguazone) *chemotherapy protocol* [also see: DFMO; MGBG]

DFP (diisopropyl flurophosphate) [see: isoflurophate]

DFV (DDP, fluorouracil, VePesid) *chemotherapy protocol*

DHA (docosahexaenoic acid) [see: doconexent]

DHAP (dexamethasone, high-dose ara-C, Platinol) *chemotherapy protocol*

DHC Plus capsules ℞ *narcotic analgesic* [dihydrocodeine bitartrate; acetaminophen; caffeine] 16•356.4•30 mg

DHE (dihydroergotamine) [see: dihydroergotamine mesylate]

D.H.E. 45 IV or IM injection ℞ *migraine prophylaxis or treatment* [dihydroergotamine mesylate] 1 mg/mL

DHEA (dehydroepiandrosterone) [q.v.]

DHPG (dihydroxy propoxymethyl guanine) [see: ganciclovir]

DHS Tar liquid shampoo, gel shampoo OTC *antiseborrheic; antipsoriatic; antipruritic; antibacterial* [coal tar] 0.5%

DHS Zinc shampoo OTC *antiseborrheic; antibacterial; antifungal* [pyrithione zinc] 2%

DHT tablets, Intensol (concentrated oral solution) ℞ *antihypocalcemic for tetany* [dihydrotachysterol] 0.125, 0.2, 0.4 mg; 0.2 mg/mL

DHT (dihydrotachysterol) [q.v.]

DHT (dihydrotestosterone) [see: androstanolone; stanolone]

DI (doxorubicin, ifosfamide [with mesna rescue]) *chemotherapy protocol*

Diaβeta (or DiaBeta) tablets ℞ *sulfonylurea antidiabetic* [glyburide] 1.25, 2.5, 5 mg

Diabetic Tussin liquid OTC *antitussive; decongestant; expectorant* [dextromethorphan hydrobromide; phenylephrine HCl; guaifenesin] 10•5•100 mg/5 mL

Diabetic Tussin DM liquid OTC *antitussive; expectorant* [dextromethorphan hydrobromide; guaifenesin] 10•100 mg/5 mL

Diabetic Tussin EX liquid OTC *expectorant* [guaifenesin] 100 mg/5 mL

Diabinese tablets ℞ *antidiabetic* [chlorpropamide] 100, 250 mg

diacerein INN

diacetamate INN, BAN

diacetolol INN, BAN *antiadrenergic (β-receptor)* [also: diacetolol HCl]

diacetolol HCl USAN *antiadrenergic (β-receptor)* [also: diacetolol]
diacetoxyphenylisatin [see: oxyphenisatin acetate]
diacetoxyphenyloxindol [see: oxyphenisatin acetate]
diacetrizoate sodium [see: diatrizoate sodium]
diacetyl diaminodiphenylsulfone (DADDS) [see: acedapsone]
diacetylated monoglycerides NF *plasticizer*
diacetylcholine chloride [see: succinylcholine chloride]
diacetyl-dihydroxydiphenylisatin [see: oxyphenisatin acetate]
diacetyldioxphenylisatin [see: oxyphenisatin acetate]
diacetylmorphine HCl USP *(heroin; banned in USA)* [also: diamorphine]
diacetylmorphine salts *(heroin; banned in USA)*
diacetylsalicylic acid [see: dipyrocetyl]
diacetyltannic acid [see: acetyltannic acid]
diacetylthiamine [see: acetiamine]
Diachlor tablets (discontinued 1993) ℞ *diuretic* [chlorothiazide]
diagniol [see: sodium acetrizoate]
Dia-Kit ℞ *allergic hypersensitivity testing* [allergenic mold extracts]
diallybarbituric acid [see: allobarbital]
diallylbarbituric acid [now: allobarbital]
diallylnortoxiferene dichloride [see: alcuronium chloride]
diallymal [see: allobarbital]
Dialose capsules (discontinued 1995) OTC *stool softener* [docusate potassium] 100 mg
Dialose tablets OTC *stool softener* [docusate sodium] 100 mg
Dialose Plus tablets, capsules OTC *laxative; stool softener* [yellow phenolphthalein; docusate sodium] 65•100 mg
Dialpak (trademarked packaging form) *patient compliance package*
Dialume capsules ℞ *antacid* [aluminum hydroxide gel] 500 mg ☒ Dalmane
Dialyte Pattern LM solution ℞ *peritoneal dialysis solution* [multiple electrolytes; dextrose] 1.5%•±, 2.5%•±, 4.5%•±

dia-mer-sulfonamides (sulfadiazine & sulfamerazine) [q.v.]
diamethine [see: dimethyltubocurarinium chloride; dimethyltubocurarine]
diamfenetide INN [also: diamphenethide]
Diamine T.D. timed-release tablets ℞ *antihistamine* [brompheniramine maleate] 8, 12 mg
diaminedipenicillin G [see: penicillin G benzathine]
diaminodiphenylsulfone (DDS) [now: dapsone]
3,4-diaminopyridine *(orphan: Lambert-Eaton myasthenic syndrome)*
cis-diamminedichloroplatinum (DDP) [see: cisplatin]
diammonium phosphate [see: ammonium phosphate]
diamocaine INN, BAN *local anesthetic* [also: diamocaine cyclamate]
diamocaine cyclamate USAN *local anesthetic* [also: diamocaine]
diamorphine BAN *(heroin; banned in USA)* [also: diacetylmorphine HCl]
Diamox powder for IV injection ℞ *anticonvulsant; diuretic* [acetazolamide sodium] 500 mg
Diamox tablets, Sequels (sustained-release capsules) ℞ *anticonvulsant; diuretic* [acetazolamide] 125, 250 mg; 500 mg
diamphenethide BAN [also: diamfenetide]
diampromide INN, BAN
diampron [see: amicarbalide]
diamthazole BAN [also: dimazole]
diamthazole dihydrochloride [see: diamthazole]
Dianeal; Dianeal 137 solution (discontinued 1996) ℞ *peritoneal dialysis solution* [multiple electrolytes; dextrose] ±•1.5%, ±•4.25%
Dianeal PD-2 peritoneal dialysis solution with 1.1% amino acids *(orphan: malnourishment of continuous ambulatory peritoneal dialysis)*
diapamide USAN *diuretic; antihypertensive* [also: tiamizide]

Diaparene Baby cream OTC *topical diaper rash treatment*

Diaparene Cornstarch Baby powder OTC *topical diaper rash treatment* [corn starch; aloe]

Diaparene Cradol liquid (discontinued 1994) OTC *antimicrobial hair dressing* [methylbenzethonium chloride] 0.07%

Diaparene Diaper Rash ointment OTC *topical diaper rash treatment* [zinc oxide]

Diaparene Medicated powder, cream (discontinued 1993) OTC *topical diaper rash treatment* [methylbenzethonium chloride]

Diaparene Peri-Anal Medicated ointment (discontinued 1993) OTC *topical diaper rash treatment* [methylbenzethonium chloride; zinc oxide]

Diaper Guard ointment OTC *topical diaper rash treatment* [dimethicone; vitamins A, D, and E; zinc oxide] 1% • ± • ?

Diaper Rash ointment OTC *topical diaper rash treatment* [zinc oxide]

diaphene [see: dibromsalan]

diaphenylsulfone [see: dapsone]

Diapid nasal spray ℞ *pituitary antidiuretic hormone for diabetes insipidus* [lypressin] 50 U/mL

Diaqua tablets (discontinued 1993) ℞ *diuretic; antihypertensive* [hydrochlorothiazide]

Diar-Aid tablets OTC *antidiarrheal; GI adsorbent* [loperamide HCl] 2 mg

diarbarone INN

Diascan reagent strips for home use OTC *in vitro diagnostic aid for blood glucose*

Diasorb tablets, liquid OTC *antidiarrheal; GI adsorbent* [activated attapulgite] 750 mg; 750 mg/5 mL

diaspirin crosslinked hemoglobin (DCL Hb) *investigational blood substitute*

Diastat viscous solution for rectal administration ℞ *(orphan: acute repetitive seizures)* [diazepam]

Diastix reagent strips for home use OTC *in vitro diagnostic aid for urine glucose*

diathymosulfone INN

diatrizoate meglumine USP *GI radiopaque medium* [also: meglumine diatrizoate] 76% injection

diatrizoate methylglucamine [see: diatrizoate meglumine]

diatrizoate sodium USP *GI radiopaque medium* [also: sodium amidotrizoate; sodium diatrizoate]

diatrizoate sodium I 125 USAN *radioactive agent*

diatrizoate sodium I 131 USAN *radioactive agent*

diatrizoic acid USAN, USP, BAN *radiopaque medium* [also: amidotrizoic acid]

Diatrol tablets OTC *antacid; antidiarrheal* [calcium carbonate; pectin]

diaveridine USAN, INN, BAN *antibacterial*

diazacholesterol dihydrochloride [see: azacosterol HCl]

diazepam USAN, USP, INN, BAN, JAN *anxiolytic; sedative; skeletal muscle relaxant; (orphan: acute repetitive seizures)* 2, 5, 10 mg oral; 5 mg/5 mL oral; 5 mg/mL oral; 5 mg/mL injection

diazinon BAN [also: dimpylate]

diaziquone USAN, INN *antineoplastic; (orphan: primary brain malignancies; grade III-IV astrocytomas)*

diazoxide USAN, USP, INN, BAN *emergency antihypertensive; glucose-elevating agent*

dibasic calcium phosphate [see: calcium phosphate, dibasic]

dibasic potassium phosphate [see: potassium phosphate, dibasic]

dibasic sodium phosphate [see: sodium phosphate, dibasic]

dibasol [see: bendazol]

dibazol [see: bendazol]

dibekacin INN, BAN

dibemethine INN

dibencil [see: penicillin G benzathine]

dibencozide [see: cobamamide]

Dibent IM injection ℞ *gastrointestinal antispasmodic* [dicyclomine HCl] 10 mg/mL

dibenthiamine [see: bentiamine]

dibenzathione [see: sulbentine]

dibenzepin INN, BAN *antidepressant* [also: dibenzepin HCl]

dibenzepin HCl USAN *antidepressant* [also: dibenzepin]
dibenzothiazine [see: phenothiazine]
dibenzothiophene USAN *keratolytic*
dibenzoyl peroxide [see: benzoyl peroxide]
dibenzoylthiamin [see: bentiamine]
dibenzthion [see: sulbentine]
dibenzylethylenediamine dipenicillin G (DBED) [see: penicillin G benzathine]
Dibenzyline capsules ℞ *antihypertensive for pheochromocytoma* [phenoxybenzamine HCl] 10 mg
N,N-dibenzylmethylamine [see: dibemethine]
dibromodulcitol [see: mitolactol]
dibromohydroxyquinoline [see: broxyquinoline]
dibromomannitol (DBM) [see: mitobronitol]
dibromopropamidine BAN [also: dibrompropamidine]
dibrompropamidine INN [also: dibromopropamidine]
dibromsalan USAN, INN *disinfectant*
dibrospidium chloride INN
dibucaine USP *topical local anesthetic* [also: cinchocaine] 1% topical
dibucaine HCl USP *local anesthetic* [also: cinchocaine HCl]
dibudinate INN *combining name for radicals or groups*
dibunate INN *combining name for radicals or groups*
dibuprol INN
dibupyrone INN, BAN
dibusadol INN
dibutoline sulfate
DIC (dimethyl imidazole carboxamide) [see: dacarbazine]
Dical CapTabs (capsule-shaped tablets) OTC *dietary supplement* [dibasic calcium phosphate; vitamin D] 117 mg (Ca)•90 mg (P)•133 IU
dicalcium phosphate [see: calcium phosphate, dibasic]
Dical-D tablets, chewable wafers OTC *dietary supplement* [dibasic calcium phosphate; vitamin D] 117 mg (Ca)•90 mg (P)•133 IU; 232 mg (Ca)•180 mg (P)•200 IU

dicarbine INN
Dicarbosil chewable tablets OTC *antacid* [calcium carbonate] 500 mg ⊇ dacarbazine
dicarfen INN
dichlofenthion BAN
dichloralantipyrine [see: dichloralphenazone]
dichloralphenazone (chloral hydrate + phenazone) BAN *mild sedative*
dichloralpyrine [see: dichloralphenazone]
dichloramine-T NF
dichloranilino imidazolin [see: clonidine HCl]
dichloren [see: mechlorethamine HCl]
dichlorisone INN
dichlorisone acetate [see: dichlorisone]
dichlormethazanone [see: dichlormezanone]
dichlormezanone INN
dichloroacetate sodium (*orphan: congenital lactic acidosis; familial hypercholesterolemia*)
dichloroacetic acid *strong keratolytic/cauterant* ⊇ Bichloracetic acid
dichlorodifluoromethane NF *aerosol propellant*
dichlorodiphenyl trichloroethane (DDT) [see: chlorophenothane]
dichlorometaxylenol [see: dichloroxylenol]
dichloromethane [see: methylene chloride]
dichlorophen INN, BAN
dichlorophenarsine INN, BAN [also: dichlorophenarsine HCl]
dichlorophenarsine HCl USP [also: dichlorophenarsine]
dichlorotetrafluoroethane NF *aerosol propellant* [also: cryofluorane]
dichlorovinyl dimethyl phosphate (DDVP) [see: dichlorvos]
dichloroxylenol INN, BAN
dichlorphenamide USP, BAN *carbonic anhydrase inhibitor* [also: diclofenamide]
dichlorvos USAN, INN, BAN *anthelmintic*
dichysterol [see: dihydrotachysterol]
diciferron INN
dicirenone USAN, INN *hypotensive; aldosterone antagonist*

Dick test (scarlet fever streptococcus toxin)

diclazuril USAN, INN, BAN *coccidiostat for poultry; investigational for cryptosporidiosis in AIDS*

diclofenac INN, BAN *antiarthritic; nonsteroidal anti-inflammatory drug (NSAID); analgesic* [also: diclofenac potassium] 25, 50, 75 mg oral

diclofenac potassium USAN *antiarthritic; nonsteroidal anti-inflammatory drug (NSAID); analgesic* [also: diclofenac]

diclofenac sodium USAN, JAN *antiarthritic; nonsteroidal anti-inflammatory drug (NSAID); analgesic*

diclofenamide INN *carbonic anhydrase inhibitor* [also: dichlorphenamide]

diclofensine INN

diclofibrate [see: simfibrate]

diclofurime INN

diclometide INN

diclonixin INN

dicloralurea USAN, INN *veterinary food additive*

dicloxacillin USAN, INN, BAN *antibacterial*

dicloxacillin sodium USAN, USP, BAN *bactericidal antibiotic* 250, 500 mg oral

dicobalt edetate INN, BAN

dicolinium iodide INN

dicophane BAN [also: chlorophenothane; clofenotane]

dicoumarin [see: dicumarol]

dicoumarol INN [also: dicumarol]

dicresulene INN

DTIC-ACTD; DICT-ACT-D (DTIC, actinomycin D) *chemotherapy protocol*

dicumarol USAN, USP *anticoagulant* [also: dicoumarol] 25 mg oral ⑨ Demerol

dicyclomine BAN *anticholinergic* [also: dicyclomine HCl; dicycloverine]

dicyclomine HCl USP *GI antispasmodic; anticholinergic* [also: dicycloverine; dicyclomine] 10, 20 mg oral; 10 mg/5 mL oral; 10 mg/mL injection

dicycloverine INN *anticholinergic* [also: dicyclomine HCl; dicyclomine]

dicycloverine HCl [see: dicyclomine HCl]

dicysteine [see: cystine]

didanosine USAN, INN, BAN *antiviral for AIDS*

didehydrodideoxythymidine [see: stavudine]

Di-Delamine gel, spray OTC *topical antihistamine; bacteriostatic* [diphenhydramine HCl; tripelennamine HCl] 1%•0.5%•

2'-3'-dideoxyadenosine *(orphan: AIDS)*

dideoxycytidine (DDC; ddC) [see: zalcitabine]

dideoxyinosine (DDI; ddI) [see: didanosine]

Didrex tablets ℞ *anorexiant* [benzphetamine HCl] 25, 50 mg

Didrocal ℞ *investigational treatment for osteoporosis* [etidronate]

Didro-Kit (Italian name for U.S. product Didronel)

Didronel tablets, IV infusion ℞ *bone resorption suppressant; (orphan: hypercalcemia of malignancy; metabolic bone disease)* [etidronate disodium] 200, 400 mg; 50 mg/mL

didrovaltrate INN

didroxane [see: dichlorophen]

dieldrin INN, BAN

diemal [see: barbital]

dienestrol USP, INN *estrogen* [also: dienoestrol]

dienoestrol BAN *estrogen* [also: dienestrol]

dienogest INN

Diet Ayds candy OTC *decrease taste perception of sweetness* [benzocaine] 6 mg

Diet-Aid timed-release capsules (discontinued 1992) OTC *diet aid* [phenylpropanolamine HCl]

Diet-Aid Plus Vitamin C timed-release capsules (discontinued 1992) OTC *diet aid* [phenylpropanolamine HCl; vitamin C]

dietamiphylline [see: etamiphyllin]

dietamiverine HCl [see: bietamiverine HCl]

diethadione INN, BAN

diethanolamine NF *alkalizing agent*

diethazine INN, BAN

diethazine HCl [see: diethazine]

diethyl phthalate NF *plasticizer*

diethylamine p-aminobenzenestibonate [see: stibosamine]
3-diethylaminobutyranilide [see: octacaine]
diethylbarbiturate monosodium [see: barbital sodium]
diethylbarbituric acid [see: barbital]
diethylcarbamazine INN, BAN *anthelmintic* [also: diethylcarbamazine citrate]
diethylcarbamazine citrate USP *anthelmintic* [also: diethylcarbamazine]
diethylcarbamazine dihydrogen citrate [see: diethylcarbamazine citrate]
diethyldithiocarbamate *investigational (Phase II/III) immunomodulator for AIDS/ARC/HIV (orphan)*
diethyldixanthogen [see: dixanthogen]
diethylenediamine citrate [see: piperazine citrate]
diethylenetriaminepentaacetic acid (DTPA) [see: pentetic acid]
N,N-diethyllysergamide [see: lysergide]
diethylmalonylurea [see: barbital]
diethylmalonylurea sodium [see: barbital sodium]
N,N-diethylnicotinamide [see: nikethamide]
diethylpropion BAN *anorexiant* [also: diethylpropion HCl; amfepramone] 75 mg oral
diethylpropion HCl USP *anorexiant; CNS stimulant* [also: amfepramone; diethylpropion] 25 mg oral
diethylstilbestrol (DES) USP, INN *estrogen for inoperable breast and prostate cancer* [also: stilboestrol] 1, 5 mg oral
diethylstilbestrol diphosphate USP *antineoplastic; estrogen* [also: fosfestrol]
diethylstilbestrol dipropionate NF
p-diethylsulfamoylbenzoic acid [see: etebenecid; ethebenecid]
diethylthiambutene INN, BAN
diethyltoluamide (DEET) USP, BAN *arthropod repellent*
diethyltryptamine (DET)
N,N-diethylvanillamide [see: ethamivan]
dietifen INN
dietroxine [see: diethadione]

Dieutrim T.D. timed-release capsules OTC *diet aid; decrease perception of sweetness* [phenylpropanolamine HCl; benzocaine] 75•9 mg
diexanthogen [see: dixanthogen]
difebarbamate INN
difemerine INN [also: difemerine HCl]
difemerine HCl [also: difemerine]
difemetorex INN
difenamizole INN
difencloxazine INN
difencloxazine HCl [see: difencloxazine]
difenidol INN *antiemetic; antivertigo* [also: diphenidol]
difenoximide INN *antiperistaltic* [also: difenoximide HCl]
difenoximide HCl USAN *antiperistaltic* [also: difenoximide]
difenoxin USAN, INN, BAN *antiperistaltic*
difenoxin HCl *antiperistaltic*
difetarsone INN, BAN
difeterol INN
Differin gel ℞ *synthetic retinoid analog for acne* [adapalene] 0.1%
diflorasone INN, BAN *topical corticosteroidal anti-inflammatory* [also: diflorasone diacetate]
diflorasone diacetate USAN, USP *topical corticosteroidal anti-inflammatory* [also: diflorasone]
difloxacin INN *anti-infective; DNA gyrase inhibitor* [also: difloxacin HCl]
difloxacin HCl USAN *anti-infective; DNA gyrase inhibitor* [also: difloxacin]
difluanazine INN *CNS stimulant* [also: difluanine HCl]
difluanazine HCl [see: difluanine HCl]
difluanine HCl USAN *CNS stimulant* [also: difluanazine]
Diflucan tablets, powder for oral suspension, IV infusion ℞ *systemic antifungal* [fluconazole] 50, 100, 150, 200 mg; 10, 40 mg/mL; 2 mg/mL
diflucortolone USAN, INN, BAN *glucocorticoid*
diflucortolone pivalate USAN *glucocorticoid*
diflumidone INN, BAN *anti-inflammatory* [also: diflumidone sodium]
diflumidone sodium USAN *anti-inflammatory* [also: diflumidone]

diflunisal USAN, USP, INN, BAN *anti-inflammatory; analgesic; antipyretic; antiarthritic; antirheumatic* 250, 500 mg oral

difluoromethylornithine (DFMO) [see: eflornithine]

difluoromethylornithine HCl [see: eflornithine HCl]

difluprednate USAN, INN *anti-inflammatory*

difolliculin [see: estradiol benzoate]

diftalone USAN, INN *anti-inflammatory*

digalloyl trioleate USAN

Di-Gel liquid OTC *antacid; antiflatulent* [aluminum hydroxide; magnesium hydroxide; simethicone] 200•200•20 mg/5 mL

Di-Gel, Advanced Formula chewable tablets OTC *antacid; antiflatulent* [magnesium hydroxide; calcium carbonate; simethicone] 128•280•20 mg

Digepepsin dual-coated tablets ℞ *digestive enzymes* [pancreatin; pepsin; bile salts] 300•250•150 mg

Digestalin tablets (discontinued 1992) OTC *digestive enzymes; antiflatulent; antacid; antidiarrheal* [pancreatin; papain; pepsin; activated charcoal; bismuth subsalicylate; berberis; hydrastis]

Digestant II tablets OTC *digestive enzymes* [pepsin; pancreatin; bile salts]

Digestozyme tablets ℞ *digestive enzymes; laxative* [pancreatin; pepsin; dehydrocholic acid] 300•250•25 mg

Digibind powder for IV injection ℞ *antidote to digoxin/digitoxin overdose* (orphan) [digoxin immune Fab (ovine)] 38 mg/vial

Digidote ℞ *antidote to digitalis/digitoxin overdose* (orphan) [digoxin immune Fab (ovine)]

digitalis USP *cardiotonic*

digitoxin USP, INN, BAN *cardiotonic; cardiac glycoside* ② Desoxyn; digoxin

digitoxin, acetyl [see: acetyldigitoxin]

α-digitoxin monoacetate [see: acetyldigitoxin]

digitoxoside [see: digitoxin]

digolil INN *combining name for radicals or groups*

digoxin USP, INN, BAN *cardiotonic; cardiac glycoside* 0.125, 0.25, 0.5 mg oral, 0.05 mg/mL oral, 0.15 mg/mL injection ② Desoxyn; digitoxin

digoxin antibody [see: digoxin immune Fab]

digoxin immune Fab (ovine) *antidote to digoxin/digitoxin intoxication* (orphan)

dihematoporphyrin ethers (orphan: *bladder carcinoma; esophageal carcinoma*)

dihexyverine INN *anticholinergic* [also: dihexyverine HCl]

dihexyverine HCl USAN *anticholinergic* [also: dihexyverine]

Dihistine elixir (discontinued 1993) OTC *decongestant; antihistamine* [phenylephrine HCl; chlorpheniramine maleate]

Dihistine DH liquid OTC *narcotic antitussive; decongestant; antihistamine* [codeine phosphate; pseudoephedrine HCl; chlorpheniramine maleate; alcohol] 10•30•2 mg/5 mL

Dihistine Expectorant liquid ℞ *narcotic antitussive; decongestant; expectorant* [codeine phosphate; pseudoephedrine HCl; guaifenesin; alcohol] 10•30•100 mg/5 mL

dihydan soluble [see: phenytoin sodium]

dihydralazine INN, BAN

dihydralazine sulfate [see: dihydralazine]

dihydrobenzthiazide [see: hydrobentizide]

dihydrocodeine INN, BAN *analgesic* [also: dihydrocodeine bitartrate]

dihydrocodeine bitartrate USP *analgesic* [also: dihydrocodeine]

dihydrocodeinone bitartrate [see: hydrocodone bitartrate]

dihydroergocornine [see: ergoloid mesylates]

dihydroergocristine [see: ergoloid mesylates]

dihydroergocryptine [see: ergoloid mesylates]

dihydroergotamine (DHE) INN, BAN *antiadrenergic; anticoagulant; rapid* *control of migraines* [also: dihydroergotamine mesylate]

dihydroergotamine mesylate USAN, USP *antiadrenergic; anticoagulant; rapid control of migraines* [also: dihydroergotamine]

dihydroergotamine methanesulfonate [see: dihydroergotamine mesylate]

dihydroergotoxine mesylate [now: ergoloid mesylates]

dihydroergotoxine methanesulfonate [now: ergoloid mesylates]

dihydroethaverine [see: drotaverine]

dihydrofollicular hormone [see: estradiol]

dihydrofolliculine [see: estradiol]

dihydrogenated ergot alkaloids [now: ergoloid mesylates]

dihydrohydroxycodeinone [see: oxycodone]

dihydrohydroxycodeinone HCl [see: oxycodone HCl]

6-dihydro-6-iminopurine [see: adenine]

dihydroisoperparine [see: drotaverine]

dihydromorphinone HCl [now: hydromorphone HCl]

dihydroneopine [see: dihydrocodeine bitartrate]

dihydrostreptomycin (DST) INN *antibacterial* [also: dihydrostreptomycin sulfate]

dihydrostreptomycin sulfate USP *antibacterial* [also: dihydrostreptomycin]

dihydrostreptomycin-streptomycin [see: streptoduocin]

dihydrotachysterol (DHT) USP, INN, BAN *calcium regulator; vitamin D_1* 0.125, 0.2, 0.4 mg oral; 0.2 mg/mL oral

dihydrotestosterone (DHT) [see: androstanolone; stanolone]

dihydrotheelin [see: estradiol]

dihydroxy(stearato)aluminum [see: aluminum monostearate]

dihydroxy propoxymethyl guanine (DHPG) [see: gancyclovir]

dihydroxyacetone *skin darkener for vitiligo and hypopigmented areas*

dihydroxyaluminum aminoacetate (DAA) USP *antacid*

dihydroxyaluminum sodium carbonate USP *antacid*

dihydroxyanthranol [see: anthralin]

dihydroxyanthraquinone (*withdrawn from market*) [see: danthron]

1,25-dihydroxycholecalciferol [see: calcitriol]

24,25-dihydroxycholecalciferol (*orphan: uremic osteodystrophy*)

dihydroxyestrin [see: estradiol]

dihydroxyfluorane [see: fluorescein]

dihydroxyphenylalanine (DOPA) [see: levodopa]

dihydroxyphenylisatin [see: oxyphenisatin acetate]

dihydroxyphenyloxindol [see: oxyphenisatin acetate]

dihydroxyprogesterone acetophenide [see: algestone acetophenide]

dihydroxypropyl theophylline [see: dyphylline]

diiodobuphenine [see: bufeniode]

diiodohydroxyquin [now: iodoquinol]

diiodohydroxyquinoline INN, BAN *antiamebic* [also: iodoquinol]

diisopromine INN

diisopromine HCl [see: diisopromine]

diisopropanolamine NF *alkalizing agent*

diisopropyl flurophosphate (DFP) [see: isoflurophate]

diisopropyl flurophosphonate [see: isoflurophate]

diisopropyl phosphorofluoridate [see: isoflurophate]

2,6-diisopropylphenol [see: propofol]

Dilacor XR sustained-release capsules ℞ *antihypertensive; antianginal; calcium channel blocker* [diltiazem HCl] 120, 180, 240 mg

Dilantin Infatabs (chewable tablets) ℞ *hydantoin-type anticonvulsant* [phenytoin] 50 mg ② Dilaudid

Dilantin Kapseals (capsules), IV or IM injection ℞ *hydantoin-type anticonvulsant* [phenytoin sodium] 30, 100 mg; 50 mg/mL

Dilantin Oros ℞ *investigational controlled-release form of Dilantin* [osmotic phenytoin]

Dilantin with Phenobarbital Kapseals (capsules) (discontinued 1996) ℞ *hydantoin-type anticonvulsant; sedative* [phenytoin sodium; phenobarbital] 100•16, 100•32 mg

Dilantin-30 Pediatric oral suspension (discontinued 1996) ℞ *hydantoin-type anticonvulsant* [phenytoin] 30 mg/5 mL

Dilantin-125 oral suspension ℞ *hydantoin-type anticonvulsant* [phenytoin] 125 mg/5 mL

Dilatrate-SR sustained-release capsules ℞ *antianginal* [isosorbide dinitrate] 40 mg

Dilaudid tablets, subcu or IM injection, suppositories ℞ *narcotic analgesic* [hydromorphone HCl] 2, 4, 8 mg; 1, 2, 4 mg/mL; 3 mg ② Dilantin

Dilaudid Cough syrup ℞ *narcotic antitussive; expectorant* [hydromorphone HCl; guaifenesin; alcohol 5%] 1•100 mg/5 mL

Dilaudid-5 oral liquid ℞ *narcotic analgesic* [hydromorphone HCl] 5 mg/5 mL

Dilaudid-HP subcu or IM injection ℞ *narcotic analgesic* [hydromorphone HCl] 10 mg/mL (250 mg/vial)

dilazep INN

dilevalol INN, BAN *antihypertensive; antiadrenergic (β-receptor)* [also: dilevalol HCl]

dilevalol HCl USAN, JAN *antihypertensive; antiadrenergic (β-receptor)* [also: dilevalol]

dilithium carbonate [see: lithium carbonate]

dilmefone INN

Dilocaine injection ℞ *injectable local anesthetic* [lidocaine HCl] 1%, 2%

Dilor elixir, injection ℞ *bronchodilator* [dyphylline] 160 mg/15 mL; 250 mg/mL

Dilor 200; Dilor 400 tablets ℞ *bronchodilator* [dyphylline] 200 mg; 400 mg

Dilor-G tablets, liquid ℞ *antiasthmatic; bronchodilator; expectorant* [dyphylline; guaifenesin] 200•200 mg; 300•300 mg/15 mL

diloxanide INN, BAN, DCF

diloxanide furoate *investigational anti-infective for amebiasis*

diltiazem INN, BAN *coronary vasodilator; calcium channel blocker; antianginal; antihypertensive* [also: diltiazem HCl]

diltiazem HCl USAN, USP, JAN *coronary vasodilator; calcium channel blocker; antianginal; antihypertensive* [also: diltiazem] 30, 60, 90, 120 mg oral; 5 mg/mL injection

diltiazem malate USAN *antihypertensive*

diluted acetic acid [see: acetic acid, diluted]

diluted alcohol [see: alcohol, diluted]

diluted hydrochloric acid [see: hydrochloric acid, diluted]

diluted sodium hypochlorite [see: sodium hypochlorite, diluted]

dimabefylline INN

Dimacid chewable tablets (discontinued 1994) OTC *antacid* [calcium carbonate; magnesium carbonate]

Dimacol caplets OTC *antitussive; decongestant; expectorant* [dextromethorphan hydrobromide; pseudoephedrine HCl; guaifenesin] 10•30•100 mg ② dimercaprol

dimantine INN *anthelmintic* [also: dymanthine HCl]

dimantine HCl INN [also: dymanthine HCl]

Dimaphen tablets, Release-Tabs (timed-release tablets), elixir OTC *decongestant; antihistamine* [phenylpropanolamine HCl; brompheniramine maleate] 25•4 mg; 75•12 mg; 12.5•2 mg/5 mL

Dimaphen S.A. sustained-release tablets (discontinued 1993) ℞ *decongestant; antihistamine* [phenylpropanolamine HCl; phenylephrine HCl; brompheniramine maleate]

dimazole INN [also: diamthazole]

dimazole dihydrochloride [see: dimazole; diamthazole]

dimecamine INN

dimecolonium iodide INN

dimecrotic acid INN

dimedrol [see: diphenhydramine HCl]

dimefadane USAN, INN *analgesic*

dimefilcon A USAN *hydrophilic contact lens material*

dimefline INN, BAN *respiratory stimulant* [also: dimefline HCl]

dimefline HCl USAN *respiratory stimulant* [also: dimefline]
dimefocon A USAN *hydrophobic contact lens material*
dimekolin [see: dimecolonium iodide]
dimelazine INN
dimelin [see: dimecolonium iodide]
dimemorfan INN
dimenhydrinate USP, INN, BAN *antiemetic; anticholinergic; antivertigo; motion sickness prophylaxis* 50 mg oral; 12.5 mg/4 mL oral; 50 mg/mL injection ② diphenhydramine
dimenoxadol INN [also: dimenoxadole]
dimenoxadole BAN [also: dimenoxadol]
dimepheptanol INN, BAN
dimepranol INN *immunomodulator* [also: dimepranol acedoben]
dimepranol acedoben USAN *immunomodulator* [also: dimepranol]
dimepregnen INN, BAN
dimepropion BAN [also: metamfepramone]
dimeprozan INN
dimeprozinum [see: dimeprozan]
dimercaprol USP, INN *antidote to arsenic, gold and mercury poisoning; lead poisoning adjunct; chelating agent* ② Dimacol
dimercaptopropanol [see: dimercaprol]
2,3-dimercaptosuccinic acid (DMSA) [see: succimer]
dimesna INN
dimesone INN, BAN
Dimetabs tablets ℞ *anticholinergic; antiemetic; antivertigo agent; motion sickness preventative* [dimenhydrinate] 50 mg ② Dimetane; Dimetapp
dimetacrine INN
dimetamfetamine INN
Dimetane elixir (discontinued 1996) OTC *antihistamine* [brompheniramine maleate] 2 mg/5 mL ② Dimetabs
Dimetane Extentabs (long-acting tablets) OTC *antihistamine* [brompheniramine maleate] 12 mg ② Dimetabs
Dimetane tablets (name changed to Dimetapp Allergy in 1994)
Dimetane Decongestant caplets, elixir OTC *decongestant; antihistamine* [phenylephrine HCl; brompheniramine maleate] 10•4 mg; 5•2 mg/5 mL

Dimetane-DC Cough syrup ℞ *narcotic antitussive; decongestant; antihistamine* [codeine phosphate; phenylpropanolamine HCl; brompheniramine maleate; alcohol 0.95%] 10•12.5•2 mg/5 mL
Dimetane-DX Cough syrup ℞ *antitussive; decongestant; antihistamine* [dextromethorphan hydrobromide; pseudoephedrine HCl; brompheniramine maleate; alcohol 0.95%] 10•30•2 mg/5 mL
Dimetapp tablets, Extentabs (long-acting tablets), elixir OTC *decongestant; antihistamine* [phenylpropanolamine HCl; brompheniramine maleate] 25•4 mg; 75•12 mg; 12.5•2 mg/5 mL ② Dimetabs
Dimetapp 4-Hour Liqui-Gels (liquid-filled capsules) OTC *decongestant; antihistamine* [phenylpropanolamine HCl; brompheniramine maleate] 25•4 mg
Dimetapp Allergy tablets OTC *antihistamine* [brompheniramine maleate] 4 mg
Dimetapp Cold & Allergy chewable tablets OTC *pediatric decongestant and antihistamine* [phenylpropanolamine HCl; brompheniramine maleate] 6.25•1 mg
Dimetapp Cold & Flu caplets OTC *decongestant; antihistamine; analgesic* [phenylpropanolamine HCl; brompheniramine maleate; acetaminophen] 12.5•2•500 mg
Dimetapp DM elixir OTC *antitussive; decongestant; antihistamine* [dextromethorphan hydrobromide; phenylpropanolamine HCl; brompheniramine maleate] 10•12.5•2 mg/5 mL
Dimetapp Plus (name changed to Dimetapp Cold & Flu in 1992)
Dimetapp Sinus caplets OTC *decongestant; analgesic* [pseudoephedrine HCl; ibuprofen] 30•200 mg
dimethadione USAN, INN *anticonvulsant*
dimethazan
dimethazine [see: mebolazine]
dimethicone USAN, NF, BAN *lubricant and hydrophobing agent; soft tissue prosthetic aid* [also: dimeticone] ② cimetidine

dimethicone 350 USAN *soft tissue prosthetic aid*

dimethindene BAN *antihistamine* [also: dimethindene maleate; dimetindene]

dimethindene maleate USP *antihistamine* [also: dimetindene; dimethindene]

dimethiodal sodium INN

dimethisoquin BAN [also: dimethisoquin HCl; quinisocaine]

dimethisoquin HCl USAN [also: quinisocaine; dimethisoquin]

dimethisterone USAN, NF, INN, BAN *progestin*

dimetholizine INN

dimethothiazine BAN *serotonin inhibitor* [also: fonazine mesylate; dimetotiazine]

dimethoxanate INN, BAN

dimethoxanate HCl [see: dimethoxanate]

dimethoxyphenyl penicillin sodium [see: methicillin sodium]

dimethpyridene maleate [see: dimethindene maleate]

dimethyl ketone [see: acetone]

dimethyl phthalate USP

dimethyl polysiloxane [see: dimethicone]

dimethyl sulfoxide (DMSO) USAN, USP, INN *topical anti-inflammatory; solvent; (orphan status withdrawn 1993)* [also: dimethyl sulphoxide]

dimethyl sulphoxide BAN *topical anti-inflammatory; solvent* [also: dimethyl sulfoxide]

dimethyl triazeno imidazole carboxamide (DIC; DTIC) [see: dacarbazine]

dimethylaminophenazone [see: aminopyrine]

dimethylcysteine [see: penicillamine]

dimethylglycine HCl

dimethylhexestrol [see: methestrol]

1,5-dimethylhexylamine [see: octodrine]

5,5-dimethyl-2,4-oxazolidinedione (DMO) [see: dimethadione]

dimethyloxyquinazine [see: antipyrine]

o,α-dimethylphenethylamine [see: ortetamine]

dimethylsiloxane polymers [see: dimethicone]

dimethylthiambutene INN, BAN

dimethyltryptamine (DMT)

dimethyltubocurarine BAN [also: dimethyltubocurarinium chloride]

dimethyltubocurarine iodide [see: metocurine iodide]

dimethyltubocurarinium chloride INN [also: dimethyltubocurarine]

dimethylxanthine [see: theophylline]

dimeticone INN *lubricant and hydrophobing agent; soft tissue prosthetic aid* [also: dimethicone]

dimetindene INN *antihistamine* [also: dimethindene maleate; dimethindene]

dimetindene maleate [see: dimethindene maleate]

dimetipirium bromide INN

dimetofrine INN

dimetotiazine INN *serotonin inhibitor* [also: fonazine mesylate; dimethothiazine]

dimetridazole INN, BAN

dimevamide INN

dimevamide sulfate [see: dimevamide]

diminazene INN, BAN

dimoxamine HCl USAN *memory adjuvant*

dimoxaprost INN

dimoxyline INN

dimpylate INN [also: diazinon]

dinaline INN

Dinate IV or IM injection ℞ *anticholinergic; antiemetic; antivertigo agent; motion sickness preventative* [dimenhydrinate] 50 mg/mL

dinazafone INN

diniprofylline INN

dinitolmide INN, BAN

dinitrotoluamide [see: dinitolmide]

dinoprost USAN, INN, BAN *oxytocic; prostaglandin*

dinoprost trometamol BAN *oxytocic; prostaglandin* [also: dinoprost tromethamine]

dinoprost tromethamine USAN *oxytocic; prostaglandin-type abortifacient* [also: dinoprost trometamol]

dinoprostone USAN, INN, BAN *oxytocic; prostaglandin-type abortifacient; cervical ripening agent*

dinsed USAN, INN *coccidiostat for poultry*

Diocto liquid, syrup OTC *stool softener* [docusate sodium] 150 mg/15 mL; 60 mg/15 mL

Diocto-C syrup OTC *stimulant laxative; stool softener* [casanthranol; docusate sodium] 30•60 mg/15 mL

Dioctocal soft gelatin OTC *stool softener* [docusate calcium]

Diocto-K capsules OTC *stool softener* [docusate potassium] 100 mg

Diocto-K Plus capsules OTC *laxative; stool softener* [casanthranol; docusate potassium] 30•100 mg

Dioctolose Plus capsules OTC *laxative; stool softener* [casanthranol; docusate potassium] 30•100 mg

dioctyl calcium sulfosuccinate [now: docusate calcium]

dioctyl potassium sulfosuccinate [now: docusate potassium]

dioctyl sodium sulfosuccinate (DSS) [now: docusate sodium]

Diodex eye drops (available only in Canada) ℞ *ophthalmic topical corticosteroidal anti-inflammatory* [dexamethasone sodium phosphate] 0.1%

diodone INN [also: iodopyracet]

Dioeze capsules OTC *stool softener* [docusate sodium] 250 mg

diohippuric acid I 125 USAN *radioactive agent*

diohippuric acid I 131 USAN *radioactive agent*

diolamine USAN, INN *combining name for radicals or groups*

diolostene [see: methandriol]

dionin [see: ethylmorphine HCl]

Dionosil Oily suspension for intratracheal use ℞ *radiopaque agent* [propyliodone in peanut oil] 60%

diophyllin [see: aminophylline]

diosmin INN

Diostate D tablets OTC *dietary supplement* [calcium; phosphorus; vitamin D] 114 mg•88 mg•133 IU

diotyrosine I 125 USAN *radioactive agent*

diotyrosine I 131 USAN *radioactive agent*

Dioval XX; Dioval 40 IM injection ℞ *estrogen replacement therapy for postmenopausal disorders; antineoplastic for prostatic cancer* [estradiol valerate in oil] 20 mg/mL; 40 mg/mL

dioxadilol INN

dioxadrol INN *antidepressant* [also: dioxadrol HCl]

dioxadrol HCl USAN *antidepressant* [also: dioxadrol]

***d*-dioxadrol HCl** [see: dexoxadrol HCl]

dioxamate INN, BAN

dioxaphetyl butyrate INN, BAN

dioxathion BAN [also: dioxation]

dioxation INN [also: dioxathion]

dioxethedrin INN

dioxethedrin HCl [see: dioxethedrin]

dioxifedrine INN

dioxindol [see: oxyphenisatin acetate]

dioxyanthranol [see: anthralin]

dioxyanthraquinone (*withdrawn from market*) [see: danthron]

dioxybenzone USAN, USP, INN *ultraviolet screen*

dipalmitoylphosphatidylcholine (DPPC) [see: colfosceril palmitate]

dipalmitoylphosphatidylcholine & phosphatidylglycerol (*orphan: neonatal respiratory distress syndrome*)

diparcol HCl [see: diethazine HCl]

dipegyl [see: niacinamide]

dipenicillin G [see: penicillin G benzathine]

dipenine bromide BAN [also: diponium bromide]

Dipentum capsules ℞ *anti-inflammatory for ulcerative colitis* [olsalazine sodium] 250 mg

diperodon USP, INN, BAN *topical anesthetic*

diperodon HCl *topical anesthetic*

diphemanil methylsulfate USP *anticholinergic* [also: diphemanil metilsulfate; diphemanil methylsulphate]

diphemanil methylsulphate BAN *anticholinergic* [also: diphemanil methylsulfate; diphemanil metilsulfate]

diphemanil metilsulfate INN *anticholinergic* [also: diphemanil methylsulfate; diphemanil methylsulphate]

Diphen Cough Syrup OTC *antihistamine; antitussive* [diphenhydramine HCl, alcohol 5%] 12.5 mg/5 mL

Diphenacen-50 injection (discontinued 1994) ℞ *antihistamine* [diphenhydramine HCl] 50 mg/mL

diphenadione USP, INN, BAN

Diphenadryl elixir, caplets OTC *antihistamine* [diphenhydramine HCl]

diphenan INN

diphenatil [see: diphemanil methylsulfate]

diphenchloxazine HCl [see: difencloxazine HCl]

diphenesenic acid [see: xenyhexenic acid]

Diphenhist Captabs (capsule-shaped tablets), elixir OTC *antihistamine; motion sickness preventative; sleep aid; antiparkinsonian* [diphenhydramine HCl] 25 mg; 12.5 mg/5 mL

diphenhydramine INN, BAN *antihistamine; anticholinergic; antiparkinsonian; motion sickness relief* [also: diphenhydramine citrate] ⑦ dimenhydrinate

diphenhydramine citrate USP *antihistamine; anticholinergic; antiparkinsonian; motion sickness relief* [also: diphenhydramine]

diphenhydramine HCl USP, BAN *antihistamine; antitussive; motion sickness prevention; sleep aid* 25, 50 mg oral; 12.5 mg/5 mL oral; 10, 50 mg/mL injection

diphenhydramine theoclate [see: dimenhydrinate]

diphenidol USAN, BAN *antiemetic; antivertigo* [also: difenidol]

diphenidol HCl USAN *antiemetic*

diphenidol pamoate USAN *antiemetic*

diphenmethanil methylsulfate [see: diphemanil methylsulfate]

diphenoxylate INN, BAN *antiperistaltic* [also: diphenoxylate HCl]

diphenoxylate HCl USP *antiperistaltic* [also: diphenoxylate]

diphenylacetylindandione [see: diphenadione]

Diphenylan Sodium capsules ℞ *anticonvulsant* [phenytoin sodium] 30, 100 mg ⑦ Diphenylin

diphenylbutazone [see: phenylbutazone]

diphenylhydantoin [now: phenytoin]

diphenylhydantoin sodium [now: phenytoin sodium]

Diphenylin syrup OTC *antitussive* [diphenhydramine HCl] ⑦ Dyphenylan

diphenylisatin [see: oxyphenisatin]

diphenylpyraline INN, BAN *antihistamine* [also: diphenylpyraline HCl]

diphenylpyraline HCl USP *antihistamine* [also: diphenylpyraline]

diphetarsone [see: difetarsone]

diphexamide iodomethylate [see: buzepide metiodide]

diphosphonic acid [see: etidronic acid]

diphosphopyridine nucleotide (DPN) [now: nadide]

diphosphoric acid, tetrasodium salt [see: sodium pyrophosphate]

diphosphothiamin [see: co-carboxylase]

diphoxazide INN

diphtheria antitoxin USP *passive immunizing agent* [also: diphtheria toxoid] 500 U/mL injection

diphtheria equine antitoxin *passive immunizing agent*

diphtheria & tetanus toxoids, adsorbed (DT; Td) USP *active immunizing agent* 2•2, 2•5, 2•10, 6.6•5, 7.5•7.5, 10•5, 12.5•5, 15•10 LfU/0.5 mL injection

diphtheria & tetanus toxoids & acellular pertussis vaccine (DTaP) *active immunizing agent*

diphtheria & tetanus toxoids & pertussis vaccine (DTP) USP *active immunizing agent*

diphtheria & tetanus toxoids & whole-cell pertussis vaccine (DTwP) *active immunizing agent* 6.5•5•4, 10•5.5•4 LfU/0.5 mL injection

diphtheria toxin, diagnostic [now: diphtheria toxin for Schick test]

diphtheria toxin, inactivated diagnostic [now: Schick test control]

diphtheria toxin for Schick test USP *dermal diphtheria immunity test*

diphtheria toxoid USP *active immunizing agent* [also: diphtheria antitoxin]

diphtheria toxoid, adsorbed USP *active immunizing agent* 15 LfU/0.5 mL injection

dipipanone INN, BAN
dipipanone HCl [see: dipipanone]
dipiproverine INN
dipiproverine HCl [see: dipiproverine]
dipivalyl epinephrine (DPE) [now: dipivefrin]
dipivefrin USAN *ophthalmic adrenergic* [also: dipivefrine]
dipivefrin HCl USP *topical antiglaucoma agent* 0.1% eye drops
dipivefrine INN, BAN *ophthalmic adrenergic* [also: dipivefrin]
diponium bromide INN [also: dipenine bromide]
dipotassium carbonate [see: potassium carbonate]
dipotassium clorazepate INN *anxiolytic; minor tranquilizer; alcohol withdrawal relief* [also: clorazepate dipotassium]
dipotassium hydrogen phosphate [see: potassium phosphate, dibasic]
dipotassium phosphate [see: potassium phosphate, dibasic]
dipotassium pyrosulfite [see: potassium metabisulfite]
diprafenone INN
diprenorphine INN, BAN
Diprivan emulsion for IV ℞ *general anesthetic* [propofol] 10 mg/mL
diprobutine INN, BAN
diprofene INN
diprogulic acid INN
diproleandomycin INN
Diprolene ointment, gel, lotion ℞ *topical corticosteroid* [augmented betamethasone diproprionate] 0.05%
Diprolene AF cream ℞ *topical corticosteroid* [augmented betamethasone diproprionate] 0.05%
diprophylline INN, BAN *bronchodilator* [also: dyphylline]
dipropylacetic acid [see: valproic acid]
2-dipropylaminoethyl diphenylthioacetate [see: diprofene]
1,1-dipropylbutylamine [see: diprobutine]
diproqualone INN
Diprosone ointment, cream, lotion, aerosol ℞ *topical corticosteroid* [betamethasone diproprionate] 0.05%; 0.05%; 0.05%; 0.1%

diproteverine INN, BAN
diprothazine [see: dimelazine]
diprotrizoate sodium USP [also: sodium diprotrizoate]
diproxadol INN
dipyridamole USAN, USP, INN, BAN *coronary vasodilator; antiplatelet agent* 25, 50, 75 mg oral
dipyrithione USAN, INN *antibacterial; antifungal*
dipyrocetyl INN
dipyrone USAN, BAN *analgesic; antipyretic* [also: metamizole sodium]
Dirame ℞ *investigational narcotic analgesic for moderate to severe pain* [propiram]
Direct LDL Cholesterol Test kit *investigational diagnostic aid*
dirithromycin USAN, INN, BAN *macrolide antibacterial antibiotic*
disaccharide tripeptide glycerol dipalmitoyl (orphan: *pulmonary and hepatic metastases of colorectal adenocarcinoma*)
Disalcid film-coated tablets, capsules ℞ *analgesic; antipyretic; anti-inflammatory; antirheumatic* [salsalate] 500, 750 mg; 500 mg
disalicylic acid [see: salsalate]
Disanthrol capsules OTC *laxative; stool softener* [casanthranol; docusate sodium] 30•100 mg
Dis-Co Pack (trademarked packaging form) *unit-dose package*
Disinfecting Solution OTC *chemical disinfecting solution for soft contact lenses*
disiquonium chloride USAN, INN *antiseptic*
Disket (trademarked dosage form) *dispersible tablet*
Dismutec *investigational free-radical scavenger to prevent irreversible brain damage after head trauma* [pegorgotein]
Disobrom sustained-release tablets ℞ *decongestant; antihistamine* [pseudoephedrine sulfate; dexbrompheniramine maleate] 120•6 mg
disobutamide USAN, INN *antiarrhythmic*
disodium carbenicillin [see: carbenicillin disodium]
disodium carbonate [see: sodium carbonate]

disodium cefotetan [see: cefotetan disodium]

disodium chromate [see: sodium chromate]

disodium clodronate (*orphan: hypercalcemia of malignancy*)

disodium clodronate tetrahydrate (*orphan: increased bone resorption due to malignancy*)

disodium cromoglycate (DSC; DSCG) [see: cromolyn sodium]

disodium dihydrogen methylenediphosphonate [see: medronate disodium]

disodium edathamil [see: edathamil disodium]

disodium edetate BAN *metal-chelating agent* [also: edetate disodium]

disodium ethylenediamine tetraacetate [see: edetate disodium]

disodium hydrogen phosphate [see: sodium phosphate]

disodium hydrogen phosphate heptahydrate [see: sodium phosphate, dibasic]

disodium hydrogen phosphate hydrate [see: sodium phosphate, dibasic]

(disodium) methylene diphosphonate (MDP) [now: medronate disodium]

disodium phosphate [see: sodium phosphate, dibasic]

disodium phosphate heptahydrate [see: sodium phosphate]

disodium phosphonoacetate monohydrate [see: fosfonet sodium]

disodium phosphorofluoridate [see: sodium monofluorophosphate]

disodium pyrosulfite [see: sodium metabisulfite]

disodium silibinin dihemisuccinate (*orphan: Amanita phalloides [mushroom] liver poisoning*)

disodium sulfate decahydrate [see: sodium sulfate]

disodium thiosulfate pentahydrate [see: sodium thiosulfate]

disofenin USAN, INN, BAN *carrier agent in diagnostic tests*

disogluside INN

Disolan capsules OTC *laxative; stool softener* [phenolphthalein; docusate sodium] 65•100 mg

Disolan Forte capsules OTC *laxative; stool softener* [casanthranol; sodium carboxymethylcellulose; docusate sodium] 30•400•100 mg

Disonate capsules, syrup, liquid OTC *stool softener* [docusate sodium] 100, 240 mg; 60 mg/15 mL; 150 mg/15 mL

Disophrol tablets, Chronotabs (sustained-action tablets) OTC *decongestant; antihistamine* [pseudoephedrine sulfate; dexbrompheniramine maleate] 60•2 mg; 120•6 mg ⓘ Desferal; disoprofol; Stilphostrol

Disoplex capsules OTC *laxative; stool softener* [sodium carboxymethylcellulose; docusate sodium] 400•100 mg

disoprofol [see: propofol] ⓘ Disophrol

disopromine HCl [see: diisopromine HCl]

disopyramide USAN, INN, BAN *antiarrhythmic*

disopyramide phosphate USAN, USP, BAN *antiarrhythmic* 100, 150 mg oral

Disotate IV infusion ℞ *calcium-lowering agent; antiarrhythmic for digitalis toxicity* [edetate disodium] 150 mg/mL

disoxaril USAN, INN *antiviral*

Di-Spaz capsules, IM injection ℞ *gastrointestinal antispasmodic* [dicyclomine HCl] 10 mg; 10 mg/mL

Dispenserpak (trademarked packaging form) *unit-of-use package*

dispersible cellulose BAN *tablet and capsule diluent* [also: cellulose, microcrystalline]

Dispertab (trademarked dosage form) *delayed-release tablet*

Dispette (trademarked delivery system) *disposable pipette*

Dispos-a-Med (trademarked delivery form) *solution for inhalation*

distaquaine [see: penicillin V]

distigmine bromide INN, BAN

disulergine INN

disulfamide INN [also: disulphamide]

disulfiram USP, INN, BAN *deterrent to alcohol consumption* 250, 500 mg oral

disulfurous acid, dipotassium salt [see: potassium metabisulfite]

disulfurous acid, disodium salt [see: sodium metabisulfite]
disulphamide BAN [also: disulfamide]
disuprazole INN
Dital slow-release capsules ℞ *anorexiant* [phendimetrazine tartrate] 105 mg
ditazole INN
ditekiren USAN *antihypertensive; renin inhibitor*
ditercalinium chloride INN
dithiazanine BAN [also: dithiazanine iodide]
dithiazanine iodide USP, INN [also: dithiazanine]
dithranol INN, BAN *antipsoriatic* [also: anthralin]
D.I.T.I.-2 vaginal cream ℞ *bacteriostatic antibiotic; antiseptic; vulnerary* [sulfanilamide; aminacrine HCl; allantoin] 15%•0.2%•2%
ditiocarb sodium INN
ditiomustine INN
ditolamide INN
ditophal INN, BAN
Ditropan tablets, syrup ℞ *urinary antispasmodic for neurogenic bladder* [oxybutynin chloride] 5 mg; 5 mg/5 mL ⓡ Intropin
Diucardin tablets ℞ *diuretic; antihypertensive* [hydroflumethiazide] 50 mg
Diulo tablets (discontinued 1993) ℞ *diuretic; antihypertensive* [metolazone]
Diupres-250; Diupres-500 tablets (discontinued 1996) ℞ *antihypertensive* [chlorothiazide; reserpine] 250•0.125 mg; 500•0.125 mg
Diurese tablets ℞ *diuretic; antihypertensive* [trichlormethiazide] 4 mg
Diurigen tablets ℞ *diuretic* [chlorothiazide] 500 mg
Diurigen with Reserpine tablets (discontinued 1992) ℞ *antihypertensive* [chlorothiazide; reserpine]
Diuril tablets, oral suspension ℞ *diuretic* [chlorothiazide] 250, 500 mg; 250 mg/5 mL
Diutensen-R tablets ℞ *antihypertensive* [methyclothiazide; reserpine] 2.5•0.1 mg ⓡ Salutensin
divabuterol INN
divalproex sodium USAN *anticonvulsant; antipsychotic for manic episodes* [also: valproate semisodium; semisodium valproate]
divanilliden cyclohexanone [see: cyclovalone]
divaplon INN
Divide-Tab (trademarked dosage form) *scored tablet*
Dividose (trademarked dosage form) *multiple-scored tablets*
diviminol [see: viminol]
divinyl ether [see: vinyl ether]
divinyl oxide [see: vinyl ether]
dixamone bromide [see: methantheline bromide]
dixanthogen INN
dixarit [see: clonidine]
Dizac injection ℞ *anxiolytic; premedication to anesthesia* [diazepam] 5 mg/mL
dizatrifone INN
Dizmiss chewable tablets OTC *anticholinergic; antivertigo agent; motion sickness preventative* [meclizine HCl] 25 mg
dizocilpine INN *neuroprotective* [also: dizocilpine maleate]
dizocilpine maleate USAN *neuroprotective* [also: dizocilpine]
Dizymes enteric-coated tablets (discontinued 1994) OTC *digestive enzymes* [pancreatin; lipase; protease; amylase] 250 mg•6750 U•41,250 U•43,750 U
D-Lay (trademarked dosage form) *timed-release tablet*
DM Cough Syrup OTC *antitussive* [dextromethorphan hydrobromide]
DMC (dactinomycin, methotrexate, cyclophosphamide) *chemotherapy protocol*
DMCT (demethylchlortetracycline) [see: demeclocycline]
D-Med 80 intralesional, soft tissue, and IM injection (discontinued 1992) ℞ *glucocorticoids* [methylprednisolone acetate] 80 mg/mL
DMG tablets OTC *dietary supplement* [calcium gluconate; dimethylglycine HCl]
DML lotion OTC *moisturizer; emollient*
DML Forte cream OTC *moisturizer; emollient*
DMO (dimethyl oxazolidinedione) [see: dimethadione]

DMP 266 *investigational (Phase I) antiviral non-nucleoside reverse transcriptase inhibitor for HIV*

DMP 728 *investigational antiplatelet agent for angina, heart attack, and stroke*

DMSA (dimercaptosuccinic acid) [see: succimer]

DMSO (dimethyl sulfoxide) [q.v.]

DMT (dimethyltryptamine)

DNA (deoxyribonucleic acid)

DNase (recombinant human deoxyribonuclease I) [see: dornase alfa]

DNJ (deoxynojirimycin) [q.v.]

DNR (daunorubicin) [q.v.]

Doak Tar bath oil, lotion, shampoo OTC *topical antipsoriatic; antiseborrheic; antiseptic* [coal tar] 0.8%; 2%; 1.2%, 3%

Doak Tar Distillate liquid OTC *topical antipsoriatic; antiseborrheic; antiseptic* [coal tar] 40%

Doak Tar Oil liquid OTC *topical antipsoriatic; antiseborrheic; antiseptic* [coal tar] 2%

Doan's Backache Spray (discontinued 1992) OTC *counterirritant; topical antiseptic* [methyl salicylate; menthol; methyl nicotinate; isopropyl alcohol]

Doan's Pills caplets OTC *analgesic; antirheumatic* [magnesium salicylate] 325, 500 mg

Doan's P.M. caplets OTC *analgesic; antirheumatic; antihistaminic sleep aid* [magnesium salicylate; diphenhydramine HCl] 500•25 mg

DOAP (daunorubicin, Oncovin, ara-C, prednisone) *chemotherapy protocol*

dobupride INN

dobutamine USAN, INN, BAN *cardiotonic; vasopressor for shock* 2 dopamine

dobutamine HCl USAN, USP, BAN *cardiotonic; vasopressor for shock* 12.5 mg/mL injection

dobutamine lactobionate USAN *cardiotonic*

dobutamine tartrate USAN *cardiotonic*

Dobutrex IV infusion ℞ *vasopressor for cardiac shock* [dobutamine] 12.5 mg/mL

DOCA (desoxycorticosterone acetate) [q.v.]

docarpamine INN

docebenone USAN, INN *5-lipoxygenase inhibitor*

docetaxel USAN, INN *antineoplastic for breast cancer; investigational for ovarian & lung cancers; analog to paclitaxel*

doconazole USAN, INN *antifungal*

doconexent INN *omega-3 marine triglyceride*

docosahexaenoic acid (DHA) [see: doconexent]

docosil INN *combining name for radicals or groups*

Doctar shampoo OTC *antiseborrheic; antipsoriatic; antipruritic; antibacterial* [coal tar] 0.5%

Docucal-P softgels OTC *laxative; stool softener* [phenolphthalein; docusate calcium] 65•60 mg

docusate calcium USAN, USP *stool softener* 240 mg oral

docusate potassium USAN, USP *stool softener*

docusate sodium USAN, USP, BAN *stool softener; surfactant/wetting agent* [also: sodium dioctyl sulfosuccinate] 50, 100, 250 mg oral; 50, 60 mg/15 mL oral;

dodeclonium bromide INN

2-dodecylisoquinolinium bromide [see: lauryl isoquinolinium bromide]

dofamium chloride INN, BAN

dofetilide USAN, INN, BAN *antiarrhythmic; potassium channel blocker*

dofosfate INN *combining name for radicals or groups*

Dofus capsules OTC *dietary supplement* [Lactobacillus acidophilus]

DOK capsules, syrup, liquid OTC *stool softener* [docusate sodium] 100, 250 mg; 60 mg/15 mL; 150 mg/15 mL

Doktors spray (discontinued 1992) OTC *nasal decongestant* [phenylephrine HCl]

Dolacet capsules ℞ *narcotic analgesic* [hydrocodone bitartrate; acetaminophen] 5•500 mg

Dolanex elixir OTC *analgesic; antipyretic* [acetaminophen] 325 mg/5 mL

dolantal [see: meperidine HCl]

dolantin [see: meperidine HCl]

dolasetron INN *antiemetic; antimigraine* [also: dolasetron mesylate]

dolasetron mesylate USAN *antiemetic; antimigraine* [also: dolasetron]

Dolene capsules ℞ *narcotic analgesic* [propoxyphene HCl; acetaminophen] 65 mg

Dolene AP-65 tablets (discontinued 1992) ℞ *narcotic analgesic* [propoxyphene HCl; acetaminophen]

Dolfen tablets ℞ *narcotic analgesic* [hydrocodone bitartrate; acetaminophen]

doliracetam INN

Dolobid film-coated tablets ℞ *analgesic; antiarthritic; antirheumatic; antiinflammatory; antipyretic* [diflunisal] 250, 500 mg

Dolomite tablets OTC *mineral supplement* [calcium; magnesium] 130•78 mg

Dolophine HCl tablets, subcu or IM injection ℞ *narcotic analgesic; narcotic addiction detoxicant* [methadone HCl] 5, 10 mg; 10 mg/mL

dolosal [see: meperidine HCl]

Dolsed sugar-coated tablets ℞ *urinary anti-infective; analgesic; antispasmodic; acidifier* [methenamine; phenyl salicylate; atropine sulfate; methylene blue; hyoscyamine sulfate; benzoic acid] 40.8•18.1•0.03•5.4•0.03•4.5 mg

dolvanol [see: meperidine HCl]

domazoline INN *anticholinergic* [also: domazoline fumarate]

domazoline fumarate USAN *anticholinergic* [also: domazoline]

Domeboro powder packets, effervescent tablets OTC *astringent wet dressing (modified Burow solution)* [aluminum sulfate; calcium acetate]

Domeboro Otic [see: Otic Domeboro]

Dome-Paste medicated gauze bandage OTC *protection and support of extremities* [zinc oxide; calamine; gelatin]

domestrol [see: diethylstilbestrol]

domibrom [see: domiphen bromide]

domiodol USAN, INN *mucolytic*

domiphen bromide USAN, BAN *topical anti-infective*

domipizone INN

Dommanate IV or IM injection (discontinued 1994) ℞ *anticholinergic; antiemetic; antivertigo agent; motion sickness preventative* [dimenhydrinate] 50 mg/mL ② Dramanate

Domol Bath and Shower Oil OTC *bath emollient*

domoprednate INN

domoxin INN

domperidone USAN, INN, BAN, JAN *antiemetic*

Donatussin drops ℞ *pediatric decongestant, antihistamine, and expectorant* [phenylephrine HCl; chlorpheniramine maleate; guaifenesin] 2•1•20 mg/mL

Donatussin syrup ℞ *antitussive; decongestant; antihistamine; expectorant* [dextromethorphan hydrobromide; phenylephrine HCl; chlorpheniramine maleate; guaifenesin] 7.5•10•2•100 mg/5 mL

Donatussin DC syrup ℞ *narcotic antitussive; decongestant; expectorant* [hydrocodone bitartrate; phenylephrine HCl; guaifenesin] 2.5•7.5•50 mg/5 mL

Dondril tablets (discontinued 1993) OTC *decongestant; antihistamine; antitussive* [phenylephrine HCl; chlorpheniramine maleate; dextromethorphan hydrobromide]

donetidine USAN, INN, BAN *antagonist to histamine H_2 receptors*

Donnagel chewable tablets, liquid OTC *antidiarrheal; GI adsorbent* [attapulgite] 600 mg; 600 mg/15 mL ② Donnatal

Donnagel oral suspension (discontinued 1992) OTC *GI adsorbent; antidiarrheal* [kaolin; pectin; hyoscyamine sulfate; atropine sulfate; scopolamine hydrobromide]

Donnagel-PG liquid (discontinued 1993) ℞ *GI adsorbent; not generally regarded as safe and effective as an antidiarrheal* [opium; kaolin; pectin; hyoscyamine sulfate; atropine sulfate; scopolamine hydrobromide]

Donnamar tablets ℞ *anticholinergic; antispasmodic* [hyoscyamine sulfate] 0.125 mg

Donnamor elixir (discontinued 1995) ℞ GI anticholinergic; sedative [atropine sulfate; scopolamine hydrobromide; hyoscyamine hydrobromide; phenobarbital] 0.0194•0.0065•0.1037•16.2 mg/5 mL

Donnapectolin-PG liquid (discontinued 1994) ℞ GI adsorbent; not generally regarded as safe and effective as an antidiarrheal [opium; kaolin; pectin; hyoscyamine sulfate; atropine sulfate; scopolamine hydrobromide]

Donnapine tablets (discontinued 1995) ℞ GI anticholinergic; sedative [atropine sulfate; scopolamine hydrobromide; hyoscyamine hydrobromide; phenobarbital] 0.0194•0.0065•0.1037•16.2 mg

Donna-Sed elixir ℞ anticholinergic; sedative [atropine sulfate; scopolamine hydrobromide; hyoscyamine hydrobromide; phenobarbital] 0.0194•0.0065•0.1037•16.2 mg/5 mL

Donnatal capsules & tablets, elixir, Extentabs (extended-release tablets) ℞ GI anticholinergic; sedative [atropine sulfate; scopolamine hydrobromide; hyoscyamine sulfate; phenobarbital] 0.0194•0.0065•0.1037•16.2 mg; 0.0194•0.0065•0.1037•16.2 mg/5 mL; 0.0582•0.0195•0.3111•48.6 mg ⊘ Donnagel

Donnatal No. 2 tablets ℞ anticholinergic; sedative [atropine sulfate; scopolamine hydrobromide; hyoscyamine sulfate; phenobarbital] 0.0194•0.0065•0.1037•32.4 mg

Donnazyme tablets ℞ digestive enzymes [pancreatin; lipase; protease; amylase] 500 mg•1000 U•12,500 U•12,500 U ⊘ Entozyme

DOPA (dihydroxyphenylalanine) [see: levodopa]

L-dopa [see: levodopa]

dopamantine USAN, INN antiparkinsonian

dopamine INN, BAN adrenergic [also: dopamine HCl] ⊘ dobutamine; Dopram

dopamine D_1-receptor antagonist investigational antipsychotic

dopamine HCl USAN, USP adrenergic; vasopressor for shock [also: dopamine] 40, 80, 160 mg/mL injection

dopamine HCl in 5% dextrose adrenergic; vasopressor for shock 80, 160, 320 mg/100 mL injection

Dopar capsules ℞ antiparkinsonian [levodopa] 100, 250, 500 mg ⊘ Dopram

Dopastat IV (discontinued 1994) ℞ vasopressor used in shock [dopamine HCl] 40 mg/mL

dopexamine USAN, INN, BAN cardiovascular agent

dopexamine HCl USAN, BAN cardiovascular agent

Dopram IV injection or infusion ℞ CNS stimulant; analeptic; adjunct to postanesthesia "stir-up" [doxapram HCl] 20 mg/mL ⊘ dopamine; Dopar

dopropidil INN

doqualast INN

Doral tablets ℞ sedative; hypnotic [quazepam] 7.5, 15 mg

dorastine INN antihistamine [also: dorastine HCl]

dorastine HCl USAN antihistamine [also: dorastine]

Dorcol Children's Cold Formula liquid OTC pediatric decongestant and antihistamine [pseudoephedrine HCl; chlorpheniramine maleate] 15•1 mg/5 mL

Dorcol Children's Cough syrup OTC pediatric antitussive, decongestant, and expectorant [dextromethorphan hydrobromide; pseudoephedrine HCl; guaifenesin] 5•15•50 mg/5 mL

Dorcol Children's Decongestant liquid OTC nasal decongestant [pseudoephedrine HCl] 15 mg/5 mL

Dorcol Children's Fever & Pain Reducer liquid OTC analgesic; antipyretic [acetaminophen] 160 mg/5 mL

Dorcol Pediatric Cold Formula liquid (name changed to Dorcol Children's Cold Formula in 1993)

doreptide INN

doretinel USAN, INN antikeratinizing agent

Dormarex capsules (discontinued 1993) OTC antihistaminic sleep aid [pyrilamine maleate]

Dormarex 2 tablets OTC *antihistaminic sleep aid; motion sickness preventative* [diphenhydramine HCl] 50 mg

dormethan [see: dextromethorphan hydrobromide]

Dormin caplets, capsules OTC *antihistaminic sleep aid* [diphenhydramine HCl] 25 mg

dormiral [see: phenobarbital]

dormonal [see: barbital]

dornase alfa *reduces respiratory viscoelasticity of sputum; for cystic fibrosis* (orphan)

Doryx capsules ℞ *tetracycline-type antibiotic* [doxycycline hyclate] 100 mg

dorzolamide HCl USAN *carbonic anhydrase inhibitor for glaucoma*

DOS softgels OTC *stool softener* [docusate sodium] 100, 250 mg

Dosalax syrup OTC *laxative* [senna concentrate; alcohol 7%] ⓶

Dosa-Trol Pack (trademarked dosage form) *unit-of-use package*

Dosepak (trademarked dosage form) *unit-of-use package*

dosergoside INN

Dosette (trademarked dosage form) *injectable unit-of-use system (vials, ampules, syringes, etc.)*

Dospan (trademarked form) *controlled-release tablets*

Dostinex (commercially available in England and Sweden) ℞ *investigational treatment for Parkinson's disease and gynecologic disorders* [cabergoline]

dosulepin INN *antidepressant* [also: dothiepin HCl; dothiepin; dosulepin HCl]

dosulepin HCl JAN *antidepressant* [also: dothiepin HCl; dosulepin; dothiepin]

dotarizine INN

dotefonium bromide INN

dothiepin BAN *antidepressant* [also: dothiepin HCl; dosulepin; dosulepin HCl]

dothiepin HCl USAN *antidepressant* [also: dosulepin; dothiepin; dosulepin HCl]

Double Ice ArthriCare [see: ArthriCare, Double Ice]

Double-Action Toothache Kit tablets + liquid OTC *analgesic; topical oral anesthetic* [(acetaminophen) + (benzocaine; alcohol 74%)] (325 mg) + (⓶)

Dovonex ointment ℞ *topical antipsoriatic* [calcipotriene] 0.005%

doxacurium chloride USAN, INN, BAN *nondepolarizing neuromuscular blocker; muscle relaxant; adjunct to anesthesia*

doxaminol INN

doxapram INN, BAN *respiratory stimulant* [also: doxapram HCl]

doxapram HCl USAN, USP *respiratory stimulant; analeptic* [also: doxapram] 20 mg/mL injection

doxaprost USAN, INN *bronchodilator*

doxate [see: docusate sodium]

doxazosin INN, BAN *antihypertensive; α_1-adrenergic blocker* [also: doxazosin mesylate]

doxazosin mesylate USAN *antihypertensive; α_1-adrenergic blocker* [also: doxazosin]

doxefazepam INN

doxenitoin INN

doxepin INN, BAN *tricyclic antidepressant* [also: doxepin HCl] ⓶ Doxidan

doxepin HCl USAN, USP *tricyclic antidepressant; anxiolytic; topical antipruritic* [also: doxepin] 10, 25, 50, 75, 100, 150 mg oral; 10 mg/mL oral

doxibetasol INN [also: doxybetasol]

Doxidan capsules OTC *laxative; stool softener* [phenolphthalein; docusate calcium] 65•60 mg ⓶ doxepin

doxifluridine INN *investigational antineoplastic*

Doxil IV injection ℞ *antibiotic antineoplastic for Kaposi sarcoma; investigational for metastatic breast cancer* [doxorubicin HCl (liposomal formulation)] 20 mg/vial

Doxinate capsules, solution (discontinued 1994) OTC *stool softener* [docusate sodium] 240 mg; 50 mg/mL

doxofylline USAN, INN *bronchodilator*

doxorubicin USAN, INN, BAN *antibiotic antineoplastic* ⓶ daunorubicin

doxorubicin HCl USP *antibiotic antineoplastic* 10, 20, 50 mg, 2 mg/mL injection

doxpicodin HCl [now: doxpicomine HCl]

doxpicomine INN *analgesic* [also: doxpicomine HCl]

doxpicomine HCl USAN *analgesic* [also: doxpicomine]

Dox-SL ℞ *investigational antineoplastic for AIDS-related Kaposi sarcoma, leukemia, breast and ovarian cancers* [liposome formulation of doxorubicin]

Doxy 100; Doxy 200 powder for IV injection ℞ *tetracycline-type antibiotic* [doxycycline hyclate] 100 mg; 200 mg

Doxy Caps capsules ℞ *tetracycline-type antibiotic* [doxycycline hyclate] 100 mg

Doxy Tabs tablets ℞ *tetracycline-type antibiotic* [doxycycline]

doxybetasol BAN [also: doxibetasol]

Doxychel Hyclate capsules, tablets, powder for IV injection ℞ *tetracycline-type antibiotic* [doxycycline hyclate] 50, 100 mg; 50, 100 mg; 100, 200 mg

doxycycline USAN, USP, INN, BAN *bacteriostatic; antirickettsial; malaria prophylaxis*

doxycycline calcium USP *antibacterial; antiprotozoal*

doxycycline fosfatex USAN, BAN *antibacterial*

doxycycline hyclate USP *antibacterial* 50, 100 mg oral; 100, 200 mg/vial injection

doxylamine INN, BAN *antihistamine* [also: doxylamine succinate]

doxylamine succinate USP *antihistamine; sleep aid* [also: doxylamine]

Doxysom Nighttime Sleep-Aid tablets (discontinued 1993) OTC *antihistaminic sleep aid* [doxylamine succinate]

DPE (dipivalyl epinephrine) [now: dipivefrin]

DPF [see: Dermprotective Factor]

DPN (diphosphopyridine nucleotide) [now: nadide]

DPPC (dipalmitoylphosphatidylcholine) [see: colfosceril palmitate]

Dr. Caldwell Senna Laxative liquid OTC *laxative* [senna concentrate] 33.3 mg/mL

Dr. Dermi-Heal ointment OTC *vulnerary; antipruritic; astringent* [allantoin; zinc oxide; balsam Peru] 1%•?•?

Dr. Scholl's Advanced Pain Relief Corn Removers; Dr. Scholl's Callus Removers; Dr Scholl's Clear Away; Dr. Scholl's Corn Removers medicated discs OTC *topical keratolytic* [salicylic acid in a rubber-based vehicle] 40%

Dr. Scholl's Athlete's Foot powder, spray powder, spray liquid OTC *topical antifungal* [tolnaftate] 1%

Dr. Scholl's Clear Away OneStep; Dr. Scholl's OneStep Corn Removers medicated strips OTC *topical keratolytic* [salicylic acid in a rubber-based vehicle] 40%

Dr. Scholl's Corn/Callus Remover liquid OTC *topical keratolytic* [salicylic acid in flexible collodion] 17%

Dr. Scholl's Cracked Heel Relief cream OTC *topical local anesthetic; antiseptic* [lidocaine HCl; benzalkonium chloride] 2%•0.13%

Dr. Scholl's Moisturizing Corn Remover Kit medicated discs + cushions + moisturizing cream OTC *topical keratolytic* [salicylic acid in a rubber-based vehicle] 40%

Dr. Scholl's Tritin powder, spray powder OTC *topical antifungal* [tolnaftate] 1%

Dr. Scholl's Wart Remover Kit liquid + adhesive pads OTC *topical keratolytic* [salicylic acid in flexible collodion] 17%

draflazine USAN *cardioprotectant*

Dramamine IV or IM injection (discontinued 1994) ℞ *antinauseant; antiemetic; antivertigo agent; motion sickness preventative* [dimenhydrinate] 50 mg/mL

Dramamine liquid ℞ *antinauseant; antiemetic; antivertigo agent; motion sickness preventative* [dimenhydrinate] 15.62 mg/5 mL

Dramamine tablets, chewable tablets, liquid OTC *antinauseant; antiemetic;*

antivertigo agent; motion sickness preventative [dimenhydrinate] 50 mg; 50 mg; 12.5 mg/4 mL

Dramamine, Children's liquid OTC *antinauseant; antiemetic; antivertigo agent; motion sickness preventative* [dimenhydrinate; alcohol 5%] 12.5 mg/5 mL

Dramamine II tablets OTC *anticholinergic; antihistamine; antivertigo agent; motion sickness preventative* [meclizine HCl] 25 mg

Dramanate IV or IM injection ℞ *antinauseant; antiemetic; antivertigo agent; motion sickness preventative* [dimenhydrinate] 50 mg/mL ▨ Dommanate

dramarin [see: dimenhydrate]

dramedilol INN

Dramilin IV or IM injection ℞ *antinauseant; antiemetic; antivertigo agent; motion sickness preventative* [dimenhydrinate] 50 mg/mL

Dramocen IV or IM injection (discontinued 1994) ℞ *antinauseant; antiemetic; antivertigo agent; motion sickness preventative* [dimenhydrinate] 50 mg/mL

Dramoject IV or IM injection (discontinued 1996) ℞ *antinauseant; antiemetic; antivertigo agent; motion sickness preventative* [dimenhydrinate] 50 mg/mL

dramyl [see: dimenhydrate]

draquinolol INN

Drawitol Drawing Salve ointment (discontinued 1992) OTC *topical local anesthetic; antiseptic; antibacterial* [diperodon HCl; benzalkonium chloride; carbolic acid; ichthammol; thymol; camphor; juniper tar]

drazidox INN

Drepanol ℞ *(orphan: prophylactic treatment of sickle cell disease)* [OM 401 (code name—generic name not yet approved)]

dribendazole USAN, INN *anthelmintic*

dricol [see: amidephrine]

Dri/Ear ear drops OTC *antibacterial/antifungal* [boric acid] 2.75%

dried aluminum hydroxide gel [see: aluminum hydroxide gel, dried]

dried basic aluminum carbonate [see: aluminum carbonate, basic]

dried ferrous sulfate [see: ferrous sulfate, dried]

dried yeast [see: yeast, dried]

drinidene USAN, INN *analgesic*

Drisdol capsules ℞ *vitamin deficiency therapy* [ergocalciferol] 50,000 IU

Drisdol Drops OTC *vitamin supplement* [ergocalciferol] 8000 IU/mL

Dristan nasal spray OTC *nasal decongestant; antihistamine* [phenylephrine HCl; pheniramine maleate] 0.5%•0.2%

Dristan 12-Hr. nasal spray OTC *nasal decongestant* [oxymetazoline HCl] 0.05%

Dristan Advanced Formula tablets (name changed to Dristan Cold Multi-Symptom Formula in 1993)

Dristan Allergy caplets (discontinued 1995) OTC *decongestant; antihistamine* [pseudoephedrine HCl; brompheniramine maleate] 60•4 mg

Dristan Cold caplets OTC *decongestant; analgesic; antipyretic* [pseudoephedrine HCl; acetaminophen] 30•500 mg

Dristan Cold, Maximum Strength caplets OTC *decongestant; antihistamine; analgesic* [pseudoephedrine HCl; brompheniramine maleate; acetaminophen] 30•2•500 mg

Dristan Cold & Flu powder (discontinued 1995) OTC *antitussive; decongestant; antihistamine; analgesic* [dextromethorphan hydrobromide; pseudoephedrine HCl; chlorpheniramine maleate; acetaminophen] 20•60•4•500 mg/packet

Dristan Cold Multi-Symptom Formula tablets OTC *decongestant; antihistamine; analgesic* [phenylephrine HCl; chlorpheniramine maleate; acetaminophen] 5•2•325 mg

Dristan Decongestant inhaler (discontinued 1993) OTC *nasal decongestant* [propylhexedrine; camphor; eucalyptol; menthol]

Dristan Juice Mix-In powder (discontinued 1995) OTC *antitussive; decongestant; analgesic* [dextromethorphan hydrobromide; pseudoephedrine HCl; acetaminophen] 20•60•500 mg/packet

Dristan Long Lasting nasal spray (name changed to Dristan 12-Hr. in 1994)

Dristan Saline Spray OTC *nasal moisturizer* [sodium chloride (saline)]

Dristan Sinus caplets OTC *decongestant; analgesic* [pseudoephedrine HCl; ibuprofen] 30•200 mg

Dristan-AF tablets (discontinued 1993) OTC *decongestant; antihistamine; analgesic* [phenylephrine HCl; chlorpheniramine maleate; acetaminophen; caffeine]

Drithocreme; Drithocreme HP 1%; Dritho-Scalp cream ℞ *topical antipsoriatic* [anthralin] 0.1%, 0.25%, 0.5%; 1%; 0.5%

Drixomed sustained-release tablets ℞ *decongestant; antihistamine* [pseudoephedrine sulfate; dexbrompheniramine maleate] 120•6 mg

Drixoral syrup OTC *decongestant; antihistamine* [pseudoephedrine sulfate; brompheniramine maleate] 30•2 mg/5 mL

Drixoral Allergy Sinus; Drixoral Cold & Flu extended-release tablets OTC *decongestant; antihistamine; analgesic* [pseudoephedrine sulfate; dexbrompheniramine maleate; acetaminophen] 60•3•500 mg

Drixoral Cold & Allergy sustained-action tablets OTC *decongestant; antihistamine* [pseudoephedrine sulfate; dexbrompheniramine maleate] 120•6 mg

Drixoral Cough & Congestion Liquid Caps (capsules) OTC *antitussive; decongestant* [dextromethorphan hydrobromide; pseudoephedrine HCl] 30•60 mg

Drixoral Cough Liquid Caps (liquid-filled capsules) OTC *antitussive* [dextromethorphan hydrobromide] 30 mg

Drixoral Cough & Sore Throat Liquid Caps (liquid-filled capsules) OTC *antitussive; analgesic* [dextromethorphan hydrobromide; acetaminophen] 15•325 mg

Drixoral Non-Drowsy Formula extended-release tablets OTC *nasal decongestant* [pseudoephedrine sulfate] 120 mg

Drixoral Plus extended-release tablets (name changed to Drixoral Cold & Flu in 1993)

Drixoral Sinus extended-release tablets (name changed to Drixoral Allergy Sinus in 1994)

Drize sustained-release capsules ℞ *decongestant; antihistamine* [phenylpropanolamine HCl; chlorpheniramine maleate] 75•12 mg

drobuline USAN, INN *antiarrhythmic*

drocarbil NF

drocinonide USAN, INN *anti-inflammatory*

droclidinium bromide INN

drocode [see: dihydrocodeine]

drofenine INN

droloxifene INN *investigational treatment for breast cancer and osteoporosis*

droloxifene citrate USAN *investigational antineoplastic for breast cancer; antiestrogen*

drometrizole USAN, INN *ultraviolet screen*

dromostanolone propionate USAN, USP *antineoplastic* [also: drostanolone]

dronabinol USAN, USP, INN *antiemetic for chemotherapy; appetite stimulant in AIDS patients (orphan)*

drop chalk [see: calcium carbonate]

Drop-Dose (trademarked delivery system) *prefilled eye drop dispenser*

dropempine INN

droperidol USAN, USP, INN, BAN *general anesthetic; antipsychotic*

Dropperettes (delivery system) *prefilled droppers*

droprenilamine USAN, INN *coronary vasodilator*

dropropizine INN, BAN

Drop-Tainers (trademarked dosage form) *prefilled eye drop dispenser*

drostanolone INN, BAN *antineoplastic* [also: dromostanolone propionate]

drotaverine INN

drotebanol INN, BAN

Drotic ear drops ℞ *topical corticosteroidal anti-inflammatory; antibiotic* [hydrocortisone; neomycin sulfate; polymyxin B sulfate] 1%•5 mg•10,000 U per mL

droxacin INN *antibacterial* [also: droxacin sodium]

droxacin sodium USAN *antibacterial* [also: droxacin]

droxicainide INN

droxicam INN

droxidopa INN

droxifilcon A USAN *hydrophilic contact lens material*

droxinavir HCl USAN *antiviral; HIV-1 protease inhibitor*

droxypropine INN, BAN

Dry and Clear lotion (discontinued 1992) OTC *topical keratolytic for acne* [benzoyl peroxide] 5%

Dry and Clear Double Strength cream (discontinued 1992) OTC *topical keratolytic for acne* [benzoyl peroxide] 10%

Dry Eye Therapy eye drops OTC *ocular moisturizer/lubricant* [glycerin] 0.3%

Dry Eyes eye drops OTC *ocular moisturizer/lubricant* [polyvinyl alcohol] 1.4%

Dry Eyes ophthalmic ointment OTC *ocular moisturizer/lubricant* [white petrolatum; mineral oil]

Dryox 2.5; Dryox 5; Dryox 10; Dryox 20 gel OTC *topical keratolytic for acne* [benzoyl peroxide] 2.5%; 5%; 10%; 20%

Dryox 10S 5; Dryox 20S 10 gel OTC *topical keratolytic for acne* [benzoyl peroxide; sulfur] 10%•5%; 20%•10%

Dryox Wash 5; Dryox Wash 10 liquid OTC *topical keratolytic for acne* [benzoyl peroxide] 5%; 10%

Drysol solution ℞ *astringent for hyperhidrosis* [aluminum chloride] 20%

Drytergent liquid OTC *soap-free therapeutic skin cleanser*

Drytex lotion OTC *topical keratolytic cleanser for acne* [salicylic acid; acetone; isopropyl alcohol] 2•10%•40%

DSC; DSCG (disodium cromoglycate) [see: cromolyn sodium]

DSMC Plus capsules OTC *laxative; stool softener* [casanthranol; docusate potassium] 30•100 mg

D-S-S capsules OTC *stool softener* [docusate sodium] 100 mg

DSS (dioctyl sodium sulfosuccinate) [now: docusate sodium]

D-S-S Plus capsules OTC *laxative; stool softener* [casanthranol; docusate sodium] 30•100 mg

DST (dihydrostreptomycin) [q.v.]

DT; Td (diphtheria & tetanus [toxoids]) *the designation DT or TD denotes the pediatric vaccine; Td denotes the adult vaccine* [see: diphtheria & tetanus toxoids, adsorbed]

DTaP (diphtheria & tetanus [toxoids] & acellular pertussis [vaccine]) [q.v.]

DTC 101 *investigational antineoplastic for neoplastic meningitis*

DTIC (dimethyl triazeno imidazole carboxamide) [see: dacarbazine]

DTIC-Dome IV injection ℞ *alkylating antineoplastic for metastatic malignant melanoma and Hodgkin's disease* [dacarbazine] 10 mg/mL

DTP (diphtheria & tetanus [toxoids] & pertussis [vaccine]) [q.v.]

DTPA (diethylenetriaminepentaacetic acid) [see: pentetic acid]

DTPA (diethylenetriaminepentaacetic acid) technetium (^{99m}Tc), human serum albumin [see: technetium Tc 99m pentetate]

DTwP (diphtheria & tetanus [toxoids] & whole-cell pertussis [vaccine]) [q.v.]

Duadacin capsules OTC *decongestant; antihistamine; analgesic* [phenylpropanolamine HCl; chlorpheniramine maleate; acetaminophen] 12.5•2•325 mg

duazomycin USAN, INN *antineoplastic*

duazomycin A [see: duazomycin]

duazomycin B [see: azotomycin]

duazomycin C [see: ambomycin]

ducodal [see: oxycodone]

Dulcagen enteric-coated tablets OTC *stimulant laxative* [bisacodyl] 5 mg

Dulcagen suppositories OTC *stimulant laxative* [bisacodyl] 10 mg

Dulcet (trademarked dosage form) *chewable tablet*

Dulcolax enteric-coated tablets OTC *stimulant laxative* [bisacodyl] 5 mg

Dulcolax suppositories OTC *stimulant laxative* [bisacodyl] 10 mg

Dulcolax Bowel Prep Kit 4 enteric-coated tablets + 1 suppository OTC *pre-procedure bowel evacuant* [bisacodyl] 5 mg; 10 mg

Dull-C powder OTC *vitamin supplement* [ascorbic acid] 4 g/tsp.

dulofibrate INN

duloxetine INN *antidepressant* [also: duloxetine HCl]

duloxetine HCl USAN *antidepressant* [also: duloxetine]

dulozafone INN

dumorelin INN

duneryl [see: phenobarbital]

Duocet tablets ℞ *narcotic analgesic* [hydrocodone bitartrate; acetaminophen] 5•500 mg

Duo-Cyp IM injection ℞ *estrogen/androgen for menopausal vasomotor symptoms* [estradiol cypionate; testosterone cypionate] 2•50 mg/mL

DuoDerm CGF; DuoDerm Extra Thin; DuoDerm Hydroactive adhesive dressings OTC *occlusive wound dressing* [hydrocolloid gel]

DuoDerm Hydroactive paste, granules OTC *wound dressing* [hydrocolloid gel] 30 g; 5 g

DuoFilm liquid OTC *topical keratolytic* [salicylic acid in flexible collodion] 17%

DuoFilm transdermal patch OTC *topical keratolytic* [salicylic acid in a rubber-based vehicle] 40%

duo-Flow solution (discontinued 1993) OTC *cleaning and soaking solution for hard contact lenses*

Duo-K liquid (discontinued 1992) ℞ *potassium supplement* [potassium gluconate; potassium chloride]

Duolube ophthalmic ointment (discontinued 1993) OTC *ocular moisturizer/lubricant*

Duo-Medihaler inhalation aerosol ℞ *bronchodilator* [isoproterenol HCl; phenylephrine bitartrate] 0.16•0.24 mg/dose

duometacin INN

duomycin [see: chlortetracycline HCl]

duoperone INN *neuroleptic* [also: duoperone fumarate]

duoperone fumarate USAN *neuroleptic* [also: duoperone]

DuoPlant gel ℞ *topical keratolytic* [salicylic acid in flexible collodion] 17%

duotal [see: guaiacol carbonate]

Duo-Trach Kit pre-filled syringe with cannula ℞ *injectable local anesthetic* [lidocaine HCl] 4%

Duotrate; Duotrate 45 sustained-release capsules (discontinued 1995) ℞ *antianginal* [pentaerythritol tetranitrate] 30 mg; 45 mg

Duphalac syrup ℞ *laxative* [lactulose] 10 g/15 mL

Duplex liquid OTC *soap-free therapeutic skin cleanser* [sodium lauryl sulfate] 15%

Duplex T shampoo OTC *antiseborrheic; antipsoriatic; antipruritic; antibacterial* [coal tar] 10%

duponol [see: sodium lauryl sulfate]

dupracetam INN

Durabolin IM injection ℞ *anabolic steroid for metastatic breast cancer in women* [nandrolone phenpropionate] 25, 50 mg/mL

Duracaps (dosage form) *sustained-release capsules*

DURAcare solution (discontinued 1995) OTC *surfactant cleaning solution for soft contact lenses*

DURAcare II solution OTC *surfactant cleaning solution for soft contact lenses*

Duracid chewable tablets (discontinued 1994) OTC *antacid* [aluminum hydroxide; magnesium carbonate; calcium carbonate] 175•175•325 mg

Duradyne tablets (discontinued 1994) OTC *analgesic; antipyretic; anti-inflammatory* [acetaminophen; aspirin; caffeine] 180•230•15 mg

Duradyne DHC tablets (discontinued 1994) ℞ *narcotic analgesic* [hydrocodone bitartrate; acetaminophen]

Dura-Estrin IM injection (discontinued 1996) ℞ *hormone replacement therapy for postmenopausal disorders* [estradiol cypionate in oil] 5 mg/mL

Duragen-10 IM injection (discontinued 1992) ℞ *estrogen replacement therapy for postmenopausal disorders;*

antineoplastic for prostatic cancer [estradiol valerate in oil] 10 mg/mL

Duragen-20; Duragen-40 IM injection (discontinued 1996) ℞ estrogen replacement therapy for postmenopausal disorders; antineoplastic for prostatic cancer [estradiol valerate in oil] 20 mg/mL; 40 mg/mL

Duragesic-25; Duragesic-50; Duragesic-75; Duragesic-100 transdermal patch ℞ narcotic analgesic [fentanyl] 2.5 mg; 5 mg; 7.5 mg; 10 mg

Dura-Gest capsules ℞ decongestant; expectorant [phenylephrine HCl; phenylpropanolamine HCl; guaifenesin] 45•5•200 mg

Duralex sustained-release capsules ℞ decongestant; antihistamine [pseudoephedrine HCl; chlorpheniramine maleate] 120•8 mg

Duralone-40; Duralone-80 intralesional, soft tissue, and IM injection ℞ glucocorticoid; anti-inflammatory; immunosuppressant [methylprednisolone acetate] 40 mg/mL; 80 mg/mL

Duralutin IM injection (discontinued 1996) ℞ progestin for amenorrhea, metrorrhagia, and dysfunctional uterine bleeding [hydroxyprogesterone caproate in oil] 250 mg/mL

Duramist Plus nasal spray OTC nasal decongestant [oxymetazoline HCl] 0.05%

Duramorph IV, subcu or IM injection ℞ narcotic analgesic; preoperative sedative and anxiolytic [morphine sulfate] 0.5, 1 mg/mL

Duranest; Duranest MPF injection ℞ injectable local anesthetic [etidocaine HCl] 1%

Duranest; Duranest MPF injection ℞ injectable local anesthetic [etidocaine HCl; epinephrine] 1%•1:200,000, 1.5%•1:200,000

Duranest HCl injection (name changed to Duranest in 1995)

durapatite USAN prosthetic aid [also: calcium phosphate, tribasic; hydroxyapatite]

Durapro (name changed to Daypro in 1992)

Duraquin sustained-release tablets (discontinued 1992) ℞ antiarrhythmic [quinidine gluconate]

DuraSite (delivery system) polymer-based eye drops

Dura-Tab (trademarked dosage form) sustained-release tablet

Dura-Tap/PD prolonged-action capsule ℞ pediatric decongestant and antihistamine [pseudoephedrine HCl; chlorpheniramine maleate] 60•4 mg

Duratears Naturale ophthalmic ointment OTC ocular moisturizer/lubricant [white petrolatum; mineral oil; lanolin]

Duratest 100; Duratest 200 IM injection ℞ androgen replacement for delayed puberty or breast cancer [testosterone cypionate] 100 mg/mL; 200 mg/mL

Duratestrin IM injection ℞ estrogen/androgen for menopausal vasomotor symptoms [estradiol cypionate; testosterone cypionate] 2•50 mg/mL

Durathate-200 IM injection ℞ androgen replacement for delayed puberty or breast cancer [testosterone enanthate] 200 mg/mL

Duration nasal spray OTC nasal decongestant [oxymetazoline HCl] 0.05%

Duration nose drops (discontinued 1992) OTC nasal decongestant [phenylephrine HCl]

Duratuss long-acting film-coated tablets ℞ decongestant; expectorant [pseudoephedrine HCl; guaifenesin] 120•600 mg

Duratuss HD elixir ℞ narcotic antitussive; decongestant; expectorant [hydrocodone bitartrate; pseudoephedrine HCl; guaifenesin] 2.5•30•100 mg/5 mL

Dura-Vent long-acting tablets ℞ decongestant; expectorant [phenylpropanolamine HCl; guaifenesin] 75•600 mg

Dura-Vent/A continuous-release capsule ℞ decongestant; antihistamine [phenylpropanolamine HCl; chlorpheniramine maleate] 75•10 mg

Dura-Vent/DA sustained-release tablets ℞ decongestant; antihistamine; anticholinergic [phenylephrine HCl;

chlorpheniramine maleate; methscopolamine nitrate] 20•8•2.5 mg

Duricef capsules, tablets ℞ *cephalosporin-type antibiotic* [cefadroxil monohydrate] 500 mg; 1000 mg

Duricef oral suspension ℞ *cephalosporin-type antibiotic* [cefadroxil] 125, 250, 500 mg/5 mL

dusting powder, absorbable USP *surgical glove lubricant*

Dutonin (British name for U.S. product Serzone)

Duvoid tablets ℞ *postsurgical cholinergic bladder muscle stimulant* [bethanechol chloride] 10, 25, 50 mg

DV vaginal cream (discontinued 1996) ℞ *estrogen replacement therapy for postmenopausal disorders* [dienestrol] 0.01%

DVB (DDP, vindesine, bleomycin) *chemotherapy protocol*

DVP (daunorubicin, vincristine, prednisone) *chemotherapy protocol*

DVPL-ASP (daunorubicin, vincristine, prednisone, L-asparaginase) *chemotherapy protocol*

Dwelle eye drops OTC *ocular moisturizer/lubricant*

Dyazide capsules ℞ *diuretic; antihypertensive* [triamterene; hydrochlorothiazide] 37.5•25 mg ② Thiacide; thiazides

Dycill capsules ℞ *bactericidal antibiotic (penicillinase-resistant penicillin)* [dicloxacillin sodium] 250, 500 mg

dyclocaine BAN *topical anesthetic* [also: dyclonine HCl; dyclonine]

Dyclone solution ℞ *anesthetic prior to upper GI and respiratory endoscopies* [dyclonine HCl] 0.5%, 1%

dyclonine INN *topical anesthetic* [also: dyclonine HCl; dyclocaine]

dyclonine HCl USP *topical anesthetic* [also: dyclonine; dyclocaine]

dydrogesterone USAN, USP, INN, BAN *progestin*

Dyflex-200 tablets ℞ *bronchodilator* [dyphylline] 200 mg

Dyflex-400 tablets (discontinued 1993) ℞ *bronchodilator* [dyphylline] 400 mg

Dyflex-G tablets ℞ *antiasthmatic; expectorant* [dyphylline; guaifenesin] 200•200 mg

dyflos BAN *antiglaucoma agent; irreversible cholinesterase inhibitor miotic* [also: isoflurophate]

dylate [see: clonitrate]

Dyline-GG tablets, liquid ℞ *antiasthmatic; bronchodilator; expectorant* [dyphylline; guaifenesin] 200•200 mg; 300•300 mg/15 mL

dymanthine HCl USAN *anthelmintic* [also: dimantine HCl]

Dymelor tablets ℞ *sulfonylurea-type antidiabetic* [acetohexamide] 250, 500 mg ② Demerol; Pamelor

Dymenate IV or IM injection ℞ *antinauseant; antiemetic; antivertigo; motion sickness preventative* [dimenhydrinate] 50 mg/mL

Dynabac enteric-coated tablets ℞ *once-daily macrolide antibiotic for respiratory and dermatological infections* [dirithromycin] 250 mg

Dynacin capsules ℞ *tetracycline-type antibiotic* [minocycline HCl] 50, 100 mg

DynaCirc capsules ℞ *antihypertensive* [isradipine] 2.5, 5 mg

dynacoryl [see: nikethamide]

Dynafed tablets OTC *decongestant; analgesic; antipyretic* [pseudoephedrine HCl; acetaminophen] 30•500 mg

Dynafed Asthma Relief tablets OTC *decongestant; expectorant* [ephedrine HCl; guaifenesin] 25•200 mg

Dynafed Pseudo tablets OTC *nasal decongestant* [pseudoephedrine HCl] 60 mg

Dyna-Hex Skin Cleanser; Dyna-Hex 2 Skin Cleanser liquid OTC *broad-spectrum antimicrobial; germicidal* [chlorhexidine gluconate; alcohol 4%] 4%; 2%

dynamine (orphan: Lambert-Eaton myasthenic syndrome; hereditary motor and sensory neuropathy)

Dynapen capsules, powder for oral suspension ℞ *bactericidal antibiotic (penicillinase-resistant penicillin)* [dicloxacillin sodium] 125, 250, 500 mg; 62.5 mg/5 mL

dynarsan [see: acetarsone]
Dynospheres M-035 ℞ *investigational imaging agent for MRI* [ferristene]
dyphylline USP *bronchodilator* [also: diprophylline] 200, 400 mg oral
Dyphylline-GG elixir OTC *antiasthmatic; bronchodilator; expectorant* [dyphylline; guaifenesin] 100•100 mg/15 mL
Dyprotex pads OTC *topical diaper rash treatment* [zinc oxide; dimethicone] 40%•2.5%
Dyrenium capsules ℞ *potassium-sparing diuretic* [triamterene] 50, 100 mg
⑨ Pyridium
Dyrexan-OD sustained-release capsules ℞ *anorexiant* [phendimetrazine tartrate] 105 mg
Dysport ℞ *(orphan: blepharospasm and strabismus with dystonia; pediatric cerebral palsy)* [botulinum toxin, type A]
dysprosium *element (Dy)*
DZAPO (daunorubicin, azacitidine, ara-C, prednisone, Oncovin) *chemotherapy protocol*

E5 ℞ *investigational agent for gram-negative sepsis* [H65-RTA monoclonal antibody]
E-200; E-400; E-1000 softgels OTC *vitamin supplement* [vitamin E] 147 mg; 400 IU; 1000 IU
E-2020 *investigational cholinesterase inhibitor for Alzheimer's disease*
Eaase capsules (discontinued 1993) OTC *dietary supplement* [multiple amino acids, vitamins, and minerals]
EACA (epsilon-aminocaproic acid) [see: aminocaproic acid]
EAP (etoposide, Adriamycin, Platinol) *chemotherapy protocol*
Ear-Dry ear drops OTC *antibacterial/antifungal* [boric acid] 2.75%
Ear-Eze ear drops ℞ *topical corticosteroidal anti-inflammatory; antibiotic* [hydrocortisone; neomycin sulfate; polymyxin B sulfate] 1%•5 mg•10,000 U per mL
Earocol Ear Drops (discontinued 1992) ℞ *topical local anesthetic; analgesic* [benzocaine; antipyrine; glycerin]
EarSol ear drops OTC *antiseptic* [alcohol] 44%
EarSol-HC ear drops OTC *topical corticosteroidal anti-inflammatory; antiseptic* [hydrocortisone; alcohol 44%] 1%
earthnut oil [see: peanut oil]
Easprin enteric-coated delayed-release tablets ℞ *analgesic; antipyretic; anti-inflammatory; antirheumatic* [aspirin] 975 mg
Easy Eyes tablets (discontinued 1992) OTC *rinsing/storage solution for soft contact lenses* [sodium chloride for normal saline solution]
EasyClean/GP Daily Cleaner solution (discontinued 1992) OTC *cleaning solution for rigid gas permeable contact lenses*
EasyClean/GP Weekly Enzymatic Cleaner solution (discontinued 1993) OTC *cleaning solution for rigid gas permeable lenses*
E-Base delayed-release enteric-coated caplets and tablets ℞ *macrolide antibiotic* [erythromycin] 333, 500 mg
ebastine USAN, INN *antihistamine*
ebiratide INN
ebrotidine INN
ebselen INN
EC (etoposide, carboplatin) *chemotherapy protocol*
ecadotril USAN, INN *antihypertensive*
ecarazine [see: todralazine]
ecastolol INN
Ecee Plus tablets OTC *vitamin/mineral supplement* [vitamins C and E; zinc sulfate; magnesium sulfate] 100•165•80•70 mg
ECHO (etoposide, cyclophosphamide, hydroxydaunomycin, Oncovin) *chemotherapy protocol*

echothiophate iodide USP *antiglaucoma agent; irreversible cholinesterase inhibitor miotic* [also: ecothiopate iodide]

Echovist intracoronary injection ℞ *ultrasound contrast agent; investigational for gynecologic uses* [galactose]

ecipramidil INN

eclanamine INN *antidepressant* [also: eclanamine maleate]

eclanamine maleate USAN *antidepressant* [also: eclanamine]

eclazolast USAN, INN *antiallergic; mediator release inhibitor*

Eclipse After Sun lotion (discontinued 1992) OTC *moisturizer; emollient*

EC-Naprosyn enteric-coated delayed-release tablets ℞ *nonsteroidal anti-inflammatory drug (NSAID); antiarthritic; analgesic* [naproxen] 375, 500 mg

ecogramostim BAN

E-Complex-600 capsules OTC *dietary supplement* [vitamin E] 600 IU

ecomustine INN

econazole USAN, INN, BAN *antifungal*

econazole nitrate USAN, USP, BAN *antifungal*

Econo B & C caplets OTC *vitamin supplement* [multiple B vitamins; vitamin C] ≛•300 mg

Econopred; Econopred Plus Drop-Tainers (eye drop suspension) ℞ *ophthalmic topical corticosteroidal anti-inflammatory* [prednisolone acetate] 0.125%; 1%

ecostigmine iodide [see: echothiophate iodide]

ecothiopate iodide INN, BAN *antiglaucoma agent; irreversible cholinesterase inhibitor miotic* [also: echothiophate iodide]

Ecotrin enteric-coated tablets, enteric-coated caplets OTC *analgesic; antipyretic; anti-inflammatory; antiarthritic* [aspirin] 325, 500 mg ② Edecrin

Ecotrin Adult Low Strength enteric-coated tablets OTC *analgesic; antipyretic; anti-inflammatory; antiarthritic* [aspirin] 81 mg

ectylurea BAN

Ed A-Hist long-acting capsules, liquid ℞ *decongestant; antihistamine* [phenylephrine HCl; chlorpheniramine maleate] 20•8 mg; 10•4 mg/5 mL

edamine [see: ethylenediamine]

EDAP (etoposide, dexamethasone, ara-C, Platinol) *chemotherapy protocol*

edathamil [now: edetate calcium disodium]

edathamil calcium disodium [now: edetate calcium disodium]

edathamil disodium [now: edetate disodium]

edatrexate USAN, INN *antineoplastic; methotrexate analog*

Edecrin tablets ℞ *loop diuretic* [ethacrynic acid] 25, 50 mg ② Ecotrin; Ethaquin

Edecrin Sodium powder for IV injection ℞ *loop diuretic* [ethacrynate sodium] 50 mg

edelfosine INN

edetate calcium disodium USAN, USP *heavy metal chelating agent for lead poisoning* [also: sodium calcium edetate; sodium calciumedetate; calcium disodium edetate]

edetate dipotassium USAN *chelating agent*

edetate disodium USP *chelating agent; preservative; antioxidant* [also: disodium edetate] 150 mg/mL injection

edetate sodium USAN *chelating agent*

edetate trisodium USAN *chelating agent*

edetic acid NF, INN, BAN *chelating agent*

edetol USAN, INN *alkalizing agent*

edifolone INN *antiarrhythmic* [also: edifolone acetate]

edifolone acetate USAN *antiarrhythmic* [also: edifolone]

edisilate INN *combining name for radicals or groups* [also: edisylate]

edisylate USAN, BAN *combining name for radicals or groups* [also: edisilate]

edithamil [see: edetate ...]

edobacomab USAN *antiendotoxin monoclonal antibody*

edogestrone INN, BAN

edoxudine USAN, INN *antiviral*

edrofuradene [see: nifurdazil]

edrophone chloride [see: edrophonium chloride]

edrophonium chloride USP, INN, BAN *antidote to curare; myasthenia gravis diagnostic aid*

Ed-Spaz tablets ℞ *anticholinergic; antispasmodic* [hyoscyamine sulfate] 0.125 mg

EDTA (ethylenediaminetetraacetic acid) [see: edetate disodium]

EDTA calcium [see: edetate calcium disodium]

ED-TLC; ED Tuss HC liquid ℞ *narcotic antitussive; decongestant; antihistamine* [hydrocodone bitartrate; phenylephrine HCl; chlorpheniramine maleate] 1.67•5•2 mg/5 mL; 2.5•10•4 mg/5 mL

E.E.S. chewable tablets (name changed to EryPed in 1992)

E.E.S. granules for oral suspension ℞ *macrolide antibiotic* [erythromycin ethylsuccinate] 200 mg/5 mL

EES (erythromycin ethylsuccinate) [q.v.]

E.E.S. 200 oral suspension ℞ *macrolide antibiotic* [erythromycin ethylsuccinate] 200 mg/5 mL

E.E.S. 400 film-coated tablets, oral suspension ℞ *macrolide antibiotic* [erythromycin ethylsuccinate] 400 mg; 400 mg/5 mL

Efamol PMS soft gel capsules OTC *dietary supplement* [multiple vitamins & amino acids]

efaroxan INN, BAN

Efed II capsules OTC *decongestant* [phenylpropanolamine HCl]

Efedron Nasal jelly (discontinued 1992) OTC *nasal decongestant* [ephedrine]

efegatran sulfate USAN *antithrombotic*

E-Ferol ointment (discontinued 1992) OTC *emollient* [vitamin E]

efetozole INN

Effer-K effervescent tablets ℞ *potassium supplement* [potassium bicarbonate; potassium citrate] 25 mEq

Effer-Syllium effervescent powder (replaced by Mylanta Natural Fiber Supplement in 1994)

Effervescent Potassium effervescent tablets ℞ *potassium supplement* [potassium bicarbonate; potassium citrate] 25 mEq

Effexor tablets ℞ *antidepressant* [venlafaxine] 25, 37.5, 50, 75, 100 mg

Effexor SR ℞ *investigational once-daily antidepressant* [venlafaxine]

Efidac/24 extended-release tablets OTC *nasal decongestant* [pseudoephedrine HCl] 240 mg

Efidac/24 Chlorpheniramine extended-release tablets OTC *antihistamine* [chlorpheniramine maleate] 16 mg

Eflone eye drop suspension ℞ *ophthalmic topical corticosteroidal anti-inflammatory* [fluorometholone acetate] 0.1%

eflornithine INN, BAN *antineoplastic; antiprotozoal* [also: eflornithine HCl]

eflornithine HCl USAN *antineoplastic; antiprotozoal; (orphan: sleeping sickness; Pneumocystis carinii pneumonia)* [also: eflornithine]

efloxate INN

eflumast INN

Efodine ointment OTC *broad-spectrum antimicrobial* [povidone-iodine] 1%

EFP (etoposide, fluorouracil, Platinol) *chemotherapy protocol*

Efricon Expectorant liquid ℞ *narcotic antitussive; decongestant; antihistamine; expectorant* [codeine phosphate; phenylephrine HCl; chlorpheniramine maleate; ammonium chloride; potassium guaiacolsulfonate; sodium citrate]

efrotomycin USAN, INN, BAN *veterinary growth stimulant*

Efudex cream, topical solution ℞ *antimetabolic antineoplastic for actinic keratoses and basal cell carcinomas* [fluorouracil] 5%; 2%, 5%

E-Gems soft capsules, oil drops, cream, lip balm, shampoo, bar soap OTC *vitamin supplement; topical antioxidant* [vitamin E]

E-Gems Plus soft capsules OTC *vitamin supplement* [vitamin E]

E-Gems with C soft capsules OTC *vitamin supplement* [vitamins C and E]

egtazic acid USAN, INN *pharmaceutic aid*

EHDP (ethane hydroxydiphosphonate) [see: etidronate disodium]

Ehrlich 594 [see: acetarsone]

Ehrlich 606 [see: arsphenamine]
eicosapentaenoic acid (EPA) [see: icosapent]
8 in 1 (Medrol, vincristine, CCNU, procarbazine, hydroxyurea, cisplatin, ara-C, cyclophosphamide) *chemotherapy protocol*
8 in 1 (Medrol, vincristine, CCNU, procarbazine, hydroxyurea, cisplatin, ara-C, dacarbazine) *chemotherapy protocol*
882 *investigational antiviral for AIDS*
8-MOP capsules ℞ *to increase tolerance to sunlight and enhance pigmentation* [methoxsalen] 10 mg
einsteinium *element (Es)*
elantrine USAN, INN *anticholinergic*
elanzepine INN
Elase powder, ointment ℞ *topical enzyme for biochemical debridement* [fibrinolysin; desoxyribonuclease] 25•15,000 U; 1•666.6 U/g
Elase-Chloromycetin ointment ℞ *topical enzyme for biochemical debridement; antibiotic* [fibrinolysin; desoxyribonuclease; chloramphenicol] 1 U•666.6 U•10 mg per g
elastofilcon A USAN *hydrophilic contact lens material*
Elavil film-coated tablets, IM injection ℞ *tricyclic antidepressant* [amitriptyline HCl] 10, 25, 50, 75, 100, 150 mg; 10 mg/mL ⊅ Aldoril; Enovil; Equanil; Mellaril
elbanizine INN
elcatonin INN
Eldec Kapseals (discontinued 1992) ℞ *vitamin/mineral/iron therapy* [multiple vitamins & minerals; iron; folic acid]
Eldecort cream (discontinued 1995) ℞ *topical corticosteroid* [hydrocortisone] 2.5%
Eldepryl capsules ℞ *antiparkinsonian (orphan)* [selegiline HCl] 5 mg
Eldercaps capsules ℞ *vitamin/mineral supplement* [multiple vitamins & minerals; folic acid] ≐•1 mg
Eldertonic liquid OTC *vitamin/mineral supplement* [multiple B vitamins & minerals; alcohol 13.5%] ≐
eldexomer INN

Eldisine ℞ *investigational antineoplastic for leukemia, melanoma, breast and lung cancers* [vindesine sulfate]
Eldopaque; Eldopaque-Forte cream OTC *hyperpigmentation bleaching agent; sunscreen* [hydroquinone in a sunblock base] 2%; 4%
Eldoquin lotion (discontinued 1993) OTC *hyperpigmentation bleaching agent* [hydroquinone] 2%
Eldoquin; Eldoquin-Forte Sunbleaching cream OTC *hyperpigmentation bleaching agent* [hydroquinone] 2%; 4%
electrocortin [see: aldosterone]
eledoisin INN
ELF (etoposide, leucovorin [rescue], fluorouracil) *chemotherapy protocol*
elfazepam USAN, INN *veterinary appetite stimulant*
elgodipine INN
Elimite cream ℞ *pediculicide; scabicide* [permethrin] 5%
eliprodil INN *investigational treatment for ischemic stroke*
Elixomin elixir ℞ *bronchodilator* [theophylline] 80 mg/15 mL
Elixophyllin capsules, elixir ℞ *bronchodilator* [theophylline] 100, 200 mg; 80 mg/15 mL
Elixophyllin GG liquid ℞ *antiasthmatic; bronchodilator; expectorant* [theophylline; guaifenesin] 100•100 mg/15 mL
Elixophyllin SR timed-release capsules (discontinued 1994) ℞ *bronchodilator* [theophylline] 125, 250 mg
Elixophyllin-KI elixir ℞ *antiasthmatic; bronchodilator; expectorant* [theophylline; potassium iodide] 80•130 mg/15 mL
ellagic acid INN
Elliott's B solution *(orphan: acute lymphocytic leukemias and lymphoblastic lymphomas)*
ellipticine *investigational antineoplastic for breast cancer*
elliptinium acetate INN, BAN
Elmiron ℞ *anti-inflammatory; (orphan: interstitial cystitis)* [pentosan polysulfate sodium]

elmustine INN
elnadipine INN
Elobromol ℞ *investigational antineoplastic* [mitolactol]
Elocon ointment, cream, lotion ℞ *topical corticosteroid* [mometasone furoate] 0.1%
E-Lor film-coated tablets (discontinued 1995) ℞ *narcotic analgesic* [propoxyphene HCl; acetaminophen] 65•650 mg
elsamitrucin USAN, INN *antineoplastic*
Elspar powder for IV or IM injection ℞ *antineoplastic adjunct for acute lymphocytic leukemia* [asparaginase] 10,000 IU
eltanolone INN *investigational IV anesthetic*
eltenac INN
eltoprazine INN
Eltroxin tablets ℞ *thyroid hormone* [levothyroxine sodium] 50, 75, 100, 125, 150, 200, 300 μg
elucaine USAN, INN *gastric anticholinergic*
Elyzol Dentalgel ℞ *investigational treatment for periodontitis*
elziverine INN
EMA (estramustine L-alanine) [q.v.]
EMA 86 (etoposide, mitoxantrone, ara-C) *chemotherapy protocol*
EMACO (etoposide, methotrexate, actinomycin D, cyclophosphamide, Oncovin) *chemotherapy protocol*
Emagrin tablets OTC *analgesic; antipyretic; anti-inflammatory* [aspirin; salicylamide; caffeine]
Emagrin Forte tablets OTC *decongestant; expectorant; analgesic; antipyretic* [phenylephrine HCl; guaifenesin; acetaminophen]
embinal [see: barbital sodium]
embonate INN, BAN *combining name for radicals or groups* [also: pamoate]
embramine INN, BAN
embramine HCl [see: embramine]
Embutane ℞ *veterinary anesthetic; veterinary euthanasia* [embutramide]
embutramide USAN, INN, BAN *veterinary anesthetic; veterinary euthanasia*
Emcyt capsules ℞ *hormonal chemotherapy for metastatic or progressive prostatic carcinoma* [estramustine phosphate sodium] 140 mg
Emecheck liquid OTC *antinauseant; antiemetic* [phosphorated carbohydrate solution] 21.5 mg/5 mL
emedastine INN
emepronium bromide INN, BAN
emepronium carrageenate BAN
Emergent-Ez Kit ℞ *carry-kit for medical personnel* [multiple drugs and devices for emergencies] ±
Emersal emulsion ℞ *topical antipsoriatic; antiseborrheic* [ammoniated mercury; salicylic acid] 5%•2.5%
Emete-con IV or IM injection (discontinued 1994) ℞ *post-anesthesia antiemetic* [benzoquinamide HCl] 50 mg/vial
emetine BAN *antiamebic* [also: emetine HCl] ② Emetrol
emetine bismuth iodide [see: emetine HCl]
emetine HCl USP *amebicide* [also: emetine]
Emetrol solution OTC *antinauseant; antiemetic* [phosphorated carbohydrate solution] ② emetine
Emgel gel ℞ *topical antibiotic for acne* [erythromycin] 2%
emiglitate INN, BAN
emilium tosilate INN *antiarrhythmic* [also: emilium tosylate]
emilium tosylate USAN *antiarrhythmic* [also: emilium tosilate]
Eminase IV injection ℞ *thrombolytic for acute MI* [anistreplase] 30 U/vial
Emitasol intranasal ℞ *investigational anti-emetic for chemotherapy* [metoclopramide HCl]
Emko; Emko Pre-Fil vaginal foam OTC *spermicidal contraceptive* [nonoxynol 9] 8%
Emla cream ℞ *topical local anesthetic* [lidocaine; prilocaine] 2.5%•2.5%
Emollia lotion OTC *moisturizer; emollient*
emonapride INN
emopamil INN
emorfazone INN
Empirin tablets OTC *analgesic; antipyretic; anti-inflammatory; antirheumatic* [aspirin] 325 mg

Empirin with Codeine No. 2 tablets (discontinued 1992) ℞ *narcotic analgesic* [codeine phosphate; aspirin]

Empirin with Codeine No. 3 & No. 4 tablets ℞ *narcotic analgesic* [codeine phosphate; aspirin] 30•325 mg; 60•325 mg

emtryl [see: dimetridazole]

Emul-O-Balm (discontinued 1992) OTC *counterirritant* [methyl salicylate; camphor; menthol]

emulsifying wax [see: wax, emulsifying]

Emulsoil emulsion OTC *stimulant laxative* [castor oil] 95%

E-Mycin enteric-coated tablets ℞ *macrolide antibiotic* [erythromycin] 250, 333 mg

emylcamate INN, BAN

Enable ℞ *investigational anti-inflammatory for rheumatoid arthritis and osteoarthritis* [tenidap]

Enablex (foreign name for U.S. product Enable)

enalapril INN, BAN *antihypertensive; angiotensin-converting enzyme (ACE) inhibitor* [also: enalapril maleate]

enalapril maleate USAN, USP *antihypertensive; angiotensin-converting enzyme (ACE) inhibitor* [also: enalapril]

enalaprilat USAN, USP, INN, BAN *antihypertensive; angiotensin-converting enzyme inhibitor*

enalkiren USAN, INN *antihypertensive; renin inhibitor*

enallynymal sodium [see: methohexital sodium]

enantate INN *combining name for radicals or groups* [also: enanthate]

enanthate USAN, USP, BAN *combining name for radicals or groups* [also: enantate]

enbucrilate INN, BAN

encainide INN, BAN *antiarrhythmic* [also: encainide HCl]

encainide HCl USAN *antiarrhythmic* [also: encainide]

Encare vaginal suppositories OTC *spermicidal contraceptive* [nonoxynol 9] 2.27%

En-Cebrin Pulvules (capsules) OTC *vitamin/mineral/iron supplement* [multiple vitamins & minerals; iron]

enciprazine INN, BAN *minor tranquilizer* [also: enciprazine HCl]

enciprazine HCl USAN *minor tranquilizer* [also: enciprazine]

enclomifene INN [also: enclomiphene]

enclomiphene USAN [also: enclomifene]

encyprate USAN, INN *antidepressant*

End Lice liquid OTC *pediculicide* [pyrethrins; piperonyl butoxide] 0.3%•3%

Endafed sustained-release capsules ℞ *decongestant; antihistamine* [pseudoephedrine HCl; brompheniramine maleate] 120•12 mg

Endagen-HD liquid ℞ *narcotic antitussive; decongestant; antihistamine* [hydrocodone bitartrate; phenylephrine HCl; chlorpheniramine maleate] 1.67•5•2 mg/5 mL

Endal timed-release tablets ℞ *decongestant; expectorant* [phenylephrine HCl; guaifenesin] 20•300 mg ⓘ Intal

Endal Expectorant syrup ℞ *narcotic antitussive; decongestant; expectorant* [codeine phosphate; phenylpropanolamine HCl; guaifenesin; alcohol 5%] 10•12.5•100 mg/5 mL

Endal-HD; Endal-HD Plus liquid ℞ *narcotic antitussive; decongestant; antihistamine* [hydrocodone bitartrate; phenylephrine HCl; chlorpheniramine maleate] 1.7•5•2 mg/5 mL; 2.5•5•2 mg/5 mL

Endep film-coated tablets ℞ *tricyclic antidepressant* [amitriptyline HCl] 10, 50, 75, 100, 150 mg

endiemal [see: metharbital]

endixaprine INN

endobenzyline bromide

endocaine [see: pyrrocaine]

EndoCRIB ℞ *investigational treatment for type II diabetes* [cellular implants]

endolate [see: meperidine HCl]

Endolor capsules ℞ *analgesic; antipyretic; sedative* [acetaminophen; caffeine; butalbital] 325•40•50 mg

endomide INN

endomycin

Endosol solution (discontinued 1992) ℞ *irrigant for eyes, ears, nose and throat during surgery* [balanced salt solution]

endralazine INN, BAN *antihypertensive* [also: endralazine mesylate]

endralazine mesylate USAN *antihypertensive* [also: endralazine]

Endrate IV infusion ℞ *calcium-lowering agent; antiarrhythmic for digitalis toxicity* [edetate disodium] 150 mg/mL

endrisone INN *topical ophthalmic anti-inflammatory* [also: endrysone]

endrysone USAN *topical ophthalmic anti-inflammatory* [also: endrisone]

Enduret (trademarked dosage form) *prolonged-action tablet*

Enduron tablets ℞ *diuretic; antihypertensive* [methyclothiazide] 5 mg ② Imuran; Inderal

Enduronyl; Enduronyl Forte tablets ℞ *antihypertensive* [methyclothiazide; deserpidine] 5•0.25 mg; 5•0.5 mg ② Inderal

Enecat concentrated suspension ℞ *GI contrast radiopaque agent* [barium sulfate] 5%

enefexine INN

Ener-B nasal gel OTC *vitamin supplement* [cyanocobalamin] 400 μg

enestebol INN

Enfamil liquid, powder OTC *total or supplementary infant feeding*

Enfamil Human Milk Fortifier powder OTC *supplement to breast milk*

Enfamil Next Step liquid, powder OTC *total or supplementary infant feeding*

Enfamil Premature Formula liquid OTC *total or supplementary infant feeding*

Enfamil with Iron liquid, powder OTC *total or supplementary infant feeding*

enfenamic acid INN

enflurane USAN, USP, INN, BAN *inhalation general anesthetic*

Engerix-B adult IM injection, pediatric IM injection ℞ *hepatitis B vaccine* [hepatitis B virus vaccine, recombinant] 20 μg/mL, 10 μg/0.5 mL

englitazone INN *antidiabetic* [also: englitazone sodium]

englitazone sodium USAN *antidiabetic* [also: englitazone]

Engran-HP tablets (discontinued 1992) OTC *vitamin/mineral/iron supplement* [multiple vitamins & minerals; iron; folic acid]

enhexymal [see: hexobarbital]

eniclobrate INN

enilconazole USAN, INN, BAN *antifungal*

enilospirone INN

enisoprost USAN, INN *antiulcerative*; *(orphan: organ transplant rejection)*

enisoprost & cyclosporine *(orphan: organ transplant rejection)*

Enisyl tablets OTC *dietary amino acid supplement* [L-lysine] 334, 500 mg

Enlon IV or IM injection ℞ *myasthenia gravis treatment; antidote to curare-type overdose* [edrophonium chloride] 10 mg/mL

Enlon Plus IV or IM injection ℞ *muscle stimulant; neuromuscular blocker antagonist* [edrophonium chloride; atropine sulfate] 10•0.14 mg

enloplatin USAN, INN *antineoplastic*

ENO powder (discontinued 1994) OTC *antacid* [sodium tartrate; sodium citrate] 1620•1172 mg/dose

enocitabine INN

enofelast USAN, INN *antiasthmatic*

enolicam INN *anti-inflammatory; antirheumatic* [also: enolicam sodium]

enolicam sodium USAN *anti-inflammatory; antirheumatic* [also: enolicam]

Enomine capsules ℞ *decongestant; expectorant* [phenylpropanolamine HCl; phenylephrine HCl; guaifenesin] 45•5•200 mg

Enomine LA long-acting tablets (discontinued 1992) ℞ *decongestant; expectorant* [phenylpropanolamine HCl; guaifenesin]

Enovid tablets ℞ *progestin for hypermenorrhea or endometriosis* [mestranol; norethynodrel] 75 μg•5 mg; 150 μg•9.85 mg

Enovil IM injection ℞ *tricyclic antidepressant* [amitriptyline HCl] 10 mg/mL ② Elavil

enoxacin USAN, INN, BAN, JAN *antibacterial*

enoxamast INN

enoxaparin BAN *anticoagulant; antithrombotic* [also: enoxaparin sodium]

enoxaparin sodium USAN, INN *anticoagulant; antithrombotic* [also: enoxaparin]

enoximone USAN, INN, BAN *cardiotonic*

enoxolone INN, BAN

enphenemal [see: mephobarbital]

enpiprazole INN, BAN

enpiroline INN *antimalarial* [also: enpiroline phosphate]

enpiroline phosphate USAN *antimalarial* [also: enpiroline]

enprazepine INN

enprofen [now: furaprofen]

enprofylline USAN, INN *bronchodilator*

enpromate USAN, INN *antineoplastic*

enprostil USAN, INN, BAN *investigational antisecretory and antiulcerative for acute peptic ulcers*

enramycin INN

Enrich Liquid with Fiber (discontinued 1994) OTC *enteral nutritional therapy* [lactose-free formula] 8 oz., 1 qt. ready-to-use

enrofloxacin USAN, INN, BAN *veterinary antibacterial*

Enseal (trademarked dosage form) *enteric-coated tablet*

Ensure liquid, powder OTC *enteral nutritional therapy* [lactose-free formula]

Ensure pudding OTC *enteral nutritional therapy* [milk-based formula] 150 g

Ensure High Protein ready-to-use liquid OTC *enteral nutritional therapy* [lactose-free formula] 237 mL

Ensure HN; Ensure with Fiber ready-to-use liquid OTC *enteral nutritional therapy* [lactose-free formula]

Ensure Plus; Ensure Plus HN liquid OTC *enteral nutritional therapy* [lactose-free formula]

E.N.T. sustained-release tablets ℞ *decongestant; antihistamine* [phenylpropanolamine HCl; brompheniramine maleate] 75•12 mg

EN-tab (trademarked dosage form) *enteric-coated tablet*

enteramine [see: serotonin]

Entero-Test; Entero-Test Pediatric string capsules for professional use *in vitro diagnostic aid for GI disorders*

Entertainer's Secret Throat Relief spray OTC *saliva substitute*

Entex capsules, liquid ℞ *decongestant; expectorant* [phenylephrine HCl; phenylpropanolamine HCl; guaifenesin] 45•5•200 mg; 20•5•100 mg/5 mL

Entex LA long-acting tablets ℞ *decongestant; expectorant* [phenylpropanolamine HCl; guaifenesin] 75•400 mg

Entex PSE prolonged-action tablets ℞ *decongestant; expectorant* [pseudoephedrine HCl; guaifenesin] 60•120 mg

Entocort tablets for rectal suspension (available only in Canada) ℞ *steroidal anti-inflammatory for bowel disease* [budesonide]

Entozyme tablets (discontinued 1994) ℞ *digestive enzymes* [pancreatin; lipase; protease; amylase] 300 mg•600 U•7500 U•7500 U ② Donnazyme

Entri-Pak (dosage form) *liquid-filled pouch*

Entrition; Entrition RDA Entri-Pak (liquid-filled pouch) (discontinued 1994) OTC *enteral nutritional therapy* [lactose-free formula]

Entrition 0.5 liquid OTC *enteral nutritional therapy* [lactose-free formula]

Entrition Half-Strength (name changed to Entrition 0.5 in 1994)

Entrition HN Entri-Pak (liquid-filled pouch) OTC *enteral nutritional therapy* [lactose-free formula]

Entrobar suspension ℞ *GI contrast radiopaque agent* [barium sulfate] 50%

entsufon INN *detergent* [also: entsufon sodium]

entsufon sodium USAN *detergent* [also: entsufon]

Entuss Expectorant liquid ℞ *narcotic antitussive; expectorant* [hydrocodone bitartrate; potassium guaiacolsulfonate] 5•300 mg/5 mL

Entuss Expectorant tablets ℞ *narcotic antitussive; expectorant* [hydrocodone bitartrate; guaifenesin] 5•300 mg

Entuss-D liquid ℞ *narcotic antitussive; decongestant* [hydrocodone bitartrate; pseudoephedrine HCl] 5•30 mg/5 mL

Entuss-D tablets ℞ *narcotic antitussive; decongestant; expectorant* [hydrocodone bitartrate; pseudoephedrine HCl; guaifenesin] 5•30•300 mg

Entuss-D Jr. liquid ℞ *pediatric narcotic antitussive, decongestant, and expectorant* [hydrocodone bitartrate; pseudoephedrine HCl; guaifenesin; alcohol 5%] 2.5•30•100 mg/5 mL

Enuclene eye drops OTC *cleaning, wetting and lubricating agent for artificial eyes* [tyloxapol] 0.25%

Enulose syrup ℞ *prevent and treat portal-systemic encephalopathy* [lactulose] 10 g/15 mL

Enviclusive (discontinued 1992) *semi-occlusive film dressing for use with Envisan*

Envinet (discontinued 1992) *nylon net for use with Envisan*

enviomycin INN

enviradene USAN, INN *antiviral*

Enviro-Stress slow-release tablets OTC *vitamin/mineral supplement* [multiple vitamins & minerals; folic acid] ±•0.4 mg

enviroxime USAN, INN *antiviral*

Envisan Treatment Multipack beads, paste (discontinued 1992) ℞ *debrider and cleanser for wet wounds* [dextranomer]

Enzobile Improved enteric-coated tablets (discontinued 1992) OTC *digestive enzymes* [pancreatic enzyme concentrate; ox bile extract; cellulase; pepsin]

Enzone cream ℞ *topical corticosteroid; local anesthetic* [hydrocortisone acetate; pramoxine HCl] 1%•1%

Enzymatic Cleaner for Extended Wear tablets OTC *enzymatic cleaner for soft contact lenses* [pork pancreatin]

Enzyme chewable tablets OTC *digestive enzymes* [amylase; protease; lipase; cellulase] 30•6•2•25 mg

EP (etoposide, Platinol) *chemotherapy protocol*

EPA capsules OTC *dietary supplement* [omega-3 fatty acids] 1000 mg

EPA (eicosapentaenoic acid) [see: icosapent]

epalrestat INN *investigational treatment for diabetic neuropathy*

epanolol INN, BAN

eperisone INN

epervudine INN

ephedrine USP, BAN *bronchodilator; nasal decongestant; vasopressor for shock* ② Appedrine; aprindine

ephedrine HCl USP, BAN *bronchodilator; nasal decongestant; vasopressor for shock*

ephedrine sulfate USP *bronchodilator; nasal decongestant; vasopressor for acute hypotensive shock* [also: ephedrine sulphate] 25, 50 mg oral; 25, 50 mg/mL injection

ephedrine sulphate BAN *bronchodilator; nasal decongestant* [also: ephedrine sulfate]

ephedrine tannate

Epi-C concentrated suspension ℞ *GI contrast radiopaque agent* [barium sulfate] 150%

epicainide INN

epicillin USAN, INN, BAN *antibacterial*

epicriptine INN

Epiderm balm (discontinued 1994) OTC *counterirritant; topical antiseptic* [methyl salicylate; menthol; alcohol]

epidermal growth factor, human *(orphan: acceleration of corneal regeneration)*

epiestriol INN [also: epioestriol]

Epifoam aerosol foam ℞ *topical corticosteroid; local anesthetic* [hydrocortisone acetate; pramoxine] 1%•1%

Epifrin eye drops ℞ *antiglaucoma agent* [epinephrine HCl] 0.5%, 1%, 2% ② epinephrine; EpiPen

epilin [see: dietifen]

E-Pilo-1; E-Pilo-2; E-Pilo-4; E-Pilo-6 eye drops ℞ *antiglaucoma agent* [pilocarpine HCl; epinephrine bitartrate] 1%•1%; 2%•1%; 4%•1%; 6%•1%

E-Pilo-3 eye drops (discontinued 1995) ℞ *antiglaucoma agent* [pilocarpine HCl; epinephrine bitartrate] 3%•1%

Epilyt lotion concentrate OTC *moisturizer; emollient*

epimestrol USAN, INN, BAN *anterior pituitary activator*

Epinal eye drops ℞ *antiglaucoma agent* [epinephryl borate] 0.5%, 1% ② Epitol

epinastine INN

epinephran [see: epinephrine]

epinephrine USP, INN *vasoconstrictor; bronchodilator; topical antiglaucoma agent; vasopressor for shock* [also: adrenaline] 1:10,000 (0.1 mg/mL) injection ② Epifrin

epinephrine bitartrate USP *bronchodilator; ophthalmic adrenergic; topical antiglaucoma agent*

epinephrine borate *topical antiglaucoma agent*

epinephrine HCl *nasal decongestant; topical antiglaucoma agent; vasopressor for shock* 0.1% eye drops; 1:1000, 1:2000, 1:10,000 (1, 0.5, 0.1 mg/mL) injection

Epinephrine Pediatric subcu injection ℞ *bronchodilator for bronchial asthma or bronchospasm; vasopressor for shock* [epinephrine HCl] 1:100,000 (0.01 mg/mL)

epinephryl borate USAN, USP *adrenergic; topical antiglaucoma agent*

epioestriol BAN [also: epiestriol]

EpiPen; EpiPen Jr. auto-injector (automatic IM injection device) ℞ *emergency treatment of anaphylaxis; vasopressor for shock* [epinephrine] 1:1000 (1 mg/mL); 1:2000 (0.5 mg/mL) ② Epifrin

epipropidine USAN, INN *antineoplastic*

epirizole USAN, INN *analgesic; antiinflammatory*

epiroprim INN

epirubicin INN, BAN *antibiotic antineoplastic* [also: epirubicin HCl]

epirubicin HCl USAN, JAN *antibiotic antineoplastic* [also: epirubicin]

epitetracycline HCl USP *antibacterial*

epithiazide USAN, BAN *antihypertensive; diuretic* [also: epitizide]

epithioandrostanol [see: epitiostanol]

epitiostanol INN

epitizide INN *antihypertensive; diuretic* [also: epithiazide]

Epitol tablets ℞ *anticonvulsant* [carbamazepine] 200 mg ② Epinal

Epitrate eye drops (discontinued 1992) ℞ *antiglaucoma agent* [epinephrine bitartrate]

Epivir film-coated tablets, oral solution ℞ *nucleoside antiviral for HIV; reverse transcriptase inhibitor* [lamivudine] 150 mg; 10 mg/mL

EPlus tablets OTC *vitamin supplement* [multiple vitamins; lemon bioflavonoids]

EPO (epoetin alfa) [q.v.]

EPOCH (etoposide, prednisone, Oncovin, cyclophosphamide, Halotestin) *chemotherapy protocol*

epoetin alfa (EPO) USAN, INN, BAN, JAN *antianemic; hematinic; (orphan: anemia of end-stage renal disease or HIV; myelodysplastic syndrome)*

epoetin beta USAN, INN, BAN, JAN *antianemic; hematinic; (orphan: anemia of end-stage renal disease)*

Epogen IV or subcu injection ℞ *stimulates RBC production; for anemia of end-stage renal disease or HIV (orphan)* [epoetin alfa] 2000, 3000, 4000, 10,000 U/mL

Epogin ℞ *investigational blood cell growth factor* [erythropoietin]

epoprostenol USAN, INN *platelet aggregation inhibitor; vasodilator for primary pulmonary hypertension (orphan)*

epoprostenol & prostacyclin *(orphan: pulmonary hypertension; hemodialysis)*

epoprostenol sodium USAN, BAN *platelet aggregation inhibitor; vasodilator; antihypertensive*

epostane USAN, INN, BAN *interceptive*

epoxytropine tropate methylbromide [see: methscopolamine bromide]

Eppy/N ½% eye drops (discontinued 1994) ℞ *antiglaucoma agent* [epinephrine borate] 0.5%

Eppy/N 1%; Eppy/N 2% eye drops (discontinued 1995) ℞ *antiglaucoma agent* [epinephrine borate] 1%; 2%

eprazinone INN

Eprex ℞ *(orphan: anemia of AIDS and ARC)* [epoetin alfa]

eprinomectin USAN *veterinary antiparasitic*

epristeride USAN *alpha reductase inhibitor for benign prostatic hypertrophy*

Epromate tablets (discontinued 1995) ℞ *analgesic; antipyretic; anti-inflammatory; anxiolytic* [aspirin; meprobamate] 325•200 mg

eprosartan USAN *antihypertensive (angiotensin II blocker)*

eprosartan mesylate USAN *antihypertensive (angiotensin II blocker)*

eprovafen INN

eproxindine INN

eprozinol INN

epsikapron [see: aminocaproic acid]

epsilon-aminocaproic acid (EACA) [see: aminocaproic acid]

epsiprantel INN, BAN

Epsom salt [see: magnesium sulfate]

e.p.t. Quick Stick test stick for home use OTC *in vitro diagnostic aid for urine pregnancy test*

eptaloprost INN

eptamestrol [see: etamestrol]

eptaprost [see: eptaloprost]

eptastatin sodium [see: pravastatin sodium]

eptastigmine INN *investigational treatment for Alzheimer's disease*

eptazocine INN

Equagesic tablets ℞ *analgesic; antipyretic; anti-inflammatory; anxiolytic* [aspirin; meprobamate] 325•200 mg

Equalactin chewable tablets OTC *bulk laxative; antidiarrheal* [calcium polycarbophil] 500 mg

Equanil tablets ℞ *anxiolytic* [meprobamate] 200, 400 mg ⓘ Elavil

Equazine M tablets (discontinued 1995) ℞ *analgesic; antipyretic; anti-inflammatory; anxiolytic* [aspirin; meprobamate] 325•200 mg

Equilet chewable tablets OTC *antacid* [calcium carbonate] 500 mg

equilin USP *estrogen*

Eramycin film-coated tablets ℞ *macrolide antibiotic* [erythromycin stearate] 250 mg

erbium *element (Er)*

erbulozole USAN, INN *antineoplastic adjunct*

erbumine USAN, INN, BAN *combining name for radicals or groups*

Ercaf tablets ℞ *migraine-specific vasoconstrictor* [ergotamine tartrate; caffeine] 1•100 mg

erdosteine INN

Ergamisol tablets ℞ *antineoplastic adjuvant for colon cancer* [levamisole HCl] 50 mg

ergocalciferol USP, INN, BAN, JAN *vitamin D_2; antirachitic* 50,000 IU oral

ergoloid mesylates USAN, USP *cognition adjuvant for age-related mental capacity decline* [also: co-dergocrine mesylate] 0.5, 1 mg oral

Ergomar sublingual tablets ℞ *agent for migraine; vasoconstrictor* [ergotamine tartrate] 2 mg

ergometrine INN, BAN *oxytocic* [also: ergonovine maleate]

ergonovine maleate USP *oxytocic* [also: ergometrine]

Ergostat sublingual tablets (discontinued 1996) ℞ *migraine-specific vasoconstrictor* [ergotamine tartrate] 2 mg

ergosterol, activated [see: ergocalciferol]

ergot alkaloids [see: ergoloid mesylates]

ergotamine INN, BAN *migraine-specific analgesic* [also: ergotamine tartrate]

ergotamine tartrate USP *migraine-specific analgesic* [also: ergotamine]

Ergotrate Maleate IM or IV injection ℞ *prevention of postpartum and postabortal hemorrhage* [ergonovine maleate] 0.2 mg/mL

Ergotrate Maleate tablets (discontinued 1995) ℞ *prevention of postpartum and postabortal hemorrhage* [ergonovine maleate] 0.2 mg

ericolol INN

Eridium tablets (discontinued 1996) ℞ *urinary analgesic* [phenazopyridine HCl] 100 mg

eriodictyon NF

eritrityl tetranitrate INN *coronary vasodilator* [also: erythrityl tetranitrate]

erizepine INN

E-R-O Ear Drops OTC *agent to emulsify and disperse ear wax* [carbamide peroxide] 6.5%

erocainide INN

ersofermin USAN, INN *wound healing agent*

Erwinase ℞ *investigational antineoplastic; (orphan: acute lymphocytic leukemia)* [erwinia L-asparaginase]

Erwinia L-asparaginase *investigational antineoplastic; (orphan: acute lymphocytic leukemia)*
ERYC delayed-release capsules containing enteric-coated pellets ℞ *macrolide antibiotic* [erythromycin] 250 mg ② ara-C
Erycette topical solution ℞ *topical antibiotic for acne* [erythromycin] 2%
EryDerm 2% topical solution ℞ *topical antibiotic for acne* [erythromycin] 2%
Erygel gel ℞ *topical antibiotic for acne* [erythromycin; alcohol 92%] 2%
Erymax topical solution ℞ *topical antibiotic for acne* [erythromycin] 2%
EryPed chewable tablets, granules for oral suspension, drops ℞ *macrolide antibiotic* [erythromycin ethylsuccinate] 200 mg; 400 mg/5 mL; 100 mg/2.5 mL
EryPed 200; EryPed 400 oral suspension ℞ *macrolide antibiotic* [erythromycin ethylsuccinate] 200 mg/5 mL; 400 mg/5 mL
Ery-Sol topical solution (discontinued 1995) ℞ *topical antibiotic for acne* [erythromycin] 2%
Ery-Tab enteric-coated delayed-release tablets ℞ *macrolide antibiotic* [erythromycin] 250, 333, 500 mg
erythorbic acid
Erythra-Derm topical solution ℞ *topical antibiotic for acne* [erythromycin] 2%
erythrityl tetranitrate USAN, USP *coronary vasodilator; antianginal* [also: eritrityl tetranitrate]
Erythrocin Stearate Filmtabs (film-coated tablets) ℞ *antibiotic* [erythromycin stearate] 250, 500 mg
erythrol tetranitrate [now: erythrityl tetranitrate]
erythromycin USP, INN, BAN *macrolide bactericidal/bacteriostatic antibiotic* 250, 333, 500 mg oral; 2% topical; 5 mg/g topical ② clarithromycin
erythromycin 2′-acetate octadecanoate [see: erythromycin acistrate]
erythromycin 2′-acetate stearate [see: erythromycin acistrate]
erythromycin acistrate USAN, INN *antibacterial*
erythromycin B [see: berythromycin]

erythromycin estolate USAN, USP, BAN *macrolide bactericidal/bacteriostatic antibiotic* 250 mg oral; 125, 250 mg/5 mL oral
erythromycin ethyl succinate BAN *antibacterial* [also: erythromycin ethylsuccinate]
erythromycin ethylcarbonate USP
erythromycin ethylsuccinate (EES) USP *macrolide bactericidal/bacteriostatic antibiotic* [also: erythromycin ethyl succinate] 400 mg oral; 200, 400 mg/5 mL oral;
erythromycin gluceptate USP *antibacterial*
erythromycin glucoheptonate [see: erythromycin gluceptate]
erythromycin lactobionate USP *macrolide bactericidal/bacteriostatic antibiotic* 500, 1000 mg/vial injection
erythromycin lauryl sulfate, propionyl [now: erythromycin estolate]
erythromycin monoglucoheptonate [see: erythromycin gluceptate]
erythromycin octadecanoate [see: erythromycin stearate]
erythromycin 2′-propanoate [see: erythromycin propionate]
erythromycin propionate USAN *antibacterial*
erythromycin 2′-propionate dodecyl sulfate [see: erythromycin estolate]
erythromycin propionate lauryl sulfate [now: erythromycin estolate]
erythromycin salnacedin USAN *antibiotic for acne vulgaris*
erythromycin stearate USP, BAN *macrolide bactericidal/bacteriostatic antibiotic* 250, 500 mg oral
erythromycin stinoprate INN
erythropoietin, recombinant human (rEPO) [see: epoetin alfa; epoetin beta]
erythrosine sodium USP *dental disclosing agent*
Eryzole granules for oral suspension ℞ *antibiotic* [erythromycin ethylsuccinate; sulfisoxazole acetyl] 200•600 mg/5 mL
esafloxacin INN
esaprazole INN

esculamine INN
E-Sel soft capsules OTC *vitamin/mineral supplement* [vitamin E; selenium methionine]
eseridine INN
eserine [see: physostigmine]
Eserine Salicylate eye drops (discontinued 1995) ℞ *antiglaucoma agent; reversible cholinesterase inhibitor miotic* [physostigmine salicylate] 0.5%
Eserine Sulfate ophthalmic ointment ℞ *antiglaucoma agent; reversible cholinesterase inhibitor miotic* [physostigmine sulfate] 0.25%
esflurbiprofen INN, BAN
Esgic tablets, capsules ℞ *analgesic; antipyretic; sedative* [acetaminophen; caffeine; butalbital] 325•40•50 mg
Esgic-Plus tablets ℞ *analgesic; antipyretic; sedative* [acetaminophen; caffeine; butalbital] 500•40•50 mg
ESHAP (etoposide, Solu-Medrol, high-dose ara-C, Platinol) *chemotherapy protocol*
ESHAP-MINE (alternating cycles of ESHAP and MINE) *chemotherapy protocol*
Esidrix tablets ℞ *diuretic; antihypertensive* [hydrochlorothiazide] 25, 50, 100 mg ② Lasix
esilate INN *combining name for radicals or groups* [also: esylate]
Esimil tablets ℞ *antihypertensive* [hydrochlorothiazide; guanethidine monosulfate] 25•10 mg ② Estinyl; Isomil
Eskalith capsules, tablets ℞ *antipsychotic* [lithium carbonate] 300 mg
Eskalith CR controlled-release tablets ℞ *antipsychotic* [lithium carbonate] 450 mg
esmolol INN, BAN *antiadrenergic (β-receptor)* [also: esmolol HCl]
esmolol HCl USAN *antiadrenergic (β-receptor)* [also: esmolol]
E-Solve OTC *lotion base*
E-Solve 2 topical solution (discontinued 1994) ℞ *topical antibiotic for acne vulgaris* [erythromycin]
Esophotrast oral suspension ℞ *esophageal contrast medium* [barium sulfate]
esorubicin INN *antineoplastic* [also: esorubicin HCl]

esorubicin HCl USAN *antineoplastic* [also: esorubicin]
Esotérica Dry Skin Treatment lotion OTC *moisturizer; emollient*
Esotérica Facial; Esotérica Fortified; Esotérica Sunscreen cream OTC *hyperpigmentation bleaching agent; sunscreen* [hydroquinone; padimate O; oxybenzone] 2%•3.3%•2.5%
Esotérica Regular; Esotérica Sensitive Skin Formula cream OTC *hyperpigmentation bleaching agent* [hydroquinone] 2%; 1.5%
Esotérica Soap OTC *bath emollient*
E.S.P. oral suspension ℞ *anti-infective; antibacterial* [erythromycin ethylsuccinate; sulfisoxazole acetyl]
esperamycin *investigational antineoplastic*
Espotabs tablets OTC *laxative* [yellow phenolphthalein] 97.2 mg
esproquin HCl USAN *adrenergic* [also: esproquine]
esproquine INN *adrenergic* [also: esproquin HCl]
Estar gel OTC *topical antipsoriatic; antiseborrheic* [coal tar] 5%
estazolam USAN, INN *hypnotic*
Ester-C Plus capsules OTC *dietary supplement* [vitamin C; calcium; various bioflavonoids; rutin] 500•62•45•5 mg
Ester-C Plus, Extra Potency tablets OTC *dietary supplement* [vitamin C; calcium; various bioflavonoids; rutin] 1000•125•250•25 mg
Ester-C Plus Multi-Mineral capsules OTC *dietary supplement* [vitamin C; multiple minerals; various bioflavonoids; rutin] 425• ± •75•5 mg
esterified estrogens [see: estrogens, esterified]
esterifilcon A USAN *hydrophilic contact lens material*
estilben [see: diethylstilbestrol dipropionate]
Estinyl tablets ℞ *hormone for estrogen replacement therapy or inoperable prostatic and breast cancer* [ethinyl estradiol] 0.02, 0.05, 0.5 mg ② Esimil
Estivin II eye drops (discontinued 1995) OTC *topical ocular decongestant/vasoconstrictor* [naphazoline HCl] 0.012%

estolate INN *combining name for radicals or groups*

estomycin sulfate [see: paromomycin sulfate]

Estrace tablets ℞ *estrogen replacement for postmenopausal disorders; antineoplastic for prostatic and breast cancer* [estradiol] 0.5, 1, 2 mg

Estrace vaginal cream ℞ *topical estrogen replacement for postmenopausal disorders* [estradiol] 0.1 mg/g

Estra-D IM injection (discontinued 1996) ℞ *hormone replacement therapy for postmenopausal disorders* [estradiol cypionate in oil] 5 mg/mL

Estraderm transdermal patch ℞ *estrogen replacement therapy for postmenopausal disorders* [estradiol] 50, 100 μg/day ② Estradurin

estradiol USP, INN *estrogen* [also: oestradiol] 0.5, 1, 2 mg oral

estradiol benzoate USP, INN, JAN [also: oestradiol benzoate]

estradiol 17-cyclopentanepropionate [see: estradiol cypionate]

estradiol cypionate USP *estrogen for hormone replacement therapy* 5 mg/mL injection (in oil)

estradiol dipropionate NF, JAN

estradiol enanthate USAN *estrogen*

estradiol 17-heptanoate [see: estradiol enanthate]

Estradiol L.A.; Estradiol L.A. 20; Estradiol L.A. 40 IM injection (discontinued 1994) ℞ *estrogen replacement therapy; antineoplastic for prostatic cancer* [estradiol valerate] 10 mg/mL; 20 mg/mL; 40 mg/mL

estradiol monobenzoate [see: estradiol benzoate]

estradiol 17-nicotinate 3-propionate [see: estrapronicate]

estradiol phosphate polymer [see: polyestradiol phosphate]

estradiol 17-undecanoate [see: estradiol undecylate]

estradiol undecylate USAN, INN *estrogen*

estradiol valerate USP, INN, JAN *estrogen replacement; hormonal antineoplastic for prostatic carcinoma* [also: oestradiol valerate] 10, 20, 40 mg/mL IM injection

Estradurin powder for IM injection (discontinued 1993) ℞ *hormonal therapy for inoperable progressing prostatic cancer* [polyestradiol phosphate] 40 mg ② Estraderm

Estra-L 20; Estra-L 40 IM injection ℞ *estrogen replacement therapy for postmenopausal disorders; antineoplastic for prostatic cancer* [estradiol valerate in oil] 20 mg/mL; 40 mg/mL

estramustine USAN, INN, BAN *antineoplastic*

estramustine L-alanine (EMA) *investigational antineoplastic for advanced prostatic cancer*

estramustine phosphate sodium USAN, BAN, JAN *hormonal antineoplastic for prostate cancer*

estrapronicate INN

Estratab tablets ℞ *estrogen replacement therapy; hypogonadism; inoperable prostatic and breast cancer* [esterified estrogens] 0.3, 0.625, 1.25, 2.5 mg ② Ethatab

Estratest; Estratest H.S. sugar-coated tablets ℞ *estrogen/androgen for menopausal vasomotor symptoms* [esterified estrogens; methyltestosterone] 1.25•2.5 mg; 0.625•1.25 mg

Estra-Testrin IM injection (discontinued 1995) ℞ *estrogen/androgen for menopausal vasomotor symptoms* [estradiol valerate; testosterone enanthate] 4•90 mg/mL

estrazinol INN *estrogen* [also: estrazinol hydrobromide]

estrazinol hydrobromide USAN *estrogen* [also: estrazinol]

Estrinex ℞ *investigational antiestrogen* (orphan: metastatic carcinoma of the breast; desmoid tumors)

Estring vaginal ring ℞ *three-month estrogen replacement therapy* [estradiol] 2 mg

estriol USP *estrogen* [also: estriol succinate; oestriol succinate]

estriol succinate INN *estrogen* [also: estriol; oestriol succinate]

estrobene [see: diethylstilbestrol]

estrobene DP [see: diethylstilbestrol dipropionate]

Estro-Cyp IM injection ℞ *hormone replacement therapy for postmenopausal disorders* [estradiol cypionate in oil] 5 mg/mL

estrofurate USAN, INN *estrogen*

Estrogenic Substance Aqueous IM injection ℞ *estrogen replacement therapy; antineoplastic for prostatic and breast cancer* [estrone and other estrogens] 2 mg/mL

estrogenic substances, conjugated [see: estrogens, conjugated]

estrogenine [see: diethylstilbestrol]

estrogens, conjugated USP, JAN *estrogen*

estrogens, esterified USP *estrogen*

Estroject-2 IM injection (discontinued 1992) ℞ *estrogen replacement therapy; antineoplastic for prostatic and breast cancer* [estrone] 2 mg/mL

Estroject-L.A. IM injection (discontinued 1995) ℞ *hormone for estrogen replacement therapy* [estradiol cypionate in oil] 5 mg/mL

estromenin [see: diethylstilbestrol]

estrone USP, INN *estrogen* [also: oestrone]

Estrone 5 IM injection ℞ *estrogen replacement therapy; antineoplastic for prostatic and breast cancer* [estrone] 5 mg/mL

Estrone Aqueous IM injection ℞ *estrogen replacement therapy; antineoplastic for prostatic and breast cancer* [estrone] 2, 5 mg/mL

estrone hydrogen sulfate [see: estrone sodium sulfate]

estrone sodium sulfate

Estronol injection (discontinued 1993) ℞ *estrogen replacement therapy; antineoplastic for prostatic and breast cancer* [estrone] 2 mg/mL

Estronol-LA injection (discontinued 1993) ℞ *estrogen* [estradiol cypionate]

estropipate USP *estrogen replacement therapy for postmenopausal disorders* 0.75, 1.5, 3 mg oral

Estrostep ℞ *investigational oral contraceptive*

Estrovis tablets (discontinued 1996) ℞ *hormone replacement therapy for postmenopausal disorders* [quinestrol] 100 μg

esuprone INN

esylate USAN, BAN *combining name for radicals or groups* [also: esilate]

etabenzarone INN

etabonate USAN, INN *combining name for radicals or groups*

etacepride INN

etacrynic acid INN, JAN *loop diuretic* [also: ethacrynic acid]

etafedrine INN, BAN *adrenergic* [also: etafedrine HCl]

etafedrine HCl USAN *adrenergic* [also: etafedrine]

etafenone INN

etafilcon A USAN *hydrophilic contact lens material*

etamestrol INN

etaminile INN

etamiphyllin INN [also: etamiphylline]

etamiphyllin methesculetol [see: metescufylline]

etamiphylline BAN [also: etamiphyllin]

etamivan INN *central and respiratory stimulant* [also: ethamivan]

etamocycline INN

etamsylate INN *hemostatic* [also: ethamsylate]

etanidazole USAN, INN *antineoplastic; hypoxic cell radiosensitizer*

etanterol INN

etaperazine [see: perphenazine]

etaqualone INN

etarotene USAN, INN *keratolytic*

etasuline INN

etazepine INN

etazolate INN *antipsychotic* [also: etazolate HCl]

etazolate HCl USAN *antipsychotic* [also: etazolate]

etebenecid INN [also: ethebenecid]

etenzamide BAN [also: ethenzamide]

eterobarb USAN, INN, BAN *anticonvulsant*

etersalate INN

ethacridine INN [also: ethacridine lactate; acrinol] ⑨ ethacrynic

ethacridine lactate [also: ethacridine; acrinol]

ethacrynate sodium USAN, USP *diuretic*

ethacrynic acid USAN, USP, BAN *loop diuretic* [also: etacrynic acid] ☒
ethacridine
ethambutol INN, BAN *bacteriostatic; primary tuberculostatic* [also: ethambutol HCl]
ethambutol HCl USAN, USP *bacteriostatic; primary tuberculostatic* [also: ethambutol]
ethamivan USAN, USP, BAN *central and respiratory stimulant* [also: etamivan]
Ethamolin IV injection ℞ *sclerosing agent; for bleeding esophageal varices (orphan)* [ethanolamine oleate] 5%
ethamsylate USAN, BAN *hemostatic* [also: etamsylate]
ethanol JAN *topical anti-infective/antiseptic; astringent; solvent* [also: alcohol]
ethanol, dehydrated JAN *antidote* [also: alcohol, dehydrated]
ethanolamine oleate USAN *sclerosing agent; for bleeding esophageal varices (orphan)* [also: monoethanolamine oleate]
Ethaquin tablets (discontinued 1996) ℞ *peripheral vasodilator* [ethaverine HCl] 100 mg ☒ Edecrin
Ethatab tablets (discontinued 1996) ℞ *peripheral vasodilator* [ethaverine HCl] 100 mg ☒ Estratab
ethaverine INN *peripheral vasodilator*
ethaverine HCl *peripheral vasodilator* [see: ethaverine]
Ethavex-100 tablets (discontinued 1996) ℞ *peripheral vasodilator* [ethaverine HCl] 100 mg
etchlorvynol USP, INN, BAN *sedative; hypnotic*
ethebenecid BAN [also: etebenecid]
ethenzamide INN, JAN [also: etenzamide]
ether USP *inhalation anesthetic*
ethiazide INN, BAN
ethidium bromide [see: homidium bromide]
ethinamate USP, INN, BAN *sedative; hypnotic* ☒ ethionamide
ethinyl estradiol USP *estrogen for hormone replacement therapy or breast and prostate cancer; (orphan: Turner syndrome)* [also: ethinylestradiol; ethinyloestradiol]
ethinylestradiol INN *estrogen* [also: ethinyl estradiol; ethinyloestradiol]
ethinyloestradiol BAN *estrogen* [also: ethinyl estradiol; ethinylestradiol]
ethiodized oil USP *radiopaque medium*
ethiodized oil (^{131}I) INN *antineoplastic; radioactive agent* [also: ethiodized oil I 131]
ethiodized oil I 131 USAN *antineoplastic; radioactive agent* [also: ethiodized oil (^{131}I)]
Ethiodol intracavitary instillation ℞ *hysterosalpingographic and lymphographic contrast medium* [ethiodized oil] 100% ☒ ethynodiol
ethiofos *(previously used USAN)* [now: amifostine]
ethionamide USAN, USP, INN, BAN *bacteriostatic; tuberculosis retreatment* ☒ ethinamate
ethisterone NF, INN, BAN
Ethmozine film-coated tablets ℞ *antiarrhythmic* [moricizine HCl] 200, 250, 300 mg
ethodryl [see: diethylcarbamazine citrate]
ethoglucid BAN [also: etoglucid]
ethoheptazine BAN [also: ethoheptazine citrate]
ethoheptazine citrate NF, INN [also: ethoheptazine]
ethohexadiol USP
ethomoxane INN, BAN
ethomoxane HCl [see: ethomoxane]
Ethon tablets (discontinued 1993) ℞ *diuretic; antihypertensive* [methyclothiazide]
ethonam nitrate USAN *antifungal* [also: etonam]
ethopabate BAN
ethopropazine BAN *antiparkinsonian* [also: ethopropazine HCl; profenamine]
ethopropazine HCl USP *antiparkinsonian; anticholinergic* [also: profenamine; ethopropazine]
ethosalamide BAN [also: etosalamide]
ethosuximide USAN, USP, INN, BAN *anticonvulsant* 250 mg/5 mL oral
ethotoin USP, INN, BAN *hydantoin-type anticonvulsant*
ethoxarutine [see: ethoxazorutoside]

ethoxazene HCl USAN *analgesic* [also: etoxazene]

ethoxazorutoside INN

ethoxyacetanilide *(withdrawn from market)* [see: phenacetin]

***o*-ethoxybenzamide** [see: ethenzamide; etenzamide]

ethoxzolamide USP

Ethrane liquid for vaporization ℞ *inhalation general anesthetic* [enflurane]

ethybenztropine USAN, BAN *anticholinergic* [also: etybenzatropine]

ethyl acetate NF *solvent*

ethyl alcohol (EtOH; ETOH) [now: alcohol; ethanol]

ethyl aminobenzoate (ethyl *p*-aminobenzoate) JAN *topical anesthetic; nonprescription diet aid* [also: benzocaine]

ethyl 2-benzimidazolecarbamate [see: lobendazole]

ethyl N-benzylcyclopropanecarbamate [see: encyprate]

ethyl biscoumacetate NF, INN, BAN

ethyl biscumacetate [see: ethyl biscoumacetate]

ethyl carbamate [now: urethane]

ethyl carfluzepate INN

ethyl cartrizoate INN

ethyl chloride USP *topical local anesthetic; topical vapo-coolant*

ethyl dibunate USAN, INN, BAN *antitussive*

ethyl dirazepate INN

ethyl ether [see: ether]

ethyl *p*-fluorophenyl sulfone [see: fluoresone]

ethyl *p*-hydroxybenzoate [see: ethylparaben]

ethyl loflazepate INN

ethyl nitrite NF

ethyl oleate NF *vehicle*

ethyl oxide [see: ether]

ethyl vanillin NF *flavoring agent*

ethylcellulose NF *tablet binder*

ethylchlordiphene [see: etofamide]

ethyldicoumarol [see: ethyl biscoumacetate]

ethylene NF *inhalation general anesthesia*

ethylene distearate [see: glycol distearate]

ethylenediamine USP, JAN

ethylenediaminetetraacetate [see: edetate disodium]

ethylenediaminetetraacetic acid (EDTA) [see: edetate disodium]

N,N-ethylenediarsanilic acid [see: difetarsone]

ethylenedinitrilotetraacetate disodium [see: edetate disodium]

ethylestrenol USAN, INN *anabolic* [also: ethyloestrenol]

ethylhexanediol [see: ethohexadiol]

2-ethylhexyl diphenyl phosphate [see: octicizer]

ethylhydrocupreine HCl NF

ethylmethylthiambutene INN, BAN

ethylmorphine BAN [also: ethylmorphine HCl]

ethylmorphine HCl NF [also: ethylmorphine]

ethylnorepinephrine HCl USP *bronchodilator*

ethyloestradiol BAN *estrogen* [also: ethinyl estradiol]

ethyloestrenol BAN *anabolic* [also: ethylestrenol]

ethylpapaverine HCl [see: ethaverine HCl]

ethylparaben NF *antifungal agent*

ethylphenacemide [see: pheneturide]

ethylstibamine [see: stibosamine]

2-ethylthioisonicotinamide [see: ethionamide]

ethynerone USAN, INN *progestin*

ethynodiol BAN *progestin* [also: ethynodiol diacetate; etynodiol] ⑨ Ethiodol

ethynodiol diacetate USAN, USP *progestin* [also: etynodiol; ethynodiol]

Ethyol powder for IV infusion ℞ *chemoprotective agent for cisplatin and paclitaxel chemotherapy (orphan)* [amifostine] 500 mg/vial

ethypicone INN

ethypropymal sodium [see: probarbital sodium]

etibendazole USAN, INN *anthelmintic*

eticlopride INN

eticyclidine INN

etidocaine USAN, INN, BAN *injectable local anesthetic*

etidocaine HCl *injectable local anesthetic*

etidronate disodium USAN, USP *calcium regulator (orphan: hypercalcemia of malignancy; metabolic bone disease)*

etidronate monosodium

etidronate sodium (*this term used only when the form of sodium cannot be more accurately identified*)

etidronate tetrasodium

etidronate trisodium

etidronic acid USAN, INN, BAN *calcium regulator*

etifelmine INN

etifenin USAN, INN, BAN *diagnostic aid*

etifoxin BAN [also: etifoxine]

etifoxine INN [also: etifoxin]

etilamfetamine INN

etilefrine INN

etilefrine pivalate INN

etintidine INN *antagonist to histamine H_2 receptors* [also: etintidine HCl]

etintidine HCl USAN *antagonist to histamine H_2 receptors* [also: etintidine]

etipirium iodide INN

etiproston INN

etiracetam INN

etiroxate INN

etisazole INN, BAN

etisomicin INN, BAN

etisulergine INN

etizolam INN

etobedolum [see: etonitazene]

etocarlide INN

etocrilene INN *ultraviolet screen* [also: etocrylene]

etocrylene USAN *ultraviolet screen* [also: etocrilene]

etodolac USAN, INN, BAN *antiarthritic; nonsteroidal anti-inflammatory drug (NSAID); analgesic* [also: etodolic acid]

etodolic acid INN *antiarthritic; nonsteroidal anti-inflammatory drug (NSAID); analgesic* [also: etodolac]

etodroxizine INN

etofamide INN

etofenamate USAN, INN, BAN *analgesic; anti-inflammatory*

etofenprox INN

etofibrate INN

etoformin INN *antidiabetic* [also: etoformin HCl]

etoformin HCl USAN *antidiabetic* [also: etoformin]

etofuradine INN

etofylline INN

etofylline clofibrate INN *antihyperlipoproteinemic* [also: theofibrate]

etoglucid INN [also: ethoglucid]

EtOH; ETOH (ethyl alcohol) [now: alcohol]

etolorex INN

etolotifen INN

etoloxamine INN

etomidate USAN, INN, BAN *general anesthetic; hypnotic*

etomidoline INN

etomoxir INN

etonam INN *antifungal* [also: ethonam nitrate]

etonam nitrate [see: ethonam nitrate]

etonitazene INN, BAN

etonogestrel USAN, INN *progestin*

etoperidone INN *antidepressant* [also: etoperidone HCl]

etoperidone HCl USAN *antidepressant* [also: etoperidone]

etophylate [see: acepifylline]

Etopophos IV injection ℞ *antineoplastic for testicular and small cell lung cancers* [etoposide phosphate] 119.3 mg/vial

etoposide USAN, INN, BAN *antineoplastic* 20, 30 mg/mL injection

etoposide phosphate USAN *antineoplastic*

etoprindole INN

etoprine USAN *antineoplastic*

etorphine INN, BAN

etosalamide INN [also: ethosalamide]

etoxadrol INN *anesthetic* [also: etoxadrol HCl]

etoxadrol HCl USAN *anesthetic* [also: etoxadrol]

etoxazene INN *analgesic* [also: ethoxazene HCl]

etoxazene HCl [see: ethoxazene HCl]

etoxeridine INN, BAN

etozolin USAN, INN *diuretic*

etrabamine INN

Etrafon; Etrafon 2–10; Etrafon-A; Etrafon-Forte tablets ℞ *antipsychotic; antidepressant* [perphenazine;

amitriptyline HCl] 2•25 mg; 2•10 mg; 4•10 mg; 4•25 mg

etretin [see: acitretin]

etretinate USAN, INN, BAN, JAN *systemic antipsoriatic*

etryptamine INN, BAN *CNS stimulant* [also: etryptamine acetate]

etryptamine acetate USAN *CNS stimulant* [also: etryptamine]

ETS-2% topical solution (name changed to Erythra-Derm in 1994)

etybenzatropine INN *anticholinergic* [also: ethybenztropine]

etymemazine INN

etymemazine HCl [see: etymemazine]

etynodiol INN *progestin* [also: ethynodiol diacetate; ethynodiol]

etyprenaline [see: isoetharine]

eucaine HCl NF

Eucalyptamint ointment, gel OTC *counterirritant; topical antiseptic* [menthol; eucalyptus oil] 16%•?; 8%•?

eucalyptol USAN *topical bacteriostatic antiseptic/germicidal*

eucalyptus oil NF *topical antiseptic*

eucatropine INN, BAN *ophthalmic anticholinergic* [also: eucatropine HCl]

eucatropine HCl USP *ophthalmic anticholinergic* [also: eucatropine]

Eucerin cream, lotion OTC *moisturizer; emollient*

Eucerin OTC *cream base*

Eucerin Cleansing lotion (discontinued 1994) OTC *cleanser; moisturizer; emollient*

Eucerin Plus lotion OTC *moisturizer; emollient*

eucodal [see: oxycodone]

Eudal-SR sustained-release tablets ℞ *decongestant; expectorant* [pseudoephedrine HCl; guaifenesin] 120•400 mg

euflavine [see: acriflavine]

eugenol USP *dental analgesic*

eukadol [see: oxycodone]

Eulexin capsules ℞ *adjunctive hormonal chemotherapy for metastatic prostatic cancer* [flutamide] 125 mg

euprocin INN *topical anesthetic* [also: euprocin HCl]

euprocin HCl USAN *topical anesthetic* [also: euprocin]

euquinine [see: quinine ethylcarbonate]

Eurax cream, lotion ℞ *scabicide; antipruritic* [crotamiton] 10% ? Serax; Urex

europium *element (Eu)*

Euthroid tablets (discontinued 1992) ℞ *thyroid hormone therapy* [liotrix] 30, 60, 120, 180 mg ? Synthroid; thyroid

EVA (etoposide, vinblastine, Adriamycin) *chemotherapy protocol*

Evac-Q-Kit oral solution + 2 tablets + 2 suppositories OTC *pre-procedure bowel evacuant* [Evac-Q-Mag (q.v.); Evac-Q-Tabs (q.v.); Evac-Q-Sert (q.v.)] ? Evac-Q-Kwik

Evac-Q-Kwik suppositories OTC *laxative* [bisacodyl] 10 mg ? Evac-Q-Kit

Evac-Q-Kwik Kit oral solution + 2 tablets + 1 suppository OTC *pre-procedure bowel evacuant* [Evac-Q-Mag (q.v.); Evac-Q-Tabs (q.v.); Evac-Q-Kwik suppository (q.v.)]

Evac-Q-Mag carbonated oral solution OTC *laxative* [magnesium citrate; citric acid; potassium citrate]

Evac-Q-Sert suppositories OTC *laxative* [sodium bicarbonate; potassium bitartrate]

Evac-Q-Tabs tablets OTC *laxative* [phenolphthalein] 130 mg

Evac-U-Gen chewable tablets OTC *laxative* [yellow phenolphthalein] 97.2 mg

Evac-U-Lax chewable wafers OTC *laxative* [phenolphthalein] 80 mg

Evalose syrup ℞ *laxative* [lactulose] 10 g/15 mL

evandamine INN

Evans blue USP *blood volume test* [also: azovan blue] 5 mL injection

Everone 100 IM injection (discontinued 1994) ℞ *androgen replacement for delayed puberty or breast cancer* [testosterone enanthate] 100 mg/mL

Everone 200 IM injection ℞ *androgen replacement for delayed puberty or breast cancer* [testosterone enanthate] 200 mg/mL

E-Vista IM injection ℞ *anxiolytic* [hydroxyzine HCl] 50 mg/mL

E-Vital cream (discontinued 1992) OTC *moisturizer; emollient; vulnerary* [vitamins D and E; panthenol; allantoin]

E-Vitamin ointment OTC *emollient* [vitamin E] 30 mg/g

E-Vitamin Succinate capsules OTC *vitamin supplement* [vitamin E] 165, 330 mg

E-VMAC (escalated methotrexate, vinblastine, Adriamycin, cisplatin) *chemotherapy protocol*

E-VMAC (escalated methotrexate, vinblastine, Adriamycin, cyclophosphamide) *chemotherapy protocol*

Exact liquid OTC *topical keratolytic cleanser for acne* [salicylic acid] 2%

Exact vanishing cream OTC *topical keratolytic for acne* [benzoyl peroxide] 5%

exalamide INN

exametazime USAN, INN, BAN *regional cerebral perfusion imaging aid*

exaprolol INN *antiadrenergic (β-receptor)* [also: exaprolol HCl]

exaprolol HCl USAN *antiadrenergic (β-receptor)* [also: exaprolol]

Excedrin caplets, tablets, geltabs OTC *analgesic; antipyretic; anti-inflammatory* [acetaminophen; aspirin; caffeine] 250•250•65 mg

Excedrin, Aspirin Free caplets, geltabs OTC *analgesic; antipyretic* [acetaminophen; caffeine] 500•65 mg

Excedrin, Sinus tablets, caplets OTC *decongestant; analgesic; antipyretic* [pseudoephedrine HCl; acetaminophen] 30•500 mg

Excedrin Dual, Aspirin Free film-coated caplets OTC *analgesic; antipyretic; antacid* [acetaminophen; calcium carbonate; magnesium carbonate; magnesium oxide] 500•111•64•30 mg

Excedrin IB tablets, caplets (discontinued 1995) OTC *nonsteroidal anti-inflammatory drug (NSAID); antiarthritic; analgesic* [ibuprofen] 200 mg

Excedrin P.M. liquid, liquigels OTC *antihistaminic sleep aid; analgesic* [diphenhydramine HCl; acetaminophen] 50•1000 mg/30 mL; 25•500 mg

Excedrin P.M. tablets, caplets OTC *antihistaminic sleep aid; analgesic* [diphenhydramine citrate; acetaminophen] 38•500 mg

Excegran ℞ *investigational anticonvulsant* [zonisamide]

Excita Extra premedicated condom OTC *spermicidal/barrier contraceptive* [nonoxynol 9] 8%

Exelderm cream (discontinued 1993) ℞ *topical antifungal* [sulconazole nitrate] 1%

Exelderm solution ℞ *topical antifungal* [sulconazole nitrate] 1%

exemestane INN *investigational hormonal antineoplastic for advanced breast cancer*

exepanol INN

Exgest LA long-acting tablets ℞ *decongestant; expectorant* [phenylpropanolamine HCl; guaifenesin] 75•400 mg

Exidine Skin Cleanser; Exidine-2 Scrub; Exidine-4 Scrub liquid OTC *broad-spectrum antimicrobial; germicidal* [chlorhexidine gluconate; alcohol 4%] 4%; 2%; 4%

exifone INN

exiproben INN

Ex-Lax chocolated chewable tablets OTC *laxative* [yellow phenolphthalein] 90 mg

Ex-Lax Extra Gentle Pills tablets OTC *laxative; stool softener* [phenolphthalein; docusate sodium] 65•75 mg

Ex-Lax Gentle Nature tablets OTC *laxative* [sennosides] 20 mg

Ex-Lax Maximum Relief; Ex-Lax Unflavored tablets OTC *laxative* [yellow phenolphthalein] 135 mg; 90 mg

Exna tablets ℞ *diuretic; antihypertensive* [benzthiazide] 50 mg

Exocaine Medicated Rub; Exocaine Plus Rub OTC *counterirritant* [methyl salicylate] 25%; 30%

Exocaine Odor Free Creme (discontinued 1993) OTC *topical analgesic* [trolamine salicylate] 10%

Exosurf ℞ *investigational agent for adult respiratory distress syndrome* [colfosceril palmitate]

Exosurf Neonatal powder for injection; intratracheal suspension (orphan) ℞ *pulmonary surfactant; for hyaline membrane disease and respiratory distress syndrome (orphan)* [colfosceril palmitate] 108 mg

Exovir-HZ gel ℞ *investigational treatment for recurrent genital herpes*

Expidet (trademarked dosage form) *fast-dissolving dose*

Exsel lotion/shampoo ℞ *antiseborrheic; antifungal* [selenium sulfide] 2.5%

exsiccated sodium arsenate [see: sodium arsenate, exsiccated]

Extencap (trademarked dosage form) *extended-release capsule*

extended insulin zinc [see: insulin zinc, extended]

Extendryl chewable tablets, syrup ℞ *decongestant; antihistamine; anticholinergic* [phenylephrine HCl; chlorpheniramine maleate; methscopolamine nitrate] 10•2•1.25 mg; 10•2•1.25 mg/5 mL

Extendryl JR sustained-release capsules ℞ *pediatric decongestant, antihistamine, and anticholinergic* [phenylephrine HCl; chlorpheniramine maleate; methscopolamine nitrate] 10•4•1.25 mg

Extendryl SR sustained-release capsules ℞ *decongestant; antihistamine; anticholinergic* [phenylephrine HCl; chlorpheniramine maleate; methscopolamine nitrate] 20•8•2.5 mg

Extentab (trademarked dosage form) *extended-release tablet*

Extenzyme Protein Cleaner tablets (discontinued 1992) OTC *enzymatic cleaner for soft contact lenses*

Extra Action Cough syrup OTC *antitussive; expectorant* [dextromethorphan hydrobromide; guaifenesin; alcohol 1.4%] 10•100 mg/5 mL

"Extra Strength" products [see under product name]

Extreme Cold Formula caplets (discontinued 1993) OTC *decongestant; antihistamine; analgesic; antitussive* [phenylpropanolamine HCl; chlorpheniramine maleate; acetaminophen; dextromethorphan hydrobromide]

Eye Drops OTC *topical ocular decongestant/vasoconstrictor* [tetrahydrozoline HCl] 0.05%

Eye Irrigating Solution OTC *extraocular irrigating solution* [sterile isotonic solution]

Eye Irrigating Wash OTC *extraocular irrigating solution* [sterile isotonic solution]

Eye Scrub solution OTC *eyelid cleanser for blepharitis or contact lenses*

Eye Stream ophthalmic solution OTC *extraocular irrigating solution* [sterile isotonic solution]

Eye Wash ophthalmic solution OTC *extraocular irrigating solution* [sterile isotonic solution]

Eye-Lube-A eye drops OTC *ocular moisturizer/lubricant* [glycerin] 0.25%

Eye-Sed eye drops OTC *ophthalmic astringent* [zinc sulfate] 0.25%

Eyesine eye drops OTC *topical ocular decongestant/vasoconstrictor* [tetrahydrozoline HCl] 0.05%

EZ Detect test kit for home use OTC *in vitro diagnostic aid for fecal occult blood*

EZ Detect test kit for home use (discontinued 1995) OTC *in vitro diagnostic aid for urine occult blood*

EZ Detect Strep-A swab test for professional use (discontinued 1995) *in vitro diagnostic aid for streptococci*

Ezide tablets ℞ *diuretic; antihypertensive* [hydrochlorothiazide] 50 mg

F

1 + 1-F Creme ℞ *topical corticosteroid; antifungal; antibacterial; local anesthetic* [hydrocortisone; clioquinol; pramoxine] 1%•3%•1%

^{18}**F** [see: fludeoxyglucose F 18]

^{18}**F** [see: sodium fluoride F 18]

FABRase ℞ (*orphan: Fabry's disease*) [alpha-galactosidase A]

FAC (fluorouracil, Adriamycin, cyclophosphamide) *chemotherapy protocol*

FAC-LEV (fluorouracil, Adriamycin, Cytoxin, levamisole) *chemotherapy protocol*

FAC-M (fluorouracil, Adriamycin, cyclophosphamide, methotrexate) *chemotherapy protocol*

Fact Plus test kit for home use OTC *in vitro diagnostic aid for urine pregnancy test*

factor II (prothrombin)

factor III [see: thromboplastin]

factor VIIa, recombinant, DNA origin *(orphan: hemophilia A and B; von Willebrand's disease)*

factor VIII [see: antihemophilic factor]

factor VIII (rDNA) BAN *blood coagulating factor*

factor VIII, fraction A BAN *blood coagulating factor*

factor IX complex USP *hemostatic; antihemophilic; for hemophilia B (orphan)* [also: factor IX fraction]

factor IX fraction BAN *hemostatic; antihemophilic* [also: factor IX complex]

factor XIII (placenta-derived) *(orphan: congenital factor XIII deficiency)*

factor XIII, recombinant *(orphan: congenital factor XIII deficiency)*

Factrel powder for subcu or IV injection ℞ *gonadotropin releasing hormone* [gonadorelin HCl] 100, 500 μg

fadrozole INN *antineoplastic; aromatase inhibitor* [also: fadrozole HCl]

fadrozole HCl USAN *antineoplastic; aromatase inhibitor* [also: fadrozole]

falintolol INN

falipamil INN

FAM (fluorouracil, Adriamycin, mitomycin) *chemotherapy protocol*

FAM-CF (fluorouracil, Adriamycin, mitomycin, citrovorum factor) *chemotherapy protocol*

famciclovir USAN, INN, BAN *antiviral for herpes simplex and zoster*

FAME; FAMe (fluorouracil, Adriamycin, MeCCNU) *chemotherapy protocol*

Family Tabs tablets (discontinued 1995) OTC *vitamin supplement* [multiple vitamins; folic acid] ≚•0.4 mg

Familytabs with Calcium, Iron & Zinc tablets (discontinued 1995) OTC *vitamin/mineral supplement* [multiple vitamins; calcium carbonate; ferrous fumarate; zinc oxide]

Familytabs with Iron tablets (discontinued 1995) OTC *vitamin/iron supplement* [multiple vitamins; iron]

famiraprinium chloride INN

FAMMe (fluorouracil, Adriamycin, mitomycin, MeCCNU) *chemotherapy protocol*

famotidine USAN, USP, INN, BAN *treatment of GI ulcers; histamine H_2 antagonist*

famotine INN *antiviral* [also: famotine HCl]

famotine HCl USAN *antiviral* [also: famotine]

fampridine USAN *(orphan: multiple sclerosis)*

famprofazone INN, BAN

FAM-S (fluorouracil, Adriamycin, mitomycin, streptozocin) *chemotherapy protocol*

FAMTX (fluorouracil, Adriamycin, methotrexate [with leucovorin rescue]) *chemotherapy protocol*

Famvir film-coated tablets ℞ *antiviral for acute herpes zoster and genital herpes* [famciclovir] 125, 250, 500 mg

fanetizole INN, BAN *immunoregulator* [also: fanetizole mesylate]

fanetizole mesylate USAN *immunoregulator* [also: fanetizole]

Fansidar tablets (discontinued 1996) ℞ *antimalarial* [sulfadoxine; pyrimethamine] 500•25 mg

fanthridone BAN *antidepressant* [also: fantridone HCl; fantridone]

fantridone INN *antidepressant* [also: fantridone HCl; fanthridone]

fantridone HCl USAN *antidepressant* [also: fantridone; fanthridone]

FAP (fluorouracil, Adriamycin, Platinol) *chemotherapy protocol*

Farbee with Vitamin C caplets OTC *vitamin supplement* [multiple B vitamins; vitamin C] ≚•300 mg

Farmorubicin ℞ *investigational antibiotic antineoplastic for multiple*

myeloma, leukemia, lymphoma and other tumors [epirubicin HCl]

farnesil INN *combining name for radicals or groups*

fasiplon INN

Faspak (trademarked form) *flexible plastic bag*

Fastin capsules ℞ *amphetamine-type anorectic* [phentermine HCl] 30 mg

Fast-Trak (trademarked delivery system) *quick-loading syringe*

fat, hard NF *suppository base*

fat emulsion, intravenous *parenteral essential fatty acid replacement*

Father John's Medicine Plus liquid OTC *antitussive; decongestant; antihistamine; expectorant* [dextromethorphan hydrobromide; phenylephrine HCl; chlorpheniramine maleate; guaifenesin; ammonium chloride] 7.5•2.5•1•30•83.3 mg/5 mL

fazadinium bromide INN, BAN

fazarabine USAN, INN *antineoplastic*

5-FC (5-fluorocytosine) [see: flucytosine]

FCAP (fluorouracil, cyclophosphamide, Adriamycin, Platinol) *chemotherapy protocol*

FCE (fluorouracil, cisplatin, etoposide) *chemotherapy protocol*

F-CL (fluorouracil, leucovorin calcium [rescue]) *chemotherapy protocol* [also: FU/LV]

FCP (fluorouracil, cyclophosphamide, prednisone) *chemotherapy protocol*

FD&C Red No. 2 (Food, Drug & Cosmetic Act) [see: amaranth]

FD&C Red No. 3 (Food, Drug & Cosmetic Act) [see: erythrosine sodium]

[18]FDG (fludeoxyglucose) [see: fludeoxyglucose F 18]

[59]Fe [see: ferric chloride Fe 59]

[59]Fe [see: ferric citrate (^{59}Fe)]

[59]Fe [see: ferrous citrate Fe 59]

[59]Fe [see: ferrous sulfate Fe 59]

febantel USAN, INN, BAN *veterinary anthelmintic*

febarbamate INN

Febrol sugar-free liquid OTC *analgesic* [acetaminophen]

Febrol EX sugar-free liquid OTC *analgesic* [acetaminophen]

febuprol INN

febuverine INN

FEC (fluorouracil, epirubicin, cyclophosphamide) *chemotherapy protocol*

feclemine INN

feclobuzone INN

FED (fluorouracil, etoposide, DDP) *chemotherapy protocol*

Fedahist tablets OTC *decongestant; antihistamine* [pseudoephedrine HCl; chlorpheniramine maleate] 60•4 mg

Fedahist Timecaps (timed-release capsules), Gyrocaps (extended-release capsules) ℞ *decongestant; antihistamine* [pseudoephedrine HCl; chlorpheniramine maleate] 120•8 mg; 65•10 mg

Fedahist Decongestant syrup (discontinued 1994) OTC *decongestant; antihistamine* [pseudoephedrine HCl; chlorpheniramine maleate] 30•2 mg/5 mL

Fedahist Expectorant pediatric drops (discontinued 1995) OTC *decongestant; expectorant* [pseudoephedrine HCl; guaifenesin] 7.5•40 mg/mL

Fedahist Expectorant syrup OTC *decongestant; expectorant* [pseudoephedrine HCl; guaifenesin] 20•200 mg/5 mL

fedotozine INN *investigational kappa selective opioid agonist for irritable bowel syndrome*

fedrilate INN

Feen-A-Mint chocolated chewable tablets OTC *laxative* [yellow phenolphthalein] 65 mg

Feen-A-Mint tablets, chewable tablets, gum OTC *laxative* [yellow phenolphthalein] 97.2 mg

Feen-A-Mint Pills tablets OTC *laxative; stool softener* [phenolphthalein; docusate sodium] 65•100 mg

Feiba VH Immuno IV injection or drip ℞ *antihemophilic to correct factor VIII deficiency and coagulation deficiency* [anti-inhibitor coagulant complex] ≟

felbamate USAN, INN *antiepileptic; for Lennox-Gastaut syndrome* (orphan)

Felbamyl ℞ (*orphan: Lennox-Gastaut syndrome*) [felbamate]

Felbatol tablets, oral suspension (the FDA and the manufacturer recommend discontinuing use due to adverse side effects) ℞ *anticonvulsant; for Lennox-Gastaut syndrome (orphan); investigational neuroprotectant* [felbamate] 400, 600 mg; 600 mg/5 mL

felbinac USAN, INN, BAN *anti-inflammatory*

Feldene capsules ℞ *nonsteroidal anti-inflammatory drug (NSAID); antiarthritic* [piroxicam] 10, 20 mg

Feldene Melt ℞ *investigational instantaneously dissolving form* [piroxicam]

felipyrine INN

felodipine USAN, INN, BAN *vasodilator; antihypertensive; calcium channel blocker*

felypressin USAN, INN, BAN *vasoconstrictor*

Femaston ℞ *investigational treatment for menopausal symptoms* [estrogen; progestogen]

Femazole tablets (discontinued 1992) ℞ *antibiotic; antiprotozoal; amebicide* [metronidazole]

FemCal tablets OTC *calcium supplement* [calcium carbonate; vitamin D; multiple minerals] 250 mg•100 IU•≟

Femcaps tablets OTC *analgesic; muscle relaxant; for menstrual pain and cramps* [atropine sulfate; ephedrine sulfate; caffeine; acetaminophen]

FemCare vaginal cream, tablets OTC *antifungal* [clotrimazole] 1%; 100 mg

Femcet capsules ℞ *analgesic; antipyretic; sedative* [acetaminophen; caffeine; butalbital] 325•40•50 mg

Fem-Etts tablets OTC *analgesic; anti-inflammatory; diuretic* [acetaminophen; pamabrom] 325•25 mg

Femicine vaginal suppositories OTC *for vaginal irritations, itching, and burning* [pulsatilla 28x]

Femidine Douche solution (discontinued 1995) OTC *antiseptic/germicidal; vaginal cleanser and deodorizer* [povidone-iodine]

Femilax tablets OTC *laxative; stool softener* [phenolphthalein; docusate sodium] 65•100 mg

Feminique Disposable Douche solution OTC *antiseptic/antifungal; vaginal cleanser and deodorizer; acidity modifier* [sodium benzoate; sorbic acid; lactic acid]

Feminique Disposable Douche solution OTC *vaginal cleanser and deodorizer; acidity modifier* [vinegar (acetic acid)]

Feminone tablets (discontinued 1993) ℞ *estrogen deficiency; inoperable prostatic and breast cancer* [ethinyl estradiol]

Femiron tablets OTC *hematinic* [ferrous fumarate] 63 mg

Femiron Multi-Vitamins and Iron tablets OTC *vitamin/iron supplement* [multiple vitamins; ferrous fumarate; folic acid] ≟•20•0.4 mg

femoxetine INN

FemPatch transdermal patch ℞ *investigational agent for estrogen replacement therapy* [estradiol]

Femstat vaginal cream (discontinued 1995) ℞ *antifungal* [butoconazole nitrate] 2%

Femstat 3 vaginal cream in prefilled applicator OTC *antifungal* [butoconazole nitrate] 2%

Femstat Prefill (prefilled applicator) (discontinued 1993) ℞ *antifungal* [butoconazole nitrate]

fenabutene INN

fenacetinol INN

fenaclon INN

fenadiazole INN

fenaftic acid INN

fenalamide USAN, INN *smooth muscle relaxant*

fenalcomine INN

fenamifuril INN

fenamisal INN *antibacterial; tuberculostatic* [also: phenyl aminosalicylate]

fenamole USAN, INN *anti-inflammatory*

fenaperone INN

fenarsone [see: carbarsone]

fenasprate [see: benorilate]

fenbendazole USAN, INN, BAN *anthelmintic*

fenbenicillin INN [also: phenbenicillin]

fenbufen USAN, INN, BAN *anti-inflammatory*

fenbutrazate INN [also: phenbutrazate]

fencamfamin INN, BAN

fencamfamin HCl [see: fencamfamin]

fencarbamide INN *anticholinergic* [also: phencarbamide]
fenchlorphos BAN *systemic insecticide* [also: ronnel; fenclofos]
fencilbutirol USAN, INN *choleretic*
fenclexonium metilsulfate INN
fenclofenac USAN, INN, BAN *anti-inflammatory*
fenclofos INN *systemic insecticide* [also: ronnel; fenchlorphos]
fenclonine USAN, INN *serotonin inhibitor*
fenclorac USAN, INN *anti-inflammatory*
fenclozic acid INN, BAN
fendiline INN
fendizoate INN *combining name for radicals or groups*
Fendol tablets OTC *decongestant; expectorant; analgesic; antipyretic* [phenylephrine HCl; acetaminophen; salicylamide; caffeine]
fendosal USAN, INN, BAN *anti-inflammatory*
feneritrol INN
Fenesin sustained-release tablets ℞ *expectorant* [guaifenesin] 600 mg
Fenesin DM tablets ℞ *antitussive; expectorant* [dextromethorphan hydrobromide; guaifenesin] 30•600 mg
fenestrel USAN, INN *estrogen*
fenethazine INN
fenethylline BAN *CNS stimulant* [also: fenethylline HCl; fenetylline]
fenethylline HCl USAN *CNS stimulant* [also: fenetylline; fenethylline]
fenetradil INN
fenetylline INN *CNS stimulant* [also: fenethylline HCl; fenethylline]
fenflumizole INN
fenfluramine INN, BAN *anorexiant; CNS depressant* [also: fenfluramine HCl]
fenfluramine HCl USAN *anorexiant; CNS depressant* [also: fenfluramine]
fenfluthrin INN, BAN
fengabine USAN, INN, BAN *mood regulator*
fenharmane INN
fenimide USAN, INN, BAN *antipsychotic*
feniodium chloride INN
fenipentol INN
fenirofibrate INN
fenisorex USAN, INN, BAN *anorectic*
fenleuton USAN *5-lipoxygenase inhibitor*

fenmetozole INN *antidepressant; narcotic antagonist* [also: fenmetozole HCl]
fenmetozole HCl USAN *antidepressant; narcotic antagonist* [also: fenmetozole]
fenmetramide USAN, INN, BAN *antidepressant*
fennel oil NF
fenobam USAN, INN *sedative*
fenocinol INN
fenoctimine INN *gastric antisecretory* [also: fenoctimine sulfate]
fenoctimine sulfate USAN *gastric antisecretory* [also: fenoctimine]
fenofibrate INN, BAN *antihyperlipidemic for hypertriglyceridemia*
fenoldopam INN, BAN *antihypertensive; dopamine agonist* [also: fenoldopam mesylate]
fenoldopam mesylate USAN *antihypertensive; dopamine agonist* [also: fenoldopam]
fenoprofen USAN, INN, BAN *nonsteroidal anti-inflammatory drug (NSAID); analgesic*
fenoprofen calcium USAN, USP, BAN *antiarthritic; nonsteroidal anti-inflammatory drug (NSAID); analgesic* 200, 300, 600 mg oral
fenoterol USAN, INN, BAN *bronchodilator* [also: fenoterol hydrobromide]
fenoterol hydrobromide JAN *bronchodilator* [also: fenoterol]
fenoverine INN
fenoxazol [see: pemoline]
fenoxazoline INN
fenoxazoline HCl [see: fenoxazoline]
fenoxedil INN
fenoxypropazine INN [also: phenoxypropazine]
fenozolone INN
fenpentadiol INN
fenperate INN
fenpipalone USAN, INN *anti-inflammatory*
fenpipramide INN, BAN
fenpiprane INN, BAN
fenpiprane HCl [see: fenpiprane]
fenpiverinium bromide INN
fenprinast INN *bronchodilator; antiallergic* [also: fenprinast HCl]
fenprinast HCl USAN *bronchodilator; antiallergic* [also: fenprinast]

fenproporex INN
fenprostalene USAN, INN, BAN *luteolysin*
fenquizone USAN, INN *diuretic*
fenretinide USAN, INN *antineoplastic*
fenspiride INN *bronchodilator; antiadrenergic (α-receptor)* [also: fenspiride HCl]
fenspiride HCl USAN *bronchodilator; antiadrenergic (α-receptor)* [also: fenspiride]
fentanyl INN, BAN *narcotic analgesic* [also: fentanyl citrate]
fentanyl citrate USAN, USP, JAN *narcotic analgesic* [also: fentanyl] 0.05 mg/mL injection
Fentanyl Oralet lozenges ℞ *narcotic analgesic* [fentanyl] 200, 300, 400 μg
fenthion BAN
fentiazac USAN, INN, BAN *anti-inflammatory*
fenticlor USAN, INN, BAN *topical anti-infective*
fenticonazole INN, BAN *antifungal* [also: fenticonazole nitrate]
fenticonazole nitrate USAN *antifungal* [also: fenticonazole]
fentonium bromide INN
fenyramidol INN *analgesic; skeletal muscle relaxant* [also: phenyramidol HCl]
fenyripol INN *skeletal muscle relaxant* [also: fenyripol HCl]
fenyripol HCl USAN *skeletal muscle relaxant* [also: fenyripol]
Feocyte prolonged-action tablets ℞ *hematinic* [ferrous fumarate, ferrous gluconate, and ferrous sulfate; desiccated liver; vitamins B_6, B_{12}, and C; folic acid] 110 mg•15 mg•2 mg•50 μg•100 mg•0.8 mg
Fe-O.D. timed-release tablets OTC *hematinic* [ferrous fumarate; ascorbic acid] 100•500 mg
Feosol elixir OTC *hematinic* [ferrous sulfate] 220 mg/5 mL ② Feostat; Fer-In-Sol; Festal
Feosol tablets, timed-release capsules OTC *hematinic* [ferrous sulfate, dried] 200 mg; 159 mg
Feostat chewable tablets, suspension, drops OTC *hematinic* [ferrous fumarate] 100 mg; 100 mg/5 mL; 45 mg/0.6 mL ② Feosol

fepentolic acid INN
fepitrizol INN
fepradinol INN
feprazone INN, BAN
fepromide INN
feprosidnine INN
Ferancee chewable tablets OTC *hematinic* [ferrous fumarate; vitamin C] 67•150 mg
Ferancee-HP film-coated tablets OTC *hematinic* [ferrous fumarate; vitamin C] 110•600 mg
Feratab tablets OTC *hematinic* [ferrous sulfate] 300 mg
Fer-gen-sol drops OTC *hematinic* [ferrous sulfate] 75 mg/0.6 mL
Fergon tablets, elixir OTC *hematinic* [ferrous gluconate] 320 mg; 300 mg/5 mL
Fergon Iron Plus Calcium timed-release caplets (discontinued 1992) OTC *antianemic; calcium supplement* [ferrous gluconate; calcium; vitamin D]
Fergon Plus caplets (discontinued 1995) ℞ *hematinic* [ferrous gluconate; vitamin B_{12} with intrinsic factor concentrate; ascorbic acid] 58 mg•0.5 U•75 mg
Feridex ℞ *investigational contrast agent for MRI of the liver* [ferumoxides]
Fer-In-Sol capsules OTC *hematinic* [ferrous sulfate, dried] 190 mg ② Feosol
Fer-In-Sol drops, syrup OTC *hematinic* [ferrous sulfate] 75 mg/0.6 mL; 90 mg/5 mL
Fer-Iron drops OTC *hematinic* [ferrous sulfate] 75 mg/0.6 mL
Fermalox tablets (discontinued 1992) OTC *hematinic* [magnesium hydroxide; aluminum hydroxide; ferrous sulfate] 100•100•200 mg
fermium *element (Fm)*
Ferocyl sustained-release tablets OTC *hematinic* [ferrous fumarate; docusate sodium] 150•100 mg
Fero-Folic-500 controlled-release Filmtabs (film-coated tablets) ℞ *hematinic* [ferrous sulfate; ascorbic acid; folic acid] 105•500•0.8 mg
Fero-Grad-500 controlled-release Filmtabs (film-coated tablets) OTC

hematinic [ferrous sulfate; sodium ascorbate] 105•500 mg

Fero-Gradumet timed-release Filmtabs (film-coated tablets) OTC *hematinic* [ferrous sulfate] 525 mg

Ferospace capsules OTC *hematinic* [ferrous sulfate] 250 mg

Ferotrinsic capsules ℞ *hematinic* [ferrous fumarate; cyanocobalamin; ascorbic acid; intrinsic factor concentrate; folic acid] 110 mg•15 µg•75 mg•240 mg•0.5 mg

Ferralet tablets OTC *hematinic* [ferrous gluconate] 320 mg

Ferralet Plus tablets OTC *hematinic* [ferrous gluconate; cyanocobalamin; ascorbic acid; folic acid] 46 mg•25 µg•400 mg•0.8 mg

Ferralet S.R. sustained-release tablets OTC *hematinic* [ferrous gluconate] 320 mg

Ferralyn Lanacaps (timed-release capsules) OTC *hematinic* [ferrous sulfate, dried] 250 mg

Ferra-TD timed-release capsules OTC *hematinic* [ferrous sulfate, dried] 250 mg

Ferretts tablets OTC *hematinic* [ferrous fumarate] 325 mg

ferric ammonium citrate NF
ferric ammonium sulfate
ferric cacodylate NF
ferric chloride
ferric chloride Fe 59 USAN *radioactive agent*
ferric citrate (^{59}Fe) INN
ferric citrochloride NF
ferric fructose USAN, INN *hematinic*
ferric glycerophosphate NF
ferric hypophosphite NF
ferric oxide NF *coloring agent*
ferric oxide, red NF
ferric oxide, yellow NF
ferric pyrophosphate, soluble NF
ferric subsulfate NF
ferricholinate [see: ferrocholinate]
ferriclate calcium sodium USAN *hematinic* [also: calcium sodium ferriclate]
ferristene USAN *paramagnetic imaging agent for MRI*
Ferrixan ℞ *investigational contrast medium for MRI of the liver*

Ferro Dok TR timed-release capsules OTC *hematinic* [ferrous fumarate; docusate sodium] 150•100 mg

ferrocholate [see: ferrocholinate]
ferrocholinate INN

Ferro-Docusate T.R. timed-release capsules OTC *hematinic* [ferrous fumarate; docusate sodium] 150•100 mg

Ferro-DSS S.R. timed-release capsules OTC *hematinic* [ferrous fumarate; docusate sodium] 150•100 mg

Ferromar sustained-release caplets OTC *hematinic* [ferrous fumarate; vitamin C] 201.5•200 mg

ferropolimaler INN

Ferro-Sequels timed-release tablets OTC *hematinic* [ferrous fumarate] 50 mg

ferrotrenine INN

ferrous citrate Fe 59 USAN, USP *radioactive agent*

ferrous fumarate USP *hematinic (33% elemental iron)* 325 mg oral

ferrous gluconate USP *hematinic (11.6% elemental iron)* 300, 325 mg oral

ferrous lactate NF

ferrous sulfate USP *hematinic (20% elemental iron)* 250, 324 mg oral; 220 mg/5 mL oral; 75 mg/0.6 mL oral

ferrous sulfate, dried USP *antianemic*

ferrous sulfate, exsiccated [see: ferrous sulfate, dried]

ferrous sulfate Fe 59 USAN *radioactive agent*

Ferrous-S.Q.L. timed-release capsules (discontinued 1992) OTC *antianemic* [ferrous fumarate; docusate sodium]

Fertinex subcu injection ℞ *ovulation stimulant* [urofollitropin] $\underline{?}$

Fertinorm HP (commercially available in Europe) ℞ *investigational infertility therapy*

fertirelin INN, BAN *veterinary gonadotropin-releasing hormone* [also: fertirelin acetate]

fertirelin acetate USAN *veterinary gonadotropin-releasing hormone* [also: fertirelin]

ferumoxides USAN *diagnostic aid for magnetic imaging*

ferumoxsil USAN *diagnostic aid for magnetic imaging*

Festal II enteric-coated tablets (discontinued 1992) OTC *digestive enzymes* [pancrelipase] ② Feosol; Festalan

Festalan enteric-coated tablets (discontinued 1992) ℞ *digestive enzymes; antispasmodic; hypermotility reducer* [amylase; protease; lipase; atropine methylnitrate] ② Festal

fetoxilate INN *smooth muscle relaxant* [also: fetoxylate HCl; fetoxylate]

fetoxylate BAN *smooth muscle relaxant* [also: fetoxylate HCl; fetoxilate]

fetoxylate HCl USAN *smooth muscle relaxant* [also: fetoxilate; fetoxylate]

Feverall Sprinkle Caps (powder) OTC *analgesic; antipyretic* [acetaminophen] 80, 160 mg ② Fiberall

Feverall, Children's; Infant's Feverall; Junior Feverall suppositories OTC *analgesic; antipyretic* [acetaminophen] 120 mg; 80 mg; 325 mg

fexicaine INN, DCF

fexinidazole INN

fexofenadine HCl USAN *nonsedating antihistamine*

fezatione INN

fezolamine INN *antidepressant* [also: fezolamine fumarate]

fezolamine fumarate USAN *antidepressant* [also: fezolamine]

FGF-4 (fibroblast growth factor-4) [q.v.]

FGN-1 (*orphan: adenomatous polyposis coli*)

fiacitabine (FIAC) USAN, INN *antiviral; investigational (Phase I/II) for AIDS/ARC/HIV*

fialuridine (FIAU) USAN, INN *antiviral; investigational (Phase II) for HIV;* (*orphan: chronic active hepatitis B*)

Fiber Rich timed-release caplets (discontinued 1992) OTC *diet aid* [phenylpropanolamine HCl; grain and citrus fruit fiber]

Fiberall chewable tablets OTC *bulk laxative; antidiarrheal* [calcium polycarbophil] 1250 mg ② Feverall

Fiberall powder, wafers OTC *laxative* [psyllium hydrophilic mucilloid] 3.4 g/tsp.; 3.4 g

FiberCon film-coated tablets OTC *bulk laxative; antidiarrheal* [calcium polycarbophil] 500 mg

Fiberlan liquid OTC *enteral nutritional therapy* [lactose-free formula]

Fiber-Lax tablets OTC *bulk laxative; antidiarrheal* [calcium polycarbophil] 625 mg

FiberNorm tablets OTC *bulk laxative; antidiarrheal* [calcium polycarbophil] 625 mg

fibracillin INN

Fibrad powder OTC *oral dietary fiber supplement* [pea, oat and sugar beet fiber] 7 g total fiber per serving

fibrin INN

fibrinase [see: factor XIII]

fibrinogen (^{125}I) INN [also: fibrinogen I 125]

fibrinogen, human USP

fibrinogen I 125 USAN *vascular patency test; radioactive agent* [also: fibrinogen (^{125}I)]

fibrinoligase [see: factor XIII]

fibrinolysin, human INN [also: plasmin]

fibrinolysin & desoxyribonuclease *topical enzymes for necrotic tissue debridement*

fibrin-stabilizing factor (FSF) [see: factor XIII]

Fibriscint ℞ *investigational imaging aid for deep venous thrombosis* [antifibrin monoclonal antibodies]

fibroblast growth factor, basic (bFGF) [see: ersofermin]

fibroblast growth factor-4 (FGF-4) *investigational vulnerary*

Fibrogammin P ℞ (*orphan: congenital factor XIII deficiency*) [factor XIII (placenta-derived)]

fibronectin (*orphan: nonhealing corneal ulcers or epithelial defects*)

50% Dextrose with Electrolyte Pattern A (or N) IV infusion ℞ *intravenous nutritional/electrolyte therapy* [combined electrolyte solution; dextrose]

50% Dextrose with Electrolyte Pattern B IV infusion (discontinued 1994) ℞ *intravenous nutritional/electrolyte therapy* [combined electrolyte solution; dextrose]

filenadol INN

filgrastim USAN, INN, BAN *antineutropenic (orphan); hematopoietic stimulant; investigational (Phase III) cytokine for AIDS*

Filibon tablets (discontinued 1995) OTC *vitamin/calcium/iron supplement* [multiple vitamins; calcium; iron; folic acid] ≟•125•18•0.4 mg

Filibon F.A.; Filibon Forte tablets (discontinued 1995) ℞ *vitamin/calcium/iron supplement* [multiple vitamins; calcium; iron; folic acid] ≟•250•45•1 mg; 300•45•1 mg

filipin USAN, INN *antifungal*

Filmix ℞ *(orphan: neurosonographic contrast medium for intracranial tumors)* [microbubble contrast agent]

Filmlok (trademarked dosage form) *film-coated tablet*

Filmseal (trademarked dosage form) *film-coated tablet*

Filmtabs (trademarked dosage form) *film-coated tablets*

FIME (fluorouracil, ICRF-159, MeCCNU) *chemotherapy protocol*

Finac lotion OTC *topical acne treatment* [salicylic acid; isopropyl alcohol] 2%•22.5%

finasteride USAN, INN, BAN *antineoplastic; androgen hormone inhibitor for benign prostatic hypertension (BPH)*

Fiogesic tablets OTC *decongestant; antihistamine; analgesic* [phenylpropanolamine HCl; pheniramine maleate; pyrilamine maleate; aspirin]

Fiorgen PF tablets ℞ *analgesic; antipyretic; anti-inflammatory; sedative* [aspirin; caffeine; butalbital] 325•40•50 mg

Fioricet tablets ℞ *analgesic; antipyretic; sedative* [acetaminophen; caffeine; butalbital] 325•40•50 mg ⑨ Lorcet

Fioricet with Codeine capsules ℞ *narcotic analgesic; sedative* [codeine phosphate; acetaminophen; caffeine; butalbital] 30•325•40•50 mg

Fiorinal tablets, capsules ℞ *analgesic; antipyretic; anti-inflammatory; sedative* [aspirin; caffeine; butalbital] 325•40•50 mg ⑨ Florinef

Fiorinal with Codeine capsules ℞ *narcotic analgesic; sedative* [codeine phosphate; aspirin; caffeine; butalbital] 30•325•40•50 mg

Fiorpap tablets ℞ *analgesic; antipyretic; sedative* [acetaminophen; caffeine; butalbital] 325•40•50 mg

fipexide INN

fire ant venom allergenic extract *(orphan: test for and desensitize fire ant reactions)*

First Choice reagent strips for home use OTC *in vitro diagnostic aid for blood glucose*

First Response test stick for home use OTC *in vitro diagnostic aid for urine pregnancy test*

First Response Ovulation Predictor test kit for home use OTC *in vitro diagnostic aid to predict ovulation time*

fisalamine [see: mesalamine]

5 + 2 protocol (cytarabine, daunorubicin) *chemotherapy protocol*

5 + 2 protocol (cytarabine, mitoxantrone) *chemotherapy protocol*

5% Alcohol and 5% Dextrose in Water; 10% Alcohol and 5% Dextrose in Water IV infusion ℞ *for caloric replacement and rehydration* [alcohol; dextrose] 5%•5%; 10%•5%

5 Benzagel; 10 Benzagel gel ℞ *keratolytic for acne* [benzoyl peroxide] 5%; 10%

5% Dextrose and Electrolyte #48; 5% Dextrose and Electrolyte #75; 10% Dextrose and Electrolyte #48 IV infusion ℞ *intravenous nutritional/electrolyte therapy* [combined electrolyte solution; dextrose]

5% Travert and Electrolyte No. 2; 10% Travert and Electrolyte No. 2 IV infusion ℞ *intravenous nutritional/electrolyte therapy* [combined electrolyte solution; invert sugar (50% dextrose + 50% fructose)]

520C9x22 [see: bispecific antibody 520C9x22]

5A8 monoclonal antibody to CD4 *(orphan: post-exposure prophylaxis to HIV exposure)*

FK-037 *investigational cephalosporin antibiotic*

FK-143 *investigational T5 alpha reductase inhibitor for benign prostatic hypertrophy*
FK-176 *investigational treatment for pollakiuria*
FK-224 *investigational neurokinin antagonist*
FK-366 *investigational aldose reductase inhibitor for diabetic neuropathy and diabetic cataracts*
FK-409 *investigational vasodilator for angina*
FK-453 *investigational adenosine A_1 receptor antagonist for acute renal failure*
FK-480 *investigational cholecystokinin antagonist for pancreatitis*
FK-508 *investigational treatment for Alzheimer's senile dementia*
FK-565 *investigational (Phase I) immunomodulator for cancer and HIV*
FK-613 *investigational antihistamine for asthma, allergic rhinitis, and urticaria*
FK-739 *investigational angiotensin II antagonist for hypertension*
FK-780 *investigational treatment for hyperglycemia, hyperinsulinemia, and diabetes-related hirsutism*
FK-906 *investigational renin inhibitor for hypertension*
FK-1052 *investigational 5-HT3 and 5-HT4 dual antagonist for irritable bowel syndrome*
FK-3311 *investigational nonsteroidal anti-inflammatory and analgesic*
FL (flutamide, leuprolide acetate) *chemotherapy protocol*
FLAC (fluorouracil, leucovorin [rescue], Adriamycin, cyclophosphamide) *chemotherapy protocol*
Flagyl film-coated tablets, capsules ℞ *antibiotic; antiprotozoal; amebicide* [metronidazole] 250, 500 mg; 375 mg
Flagyl IV powder for injection ℞ *antibiotic; antiprotozoal; amebicide* [metronidazole HCl] 500 mg
Flagyl IV RTU (ready-to-use) injection ℞ *antibiotic; antiprotozoal; amebicide* [metronidazole] 500 mg/100 mL
flamenol INN
Flanders Buttocks ointment OTC *topical diaper rash treatment* [zinc oxide; balsam Peru]

FLAP (fluorouracil, leucovorin [rescue], Adriamycin, Platinol) *chemotherapy protocol*
Flarex Drop-Tainers (eye drop suspension) ℞ *ophthalmic topical corticosteroidal anti-inflammatory* [fluorometholone acetate] 0.1%
Flatulex drops OTC *antiflatulent* [simethicone] 40 mg/0.6 mL
Flatulex tablets OTC *adsorbent; detoxicant; antiflatulent* [activated charcoal; simethicone] 250•80 mg
flavamine INN
flavine [see: acriflavine HCl]
flavodic acid INN
flavodilol INN *antihypertensive* [also: flavodilol maleate]
flavodilol maleate USAN *antihypertensive* [also: flavodilol]
flavonoid [see: troxerutin]
Flavons-500 tablets OTC *dietary supplement* [citrus bioflavonoids and hesperidin complex] 500 mg
Flavorcee chewable tablets OTC *vitamin supplement* [ascorbic acid] 100, 250, 500 mg
flavoxate INN, BAN *smooth muscle relaxant; urinary antispasmodic* [also: flavoxate HCl]
flavoxate HCl USAN *smooth muscle relaxant; urinary antispasmodic* [also: flavoxate]
Flaxedil IV (discontinued 1996) ℞ *neuromuscular blocker* [gallamine triethiodide] 20 mg/mL ② Flexeril
flazalone USAN, INN, BAN *anti-inflammatory*
FLe (fluorouracil, levamisole) *chemotherapy protocol*
flecainide INN, BAN *antiarrhythmic* [also: flecainide acetate]
flecainide acetate USAN *antiarrhythmic* [also: flecainide]
Fleet Babylax rectal liquid OTC *hyperosmolar laxative* [glycerin] 4 mL/dose
Fleet Bagenema rectal liquid OTC *laxative* [Castile soap]
Fleet Bisacodyl Enema; Fleet Bisacodyl Prep rectal liquid OTC *stimulant laxative* [bisacodyl] 10 mg/30 mL; 10 mg/packet

Fleet Children's Enema rectal liquid OTC *saline laxative* [monobasic sodium phosphate; dibasic sodium phosphate]

Fleet Enema rectal liquid OTC *saline laxative* [monobasic sodium phosphate; dibasic sodium phosphate] 7•19 g/118 mL

Fleet Flavored Castor Oil emulsion OTC *stimulant laxative* [castor oil] 67%

Fleet Laxative enteric-coated tablets OTC *stimulant laxative* [bisacodyl] 5 mg

Fleet Laxative suppositories OTC *stimulant laxative* [bisacodyl] 10 mg

Fleet Medicated Wipes cleansing pads OTC *moisturizer and cleanser for external rectal/vaginal areas; astringent; antiseptic; antifungal* [hamamelis water; glycerin; alcohol] 50%•10%•7%

Fleet Mineral Oil Enema rectal liquid OTC *lubricant laxative* [mineral oil]

Fleet Pain Relief anorectal wipes OTC *topical local anesthetic* [pramoxine HCl; glycerin] 1%•12%

Fleet Phospho-Soda oral solution OTC *buffered saline laxative* [monobasic sodium phosphate; dibasic sodium phosphate] 18•48 g/100 mL

Fleet Prep Kits No. 1 to No. 6 OTC *pre-procedure bowel evacuant* [other Fleet products in combination kits]

Fleet Relief anorectal ointment (discontinued 1995) OTC *hemorrhoidal astringent; protectant* [zinc oxide; white petrolatum; mineral oil]

Fleet Relief Anesthetic Hemorrhoidal ointment (discontinued 1995) OTC *topical local anesthetic* [pramoxine HCl] 1%

flerobuterol INN

fleroxacin USAN, INN *antibacterial*

flesinoxan INN *investigational antidepressant and anxiolytic*

flestolol INN *antiadrenergic (β-receptor)* [also: flestolol sulfate]

flestolol sulfate USAN *antiadrenergic (β-receptor)* [also: flestolol]

fletazepam USAN, INN, BAN *skeletal muscle relaxant*

Fletcher's Castoria liquid OTC *laxative* [senna concentrate] 33.3 mg/mL

Flex-all 454 gel OTC *topical antipruritic; counterirritant; topical local anesthetic* [menthol; methyl salicylate] 16%• ?

Flexaphen capsules ℞ *skeletal muscle relaxant; analgesic* [chlorzoxazone; acetaminophen] 250•300 mg

Flex-Care Especially for Sensitive Eyes solution OTC *chemical disinfecting solution for soft contact lenses* [note: soft contact indication different from RGP contact indication for same product]

Flex-Care Especially for Sensitive Eyes solution OTC *disinfecting/wetting/soaking solution for rigid gas permeable contact lenses* [note: RGP contact indication different from soft contact indication for same product]

Flexeril film-coated tablets ℞ *skeletal muscle relaxant* [cyclobenzaprine HCl] 10 mg ? Flaxedil

Flexoject IV or IM injection ℞ *skeletal muscle relaxant* [orphenadrine citrate] 30 mg/mL

Flexon IV or IM injection ℞ *skeletal muscle relaxant* [orphenadrine citrate] 30 mg/mL

FlexPack HP test for professional use *diagnostic aid for serum IgG antibodies to H. pylori (for peptic ulcers)*

Flintstones Children's; Flintstones Plus Calcium; Flintstones Plus Extra C Children's chewable tablets OTC *vitamin supplement* [multiple vitamins; folic acid] ±•0.3 mg

Flintstones Complete chewable tablets OTC *vitamin/mineral/iron supplement* [multiple vitamins & minerals; iron; folic acid; biotin] ±•18 mg•0.4 mg•40 μg

Flintstones Plus Iron chewable tablets OTC *vitamin/iron supplement* [multiple vitamins; iron; folic acid] ±•15•0.3 mg

Flixonase (foreign name for U.S. product Flonase)

Flixotide (foreign name for U.S. product Flovent)

Flo-Coat suspension ℞ *GI contrast radiopaque agent* [barium sulfate] 100%

floctafenine USAN, INN, BAN *analgesic*

Flolan IV infusion ℞ *platelet aggregation inhibitor; vasodilator for primary pulmonary hypertension (orphan)* [epoprostenol] 0.5, 1.5 mg

flomoxef INN

Flonase nasal spray ℞ *intranasal steroidal anti-inflammatory* [fluticasone propionate] 50 μg/dose

Flo-Pack (trademarked packaging form) *vial for IV drip*

flopropione INN

florantyrone INN, BAN

flordipine USAN, INN *antihypertensive*

floredil INN

floretione [see: fluoresone]

florfenicol USAN, INN, BAN *veterinary antibacterial*

Florical capsules, tablets OTC *calcium supplement* [calcium carbonate; sodium fluoride] 364•8.3 mg

Florida Sunburn Relief lotion OTC *antipruritic; counterirritant* [benzyl alcohol; phenol; camphor; menthol] 3%•0.4%•0.2%•0.15%

florifenine INN

Florinef Acetate tablets ℞ *adrenocortical insufficiency in Addison's disease* [fludrocortisone acetate] 0.1 mg ⑨ Fiorinal

Florone cream, ointment ℞ *topical corticosteroidal anti-inflammatory* [diflorasone diacetate] 0.05%

Florone E cream ℞ *topical corticosteroidal anti-inflammatory; emollient* [diflorasone diacetate] 0.05%

floropipamide [now: pipamperone]

floropipeton [see: propyperone]

Floropryl ophthalmic ointment (discontinued 1995) ℞ *antiglaucoma agent; irreversible cholinesterase inhibitor miotic* [isoflurophate] 0.025%

Florvite drops ℞ *pediatric vitamin supplement and dental caries preventative* [multiple vitamins; sodium fluoride] ±•0.25, ±•0.5 mg/mL

Florvite; Florvite Half Strength chewable tablets ℞ *pediatric vitamin supplement and dental caries preventative* [multiple vitamins; sodium fluoride; folic acid] ±•1•0.3 mg; ±•0.5•0.3 mg

Florvite + Iron drops ℞ *pediatric vitamin/iron supplement and dental caries preventative* [multiple vitamins & minerals; sodium fluoride; ferrous sulfate] ±•0.25•10, ±•0.5•10 mg/mL

Florvite + Iron; Half Strength Florvite + Iron chewable tablets ℞ *pediatric vitamin/iron supplement and dental caries preventative* [multiple vitamins & minerals; sodium fluoride; ferrous sulfate; folic acid] ±•1•12•0.3 mg; ±•0.5•12•0.3 mg

flosequinan USAN, INN, BAN *antihypertensive; vasodilator*

flotrenizine INN

Flovent metered dose inhaler ℞ *corticosteroidal antiasthmatic* [fluticasone propionate] 44, 110, 220 μg/inhalation

floverine INN

floxacillin USAN *antibacterial* [also: flucloxacillin]

floxacrine INN

Floxin film-coated tablets, UroPak (3-day supply), IV injection ℞ *broad-spectrum fluoroquinolone-type antibiotic* [ofloxacin] 200, 300, 400 mg; 6 tablets × 200 mg; 200, 400 mg

floxuridine USAN, USP, INN *antiviral; antimetabolic antineoplastic* 100 mg/mL injection; 500 mg/vial injection

Floxyfral ℞ *investigational antidepressant and antipsychotic* [fluvoxamine]

FLT (fluorothymidine) [q.v.]

Flu, Cold & Cough Medicine powder for oral solution OTC *antitussive; decongestant; antihistamine; analgesic* [dextromethorphan hydrobromide; pseudoephedrine HCl; chlorpheniramine maleate; acetaminophen] 20•60•4•500 mg/packet

fluacizine INN

flualamide INN

fluanisone INN, BAN

fluazacort USAN, INN *anti-inflammatory*

flubanilate INN *CNS stimulant* [also: flubanilate HCl]

flubanilate HCl USAN *CNS stimulant* [also: flubanilate]

flubendazole USAN, INN, BAN *antiprotozoal*

flubenisolone [see: betamethasone]

flubepride INN

flubuperone [see: melperone]
flucarbril INN
flucetorex INN
flucindole USAN, INN *antipsychotic*
fluciprazine INN
fluclorolone acetonide INN, BAN *glucocorticoid* [also: flucloronide]
flucloronide USAN *glucocorticoid* [also: fluclorolone acetonide]
flucloxacillin INN, BAN *antibacterial* [also: floxacillin]
fluconazole USAN, INN, BAN *broad-spectrum systemic fungistatic*
flucrilate INN *tissue adhesive* [also: flucrylate]
flucrylate USAN *tissue adhesive* [also: flucrilate]
flucytosine USAN, USP, INN, BAN *fungicidal*
fludalanine USAN, INN *antibacterial*
Fludara powder for IV injection ℞ *antimetabolic antineoplastic; for chronic lymphocytic leukemia and non-Hodgkin's lymphoma (orphan)* [fludarabine phosphate] 50 mg
fludarabine INN *antimetabolic antineoplastic* [also: fludarabine phosphate]
fludarabine phosphate USAN *antimetabolic antineoplastic; for chronic lymphocytic leukemia and non-Hodgkin's lymphoma (orphan)* [also: fludarabine]
fludazonium chloride USAN, INN *topical anti-infective*
fludeoxyglucose (^{18}F) INN *diagnostic aid; radioactive agent* [also: fludeoxyglucose F 18]
fludeoxyglucose F 18 USAN, USP *diagnostic aid; radioactive agent* [also: fludeoxyglucose (^{18}F)]
fludiazepam INN
fludorex USAN, INN *anorectic; antiemetic*
fludoxopone INN
fludrocortisone INN, BAN *salt-regulating adrenocortical steroid; mineralocorticoid* [also: fludrocortisone acetate]
fludrocortisone acetate USP *salt-regulating adrenocortical steroid; mineralocorticoid* [also: fludrocortisone]
fludroxicortide [see: flurandrenolide]
fludroxycortide INN *topical corticosteroid* [also: flurandrenolide; flurandrenolone]

flufenamic acid USAN, INN, BAN *anti-inflammatory*
flufenisal USAN, INN *analgesic*
flufosal INN
flufylline INN
flugestone INN, BAN *progestin* [also: flurogestone acetate]
flugestone acetate [see: flurogestone acetate]
Fluidex tablets (discontinued 1992) OTC *mild diuretic* [buchu; couch grass; corn silk; hydrangea]
Fluidex with Pamabrom capsules (discontinued 1992) OTC *diuretic* [pamabrom]
Fluimucil ℞ *investigational (Phase I) immunomodulator for AIDS/ARC/HIV* [acetylcysteine]
Flu-Imune IM injection (discontinued 1994) ℞ *flu vaccine* [influenza purified surface antigen] 90 μg/mL
fluindarol INN
fluindione INN
Flumadine film-coated tablets, syrup ℞ *antiviral; prophylaxis and treatment for influenza A virus* [rimantadine HCl] 100 mg; 50 mg/5 mL
flumazenil USAN, INN, BAN *benzodiazepine antagonist/antidote*
flumazepil [see: flumazenil]
flumecinol INN *(orphan: neonatal hyperbilirubinemia)*
flumedroxone INN, BAN
flumequine USAN, INN, BAN *antibacterial*
flumeridone USAN, INN, BAN *antiemetic*
flumetasone INN *glucocorticoid* [also: flumethasone]
flumethasone USAN, BAN *glucocorticoid* [also: flumetasone]
flumethasone pivalate USAN, USP, BAN *glucocorticoid*
flumethiazide INN, BAN
flumethrin BAN
flumetramide USAN, INN *skeletal muscle relaxant*
flumexadol INN
flumezapine USAN, INN, BAN *antipsychotic; neuroleptic*
fluminorex USAN, INN *anorectic*
flumizole USAN, INN *anti-inflammatory*
flumoxonide USAN, INN *adrenocortical steroid*

flunamine INN
flunarizine INN, BAN *vasodilator; (orphan: alternating hemiplegia)* [also: flunarizine HCl]
flunarizine HCl USAN *vasodilator* [also: flunarizine]
flunidazole USAN, INN *antiprotozoal*
flunisolide USAN, USP, INN, BAN *corticosteroid inhalant for asthma; intranasal steroid*
flunisolide acetate USAN *anti-inflammatory*
flunitrazepam USAN, INN, BAN *hypnotic*
flunixin USAN, INN, BAN *anti-inflammatory; analgesic*
flunixin meglumine USAN *anti-inflammatory; analgesic*
flunoprost INN
flunoxaprofen INN
fluocinolide [now: fluocinonide]
fluocinolone BAN *topical corticosteroid* [also: fluocinolone acetonide]
fluocinolone acetonide USAN, USP, INN *topical corticosteroid* [also: fluocinolone] 0.01%, 0.025% topical
fluocinonide USAN, USP, INN, BAN *topical corticosteroid* 0.05% topical
fluocortin INN *anti-inflammatory* [also: fluocortin butyl]
fluocortin butyl USAN, BAN *anti-inflammatory* [also: fluocortin]
fluocortolone USAN, INN, BAN *glucocorticoid*
fluocortolone caproate USAN *glucocorticoid*
Fluogen IM injection, Steri-Vials, Steri-Dose (disposable syringes) ℞ *flu vaccine* [influenza split-virus vaccine] 0.5 mL/dose
Fluonex cream ℞ *topical corticosteroid* [fluocinonide] 0.05%
Fluonid topical solution ℞ *topical corticosteroid* [fluocinolone acetonide] 0.01%
fluopromazine BAN *antipsychotic* [also: triflupromazine]
Fluoracaine eye drops ℞ *topical ophthalmic anesthetic; corneal disclosing agent* [proparacaine HCl; fluorescein sodium] 0.5%•0.25%
fluoracizine [see: fluacizine]

fluorescein USP, BAN, JAN *corneal trauma indicator*
fluorescein, soluble [now: fluorescein sodium]
fluorescein sodium USP, BAN, JAN *corneal trauma indicator* 2% eye drops
Fluorescite IV injection ℞ *corneal disclosing agent* [fluorescein sodium] 10%, 25%
Fluoresoft eye drops ℞ *diagnostic aid in fitting contact lenses* [fluorexon] 0.35%
fluoresone INN
Fluorets ophthalmic strips OTC *corneal disclosing agent* [fluorescein sodium] 1 mg
fluorexon *diagnosis and fitting aid for contact lenses*
fluorhydrocortisone acetate [see: fludrocortisone acetate]
Fluoride tablets OTC *dental caries preventative* [sodium fluoride] 2.21 mg
Fluoride Loz lozenges ℞ *dental caries preventative* [sodium fluoride] 2.21 mg
Fluorigard oral rinse OTC *topical dental caries preventative* [sodium fluoride; alcohol 6%] 0.05%
Fluori-Methane spray ℞ *topical vapocoolant anesthetic* [trichloromonofluoromethane; dichlorodifluoromethane] 85%•15%
fluorine *element (F)*
fluorine F 18 fluorodeoxyglucose [see: fludeoxyglucose F 18]
Fluorinse oral rinse ℞ *topical dental caries preventative* [sodium fluoride] 0.2%
Fluor-I-Strip; Fluor-I-Strip A.T. ophthalmic strips ℞ *corneal disclosing agent* [fluorescein sodium] 9 mg; 1 mg
Fluoritab chewable tablets, drops ℞ *dental caries preventative* [sodium fluoride] 1.1, 2.2 mg; 0.55 mg/drop
fluormethylprednisolone [see: dexamethasone]
5-fluorocytosine (5-FC) [see: flucytosine]
fluorodeoxyglucose F 18 [see: fludeoxyglucose F 18]
fluorometholone USP, INN, BAN *glucocorticoid; ophthalmic anti-inflammatory*
fluorometholone acetate USAN *anti-inflammatory*

Fluor-Op eye drop suspension ℞ *ophthalmic topical corticosteroidal anti-inflammatory* [fluorometholone] 0.1%

Fluoroplex cream, topical solution ℞ *antimetabolic antineoplastic for actinic keratoses and basal cell carcinomas* [fluorouracil] 1%

fluorosalan USAN *disinfectant* [also: flusalan]

fluorothymidine (FLT) *investigational (Phase II) antiviral for AIDS/ARC/ARC*

fluorouracil (5-FU) USAN, USP, INN, BAN *antimetabolic antineoplastic* 50 mg/mL injection

fluorouracil & interferon alfa-2a (*orphan: esophageal and advanced colorectal carcinoma*)

fluorouracil & leucovorin (*orphan: metastatic adenocarcinoma of colon and rectum*)

fluoruridine deoxyribose [see: floxuridine]

Fluosol emulsion for intracoronary perfusion (discontinued 1995) ℞ *myocardial oxygenation during PTCA* [intravascular perfluorochemical (PFC) emulsion] 20%

fluostigmine [see: isoflurophate]

Fluothane liquid for vaporization ℞ *inhalation general anesthetic* [halothane]

fluotracen INN *antipsychotic; antidepressant* [also: fluotracen HCl]

fluotracen HCl USAN *antipsychotic; antidepressant* [also: fluotracen]

fluoxetine USAN, INN, BAN *antidepressant*

fluoxetine HCl USAN *antidepressant; selective serotonin reuptake inhibitor; used for obsessive-compulsive disorder*

fluoximesterone [see: fluoxymesterone]

Flu-Oxinate eye drops ℞ *topical ophthalmic anesthetic; corneal disclosing agent* [benoxinate HCl; fluorescein sodium] 0.4%•0.25%

fluoxiprednisolone [see: triamcinolone]

fluoxymesterone USP, INN, BAN *oral androgen* 10 mg oral

fluparoxan INN, BAN *antidepressant; investigational treatment for male sexual dysfunction* [also: fluparoxan HCl]

fluparoxan HCl USAN *antidepressant; investigational treatment for male sexual dysfunction* [also: fluparoxan]

flupenthixol BAN [also: flupentixol]

flupentixol INN [also: flupenthixol]

fluperamide USAN, INN *antiperistaltic*

fluperlapine INN

fluperolone INN, BAN *glucocorticoid* [also: fluperolone acetate]

fluperolone acetate USAN *glucocorticoid* [also: fluperolone]

fluphenazine INN, BAN *antipsychotic* [also: fluphenazine enanthate]

fluphenazine decanoate *antipsychotic; prolonged parenteral neuroleptic therapy* 25 mg/mL injection

fluphenazine enanthate USP *antipsychotic; prolonged parenteral neuroleptic therapy* [also: fluphenazine]

fluphenazine HCl USP, BAN *antipsychotic* 1, 2.5, 5, 10 mg oral; 2.5 mg/mL injection

flupimazine INN

flupirtine INN, BAN *analgesic* [also: flupirtine maleate]

flupirtine maleate USAN *analgesic* [also: flupirtine]

flupranone INN

fluprazine INN

fluprednidene INN, BAN

fluprednisolone USAN, NF, INN, BAN *glucocorticoid*

fluprednisolone valerate USAN *glucocorticoid*

fluprofen INN, BAN

fluprofylline INN

fluproquazone USAN, INN, BAN *analgesic*

fluprostenol INN, BAN *prostaglandin* [also: fluprostenol sodium]

fluprostenol sodium USAN *prostaglandin* [also: fluprostenol]

fluquazone USAN, INN *anti-inflammatory*

Flura tablets ℞ *dental caries preventative* [sodium fluoride] 2.2 mg

fluracil [see: fluorouracil]

fluradoline INN *analgesic* [also: fluradoline HCl]

fluradoline HCl USAN *analgesic* [also: fluradoline]

Flura-Drops ℞ *dental caries preventative* [sodium fluoride] 0.55 mg/drop

Flura-Loz lozenges ℞ *dental caries preventative* [sodium fluoride] 2.2 mg

flurandrenolide USAN, USP *topical corticosteroid* [also: fludroxycortide; flurandrenolone] 0.05% topical

flurandrenolone BAN *topical corticosteroid* [also: flurandrenolide; fludroxycortide]

flurantel INN

Flurate eye drops ℞ *topical ophthalmic anesthetic; corneal disclosing agent* [benoxinate HCl; fluorescein sodium] 0.4%•0.25%

flurazepam INN, BAN *anticonvulsant; hypnotic; muscle relaxant; sedative* [also: flurazepam HCl]

flurazepam HCl USAN, USP *anticonvulsant; hypnotic; muscle relaxant; sedative* [also: flurazepam] 15, 30 mg oral

flurbiprofen USAN, USP, INN, BAN *antiarthritic; nonsteroidal anti-inflammatory drug (NSAID); analgesic* 50, 100 mg oral

flurbiprofen sodium USP *prostaglandin synthesis inhibitor; antimiotic; ocular nonsteroidal anti-inflammatory drug (NSAID)* 0.03% eye drops

Fluress eye drops ℞ *topical ophthalmic anesthetic; corneal disclosing agent* [benoxinate HCl; fluorescein sodium] 0.4%•0.25%

fluretofen USAN, INN *anti-inflammatory; antithrombotic*

flurfamide [now: flurofamide]

flurithromycin INN

flurocitabine USAN, INN *antineoplastic*

Fluro-Ethyl aerosol spray ℞ *topical refrigerant anesthetic* [ethyl chloride; dichlorotetrafluoroethane] 25%•75%

flurofamide USAN, INN *urease enzyme inhibitor*

flurogestone acetate USAN *progestin* [also: flugestone]

Flurosyn ointment, cream ℞ *topical corticosteroid* [fluocinolone acetonide] 0.025%; 0.01, 0.025%

flurothyl USAN, USP, BAN *CNS stimulant* [also: flurotyl]

flurotyl INN *CNS stimulant* [also: flurothyl]

fluroxene USAN, NF, INN *inhalation anesthetic*

fluroxyspiramine [see: spiramide]

flusalan INN *disinfectant* [also: fluorosalan]

FluShield IM injection, Tubex (cartridge-needle unit) ℞ *flu vaccine* [influenza purified split-virus vaccine] 0.5 mL/dose

flusoxolol INN, BAN

fluspiperone USAN, INN *antipsychotic*

fluspirilene USAN, INN, BAN *antipsychotic*

flutamide USAN, INN, BAN *antineoplastic; antiandrogen hormone*

flutazolam INN

flutemazepam INN

Flutex ointment, cream ℞ *topical corticosteroid* [triamcinolone acetonide] 0.025%, 0.1%, 0.5%

flutiazin USAN, INN *veterinary anti-inflammatory*

fluticasone INN, BAN *topical corticosteroidal anti-inflammatory* [also: fluticasone propionate]

fluticasone propionate USAN *topical corticosteroidal anti-inflammatory* [also: fluticasone]

flutizenol INN

flutomidate INN

flutonidine INN

flutoprazepam INN

flutrimazole INN

flutroline USAN, INN *antipsychotic*

flutropium bromide INN

fluvastatin INN, BAN *antihyperlipidemic for hypercholesterolemia; HMG-CoA reductase inhibitor* [also: fluvastatin sodium]

fluvastatin sodium USAN *antihyperlipidemic for hypercholesterolemia; HMG-CoA reductase inhibitor* [also: fluvastatin]

Fluvirin IM injection, prefilled syringes ℞ *flu vaccine* [influenza purified surface antigen] 0.5 mL/dose

fluvoxamine INN, BAN *antipsychotic; selective serotonin reuptake inhibitor (SSRI) for obsessive-compulsive disorder* [also: fluvoxamine maleate]

fluvoxamine maleate USAN *antidepressant; selective serotonin reuptake inhibitor (SSRI) for obsessive-compulsive disorder* [also: fluvoxamine]

fluzinamide USAN, INN *anticonvulsant*

Fluzone IM injection, prefilled syringes ℞ *flu vaccine* [influenza split-virus/whole-virus vaccine] 0.5 mL/dose

fluzoperine INN

FML; FML Forte eye drop suspension ℞ *ophthalmic topical corticosteroidal anti-inflammatory* [fluorometholone] 0.1%; 0.25%

FML S.O.P. ophthalmic ointment ℞ *ophthalmic topical corticosteroidal anti-inflammatory* [fluorometholone] 0.1%

FML-S eye drop suspension ℞ *ophthalmic topical corticosteroidal anti-inflammatory; bacteriostatic* [fluorometholone; sulfacetamide sodium] 0.1%•10%

FMS (fluorouracil, mitomycin, streptozocin) *chemotherapy protocol*

FMV (fluorouracil, MeCCNU, vincristine) *chemotherapy protocol*

FNC (fluorouracil, Novantrone, cyclophosphamide) *chemotherapy protocol* [also: CFM; CNF]

FNM (fluorouracil, Novantrone, methotrexate) *chemotherapy protocol*

FOAM (fluorouracil, Oncovin, Adriamycin, mitomycin) *chemotherapy protocol*

Foamicon chewable tablets OTC *antacid* [aluminum hydroxide; magnesium trisilicate] 80•20 mg

Focalpak kit ℞ *fluorescein angiography* [fluorescein]

focofilcon A USAN *hydrophilic contact lens material*

Foille spray OTC *topical local anesthetic; antiseptic* [benzocaine; chloroxylenol] 5%•0.63%

Foille Medicated First Aid ointment, aerosol spray OTC *topical local anesthetic; antiseptic* [benzocaine; chloroxylenol] 5%•0.1%; 5%•0.6%

Foille Plus aerosol spray OTC *topical local anesthetic; antiseptic* [benzocaine; chloroxylenol; alcohol 57.33%] 5%•0.6%

FoilleCort cream (discontinued 1993) OTC *topical corticosteroid* [hydrocortisone acetate]

Folabee IM injection (discontinued 1994) ℞ *antianemic; vitamin supplement* [liver extracts; vitamin B_{12}; folic acid]

folacin [see: folic acid] ② Fulvicin

folate [see: folic acid]

folate sodium USP

folescutol INN

Folex powder for IV or IM injection (discontinued 1992) ℞ *antimetabolic antineoplastic for multiple leukemias; systemic antipsoriatic; antirheumatic* [methotrexate sodium] 25, 50, 100, 250 mg

Folex PFS powder for IV or IM injection ℞ *antimetabolic antineoplastic for multiple leukemias; systemic antipsoriatic; antirheumatic* [methotrexate sodium] 25 mg/mL

folic acid USP, INN, BAN *vitamin B_c; vitamin M; hematopoietic* 0.4, 0.8, 1 mg oral; 5 mg/mL injection

folinate-SF calcium [see: leucovorin calcium]

folinic acid [see: leucovorin calcium]

follicle-stimulating hormone (FSH) BAN [also: menotropins]

follidrin [see: estradiol benzoate]

follotropin [see: menotropins]

Follow-Up [see: Carnation Follow-Up]

Follutein powder for IM injection (discontinued 1995) ℞ *hormone for prepubertal cryptorchidism and hypogonadism; ovulation stimulant* [chorionic gonadotropin] 1000 U/mL

Foltrin capsules ℞ *hematinic* [ferrous fumarate; cyanocobalamin; ascorbic acid; intrinsic factor concentrate; folic acid] 110 mg•15 μg•75 mg•240 mg•0.5 mg

Folvite IM injection ℞ *antianemic* [folic acid] 5 mg/mL

Folvite tablets (discontinued 1993) ℞ *antianemic* [folic acid]

fomepizole USAN *antidote; alcohol dehydrogenase inhibitor;* (orphan: *methanol or ethylene glycol poisoning*)

FOMI; FOMi (fluorouracil, Oncovin, mitomycin) *chemotherapy protocol*

fomidacillin INN, BAN

fominoben INN

fomocaine INN, BAN

fonatol [see: diethylstilbestrol]

fonazine mesylate USAN *serotonin inhibitor* [also: dimetotiazine; dimethothiazine]

fontarsol [see: dichlorophenarsine HCl]

fopirtoline INN

Foradil ℞ *investigational long-acting antiasthmatic*

Forane liquid for vaporization ℞ *inhalation general anesthetic* [isoflurane]

forasartan USAN *antihypertensive; CHF treatment; angiotensin II receptor antagonist*

forfenimex INN

formaldehyde solution USP *disinfectant*

Formalyde-10 spray ℞ *for hyperhidrosis and bromhidrosis* [formaldehyde] 10%

formebolone INN, BAN

formetamide [see: formetorex]

formetorex INN

formidacillin [see: fomidacillin]

forminitrazole INN, BAN

formocortal USAN, INN, BAN *glucocorticoid*

formoterol INN

Formula 44 syrup (name changed to Vicks Dry Hacking Cough in 1994)

Formula 44 Cough Control Disks; Formula 44 Cough Silencers lozenges OTC *antitussive; topical oral anesthetic* [dextromethorphan hydrobromide; benzocaine] 5•1.25 mg; 2.5•1 mg

Formula 44 Cough Medicine liquid (discontinued 1992) OTC *antihistamine; antitussive* [chlorpheniramine maleate; dextromethorphan hydrobromide; alcohol]

Formula 44 Non-Drowsy Cold & Cough LiquiCaps (capsules) (name changed to Vicks 44 Non-Drowsy Cold & Cough in 1994)

Formula 44 Pediatric syrup (name changed to Vicks Pediatric 44d Dry Hacking Cough and Head Congestion in 1994)

Formula 44D Cough & Decongestant liquid (name changed to Vicks Formula 44D Cough & Decongestant in 1994)

Formula 44d Cough & Decongestant, Pediatric liquid (name changed to Vicks Pediatric Formula 44d Cough & Decongestant in 1994)

Formula 44D Cough & Head Congestion liquid (name changed to Vicks 44D Cough & Head Congestion in 1994)

Formula 44E liquid (name changed to Vicks 44E in 1994)

Formula 44e, Pediatric liquid (name changed to Vicks Pediatric Formula 44e in 1994)

Formula 44M Cold, Flu & Cough LiquiCaps (capsules) (name changed to Vicks 44M Cold, Flu & Cough LiquiCaps in 1994)

Formula 44M Cough and Cold liquid (discontinued 1994) OTC *antitussive; decongestant; antihistamine; analgesic* [dextromethorphan hydrobromide; pseudoephedrine HCl; chlorpheniramine maleate; acetaminophen; alcohol]

Formula 44m Multi-Symptom Cough and Cold, Pediatric liquid (name changed to Vicks Pediatric Formula 44m Multi-Symptom Cough & Cold in 1994)

Formula 405 cleansing bar OTC *therapeutic skin cleanser*

Formula B tablets ℞ *vitamin supplement* [multiple B vitamins; vitamin C; folic acid] ≐•500•0.5 mg

Formula B Plus tablets ℞ *vitamin/mineral/iron supplement* [multiple vitamins & minerals; ferrous fumarate; folic acid; biotin] ≐•27•0.8•0.15 mg

Formula E 400; Formula E 1000 perles OTC *vitamin supplement* [vitamin E] 400 IU; 1000 IU

Formula N sustained-release tablets OTC *vitamin supplement* [niacin]

Formula N-AM sustained-release tablets OTC *vitamin supplement* [niacinamide]

Formula Q capsules (discontinued 1996) OTC *prevention and treatment of nocturnal leg cramps* [quinine sulfate] 65 mg

Formula VM-2000 tablets OTC *dietary supplement* [multiple vitamins, minerals, and amino acids; iron; folic acid; biotin] ≐•5 mg•0.2 mg•50 µg

4′-formylacetanilide thiosemicarbazone [see: thioacetazone; thiacetazone]

forskolin [see: colforsin]

Forta Cereal (discontinued 1993) OTC *oral nutritional supplement*

Forta Drink powder OTC *enteral nutritional therapy* [lactose-free formula]

Forta Shake powder OTC *enteral nutritional therapy* [milk-based formula]

Fortaz powder for IV or IM injection ℞ *cephalosporin-type antibiotic* [ceftazidime] 0.5, 1, 2, 6 g

Forte L.I.V. IM injection ℞ *antianemic* [ferrous gluconate; multiple B vitamins; procaine]

Fortel Home Ovulation Test kit for home use (discontinued 1995) OTC *in vitro diagnostic aid to predict ovulation time*

Fortel Midstream test stick for professional use *in vitro diagnostic aid for urine pregnancy test*

Fortel Plus test kit for home use OTC *in vitro diagnostic aid for urine pregnancy test*

fortimicin A [now: astromicin sulfate]

40 winks capsules OTC *antihistaminic sleep aid* [diphenhydramine HCl] 50 mg

Fosamax tablets ℞ *biphosphonate for postmenopausal osteoporosis and Paget's disease* [alendronate sodium] 10, 40 mg

fosarilate USAN, INN *antiviral*

fosazepam USAN, INN, BAN *hypnotic*

foscarnet sodium USAN, INN, BAN *antiviral for cytomegalovirus (CMV), various herpesvirus types, and Epstein-Barr virus (EBV)*

Foscavir IV injection ℞ *antiviral for cytomegalovirus retinitis and herpes simplex infections in AIDS* [foscarnet sodium] 24 mg/mL

Foscavir topical ℞ *investigational (Phase I) antiviral for herpes simplex infections in AIDS* [foscarnet sodium]

foscolic acid INN

fosenazide INN

fosenopril sodium [see: fosinopril sodium]

fosfestrol INN, BAN *antineoplastic; estrogen* [also: diethylstilbestrol diphosphate]

fosfocreatinine INN

fosfomycin USAN, INN, BAN *antibacterial*

fosfomycin tromethamine USAN *antibacterial*

fosfonet sodium USAN, INN *antiviral*

fosfosal INN

Fosfree tablets OTC *vitamin/iron supplement* [multiple vitamins; iron] ± •14.5 mg

fosinopril INN, BAN *antihypertensive; angiotensin-converting enzyme (ACE) inhibitor* [also: fosinopril sodium]

fosinopril sodium USAN *antihypertensive; angiotensin-converting enzyme (ACE) inhibitor* [also: fosinopril]

fosinoprilat USAN, INN *antihypertensive*

fosmenic acid INN

fosmidomycin INN

fosphenytoin INN (*orphan: grand mal status epilepticus*)

fosphenytoin sodium USAN, INN *hydantoin-type anticonvulsant*

fospirate USAN, INN *veterinary anthelmintic*

fosquidone USAN, INN, BAN *antineoplastic*

fostedil USAN, INN *vasodilator; calcium channel blocker*

Fostex cleansing bar OTC *topical keratolytic for acne* [benzoyl peroxide] 10% ② pHisoHex

Fostex 5% BPO gel (discontinued 1994) OTC *topical keratolytic for acne* [benzoyl peroxide] 5%

Fostex 10% BPO gel OTC *topical keratolytic for acne* [benzoyl peroxide] 10%

Fostex 10% BPO tinted cream (discontinued 1994) OTC *topical keratolytic for acne* [benzoyl peroxide] 10%

Fostex 10% BPO wash (name changed to Fostex 10% Wash in 1994)

Fostex 10% Wash liquid OTC *topical keratolytic for acne* [benzoyl peroxide] 10%

Fostex Acne Cleansing cream OTC *topical keratolytic for acne* [salicylic acid] 2%

Fostex Acne Medication Cleansing bar OTC *medicated cleanser for acne* [salicylic acid] 2%

Fostex Medicated Cleansing Shampoo OTC *antiseborrheic; keratolytic* [sulfur; salicylic acid] 2%•2%

Fostex Medicated Cover-Up cream (discontinued 1994) OTC *antibacterial and exfoliant for acne* [sulfur] 2%

fostriecin INN *antineoplastic* [also: fostriecin sodium]

fostriecin sodium USAN *antineoplastic* [also: fostriecin]

Fostril lotion OTC *topical acne treatment* [sulfur; zinc oxide]

fotemustine INN, BAN

Fototar cream OTC *topical antipsoriatic; antiseborrheic* [coal tar] 2%

fotretamine INN

Fouchet's reagent (solution)

4 Hair softgel capsules OTC *vitamin/mineral/iron supplement* [multiple vitamins & minerals; iron; folic acid; biotin] ≐•2.5•33.3•0.25 mg

4 Nails softgel capsules OTC *vitamin/mineral/calcium/iron supplement* [multiple vitamins & minerals; calcium; iron; folic acid; biotin] ≐•167•3•0.333•0.0083 mg

4-Way Cold tablets (discontinued 1995) OTC *decongestant; antihistamine; analgesic* [phenylpropanolamine HCl; chlorpheniramine maleate; acetaminophen] 12.5•2•325 mg

4-Way Fast Acting nasal spray OTC *nasal decongestant; antihistamine* [phenylephrine HCl; naphazoline HCl; pyrilamine maleate] 0.5%•0.05%•0.2%

4-Way Long Lasting nasal spray OTC *nasal decongestant* [oxymetazoline HCl] 0.05%

403U *investigational antidepressant*

4197X-RA *investigational cataract preventative*

447C *investigational ACAT inhibitor to reduce serum cholesterol*

4MRTA *investigational antineoplastic for T-cell malignancies*

Fourneau 309 (available only from the Centers for Disease Control) ℞ *investigational anti-infective for trypanosomiasis and onchocerciasis* [suramin sodium]

FPL64170 *investigational treatment for psoriasis and ulcerative colitis*

FPL67085 *investigational treatment for acute thrombotic events*

frabuprofen INN

Fractar (trademarked ingredient) OTC *antipsoriatic; antiseborrheic* [crude coal tar]

Fragmin subcu injection ℞ *anticoagulant for prevention of deep vein thrombosis* [dalteparin sodium] 2500, 5000 IU/0.2 mL (16, 32 mg/0.2 mL)

framycetin INN, BAN

francium *element (Fr)*

FreAmine III 3% IV infusion (discontinued 1992) ℞ *peripheral parenteral nutrition* [multiple essential and nonessential amino acids]

FreAmine III 3% (8.5%) with Electrolytes IV infusion ℞ *total parenteral nutrition (8.5% only); peripheral parenteral nutrition (both)* [multiple essential and nonessential amino acids & electrolytes]

FreAmine III 8.5%; FreAmine III 10% IV infusion ℞ *total parenteral nutrition; peripheral parenteral nutrition* [multiple essential and nonessential amino acids]

FreAmine HBC 6.9% IV infusion ℞ *nutritional therapy for high metabolic stress* [multiple branched-chain essential and nonessential amino acids; electrolytes]

Free & Clear shampoo OTC *soap-free therapeutic cleanser*

Freedavite tablets OTC *vitamin/mineral/iron supplement* [multiple vitamins & minerals; ferrous fumarate] ≐•10 mg

Freedox solution ℞ *investigational lazaroid for subarachnoid hemorrhage, ischemic stroke, spinal cord and head injury* [tirilazad mesylate]

Freezone liquid OTC *topical keratolytic* [salicylic acid in a collodion-like vehicle] 13.6%

frentizole USAN, INN, BAN *immunoregulator*

Frisium ℞ *investigational benzodiazepine-type tranquilizer; anxiolytic* [clobazam]

Frone (commercially available in Europe, Asia, and Latin America) ℞ *investigational treatment for multiple sclerosis, herpes, leukemia, cervical neoplasia and hepatitis* [natural beta interferon]

fronepidil INN

froxiprost INN

fructose (D-fructose) USP *nutrient; caloric replacement* [also: levulose]

Fruity Chews chewable tablets OTC *vitamin supplement* [multiple vitamins; folic acid] ≛•0.3 mg

Fruity Chews with Iron chewable tablets OTC *vitamin/iron supplement* [multiple vitamins; iron; folic acid] ≛•12•0.3 mg

frusemide BAN *diuretic* [also: furosemide]

FS Shampoo ℞ *topical corticosteroid; antiseborrheic* [fluocinolone acetonide] 0.01%

FSF (fibrin-stabilizing factor) [see: factor XIII]

FSH (follicle-stimulating hormone) [see: menotropins]

ftalofyne INN *veterinary anthelmintic* [also: phthalofyne]

ftaxilide INN

ftivazide INN

ftormetazine INN

ftorpropazine INN

5-FU (5-fluorouracil) [see: fluorouracil]

fubrogonium iodide INN

fuchsin, basic USP *topical antibacterial/antifungal*

Fucidin *investigational topical antibacterial for impetigo and folliculitis* [fusidate sodium]

FUDR powder for IV injection ℞ *antimetabolic antineoplastic for brain, breast, head, neck, liver, gallbladder, and bile duct cancer* [floxuridine] 500 mg

FUDR; FUdR (5-fluorouracil deoxyribonucleoside) [see: floxuridine]

Ful-Glo ophthalmic strips ℞ *corneal disclosing agent* [fluorescein sodium] 0.6 mg

fulmicoton [see: pyroxylin]

FU/LV (fluorouracil, leucovorin calcium [rescue]) *chemotherapy protocol* [also: F-CL]

Fulvicin P/G tablets ℞ *systemic antifungal* [griseofulvin (ultramicrosize)] 125, 165, 250, 330 mg ⊡ folacin; Furacin

Fulvicin U/F tablets ℞ *systemic antifungal* [griseofulvin (microsize)] 250, 500 mg

FUM (fluorouracil, methotrexate) *chemotherapy protocol*

fumagillin INN, BAN

Fumaral Spancaps (timed-release capsules) (discontinued 1992) OTC *antianemic* [ferrous fumarate; ascorbic acid]

fumaric acid NF *acidifier*

Fumasorb tablets OTC *hematinic* [ferrous fumarate] 200 mg

Fumatinic sustained-release capsules ℞ *hematinic* [ferrous fumarate; cyanocobalamin; ascorbic acid; folic acid] 90 mg•15 µg•100 mg•1 mg

Fumerin sugar-coated tablets OTC *hematinic* [ferrous fumarate] 195 mg

Fumide tablets (discontinued 1993) ℞ *loop diuretic* [furosemide]

fumoxicillin USAN, INN *antibacterial*

Funduscein-10; Funduscein-25 IV injection ℞ *corneal disclosing agent* [fluorescein sodium] 10%; 25%

Fungatin cream OTC *topical antifungal* [tolnaftate]

fungicidin [see: nystatin]

fungimycin USAN *antifungal*

Fungi-Nail liquid OTC *topical antifungal; keratolytic; anesthetic* [resorcinol; salicylic acid; chloroxylenol; benzocaine; alcohol 50%] 1%•2%•2%•0.5%

Fungizone cream, lotion, ointment ℞ *topical antifungal* [amphotericin B] 3%

Fungizone oral solution, IV infusion ℞ *systemic antifungal* [amphotericin B] 100 mg/mL; 50 mg/vial

Fungoid cream, tincture ℞ *topical antifungal* [miconazole nitrate] 2%

Fungoid solution ℞ *topical antifungal* [undecylenic acid] 25%

Fungoid-HC cream ℞ *topical corticosteroid; antipruritic; antifungal; antibacterial* [miconazole nitrate; hydrocortisone] 2%•1%

fuprazole INN

furacilin [see: nitrofurazone]

Furacin topical solution, cream ℞ broad-spectrum antibacterial for adjunctive burn therapy [nitrofurazone] 0.2% ② Fulvicin

Furacin Soluble Dressing ointment ℞ broad-spectrum antibacterial for adjunctive burn therapy [nitrofurazone] 2%

furacrinic acid INN, BAN

Furadantin oral suspension ℞ urinary bacteriostatic [nitrofurantoin] 25 mg/5 mL

Furadantin tablets (discontinued 1993) ℞ urinary bacteriostatic [nitrofurantoin] 50, 100 mg

furafylline INN

Furalan tablets ℞ urinary bacteriostatic [nitrofurantoin] 50, 100 mg

furalazine INN

furaltadone INN, BAN

Furamide (available only from the Centers for Disease Control) ℞ investigational anti-infective for amebiasis [diloxanide furoate]

Furan tablets (discontinued 1992) ℞ urinary bacteriostatic [nitrofurantoin] 50, 100 mg

Furanite tablets ℞ urinary bacteriostatic [nitrofurantoin] 50, 100 mg

furaprofen USAN, INN anti-inflammatory

furazabol INN

furazolidone USP, INN, BAN bactericidal; antiprotozoal (Trichomonas); antidiarrheal

furazolium chloride USAN, INN antibacterial

furazolium tartrate USAN antibacterial

furbucillin INN

furcloprofen INN

furegrelate INN thromboxane synthetase inhibitor [also: furegrelate sodium]

furegrelate sodium USAN thromboxane synthetase inhibitor [also: furegrelate]

furethidine INN, BAN

furfenorex INN

furfuryltrimethylammonium iodide [see: furtrethonium iodide]

furidarone INN

furmethoxadone INN

furobufen USAN, INN anti-inflammatory

furodazole USAN, INN anthelmintic

furofenac INN

furomazine INN

Furomide M.D. injection (discontinued 1993) ℞ loop diuretic [furosemide]

Furonatal F.A. tablets (discontinued 1992) ℞ antianemic [multiple vitamins & minerals]

furosemide USAN, USP, INN, JAN loop diuretic [also: frusemide] 20, 40, 80 mg oral; 10 mg/mL oral; 40 mg/5 mL oral; 10 mg/mL injection

furostilbestrol INN

furoxicillin [see: fumoxicillin]

Furoxone tablets, liquid ℞ antibacterial [furazolidone] 100 mg; 50 mg/15 mL

fursalan USAN, INN disinfectant

fursultiamine INN

furterene INN

furtrethonium iodide INN

furtrimethonium iodide [see: furtrethonium iodide]

Furtulon (commercially available in Japan and Korea) ℞ investigational antineoplastic [doxifluridine]

fusafungine INN, BAN

fusidate sodium USAN antibacterial

fusidic acid USAN, INN, BAN antibacterial

fusidic acid, sodium salt [see: fusidate sodium]

FUVAC (5-FU, vinblastine, Adriamycin, cyclophosphamide) chemotherapy protocol

fuzlocillin INN, BAN

fytic acid INN

FZ (flutamide, Zoladex) chemotherapy protocol

G

G-201 *investigational topical nonsteroidal anti-inflammatory drug (NSAID) for skin disorders*

G-203 *investigational topical corticosteroidal wipe for eczema and atopic dermatitis* [fluocinonide]

^{67}Ga [see: gallium citrate Ga 67]

gabapentin USAN, INN *anticonvulsant*

Gabbromicina ℞ *(orphan: Mycobacterium avium complex)* [aminosidine]

gabexate INN

gaboxadol INN

gadobenate dimeglumine USAN *MRI diagnostic aid* [also: gadobenic acid]

gadobenic acid INN *MRI diagnostic aid* [also: gadobenate dimeglumine]

gadobutrol INN *investigational aid for MRI*

gadodiamide USAN, INN, BAN *diagnostic aid for magnetic imaging*

gadolinium *element (Gd)*

gadopenamide INN

gadopentetate dimeglumine USAN *radiopaque medium* [also: gadopentetic acid]

gadopentetic acid INN, BAN *diagnostic aid* [also: gadopentetate dimeglumine]

gadoteric acid INN

gadoteridol USAN, INN, BAN *diagnostic aid for magnetic imaging*

gadoversetamide USAN, INN *paramagnetic MRI contrast agent for brain, head, and spine*

gaiactamine [see: guaiactamine]

gaietamine [see: guaiactamine]

galamustine INN

galantamine INN

galantamine hydrobromide

galanthamine [see: galantamine]

Galardin ℞ *(orphan: treatment for corneal ulcers)* [matrix metalloproteinase inhibitor]

galdansetron INN, BAN *antiemetic* [also: galdansetron HCl]

galdansetron HCl USAN *antiemetic* [also: galdansetron]

gallamine BAN *neuromuscular blocker* [also: gallamine triethiodide]

gallamine triethiodide USP, INN *neuromuscular blocker; muscle relaxant* [also: gallamine]

gallamone triethiodide [see: gallamine triethiodide]

gallic acid NF

gallic acid, bismuth basic salt [see: bismuth subgallate]

gallium *element (Ga)*

gallium (^{67}Ga) citrate INN *radiopaque medium; radioactive agent* [also: gallium citrate Ga 67]

gallium citrate Ga 67 USAN, USP *radiopaque medium; radioactive agent* [also: gallium (^{67}Ga) citrate]

gallium nitrate USAN *calcium regulator; for hypercalcemia of malignancy (orphan)*

gallium nitrate nonahydrate [see: gallium nitrate]

gallopamil INN, BAN

gallotannic acid [see: tannic acid]

galosemide INN

galtifenin INN

Gamastan IM injection ℞ *passive immunizing agent* [immune globulin] 2, 10 mL ⚕ Garamycin

gamfexine USAN, INN *antidepressant*

Gamimune N IV infusion ℞ *passive immunizing agent; immunomodulator for AIDS/ARC (orphan: acute myocarditis)* [immune globulin] 5%, 10%

gamma benzene hexachloride [now: lindane]

gamma globulin [see: globulin, immune]

Gammagard powder for IV infusion (discontinued 1994; replaced by Gammagard S/D) ℞ *passive immunizing agent* [immune globulin]

Gammagard S/D freeze-dried powder for IV infusion ℞ *passive immunizing agent; immunomodulator for AIDS/ARC* [immune globulin, solvent/detergent treated] 50 mg/mL

gamma-hydroxybutyrate sodium [see: hydroxybutyrate sodium, gamma]

gamma-linolenic acid (GLA) *(orphan: juvenile rheumatoid arthritis)*

gammaphos [now: ethiofos]

Gammar IM injection ℞ *immunizing agent* [immune globulin] 2, 10 mL

Gammar-IV powder for IV infusion (replaced with Gammar-P IV in 1996; P is for "pasteurized") ℞ *immunizing agent* [immune globulin] 5%

Gammar-P IV powder for IV infusion ℞ *passive immunizing agent; immunomodulator for AIDS/ARC* [immune globulin, pasteurized] 5%

gamma-vinyl GABA (gamma-aminobutyric acid) [see: vigabatrin]

gamolenic acid INN, BAN

Gamulin Rh IM injection ℞ *obstetric Rh factor immunity suppressant* [Rh$_0$(D) immune globulin] 300 μg

ganciclovir USAN, INN, BAN *antiviral* [also: ganciclovir sodium]

ganciclovir sodium USAN *antiviral; (orphan: cytomegalovirus retinitis in AIDS)* [also: ganciclovir]

ganglefene INN

gangliosides, sodium salts *(orphan: retinitis pigmentosa)*

ganirelix INN *gonad-stimulating principle* [also: ganirelix acetate]

ganirelix acetate USAN *gonad-stimulating principle* [also: ganirelix]

Ganite IV infusion ℞ *calcium resorption inhibitor for hypercalcemia of malignancy (orphan)* [gallium nitrate] 25 mg/mL

Gantanol oral suspension (discontinued 1994) ℞ *broad-spectrum bacteriostatic* [sulfamethoxazole] 500 mg/5 mL ⊡ Gantrisin

Gantanol tablets ℞ *broad-spectrum bacteriostatic* [sulfamethoxazole] 500 mg

Gantrisin eye drops (discontinued 1995) ℞ *ophthalmic bacteriostatic* [sulfisoxazole diolamine] 4% ⊡ Gantanol

Gantrisin ophthalmic ointment (discontinued 1992) ℞ *ophthalmic bacteriostatic* [sulfisoxazole diolamine]

Gantrisin pediatric suspension (discontinued 1996) ℞ *broad-spectrum bacteriostatic* [sulfisoxazole acetyl] 500 mg/5 mL

Gantrisin syrup (discontinued 1994) ℞ *broad-spectrum bacteriostatic* [sulfisoxazole acetyl] 500 mg/5 mL

Gantrisin tablets (discontinued 1996) ℞ *broad-spectrum bacteriostatic* [sulfisoxazole] 500 mg

gapicomine INN

gapromidine INN

Garamicina (Mexican name for U.S. product Garamycin)

Garamycin cream, ointment ℞ *topical antibiotic* [gentamicin sulfate] 0.1% ⊡ Gamastan; kanamycin; Terramycin

Garamycin eye drops, ophthalmic ointment ℞ *ophthalmic antibiotic* [gentamicin sulfate] 3 mg/mL; 3 mg/g

Garamycin IV or IM injection, intrathecal injection ℞ *aminoglycoside-type antibiotic* [gentamicin sulfate] 40 mg/mL; 2 mg/mL

Garamycin Pediatric IV or IM injection ℞ *aminoglycoside-type antibiotic* [gentamicin sulfate] 10 mg/mL

Garden Fresh bar soap OTC *cleanser* [vegetable-based]

Gardrin ℞ *investigational treatment for acute peptic ulcers* [enprostil]

Garfield; Garfield Plus Extra C chewable tablets OTC *vitamin supplement* [multiple vitamins; folic acid] ±•0.3 mg

Garfield Complete with Minerals chewable tablets OTC *vitamin/mineral/iron supplement* [multiple vitamins & minerals; iron; folic acid; biotin] ±•18•0.4•0.04 mg

Garfield Plus Iron chewable tablets OTC *vitamin/iron supplement* [multiple vitamins; iron; folic acid] ±•15•0.3 mg

gas gangrene antitoxin, pentavalent

gas gangrene antitoxin, polyvalent [see: gas gangrene antitoxin, pentavalent]

Gas Permeable Daily Cleaner solution OTC *cleaning solution for rigid gas permeable contact lenses*

Gas Permeable Wetting and Soaking solution (discontinued 1993) OTC *disinfecting/wetting/soaking solution for rigid gas permeable contact lenses*

Gas Relief chewable tablets, drops OTC *antiflatulent* [simethicone] 80, 125 mg; 40 mg/0.6 mL

Gas-Ban tablets OTC *antacid; antiflatulent* [calcium carbonate; simethicone] 300•40 mg

Gas-Ban DS liquid OTC *antacid; antiflatulent* [aluminum hydroxide; magnesium hydroxide; simethicone] 400•400•40 mg/5 mL

gastric mucin BAN

Gastroccult slide test for professional use *in vitro diagnostic aid for gastric occult blood*

Gastrocrom capsules ℞ *bronchodilator for bronchial asthma; for mastocytosis (orphan)* [cromolyn sodium] 100 mg

Gastrografin solution ℞ *GI contrast radiopaque agent* [diatrizoate meglumine; diatrizoate sodium] 66%•10%

Gastromark ℞ *investigational bowel imaging agent for MRI* [ferumoxsil]

Gastronol ℞ *investigational antiulcerative* [proglumide]

Gastrosed drops, tablets ℞ *anticholinergic* [hyoscyamine sulfate] 0.125 mg/mL; 0.125 mg

Gastro-Test string capsules for professional use *in vitro diagnostic aid for GI disorders*

Gastrozepine ℞ *investigational antiulcerative* [pirenzepine HCl]

Gas-X chewable tablets OTC *antiflatulent* [simethicone] 80, 125 mg

gaultheria oil [see: methyl salicylate]

gauze, absorbent USP *surgical aid*

gauze, petrolatum USP *surgical aid*

gauze bandage [see: bandage, gauze]

Gaviscon liquid OTC *antacid* [aluminum hydroxide; magnesium carbonate] 31.7•119.3 mg/5 mL

Gaviscon; Gaviscon-2 chewable tablets OTC *antacid* [aluminum hydroxide; magnesium trisilicate] 80•20 mg; 160•40 mg

Gaviscon Relief Formula chewable tablets, liquid OTC *antacid* [aluminum hydroxide; magnesium carbonate] 160•105 mg; 254•237.5 mg/5 mL

G.B.S. tablets (discontinued 1992) ℞ *laxative; hydrocholeretic; sedative* [dehydrocholic acid; homatropine methylbromide; phenobarbital]

G-CSF (granulocyte colony-stimulating factor) [see: filgrastim]

gedocarnil INN *investigational treatment of central nervous system disorders*

Gee-Gee tablets OTC *expectorant* [guaifenesin] 200 mg

gefarnate INN, BAN

Gel Clean (discontinued 1992) OTC *cleaning gel for hard contact lenses*

gelatin NF *encapsulating, suspending, binding and coating agent*

gelatin film, absorbable USP *topical local hemostatic*

gelatin powder, absorbable *topical local hemostatic*

gelatin solution, special intravenous [see: polygeline]

gelatin sponge, absorbable USP *topical local hemostatic*

gelcaps (dosage form) *soft gelatin capsules*

Gelfilm; Gelfilm Ophthalmic ℞ *topical local hemostat for surgery* [absorbable gelatin film]

Gelfoam powder ℞ *topical local hemostat for surgery* [absorbable gelatin powder] ② Ger-O-Foam

Gelfoam sponge, packs, dental packs, prostatectomy cones ℞ *topical local hemostat for surgery* [absorbable gelatin sponge] ② Ger-O-Foam

Gel-Kam gel ℞ *topical dental caries preventative* [stannous fluoride] 0.4%

Gelpirin tablets OTC *analgesic; antipyretic; anti-inflammatory* [acetaminophen; buffered aspirin; caffeine] 125•240•32 mg

Gelpirin-CCF tablets OTC *decongestant; antihistamine; analgesic; expectorant* [phenylpropanolamine HCl; chlorpheniramine maleate; acetaminophen; guaifenesin] 12.5•1•325•25 mg

Gelseal (trademarked dosage form) *soft gelatin capsule*

gelsolin, recombinant human (*orphan: respiratory symptoms of cystic fibrosis*)

Gel-Tin gel OTC *topical dental caries preventative* [stannous fluoride] 0.4%

Gelusil chewable tablets OTC *antacid; antiflatulent* [aluminum hydroxide; magnesium hydroxide; simethicone] 200•200•25 mg

Gelusil liquid (discontinued 1996) OTC *antacid; antiflatulent* [aluminum hydroxide; magnesium hydroxide; simethicone] 200•200•25 mg/5 mL

Gelusil-II chewable tablets, liquid (discontinued 1994) OTC *antacid; antiflatulent* [aluminum hydroxide; magnesium hydroxide; simethicone] 400•400•30 mg; 80•80•6 mg/mL

GEM 91 *investigational (phase I) antiviral for HIV*

gemazocine INN

gemcadiol USAN, INN *antihyperlipoproteinemic*

gemcitabine USAN, INN, BAN *antineoplastic*

gemcitabine HCl USAN *antineoplastic for pancreatic cancer*

Gemcor film-coated tablets ℞ *antihyperlipidemic agent (cholesterol-lowering)* [gemfibrozil] 600 mg

gemeprost USAN, INN, BAN *prostaglandin*

gemfibrozil USAN, USP, INN, BAN *antihyperlipoproteinemic* 300, 600 mg oral

Gemnisyn tablets (discontinued 1994) OTC *analgesic; antipyretic; antiinflammatory* [acetaminophen; aspirin] 325•325 mg

Gemzar powder for IV infusion ℞ *antineoplastic for advanced or metastatic pancreatic cancer; investigational for lung cancer* [gemcitabine HCl] 20 mg/mL

Genabid timed-release capsules ℞ *peripheral vasodilator* [papaverine HCl] 150 mg

Genac tablets OTC *decongestant; antihistamine* [pseudoephedrine HCl; triprolidine HCl] 60•2.5 mg

Genacol tablets OTC *antitussive; decongestant; antihistamine; analgesic* [dextromethorphan hydrobromide; phenylpropanolamine HCl; chlorpheniramine maleate; acetaminophen] 10•30•2•325 mg

Genagesic tablets (discontinued 1995) ℞ *narcotic analgesic* [propoxyphene HCl; acetaminophen] 65•650 mg

Genahist capsules, tablets, elixir ℞ *antihistamine; motion sickness preventative; sleep aid; antiparkinsonian* [diphenhydramine HCl] 25 mg; 25 mg; 12.5 mg/5 mL

Genalac chewable tablets (discontinued 1994) OTC *antacid* [calcium carbonate; glycine]

Gen-Allerate tablets OTC *antihistamine* [chlorpheniramine maleate] 4 mg

Genamin Cold syrup OTC *decongestant; antihistamine* [phenylpropanolamine HCl; chlorpheniramine maleate] 6.25•1 mg/5 mL

Genapap tablets OTC *analgesic; antipyretic* [acetaminophen] 500 mg

Genapap, Children's chewable tablets, elixir OTC *analgesic; antipyretic* [acetaminophen] 80 mg; 160 mg/5 mL

Genapap, Infants' drops OTC *analgesic; antipyretic* [acetaminophen] 100 mg/mL

Genapax medicated tampons (discontinued 1994) ℞ *antifungal* [gentian violet]

Genaphed tablets OTC *nasal decongestant* [pseudoephedrine HCl] 30 mg

Genasal nasal spray OTC *nasal decongestant* [oxymetazoline HCl] 0.05%

Genasoft Plus softgels OTC *laxative; stool softener* [casanthranol; docusate sodium] 30•100 mg

Genaspor cream OTC *topical antifungal* [tolnaftate] 1%

Genatap elixir OTC *decongestant; antihistamine* [phenylpropanolamine HCl; brompheniramine maleate] 12.5•2 mg/5 mL 🔊 Genapap

Genaton chewable tablets OTC *antacid* [aluminum hydroxide; magnesium trisilicate] 80•20 mg

Genaton liquid OTC *antacid* [aluminum hydroxide; magnesium carbonate] 31.7•137.3 mg/5 mL

Genaton, Extra Strength chewable tablets OTC *antacid* [aluminum hydroxide; magnesium carbonate] 160•105 mg

Genatuss syrup OTC *expectorant* [guaifenesin; alcohol 3.5%] 100 mg/5 mL

Genatuss DM syrup OTC *antitussive; expectorant* [dextromethorphan hydrobromide; guaifenesin] 10•100 mg/5 mL

Gen-bee with C caplets OTC *vitamin supplement* [multiple B vitamins; vitamin C] ±•300 mg

Gencalc 600 film-coated tablets OTC *calcium supplement* [calcium carbonate] 1.5 g

GenCept tablets (discontinued 1994) ℞ *oral contraceptive* [norethindrone; ethinyl estradiol]

Gencold sustained-release capsules OTC *decongestant; antihistamine* [phenylpropanolamine HCl; chlorpheniramine maleate] 75•8 mg

Gendecon tablets OTC *decongestant; antihistamine; analgesic* [phenylephrine HCl; chlorpheniramine maleate; acetaminophen] 5•2•325 mg

Gendex 75 IV infusion ℞ *plasma volume expander for shock due to hemorrhage, burns, or surgery* [dextran 75] 6%

Gen-D-Phen syrup (discontinued 1994) OTC *antihistamine; antitussive* [diphenhydramine HCl; alcohol 5%] 12.5 mg/5 mL

Genebs tablets OTC *analgesic; antipyretic* [acetaminophen] 325, 500 mg

Generet-500 timed-release tablets OTC *hematinic* [ferrous sulfate; multiple B vitamins; sodium ascorbate] 105•±•500 mg ⑨ Gentap

Generix-T tablets OTC *vitamin/mineral/iron supplement* [multiple vitamins & minerals; iron] ±•15 mg

GenESA System ℞ *investigational stress test for coronary artery disease, with a computer-controlled delivery system* [arbutamine]

Genevax-HIV ℞ *investigational (Phase I) vaccine for HIV*

Gcnex capsules (discontinued 1993) OTC *decongestant; analgesic* [phenylpropanolamine HCl; acetaminophen]

Geneye eye drops OTC *topical ocular decongestant/vasoconstrictor* [tetrahydrozoline HCl] 0.05%

Geneye AC Allergy Formula eye drops OTC *topical ocular decongestant; astringent* [tetrahydrozoline HCl; zinc sulfate] 0.05%•0.25%

Geneye Extra eye drops OTC *topical ocular decongestant/vasoconstrictor; emollient* [tetrahydrozoline HCl; PEG 400] 0.05%•1%

Genite liquid OTC *antitussive; decongestant; antihistamine; analgesic* [dextromethorphan hydrobromide; pseudoephedrine HCl; doxylamine succinate; acetaminophen; alcohol 25%] 5•10•1.25•167 mg/5 mL

Gen-K powder ℞ *potassium supplement* [potassium chloride] 20 mEq/packet

genophyllin [see: aminophylline]

Genoptic eye drops ℞ *ophthalmic antibiotic* [gentamicin sulfate] 3 mg/mL

Genoptic S.O.P. ophthalmic ointment ℞ *ophthalmic antibiotic* [gentamicin sulfate] 3 mg/g

Genora 0.5/35; Genora 1/35 tablets ℞ *monophasic oral contraceptive* [norethindrone; ethinyl estradiol] 0.5 mg•35 μg; 1 mg•35 μg

Genora 1/50 tablets ℞ *monophasic oral contraceptive* [norethindrone; mestranol] 1 mg•50 μg

Genotonorm ℞ *investigational human growth hormone (orphan: growth hormone deficiency)* [somatropin]

Genotropin injection ℞ *(orphan: growth hormone deficiency)* [somatropin] 1.5, 5.8 mg

Genpril film-coated tablets, film-coated caplets OTC *nonsteroidal anti-inflammatory drug (NSAID); antiarthritic; analgesic* [ibuprofen] 200 mg

Genprin tablets OTC *analgesic; antipyretic; anti-inflammatory; antirheumatic* [aspirin] 325 mg

Gensan tablets OTC *analgesic; antipyretic; anti-inflammatory* [aspirin; caffeine] 400•32 mg

Gentab-LA long-acting tablets (discontinued 1994) ℞ *decongestant; expectorant* [phenylpropanolamine HCl; guaifenesin]

Gentacidin eye drops, ophthalmic ointment ℞ *ophthalmic antibiotic* [gentamicin sulfate] 3 mg/mL; 3 mg/g

Gentak eye drops, ophthalmic ointment ℞ *ophthalmic antibiotic* [gentamicin sulfate] 3 mg/mL; 3 mg/g

gentamicin BAN *aminoglycoside bactericidal antibiotic* [also: gentamicin sulfate] ⑨ Jenamicin; kanamycin

gentamicin liposome *(orphan: disseminated Mycobacterium avium-intracellulare)*

gentamicin sulfate USAN, USP *aminoglycoside bactericidal antibiotic* [also: gentamicin] 3 mg/mL eye drops; 3 mg/g topical; 0.1% topical; 10, 40 mg/mL injection

gentamicin-impregnated PMMA beads *(orphan: chronic osteomyelitis)*

gentian violet USP *topical anti-infective/antifungal* [also: methylrosanilinium chloride]

gentisic acid ethanolamine NF *complexing agent*

Gentlax granules OTC *laxative* [senna concentrate] 326 mg/tsp.

Gentlax S tablets OTC *laxative; stool softener* [docusate sodium; sennosides] 50•8.6 mg

Gentran 40 IV injection ℞ *plasma volume expander for shock due to hemorrhage, burns, or surgery* [dextran 40] 10%

Gentran 70 IV infusion ℞ *plasma volume expander for shock due to hemorrhage, burns, or surgery* [dextran 70] 6%

Gentran 75 IV infusion (discontinued 1996) ℞ *plasma volume expander for shock due to hemorrhage, burns, or surgery* [dextran 75] 6%

Gentrasul eye drops, ophthalmic ointment (discontinued 1993) ℞ *ophthalmic antibiotic* [gentamicin]

Gentz anorectal wipes (discontinued 1995) OTC *topical local anesthetic; astringent* [pramoxine HCl; alcloxa; hamamelis water; propylene glycol] 1%•0.2%•50%•10%

Genvite tablets OTC *antianemic* [ferrous fumarate; multiple vitamins]

Gen-Xene tablets ℞ *anxiolytic; minor tranquilizer; anticonvulsant adjunct* [chlorazepate dipotassium] 3.75, 7.5, 15 mg

Geocillin film-coated tablets ℞ *extended-spectrum penicillin-type antibiotic* [carbenicillin indanyl sodium] 382 mg

gepefrine INN

gepirone INN *tranquilizer; anxiolytic; antidepressant* [also: gepirone HCl]

gepirone HCl USAN *tranquilizer; anxiolytic; antidepressant* [also: gepirone]

2-geranylhydroquinone [see: geroquinol]

Geravim elixir OTC *vitamin/mineral supplement* [multiple B vitamins & minerals] ±

Geravite elixir OTC *geriatric vitamin supplement* [multiple B vitamins] ±

Gerber Baby Formula with Iron liquid, powder OTC *total or supplementary infant feeding*

Gerber Baby Low Iron Formula liquid, powder OTC *total or supplementary infant feeding*

Gerber Soy Formula liquid, powder OTC *hypoallergenic infant formula* [soy protein formula]

Geref powder for IV injection ℞ *pituitary diagnostic aid; (orphan: growth hormone deficiency; anovulation; AIDS-related weight loss)* [sermorelin acetate] 50 μg

Geriamic tablets (discontinued 1992) OTC *antianemic* [ferrous sulfate; multiple B vitamins; vitamin C]

Geridium tablets ℞ *urinary analgesic* [phenazopyridine HCl] 100, 200 mg

Gerimal sublingual tablets, tablets ℞ *for age-related mental capacity decline* [ergoloid mesylates] 0.5, 1 mg; 1 mg

Gerimed film-coated tablets OTC *geriatric vitamin/mineral supplement* [multiple vitamins & minerals] ±

Geriot film-coated tablets OTC *hematinic; vitamin/mineral supplement* [carbonyl iron; multiple vitamins & minerals; folic acid; biotin] 50 mg•±•0.4 mg•45 μg

Geriplex-FS Kapseals (capsules) (discontinued 1995) OTC *geriatric dietary supplement* [multiple vitamins & minerals] ±

Geritol Complete tablets OTC *vitamin/mineral/iron supplement* [multiple vitamins & minerals; ferrous fumarate; folic acid; biotin] ±•18 mg•0.4 mg•45 μg

Geritol Extend caplets OTC *vitamin/mineral/iron supplement* [multiple vitamins & minerals; ferrous fumarate; folic acid] ±•10•0.2 mg

Geritol Tonic liquid OTC *hematinic* [ferric pyrophosphate; multiple B vitamins; alcohol 12%] 18•≛ mg/15 mL

Geritonic liquid OTC *hematinic* [ferric ammonium citrate; liver fraction 1; multiple B vitamins and minerals; alcohol 20%] 105•375•≛ mg/15 mL

Gerivite liquid OTC *geriatric vitamin/mineral supplement* [multiple B vitamins & minerals; alcohol 18%] ≛

Gerivites tablets OTC *hematinic; vitamin/mineral supplement* [ferrous sulfate; multiple vitamins and minerals; folic acid] 50•≛•0.4 mg

Germanin (available only from the Centers for Disease Control) ℞ *investigational anti-infective for trypanosomiasis and onchocerciasis* [suramin sodium]

germanium *element (Ge)*

Germicin solution (discontinued 1992) OTC *topical antiseptic* [benzalkonium chloride]

Ger-O-Foam aerosol (discontinued 1992) OTC *counterirritant; topical anesthetic* [methyl salicylate; benzocaine] 🗓 Gelfoam

geroquinol INN

Geroton Forte liquid OTC *geriatric vitamin/mineral supplement* [multiple B vitamins & minerals; alcohol 13.5%] ≛

gesarol [see: chlorophenothane]

gestaclone USAN, INN *progestin*

gestadienol INN

gestanin [see: allyloestrenol]

Gesterol 50 IM injection (discontinued 1994) ℞ *progestin for amenorrhea or functional uterine bleeding* [progesterone] 50 mg/mL

Gesterol L.A. 250 IM injection (discontinued 1994) ℞ *progestin for amenorrhea, metrorrhagia, and dysfunctional uterine bleeding* [hydroxyprogesterone caproate in oil] 250 mg/mL

gestodene USAN, INN, BAN *progestin*

gestonorone caproate USAN, INN *progestin* [also: gestronol]

gestrinone USAN, INN *progestin*

gestronol BAN *progestin* [also: gestonorone caproate]

Gets-It liquid OTC *topical keratolytic* [salicylic acid; zinc chloride; alcohol 28%]

gevotroline INN *antipsychotic* [also: gevotroline HCl]

gevotroline HCl USAN *antipsychotic* [also: gevotroline]

Gevrabon liquid OTC *vitamin/mineral supplement* [multiple B vitamins & minerals; alcohol 18%] ≛

Gevral tablets OTC *vitamin/mineral/iron supplement* [multiple vitamins & minerals; ferrous fumarate; folic acid] ≛•18 mg•0.4 mg

Gevral Protein powder OTC *oral protein supplement* [calcium caseinate; sucrose]

Gevral T film-coated tablets (discontinued 1995) OTC *vitamin/mineral/iron supplement* [ferrous fumarate; multiple vitamins & minerals; folic acid] 27•≛•0.4 mg

GG-Cen capsules OTC *expectorant* [guaifenesin] 200 mg

GHRF; GH-RF (growth hormone-releasing factor) [q.v.]

giparmen INN

giractide INN

gitalin NF [also: gitalin amorphous]

gitalin amorphous INN [also: gitalin]

gitaloxin INN

gitoformate INN

gitoxin 16-formate [see: gitaloxin]

gitoxin pentaacetate [see: pengitoxin]

GLA (gamma-linolenic acid)

glacial acetic acid [see: acetic acid, glacial]

glafenine INN

Glandosane oral spray OTC *saliva substitute*

glaphenine [see: glafenine]

Glauber salt [see: sodium sulfate]

glaucarubin

Glaucon Drop-Tainers (eye drops) ℞ *antiglaucoma agent* [epinephrine HCl] 1%, 2%

GlaucTabs tablets ℞ *carbonic anhydrase inhibitor; diuretic* [methazolamide] 25, 50 mg

Glaxal cream OTC *investigational moisturizing cream base*

glaze, pharmaceutical NF *tablet-coating agent*

glaziovine INN

glemanserin USAN, INN *anxiolytic*

gleptoferron USAN, INN, BAN *veterinary hematinic*

Gliadel wafers ℞ *investigational antineoplastic cerebral implants for excised brain tumors* [carmustine]

gliamilide USAN, INN *antidiabetic*

glibenclamide INN, BAN *sulfonylurea-type antidiabetic* [also: glyburide]

glibornuride USAN, INN, BAN *antidiabetic*

glibutimine INN

glicaramide INN

glicetanile INN *antidiabetic* [also: glicetanile sodium]

glicetanile sodium USAN *antidiabetic* [also: glicetanile]

gliclazide INN, BAN

glicondamide INN

glidazamide INN

gliflumide USAN, INN *antidiabetic*

glimepiride USAN, INN, BAN *sulfonylurea-type antidiabetic*

glipentide [see: glisentide]

glipizide USAN, INN, BAN *sulfonylurea-type antidiabetic* 5, 10 mg oral

gliquidone INN, BAN

glisamuride INN

glisentide INN

glisindamide INN

glisolamide INN

glisoxepide INN, BAN

globin zinc insulin INN [also: insulin, globin zinc]

globulin, aerosolized pooled immune (orphan: *respiratory syncytial virus*)

globulin, immune USP *passive immunizing agent; investigational immunomodulator for AIDS/ARC*; (orphan: *acute myocarditis*)

globulin, immune human serum [now: globulin, immune]

Glossets (trademarked form) *sublingual or rectal administration*

gloxazone USAN, INN, BAN *veterinary anaplasmodastat*

gloximonam USAN, INN *antibacterial*

glucagon USP, INN, BAN *antidiabetic; glucose elevating agent* 1, 10 mg/vial injection

Glucagon Emergency Kit Hyporets (prefilled disposable syringes) ℞ *emergency treatment for hypoglycemic crisis* [glucagon; lactose] 1•49 mg/mL

glucalox INN [also: glycalox]

glucametacin INN

D-glucaric acid, calcium salt tetrahydrate [see: calcium saccharate]

gluceptate USAN, USP, INN, BAN *combining name for radicals or groups*

gluceptate sodium USAN *pharmaceutic aid*

Glucerna ready-to-use liquid OTC *enteral nutritional therapy for abnormal glucose tolerance*

D-glucitol [see: sorbitol]

D-glucitol hexanicotinate [see: sorbinicate]

Glucobay (commercially available in Europe and Japan) ℞ *investigational antidiabetic* [acarbose]

β-glucocerebrosidase, macrophage-targeted [see: alglucerase]

glucocerebrosidase recombinant retroviral vector (orphan: *enzyme replacement in Gaucher's disease*)

glucocerebrosidase-β-glucosidase [see: alglucerase]

Glucofilm reagent strips for home use OTC *in vitro diagnostic aid for blood glucose*

glucoheptonic acid, calcium salt [see: calcium gluceptate]

Glucometer Encore; Glucometer Elite reagent strips for home use OTC *in vitro diagnostic aid for blood glucose*

D-gluconic acid, calcium salt [see: calcium gluconate]

D-gluconic acid, magnesium salt [see: magnesium gluconate]

D-gluconic acid, monopotassium salt [see: potassium gluconate]

D-gluconic acid, monosodium salt [see: sodium gluconate]

Glucophage film-coated tablets ℞ *biguanide antidiabetic* [metformin HCl] 500, 850 mg

β-D-glucopyranuronamide [see: glucuronamide]

glucosamine USAN, INN *pharmaceutic aid*

d-glucose [see: dextrose]

glucose, liquid NF *tablet binder and coating agent; antihypoglycemic* ⊡ Glutose

Glucose & Ketone Urine Test reagent strips (discontinued 1995) *in vitro diagnostic aid for multiple urine products*

d-glucose monohydrate [see: dextrose]

glucose oxidase

glucose polymers *caloric replacement*

Glucose-40 ophthalmic ointment ℞ *corneal edema-reducing agent* [glucose] 40%

Glucostix reagent strips for home use OTC *in vitro diagnostic aid for blood glucose*

glucosulfamide INN

glucosulfone INN

glucosylceramidase [see: alglucerase]

Glucotrol tablets ℞ *sulfonylurea-type antidiabetic* [glipizide] 5, 10 mg

Glucotrol XL extended-release tablets ℞ *sulfonylurea-type antidiabetic* [glipizide] 5, 10 mg

glucurolactone INN

glucuronamide INN, BAN

Glukor powder for IM injection (discontinued 1995) ℞ *hormone for prepubertal cryptorchidism and hypogonadism; ovulation stimulant* [chorionic gonadotropin] 200 U/mL

glunicate INN

gluside [see: saccharin]

gluside, soluble [see: saccharin sodium]

glusoferron INN

glutamic acid (L-glutamic acid) USAN, INN *nonessential amino acid; symbols:* Glu, E 340, 500 mg oral

glutamic acid HCl *gastric acidifier*

glutamine (L-glutamine) *nonessential amino acid; symbols:* Gln, Q [see: levoglutamide]

glutaral USAN, USP, INN *disinfectant*

glutaraldehyde [see: glutaral]

Glutarex-1 powder OTC *formula for infants with glutaric aciduria type I*

Glutarex-2 powder OTC *enteral nutritional therapy for glutaric aciduria type I*

glutasin [see: glutamic acid HCl]

L-glutathione, reduced (*orphan: cachexia of AIDS*)

glutaurine INN

glutethimide USP, INN, BAN *sedative* 250, 500 mg oral

Glutofac tablets OTC *vitamin/mineral supplement* [multiple vitamins & minerals] ±

Glutose gel OTC *glucose elevating agent* [glucose] 40% ② glucose

Glyate syrup OTC *expectorant* [guaifenesin; alcohol 3.5%] 100 mg/5 mL

glyburide USAN *sulfonylurea-type antidiabetic* [also: glibenclamide] 1.25, 2.5, 5 mg oral

glybutamide [see: carbutamide]

glybuthiazol INN

glybuthizol [see: glybuthiazol]

glybuzole INN

glycalox BAN [also: glucalox]

Glycate chewable tablets (discontinued 1992) OTC *antacid* [calcium carbonate; glycine]

glycerides oleiques polyoxyethylenes [see: peglicol 5 oleate]

glycerin USP *humectant; solvent; osmotic diuretic; laxative; emollient/protectant* [also: glycerol]

glycerol INN *humectant; solvent; osmotic diuretic; laxative; emollient/protectant; monoctanoin component D* [also: glycerin]

glycerol, iodinated USAN, BAN (*disapproved for use as an expectorant in 1991*)

glycerol 1-decanoate *monoctanoin component B* [see: monoctanoin]

glycerol 1,2-dioctanoate *monoctanoin component C* [see: monoctanoin]

glycerol 1-octanoate *monoctanoin component A* [see: monoctanoin]

glycerol phosphate, manganese salt [see: manganese glycerophosphate]

glyceryl behenate NF *tablet and capsule lubricant*

glyceryl borate [see: boroglycerin]

glyceryl guaiacolate [now: guaifenesin]

glyceryl monostearate NF *emulsifying agent*

glyceryl triacetate [now: triacetin]

glyceryl trinitrate BAN *coronary vasodilator* [also: nitroglycerin]

glycerylaminophenaquine [see: glafenine]

Glyceryl-T capsules, liquid ℞ *antiasthmatic; bronchodilator; expectorant* [theophylline; guaifenesin] 150•90 mg; 150•90 mg/15 mL

glycinato dihydroxyaluminum hydrate [see: dihydroxyaluminum aminoacetate]

glycine USP, INN *nonessential amino acid; urologic irrigant; symbols: Gly, G* [also: aminoacetic acid] 1.5%

glycine aluminum-zirconium complex [see: aluminum zirconium tetrachlorohydrex gly; aluminum zirconium trichlorohydrex gly]

glyclopyramide INN

glycobiarsol USP, INN [also: bismuth glycollylarsanilate]

glycocholate sodium [see: sodium glycocholate]

glycocoll [see: glycine]

Glycofed tablets OTC *decongestant; expectorant* [pseudoephedrine HCl; guaifenesin] 30•100 mg

glycol distearate USAN *thickening agent*

glycolic acid *mild exfoliant and keratolytic*

***p*-glycolophenetidide** [see: fenacetinol]

glycophenylate [see: mepenzolate bromide]

glycopyrrolate USAN, USP *peptic ulcer adjunct* [also: glycopyrronium bromide] 0.2 mg/mL injection

glycopyrrone bromide [see: glycopyrrolate]

glycopyrronium bromide INN, BAN *anticholinergic* [also: glycopyrrolate]

Glycotuss tablets OTC *expectorant* [guaifenesin] 100 mg ② Glytuss

Glycotuss-dM tablets OTC *antitussive; expectorant* [dextromethorphan hydrobromide; guaifenesin] 10•100 mg

glycyclamide INN, BAN

glycyrrhetinic acid [see: enoxolone]

glycyrrhiza NF

glydanile sodium [now: glicetanile sodium]

glyhexamide USAN, INN *antidiabetic*

glyhexylamide [see: metahexamide]

Glylorin ℞ *(orphan: congenital primary ichthyosis)* [monolaurin]

glymidine BAN *antidiabetic* [also: glymidine sodium]

glymidine sodium USAN, INN *antidiabetic* [also: glymidine]

glymol [see: mineral oil]

Glynase PresTabs (micronized tablets) ℞ *sulfonylurea antidiabetic* [glyburide] 1.5, 3, 6 mg

glyoctamide USAN, INN *antidiabetic*

Gly-Oxide oral solution OTC *oral anti-inflammatory/anti-infective* [carbamide peroxide] 10%

glyparamide USAN *antidiabetic*

glyphylline [see: dyphylline]

glypinamide INN

Glypressin ℞ *investigational treatment for epistaxis (orphan: bleeding esophageal ulcers)* [terlipressin]

glyprothiazol INN

glyprothizol [see: glyprothiazol]

glysobuzole INN [also: isobuzole]

Glytuss film-coated tablets OTC *expectorant* [guaifenesin] 200 mg ② Glycotuss

GM 6001 *(orphan: corneal ulcers)*

GM-CSF (granulocyte-macrophage colony-stimulating factor) [see: regramostim; sargramostim; molgramostim]

G-myticin cream, ointment ℞ *topical antibiotic* [gentamicin sulfate] 1 mg

Go-Evac powder for oral solution ℞ *pre-procedure bowel evacuant* [polyethylene glycol-electrolyte solution] 59 g/L

gold *element (Au)*

gold Au 198 USAN, USP *antineoplastic; liver imaging aid; radioactive agent*

gold sodium thiomalate USP *antirheumatic (50% gold)* [also: sodium aurothiomalate] 50 mg/mL injection

gold sodium thiosulfate NF [also: sodium aurotiosulfate]

gold thioglucose [see: aurothioglucose]

GoLYTELY powder for oral solution ℞ *pre-procedure bowel evacuant* [polyethylene glycol-electrolyte solution]

gonacrine [see: acriflavine]

gonadorelin INN, BAN *gonad-stimulating principle* [also: gonadorelin acetate]

gonadorelin acetate USAN *gonad-stimulating principle; for hypothalamic amenorrhea (orphan)* [also: gonadorelin]

gonadorelin HCl USAN *gonad-stimulating principle*

gonadotrophin, chorionic INN, BAN *gonad-stimulating principle* [also: gonadotropin, chorionic]

gonadotrophin, serum INN

gonadotropin, chorionic USP *gonad-stimulating principle* [also: gonadotrophin, chorionic] 500, 1000, 2000 U/mL injection

gonadotropin, serum [see: gonadotrophin, serum]

Gonak ophthalmic solution OTC *gonioscopic examination aid* [hydroxypropyl methylcellulose] 2.5% ☒ Gonic

Gonal-F ℞ *investigational fertility stimulant* [recombinant human follicle-stimulating hormone (rhFSH)]

Gonic powder for IM injection ℞ *hormone for prepubertal cryptorchidism and hypogonadism; ovulation stimulant* [chorionic gonadotropin] 1000 U/mL ☒ Gonak

Gonioscopic Prism Solution Drop-Tainers (eye drops) OTC *agent for bonding gonioscopic prisms to eye* [hydroxyethyl cellulose]

Goniosol ophthalmic solution OTC *gonioscopic examination aid* [hydroxypropyl methylcellulose] 2.5%

Gonodecten Test Kit tube test for professional use (discontinued 1995) *in vitro diagnostic aid for Neisseria gonorrhoeae*

Gonozyme Diagnostic reagent kit for professional use *in vitro diagnostic aid for Neisseria gonorrhoeae*

GoodStart [see: Carnation GoodStart]

Goody's Headache powder OTC *analgesic; antipyretic; anti-inflammatory* [acetaminophen; aspirin; caffeine] 250•520•32.5 mg/dose

Gordobalm OTC *counterirritant; topical antiseptic* [methyl salicylate; menthol; camphor; alcohol 16%]

Gordochom solution ℞ *topical antifungal; antiseptic* [undecylenic acid; chloroxylenol] 25%•3%

Gordofilm liquid ℞ *topical keratolytic* [salicylic acid in flexible collodion] 16.7%

Gordogesic Creme OTC *counterirritant* [methyl salicylate] 10%

Gordon's Urea 40% cream ℞ *for removal of dystrophic nails* [urea] 40%

Gordo-Vite E cream (discontinued 1992) OTC *emollient* [vitamin E]

Gormel Creme OTC *moisturizer; emollient; keratolytic* [urea] 20%

goserelin USAN, INN, BAN *antineoplastic; luteinizing hormone-releasing hormone (LHRH) agonist* [also: goserelin acetate]

goserelin acetate JAN *antineoplastic; luteinizing hormone-releasing hormone (LHRH) agonist* [also: goserelin]

gossypol (orphan: *adrenal cortex cancer*)

govafilcon A USAN *hydrophilic contact lens material*

gp120 (glycoprotein) *investigational (Phase III) antiviral AIDS vaccine* [also: AIDS vaccine]

gp160 (glycoprotein) *investigational antiviral (therapeutic, Phase II) and vaccine (preventative, Phase I) for HIV*

GP-500 tablets ℞ *decongestant; expectorant* [pseudoephedrine HCl; guaifenesin] 120•500 mg

GR 85478 *investigational antiviral*

Gradumet (trademarked dosage form) *controlled-release tablet*

gramicidin USP, INN *antibacterial antibiotic*

gramicidin S INN

granisetron USAN, INN, BAN *antiemetic*

granisetron HCl USAN *antiemetic/antinauseant for chemotherapy*

Granocyte ℞ *investigational treatment for chemotherapy-induced neutropenia* [lenograstim]

Granulderm aerosol spray ℞ *topical enzyme for wound debridement* [trypsin; balsam Peru] 0.1•72.5 mg/0.82 mL

Granulex aerosol spray ℞ *topical enzyme for wound debridement* [trypsin; balsam Peru] 0.1•72.5 mg/0.82 mL

granulocyte colony-stimulating factor (G-CSF), recombinant [see: filgrastim]

granulocyte-macrophage colony-stimulating factor (GM-CSF) [see: regramostim; sargramostim; molgramostim]

GranuMed aerosol spray ℞ *topical enzyme for wound debridement* [trypsin; balsam Peru] 0.1•72.5 mg/0.82 mL

Grapefruit Diet Plan with Diadax sustained-release capsules, chewable tablets (discontinued 1992) OTC *diet*

aid [phenylpropanolamine HCl; grapefruit extract] 30•⅖, 75•⅖ mg; 12.5•⅖ mg

green soap [see: soap, green]

grepafloxacin INN

grepafloxacin HCl USAN *antibacterial*

Grifulvin V tablets, oral suspension ℞ *systemic antifungal* [griseofulvin (microsize)] 250, 500 mg; 125 mg/5 mL

Grisactin; Grisactin 250 capsules (discontinued 1996) ℞ *systemic antifungal* [griseofulvin (microsize)] 125 mg; 250 mg

Grisactin 500 tablets ℞ *systemic antifungal* [griseofulvin (microsize)] 500 mg

Grisactin Ultra tablets ℞ *systemic antifungal* [griseofulvin (ultramicrosize)] 125, 250, 330 mg

griseofulvin USP, INN, BAN *fungistatic* 165, 330 mg oral

Gris-PEG film-coated tablets ℞ *systemic antifungal* [griseofulvin (ultramicrosize)] 125, 250 mg

growth hormone, human (hGH) [see: somatropin]

growth hormone, human recombinant (rhGH) with insulin-like growth factor, human recombinant (rhIGF) *investigational (Phase II) cytokine for AIDS wasting syndrome*

growth hormone-releasing factor (GHRF; GH-RF) *(orphan: inadequate endogenous growth hormone)*

GS 393 *investigational antiviral for AIDS* [PMEA]

GS 504 *investigational treatment for peripheral retinitis due to cytomegalovirus*

GS 840 *investigational (Phase I/II) oral antiviral for HIV and AIDS*

G-strophanthin [see: ouabain]

guabenxan INN

guacetisal INN

guafecainol INN

guaiac

guaiacol NF

guaiacol carbonate NF

guaiacol glyceryl ether [see: guaifenesin]

guaiactamine INN

guaiapate USAN, INN *antitussive*

guaiazulene soluble [see: sodium guaiaenate]

guaietolin INN

Guaifed syrup OTC *decongestant; expectorant* [pseudoephedrine HCl; guaifenesin] 30•200 mg

Guaifed timed-release capsules ℞ *decongestant; expectorant* [pseudoephedrine HCl; guaifenesin] 120•250 mg

Guaifed-PD timed-release capsules ℞ *pediatric decongestant and expectorant* [pseudoephedrine HCl; guaifenesin] 60•300 mg

guaifenesin USAN, USP, INN *expectorant* [also: guaiphenesin] 100 mg/5 mL oral ② guanfacine

Guaifenex liquid ℞ *decongestant; expectorant* [phenylpropanolamine HCl; phenylephrine HCl; guaifenesin] 20•5•100 mg/5 mL

Guaifenex DM extended-release tablets ℞ *antitussive; expectorant* [dextromethorphan hydrobromide; guaifenesin] 30•600 mg

Guaifenex LA extended-release tablets ℞ *expectorant* [guaifenesin] 600 mg

Guaifenex PPA 75 extended-release tablets ℞ *decongestant; expectorant* [phenylpropanolamine HCl; guaifenesin] 75•600 mg

Guaifenex PSE 60; Guaifenex PSE 120 extended-release tablets ℞ *decongestant; expectorant* [pseudoephedrine HCl; guaifenesin] 60•600 mg; 120•600 mg

guaifylline INN *bronchodilator; expectorant* [also: guaithylline]

GuaiMAX-D extended-release tablets ℞ *decongestant; expectorant* [pseudoephedrine HCl; guaifenesin] 120•600 mg

guaimesal INN

Guaipax sustained-release tablets ℞ *decongestant; expectorant* [phenylpropanolamine HCl; guaifenesin] 75•400 mg

guaiphenesin BAN *expectorant* [also: guaifenesin]

guaisteine INN

Guaitab tablets OTC *decongestant; expectorant* [pseudoephedrine HCl; guaifenesin] 60•400 mg

guaithylline USAN *bronchodilator; expectorant* [also: guaifylline]

Guaivent capsules ℞ *decongestant; expectorant* [pseudoephedrine HCl; guaifenesin] 120•250 mg

Guaivent PD capsules ℞ *pediatric decongestant and expectorant* [pseudoephedrine HCl; guaifenesin] 60•300 mg

Guai-Vent/PSE sustained-release tablets ℞ *decongestant; expectorant* [pseudoephedrine HCl; guaifenesin] 120•600 mg

guamecycline INN, BAN

guanabenz USAN, INN *antihypertensive*

guanabenz acetate USAN, USP *antihypertensive* 4, 8 mg oral

guanacline INN, BAN *antihypertensive* [also: guanacline sulfate]

guanacline sulfate USAN *antihypertensive* [also: guanacline]

guanadrel INN *antihypertensive* [also: guanadrel sulfate]

guanadrel sulfate USAN, USP *antihypertensive* [also: guanadrel]

guanatol HCl [see: chloroguanide HCl]

guanazodine INN

guancidine INN *antihypertensive* [also: guancydine]

guancydine USAN *antihypertensive* [also: guancidine]

guanethidine INN, BAN *antihypertensive* [also: guanethidine monosulfate] ⊇ guanidine

guanethidine monosulfate USAN, USP *antihypertensive; (orphan: reflex sympathetic dystrophy and causalgia)* [also: guanethidine]

guanethidine sulfate USAN, USP, JAN *antihypertensive*

guanfacine INN, BAN *antihypertensive; antiadrenergic* [also: guanfacine HCl] ⊇ guaifenesin

guanfacine HCl USAN *antihypertensive; antiadrenergic* [also: guanfacine]

guanidine HCl *cholinergic muscle stimulant* 125 mg oral ⊇ guanethidine

guanisoquin sulfate USAN *antihypertensive* [also: guanisoquine]

guanisoquine INN *antihypertensive* [also: guanisoquin sulfate]

guanoclor INN, BAN *antihypertensive* [also: guanoclor sulfate]

guanoclor sulfate USAN *antihypertensive* [also: guanoclor]

guanoctine INN *antihypertensive* [also: guanoctine HCl]

guanoctine HCl USAN *antihypertensive* [also: guanoctine]

guanoxabenz USAN, INN *antihypertensive*

guanoxan INN, BAN *antihypertensive* [also: guanoxan sulfate]

guanoxan sulfate USAN *antihypertensive* [also: guanoxan]

guanoxyfen INN *antihypertensive; antidepressant* [also: guanoxyfen sulfate]

guanoxyfen sulfate USAN *antihypertensive; antidepressant* [also: guanoxyfen]

guar gum NF *tablet binder and disintegrant*

guaranine [see: caffeine]

GuiaCough syrup OTC *expectorant* [guaifenesin]

GuiaCough CF liquid OTC *antitussive; decongestant; expectorant* [dextromethorphan hydrobromide; phenylpropanolamine HCl; guaifenesin; alcohol 4.75%] 10•12.5•100 mg/5 mL

GuiaCough DM syrup OTC *expectorant; antitussive* [guaifenesin; dextromethorphan hydrobromide]

GuiaCough PE syrup OTC *decongestant; expectorant* [pseudoephedrine HCl; guaifenesin; alcohol 1.4%] 30•100 mg/5 mL

Guiafenesin-DAC syrup (discontinued 1993) ℞ *narcotic antitussive; decongestant; expectorant* [codeine phosphate; pseudoephedrine HCl; guaifenesin; alcohol]

Guiaphed elixir (discontinued 1993) OTC *antiasthmatic; bronchodilator; decongestant; expectorant; sedative* [theophylline; ephedrine sulfate; guaifenesin; phenobarbital]

Guiatuss syrup OTC *expectorant* [guaifenesin] 100 mg/5 mL ⊇ Guiatussin

Guiatuss AC syrup ℞ *narcotic antitussive; expectorant* [codeine phosphate; guaifenesin; alcohol] 10•100 mg/5 mL

Guiatuss CF liquid OTC *antitussive; decongestant; expectorant* [dextromethorphan hydrobromide; phenylpropanolamine HCl; guaifenesin; alcohol 4.75%] 10•12.5•100 mg/5 mL

Guiatuss DAC liquid ℞ *narcotic antitussive; decongestant; expectorant* [codeine phosphate; pseudoephedrine HCl; guaifenesin; alcohol] 10•30•100 mg/5 mL

Guiatuss DM liquid OTC *antitussive; expectorant* [dextromethorphan hydrobromide; guaifenesin] 10•100 mg/5 mL

Guiatuss PE liquid OTC *decongestant; expectorant* [pseudoephedrine HCl; guaifenesin; alcohol 1.4%] 30•100 mg/5 mL

Guiatussin DAC syrup ℞ *narcotic antitussive; decongestant; expectorant* [codeine phosphate; pseudoephedrine HCl; guaifenesin; alcohol 1.6%] 10•30•100 mg/5 mL ② Guiatuss

Guiatussin with Codeine Expectorant liquid ℞ *narcotic antitussive; expectorant* [codeine phosphate; guaifenesin; alcohol 3.5%] 10•100 mg/5 mL

Guiatussin with Dextromethorphan liquid OTC *antitussive; expectorant* [dextromethorphan hydrobromide; guaifenesin; alcohol 1.4%] 15•100 mg/5 mL

Guipax tablets ℞ *decongestant; expectorant* [phenylpropanolamine HCl; guaifenesin]

gum arabic [see: acacia]
gum senegal [see: acacia]
guncotton, soluble [see: pyroxylin]
gusperimus INN
gusperimus trihydrochloride USAN *immunosuppressant*

Gustase tablets OTC *digestive enzymes* [amylase; protease; cellulase] 30•6•2 mg

Gustase Plus tablets ℞ *digestive enzymes; sedative* [amylase; protease; cellulase; homatropine methylbromide; phenobarbital] 30•6•2•2.5•8 mg

gutta percha USP *dental restoration agent*

G-Well lotion, shampoo ℞ *scabicide; pediculicide* [lindane] 1%

Gynecort 5; Gynecort 10 cream OTC *topical corticosteroid* [hydrocortisone acetate] 0.5%; 1%

Gyne-Lotrimin vaginal cream, vaginal tablets, combination pack (vaginal tablets + cream) OTC *antifungal* [clotrimazole] 1%; 100 mg

Gyne-Lotrimin 3 vaginal tablets, combination pack (vaginal tablets + cream) OTC *antifungal* [clotrimazole] 100 mg; 1%

Gyne-Moistrin vaginal gel OTC *lubricant* [propylene glycol]

gynergon [see: estradiol]

Gyne-Sulf vaginal cream ℞ *broad-spectrum bacteriostatic* [sulfathiazole; sulfacetamide; sulfabenzamide] 3.42%•2.86%•3.7%

gynoestryl [see: estradiol]

Gynogen IM injection (discontinued 1992) ℞ *estrogen replacement therapy; antineoplastic for prostatic and breast cancer* [estrone] 2 mg/mL

Gynogen L.A. "10" IM injection (discontinued 1992) ℞ *estrogen replacement therapy for postmenopausal disorders; antineoplastic for prostatic cancer* [estradiol valerate in oil] 10 mg/mL

Gynogen L.A. "20" IM injection ℞ *estrogen replacement therapy for postmenopausal disorders; antineoplastic for prostatic cancer* [estradiol valerate in oil] 20 mg/mL

Gynogen L.A. "40" IM injection (discontinued 1996) ℞ *estrogen replacement therapy for postmenopausal disorders; antineoplastic for prostatic cancer* [estradiol valerate in oil] 40 mg/mL

Gynol II Contraceptive vaginal gel, vaginal jelly OTC *spermicidal contraceptive (for use with a diaphragm)* [nonoxynol 9] 2%; 3%

Gynovite Plus tablets OTC *vitamin/mineral/calcium/iron supplement* [multiple vitamins & minerals; calcium; iron; folic acid; biotin] ≟•83•3•0.067•≟ mg

Gy-Pak (trademarked packaging form) *unit-of-issue package*

Gyrocap (trademarked dosage form) *timed-release capsule*

²H (deuterium) [see: deuterium oxide]
H₂¹⁵O [see: water O 15]
³H (tritium) [see: tritiated water]
Habitrol transdermal patch ℞ *smoking deterrent; nicotine withdrawal aid* [nicotine] 17.5, 35, 52.5 mg
hachimycin INN, BAN
HAD (hexamethylmelamine, Adriamycin, DDP) *chemotherapy protocol*
hafnium *element* (Hf)
Hair Booster Vitamin tablets OTC *vitamin/mineral/iron supplement* [multiple B vitamins & minerals; iron; folic acid] ≛•18•0.4 mg
halarsol [see: dichlorophenarsine HCl]
halazepam USAN, USP, INN, BAN *anxiolytic; sedative*
halazone USP, INN *disinfectant; water purifier*
Halazone tablets (discontinued 1996) OTC *water purifier*
Hal-C ℞ *investigational coating agent for abdominal procedures (orphan: gynecologic surgery)* [hyaluronic acid]
halcinonide USAN, USP, INN, BAN *topical corticosteroidal anti-inflammatory*
Halcion tablets ℞ *sedative; hypnotic* [triazolam] 0.125, 0.25 mg
Haldol oral concentrate, IM injection ℞ *antipsychotic; control manifestations of Tourette syndrome* [haloperidol lactate] 2 mg/mL; 5 mg/mL ② Halenol; Halog
Haldol tablets ℞ *antipsychotic; control manifestations of Tourette syndrome* [haloperidol] 0.5, 1, 2, 5, 10, 20 mg
Haldol Decanoate 50; Haldol Decanoate 100 long-acting IM injection ℞ *antipsychotic* [haloperidol decanoate] 50 mg/mL; 100 mg/mL
Halenol tablets (discontinued 1992) OTC *analgesic; antipyretic* [acetaminophen] 325, 500 mg ② Haldol
Halenol Children's liquid OTC *analgesic; antipyretic* [acetaminophen] 160 mg/5 mL
Halercol capsules OTC *vitamin supplement* [multiple vitamins]
haletazole INN [also: halethazole]
halethazole BAN [also: haletazole]

Haley's M-O liquid OTC *laxative* [magnesium hydroxide; mineral oil] 900 mg•3.75 mL per 15 mL
Hal-F *investigational resorbable film for abdominal surgery* [hyaluronic acid]
Halfan ℞ *investigational antimalarial (orphan) (approved by the FDA but not marketed by the manufacturer)* [halofantrine HCl]
Halfprin; Halfprin 81 enteric-coated tablets OTC *analgesic; antipyretic; anti-inflammatory; antirheumatic* [aspirin] 165 mg; 81 mg
Hal-G *investigational gel to prevent adhesions in minor surgery* [hyaluronic acid]
Hall's Mentho-Lyptus lozenges (discontinued 1994) OTC *antipruritic/counterirritant; mild local anesthetic; antiseptic* [menthol; eucalyptus oil]
Hall's Plus lozenges OTC *antipruritic/counterirritant; mild local anesthetic; antiseptic* [menthol] 10 mg
Hall's Sugar Free Mentho-Lyptus lozenges OTC *antipruritic/counterirritant; mild local anesthetic; antiseptic* [menthol; eucalyptus oil] 5•2.8, 6•2.8 mg
halobetasol propionate USAN *topical corticosteroidal anti-inflammatory* [also: ulobetasol]
halocarban INN *disinfectant* [also: cloflucarban]
halocortolone INN
halocrinic acid [see: brocrinat]
Halodrin tablets (discontinued 1994) ℞ *estrogen/androgen for menopausal vasomotor symptoms* [ethinyl estradiol; fluoxymesterone] 0.02•1 mg
halofantrine INN, BAN *antimalarial (orphan)* [also: halofantrine HCl]
halofantrine HCl USAN *antimalarial* [also: halofantrine]
Halofed syrup (discontinued 1993) OTC *nasal decongestant* [pseudoephedrine HCl]
Halofed tablets OTC *nasal decongestant* [pseudoephedrine HCl] 30, 60 mg
halofenate USAN, INN, BAN *antihyperlipoproteinemic; uricosuric*
halofuginone INN, BAN *antiprotozoal* [also: halofuginone hydrobromide]

halofuginone hydrobromide USAN *antiprotozoal* [also: halofuginone]
Halog ointment, cream, solution ℞ *topical corticosteroidal anti-inflammatory* [halcinonide] 0.1%; 0.025%, 0.1%; 0.1% ⓓ Haldol
Halog-E cream ℞ *topical corticosteroidal anti-inflammatory; emollient* [halcinonide] 0.1%
halometasone INN
halonamine INN
halopemide USAN, INN *antipsychotic*
halopenium chloride INN, BAN
haloperidol USAN, USP, INN, BAN *antidyskinetic for Tourette's disease; antipsychotic* 0.5, 1, 2, 5, 10, 20 mg oral
haloperidol decanoate USAN, BAN *antipsychotic*
haloperidol lactate *antidyskinetic for Tourette's disease; antipsychotic* 2 mg/mL oral; 5 mg/mL injection
halopone chloride [see: halopenium chloride]
halopredone INN *topical anti-inflammatory* [also: halopredone acetate]
halopredone acetate USAN *topical anti-inflammatory* [also: halopredone]
haloprogesterone USAN, INN *progestin*
haloprogin USAN, USP, INN, JAN *antibacterial; antifungal*
halopyramine BAN [also: chloropyramine]
Halotestin tablets ℞ *androgenic hormone for male hypogonadism and female breast cancer* [fluoxymesterone] 2, 5, 10 mg ⓓ Halotex; Halotussin
Halotex cream, solution ℞ *topical antifungal* [haloprogin] 1% ⓓ Halotestin
halothane USP, INN, BAN *inhalation general anesthetic*
Halotussin syrup OTC *expectorant* [guaifenesin; alcohol 3.5%] 100 mg/5 mL ⓓ Halotestin
Halotussin AC liquid ℞ *narcotic antitussive; expectorant* [codeine phosphate; guaifenesin]
Halotussin PE liquid OTC *expectorant; decongestant* [guaifenesin; pseudoephedrine HCl]
Halotussin-DAC liquid ℞ *narcotic antitussive; decongestant; expectorant* [codeine; pseudoephedrine HCl; guaifenesin]
Halotussin-DM liquid, sugar-free liquid OTC *antitussive; expectorant* [dextromethorphan hydrobromide; guaifenesin] 10•100 mg/5 mL
haloxazolam INN
haloxon INN, BAN
halquinol BAN *topical anti-infective* [also: halquinols]
halquinols USAN *topical anti-infective* [also: halquinol]
Hal-S *investigational synovial fluid replacement for arthroscopic surgery of meniscal tear* [hyaluronic acid]
Haltran tablets OTC *nonsteroidal anti-inflammatory drug (NSAID); antiarthritic; analgesic* [ibuprofen] 200 mg
HAM (hexamethylmelamine, Adriamycin, melphalan) *chemotherapy protocol*
HAM (hexamethylmelamine, Adriamycin, methotrexate) *chemotherapy protocol*
hamamelis water *astringent*
hamycin USAN, INN *antifungal*
hard fat [see: fat, hard]
Havrix IM injection, prefilled syringe ℞ *immunization against hepatitis A* [hepatitis A vaccine, inactivated] 360, 720 ELISA units (EL.U.)/0.5 mL (pediatric), 1440 EL.U./mL (adult)
Hawaiian Tropic Cool Aloe with I.C.E. gel OTC *topical local anesthetic; counterirritant* [lidocaine; menthol] 2•2
Hayfebrol liquid OTC *decongestant; antihistamine* [pseudoephedrine HCl; chlorpheniramine maleate] 30•2 mg/5 mL
H-BIG IM injection ℞ *hepatitis B immunizing agent* [hepatitis B immune globulin] 4, 5 mL
HBIG (hepatitis B immune globulin) [q.v.]
HBY097 *investigational (Phase II) antiviral non-nucleoside reverse transcriptase inhibitor for HIV*
1% HC ointment ℞ *topical corticosteroid* [hydrocortisone] 1%
HC (hydrocortisone) [q.v.]

4-HC (4-hydroperoxycyclophosphamide) [q.v.]

HC Derma-Pax liquid OTC *topical corticosteroid; antihistamine; antiseptic* [hydrocortisone; pyrilamine maleate; chlorpheniramine maleate; chlorobutanol] 0.5%•0.44%•0.06%•25%

HCA (hydrocortisone acetate) [q.v.]

H-CAP (hexamethylmelamine, cyclophosphamide, Adriamycin, Platinol) *chemotherapy protocol*

hCG (human chorionic gonadotropin) [see: gonadotropin, chorionic]

HCG-nostick test kit for professional use (discontinued 1995) *in vitro diagnostic aid for urine pregnancy test* [sol particle immunoassay (SPIA)]

HCP-30 *Investigational (Phase I) vaccine for HIV*

HCT (hydrochlorothiazide) [q.v.]

HCTZ (hydrochlorothiazide) [q.v.]

HD 85 suspension ℞ *GI contrast radiopaque agent* [barium sulfate] 85%

HD 200 Plus powder for suspension ℞ *GI contrast radiopaque agent* [barium sulfate] 98%

HDCV (human diploid cell vaccine) [see: rabies vaccine]

HDMTX (high-dose methotrexate [with leucovorin rescue]) *chemotherapy protocol*

HDMTX-CF (high-dose methotrexate, citrovorum factor) *chemotherapy protocol*

HDMTX/LV (high-dose methotrexate, leucovorin [rescue]) *chemotherapy protocol*

HDPEB (high-dose PEB protocol) *chemotherapy protocol* [see: PEB]

HD-VAC (high-dose [methotrexate], vinblastine, Adriamycin, cisplatin) *chemotherapy protocol*

Head & Shoulders cream shampoo, lotion shampoo OTC *antiseborrheic; antibacterial; antifungal* [pyrithione zinc] 1%

Head & Shoulders Dry Scalp shampoo OTC *antiseborrheic; antibacterial; antifungal* [pyrithione zinc] 1%

Head & Shoulders Intensive Treatment Dandruff Shampoo OTC *antiseborrheic* [selenium sulfide] 1%

Healon; Healon GV intraocular injection ℞ *viscoelastic agent for ophthalmic surgery* [hyaluronate sodium] 10 mg/mL; 14 mg/mL

Healon Yellow intraocular injection ℞ *viscoelastic agent for ophthalmic surgery; corneal disclosing agent* [sodium hyaluronate; fluorescein sodium] 10•0.005 mg/mL

Heatrol tablets (discontinued 1992) OTC *salt replacement; electrolyte replacement* [sodium chloride; potassium chloride; calcium phosphate; magnesium carbonate]

heavy liquid petrolatum [see: mineral oil]

heavy water (D_2O) [see: deuterium oxide]

Heb Cream Base OTC *cream base*

hedaquinium chloride INN, BAN

Heet Liniment OTC *counterirritant; topical antiseptic* [methyl salicylate; camphor; capsaicin; alcohol 70%] 15%•3.6%•0.025%

Heet Spray (discontinued 1994) OTC *counterirritant; topical antiseptic* [methyl salicylate; camphor; menthol; methyl nicotinate; alcohol] 25%•3%•3%•1%

hefilcon A USAN *hydrophilic contact lens material*

hefilcon B USAN *hydrophilic contact lens material*

helenien [see: xantofyl palmitate]

helicon [see: aspirin]

Helidac 14-day dose-pack ℞ *combination treatment for active duodenal ulcer with H. pylori infection* [bismuth subsalicylate (tablets); metronidazole (tablets); tetracycline HCl (capsules)] 262.4 mg; 250 mg; 500 mg

heliomycin INN

Helistat sponge ℞ *hemostasis adjunct during surgery* [absorbable collagen hemostatic sponge]

helium USP *diluent for gases; element (He)*

Helixate powder for IV injection ℞ *antihemophilic to correct coagulation deficiency* [antihemophilic factor VIII, recombinant] 250, 500, 1000 IU

Hem Fe capsules (discontinued 1996) ℞ *hematinic* [ferrous fumarate; cyanocobalamin; ascorbic acid; docusate sodium] 100 mg•5 μg•125 mg•25 mg

HEMA (2-hydroxyethyl methacrylate) *contact lens material*

Hemabate IM injection ℞ *prostaglandin-type abortifacient; for postpartum uterine bleeding* [carboprost tromethamine] 250 μg/mL

Hema-Check slide tests for home use OTC *in vitro diagnostic aid for fecal occult blood*

Hema-Combistix reagent strips *in vitro diagnostic aid for multiple urine products*

Hemaspan timed-release tablets OTC *hematinic* [ferrous fumarate; vitamin C; docusate sodium] 110•200•20 mg

Hemastix reagent strips for professional use *in vitro diagnostic aid for urine occult blood*

Hematest reagent tablets for professional use *in vitro diagnostic aid for fecal occult blood*

heme arginate (*orphan: acute symptomatic porphyria; myelodysplastic syndromes*)

HemeSelect Collection kit for home use *in vitro diagnostic aid for fecal occult blood* [for use with HemeSelect Reagent kit]

HemeSelect Reagent kit for professional use *in vitro diagnostic aid for fecal occult blood* [for use with HemeSelect Collection kit]

Hemet Rectal ointment (discontinued 1993) OTC *topical anesthetic; vasoconstrictor; astringent* [diperodon HCl; pyrilamine maleate; phenylephrine HCl; bismuth subcarbonate; zinc oxide] 0.25%•0.1%•0.25%•0.2%•5%

Hemex ℞ (*orphan: acute porphyric syndromes*) [hemin; zinc mesoporphyrin]

hemiacidrin [see: citric acid, glucono-delta-lactone & magnesium carbonate]

hemin *for acute intermittent porphyria and hereditary coproporphyria* (*orphan*)

hemin & zinc mesoporphyrin (*orphan: acute porphyric syndromes*)

Hemocaine anorectal ointment (discontinued 1995) OTC *topical anesthetic; vasoconstrictor; astringent* [diperodon HCl; pyrilamine maleate; phenylephrine HCl; bismuth subcarbonate; zinc oxide] 0.25%•0.1%•0.25%•0.2%•5%

Hemoccult slide tests for professional use, test tape for professional use *in vitro diagnostic aid for fecal occult blood*

Hemoccult II slide tests for professional use *in vitro diagnostic aid for fecal occult blood*

Hemoccult II Dispenserpak; Hemoccult II Dispenserpak Plus slide tests for home use OTC *in vitro diagnostic aid for fecal occult blood*

Hemoccult SENSA; Hemoccult II SENSA slide tests for professional use *in vitro diagnostic aid for fecal occult blood*

Hemocyte IM injection (discontinued 1995) ℞ *hematinic* [ferrous gluconate; multiple B vitamins; procaine HCl] 3 mg/mL• ± •2%

Hemocyte tablets OTC *hematinic* [ferrous fumarate] 324 mg

Hemocyte Plus elixir ℞ *hematinic* [polysaccharide iron complex; multiple B vitamins and minerals; folic acid] 12• ± •0.33 mg

Hemocyte Plus tablets ℞ *hematinic* [ferrous fumarate; multiple B vitamins and minerals; sodium ascorbate; folic acid] 106• ± •200•1 mg

Hemocyte-F tablets ℞ *hematinic* [ferrous fumarate; folic acid] 106•1 mg

Hemocyte-V IM injection (discontinued 1995) ℞ *hematinic* [ferrous gluconate; multiple B vitamins] 3.6• ± mg/mL

Hemofil M IV injection ℞ *antihemophilic to correct coagulation deficiency* [antihemophilic factor VIII] 10, 20, 30 mL

Hemonyne IV infusion ℞ *antihemophilic to correct factor IX deficiency and anticoagulant-induced hemorrhage* [factor IX complex, human, heat treated] 20, 40 mL

Hemopad fiber ℞ *topical hemostatic aid in surgery* [microfibrillar collagen hemostat]

Hemophilus b conjugate vaccine *active bacterin for Haemophilus influenzae type b*

Hemopure; Hemopure 2 ℞ *investigational blood substitute*

Hemorid for Women cream OTC *topical local anesthetic; vasoconstrictor* [pramoxine HCl; phenylephrine HCl] 1%•0.25%

Hemorid for Women lotion OTC *emollient/protectant* [mineral oil; petrolatum; glycerin]

Hemorid for Women rectal suppositories OTC *astringent; topical vasoconstrictor* [zinc oxide; phenylephrine HCl] 11%•0.25%

Hemorrhoidal HC rectal suppositories ℞ *topical corticosteroidal anti-inflammatory* [hydrocortisone acetate] 25 mg

Hemotene fiber ℞ *topical hemostatic aid in surgery* [microfibrillar collagen hemostat] 1 g

Hemo-Vite liquid (discontinued 1992) ℞ *antianemic* [ferric pyrophosphate; multiple B vitamins; folic acid]

Hemo-Vite tablets (discontinued 1992) ℞ *antianemic* [ferrous fumarate; intrinsic factor; vitamin C; multiple B vitamins; folic acid]

Hem-Prep anorectal ointment, rectal suppositories OTC *temporary relief of hemorrhoidal symptoms; topical vasoconstrictor; astringent* [phenylephrine HCl; zinc oxide] 0.025%•11%; 0.25%•11%

Hemril Uniserts (rectal suppositories) OTC *temporary relief of hemorrhoidal symptoms* [bismuth subgallate; bismuth resorcin compound; benzyl benzoate; peruvian balsam; zinc oxide] 2.25%•1.75%•1.2%•1.8%•11%

Hemril-HC Uniserts (suppositories) ℞ *topical corticosteroidal anti-inflammatory; antipruritic* [hydrocortisone acetate] 25 mg

heneicosafluorotripropylamine [see: perfluamine]

HEOD (hexachloro-epoxy-octahydro-dimethanonaththalene) [see: dieldrin]

Hepandrin ℞ *(orphan: alcoholic hepatitis; protein calorie malnutrition)* [oxandrolone]

heparin BAN *anticoagulant* [also: heparin calcium]

heparin, 2-0-desulfated *(orphan: cystic fibrosis)*

heparin calcium USP *anticoagulant* [also: heparin]

heparin sodium USP, INN, BAN *anticoagulant* 1000, 5000, 10,000, 20,000, 40,000 U/mL injection

heparin sulfate [see: danaparoid sodium]

heparin whole blood [see: blood, whole]

heparin-binding neurotrophic factor *investigational protectant for nerve calls*

HepatAmine IV infusion ℞ *nutritional therapy for hepatic failure and hepatic encephalopathy* [multiple branched-chain essential and nonessential amino acids; electrolytes]

Hepatic-Aid II Instant Drink powder OTC *enteral nutritional treatment for chronic liver disease* [branched chain amino acids]

hepatitis A and B combination vaccine *investigational immunizing agent*

hepatitis A vaccine, inactivated *active immunizing agent for hepatitis A virus*

hepatitis B immune globulin (HBIG) USP *passive immunizing agent*

hepatitis B surface antigen [see: hepatitis B virus vaccine, inactivated]

hepatitis B virus vaccine, inactivated USP *active immunizing agent*

Hep-B-Gammagee IM injection (discontinued 1996) ℞ *hepatitis B immunizing agent* [hepatitis B immune globulin] 5 mL

Hepfomin-R IM injection (discontinued 1994) ℞ *antianemic; vitamin supplement* [liver extracts; vitamin B_{12}; folic acid]

Hep-Forte capsules OTC *geriatric dietary supplement* [multiple vitamins & food products; folic acid; biotin] ±• 60•±̲ μg

Hep-Lock; Hep-Lock U/P solution ℞ *IV flush for catheter patency (not therapeutic)* [heparin sodium] 10, 100 U/mL

Hep-Lock PF solution (discontinued 1992) ℞ *IV flush for catheter patency (not therapeutic)* [heparin sodium]

HEPP (H-chain [see: pentigetide]

hepronicate INN

hepsulfam *investigational antineoplastic*

heptabarb INN [also: heptabarbitone]

heptabarbital [see: heptabarb; heptabarbitone]

heptabarbitone BAN [also: heptabarb]

Heptalac syrup ℞ *laxative* [lactulose] 10 g/15 mL

heptaminol INN, BAN

heptaminol HCl [see: heptaminol]

2-heptanamine [see: tuaminoheptane]

2-heptanamine sulfate [see: tuaminoheptane sulfate]

heptaverine INN

heptolamide INN

Heptuna Plus capsules (discontinued 1995) ℞ *hematinic* [ferrous sulfate; multiple B vitamins; multiple minerals; vitamin C; intrinsic factor concentrate] 100•≚•≚•150•25 mg

hepzidine INN

HER2 humanized monoclonal antibody *investigational antineoplastic for breast and ovarian cancer*

Herbal Cellulex tablets (discontinued 1992) OTC *dietary supplement* [vitamin C; multiple minerals]

Herbal Laxative tablets OTC *laxative* [senna leaves; cascara sagrada bark] 125•20 mg

heroin *(banned in the USA)*

heroin HCl *(banned in the USA)* [see: diacetylmorphine HCl]

Herpecin-L lip balm OTC *vulnerary; sunblock* [allantoin; padimate O]

herpes simplex virus gene *(orphan: primary and metastatic brain tumors)*

Herpetrol tablets OTC *dietary supplement; claimed to prevent and treat herpes simplex infections* [L-lysine; multiple vitamins; zinc]

Herplex eye drops ℞ *ophthalmic antiviral* [idoxuridine] 0.1%

Herrick Lacrimal Plug ℞ *blocks the puncta and canaliculus to eliminate tear loss in keratitis sicca* [silicone plug]

HES (hydroxyethyl starch) [see: hetastarch]

Hespan IV infusion ℞ *plasma volume expander for shock due to hemorrhage, burns, surgery* [hetastarch] 6 g/100 mL ⑨ Histatan

hesperidin

hesperidin methyl chalcone [see: bioflavonoids]

hetacillin USAN, USP, INN, BAN *antibacterial*

hetacillin potassium USAN, USP *antibacterial*

hetaflur USAN, INN, BAN *dental caries prophylactic*

hetastarch USAN, BAN *plasma volume extender* [also: hydroxyethylstarch]

heteronium bromide USAN, INN, BAN *anticholinergic*

hexaammonium molybdate tetrahydrate [see: ammonium molybdate]

Hexabrix injection ℞ *parenteral radiopaque agent* [ioxaglate meglumine; ioxaglate sodium] 39.3%•19.6%

HexaCAF; Hexa-CAF (hexamethylmelamine, cyclophosphamide, amethopterin, fluorouracil) *chemotherapy protocol*

hexacarbacholine bromide INN [also: carbolonium bromide]

hexachlorane [see: lindane]

hexachlorocyclohexane [see: lindane]

hexachlorophane BAN *topical anti-infective; detergent* [also: hexachlorophene]

hexachlorophene USP, INN *topical anti-infective; detergent* [also: hexachlorophane]

hexacyclonate sodium INN

hexacyprone INN

hexadecanoic acid, methylethyl ester [see: isopropyl palmitate]

hexadecanol [see: cetyl alcohol]

hexadecylamine hydrofluoride [see: hetaflur]

hexadecylpyridinium chloride [see: cetylpyridinium chloride]

hexadecyltrimethylammonium bromide [see: cetrimonium bromide]

hexadecyltrimethylammonium chloride [see: cetrimonium chloride]
2,4-hexadienoic acid, potassium salt [see: potassium sorbate]
hexadiline INN
hexadimethrine bromide INN, BAN
hexadiphane [see: prozapine]
Hexadrol tablets, elixir ℞ *glucocorticoids* [dexamethasone] 1.5, 4 mg; 0.5 mg/5 mL ⓓ Hexalol
Hexadrol Phosphate intra-articular, intralesional, soft tissue, or IM injection ℞ *glucocorticoids* [dexamethasone sodium phosphate] 4, 10, 20 mg/mL
hexadylamine [see: hexadiline]
hexafluorenium bromide USAN, USP *skeletal muscle relaxant; succinylcholine synergist* [also: hexafluronium bromide]
hexafluorodiethyl ether [see: flurothyl]
hexaflurone bromide [see: hexafluorenium bromide]
hexafluronium bromide INN *skeletal muscle relaxant; succinylcholine synergist* [also: hexafluorenium bromide]
Hexalen capsules ℞ *antineoplastic; for ovarian adenocarcinoma (orphan)* [altretamine] 50 mg ⓓ Hexalol
Hexalol sugar-coated tablets (discontinued 1994) ℞ *urinary anti-infective; analgesic; antispasmodic; acidifier* [methenamine; phenyl salicylate; atropine sulfate; methylene blue; hyoscyamine; benzoic acid] 40.8•18.1•0.03•5.4•0.03•4.5 mg ⓓ Hexadrol; Hexalen
hexamarium bromide [see: distigmine bromide]
hexametazime BAN
hexamethone bromide [see: hexamethonium bromide]
hexamethonium bromide INN, BAN
hexamethylenamine [now: methenamine]
hexamethylenamine mandelate [see: methenamine mandelate]
hexamethylenetetramine [see: methenamine]
hexamethylmelamine (HMM; HXM) [see: altretamine]
hexamidine INN

hexamine hippurate BAN *urinary antibacterial* [also: methenamine hippurate]
hexamine mandelate [see: methenamine mandelate]
hexapradol INN
hexaprofen INN, BAN
hexapropymate INN, BAN
hexasonium iodide INN
Hexastat capsules ℞ *antineoplastic for ovarian adenocarcinoma (orphan)* [altretamine]
hexavitamin USP
Hexavitamin tablets OTC *vitamin supplement* [multiple vitamins] ±
hexcarbacholine bromide INN [also: carbolonium bromide]
hexedine USAN, INN *antibacterial*
hexemal [see: cyclobarbital]
hexestrol NF, INN
hexetidine BAN
hexicide [see: lindane]
hexinol [see: cyclomenol]
hexobarbital USP, INN
hexobarbital sodium NF
hexobendine USAN, INN, BAN *vasodilator*
hexocyclium methylsulfate *peptic ulcer adjunct* [also: hexocyclium metilsulfate; hexocyclium methylsulphate]
hexocyclium methylsulphate BAN [also: hexocyclium methylsulfate; hexocyclium metilsulfate]
hexocyclium metilsulfate INN [also: hexocyclium methylsulfate; hexocyclium methylsulphate]
hexoprenaline INN, BAN *tocolytic; bronchodilator* [also: hexoprenaline sulfate]
hexoprenaline sulfate USAN, JAN *tocolytic; bronchodilator* [also: hexoprenaline]
hexopyrimidine [see: hexetidine]
hexopyrrolate [see: hexopyrronium bromide]
hexopyrronium bromide INN
hexydaline [see: methenamine mandelate]
hexylcaine INN *local anesthetic* [also: hexylcaine HCl]
hexylcaine HCl USP *local anesthetic* [also: hexylcaine]

hexylene glycol NF *humectant; solvent*
hexylresorcinol USP *anthelmintic; topical antiseptic*
1-hexyltheobromine [see: pentifylline]
H-F Gel ℞ *(orphan: hydrofluoric acid burns)* [calcium gluconate]
hFSH (human follicle-stimulating hormone) [now: menotropins]
HFZ (homofenazine) [q.v.]
^{197}**Hg** [see: chlormerodrin Hg 197]
^{197}**Hg** [see: merisoprol acetate Hg 197]
^{197}**Hg** [see: merisoprol Hg 197]
^{203}**Hg** [see: chlormerodrin Hg 203]
^{203}**Hg** [see: merisoprol acetate Hg 203]
hGH (human growth hormone) [see: somatropin]
HGP-30 *investigational (Phase I) vaccine for HIV*
H-H-R tablets (discontinued 1993) ℞ *antihypertensive* [hydralazine HCl; hydrochlorothiazide; reserpine]
hibenzate INN *combining name for radicals or groups* [also: hybenzate]
Hibiclens sponge/brush OTC *broad-spectrum antimicrobial; germicidal* [chlorhexidine gluconate; alcohol 4%] 4%
Hibiclens Antiseptic/AntiMicrobial Skin Cleanser liquid OTC *broad-spectrum antimicrobial; germicidal* [chlorhexidine gluconate; alcohol 4%] 4%
Hibistat Germicidal Hand Rinse liquid OTC *broad-spectrum antimicrobial; germicidal* [chlorhexidine gluconate; alcohol 70%] 0.5%
Hibistat Towelette OTC *broad-spectrum antimicrobial; germicidal* [chlorhexidine gluconate; alcohol 70%] 0.5%
HibTITER IM injection ℞ *Haemophilus influenzae type b (HIB) vaccine* [Hemophilus b conjugate vaccine] 0.5 mL
Hi-Cal VM nutrition bar OTC *enteral nutritional therapy for HIV and AIDS*
Hi-Cor 1.0; Hi-Cor 2.5 cream ℞ *topical corticosteroid* [hydrocortisone] 1%; 2.5%
HIDA (hepatoiminodiacetic acid) [see: lidofenin]
HiDAC (high-dose ara-C) *chemotherapy protocol*
high molecular weight dextran [see: dextran 70]

High Potency N-Vites tablets OTC *vitamin supplement* [multiple B vitamins; vitamin C] ±•500 mg
High Potency Tar gel shampoo OTC *antiseborrheic; antipsoriatic; antipruritic; antibacterial* [coal tar] 25%
hioxifilcon A USAN *hydrophilic contact lens material*
Hipotest tablets OTC *dietary supplement* [multiple vitamins, minerals, and food products; calcium; iron; biotin] ±•53.5•50•0.001 mg
Hi-Po-Vites tablets OTC *dietary supplement* [multiple vitamins, minerals, and food products; iron; folic acid; biotin] ±•6•0.4•1 mg
Hiprex tablets ℞ *urinary bactericidal* [methenamine hippurate] 1 g
hirudin, recombinant *investigational anticoagulant and antithrombotic*
Hirulog ℞ *investigational agent for DVT and unstable angina, and to prevent reocclusion in MI and angioplasty* [bivalirudin]
Hismanal tablets ℞ *nonsedating antihistamine* [astemizole] 10 mg
Hismanal-D ℞ *investigational antihistamine/decongestant combination* [astemizole; pseudoephedrine HCl]
Histagesic Modified tablets OTC *decongestant; antihistamine; analgesic* [phenylephrine HCl; chlorpheniramine maleate; acetaminophen] 10•4•324 mg
Histaject subcu or IM injection (discontinued 1996) ℞ *antihistamine; anaphylaxis* [brompheniramine maleate] 10 mg/mL
Histalet syrup ℞ *decongestant; antihistamine* [pseudoephedrine HCl; chlorpheniramine maleate] 45•3 mg/5 mL
Histalet Forte tablets ℞ *decongestant; antihistamine* [phenylpropanolamine HCl; phenylephrine HCl; chlorpheniramine maleate; pyrilamine maleate] 50•10•4•25 mg
Histalet X tablets, syrup ℞ *decongestant; expectorant* [pseudoephedrine HCl; guaifenesin] 120•400 mg; 45•200 mg/5 mL
Histamic sustained-release capsules ℞ *decongestant; antihistamine* [phenyl-

propanolamine HCl; phenylephrine HCl; chlorpheniramine maleate; phenyltoloxamine citrate]

histamine dihydrochloride USAN

histamine phosphate USP *gastric secretory stimulant; diagnostic aid for pheochromocytoma*

histantin [see: chlorcyclizine HCl]

histapyrrodine INN

Histatab Plus tablets OTC *decongestant; antihistamine* [phenylephrine HCl; chlorpheniramine maleate] 5•2 mg

Histatan Pediatric suspension (discontinued 1992) ℞ *decongestant; antihistamine* [phenylephrine tannate; chlorpheniramine tannate; pyrilamine tannate] ② Hespan; Histatime

Histatime Forte tablets (discontinued 1993) ℞ *decongestant; antihistamine* [phenylpropanolamine HCl; phenylephrine HCl; chlorpheniramine maleate; pyrilamine maleate] ② Histatan

Histatrol intracutaneous injection, topical solution ℞ *intradermal or prick, puncture and scratch allergenic skin test* [histamine phosphate]

Hista-Vadrin tablets ℞ *decongestant; antihistamine* [phenylpropanolamine HCl; phenylephrine HCl; chlorpheniramine maleate] 40•5•6 mg

Histerone 50 IM injection (discontinued 1994) ℞ *androgen replacement for delayed puberty or breast cancer* [testosterone] 50 mg/mL

Histerone 100 IM injection ℞ *androgen replacement for delayed puberty or breast cancer* [testosterone] 100 mg/mL

histidine (L-histidine) USAN, USP, INN *amino acid (essential in infants and in renal failure, nonessential otherwise); symbols: His, H*

histidine monohydrochloride NF

495-L-histidineglucosylceramidase [see: imiglucerase]

Histine DM syrup ℞ *antitussive; decongestant; antihistamine* [dextromethorphan hydrobromide; phenylpropanolamine HCl; brompheniramine maleate] 10•12.5•2 mg/5 mL

Histinex HC syrup ℞ *narcotic antitussive; decongestant; antihistamine* [hydrocodone bitartrate; phenylephrine HCl; chlorpheniramine maleate] 2•5•2 mg/5 mL

Histinex PV syrup ℞ *narcotic antitussive; decongestant; antihistamine* [hydrocodone bitartrate; pseudoephedrine HCl; chlorpheniramine maleate] 2.5•30•2 mg/5 mL

Histodrix sustained-release tablets (discontinued 1993) OTC *decongestant; antihistamine* [pseudoephedrine sulfate; dexbrompheniramine maleate]

Histolyn-CYL intradermal injection ℞ *diagnostic aid for histoplasmosis* [histoplasmin (mycelial derivative)] 1:100

histoplasmin USP *dermal histoplasmosis test; Histoplasma capsulatum cultures in mycelial or yeast lysate form* 1:100 injection (yeast lysate form)

Histor-D syrup ℞ *decongestant; antihistamine* [phenylephrine HCl; chlorpheniramine maleate; alcohol 2%] 5•2 mg/5 mL

Histor-D Timecelles (sustained-release capsules) (discontinued 1995) ℞ *decongestant; antihistamine; anticholinergic* [phenylephrine HCl; chlorpheniramine maleate; methscopolamine nitrate] 20•8•2.5 mg

Histosal tablets OTC *decongestant; antihistamine; analgesic* [phenylpropanolamine HCl; pyrilamine maleate; acetaminophen; caffeine] 20•12.5•324•30 mg

histrelin USAN, INN *LHRH agonist (orphan: acute intermittent porphyria; hereditary coproporphyria; variegate porphyria)*

histrelin acetate *LHRH agonist; for central precocious puberty (orphan)*

Histussin HC syrup ℞ *narcotic antitussive; decongestant; antihistamine* [hydrocodone bitartrate; phenylephrine HCl; chlorpheniramine maleate] 2.5•5•2 mg/5 mL

HIV immune globulin (HIVIG) [see: human immunodeficiency virus immune globulin]

HIV immunotherapeutic (HIV-IT) *investigational (Phase II/III) gene therapy for HIV infection*

HIV vaccine [see: AIDS vaccine]

HIV-1 LA test [see: Recombigen HIV-1 LA]
HIV-1 peptide vaccine *investigational (Phase I) vaccine for HIV*
HIVAB HIV-1 EIA; HIVAB HIV-1/HIV-2 EIA; HIVAB HIV-2 EIA reagent kit for professional use *in vitro diagnostic aid for HIV antibodies* [enzyme immunoassay (EIA)]
HIVAG-1 reagent kit for professional use *in vitro diagnostic aid for HIV antibodies* [enzyme immunoassay (EIA)]
Hi-Value III; Hi-Value V ℞ *investigational in vitro diagnostic aid for glucose levels*
Hi-Vegi-Lip tablets OTC *digestive enzymes* [pancreatin; lipase; protease; amylase] 2400 mg•4800 U•60,000 U•60,000 U
Hivid film-coated tablets ℞ *antiviral for advanced HIV infection; and AIDS (orphan)* [zalcitabine] 0.375, 0.75 mg
HIV-IG ℞ *investigational (Phase III) immunomodulator for maternal/fetal HIV transfer* [HIV immune globulin]
HIV-neutralizing antibodies *(orphan: AIDS)*
HMB (homatropine methylbromide) [q.v.]
HMDP (hydroxymethylene diphosphonate) [see: oxidronic acid]
hMG (human menopausal gonadotropin) [see: menotropins]
HMM (hexamethylmelamine) [see: altretamine]
HMS eye drop suspension ℞ *ophthalmic topical corticosteroidal anti-inflammatory* [medrysone] 1%
HN₂ (nitrogen mustard) [see: mechlorethamine HCl]
hNGF (human nerve growth factor) [see: nerve growth factor]
HOAP-BLEO (hydroxydaunomycin, Oncovin, ara-C, prednisone, bleomycin) *chemotherapy protocol*
Hold DM; Children's Hold lozenges OTC *antitussive* [dextromethorphan hydrobromide] 5 mg
holmium *element (Ho)*
homarylamine INN

homatropine BAN *ophthalmic anticholinergic* [also: homatropine hydrobromide]
homatropine hydrobromide USP *ophthalmic anticholinergic; cycloplegic; mydriatic* [also: homatropine] 5% eye drops
homatropine methylbromide USP, INN, BAN *GI anticholinergic/antispasmodic*
Home Access; Home Access Express test kit for home use OTC *in vitro diagnostic aid for HIV in the blood*
Home Treatment Fluoride Gelution gel (discontinued 1992) ℞ *topical dental caries preventative* [acidulated phosphate fluoride]
Homicebrin liquid (discontinued 1992) OTC *vitamin supplement* [multiple vitamins]
homidium bromide INN, BAN
Hominex-1 powder OTC *formula for infants with homocystinuria or hypermethioninemia*
Hominex-2 powder OTC *enteral nutritional therapy for homocystinuria or hypermethioninemia*
homochlorcyclizine INN, BAN
homofenazine (HFZ) INN
homomenthyl salicylate [now: homosalate]
homopipramol INN
homosalate USAN, INN *ultraviolet screen*
4-homosulfanilamide [see: mafenide]
homprenorphine INN, BAN
HOP (hydroxydaunomycin, Oncovin, prednisone) *chemotherapy protocol*
hopantenic acid INN
hoquizil INN *bronchodilator* [also: hoquizil HCl]
hoquizil HCl USAN *bronchodilator* [also: hoquizil]
H.P. Acthar Gel IM or subcu injectable gel ℞ *steroid* [repository corticotropin] 40, 80 U/mL
HPA-23 *(orphan status withdrawn 1994)*
HPMCP (hydroxypropyl methylcellulose phthalate) [q.v.]
HPMPC (3-hydroxy-2-phosphonomethoxypropyl cytosine [dihydrate]) [see: cidofovir]

H-R Lubricating vaginal jelly OTC *lubricant* [hydroxypropyl methylcellulose]

HRT ℞ *investigational hormone replacement therapy for osteoporosis* [norethindrone acetate; ethinyl estradiol]

5-HT (5-hydroxytryptamine) [see: serotonin]

HT (human thrombin) [see: thrombin]

HT; 3-HT (3-hydroxytyramine) [see: dopamine]

HU-211 *investigational antiglaucoma agent*

Hulk Hogan Complete Multi-Vitamins chewable tablets (discontinued 1993) OTC *vitamin/mineral supplement* [multiple vitamins & minerals; folic acid; biotin]

Hulk Hogan Multi-Vitamins Plus Extra C chewable tablets (discontinued 1993) OTC *vitamin supplement* [multiple vitamins; folic acid]

Hulk Hogan Multi-Vitamins Plus Iron chewable tablets (discontinued 1993) OTC *vitamin/iron supplement* [multiple vitamins; iron; folic acid]

Humalog subcu injection, prefilled syringe cartridges ℞ *human insulin analog for diabetes* [insulin lispro (rDNA)] 100 U/mL; 1.5 mL

human albumin [see: albumin, human]

human amniotic fluid-derived surfactant [see: surfactant, human amniotic fluid derived]

human antihemophilic factor [see: antihemophilic factor]

human chorionic gonadotropin (hCG) [see: gonadotropin, chorionic]

human cytomegalovirus immune globulin [see: cytomegalovirus immune globulin, human]

human diploid cell vaccine (HDCV) [see: rabies vaccine]

human epidermal growth factor [see: epidermal growth factor, human]

human fibrinogen [see: fibrinogen, human]

human fibrinolysin [see: fibrinolysin, human]

human follicle-stimulating hormone (hFSH) [now: menotropins]

human growth hormone (hGH) JAN *growth hormone* [also: somatropin]

human growth hormone, recombinant (rhGH) *(orphan status withdrawn 1993)* [see: somatropin]

human growth hormone releasing factor [see: growth hormone-releasing factor]

human IgM monoclonal antibody (C-58) to cytomegalovirus (CMV) *(orphan status withdrawn 1994)*

human immunodeficiency virus (HIV-1) immune globulin (HIVIG) *investigational (Phase III) immunomodulator for maternal/fetal HIV transfer (orphan)*

human insulin [see: insulin, human]

human luteinizing hormone, recombinant *(orphan: chronic anovulation due to hypogonadism)*

human menopausal gonadotropin (hMG) [see: menotropins]

human nerve growth factor (hNGF) [see: nerve growth factor]

human respiratory syncytial virus immune globulin [see: respiratory syncytial virus immune globulin, human]

human serum albumin diethylenetriaminepentaacetic acid (DTPA) technetium (^{99m}Tc) JAN *radioactive agent* [also: technetium Tc 99m pentetate]

human superoxide dismutase (SOD) [see: superoxide dismutase, human]

Human Surf *(orphan status withdrawn 1994)* [surfactant, human amniotic fluid derived]

human T-cell inhibitor [see: muromonab-CD3]

human T-cell lymphotrophic virus type III (HTLV-III) [now: human immunodeficiency virus (HIV)]

Human T-Lymphotropic Virus Type I EIA reagent kit for professional use *in vitro diagnostic aid for HTLV I antibody in serum or plasma* [enzyme immunoassay (EIA)]

Humate-P IV injection ℞ *antihemophilic to correct coagulation deficiency* [antihemophilic factor VIII] ⚠

Humatin capsules ℞ *aminoglycoside-type antibiotic; amebicide* [paromomycin sulfate] 250 mg

Humatrope powder for subcu or IM injection ℞ *growth hormone; (orphan: growth failure; Turner syndrome; anovulation; severe burns)* [somatropin] 5 mg (13 IU)

Humegon powder for IM injection ℞ *ovulation stimulant for women; spermatogenesis stimulant for men* [menotropins] 75, 150 IU

Humibid DM sustained-release tablets ℞ *antitussive; expectorant* [dextromethorphan hydrobromide; guaifenesin] 30•600 mg

Humibid DM Sprinkle sustained-release capsules ℞ *antitussive; expectorant* [dextromethorphan hydrobromide; guaifenesin] 15•300 mg

Humibid L.A. sustained-release tablets ℞ *expectorant* [guaifenesin] 600 mg

Humibid Sprinkle sustained-release capsules ℞ *expectorant* [guaifenesin] 300 mg

HuMist nasal mist OTC *nasal moisturizer* [sodium chloride (saline)] 0.65%

Humorphan H.P. ℞ *(orphan: narcotic-tolerant pain)* [oxymorphone HCl]

Humorsol Ocumeter (eye drops) ℞ *antiglaucoma agent; reversible cholinesterase inhibitor miotic* [demecarium bromide] 0.125%, 0.25%

Humulin 50/50 subcu injection OTC *antidiabetic* [isophane insulin (human recombinant); human insulin (recombinant)] 100 U/mL

Humulin 70/30 subcu injection, prefilled syringe cartridges OTC *antidiabetic* [isophane insulin (human recombinant); human insulin (recombinant)] 100 U/mL; 1.5 mL

Humulin BR subcu injection (discontinued 1994) OTC *antidiabetic* [buffered human insulin (recombinant)] 100 U/mL

Humulin L subcu injection OTC *antidiabetic* [insulin zinc (human recombinant)] 100 U/mL

Humulin N subcu injection, prefilled syringe cartridges OTC *antidiabetic* [isophane insulin (human recombinant)] 100 U/mL; 1.5 mL

Humulin R subcu injection, prefilled syringe cartridges OTC *antidiabetic* [human insulin (recombinant)] 100 U/mL; 1.5 mL

Humulin U Ultralente subcu injection OTC *antidiabetic* [extended insulin zinc (human recombinant)] 100 U/mL

Hurricaine spray, liquid, gel OTC *mucous membrane anesthetic* [benzocaine] 20%

HVS 1+2 solution (discontinued 1994) OTC *oral antibacterial* [benzalkonium chloride]

HXM (hexamethylmelamine) [see: altretamine]

Hyal-ct 1101 *investigational antineoplastic for basal cell carcinoma*

Hyalex tablets OTC *vitamin/mineral supplement* [multiple vitamins; magnesium salicylate; magnesium PABA; zinc]

hyalosidase INN, BAN

hyaluronate sodium USAN, JAN *veterinary synovitis agent; ophthalmic surgical aid* [also: hyaluronic acid]

hyaluronic acid BAN *veterinary synovitis agent; ophthalmic surgical aid* [also: hyaluronate sodium]

hyaluronidase USP, INN, BAN *dispersion aid; absorption facilitator*

hyaluronoglucosaminidase [see: hyalosidase]

hyamate [see: buramate]

hybenzate USAN *combining name for radicals or groups* [also: hibenzate]

Hybolin Decanoate-50; Hybolin Decanoate-100 IM injection ℞ *anabolic steroid for anemia of renal insufficiency* [nandrolone decanoate] 50 mg/mL; 100 mg/mL

Hybolin Improved IM injection ℞ *anabolic steroid for metastatic breast cancer in women* [nandrolone phenpropionate] 50 mg/mL

Hybri-CEAker *(orphan: diagnostic aid in colorectal carcinoma)* [indium In 111 altumomab pentetate]

Hycamtin powder for IV injection ℞ *topoisomerase I inhibitor; antineoplastic*

for ovarian cancer [topotecan HCl] 4 mg/vial

hycanthone USAN, INN *antischistosomal*

hycanthone mesylate

hyclate INN *combining name for radicals or groups*

HycoClear Tuss syrup ℞ *narcotic antitussive; expectorant* [hydrocodone bitartrate; guaifenesin] 5•100 mg/5 mL

Hycodan tablets, syrup ℞ *narcotic antitussive; GI anticholinergic/antispasmodic* [hydrocodone bitartrate; homatropine methylbromide] 5•1.5 mg; 5•1.5 mg/5 mL ⓘ Hycomine; Vicodin

Hycomine syrup, pediatric syrup ℞ *narcotic antitussive; decongestant* [hydrocodone bitartrate; phenylpropanolamine HCl] 5•25 mg/5 mL; 2.5•12.5 mg/5 mL ⓘ Byclomine; Hycodan; Vicodin

Hycomine Compound tablets ℞ *narcotic antitussive; decongestant; antihistamine; analgesic* [hydrocodone bitartrate; phenylephrine HCl; chlorpheniramine maleate; acetaminophen; caffeine] 5•10•2•250•30 mg

Hycort cream, ointment ℞ *topical corticosteroid* [hydrocortisone] 1%

Hycotuss Expectorant syrup ℞ *narcotic antitussive; expectorant* [hydrocodone bitartrate; guaifenesin; alcohol 10%] 5•100 mg/5 mL

Hydeltrasol IV, IM injection ℞ *glucocorticoids* [prednisolone sodium phosphate] 20 mg/mL

Hydelta-T.B.A. intra-articular, intralesional, or soft tissue injection ℞ *glucocorticoids* [prednisolone tebutate] 20 mg/mL

Hydergine sublingual tablets, tablets, liquid ℞ *for age-related mental capacity decline* [ergoloid mesylates] 0.5, 1 mg; 1 mg; 1 mg/mL ⓘ Hydramine

Hydergine LC liquid capsules ℞ *for age-related mental capacity decline* [ergoloid mesylates] 1 mg

hydracarbazine INN

hydralazine INN, BAN *antihypertensive; peripheral vasodilator* [also: hydralazine HCl]

hydralazine HCl USP, JAN *antihypertensive; peripheral vasodilator* [also: hydralazine] 10, 25, 50, 100 mg oral; 20 mg/mL injection

hydralazine polistirex USAN *antihypertensive*

Hydramine syrup, elixir (discontinued 1994) ℞ *antitussive* [diphenhydramine HCl] 12.5 mg/5 mL ⓘ Bydramine; Hydergine; Hydramyn; Hytramyn

Hydramyn syrup ℞ *antihistamine; antitussive* [diphenhydramine HCl; alcohol 5%] 12.5 mg/5 mL ⓘ Hydramine; Hytramyn

Hydrap-ES tablets ℞ *antihypertensive* [hydrochlorothiazide; reserpine; hydralazine HCl] 15•0.1•25 mg

hydrargaphen INN, BAN

hydrastine USP

hydrastine HCl USP

hydrastinine HCl NF

Hydrate IV or IM injection ℞ *antinauseant; antiemetic; antivertigo; motion sickness preventative* [dimenhydrinate] 50 mg/mL

Hydra-Zide capsules ℞ *antihypertensive* [hydrochlorothiazide; hydralazine HCl]

Hydrazide 25/25; Hydrazide 50/50 capsules (discontinued 1995) ℞ *antihypertensive* [hydrochlorothiazide; hydralazine HCl] 25•25 mg; 50•50 mg

hydrazinecarboximidamide monohydrochloride [see: pimagedine HCl]

hydrazinoxane [see: domoxin]

Hydrea capsules ℞ *antineoplastic for melanoma, ovarian carcinoma and myelocytic leukemia; (orphan: sickle cell anemia)* [hydroxyurea] 500 mg

Hydrex tablets (discontinued 1993) ℞ *diuretic; antihypertensive* [benzthiazide]

Hydrisalic gel (discontinued 1994) ℞ *topical keratolytic* [salicylic acid] 6%

Hydrisea lotion OTC *moisturizer; emollient* [Dead Sea salts]

Hydrisinol cream, lotion OTC *moisturizer; emollient*

Hydro Cobex IM injection ℞ *antianemic; vitamin B_{12} supplement* [hydroxocobalamin] 1000 μg/mL

hydrobentizide INN

Hydrobexan IM injection (discontinued 1995) ℞ *antianemic; vitamin B_{12} supplement* [hydroxocobalamin] 1000 μg/mL

hydrobutamine [see: butidrine]

Hydrocare Cleaning and Disinfecting solution OTC *chemical disinfecting solution for soft contact lenses*

Hydrocare Preserved Saline solution OTC *rinsing/storage solution for soft contact lenses* [preserved saline solution]

Hydrocet capsules ℞ *narcotic analgesic* [hydrocodone bitartrate; acetaminophen] 5•500 mg

Hydro-Chlor tablets (discontinued 1993) ℞ *diuretic; antihypertensive* [hydrochlorothiazide]

hydrochloric acid NF *acidifying agent*

hydrochloric acid, diluted NF *acidifying agent*

hydrochlorothiazide (HCT; HCTZ) USP, INN, BAN *diuretic; antihypertensive* 25, 50, 100 mg oral; 50 mg/5 mL oral; 100 mg/mL oral

Hydrocil Instant powder OTC *bulk laxative* [psyllium hydrophilic mucilloid] 3.5 g/scoop or packet

hydrocodone INN, BAN *antitussive* [also: hydrocodone bitartrate]

hydrocodone bitartrate USAN, USP *antitussive* [also: hydrocodone]

Hydrocodone Compound syrup ℞ *narcotic antitussive; GI anticholinergic/ antispasmodic* [hydrocodone bitartrate; homatropine hydrobromide] 5•1.5 mg/5 mL

hydrocodone polistirex USAN *antitussive*

hydrocolloid gel *dressings for wet wounds*

Hydrocort cream ℞ *topical corticosteroid* [hydrocortisone] 2.5%

hydrocortamate INN

hydrocortamate HCl [see: hydrocortamate]

hydrocortisone (HC) USP, INN, BAN *corticosteroid* 5, 10, 20 mg oral; 0.5%, 1%, 2.5% topical

hydrocortisone aceponate INN

hydrocortisone acetate (HCA) USP, BAN *corticosteroid* 25, 50 mg/mL injection

hydrocortisone buteprate USAN *corticosteroid*

hydrocortisone butyrate USAN, USP, BAN *topical corticosteroid*

hydrocortisone cyclopentylpropionate [see: hydrocortisone cypionate]

hydrocortisone cypionate USP *glucocorticoid*

hydrocortisone hemisuccinate USP *adrenocortical steroid*

hydrocortisone sodium phosphate USP, BAN *glucocorticoid*

hydrocortisone sodium succinate USP, BAN *glucocorticoid*

hydrocortisone valerate USAN, USP *topical corticosteroid*

Hydrocortone tablets ℞ *glucocorticoids* [hydrocortisone] 10, 20 mg

Hydrocortone Acetate intralesional, intra-articular, or soft tissue injection ℞ *glucocorticoids* [hydrocortisone acetate] 25, 50 mg/mL

Hydrocortone Phosphate IV, subcu, or IM injection ℞ *glucocorticoids* [hydrocortisone sodium phosphate] 50 mg/mL

Hydrocream Base OTC *cream base*

Hydro-Crysti 12 IM injection ℞ *antianemic; vitamin B_{12} supplement* [hydroxocobalamin] 1000 μg/mL

HydroDIURIL tablets ℞ *diuretic; antihypertensive* [hydrochlorothiazide] 25, 50, 100 mg

Hydro-Ergoloid oral tablets, sublingual tablets ℞ *cognition adjuvant* [ergoloid mesylates]

hydrofilcon A USAN *hydrophilic contact lens material*

hydroflumethiazide USP, INN, BAN *antihypertensive; diuretic* 50 mg oral

hydrofluoric acid *dental caries prophylactic*

Hydro-Fluserpine #2 tablets ℞ *antihypertensive* [hydroflumethiazide; reserpine]

hydrogen *element (H)*

hydrogen peroxide USP *topical anti-infective*

hydrogen tetrabromoaurate [see: bromauric acid]

hydrogenated ergot alkaloids [now: ergoloid mesylates]

hydrogenated vegetable oil [see: vegetable oil, hydrogenated]

Hydrogesic capsules ℞ *narcotic analgesic* [hydrocodone bitartrate; acetaminophen] 5•500 mg

hydromadinone INN

Hydromal tablets (discontinued 1993) ℞ *diuretic; antihypertensive* [hydrochlorothiazide]

Hydromet syrup ℞ *narcotic antitussive; GI anticholinergic/antispasmodic* [hydrocodone bitartrate; homatropine methylbromide] 5•1.5 mg/5 mL

hydromorphinol INN, BAN

hydromorphone INN, BAN *narcotic analgesic* [also: hydromorphone HCl]

hydromorphone HCl USP *narcotic analgesic* [also: hydromorphone] 2, 4 mg oral; 1, 2, 3, 4, 10 mg/mL injection

hydromorphone sulfate

Hydromox tablets ℞ *diuretic; antihypertensive* [quinethazone] 50 mg

Hydromox R tablets (discontinued 1992) ℞ *antihypertensive* [quinethazone; reserpine]

Hydromycin ophthalmic suspension, otic suspension ℞ *topical antibiotic* [neomycin sulfate; polymyxin B sulfate; hydrocortisone]

Hydropane syrup (name changed to Hydrocodone Compound in 1995)

Hydro-Par tablets ℞ *diuretic; antihypertensive* [hydrochlorothiazide] 25, 50 mg

Hydropel ointment OTC *skin protectant* [silicone; hydrophobic starch derivative] 30%•10%

4-hydroperoxycyclophosphamide (4-HC) *(orphan: ex vivo treatment of autologous bone marrow for acute myelogenous leukemia)*

Hydrophed tablets ℞ *antiasthmatic; bronchodilator; decongestant; anxiolytic* [theophylline; ephedrine sulfate; hydroxyzine HCl] 130•25•10 mg

Hydrophen Pediatric liquid (discontinued 1992) ℞ *narcotic antitussive; decongestant* [hydrocodone bitartrate; phenylpropanolamine HCl;] ⑨ Hydropine

Hydrophilic OTC *ointment base*

hydrophilic ointment [see: ointment, hydrophilic]

hydrophilic petrolatum [see: petrolatum, hydrophilic]

Hydropine; Hydropine H.P. tablets (discontinued 1993) ℞ *antihypertensive* [hydroflumethiazide; reserpine] ⑨ Hydropane; Hydrophen

Hydropres-25 tablets (discontinued 1996) ℞ *antihypertensive* [hydrochlorothiazide; reserpine] 25•0.125 mg

Hydropres-50 tablets ℞ *antihypertensive* [hydrochlorothiazide; reserpine] 50•0.125 mg

Hydro-Propanolamine syrup ℞ *narcotic antitussive; decongestant* [hydrocodone bitartrate; phenylpropanolamine HCl]

hydroquinone USP *hyperpigmentation bleaching agent*

Hydro-Serp tablets ℞ *antihypertensive* [hydrochlorothiazide; reserpine] 50•0.125 mg

Hydroserpine #1; Hydroserpine #2 tablets ℞ *antihypertensive* [hydrochlorothiazide; reserpine] 25•0.125 mg; 50•0.125 mg

Hydrosine 25, Hydrosine 50 tablets ℞ *antihypertensive* [hydrochlorothiazide; reserpine]

HydroStat IR tablets ℞ *narcotic analgesic* [hydromorphone HCl] 1, 2, 3, 4 mg

Hydro-T tablets (discontinued 1993) ℞ *diuretic; antihypertensive* [hydrochlorothiazide]

hydrotalcite INN, BAN

HydroTex cream ℞ *topical corticosteroid* [hydrocortisone] 0.5%

HydroTex ointment (discontinued 1993) ℞ *topical corticosteroid* [hydrocortisone]

Hydroxacen injection (discontinued 1994) ℞ *anxiolytic; antihistamine* [hydroxyzine HCl] 50 mg/mL

hydroxamethocaine BAN [also: hydroxytetracaine]

hydroxidione sodium succinate [see: hydroxydione sodium succinate]

hydroxindasate INN

hydroxindasol INN
hydroxizine chloride [see: hydroxyzine HCl]
Hydroxo-12 IM injection (discontinued 1992) ℞ *antianemic; vitamin supplement* [hydroxocobalamin]
hydroxocobalamin USAN, USP, INN, BAN, JAN *vitamin B_{12}; hematopoietic* [also: hydroxocobalamin acetate] 1 mg/mL injection
hydroxocobalamin acetate JAN *vitamin B_{12}; hematopoietic* [also: hydroxocobalamin]
hydroxocobemine [see: hydroxocobalamin]
3-hydroxy-2-phosphonomethoxypropyl cytosine (HPMPC) dihydrate [see: cidofovir]
N-hydroxyacetamide [see: acetohydroxamic acid]
4′-hydroxyacetanilide [see: acetaminophen]
4′-hydroxyacetanilide salicylate [see: acetaminosalol]
hydroxyamfetamine INN *ophthalmic adrenergic; mydriatic* [also: hydroxyamphetamine hydrobromide; hydroxyamphetamine]
hydroxyamphetamine BAN *ophthalmic adrenergic; mydriatic* [also: hydroxyamphetamine hydrobromide; hydroxyamfetamine]
hydroxyamphetamine hydrobromide USP *ophthalmic adrenergic/vasoconstrictor; mydriatic* [also: hydroxyamfetamine; hydroxyamphetamine]
hydroxyapatite BAN *prosthetic aid* [also: durapatite; calcium phosphate, tribasic]
2-hydroxybenzamide [see: salicylamide]
2-hydroxybenzoic acid [see: salicylic acid]
o-hydroxybenzyl alcohol [see: salicyl alcohol]
hydroxybutanedioic acid [see: malic acid]
hydroxybutyrate sodium, gamma [see: sodium oxybate]
hydroxycarbamide INN *antineoplastic* [also: hydroxyurea]

hydroxychloroquine INN, BAN *antimalarial; lupus erythematosus suppressant* [also: hydroxychloroquine sulfate]
hydroxychloroquine sulfate USP *antimalarial; antirheumatic; lupus erythematosus suppressant* [also: hydroxychloroquine] 200 mg oral
25-hydroxycholecalciferol [see: calcifediol]
hydroxycincophene [see: oxycinchophen]
hydroxycobalamin & sodium thiosulfate (*orphan: severe acute cyanide poisoning*)
hydroxydaunomycin [see: doxorubicin]
14-hydroxydihydromorphine [see: hydromorphinol]
hydroxydione sodium succinate INN, BAN
hydroxyethyl cellulose NF *suspending and viscosity-increasing agent; ophthalmic aid*
2-hydroxyethyl methacrylate (HEMA) *contact lens material*
hydroxyethyl starch (HES) [see: hetastarch]
hydroxyethylstarch JAN *plasma volume extender* [also: hetastarch]
hydroxyhexamide
hydroxylapatite [see: durapatite; calcium phosphate, tribasic]
hydroxymagnesium aluminate [see: magaldrate]
hydroxymesterone [see: medrysone]
hydroxymethylene diphosphonate (HMDP) [see: oxidronic acid]
hydroxymethylgramicidin [see: methocidin]
N-hydroxynaphthalimide diethyl phosphate [see: naftalofos]
hydroxypethidine INN, BAN
hydroxyphenamate USAN *minor tranquilizer* [also: oxyfenamate]
hydroxyprocaine INN, BAN
hydroxyprogesterone INN, BAN *progestin* [also: hydroxyprogesterone caproate]
hydroxyprogesterone caproate USP, INN, JAN *progestin for amenorrhea, metrorrhagia, and dysfunctional uterine*

bleeding [also: hydroxyprogesterone] 125, 250 mg/mL IM injection (in oil)

2-hydroxypropanoic acid, calcium salt, hydrate [see: calcium lactate]

hydroxypropyl cellulose NF *topical protectant; emulsifying and coating agent* [also: hydroxypropylcellulose]

hydroxypropyl methylcellulose USP *suspending and viscosity-increasing agent; ophthalmic surgical aid* [also: hypromellose; hydroxypropylmethylcellulose]

hydroxypropyl methylcellulose 1828 USP

hydroxypropyl methylcellulose phthalate (HPMCP) NF *tablet-coating agent* [also: hydroxypropylmethylcellulose phthalate]

hydroxypropyl methylcellulose phthalate 200731 NF *tablet-coating agent*

hydroxypropyl methylcellulose phthalate 220824 NF *tablet-coating agent*

hydroxypropylcellulose JAN *topical protectant; emulsifying and coating agent* [also: hydroxypropyl cellulose]

hydroxypropylmethylcellulose JAN *suspending and viscosity-increasing agent; ophthalmic surgical aid* [also: hydroxypropyl methylcellulose; hypromellose]

hydroxypropylmethylcellulose phthalate JAN *tablet-coating agent* [also: hydroxypropyl methylcellulose phthalate]

hydroxypyridine tartrate INN

hydroxyquinoline *topical antiseptic*

4′-hydroxysalicylanilide [see: osalmid]

hydroxystearin sulfate NF

hydroxystenozole INN

hydroxystilbamidine INN, BAN *antileishmanial* [also: hydroxystilbamidine isethionate]

hydroxystilbamidine isethionate USP *antileishmanial* [also: hydroxystilbamidine]

hydroxysuccinic acid [see: malic acid]

hydroxytetracaine INN [also: hydroxamethocaine]

hydroxytoluic acid INN, BAN

5-hydroxytryptamine (5-HT) [see: serotonin]

hydroxytryptophan [see: L-5 hydroxytryptophan]

3-hydroxytyramine (HT; 3-HT) [see: dopamine]

hydroxyurea USAN, USP, BAN *antineoplastic; (orphan: sickle cell anemia)* [also: hydroxycarbamide]

hydroxyzine INN, BAN *anxiolytic; minor tranquilizer; antihistamine; antipruritic* [also: hydroxyzine HCl]

hydroxyzine HCl USP *anxiolytic; minor tranquilizer; antihistamine; antipruritic* [also: hydroxyzine] 10, 25, 50 mg oral; 10 mg/5 mL oral; 25, 50 mg/mL injection

hydroxyzine pamoate USP *minor tranquilizer* 25, 50, 100 mg oral

Hydro-Z-50 tablets (discontinued 1992) R *diuretic; antihypertensive* [hydrochlorothiazide]

Hydrozide-50 tablets (discontinued 1993) R *diuretic; antihypertensive* [hydrochlorothiazide]

hy-Flow solution (discontinued 1993) OTC *wetting solution for hard contact lenses*

Hygenic Cleansing anorectal pads OTC *moisturizer and cleanser for external rectal/vaginal areas; astringent* [witch hazel] 50%

Hygroton tablets R *diuretic; antihypertensive* [chlorthalidone] 25, 50, 100 mg ▣ Regroton

Hylidone tablets (discontinued 1993) R *antihypertensive* [chlorthalidone]

Hyliver Plus IM injection (discontinued 1994) R *antianemic; vitamin supplement* [liver extracts; vitamin B_{12}; folic acid]

Hylorel tablets R *antihypertensive* [guanadrel sulfate] 10, 25 mg

Hylutin IM injection R *progestin for amenorrhea, metrorrhagia, and dysfunctional uterine bleeding* [hydroxyprogesterone caproate in oil] 250 mg/mL

hymecromone USAN, INN *choleretic*

hyoscine hydrobromide BAN *GI antispasmodic; prevent motion sickness; cycloplegic; mydriatic* [also: scopolamine hydrobromide]

hyoscine methobromide BAN *anticholinergic* [also: methscopolamine bromide]

hyoscyamine (L-hyoscyamine) USP, BAN *anticholinergic*

hyoscyamine hydrobromide USP *anticholinergic*

hyoscyamine sulfate USP *GI anticholinergic/antispasmodic* [also: hyoscyamine sulphate] 0.375 mg oral

hyoscyamine sulphate BAN *GI anticholinergic/antispasmodic* [also: hyoscyamine sulfate]

Hyosophen tablets, elixir ℞ *GI anticholinergic; sedative* [atropine sulfate; scopolamine hydrobromide; hyoscyamine hydrobromide; phenobarbital] 0.0194•0.0065•0.1037•16.2 mg; 0.0194•0.0065•0.1037•16.2 mg/5 mL

Hypaque Meglumine injection ℞ *parenteral radiopaque agent* [diatrizoate meglumine] 30%, 60%

Hypaque Sodium injection ℞ *GI contrast radiopaque agent* [diatrizoate sodium] 20%, 25%, 50%

Hypaque Sodium solution, powder ℞ *GI contrast radiopaque agent* [diatrizoate sodium] 41.66%; 100%

Hypaque-Cysto intracavitary instillation ℞ *cholecystographic radiopaque agent* [diatrizoate meglumine] 30%

Hypaque-M 75; Hypaque-M 90; Hypaque-76 injection ℞ *parenteral radiopaque agent* [diatrizoate meglumine; diatrizoate sodium] 50%•25%; 60%•30%; 66%•10%

Hyperab IM injection ℞ *rabies prophylaxis* [rabies immune globulin] 150 IU/mL

HyperGAM+CF ℞ *investigational vaccine for Pseudomonas aeruginosa lung infections associated with cystic fibrosis* [polyclonal antibodies]

HyperHep IM injection ℞ *hepatitis B immunizing agent* [hepatitis B immune globulin] 0.5, 1, 5 mL ② Hyper-Tet; Hyperstat

hypericin *investigational (Phase I) antiviral for AIDS/HIV*

Hyperlyte; Hyperlyte CR; Hyperlyte R IV admixture ℞ *intravenous electrolyte therapy* [combined electrolyte solution]

Hypermune RSV ℞ *(orphan: prophylaxis and treatment of respiratory syncytial virus)* [respiratory syncytial virus immune globulin, human]

Hyperstat IV injection ℞ *antihypertensive for hypertensive emergencies* [diazoxide] 15 mg/mL ② Hyper-Tet; HyperHep; Nitrostat

Hyper-Tet IM injection ℞ *tetanus immunizing agent* [tetanus immune globulin] 250 U ② HyperHep; Hyperstat

Hypervax ℞ *investigational anti-infective for renal dialysis patients* [Staphylococcus aureus vaccine]

Hy-Phen tablets ℞ *narcotic analgesic* [hydrocodone bitartrate; acetaminophen] 5•500 mg

hyphylline [see: dyphylline]

hypnogene [see: barbital]

hypochlorous acid, sodium salt [see: sodium hypochlorite]

Hypo-Clear solution (discontinued 1992) OTC *rinsing/storage solution for soft contact lenses* [saline solution]

β-hypophamine [see: vasopressin]

α-hypophamine [see: oxytocin]

hypophosphorous acid NF *antioxidant*

Hyporet (trademarked delivery system) *prefilled disposable syringe*

HypoTears ophthalmic ointment OTC *ocular moisturizer/lubricant* [white petrolatum; mineral oil]

HypoTears; HypoTears PF eye drops OTC *ocular moisturizer/lubricant* [polyvinyl alcohol] 1%

HypoTears PF ophthalmic ointment (discontinued 1993) OTC *ocular moisturizer/lubricant*

HypRho-D; HypRho-D Mini-Dose IM injection ℞ *obstetric Rh factor immunity suppressant* [Rh$_0$(D) immune globulin] 300 μg; 50 μg

Hyprogest 250 IM injection ℞ *progestin for amenorrhea, metrorrhagia, and dysfunctional uterine bleeding* [hydroxyprogesterone caproate in oil] 250 mg/mL

hyprolose [see: hydroxypropyl cellulose]

hypromellose INN, BAN *suspending and viscosity-increasing agent* [also: hydroxypropyl methylcellulose; hydroxypropylmethylcellulose]

Hyrexin-50 injection ℞ *antihistamine; motion sickness preventative; sleep aid; antiparkinsonian* [diphenhydramine HCl] 50 mg/mL

Hyskon uterine infusion ℞ *hysteroscopy aid* [dextran 70; dextrose] 32%•10%

Hysone cream OTC *topical corticosteroid; antifungal; antibacterial* [hydrocortisone; clioquinol] 10•30 mg/g

Hytakerol capsules, oral solution ℞ *vitamin deficiency therapy* [dihydrotachysterol] 0.125 mg; 0.25 mg/mL

Hytinic capsules OTC *hematinic* [polysaccharide-iron complex] 150 mg

Hytinic IM injection ℞ *hematinic* [ferrous gluconate; multiple B vitamins; procaine HCl] 3 mg/mL•≚•2%

Hytone cream, lotion, ointment ℞ *topical corticosteroid* [hydrocortisone] 1%, 2.5%; 1%, 2.5%; 2.5% ⑨ Vytone

Hytone 1% ointment, spray ℞ *topical corticosteroid* [hydrocortisone] 1%

Hytrin soft capsules ℞ *antihypertensive; antiadrenergic; treatment for benign prostatic hyperplasia* [terazosin HCl] 1, 2, 5, 10 mg

Hytrin tablets (discontinued 1995) ℞ *antihypertensive; antiadrenergic; treatment for benign prostatic hyperplasia* [terazosin HCl] 1, 2, 5, 10 mg

Hytuss tablets OTC *expectorant* [guaifenesin] 100 mg

Hytuss 2X capsules OTC *expectorant* [guaifenesin] 200 mg

Hyzaar film-coated tablets ℞ *antihypertensive; angiotensin II blocker; diuretic* [losartan potassium; hydrochlorothiazide] 50•12.5 mg

Hyzine-50 IM injection ℞ *anxiolytic* [hydroxyzine HCl] 50 mg/mL

I

^{123}**I** [see: iodohippurate sodium I 123]
^{123}**I** [see: sodium iodide I 123]
^{125}**I** [see: albumin, iodinated I 125 serum]
^{125}**I** [see: diatrizoate sodium I 125]
^{125}**I** [see: diohippuric acid I 125]
^{125}**I** [see: diotyrosine I 125]
^{125}**I** [see: fibrinogen I 125]
^{125}**I** [see: insulin I 125]
^{125}**I** [see: iodohippurate sodium I 125]
^{125}**I** [see: iodopyracet I 125]
^{125}**I** [see: iomethin I 125]
^{125}**I** [see: iothalamate sodium I 125]
^{125}**I** [see: liothyronine I 125]
^{125}**I** [see: oleic acid I 125]
^{125}**I** [see: povidone I 125]
^{125}**I** [see: rose bengal sodium I 125]
^{125}**I** [see: sodium iodide I 125]
^{125}**I** [see: thyroxine I 125]
^{125}**I** [see: triolein I 125]
^{131}**I** [see: albumin, aggregated iodinated I 131 serum]
^{131}**I** [see: albumin, iodinated I 131 serum]
^{131}**I** [see: diatrizoate sodium I 131]
^{131}**I** [see: diohippuric acid I 131]
^{131}**I** [see: diotyrosine I 131]
^{131}**I** [see: ethiodized oil I 131]
^{131}**I** [see: insulin I 131]
^{131}**I** [see: iodipamide sodium I 131]
^{131}**I** [see: iodoantipyrine I 131]
^{131}**I** [see: iodocholesterol I 131]
^{131}**I** [see: iodohippurate sodium I 131]
^{131}**I** [see: iodopyracet I 131]
^{131}**I** [see: iomethin I 131]
^{131}**I** [see: iothalamate sodium I 131]
^{131}**I** [see: iotyrosine I 131]
^{131}**I** [see: liothyronine I 131]
^{131}**I** [see: macrosalb (^{131}I)]
^{131}**I** [see: oleic acid I 131]
^{131}**I** [see: povidone I 131]
^{131}**I** [see: rose bengal sodium I 131]
^{131}**I** [see: sodium iodide I 131]
^{131}**I** [see: thyroxine I 131]
^{131}**I** [see: tolpovidone I 131]

131I [see: triolein I 131]

I-131 radiolabeled B1 monoclonal antibody (orphan: non-Hodgkin's B-cell lymphoma)

Iamin ℞ investigational treatment for peptic ulcers, surgical wound repair, and bone healing [peptide copper compound]

ibacitabine INN

ibafloxacin USAN, INN, BAN antibacterial

ibazocine INN

IBC (isobutyl cyanoacrylate) [see: bucrylate]

Iberet; Iberet-500 controlled-release Filmtabs (film-coated tablets) OTC hematinic [ferrous sulfate; multiple B vitamins; sodium ascorbate] 105•≜•150 mg; 105•≜•500 mg

Iberet; Iberet-500 liquid OTC hematinic [ferrous sulfate; multiple B vitamins] 78.75•≜ mg/15 mL

Iberet-Folic-500 controlled-release Filmtabs (film-coated tablets) ℞ hematinic [ferrous sulfate; multiple B vitamins; sodium ascorbate; folic acid] 105•≜•500•0.8 mg

ibopamine USAN, INN, BAN peripheral dopaminergic agent; vasodilator

ibrotal [see: ibrotamide]

ibrotamide INN

Ibu film-coated tablets ℞ nonsteroidal anti-inflammatory drug (NSAID); antiarthritic; analgesic [ibuprofen] 400, 600, 800 mg

ibudilast INN

ibufenac USAN, INN, BAN analgesic; anti-inflammatory

Ibuprin tablets OTC nonsteroidal anti-inflammatory drug (NSAID); antiarthritic; analgesic [ibuprofen] 200 mg

ibuprofen USAN, USP, INN, BAN antiarthritic; nonsteroidal anti-inflammatory drug (NSAID); analgesic 200, 300, 400, 600, 800 mg oral

ibuprofen aluminum USAN anti-inflammatory

ibuprofen piconol USAN topical anti-inflammatory

Ibuprohm caplets, tablets OTC nonsteroidal anti-inflammatory drug (NSAID); antiarthritic; analgesic [ibuprofen] 200 mg

Ibuprohm tablets ℞ nonsteroidal anti-inflammatory drug (NSAID); antiarthritic; analgesic [ibuprofen] 400 mg

ibuproxam INN

Ibu-Tab film-coated tablets (discontinued 1996) OTC nonsteroidal anti-inflammatory drug (NSAID); antiarthritic; analgesic [ibuprofen] 200 mg

Ibu-Tab film-coated tablets (discontinued 1996) ℞ nonsteroidal anti-inflammatory drug (NSAID); antiarthritic; analgesic [ibuprofen] 400, 600, 800 mg

ibuterol INN

ibutilide INN antiarrhythmic [also: ibutilide fumarate]

ibutilide fumarate USAN antiarrhythmic for atrial fibrillation/flutter [also: ibutilide]

ibuverine INN

ibylcaine chloride [see: butethamine HCl]

ICAPS timed-release tablets OTC vitamin/mineral supplement [multiple vitamins & minerals] ≜

ICAPS Plus tablets OTC vitamin/mineral supplement [multiple vitamins & minerals] ≜

icatibant acetate USAN antiasthmatic

ICE (ifosfamide [with mesna rescue], carboplatin, etoposide) chemotherapy protocol [also: MICE]

ichthammol USP, BAN topical anti-infective 10%, 20%

iclazepam INN

icosapent INN omega-3 marine triglyceride

icospiramide INN

icotidine USAN antagonist to histamine H_1 and H_2 receptors

ictasol USAN disinfectant

Ictotest reagent tablets for professional use in vitro diagnostic aid for bilirubin in the urine

Icy Hot balm, cream, stick OTC counterirritant [methyl salicylate; menthol] 29%•7.6%; 30%•10%; 30%•10%

Idamycin powder for IV injection ℞ antibiotic antineoplastic; for acute myelogenous and other leukemias (orphan) [idarubicin HCl] 5, 10, 20 mg

Idarac ℞ investigational nonsteroidal anti-inflammatory drug (NSAID); analgesic [floctafenine]

idarubicin INN, BAN *antibiotic antineoplastic* [also: idarubicin HCl]

idarubicin HCl USAN, INN *antibiotic antineoplastic (orphan: various leukemias)* [also: idarubicin]

idaverine INN

idazoxan INN, BAN

idebenone INN *investigational treatment for Alzheimer's disease*

idenast INN

Identi-Dose (trademarked dosage form) *unit dose package*

idoxuridine (IDU) USAN, USP, INN, BAN *ophthalmic antiviral*

idralfidine INN

idrobutamine [see: butidrine]

idrocilamide INN

idropranolol INN

IDU (idoxuridine) [q.v.]

IE (ifosfamide [with mesna rescue], etoposide) *chemotherapy protocol*

ifenprodil INN

ifetroban USAN *antithrombotic; anti-ischemic; antivasospastic*

ifetroban sodium USAN *antithrombotic; anti-ischemic; antivasospastic*

Ifex powder for IV injection ℞ *alkylating antineoplastic; (orphan: testicular cancer; bone and soft tissue sarcomas)* [ifosfamide] 1, 3 g

IFN (interferon) [q.v.]

IFN-alpha 2 (interferon alfa-2) [see: interferon alfa-2b, recombinant]

ifosfamide USAN, USP, INN, BAN *alkylating antineoplastic; (orphan: testicular cancer; bone and soft tissue sarcomas)*

IfoVP (ifosfamide [with mesna rescue], VePesid) *chemotherapy protocol*

ifoxetine INN

IG (immune globulin) [see: globulin, immune]

IgE pentapeptide [see: pentigetide]

Igef ℞ *investigational treatment for growth hormone receptor impairment (Laron syndrome)* [recombinant human insulin-like growth factor]

IGF-1 (insulin-like growth factor-1) [q.v.]

IgG 1 [see: immunoglobulin G 1]

IGIV (immune globulin intravenous) [see: globulin, immune]

Ikorel ℞ *investigational treatment for angina and congestive heart failure* [nicorandil]

IL-1, IL-2, etc. [see: interleukin-1, interleukin-2, etc.]

IL-1R (interleukin-1 receptor) [q.v.]

IL-2 (interleukin-2) [see: aldesleukin; teceleukin; celmoleukin]

IL-2 fusion toxin *investigational (Phase I/II) agent for HIV; investigational antipsoriatic*

IL-4R (interleukin-4 receptor) [q.v.]

ilepcimide USAN *anticonvulsant; (orphan: generalized tonic-clonic epilepsy)*

Iletin *insulin* [see under: Regular, NPH, Protamine, Lente, Semilente, and Ultralente]

ilmofosine USAN, INN *antineoplastic*

ilonidap USAN *anti-inflammatory*

Ilopan IM injection, IV infusion ℞ *postoperative ileus prophylactic* [dexpanthenol] 250 mg/mL

Ilopan-Choline tablets ℞ *antiflatulent for splenic flexure syndrome* [dexpanthenol; choline bitartrate] 50•25 mg

iloperidone USAN *antipsychotic*

iloprost INN, BAN *investigational prostacyclin analog for cardiovascular disorders (orphan: Raynaud's phenomenon)*

Ilosone tablets, Pulvules (capsules), oral suspension ℞ *macrolide antibiotic* [erythromycin estolate] 500 mg; 250 mg; 125, 250 mg/5 mL ⊡ inosine

Ilotycin ophthalmic ointment ℞ *ophthalmic antibiotic* [erythromycin] 5 mg/g

Ilotycin Gluceptate injection ℞ *macrolide antibiotic* [erythromycin gluceptate] 33.33 mg/mL

Ilozyme tablets ℞ *digestive enzymes* [lipase; protease; amylase] 11,000•30,000•30,000 U

I-L-X elixir OTC *hematinic* [ferrous gluconate; liver concentrate 1:20; multiple B vitamins] 70•98• ± mg/15 mL

I-L-X B$_{12}$ caplets OTC *hematinic* [carbonyl iron; desiccated liver; multiple B vitamins; ascorbic acid] 37.5•130• ± •120 mg

I-L-X B$_{12}$ elixir OTC *hematinic* [ferric ammonium citrate; liver fraction 1;

multiple B vitamins] 102•98• ± mg/15 mL

imafen INN *antidepressant* [also: imafen HCl]

imafen HCl USAN *antidepressant* [also: imafen]

Imagent BP ℞ *investigational imaging agent for CT and ultrasound scans of the liver and spleen*

Imagent GI oral liquid ℞ *oral GI contrast agent for MRI and x-ray imaging* [perflubron] 200 mL

Imagent LN ℞ *investigational lymph node imaging agent for CT scans*

Imagent US ℞ *investigational imaging agent for ultrasound procedures*

imanixil INN

imazodan INN *cardiotonic* [also: imazodan HCl]

imazodan HCl USAN *cardiotonic* [also: imazodan]

imcarbofos USAN, INN *veterinary anthelmintic*

imciromab INN *antimyosin monoclonal antibody* [also: imciromab pentetate]

imciromab pentetate USAN, BAN *antimyosin monoclonal antibody (orphan: diagnostic aid for cardiac transplant rejection)* [also: imciromab]

Imdur extended-release tablets ℞ *angina preventative* [isosorbide mononitrate] 30, 120 mg

imexon INN

IMF (ifosfamide [with mesna rescue], methotrexate, fluorouracil) *chemotherapy protocol*

Imferon IM injection (discontinued 1992) ℞ *antianemic* [iron dextran] ② imipramine; Imuran

imiclopazine INN

imidapril INN, BAN

imidazole carboxamide [see: dacarbazine]

imidazole salicylate INN

imidecyl iodine USAN *topical anti-infective*

imidocarb INN, BAN *antiprotozoal (Babesia)* [also: imidocarb HCl]

imidocarb HCl USAN *antiprotozoal (Babesia)* [also: imidocarb]

imidoline INN *antipsychotic* [also: imidoline HCl]

imidoline HCl USAN *antipsychotic* [also: imidoline]

imidurea NF *antimicrobial*

imiglucerase USAN, INN *glucocerebrosidase enzyme replacement for type I Gaucher's disease*

Imigran (foreign name for U.S. product Imitrex)

imiloxan INN *antidepressant* [also: imiloxan HCl]

imiloxan HCl USAN *antidepressant* [also: imiloxan]

iminophenimide INN

iminostilbene [see: carbamazepine]

imipemide [now: imipenem]

imipenem USAN, USP, INN, BAN, JAN *bactericidal antibiotic*

imipramine INN, BAN *tricyclic antidepressant* [also: imipramine HCl] ② Imferon; Norpramin; trimipramine

imipramine HCl USP *tricyclic antidepressant; treatment of childhood enuresis* [also: imipramine] 10, 25, 50 mg oral

imipramine pamoate *tricyclic antidepressant*

imipraminoxide INN

imiquimod USAN *immunomodulator; investigational cream for anal and genital warts*

imirestat INN

Imitrex film-coated tablets ℞ *antimigraine agent* [sumatriptan succinate] 25, 50 mg

Imitrex subcu injection in vials, prefilled syringes, or SELFdose kits (two prefilled syringes) ℞ *serotonin agonist to relieve migraine attacks and cluster headaches* [sumatriptan succinate] 12 mg/mL

ImmTher ℞ *(orphan: pulmonary and hepatic metastases of colorectal adenocarcinoma)* [disaccharide tripeptide glycerol dipalmitoyl]

Immun-Aid powder OTC *enteral nutritional therapy for immunocompromised patients*

immune globulin (IG) [see: globulin, immune]

immune globulin intramuscular [see: globulin, immune]

immune globulin intravenous (IGIV) [see: globulin, immune]

immune serum globulin (ISG) [see: globulin, immune]

Immuneron ℞ *investigational anti-infective for granulomatous disease, rheumatoid arthritis, and venereal warts* [interferon gamma]

Immunex CRP test kit for professional use *in vitro diagnostic aid for C-reactive protein (CRP) in blood to diagnose inflammatory conditions* [latex agglutination test]

Immuno-C ℞ *investigational (Phase II) treatment of cryptosporidiosis in immunocompromised patients (orphan)* [bovine whey protein concentrate]

immunoglobulin G 1 (mouse monoclonal 7E11-C5.3 antihuman prostatic carcinoma cell) disulfide [see: capromab pendetide]

immunoglobulin G 1 (mouse monoclonal ZCE025 antihuman antigen CEA) disulfide [see: indium In 111 altumomab pentetate; altumomab]

Immunovir ℞ *investigational treatment for HIV infection* [isoprinosine]

Immupath ℞ *(orphan: AIDS)* [HIV-neutralizing antibodies]

ImmuRAID-AFP ℞ *(orphan: diagnostic aid for hepatic cancer in AFP-producing tumors)* [technetium Tc 99m murine monoclonal antibody to human alpha-fetoprotein (AFP)]

ImmuRAID-CEA ℞ *investigational monoclonal antibody-based diagnostic aid for colorectal cancer*

ImmuRAID-hCG ℞ *(orphan: diagnostic aid for hCG-producing tumors)* [technetium Tc 99m murine monoclonal antibody to human chorionic gonadotropin (hCG)]

ImmuRAID-LL2 ℞ *(orphan: diagnostic aid for B-cell leukemia and lymphoma)* [technetium Tc 99m murine monoclonal antibody IgG$_2$a to B cell]

ImmuRAID-MN3 ℞ *investigational monoclonal antibody-based diagnostic aid for infectious diseases*

ImmuRAIT-CEA ℞ *investigational treatment for colorectal cancer* [iodine I 131 murine monoclonal antibody IgG]

ImmuRAIT-LL2 ℞ *(orphan: B-cell leukemia and lymphoma therapy)* [iodine I 131 murine monoclonal antibody IgG$_2$a to B cell]

IM-Nutrients soft capsules OTC *vitamin/mineral supplement* [vitamins A and E; buffered vitamin C; selenium methionine; zinc citrate]

Imodium capsules ℞ *antidiarrheal* [loperamide HCl] 2 mg

Imodium A-D caplets, liquid OTC *antidiarrheal* [loperamide HCl] 1 mg; 1 mg/5 mL

Imogam IM injection ℞ *rabies prophylaxis* [rabies immune globulin] 150 IU/mL (300 IU/mL available in Canada)

imolamine INN, BAN

Imovane tablets (available only in Canada) ℞ *sedative; hypnotic* [zopiclone] 7.5 mg

Imovax intradermal (ID) injection, IM injection ℞ *rabies prophylaxis* [rabies vaccine (HDCV)] 0.25 IU/0.1 mL; 2.5 IU/mL

imoxiterol INN

impacarzine INN

Impact ready-to-use liquid OTC *enteral nutritional therapy* [lactose-free formula]

Impact Rubella slide test for professional use *in vitro diagnostic aid for detection of rubella virus antibodies in serum* [latex agglutination test]

IMPE [see: etipirium iodide]

impromidine INN, BAN *gastric secretion indicator* [also: impromidine HCl]

impromidine HCl USAN *gastric secretion indicator* [also: impromidine]

improsulfan INN

Improved Analgesic ointment OTC *counterirritant* [methyl salicylate; menthol] 18.3%•16%

Improved Congestant tablets OTC *antihistamine; analgesic* [chlorpheniramine maleate; acetaminophen] 2•325 mg

Imreg-1 ℞ *investigational (Phase III) immunomodulator for HIV*

Imreg-2 ℞ *investigational immunomodulator for AIDS (clinical trials discontinued 1994)*

imuracetam INN

Imuran IV injection ℞ *immunosuppressant for organ transplantation and rheumatoid arthritis* [azathioprine sodium] 100 mg ② Enduron; Imferon

Imuran tablets ℞ *immunosuppressant for organ transplantation and rheumatoid arthritis* [azathioprine] 50 mg

Imuthiol ℞ *investigational (Phase II/III) immunomodulator for AIDS/ARC/HIV (orphan)* [diethyldithiocarbamate]

Imuvert ℞ *investigational antineoplastic for breast and ovarian cancers (orphan: primary brain malignancies)* [Serratia marcescens extract (polyribosomes)]

^{111}**In** [see: indium In 111 altumomab pentetate]

^{111}**In** [see: indium In 111 imciromab pentetate]

^{111}**In** [see: indium In 111 murine anti-CEA monoclonal antibody]

^{111}**In** [see: indium In 111 murine monoclonal antibody]

^{111}**In** [see: indium In 111 oxyquinoline]

^{111}**In** [see: indium In 111 pentetate]

^{111}**In** [see: indium In 111 pentetreotide]

^{111}**In** [see: indium In 111 satumomab pendetide]

^{111}**In** [see: pentetate indium disodium In 111]

^{113m}**In** [see: indium chlorides In 113m]

inactivated mumps vaccine [see: mumps virus vaccine, inactivated]

inactivated poliomyelitis vaccine (IPV) [see: poliovirus vaccine inactivated]

inactivated poliovirus vaccine (IPV) [see: poliovirus vaccine, inactivated]

inaperisone INN

Inapsine IV or IM injection ℞ *general anesthetic* [droperidol] 2.5 mg/mL

Incremin with Iron syrup (discontinued 1995) OTC *hematinic* [ferric pyrophosphate; multiple B vitamins; lysine; alcohol 0.75%] 90•±•900 mg/15 mL

Incystene ℞ *investigational oral treatment for interstitial cystitis and stroke* [nalmefene]

indacrinic acid [see: indacrinone]

indacrinone USAN, INN *antihypertensive; diuretic*

indalpine INN, BAN

indanazoline INN

indandione *anticoagulant*

indanidine INN

indanorex INN

indapamide USAN, INN, BAN *antihypertensive; diuretic* 2.5 mg oral

indatraline INN

indecainide INN *antiarrhythmic* [also: indecainide HCl]

indecainide HCl USAN *antiarrhythmic* [also: indecainide]

indeloxazine INN *antidepressant* [also: indeloxazine HCl]

indeloxazine HCl USAN *antidepressant* [also: indeloxazine]

indenolol INN, BAN

Inderal tablets, IV injection ℞ *antianginal; antihypertensive; migraine preventative* [propranolol HCl] 10, 20, 40, 60, 80 mg; 1 mg/mL ② Enduron; Enduronyl; Inderide

Inderal LA long-acting capsules ℞ *antianginal; antihypertensive; migraine preventative* [propranolol HCl] 60, 80, 120, 160 mg

Inderide 40/25; Inderide 80/25 tablets ℞ *antihypertensive* [propranolol HCl; hydrochlorothiazide] 40•25 mg; 80•25 mg ② Inderal

Inderide LA 80/50; Inderide LA 120/50; Inderide LA 160/50 long-acting capsules ℞ *antihypertensive* [propranolol HCl; hydrochlorothiazide] 80•50 mg; 120•50 mg; 160•50 mg

indigo carmine BAN *cystoscopy aid* [also: indigotindisulfonate sodium]

indigotindisulfonate sodium USP *cystoscopy aid* [also: indigo carmine]

indinavir sulfate USAN *investigational antiviral; HIV-1 protease inhibitor*

indium *element (In)*

indium (^{111}In) diethylenetriamine pentaacetate JAN *radionuclide cisternography aid; radioactive agent* [also: indium In 111 pentetate]

indium chlorides In 113m USAN, USP *radioactive agent*

indium In 111 altumomab pentetate USAN *radiodiagnostic monoclonal antibody for colorectal carcinoma (orphan); anticarcinoembryonic antigen* [also: altumomab]

indium In 111 antimelanoma antibody XMMME-0001-DTPA [see: antimelanoma antibody]

indium In 111 CYT-103 [now: indium In 111 satumomab pendetide]

indium In 111 imciromab pentetate *radioactive diagnostic aid for cardiac imaging*

indium In 111 murine anti-CEA monoclonal antibody type ZCE 025 (*orphan: diagnostic aid in colorectal carcinoma*)

indium In 111 murine monoclonal antibody 2B8-MX-DTPA & Y-90 murine monoclonal antibody 2B8-MX-DTPA (*orphan: non-Hodgkin's B-cell lymphoma*)

indium In 111 murine monoclonal antibody B72.3 (*orphan: diagnostic aid in ovarian carcinoma*)

indium In 111 murine monoclonal antibody Fab to myosin (*orphan: diagnostic aid for cardiac necrosis and myocarditis*)

indium In 111 oxyquinoline USAN, USP *radioactive agent; diagnostic aid*

indium In 111 pentetate USP *radionuclide cisternography aid; radioactive agent* [also: indium (^{111}In) diethylenetriamine pentaacetate]

indium In 111 pentetreotide USAN *tumor imaging agent for SPECT scans*

indium In 111 satumomab pendetide USAN *radiodiagnostic monoclonal antibody for ovarian and colorectal carcinoma*

indobufen INN

indocate INN

Indochron E-R extended-release tablets ℞ *nonsteroidal anti-inflammatory drug (NSAID); antiarthritic; analgesic* [indomethacin] 75 mg

Indocin capsules, oral suspension, suppositories ℞ *nonsteroidal anti-inflammatory drug (NSAID); antiarthritic; analgesic* [indomethacin] 25, 50 mg; 25 mg/5 mL; 50 mg ⑨ Lincocin; Minocin

Indocin I.V. powder for IV injection ℞ *prostaglandin synthesis inhibitor for patent ductus arteriosus* [indomethacin sodium trihydrate] 1 mg

Indocin SR sustained-release capsules ℞ *nonsteroidal anti-inflammatory drug (NSAID); antiarthritic; analgesic* [indomethacin] 75 mg

indocyanine green USP, JAN *cardiac output test; hepatic function test; ophthalmic angiography*

indolapril INN *antihypertensive* [also: indolapril HCl]

indolapril HCl USAN *antihypertensive* [also: indolapril]

indolidan USAN, INN, BAN *cardiotonic*

indometacin INN, JAN *nonsteroidal anti-inflammatory drug (NSAID); antiarthritic; analgesic* [also: indomethacin]

indometacin farnesil JAN *nonsteroidal anti-inflammatory drug (NSAID); antiarthritic; analgesic* [also: indomethacin]

indomethacin USAN, USP, BAN *nonsteroidal anti-inflammatory drug (NSAID); antiarthritic; analgesic* [also: indometacin; indometacin farnesil] 25, 50, 75 mg oral; 25 mg/5 mL oral

indomethacin sodium USAN *anti-inflammatory*

indomethacin sodium trihydrate *neonatal closure of patent ductus arteriosus*

indopanolol INN

indopine INN

indoprofen USAN, INN, BAN *analgesic; anti-inflammatory*

indoramin USAN, INN, BAN *antihypertensive*

indoramin HCl USAN, BAN *antihypertensive*

indorenate INN *antihypertensive* [also: indorenate HCl]

indorenate HCl USAN *antihypertensive* [also: indorenate]

indoxole USAN, INN *antipyretic; anti-inflammatory*

indriline INN *CNS stimulant* [also: indriline HCl]

indriline HCl USAN *CNS stimulant* [also: indriline]

inductin [see: diphoxazide]

Infalyte oral solution OTC *electrolyte replacement* [sodium, potassium, and chloride electrolytes]

Infasurf ℞ (*orphan: respiratory failure in premature infants*) [surface active extract of saline lavage of bovine lungs]

Infatab (trademarked dosage form) *pediatric chewable tablet*

Infectrol eye drop suspension, ophthalmic ointment (discontinued 1993) ℞ *topical ophthalmic corticosteroidal anti-inflammatory; antibiotic* [dexamethasone; neomycin sulfate; polymyxin B sulfate]

InFeD IV injection ℞ *hematinic* [iron dextran] 50 mg/mL

Infergen ℞ *investigational treatment for hepatitis C* [consensus interferon]

Inflamase Mild; Inflamase Forte eye drops ℞ *ophthalmic topical corticosteroidal anti-inflammatory* [prednisolone sodium phosphate] 0.125%; 1%

influenza purified split-virus vaccine *subcategory of influenza virus vaccine*

influenza purified surface antigen *subcategory of influenza virus vaccine*

influenza split-virus vaccine *subcategory of influenza virus vaccine*

influenza subvirion vaccine [see: influenza split-virus vaccine]

influenza virus vaccine USP *active immunizing agent for influenza*

influenza whole-virus vaccine *subcategory of influenza virus vaccine*

infraRUB cream OTC *counterirritant* [methyl salicylate; menthol] 35% • 10%

Infumorph 200; Infumorph 500 concentrate for continuous microinfusion ℞ *narcotic analgesic; intraspinal microinfusion for intractable chronic pain (orphan)* [morphine sulfate] 10 mg/mL (200 mg/vial); 25 mg/mL (500 mg/vial)

INH (isonicotinic acid hydrazide) [see: isoniazid]

Inhal-Aid (trademarked form) *portable inhalation device*

Inhibace (commercially available in Latin America) ℞ *antihypertensive; ACE inhibitor (approved by the FDA, but not being marketed by the manufacturer)* [cilazapril]

Inhibace Plus ℞ *investigational antihypertensive* [cilazapril; hydrochlorothiazide]

inicarone INN

Inject-all (trademarked delivery system) *prefilled disposable syringe*

Inlay-Tab (trademarked dosage form) *tablets with contrasting inlay*

InnoGel Plus gel packs + comb OTC *pediculicide* [pyrethrins; piperonyl butoxide technical] 3% • 3%

Innovar injection ℞ *narcotic analgesic; major tranquilizer* [fentanyl citrate; droperidol] 0.05 • 2.5 mg/mL

Inocor IV injection ℞ *vasodilator for congestive heart failure* [amrinone lactate] 5 mg/mL

inocoterone INN *anti-acne* [also: inocoterone acetate]

inocoterone acetate USAN *anti-acne* [also: inocoterone]

inosine INN, JAN ② Ilosone

inosine pranobex BAN, JAN *investigational antiviral/immunomodulator for AIDS; (orphan: subacute sclerosing panencephalitis)*

inosiplex [now: inosine pranobex]

inositol NF *dietary lipotropic supplement* 250, 500, 650 mg oral

inositol niacinate USAN *peripheral vasodilator* [also: inositol nicotinate]

inositol nicotinate INN, BAN *peripheral vasodilator* [also: inositol niacinate]

Inpersol; Inpersol-LM solution (discontinued 1996) ℞ *peritoneal dialysis solution* [multiple electrolytes; dextrose] ± • 1.5%, ± • 2.5%, ± • 4.5%

inprochone [see: inproquone]

inproquone INN, BAN

INSH (isonicotinoyl-salicylidenehydrazine) [see: salinazid]

InspirEase (trademarked form) *portable inhalation device*

Insta-Glucose gel OTC *glucose elevating agent* [glucose] 40%

Insulatard NPH subcu injection (discontinued 1994) OTC *antidiabetic* [isophane insulin (pork)]

Insulatard NPH Human subcu injection (discontinued 1994) OTC *antidiabetic* [isophane insulin (human semisynthetic)]

insulin USP *antidiabetic* ② inulin

insulin, biphasic INN, BAN

insulin, dalanated USAN, INN *antidiabetic*

insulin, globin zinc USP [also: globin zinc insulin]

insulin, human USAN, USP, INN, BAN *antidiabetic*

insulin, isophane USP, INN *antidiabetic* [also: isophane insulin]

insulin, neutral USAN *antidiabetic* [also: neutral insulin]

insulin, NPH (neutral protamine Hagedorn) [see: insulin, isophane]

insulin, protamine zinc USP *antidiabetic* [also: protamine zinc insulin]

insulin argine INN

insulin defalan INN

insulin I 125 USAN *radioactive agent*

insulin I 131 USAN *radioactive agent*

insulin lispro USAN *antidiabetic*

Insulin Reaction gel OTC *glucose elevating agent* [glucose] 40%

insulin zinc USP, BAN *antidiabetic* [also: compound insulin zinc suspension]

insulin zinc, extended USP *antidiabetic* [also: insulin zinc suspension (crystalline)]

insulin zinc, prompt USP *antidiabetic* [also: insulin zinc suspension (amorphous)]

insulin zinc suspension (amorphous) INN, BAN *antidiabetic* [also: insulin zinc, prompt]

insulin zinc suspension (crystalline) INN, BAN *antidiabetic* [also: insulin zinc, extended]

insulin-like growth factor-1, recombinant human (rhIGF) *investigational cytokine for AIDS and antidiabetic agent (orphan: amyotrophic lateral sclerosis)*

insulinotropin *investigational blood glucose regulating agent*

Intal capsules for inhalation (discontinued 1995) ℞ *bronchodilator for bronchial asthma and bronchospasm* [cromolyn sodium] 20 mg ⓘ Endal

Intal solution for nebulization, aerosol spray ℞ *bronchodilator for bronchial asthma and bronchospasm* [cromolyn sodium] 20 mg/ampule; 800 μg/dose ⓘ Endal

Integrelin ℞ *investigational antithrombotic for unstable angina*

Intensol (trademarked form) *concentrated oral solution*

Intercept Contraceptive Inserts vaginal suppositories (discontinued 1992) OTC *spermicidal contraceptive* [nonoxynol 9] 100 mg

α-2-interferon [see: interferon alfa-2b, recombinant]

interferon α2b [see: interferon alfa-2b]

interferon αA [see: interferon alfa-2a]

interferon alfa JAN

interferon alfa (BALL-1) JAN

interferon alfa-2a (IFN-αA) USAN, INN, BAN, JAN *antineoplastic; antiviral; investigational (Phase I) cytokine for ARC; (orphan: various cancers)*

interferon alfa-2b (IFN-α2) USAN, INN, BAN *antineoplastic for various cancers and AIDS-related Kaposi sarcoma; antiviral for hepatitis (orphan)*

interferon alfa-n1 USAN, INN, BAN *antineoplastic; investigational cytokine for HIV; (orphan: Kaposi sarcoma; human papillomavirus)*

interferon alfa-n3 USAN *antineoplastic; antiviral; investigational (Phase I/II) cytokine for AIDS/ARC*

interferon beta (IFN-B) JAN *antineoplastic; antiviral; immunomodulator; (orphan: multiple carcinomas; hepatitis; AIDS)*

interferon beta-1a USAN *antineoplastic; immunomodulator for multiple sclerosis; biological response modifier*

interferon beta-1b USAN *immunomodulator for multiple sclerosis; investigational (Phase II/III) cytokine for AIDS/ARC*

interferon beta-2 *investigational treatment for multiple sclerosis*

interferon gamma-1a JAN

interferon gamma-1b USAN, INN, BAN *antineoplastic; antiviral; immunoregulator; for chronic granulomatous disease (orphan)*

interferon gamma-2a [see: interferon gamma-1b]

α-interferons [see: interferon alfa-n1 and -n3]

interleukin-1 alpha, recombinant human (orphan: bone marrow transplants; aplastic anemia)

interleukin-1 beta investigational antineoplastic for melanoma

interleukin-1 receptor (IL-1R) investigational treatment for rheumatoid arthritis, sepsis, GVH disease, AML, asthma, and allergy

interleukin-1 receptor, soluble investigational (Phase I) antiviral for HIV

interleukin-1 receptor antagonist, recombinant human (orphan: juvenile rheumatoid arthritis; transplant graft vs. host disease)

interleukin-2, liposome-encapsulated recombinant (orphan: brain and central nervous system tumors; kidney and renal pelvis cancers)

interleukin-2, recombinant (IL-2) [see: aldesleukin; teceleukin; celmoleukin]

interleukin-2 PEG [see: PEG-interleukin-2]

interleukin-3, recombinant human investigational HIV drug and adjunct to bone marrow transplants; (orphan: Diamond-Blackfan anemia)

interleukin-3, recombinant human & sargramostim (orphan: bone marrow transplants for Hodgkin's disease and non-Hodgkin's lymphoma)

interleukin-4 (IL-4) investigational immunomodulator for life-threatening immunodeficiency diseases and cancer

interleukin-4 receptor (IL-4R) investigational treatment for allergy, asthma, transplant rejection, and infectious disease

interleukin-6 (IL-6) investigational bone marrow/platelet stimulant following chemotherapy

interleukin-6 mutein investigational treatment for thrombocytopenia

interleukin-7 (IL-7) investigational antineoplastic and lymphocyte stimulant

interleukin-9 (IL-9) investigational treatment for anemia and red blood cell disorders

interleukin-10 (IL-10) investigational immunomodulator for solid tumors, organ transplants, and autoimmune disorders

interleukin-11 (IL-11) investigational biological response modifier for cancer chemotherapy and bone marrow transplantation

interleukin-11, recombinant human (rhIL-11) investigational adjunct to chemotherapy for breast cancer

interleukin-12 (IL-12) investigational (Phase I) immunomodulator for HIV

intermedine INN

Interquim ℞ investigational treatment for stroke and head trauma [citicoline sodium]

intoplicine INN investigational antineoplastic

Intralipid 10%; Intralipid 20% IV infusion ℞ nutritional therapy [intravenous fat emulsion]

IntraSite gel OTC wound dressing [graft T starch copolymer] 2%

intravascular perfluorochemical emulsion synthetic blood oxygen carrier for PTCA

intravenous fat emulsion [see: fat emulsion, intravenous]

intravenous immunoglobulin (IVIG) investigational IV solution of concentrated antibodies for AIDS

intrazole USAN, INN anti-inflammatory

Intrinsitinic capsules ℞ dietary supplement [liver-stomach concentrate; multiple vitamins; ferrous fumarate]

intriptyline INN antidepressant [also: intriptyline HCl]

intriptyline HCl USAN antidepressant [also: intriptyline]

Introlan Half-Strength liquid OTC enteral nutritional therapy [lactose-free formula]

Introlite liquid OTC enteral nutritional therapy [lactose-free formula]

Intron A subcu or IM injection ℞ antineoplastic for hairy cell leukemia and Kaposi sarcoma; antiviral for chronic hepatitis (orphan) [interferon alfa-2b] 3, 5, 10, 18, 25, 50 million IU/vial

Intropin IV injection ℞ vasopressor for cardiac, pulmonary, traumatic, septic, or renal shock [dopamine HCl] 40, 80, 160 mg/mL ⓓ Ditropan; Isoptin

inulin USP *renal function test* 100 mg/mL injection ☒ insulin

invenol [see: carbutamide]

Inversine tablets ℞ *antihypertensive* [mecamylamine HCl] 2.5 mg

invert sugar [see: sugar, invert]

Invirase capsules ℞ *antiviral protease inhibitor for HIV* [saquinavir mesylate] 200 mg

iobenguane (^{131}I) INN

iobenguane sulfate I 123 USAN *diagnostic radiopharmaceutical*

iobenzamic acid USAN, INN, BAN *cholecystographic radiopaque medium*

Iobid DM sustained-release tablets ℞ *antitussive; expectorant* [dextromethorphan hydrobromide; guaifenesin] 30•600 mg

iobutoic acid INN

Iocare Balanced Salt ophthalmic solution OTC *intraocular irrigating solution* [balanced saline solution]

iocarmate meglumine USAN *radiopaque medium* [also: meglumine iocarmate]

iocarmic acid USAN, INN, BAN *radiopaque medium*

iocetamic acid USAN, USP, INN, BAN *cholecystographic radiopaque medium*

Iocon shampoo OTC *antiseborrheic; antipsoriatic; antipruritic; antibacterial* [coal tar; alcohol]

Iodal HD liquid ℞ *narcotic antitussive; decongestant; antihistamine* [hydrocodone bitartrate; phenylephrine HCl; chlorpheniramine maleate] 1.67•5•2 mg/5 mL

iodamide USAN, INN, BAN *radiopaque medium*

iodamide meglumine USAN *radiopaque medium*

iodecimol INN

iodecol [see: iodecimol]

iodetryl INN

Iodex; Iodex-P ointment OTC *broad-spectrum antimicrobial* [povidone-iodine] 4.7%; 10%

Iodex M/S (name changed to Iodex with Methyl Salicylate in 1992)

Iodex with Methyl Salicylate salve OTC *counterirritant; topical anti-infective* [methyl salicylate; iodine; oil of wintergreen] ≜•4.7%•4.8%

iodinated (^{125}I) human serum albumin INN *radioactive agent; blood volume test* [also: albumin, iodinated I 125 serum]

iodinated (^{131}I) human serum albumin INN, JAN *radioactive agent; intrathecal imaging agent; blood volume test* [also: albumin, iodinated I 131 serum]

iodinated glycerol [see: glycerol, iodinated]

Iodinated Glycerol DM liquid (discontinued 1993) ℞ *antitussive; expectorant* [iodinated glycerol; dextromethorphan hydrobromide]

iodinated I 125 albumin [see: albumin, iodinated I 125]

iodinated I 131 aggregated albumin [see: albumin, iodinated I 131 aggregated]

iodinated I 131 albumin [see: albumin, iodinated I 131]

iodine USP *broad-spectrum topical anti-infective; element (I)* 2% topical

iodine I 123 murine monoclonal antibody to alpha-fetoprotein (AFP) (orphan: *diagnostic aid in AFP-producing tumors and hepatic cancer*)

iodine I 123 murine monoclonal antibody to human chorionic gonadotropin (hCG) (orphan: *diagnostic aid in hCG-producing tumors*)

iodine I 131 6B-iodomethyl-19-norcholesterol (orphan: *adrenal cortical imaging*)

iodine I 131 Lym-1 monoclonal antibody (orphan: *B-cell lymphoma*)

iodine I 131 metaiodobenzylguanidine sulfate (orphan: *diagnostic aid in pheochromocytoma*)

iodine I 131 murine monoclonal antibody IgG$_2$a to B cell (orphan: *B-cell leukemia and lymphoma*)

iodine I 131 murine monoclonal antibody to alpha-fetoprotein (AFP) (orphan: *AFP-producing tumors; hepatocellular carcinoma; hepatoblastoma*)

iodine I 131 murine monoclonal antibody to human chorionic

gonadotropin (hCG) *(orphan: hCG-producing tumors)*
iodipamide USP, BAN [also: adipiodone]
iodipamide meglumine USP, BAN *radiopaque medium* [also: adipiodone meglumine]
iodipamide methylglucamine [see: iodipamide meglumine]
iodipamide sodium USP
iodipamide sodium I 131 USAN *radioactive agent*
iodisan [see: prolonium iodide]
iodixanol USAN, INN, BAN *radiopaque medium*
iodized oil NF
iodoalphionic acid NF [also: pheniodol sodium]
iodoantipyrine I 131 USAN *radioactive agent*
iodobehenate calcium NF
iodobenzylguaninine sulfate I 123 [see: iobenguane sulfate I 123]
iodocetylic acid (^{123}I) INN *diagnostic aid* [also: iodocetylic acid I 123]
iodocetylic acid I 123 USAN *diagnostic aid* [also: iodocetylic acid (^{123}I)]
iodochlorhydroxyquin [now: clioquinol]
iodocholesterol (^{131}I) INN *radioactive agent* [also: iodocholesterol I 131]
iodocholesterol I 131 USAN *radioactive agent* [also: iodocholesterol (^{131}I)]
iodoform NF
iodohippurate sodium I 123 USAN, USP *renal function test; radioactive agent*
iodohippurate sodium I 125 USAN *radioactive agent*
iodohippurate sodium I 131 USAN, USP *renal function test; radioactive agent* [also: sodium iodohippurate (^{131}I)]
iodohydroxyquin [see: clioquinol]
iodol USP
iodomethamate sodium NF
Iodo-Niacin controlled-action tablets (discontinued 1994) ℞ *expectorant* [potassium iodide; niacinamide hydroiodide] 135•25 mg
Iodo-Pak IV injection ℞ *intravenous nutritional therapy* [sodium iodide]
iodopanoic acid [see: iopanoic acid]

Iodopen IV injection ℞ *intravenous nutritional therapy* [sodium iodide] 118 μg/mL
iodophthalein, soluble [now: iodophthalein sodium]
iodophthalein sodium NF, INN
iodopyracet NF [also: diodone]
iodopyracet I 125 USAN *radioactive agent*
iodopyracet I 131 USAN *radioactive agent*
iodoquinol USAN, USP *amebicide; antimicrobial* [also: diiodohydroxyquinoline]
Iodosorb gel ℞ *investigational treatment of skin ulcers* [cadexomer iodine]
iodothiouracil INN, BAN
iodothymol [see: thymol iodide]
Iodotope capsules, oral solution ℞ *radioactive agent for hyperthyroidism and thyroid carcinoma* [sodium iodide I 131] 1–50 mCi; 7.05 mCi/mL
iodoxamate meglumine USAN, BAN *radiopaque medium*
iodoxamic acid USAN, INN, BAN *radiopaque medium*
iodoxyl [see: iodomethamate sodium]
Iofed extended-release capsules ℞ *decongestant; antihistamine* [pseudoephedrine HCl; brompheniramine maleate] 120•12 mg
Iofed PD extended-release capsules ℞ *pediatric decongestant and antihistamine* [pseudoephedrine HCl; brompheniramine maleate] 60•6 mg
iofendylate INN *radiopaque medium* [also: iophendylate]
iofetamine (^{123}I) INN *diagnostic aid; radioactive agent* [also: iofetamine HCl I 123]
iofetamine HCl I 123 USAN *diagnostic aid; radioactive agent* [also: iofetamine (^{123}I)]
Iofoam (trademarked form) *foaming skin cleanser*
ioglicic acid USAN, INN, BAN *radiopaque medium*
ioglucol USAN, INN *radiopaque medium*
ioglucomide USAN, INN *radiopaque medium*
ioglunide INN
ioglycamic acid USAN, INN, BAN *cholecystographic radiopaque medium*

iogulamide USAN *radiopaque medium*

iohexol USAN, INN, BAN *radiopaque medium*

Iohist D elixir ℞ *decongestant; antihistamine* [phenylpropanolamine HCl; phenyltoloxamine citrate; pyrilamine maleate; pheniramine maleate] 12.5•4•4•4 mg/5 mL

Iohist DM syrup ℞ *antitussive; decongestant; antihistamine* [dextromethorphan hydrobromide; phenylpropanolamine HCl; brompheniramine maleate] 10•12.5•2 mg/5 mL

iolidonic acid INN

iolixanic acid INN

iomeglamic acid INN

iomeprol USAN, INN, BAN *radiopaque medium*

iomethin I 125 USAN *neoplasm test; radioactive agent* [also: iometin (^{125}I)]

iomethin I 131 USAN *neoplasm test; radioactive agent* [also: iometin (^{131}I)]

iometin (^{125}I) INN *neoplasm test; radioactive agent* [also: iomethin I 125]

iometin (^{131}I) INN *neoplasm test; radioactive agent* [also: iomethin I 131]

iomorinic acid INN

Ionamin capsules ℞ *anorexiant* [phentermine HCl resin complex] 15, 30 mg

Ionax foam OTC *topical cleanser for acne* [benzalkonium chloride]

Ionax Astringent Skin Cleanser liquid OTC *topical keratolytic cleanser for acne* [salicylic acid; isopropyl alcohol]

Ionax Scrub OTC *abrasive cleanser for acne* [benzalkonium chloride]

Ionil shampoo OTC *antiseborrheic; keratolytic; antiseptic* [salicylic acid; benzalkonium chloride]

Ionil Plus shampoo OTC *antiseborrheic; keratolytic* [salicylic acid] 2%

Ionil T shampoo OTC *antiseborrheic; antipsoriatic; keratolytic; antiseptic* [coal tar; salicylic acid; benzalkonium chloride]

Ionil-T Plus shampoo OTC *antiseborrheic; antipsoriatic; antipruritic; antibacterial* [coal tar] 2%

ionphylline [see: aminophylline]

iopamidol USAN, USP, INN, BAN *radiopaque medium*

iopanoic acid USP, INN, BAN *cholecystographic radiopaque medium*

iopentol USAN, INN, BAN *radiopaque medium*

Iophen tablets, elixir, drops ℞ *expectorant* [iodinated glycerol] 30 mg; 60 mg/5 mL; 50 mg/mL

Iophen-C liquid ℞ *narcotic antitussive; expectorant* [codeine phosphate; iodinated glycerol] 10•30 mg/5 mL

Iophen-DM liquid ℞ *antitussive; expectorant* [dextromethorphan hydrobromide; iodinated glycerol] 10•30 mg/5 mL

iophendylate USP, BAN *radiopaque medium* [also: iofendylate]

iophenoic acid INN [also: iophenoxic acid]

iophenoxic acid USP [also: iophenoic acid]

Iophylline elixir ℞ *antiasthmatic; bronchodilator; expectorant* [theophylline; iodinated glycerol] 120•30 mg/15 mL

Iopidine Drop-Tainer (eye drops) ℞ *topical antiglaucoma agent (sympathomimetic)* [apraclonidine HCl] 0.5%, 1%

ioprocemic acid USAN, INN *radiopaque medium*

iopromide USAN, INN, BAN *radiopaque imaging agent; source of iodine*

iopronic acid USAN, INN, BAN *cholecystographic radiopaque medium*

iopydol USAN, INN, BAN *bronchographic radiopaque medium*

iopydone USAN, INN, BAN *bronchographic radiopaque medium*

Iosal II extended-release tablets ℞ *decongestant; expectorant* [pseudoephedrine HCl; guaifenesin] 60•600 mg

iosarcol INN

iosefamic acid USAN, INN *radiopaque medium*

ioseric acid USAN, INN *radiopaque medium*

iosimide INN

iosulamide INN *radiopaque medium* [also: iosulamide meglumine]

iosulamide meglumine USAN *radiopaque medium* [also: iosulamide]

iosulfan blue *lymphography radiopaque medium*
iosumetic acid USAN, INN *radiopaque medium*
iotalamic acid INN *radiopaque medium* [also: iothalamic acid]
iotasul USAN, INN *radiopaque medium*
iotetric acid USAN, INN *radiopaque medium*
iothalamate meglumine USP *radiopaque medium* [also: meglumine iothalamate]
iothalamate sodium USP *radiopaque medium* [also: sodium iothalamate]
iothalamate sodium I 125 USAN *radioactive agent* [also: sodium iotalamate (^{125}I)]
iothalamate sodium I 131 USAN *radioactive agent* [also: sodium iotalamate (^{131}I)]
iothalamic acid USP, BAN *radiopaque medium* [also: iotalamic acid]
iothiouracil sodium
iotranic acid INN
iotriside INN
iotrizoic acid INN
iotrol [now: iotrolan]
iotrolan USAN, INN, BAN *radiopaque medium*
iotroxic acid USAN, INN, BAN *radiopaque medium*
IoTuss liquid (discontinued 1994) ℞ *narcotic antitussive; expectorant* [codeine phosphate; iodinated glycerol]
IoTuss-DM liquid (discontinued 1994) ℞ *antitussive; expectorant* [dextromethorphan hydrobromide; iodinated glycerol]
Iotussin HC syrup ℞ *narcotic antitussive; decongestant; antihistamine* [hydrocodone bitartrate; phenylephrine HCl; chlorpheniramine maleate] 2.5•5•2 mg/5 mL
iotyrosine I 131 USAN *radioactive agent*
ioversol USAN, INN, BAN *radiopaque medium*
ioxabrolic acid INN
ioxaglate meglumine USAN *radiopaque medium* [also: meglumine ioxaglate]
ioxaglate sodium USAN *radiopaque medium* [also: sodium ioxaglate]
ioxaglic acid USAN, INN, BAN *radiopaque medium*
ioxilan USAN, INN *diagnostic aid*
ioxitalamic acid INN
ioxotrizoic acid USAN, INN *radiopaque medium*
iozomic acid INN
IP 456 *investigational anxiolytic*
ipazilide fumarate USAN *antiarrhythmic*
ipecac USP *emetic* ⚠
ipecac, powdered USP
ipexidine INN *dental caries prophylactic* [also: ipexidine mesylate]
ipexidine mesylate USAN, INN *dental caries prophylactic* [also: ipexidine]
I-Pilopine eye drops (discontinued 1992) ℞ *antiglaucoma agent; miotic* [pilocarpine HCl]
ipodate calcium USP *cholecystographic radiopaque medium*
ipodate sodium USAN, USP *cholecystographic radiopaque medium* [also: sodium iopodate]
IPOL subcu injection ℞ *poliomyelitis vaccine* [poliovirus vaccine, inactivated] 0.5 mL
ipragratine INN
ipramidil INN
Ipran tablets ℞ *antianginal; antihypertensive; antimigrainal* [propranolol HCl]
ipratropium bromide USAN, INN, BAN *bronchodilator; anticholinergic*
Ipravent [see: Apo-Ipravent]
iprazochrome INN
iprazone [see: isoprazone]
ipriflavone INN
iprindole USAN, INN, BAN *antidepressant*
iprocinodine HCl USAN, BAN *veterinary antibacterial*
iproclozide INN, BAN
iprocrolol INN
iprofenin USAN *hepatic function test*
iproheptine INN
iproniazid INN, BAN
ipronidazole USAN, INN, BAN *antiprotozoal (Histomonas)*
ipropethidine [see: properidine]
iproplatin USAN, INN, BAN *antineoplastic*
iprotiazem INN

iproxamine INN *vasodilator* [also: iproxamine HCl]
iproxamine HCl USAN *vasodilator* [also: iproxamine]
iprozilamine INN
ipsalazide INN, BAN
ipsapirone INN, BAN *anxiolytic; investigational antidepressant* [also: ipsapirone HCl]
ipsapirone HCl USAN *anxiolytic; investigational antidepressant* [also: ipsapirone]
Ipsatol Cough Formula for Children; Ipsatol Cough Formula for Adults liquid OTC *antitussive; decongestant; expectorant* [dextromethorphan hydrobromide; phenylpropanolamine HCl; guaifenesin] 10•9•100 mg/5 mL
IPTD (isopropyl-thiadiazol) [see: glyprothiazol]
IPV (inactivated poliomyelitis vaccine) [see: poliovirus vaccine, inactivated]
IPV (inactivated poliovaccine) [see: poliovirus vaccine, inactivated]
iquindamine INN
^{192}**Ir** [see: iridium Ir 192]
Ircon tablets OTC *hematinic* [ferrous fumarate] 200 mg
Ircon-FA tablets OTC *hematinic* [ferrous fumarate; folic acid] 82•0.8 mg
irgasan [see: triclosan]
iridium *element (Ir)*
iridium Ir 192 USAN *radioactive agent*
irindalone INN
irinotecan INN *antineoplastic for cervical, colon, and rectal cancers; topoisomerase I inhibitor* [also: irinotecan HCl]
irinotecan HCl USAN, JAN *antineoplastic for cervical, colon, and rectal cancers; topoisomerase I inhibitor* [also: irinotecan]
irloxacin INN
Irodex IV, IM injection (discontinued 1992) ℞ *antianemic* [iron dextran]
irolapride INN
Iromin-G tablets OTC *vitamin/iron supplement* [multiple vitamins; ferrous gluconate; folic acid] ± •30•0.8 mg
iron *element (Fe)*
iron carbohydrate complex [see: polyferose]

iron dextran USP *hematinic*
iron heptonate [see: gleptoferron]
iron perchloride [see: ferric chloride]
iron polymalether [see: ferropolimaler]
iron sorbitex USAN, USP *hematinic*
Iron-Folic 500 timed-release tablets OTC *hematinic* [ferrous sulfate; multiple B vitamins; sodium ascorbate; folic acid] 105• ± •500•0.8 mg
Irospan timed-release capsules, timed-release tablets OTC *hematinic* [ferrous sulfate; ascorbic acid] 60•150 mg
Irrigate eye wash OTC *extraocular irrigating solution* [sterile isotonic solution]
irsogladine INN
irtemazole USAN, INN, BAN *uricosuric*
IS 5-MN (isosorbide 5-mononitrate) [see: isorbide mononitrate]
isaglidole INN
isamfazone INN
isamoltan INN
isamoxole USAN, INN, BAN *antiasthmatic*
isaxonine INN
isbogrel INN
iscador *investigational (Phase I) antiviral for AIDS/ARC/HIV*
I-Scrub solution (name changed to Eye Scrub in 1996)
Iselan ℞ *investigational antianginal* [isosorbide mononitrate]
Isepacin injection ℞ *investigational aminoglycoside antibiotic for gram-positive and gram-negative infections* [isepamicin]
isepamicin USAN, INN, BAN *antibacterial; aminoglycoside*
isethionate USAN, BAN *combining name for radicals or groups* [also: isetionate]
isetionate INN *combining name for radicals or groups* [also: isethionate]
ISG (immune serum globulin) [see: globulin, immune]
ISIS 2105 ℞ *investigational antiviral for genital warts*
ISIS 2922 *investigational (Phase III) antiviral for AIDS-related cytomegalovirus retinitis*
Ismelin tablets ℞ *antihypertensive; (orphan: reflex sympathetic dystrophy and causalgia)* [guanethidine monosulfate] 25 mg ▣ Ritalin

Ismelin Sulfate tablets (name changed to Ismelin in 1993)
Ismo film-coated tablets ℞ *angina preventative* [isosorbide mononitrate] 20 mg
Ismotic solution ℞ *osmotic diuretic* [isosorbide] 45%
iso-alcoholic elixir NF
isoaminile INN, BAN
isoamyl nitrate [see: amyl nitrite]
Iso-B capsules OTC *vitamin supplement* [multiple B vitamins; folic acid; biotin] ±•200•100 µg
Iso-Bid sustained-release capsules (discontinued 1995) ℞ *antianginal* [isosorbide dinitrate] 40 mg
isobromindione INN
isobucaine HCl USP
isobutamben USAN, INN *topical anesthetic*
isobutane NF *aerosol propellant*
isobutyl *p*-aminobenzoate [see: isobutamben]
isobutyl α-phenylcyclohexaneglycolate [see: ibuverine]
isobutyl 2-cyanoacrylate (IBC) [see: bucrylate]
***p*-isobutylhydratropohydroxamic acid** [see: ibuproxam]
isobutylhydrochlorothiazide [see: buthiazide]
isobutyramide (*orphan: sickle cell disease; beta-thalassemia syndrome; beta-hemoglobinopathies*)
isobuzole BAN [also: glysobuzole]
Isocaine HCl injection ℞ *injectable local anesthetic* [mepivacaine HCl] 3%
Isocaine HCl injection ℞ *injectable local anesthetic* [mepivacaine HCl; levonordefrin] 2%•1:20,000
Isocal liquid OTC *enteral nutritional therapy* [lactose-free formula]
Isocal HCN ready-to-use liquid OTC *enteral nutritional therapy* [lactose-free formula]
Isocal HN liquid OTC *enteral nutritional therapy* [lactose-free formula]
isocarboxazid USP, INN, BAN *antidepressant; MAO inhibitor*
Isocet tablets ℞ *analgesic; anti-inflammatory; sedative* [acetaminophen; caffeine; butalbital] 325•40•50 mg

Isoclor Timesules (sustained-release capsules), tablets, liquid (discontinued 1995) OTC *decongestant; antihistamine* [pseudoephedrine HCl; chlorpheniramine maleate] 120•8 mg; 60•4 mg; 30•2 mg/5 mL
Isoclor Expectorant liquid ℞ *narcotic antitussive; decongestant; expectorant* [codeine phosphate; pseudoephedrine HCl; guaifenesin; alcohol 5%] 10•30•100 mg/5 mL
Isocom capsules ℞ *vasoconstrictor; sedative; analgesic (for migraine)* [isometheptene mucate; dichloralphenazone; acetaminophen] 65•100•325 mg
isoconazole USAN, INN, BAN *antibacterial; antifungal*
isocromil INN
Isocult for Bacteriuria culture paddles for professional use *in vitro diagnostic aid for nitrate, uropathogens, or bacteria in the urine*
Isocult for Candida culture paddles for professional use *in vitro diagnostic aid for Candida albicans in the vagina*
Isocult for N gonorrhoeae and Candida culture test for professional use OTC *in vitro diagnostic aid for gonorrhea and Candida in various specimens*
Isocult for Neisseria gonorrhoeae culture paddles for professional use *in vitro diagnostic aid for Neisseria gonorrhoeae*
Isocult for Pseudomonas aeruginosa culture test for professional use (discontinued 1995) *in vitro diagnostic aid for Pseudomonas aeruginosa in exudate or urine*
Isocult for Staphylococcus aureus culture paddles for professional use *in vitro diagnostic aid for Staphylococcus aureus in exudate*
Isocult for Streptococcal pharyngitis culture paddles for professional use *in vitro diagnostic test for streptococcal pharyngitis in throat swabs*
Isocult for T vaginalis and Candida culture test for professional use *in vitro diagnostic aid for Trichomonas and Candida in vaginal or urethral cultures*
Isocult for Trichomonas vaginalis culture test for professional use (dis-

continued 1995) *in vitro diagnostic aid for Trichomonas vaginalis in urethra or vagina*

Isocult Throat Streptococci test (name changed to Isocult for Streptococcal pharyngitis in 1995)

isodapamide [see: zidapamide]

d-isoephedrine HCl [see: pseudoephedrine HCl]

isoetarine INN *bronchodilator* [also: isoetharine]

isoethadione [see: paramethadione]

isoetharine USAN, BAN *bronchodilator* [also: isoetarine]

isoetharine HCl USP, BAN *bronchodilator* 0.08%, 0.1%, 0.125%, 0.167%, 0.17%, 0.2%, 0.25%, 1% inhalation

isoetharine mesylate USP, BAN *bronchodilator*

isofezolac INN

isoflupredone INN, BAN *anti-inflammatory* [also: isoflupredone acetate]

isoflupredone acetate USAN *anti-inflammatory* [also: isoflupredone]

isoflurane USAN, USP, INN, BAN *inhalation general anesthetic*

isoflurophate USP *antiglaucoma agent; irreversible cholinesterase inhibitor miotic* [also: dyflos]

Isoject (trademarked delivery system) *prefilled disposable syringe*

I-Sol ophthalmic solution (discontinued 1992) OTC *extraocular irrigating solution* [balanced saline solution]

Isolan liquid OTC *enteral nutritional therapy* [lactose-free formula]

isoleucine (L-isoleucine) USAN, USP, INN, JAN *essential amino acid; symbols: Ile, I*

Isollyl Improved tablets, capsules ℞ *analgesic; antipyretic; anti-inflammatory; sedative* [aspirin; caffeine; butalbital] 325•40•50 mg

Isolyte E (G; H; M; P; R; S) with 5% Dextrose IV infusion ℞ *intravenous nutritional/electrolyte therapy* [combined electrolyte solution; dextrose]

Isolyte E; Isolyte S; Isolyte S pH 7.4 IV infusion ℞ *intravenous electrolyte therapy* [combined electrolyte solution]

Isolyte S pH 7.4 IV infusion ℞ *intravenous electrolyte therapy* [combined electrolyte solution]

isomazole INN *cardiotonic* [also: isomazole HCl]

isomazole HCl USAN *cardiotonic* [also: isomazole]

isomeprobamate [see: carisoprodol]

isomerol USAN *antiseptic*

isometamidium BAN [also: isometamidium chloride]

isometamidium chloride INN [also: isometamidium]

isomethadone INN, BAN

isomethepdrine chloride [see: isometheptene]

isometheptene INN, BAN

isometheptene HCl [see: isometheptene]

isometheptene mucate USP *cerebral vasoconstrictor; "possibly effective" for migraine headaches*

Isomil liquid, powder OTC *hypoallergenic infant food* [soy protein formula] ⓘ Esimil

Isomil DF ready-to-use liquid OTC *hypoallergenic infant food for management of diarrhea* [soy protein formula]

Isomil SF liquid OTC *hypoallergenic infant food* [soy protein formula, sucrose free]

isomylamine HCl USAN *smooth muscle relaxant*

isoniazid USP, INN, BAN *bactericidal; primary tuberculostatic* 50, 100, 300 mg oral; 50 mg/5 mL oral; 100 mg/mL injection

isonicophen [see: aconiazide]

isonicotinic acid hydrazide (INH) [see: isoniazid]

isonicotinic acid vanillylidenehydrazide [see: ftivazide]

1-isonicotinoyl-2-salicylidenehydrazine (INSH) [see: salinazid]

isonicotinylhydrazine [see: isoniazid]

isonixin INN

isooctadecanol [see: isostearyl alcohol]

isooctadecyl alcohol [see: isostearyl alcohol]

Isopan liquid OTC *antacid* [magaldrate] 540 mg/5 mL

Isopan Plus liquid OTC *antacid; antiflatulent* [magaldrate; simethicone] 540•40 mg/5 mL

Isopap capsules ℞ *vasoconstrictor; sedative; analgesic (for migraine)* [isometheptene mucate; dichloralphenazone; acetaminophen] 65•100•325 mg

isopentyl nitrite [see: amyl nitrite]

Iso-PH tablets OTC *dietary supplement* [plum pulp]

isophane insulin BAN *antidiabetic* [also: insulin, isophane]

isophenethanol [see: nifenalol]

isoprazone INN, BAN

isoprednidene INN, BAN

isopregnenone [see: dydrogesterone]

isoprenaline INN, BAN *bronchodilator; vasopressor for shock* [also: isoproterenol HCl]

L-isoprenaline [see: levisoprenaline]

isoprenaline HCl [see: isoproterenol HCl]

Isoprinosine ℞ *investigational antiviral/immunomodulator for AIDS; (orphan: subacute sclerosing panencephalitis)* [inosine pranobex]

isoprofen INN

isopropamide iodide USP, INN, BAN *peptic ulcer adjunct*

isopropanol [see: isopropyl alcohol]

isopropicillin INN

isoproponum iodide [see: isopropamide iodide]

7-isopropoxyisoflavone [see: ipriflavone]

isopropyl alcohol USP *topical anti-infective/antiseptic; solvent*

isopropyl alcohol, rubbing USP *rubefacient*

N-isopropyl meprobamate [see: carisoprodol]

isopropyl myristate NF *emollient*

isopropyl palmitate NF *oleaginous vehicle*

isopropyl sebacate

isopropylantipyrine [see: propyphenazone]

isopropylarterenol HCl [see: isoproterenol HCl]

isopropylarterenol sulfate [see: isoproterenol sulfate]

isoproterenol HCl USP *bronchodilator; vasopressor for shock* [also: isoprenaline] 0.25%, 0.5%, 1% (1:400, 1:200, 1:100) inhalation; 0.25% aerosol; 0.2 mg/mL (1:5000) injection

isoproterenol sulfate USP *bronchodilator*

Isoptin film-coated tablets ℞ *antianginal; antiarrhythmic; antihypertensive; calcium channel blocker* [verapamil HCl] 40, 80, 120 mg ⊇ Intropin

Isoptin IV injection ℞ *antitachyarrhythmic; calcium channel blocker* [verapamil HCl] 5 mg/2 mL

Isoptin SR film-coated sustained-release tablets ℞ *antihypertensive; calcium channel blocker* [verapamil HCl] 120, 180, 240 mg

Isopto Alkaline Drop-Tainers (eye drops) (discontinued 1995) OTC *ocular moisturizer/lubricant* [hydroxypropyl methylcellulose] 1%

Isopto Atropine Drop-Tainers (eye drops) ℞ *cycloplegic; mydriatic* [atropine sulfate] 0.5%, 1%

Isopto Carbachol Drop-Tainers (eye drops) ℞ *antiglaucoma agent; direct-acting miotic* [carbachol] 0.75%, 1.5%, 2.25%, 3%

Isopto Carpine Drop-Tainers (eye drops) ℞ *antiglaucoma agent; direct-acting miotic* [pilocarpine HCl] 0.25%, 0.5%, 1%, 2%, 3%, 4%, 5%, 6%, 8%, 10% ⊇ Isopto Eserine

Isopto Cetamide Drop-Tainers (eye drops) ℞ *ophthalmic bacteriostatic* [sulfacetamide sodium] 15%

Isopto Cetapred eye drop suspension ℞ *ophthalmic topical corticosteroidal anti-inflammatory; bacteriostatic* [prednisolone acetate; sulfacetamide sodium] 0.25%•10%

Isopto Eserine eye drops (discontinued 1994) ℞ *antiglaucoma agent; reversible cholinesterase inhibitor miotic* [physostigmine salicylate] 0.25%, 0.5% ⊇ Isopto Carpine

Isopto Frin eye drops (discontinued 1995) OTC *topical ocular decongestant* [phenylephrine HCl] 0.12%

Isopto Homatropine Drop-Tainers (eye drops) ℞ *cycloplegic; mydriatic* [homatropine hydrobromide] 2%, 5%

Isopto Hyoscine Drop-Tainers (eye drops) ℞ *cycloplegic; mydriatic* [scopolamine hydrobromide] 0.25%

Isopto P-ES Drop-Tainers (eye drops) (discontinued 1994) ℞ *antiglaucoma agent* [pilocarpine HCl; physostigmine salicylate] 2%•0.25%

Isopto Plain; Isopto Tears Drop-Tainers (eye drops) OTC *ocular moisturizer/lubricant* [hydroxypropyl methylcellulose] 0.5%

Isordil Titradose (tablets), Tembid (sustained-release capsules and tablets), sublingual ℞ *antianginal* [isosorbide dinitrate] 5, 10, 20, 30, 40 mg; 40 mg; 2.5, 5, 10 mg ⊡ Isuprel

isosorbide USAN, USP, INN, BAN *osmotic diuretic*

isosorbide dinitrate USAN, USP, INN, BAN *coronary vasodilator; antianginal* 2.5, 5, 10, 20, 30, 40 mg oral

isosorbide mononitrate USAN, INN, BAN *coronary vasodilator*

Isosource; Isosource HN liquid OTC *enteral nutritional therapy* [lactose-free formula]

isospaglumic acid INN

isospirilene [see: spirilene]

isostearyl alcohol USAN *emollient; solvent*

isosulfamerazine [see: sulfaperin]

isosulfan blue USAN *lymphangiography aid* [also: sulphan blue]

isosulpride INN

Isotein HN powder OTC *enteral nutritional therapy* [lactose-free formula]

3-isothiocyanato-1-propene [see: allyl isothiocyanate]

isothiocyanic acid, allyl ester [see: allyl isothiocyanate]

isothipendyl INN, BAN

isothipendyl HCl [see: isothipendyl]

isotiquimide USAN, INN, BAN *antiulcerative*

Isotrate Timecelles (sustained-release capsules) (discontinued 1995) ℞ *antianginal* [isosorbide dinitrate] 40 mg

isotretinoin USAN, USP, INN, BAN *keratolytic*

Isotrex ℞ *investigational keratolytic for acne* [isotretinoin]

Isovex capsules (discontinued 1996) ℞ *peripheral vasodilator* [ethaverine HCl] 100 mg

Isovist ℞ *investigational contrast medium for urography and angiography* [iotrolan]

Isovorin ℞ *investigational chemotherapy rescue (orphan: adjunct to colorectal adenocarcinoma and osteosarcoma)* [L-leucovorin]

Isovue-128; Isovue-200; Isovue-300; Isovue-370 injection ℞ *parenteral radiopaque agent* [iopamidol] 26%; 41%; 61%; 76%

Isovue-M 200; Isovue-M 300 intrathecal injection ℞ *parenteral myelographic radiopaque agent* [iopamidol] 41%; 61%

isoxaprolol INN

isoxepac USAN, INN, BAN *anti-inflammatory*

isoxicam USAN, INN, BAN *nonsteroidal anti-inflammatory drug (NSAID); antiarthritic; analgesic; antipyretic*

isoxsuprine INN, BAN *peripheral vasodilator* [also: isoxsuprine HCl]

isoxsuprine HCl USP *peripheral vasodilator* [also: isoxsuprine] 10, 20 mg oral

I-Soyalac liquid OTC *hypoallergenic infant food* [soybean protein formula]

isradipine USAN, INN, BAN *antihypertensive; calcium channel antagonist; calcium channel blocker*

isrodipine [see: isradipine]

Istin (European name for U.S. product Norvasc)

Isuprel Glossets (sublingual tablets) (discontinued 1996) ℞ *bronchodilator for bronchial asthma and bronchospasm* [isoproterenol HCl] 10, 15 mg

Isuprel intracardiac, IV, IM, or subcu injection ℞ *vasopressor for cardiac, hypovolemic, or septic shock* [isoproterenol HCl] 1:5000 (0.2 mg/mL), 1:50,000 (0.02 mg/mL) ⊡ Isordil

Isuprel Mistometer (metered-dose inhalation aerosol), solution for inhalation ℞ *bronchodilator for bronchial asthma and bronchospasm* [isoproterenol HCl] 131 μg/dose; 1:200 (0.5%)

itanoxone INN

itazigrel USAN, INN *platelet antiaggregatory agent*
itazogrel [see: itazigrel]
Itch-X spray, gel OTC *topical local anesthetic* [pramoxine HCl] 1%
itobarbital [see: butalbital]
itraconazole USAN, INN, BAN *systemic antifungal*
itramin tosilate INN [also: itramin tosylate]
itramin tosylate BAN [also: itramin tosilate]
itrocainide INN
I-Valex-1 powder OTC *formula for infants with leucine catabolism disorder*
I-Valex-2 powder OTC *enteral nutritional therapy for leucine catabolism disorder*
Ivarest cream, lotion OTC *topical poison ivy treatment* [calamine; benzocaine] 14%•5%
ivarimod INN

Iveegam freeze-dried powder for IV infusion ℞ *passive immunizing agent; immunomodulator for AIDS/ARC* [immune globulin] 50 mg/mL
ivermectin USAN, INN, BAN *antiparasitic*
ivermectin component B$_{1a}$
ivermectin component B$_{1b}$
IVIG (intravenous immunoglobulin) [q.v.]
Ivomec-SR bolus ℞ *investigational antiparasitic* [ivermectin]
ivoqualine INN
Ivy Block OTC *topical poison ivy treatment* [quaternium-18 bentonite] ⚠
Ivy Shield cream OTC *skin protectant*
Ivy-Chex spray OTC *topical poison ivy treatment* [polyvinylpyrrolidone-vinylacetate copolymers; methyl salicylate; benzalkonium chloride]
Ivy-Rid spray OTC *topical poison ivy treatment* [polyvinylpyrrolidone-vinylacetate copolymers; benzalkonium chloride]

Janimine Filmtabs (film-coated tablets) ℞ *tricyclic antidepressant; treatment for childhood enuresis* [imipramine HCl] 10, 25, 50 mg
Japanese encephalitis (JE) virus vaccine *active immunization vaccine*
Jenamicin IV or IM injection ℞ *aminoglycoside-type antibiotic* [gentamicin sulfate] 40 mg/mL
Jenest-28 tablets ℞ *biphasic oral contraceptive* [norethindrone; ethinyl estradiol] Phase 1: 0.5 mg•35 μg; Phase 2: 1 mg•35 μg
Jeri-Bath Oil (discontinued 1992) OTC *bath emollient*
Jets chewable tablets OTC *dietary supplement* [lysine; multiple vitamins] 300•≐ mg

JE-VAX powder for subcu injection ℞ *active immunizing agent* [Japanese encephalitis virus vaccine] 0.5 mL
Jevity liquid OTC *enteral nutritional therapy* [lactose-free formula]
Jiffy Toothache Drops (discontinued 1994) OTC *topical oral anesthetic; analgesic; antipruritic/counterirritant* [benzocaine; eugenol; menthol; alcohol 76%] 5%•9%•2%
jodphthalein sodium [see: iodophthalein sodium]
jofendylate [see: iophendylate]
jopanoic acid [see: iopanoic acid]
josamycin USAN, INN *antibacterial*
jotrizoic acid [see: iotrizoic acid]
juniper tar USP *antieczematic*
Just Tears eye drops OTC *ocular moisturizer/lubricant* [polyvinyl alcohol] 1.4%

K+ 8; K+ 10 film-coated extended-release tablets ℞ *potassium supplement* [potassium chloride] 8 mEq (600 mg); 10 mEq (750 mg)

K+ Care powder ℞ *potassium supplement* [potassium chloride] 15, 20, 25 mEq/packet

K+ Care ET effervescent tablets ℞ *potassium supplement* [potassium bicarbonate] 20, 25 mEq

^{42}K [see: potassium chloride K 42]

Kabi 2234 *investigational treatment for urge incontinence*

Kabikinase powder for IV or intracoronary infusion ℞ *thrombolytic enzyme for lysis of thrombi and catheter clearance* [streptokinase] 250,000, 600,000, 750,000, 1,500,000 IU

Kadian polymer-coated sustained-release pellets in capsules ℞ *narcotic analgesic* [morphine sulfate] 20, 50, 100 mg

Kainair eye drops (discontinued 1994) ℞ *topical ophthalmic anesthetic* [proparacaine HCl]

kainic acid INN

Kala tablets OTC *dietary supplement; fever blister treatment; not generally regarded as safe and effective as an antidiarrheal* [Lactobacillus acidophilus (soy-based)] 200 million U

kalafungin USAN, INN *antifungal*

Kalcinate IV injection or infusion (discontinued 1992) ℞ *calcium replenisher for hypocalcemia or hyperkalemia* [calcium gluconate]

kallidinogenase INN, BAN

kalmopyrin [see: calcium acetylsalicylate]

kalsetal [see: calcium acetylsalicylate]

Kaltostat; Kaltostat Fortex pads OTC *wound dressing* [calcium alginate fiber]

kanamycin INN, BAN *aminoglycoside bactericidal antibiotic; tuberculosis retreatment* [also: kanamycin sulfate] ☒ Garamycin; gentamicin

kanamycin B [see: bekanamycin]

kanamycin sulfate USP *aminoglycoside bactericidal antibiotic; tuberculosis retreatment* [also: kanamycin] 75, 500, 1000 mg/vial injection

Kank-a liquid/film OTC *topical oral anesthetic* [benzocaine] 20%

Kantrex capsules, IV or IM injection, pediatric injection ℞ *aminoglycoside-type antibiotic* [kanamycin sulfate] 500 mg; 500, 1000 mg; 75 mg

Kaochlor 10%; Kaochlor S-F liquid ℞ *potassium supplement* [potassium chloride; alcohol 5%] 20 mEq/15 mL ☒ K-Lor

Kaodene Non-Narcotic liquid OTC *antidiarrheal; GI adsorbent; antacid* [kaolin; pectin; bismuth subsalicylate] 3.9 g•194.4 mg•$\frac{2}{}$ per 30 mL ☒ codeine

Kaodene Non-Narcotic oral liquid OTC *antidiarrheal; GI adsorbent; antacid* [kaolin; pectin; bismuth subsalicylate] 130•6.48•$\frac{2}{}$ mg/mL

kaolin USP *GI adsorbent* ☒ Kaon

Kaon elixir ℞ *potassium supplement* [potassium gluconate] 20 mEq/15 mL ☒ kaolin

Kaon-Cl; Kaon-Cl 10 extended-release tablets ℞ *potassium supplement* [potassium chloride] 500 mg (6.7 mEq); 750 mg (10 mEq)

Kaon-Cl 20% liquid ℞ *potassium supplement* [potassium chloride; alcohol 5%] 40 mEq/15 mL

Kaopectate, Children's chewable tablets (discontinued 1995) OTC *antidiarrheal; GI adsorbent* [attapulgite] 300 mg ☒ Kapectalin

Kaopectate, Children's liquid OTC *antidiarrheal; GI adsorbent* [attapulgite] 600 mg/15 mL ☒ Kapectalin

Kaopectate II caplets OTC *antidiarrheal* [loperamide HCl] 2 mg

Kaopectate Advanced Formula oral liquid OTC *antidiarrheal; GI adsorbent* [attapulgite] 750 mg/15 mL

Kaopectate Maximum Strength caplets OTC *antidiarrheal; GI adsorbent* [attapulgite] 750 mg

Kao-Spen oral suspension OTC *GI adsorbent; antidiarrheal* [kaolin; pectin] 5.2 g•260 mg per 30 mL

Kapectolin liquid OTC *GI adsorbent; antidiarrheal* [kaolin; pectin] 90•2 g/30 mL ⓓ Kaopectate

Kapectolin PG liquid (discontinued 1994) ℞ *GI adsorbent; not generally regarded as safe and effective as an antidiarrheal* [opium; kaolin; pectin; hyoscyamine sulfate; atropine sulfate; scopolamine hydrobromide]

Kapectolin with Paregoric liquid (discontinued 1992) ℞ *GI adsorbent; (not generally regarded as safe and effective as an antidiarrheal)* [opium (paregoric); kaolin; pectin]

Kapseal (trademarked dosage form) *capsules sealed with a band*

Karbozyme enteric-coated tablets OTC *dietary supplement* [pancreatin; sodium bicarbonate; potassium bicarbonate]

Karidium tablets, chewable tablets, drops ℞ *dental caries preventative* [sodium fluoride] 2.2 mg; 2.2 mg; 0.275 mg/drop

Karigel; Karigel-N gel ℞ *topical dental caries preventative* [sodium fluoride] 1.1%

kasal USAN *food additive*

Kasdenol powder OTC *germicidal mouthwash* [monoxychlorosene]

Kasof capsules OTC *stool softener* [docusate potassium] 240 mg

Katadolon ℞ *investigational narcotic analgesic and muscle relaxant* [flupirtine]

Kato powder (discontinued 1995) ℞ *potassium supplement* [potassium chloride] 20 mEq/packet

Kay Ciel liquid, powder ℞ *potassium supplement* [potassium chloride] 20 mEq/15 mL; 20 mEq/packet ⓓ KCl

Kaybovite-1000 IM or subcu injection (discontinued 1994) ℞ *antianemic; vitamin B_{12} supplement* [cyanocobalamin] 1000 μg/mL

Kayexalate powder ℞ *potassium-removing agent for hyperkalemia* [sodium polystyrene sulfonate]

Kaylixir liquid ℞ *potassium supplement* [potassium gluconate; alcohol 5%] 20 mEq/15 mL

Kaysine injection (discontinued 1995) ℞ *treatment for varicose veins* with stasis dermatitis [adenosine phosphate] 25 mg/mL

K-C oral suspension OTC *antidiarrheal; GI adsorbent; antacid* [kaolin; pectin; bismuth subcarbonate] 5 g•260 mg•260 mg per 30 mL

KCl (potassium chloride) [q.v.] ⓓ Kay Ciel

K-DEC tablets (discontinued 1994) OTC *vitamin/mineral/iron supplement* [multiple vitamins & minerals; ferrous fumarate; folic acid; biotin] ≛•18 mg•0.4 mg•30 μg

K-Dur 10; K-Dur 20 controlled-release tablets ℞ *potassium supplement* [potassium chloride] 750 mg (10 mEq); 1500 mg (20 mEq)

kebuzone INN

Keflet tablets (discontinued 1993) ℞ *cephalosporin-type antibiotic* [cephalexin monohydrate] 250, 500, 1000 mg ⓓ Keflex; Keflin

Keflex pediatric drops (discontinued 1995) ℞ *cephalosporin-type antibiotic* [cephalexin monohydrate] 100 mg/mL ⓓ Keflet; Keflin

Keflex Pulvules (capsules), oral suspension ℞ *cephalosporin-type antibiotic* [cephalexin monohydrate] 250, 500 mg; 125, 250 mg/5 mL ⓓ Keflet; Keflin

Keflin, Neutral powder for IV or IM injection (discontinued 1996) ℞ *cephalosporin-type antibiotic* [cephalothin sodium] 1, 2 g ⓓ Keflet; Keflex

Keftab tablets ℞ *cephalosporin-type antibiotic* [cephalexin HCl monohydrate] 500 mg

Kefurox powder for IV or IM injection ℞ *cephalosporin-type antibiotic* [cefuroxime sodium] 0.75, 1.5, 7.5 g

Kefzol powder for IV or IM injection ℞ *cephalosporin-type antibiotic* [cefazolin sodium] 0.25, 0.5, 1, 10, 20 g ⓓ Cefzil

K-Electrolyte effervescent tablets ℞ *potassium supplement* [potassium bicarbonate; potassium citrate]

K-Electrolyte/Cl effervescent tablets ℞ *potassium supplement* [potassium chloride]

kellofylline [see: visnafylline]

Kemadrin tablets ℞ *anticholinergic; antiparkinsonian agent* [procyclidine HCl] 5 mg ⓟ Coumadin

Kemron ℞ *investigational oral treatment for AIDS* [interferon alfa]

Kenacort tablets, syrup ℞ *glucocorticoids* [triamcinolone] 4, 8 mg; 4 mg/5 mL

Kenaject-40 IM, intra-articular, intrabursal, intradermal injection ℞ *glucocorticoids* [triamcinolone acetonide] 40 mg/mL

Kenalog ointment, cream, lotion, aerosol spray ℞ *topical corticosteroid* [triamcinolone acetonide] 0.025%, 0.1%, 0.5%; 0.025%, 0.1%, 0.5%; 0.025%, 0.1%; ≟ ⓟ Ketalar

Kenalog in Orabase oral paste ℞ *topical corticosteroid* [triamcinolone acetonide] 0.1%

Kenalog-10; Kenalog-40 IM, intra-articular, intrabursal, intradermal injection ℞ *glucocorticoids* [triamcinolone acetonide] 10 mg/mL; 40 mg/mL

Kenalog-H cream ℞ *topical corticosteroid* [triamcinolone acetonide] 0.1%

Kendall's compound A [see: dehydrocorticosterone]

Kendall's compound B [see: corticosterone]

Kendall's compound E [see: cortisone acetate]

Kendall's compound F [see: hydrocortisone]

Kendall's desoxy compound B [see: desoxycorticosterone acetate]

Kenicef ℞ *investigational cephalosporin antibiotic* [cefodizime]

Kenonel cream ℞ *topical corticosteroid* [triamcinolone acetonide] 1%

Kenwood Therapeutic liquid OTC *vitamin/mineral supplement* [multiple vitamins & minerals] ±

keoxifene HCl [now: raloxifene HCl]

keracyanin INN

Keralyte gel (discontinued 1994) ℞ *topical keratolytic* [salicylic acid] 6%

keratinocyte growth factor *investigational GI protective agent*

Keri; Keri Light lotion OTC *moisturizer; emollient*

Keri Creme OTC *moisturizer; emollient*

Keri Facial Cleanser liquid (discontinued 1994) OTC *soap-free therapeutic skin cleanser*

KeriCort-10 cream OTC *topical corticosteroid* [hydrocortisone] 1%

Kerledex ℞ *investigational antihypertensive β-blocker and diuretic combination* [betaxolol HCl; chlorthalidone]

Kerlone tablets ℞ *antihypertensive; β-blocker* [betaxolol HCl] 10, 20 mg

Kerodex #51 cream OTC *skin protectant for dry or oily work*

Kerodex #71 cream OTC *water repellant skin protectant for wet work*

Kestrone 5 IM injection ℞ *estrogen replacement therapy; antineoplastic for prostatic and breast cancer* [estrone] 5 mg/mL

Ketalar IV or IM injection ℞ *general anesthetic* [ketamine HCl] 10, 50, 100 mg/mL ⓟ Kenalog

ketamine INN, BAN *anesthetic* [also: ketamine HCl]

ketamine HCl USAN, USP *general anesthetic* [also: ketamine]

ketanserin USAN, INN, BAN *serotonin antagonist*

ketazocine USAN, INN *analgesic*

ketazolam USAN, INN, BAN *minor tranquilizer*

kethoxal USAN *antiviral* [also: ketoxal]

ketimipramine INN *antidepressant* [also: ketipramine fumarate]

ketimipramine fumarate [see: ketipramine fumarate]

ketipramine fumarate USAN *antidepressant* [also: ketimipramine]

ketobemidone INN, BAN

ketocaine INN

ketocainol INN

ketocholanic acid [see: dehydrocholic acid]

ketoconazole USAN, USP, INN, BAN *broad-spectrum antifungal; (orphan: diminish cyclosporine-induced nephrotoxicity of transplants)*

Keto-Diastix reagent strips *in vitro diagnostic aid for multiple urine products*

ketohexazine [see: cetohexazine]

Ketonex-1 powder OTC *formula for infants with maple syrup urine disease*

Ketonex-2 powder OTC *enteral nutritional therapy for maple syrup urine disease*

ketoprofen USAN, INN, BAN, JAN *antiarthritic; nonsteroidal anti-inflammatory drug (NSAID); analgesic* 25, 50, 75 mg oral

ketorfanol USAN, INN *analgesic*

ketorolac INN, BAN *analgesic; nonsteroidal anti-inflammatory drug (NSAID); antipyretic* [also: ketorolac tromethamine]

ketorolac tromethamine USAN *analgesic; nonsteroidal anti-inflammatory drug (NSAID); antipyretic* [also: ketorolac]

Ketostix reagent strips for home use OTC *in vitro diagnostic aid for acetone (ketones) in the urine*

ketotifen INN, BAN *antiasthmatic* [also: ketotifen fumarate]

ketotifen fumarate USAN, JAN *antiasthmatic* [also: ketotifen]

ketotrexate INN

ketoxal INN *antiviral* [also: kethoxal]

Kevadon ℞ *investigational treatment for graft vs. host disease* [thalidomide]

Key-E tablets, caplets, cream, ointment, suppositories, powder, spray OTC *vitamin supplement; topical antioxidant* [vitamin E]

Key-E Kaps capsules OTC *vitamin supplement* [vitamin E]

Key-Min cellulose-coated caplet OTC *mineral supplement* [multiple minerals; vitamin D_3]

Key-Plex injection ℞ *parenteral vitamin therapy* [multiple B vitamins; vitamin C] $\pm$ •50 mg/mL

Key-Pred 25; Key-Pred 50 IM injection ℞ *glucocorticoids* [prednisolone acetate] 25 mg/mL; 50 mg/mL

Key-Pred-SP IV or IM injection ℞ *glucocorticoids* [prednisolone sodium phosphate] 20 mg/mL

Key-Ron cellulose-coated caplet OTC *iron supplement* [ferrous fumarate; vitamin B_{12}; vitamin C; bovine liver]

K-Feron IV, IM injection (discontinued 1992) ℞ *antianemic* [iron dextran]

K-Flex IV or IM injection (discontinued 1993) ℞ *skeletal muscle relaxant* [orphenadrine citrate]

K-G Elixir ℞ *potassium supplement* [potassium gluconate] 20 mEq/15 mL

khellin INN

khelloside INN

Kiddy Chews chewable tablets (discontinued 1995) OTC *vitamin supplement* [multiple vitamins; folic acid] $\pm$ •0.3 mg

Kiddy Chews with Iron chewable tablets (discontinued 1995) OTC *vitamin/iron supplement* [multiple vitamins; iron; folic acid] $\pm$ •15•0.3 mg

KIE syrup ℞ *decongestant; expectorant* [ephedrine HCl; potassium iodide] 8•150 mg/5 mL

Kinedak ℞ *investigational treatment for diabetic neuropathy* [epalrestat]

Kinesed chewable tablets (discontinued 1995) ℞ *GI anticholinergic; sedative* [atropine sulfate; scopolamine hydrobromide; hyoscyamine hydrobromide; phenobarbital] 0.12•0.007•0.12•16 mg

Kinevac powder for IV injection ℞ *in vivo gallbladder function test* [sincalide] 1 μg/mL

kitasamycin USAN, INN, BAN, JAN *antibacterial* [also: acetylkitasamycin; kitasamycin tartrate]

kitasamycin tartrate JAN *antibacterial* [also: kitasamycin; acetylkitasamycin]

KLB6; Ultra KLB6 softgels OTC *dietary supplement* [vitamin B_6; multiple food supplements] 3.5• $\pm$ mg; 16.7• $\pm$ mg

KLB6 Complete tablets (discontinued 1992) OTC *dietary supplement* [multiple vitamins & food supplements]

K-Lease extended-release capsules ℞ *potassium supplement* [potassium chloride] 750 mg (10 mEq)

Klerist-D tablets, sustained-release capsules ℞ *decongestant; antihistamine* [pseudoephedrine HCl; chlorpheniramine maleate] 60•4 mg; 120•8 mg

Klonopin tablets, Rx Pak (prescription package), Tel-E-Dose (unit dose package) ℞ *anticonvulsant; (orphan:*

hyperexplexia) [clonazepam] 0.5, 1, 2 mg ⊇ clonidine

K-Lor powder ℞ *potassium supplement* [potassium chloride] 15, 20 mEq/packet ⊇ Kaochlor

Klor-Con; Klor-Con/25 powder ℞ *potassium supplement* [potassium chloride] 20 mEq/packet; 25 mEq/packet

Klor-Con 8; Klor-Con 10 film-coated extended-release tablets ℞ *potassium supplement* [potassium chloride] 600 mg (8 mEq); 750 mg (10 mEq)

Klor-Con/EF effervescent tablets ℞ *potassium supplement* [potassium bicarbonate; potassium citrate] 25 mEq (K)

Kloromin tablets OTC *antihistamine* [chlorpheniramine maleate]

Klorvess liquid, effervescent granules, effervescent tablets ℞ *potassium supplement* [potassium chloride] 20 mEq/15 mL; 20 mEq/packet; 20 mEq

Klotrix film-coated controlled-release tablets ℞ *potassium supplement* [potassium chloride] 750 mg (10 mEq) ⊇ Liotrix

K-Lyte; K-Lyte DS effervescent tablets ℞ *potassium supplement* [potassium bicarbonate; potassium citrate] 25 mEq; 50 mEq (K)

K-Lyte/Cl powder ℞ *potassium supplement* [potassium chloride] 25 mEq/dose

K-Lyte/Cl; K-Lyte/Cl 50 effervescent tablets ℞ *potassium supplement* [potassium chloride] 25 mEq; 50 mEq

KNI-272 *investigational (Phase I) antiviral for pediatric and adult HIV*

K-Norm controlled-release capsules ℞ *potassium supplement* [potassium chloride] 750 mg (10 mEq)

Koāte-HP powder for IV injection ℞ *antihemophilic to correct coagulation deficiency* [antihemophilic factor VIII] 250, 500, 1000, 1500 IU

Koāte-HS powder for IV injection (discontinued 1994) ℞ *antihemophilic to correct coagulation deficiency* [antihemophilic factor VIII] ⊇

Kof-Eze lozenges OTC *topical antipruritic/counterirritant; mild local anesthetic* [menthol] 6 mg

KoGENate powder for IV injection ℞ *antihemophilic to correct coagulation deficiency* [antihemophilic factor VIII, recombinant] ⊇

KOH (potassium hydroxide) [q.v.]

Kolephrin caplets OTC *decongestant; antihistamine; analgesic* [pseudoephedrine HCl; chlorpheniramine maleate; acetaminophen] 30•2•325 mg

Kolephrin GG/DM liquid OTC *antitussive; expectorant* [dextromethorphan hydrobromide; guaifenesin] 10•150 mg/5 mL

Kolephrin/DM caplets OTC *antitussive; decongestant; antihistamine; analgesic* [dextromethorphan hydrobromide; pseudoephedrine HCl; chlorpheniramine maleate; acetaminophen] 10•30•2•325 mg

kolfocon A USAN *hydrophobic contact lens material*

kolfocon B USAN *hydrophobic contact lens material*

kolfocon C USAN *hydrophobic contact lens material*

kolfocon D USAN *hydrophobic contact lens material*

Kolyum liquid ℞ *potassium supplement* [potassium gluconate; potassium chloride] 20 mEq/15 mL (K)

Kolyum powder (discontinued 1993) ℞ *potassium supplement* [potassium gluconate; potassium chloride] 20 mEq/packet (K)

Komed lotion (discontinued 1994) OTC *topical acne treatment* [salicylic acid; sodium thiosulfate; isopropyl alcohol] 2%•8%•25%

Komex scrub (discontinued 1992) OTC *abrasive cleanser for acne* [sodium tetraborate decahydrate dissolving particles] ⊇ Koromex

Konakion IM injection ℞ *coagulant; correct anticoagulant-induced prothrombin deficiency; vitamin K supplement* [phytonadione] 2, 10 mg/mL

Kondon's Nasal jelly OTC *nasal decongestant* [ephedrine] 1%

Kondremul Plain emulsion OTC *emollient laxative* [mineral oil]
Kondremul with Phenolphthalein emulsion OTC *laxative* [mineral oil; phenolphthalein] 55%•150 mg/15 mL
Konsyl powder OTC *bulk laxative* [psyllium] 100%
Konsyl Fiber tablets OTC *bulk laxative; antidiarrheal* [calcium polycarbophil] 625 mg
Konsyl-D; Konsyl Orange powder OTC *bulk laxative* [psyllium hydrophilic mucilloid] 3.4 g/tbsp.
Konȳne 80 IV infusion ℞ *antihemophilic to correct factor IX deficiency and anticoagulant-induced hemorrhage* [factor IX complex, human, heat treated] 20, 40 mL
Konȳne-HT (name changed to Konȳne 80 in 1992)
Kophane Cough & Cold Formula liquid OTC *antitussive; decongestant; antihistamine* [dextromethorphan hydrobromide; phenylpropanolamine HCl; chlorpheniramine maleate] 10•12.5•2 mg/5 mL
Korigesic tablets (discontinued 1993) ℞ *decongestant; antihistamine; analgesic* [phenylephrine HCl; chlorpheniramine maleate; acetaminophen; caffeine]
Koromex premedicated condom (discontinued 1995) OTC *spermicidal/barrier contraceptive* [nonoxynol 9] 5.6%
Koromex vaginal cream OTC *spermicidal contraceptive (for use with a diaphragm)* [octoxynol 9] 3%
Koromex vaginal foam, vaginal jelly OTC *spermicidal contraceptive* [nonoxynol 9] 12.5%; 3% ② Komex
Koromex Crystal Clear vaginal gel OTC *spermicidal contraceptive (for use with a diaphragm)* [nonoxynol 9] 2%
Kovitonic liquid OTC *hematinic* [ferric pyrophosphate; multiple B vitamins; lysine; folic acid] 42•±•10•0.1 mg/15 mL
K-P suspension (discontinued 1992) OTC *antidiarrheal; GI adsorbent* [kaolin; pectin]

K-Pek oral suspension OTC *antidiarrheal; GI adsorbent* [attapulgite] 600 mg/15 mL
K-Phen-50 injection ℞ *antihistamine; motion sickness; sleep aid; antiemetic; sedative* [promethazine HCl] 50 mg/mL
K-Phos Neutral film-coated tablets ℞ *phosphorus supplement* [dibasic potassium phosphate; monobasic sodium phosphate; monobasic potassium phosphate] 250 mg (P)
K-Phos No. 2; K-Phos M.F. tablets ℞ *urinary acidifier* [potassium acid phosphate; sodium acid phosphate] 305•700 mg; 155•350 mg
K-Phos Original tablets ℞ *urinary acidifier* [potassium acid phosphate] 500 mg
K.P.N. tablets OTC *vitamin/mineral/calcium/iron supplement* [multiple vitamins & minerals; calcium; iron; folic acid] ±•333•11•0.27 mg
^{81m}**Kr** [see: krypton Kr 81m]
^{85}**Kr** [see: krypton clathrate Kr 85]
Kredex (European name for U.S. product Coreg)
Kronocap (trademarked dosage form) *sustained-release capsule*
Kronofed-A sustained-release capsules ℞ *decongestant; antihistamine* [pseudoephedrine HCl; chlorpheniramine maleate] 120•8 mg
Kronofed-A Jr. Kronocaps (sustained-release capsules) ℞ *pediatric decongestant and antihistamine* [pseudoephedrine HCl; chlorpheniramine maleate] 60•4 mg
krypton *element (Kr)*
krypton clathrate Kr 85 USAN *radioactive agent*
krypton Kr 81m USAN, USP *radioactive agent*
K-Tab film-coated extended-release tablets ℞ *potassium supplement* [potassium chloride] 750 mg (10 mEq)
Kudrox oral suspension OTC *antacid* [aluminum hydroxide; magnesium hydroxide; simethicone] 500•450•40 mg/5 mL
Kutapressin subcu or IM injection ℞ *claimed to be an anti-inflammatory for*

multiple dermatoses [liver derivative complex] 25.5 mg/mL

Kutrase capsules ℞ *digestive enzymes; antispasmodic; sedative* [amylase; protease; lipase; cellulase; hyoscyamine sulfate; phenyltoloxamine citrate] 30•6•75•2•0.0625•15 mg

Ku-Zyme capsules ℞ *digestive enzymes* [amylase; protease; lipase; cellulase] 30•6•75•2 mg

Ku-Zyme HP capsules ℞ *digestive enzymes* [lipase; protease; amylase] 8000•30,000•30,000 U

Kwelcof liquid ℞ *narcotic antitussive; expectorant* [hydrocodone bitartrate; guaifenesin] 5•100 mg/5 mL

Kwell cream, lotion, shampoo (discontinued 1996) ℞ *scabicide; pediculicide* [lindane] 1%

Kwildane lotion, shampoo ℞ *scabicide; pediculicide* [lindane]

K-Y vaginal jelly OTC *lubricant* [glycerin; hydroxyethyl cellulose]

K-Y Plus vaginal gel OTC *spermicidal contraceptive (for use with a diaphragm)* [nonoxynol 9] 2.2%

kyamepromazin [see: cyamemazine]

Kybernin ℞ *(orphan: prevent and treat thromboembolism in genetic AT-III deficiency)* [antithrombin III concentrate IV]

Kynac ℞ *investigational treatment for psoriasis and eczema*

Kynacyte ℞ *investigational cancer chemotherapy enhancer*

Kytril IV infusion, film-coated tablets ℞ *antiemetic/antinauseant for chemotherapy* [granisetron HCl] 1 mg/mL; 1 mg

L-5 hydroxytryptophan (L-5HTP) *(orphan: postanoxic intention myoclonus)*

L-696,229 [see: non-nucleoside reverse transcriptase inhibitor]

L-697,661 *investigational non-nucleoside antiviral for AIDS (clinical trials discontinued 1994)*

LA-12 IM injection ℞ *antianemic; vitamin B_{12} supplement* [hydroxocobalamin] 1000 μg/mL

LAAM (l-acetyl-α-methadol [or] l-alpha-acetyl-methadol) [see: levomethadyl acetate]

labetalol INN, BAN *antiadrenergic (α- and β-receptor)* [also: labetalol HCl]

labetalol HCl USAN, USP *antiadrenergic (α- and β-receptor)* [also: labetalol]

Labstix reagent strips *in vitro diagnostic aid for multiple urine products*

Lac-Hydrin lotion ℞ *moisturizer; emollient* [ammonium lactate] 12%

Lac-Hydrin Five lotion OTC *moisturizer; emollient* [lactic acid]

lacidipine USAN, INN, BAN *antihypertensive; calcium channel blocker*

Lacipil (commercially available in Europe) ℞ *investigational antihypertensive; calcium channel blocker* [lacidipine]

Lacril eye drops OTC *ocular moisturizer/lubricant* [hydroxypropyl methylcellulose] 0.5%

Lacri-Lube NP; Lacri-Lube S.O.P. ophthalmic ointment OTC *ocular moisturizer/lubricant* [white petrolatum; mineral oil; lanolin]

Lacrisert ophthalmic insert OTC *ocular moisturizer/lubricant* [hydroxypropyl cellulose] 5 mg

LactAid liquid, tablets OTC *digestive aid for lactose intolerance* [lactase enzyme] 250 U/drop; 3000 U

lactalfate INN

lactase enzyme *digestive enzyme for lactose intolerance*

lactated potassic saline [see: potassic saline, lactated]

lactated Ringer's (LR) injection [see: Ringer's injection, lactated]

lactated Ringer's (LR) solution [see: Ringer's injection, lactated]

lactic acid USP *pH adjusting agent*

LactiCare lotion OTC *emollient; moisturizer* [lactic acid]

LactiCare-HC lotion ℞ *topical corticosteroid* [hydrocortisone] 1%, 2.5%

Lactinex granules, chewable tablets OTC *dietary supplement; fever blister treatment; not generally regarded as safe and effective as an antidiarrheal* [Lactobacillus acidophilus; Lactobacillus bulgaricus]

Lactinol lotion ℞ *emollient; moisturizer* [lactic acid] 10%

Lactinol-E cream ℞ *emollient; moisturizer* [lactic acid; vitamin E] 10%•116.67 IU/g

Lactisol; Lactisol-Forte liquid (discontinued 1994) ℞ *topical keratolytic* [salicylic acid in a collodion base; lactic acid] 16.7%•16.7%; 20%•20%

lactitol INN, BAN

Lactobacillus acidophilus *dietary supplement; not generally regarded as safe and effective as an antidiarrheal*

Lactobacillus bulgaricus *dietary supplement; not generally regarded as safe and effective as an antidiarrheal*

lactobin (orphan: AIDS-related diarrhea)

lactobionic acid, calcium salt, dihydrate [see: calcium lactobionate]

Lactocal-F film-coated tablets ℞ *vitamin/mineral/calcium/iron supplement* [multiple vitamins & minerals; calcium; iron; folic acid] ≟•200•65•1 mg

lactoflavin [see: riboflavin]

Lactofree liquid, powder OTC *hypoallergenic infant formula* [milk-based formula, lactose free]

Lactogest soft gel capsules (discontinued 1994) OTC *digestive aid for lactose intolerance* [lactase enzyme]

β-lactone [see: propiolactone]

γ-lactone D-glucofuranuronic acid [see: glucurolactone]

lactose NF *tablet and capsule diluent; dietary supplement*

Lactrase capsules OTC *digestive aid for lactose intolerance* [lactase enzyme] 250 mg

lactulose USAN, USP, INN, BAN *laxative*

ladakamycin [now: azacitidine]

Lady Esther cream OTC *moisturizer; emollient* [mineral oil] ≟

L.A.E. 20 IM injection (discontinued 1992) ℞ *estrogen replacement therapy; antineoplastic for prostatic cancer* [estradiol valerate in oil]

laidlomycin INN *veterinary growth stimulant* [also: laidlomycin propionate potassium]

laidlomycin propionate potassium USAN *veterinary growth stimulant* [also: laidlomycin]

Laki-Lorand factor [see: factor XIII]

Lamictal tablets ℞ *anticonvulsant* [lamotrigine] 25, 100, 150, 200 mg

lamifiban USAN, INN *fibrinogen receptor antagonist*

Lamisil cream ℞ *topical antifungal* [terbinafine HCl] 1%

Lamisil tablets ℞ *systemic antifungal for onychomycosis* [terbinafine HCl] 250 mg

lamivudine USAN, INN, BAN *antiviral for HIV; investigational (Phase II/III) for hepatitis B*

lamotrigine USAN, INN, BAN *phenyltriazine anticonvulsant*

Lampit (available only from the Centers for Disease Control) ℞ *investigational anti-infective for Chagas disease* [nifurtimox]

Lamprene capsules ℞ *bactericidal; tuberculostatic; leprostatic* (orphan) [clofazimine] 50, 100 mg

lamtidine INN, BAN

Lanabiotic ointment OTC *topical antibiotic; anesthetic* [polymyxin B sulfate; neomycin sulfate; bacitracin; lidocaine] 10,000 U•3.5 mg•500 U•40 mg per g

Lanacaine spray, cream OTC *topical local anesthetic; antiseptic* [benzocaine; benzethonium chloride] 20%•0.1%; 6%•0.1%

Lanacaps (dosage form) *timed-release capsules*

Lanacort 5; Lanacort 10 cream, ointment OTC *topical corticosteroid* [hydrocortisone acetate] 0.5%; 1%

Lanaphilic cream OTC *moisturizer; emollient; keratolytic* [urea] 20%

Lanaphilic OTC *ointment base*

Lanaphilic with Urea OTC *ointment base* [urea] 10%

Lanatabs (dosage form) *sustained-release tablets*

lanatoside NF, INN, BAN

Lanatuss Expectorant liquid (discontinued 1994) OTC *decongestant; antihistamine; expectorant* [phenylpropanolamine HCl; chlorpheniramine maleate; guaifenesin]

Lanazets Improved lozenges (discontinued 1993) OTC *topical oral anesthetic; antiseptic* [benzocaine; cetylpyridinium chloride] 5•1 mg

Laniazid tablets, syrup ℞ *tuberculostatic* [isoniazid] 50, 100 mg; 50 mg/5 mL

Laniazid C.T. tablets ℞ *tuberculostatic* [isoniazid] 300 mg

lanolin USP *ointment base; water-in-oil emulsion; emollient/protectant* ② Lanoline

lanolin, anhydrous USP *absorbent ointment base*

lanolin alcohols *ointment base ingredient*

Lanoline cream (discontinued 1992) OTC *moisturizer; emollient* ② lanolin

Lanolor cream OTC *moisturizer; emollient*

Lanophyllin elixir ℞ *bronchodilator* [theophylline] 80 mg/15 mL

Lanophyllin-GG capsules (discontinued 1993) ℞ *antiasthmatic; expectorant* [theophylline; bronchodilator; guaifenesin]

Lanoplex elixir (discontinued 1993) OTC *vitamin supplement* [multiple B vitamins]

Lanorinal tablets, capsules ℞ *analgesic; antipyretic; anti-inflammatory; sedative* [aspirin; caffeine; butalbital] 325•40•50 mg

Lanoxicaps capsules ℞ *cardiac glycoside to increase cardiac output; antiarrhythmic* [digoxin] 0.05, 0.1, 0.2 mg

Lanoxin tablets, pediatric elixir, IV or IM injection ℞ *cardiac glycoside to increase cardiac output; antiarrhythmic* [digoxin] 0.125, 0.25, 0.5 mg; 0.05 mg/mL; 0.1, 0.25 mg/mL ② Levoxine

lanreotide acetate USAN *antineoplastic*

lansoprazole USAN, INN, BAN *antiulcerative; antisecretory; proton pump inhibitor*

lanthanum *element (La)*

Lanvisone cream (discontinued 1993) ℞ *topical corticosteroid; antifungal; antibacterial* [hydrocortisone; clioquinol]

lapirium chloride INN *surfactant* [also: lapyrium chloride]

LAPOCA (L-asparaginase, Oncovin, cytarabine, Adriamycin) *chemotherapy protocol*

laprafylline INN

lapyrium chloride USAN *surfactant* [also: lapirium chloride]

laramycin [see: zorbamycin]

Largon IV or IM injection ℞ *sedative; analgesic adjunct* [propiomazine HCl] 20 mg/mL

Lariam tablets ℞ *antimalarial; for acute chloroquine-resistant malaria (orphan)* [mefloquine HCl] 250 mg

Larobec tablets (discontinued 1994) ℞ *vitamin supplement* [multiple B vitamins; vitamin C; folic acid] ±• 500•0.5 mg

Larodopa capsules ℞ *antiparkinsonian* [levodopa] 100, 250, 500 mg

Larodopa tablets ℞ *antiparkinsonian* [levodopa] 100, 250, 500 mg

laroxyl [see: amitriptyline]

lasalocid USAN, INN, BAN *coccidiostat for poultry*

Lasan cream, ointment ℞ *topical antipsoriatic* [anthralin] 0.1%, 0.2%, 0.4%; 0.4%

Lasan HP-1 cream ℞ *topical antipsoriatic* [anthralin] 1%

Lasix tablets, oral solution, IM or IV injection ℞ *loop diuretic* [furosemide] 20, 40, 80 mg; 10 mg/mL; 10 mg/mL ② Esidrix; Lidex

Lassar's paste [betanaphthol (q.v.) + zinc oxide (q.v.)]

latamoxef INN, BAN *anti-infective* [also: moxalactam disodium]

latamoxef disodium [see: moxalactam disodium]

latanoprost INN *prostaglandin agonist for glaucoma and ocular hypertension*

laudexium methylsulfate [see: laudexium metilsulfate; laudexium methylsulphate]

laudexium methylsulphate BAN [also: laudexium metilsulfate]

laudexium metilsulfate INN [also: laudexium methylsulphate]
lauralkonium chloride INN
laureth 10S USAN *spermaticide*
laureth 4 USAN *surfactant*
laureth 9 USAN *spermaticide; surfactant*
lauril INN *combining name for radicals or groups*
laurilsulfate INN *combining name for radicals or groups* [also: sodium lauryl sulfate]
laurixamine INN
laurocapram USAN, INN *excipient*
lauroguadine INN
laurolinium acetate INN, BAN
lauromacrogol 400 INN
lauryl isoquinolinium bromide USAN *anti-infective*
lavender oil NF
lavoltidine INN *antiulcerative; histamine H_2-receptor blocker* [also: lavoltidine succinate; loxtidine]
lavoltidine succinate USAN *antiulcerative; histamine H_2-receptor blocker* [also: lavoltidine; loxtidine]
Lavoptik Eye Wash ophthalmic solution OTC *extraocular irrigating solution* [balanced saline solution]
lawrencium *element (Lr)*
Lax Pills tablets OTC *laxative* [yellow phenolphthalein] 90 mg
Laxative Pills tablets OTC *laxative* [yellow phenolphthalein] 90 mg
lazabemide USAN, INN *antiparkinsonian; investigational MAO B inhibitor for Alzheimer's disease*
Lazer Creme OTC *moisturizer; emollient* [vitamins A and E] 3333.3•116.67 U/g
Lazer Formalyde solution Ŗ *for hyperhidrosis and bromhidrosis* [formaldehyde] 10%
LazerSporin-C ear drops Ŗ *topical corticosteroidal anti-inflammatory; antibiotic* [hydrocortisone; neomycin sulfate; polymyxin B sulfate] 1%•5 mg•10,000 U per mL
LC-65 solution OTC *cleaning solution for hard, soft, or rigid gas permeable contact lenses*

L-Caine injection (discontinued 1995) Ŗ *injectable local anesthetic* [lidocaine HCl] 1%
LCD (liquor carbonis detergens) [see: coal tar]
LCR (leurocristine) [see: vincristine]
LCx Neisseria gonorrhoeae Assay reagent kit for professional use *in vitro diagnostic aid for Neisseria gonorrhoeae*
lead *element (Pb)*
lecimibide USAN *hypocholesterolemic; antihyperlipidemic*
lecithin NF *emulsifying agent; dietary lipotropic supplement* 420, 1200 mg oral
Ledercillin VK tablets, powder for oral solution Ŗ *bactericidal antibiotic* [penicillin V potassium] 250, 500 mg; 250 mg/5 mL
Lederject (trademarked delivery system) *prefilled disposable syringe*
Lederplex capsules (discontinued 1995) OTC *vitamin supplement* [multiple B vitamins]
Lederplex liquid (discontinued 1992) OTC *vitamin supplement* [multiple B vitamins]
lefetamine INN
leflunomide INN *investigational antiarthritic*
Legalon Ŗ *(orphan: Amanita phalloides [mushroom] liver poisoning)* [disodium silibinin dihemisuccinate]
Legatrin tablets (discontinued 1995) OTC *prevention and treatment of nocturnal leg cramps* [quinine sulfate] 162.5 mg
Legatrin PM caplets OTC *prevention and treatment of nocturnal leg cramps* [diphenhydramine HCl; acetaminophen] 50•500 mg
Legatrin Rub gel (discontinued 1994) OTC *counterirritant; topical anesthetic* [menthol; benzocaine; alcohol 44%] 4%•2%
leiopyrrole INN
lemidosul INN
lemon oil NF
lenampicillin INN
Lenate oral solution (discontinued 1993) OTC *expectorant; oral anti-infective; minor topical anesthetic*

[menthol; guaifenesin; strong iodine tincture; phenol]
leniquinsin USAN, INN *antihypertensive*
lenitzol [see: amitriptyline]
lenograstim USAN, INN *immunomodulator; investigational treatment for chemotherapy-induced neutropenia*
Lenoxin ℞ *investigational topical ophthalmic corticosteroidal anti-inflammatory*
lenperone USAN, INN *antipsychotic*
Lens Clear solution (discontinued 1995) OTC *surfactant cleaning solution for soft contact lenses*
Lens Drops solution OTC *rewetting solution for hard or soft contact lenses*
Lens Fresh solution (discontinued 1995) OTC *rewetting solution for hard or soft contact lenses*
Lens Lubricant solution OTC *rewetting solution for hard or soft contact lenses*
Lens Plus Daily Cleaner solution OTC *surfactant cleaning solution for soft contact lenses*
Lens Plus Oxysept products [see: Oxysept]
Lens Plus Rewetting Drops OTC *rewetting solution for soft contact lenses*
Lens Plus Sterile Saline aerosol solution OTC *rinsing/storage solution for soft contact lenses* [preservative-free saline solution]
Lensept solutions (discontinued 1995) OTC *two-step chemical disinfecting system for soft contact lenses* [hydrogen peroxide based] 3%
Lensine solution (discontinued 1992) OTC *cleaning solution for hard contact lenses*
Lensrins solution (discontinued 1992) OTC *rinsing/storage solution for soft contact lenses* [preserved saline solution]
Lens-Wet solution (discontinued 1993) OTC *rewetting solution for soft or hard contact lenses*
Lentaron ℞ *investigational aromatase inhibitor for the treatment of breast cancer*
Lente Iletin I subcu injection OTC *antidiabetic* [insulin zinc (beef-pork)] 100 U/mL

Lente Iletin II (beef) subcu injection (discontinued 1994) OTC *antidiabetic* [insulin zinc] 100 U/mL
Lente Iletin II (pork) subcu injection OTC *antidiabetic* [insulin zinc] 100 U/mL
Lente Insulin subcu injection OTC *antidiabetic* [insulin zinc (beef)] 100 U/mL
Lente L subcu injection OTC *antidiabetic* [insulin zinc (pork)] 100 U/mL
Lente Purified Pork Insulin subcu injection (name changed to Lente L in 1994)
lentin [see: carbachol]
lentinan JAN *investigational (Phase II/III) immunomodulator for AIDS/ARC/HIV*
leptacline INN
lergotrile USAN, INN *prolactin enzyme inhibitor*
lergotrile mesylate USAN *prolactin enzyme inhibitor*
Lescol capsules ℞ *cholesterol-lowering antihyperlipidemic* [fluvastatin sodium] 20, 40 mg
lesopitron INN *investigational anxiolytic*
letimide INN *analgesic* [also: letimide HCl]
letimide HCl USAN *analgesic* [also: letimide]
letosteine INN
letrazuril INN *investigational treatment for AIDS-related cryptosporidial diarrhea*
letrozole USAN *antineoplastic; aromatase inhibitor*
leucarsone [see: carbarsone]
leucine (L-leucine) USAN, USP, INN, JAN *essential amino acid; symbols: Leu, L*
leucinocaine INN
leucocianidol INN
Leucomax (commercially available in 36 foreign countries) ℞ *investigational cytokine for AIDS (orphan: neutropenia; myelodysplastic syndrome; aplastic anemia)* [molgramostim]
leucomycin [see: kitasamycin; spiramycin]
Leucotropin ℞ *investigational antineoplastic* [blood cell growth factor]

L-leucovorin *investigational chemotherapy rescue; (orphan: adjunct to metastatic adenocarcinoma and osteosarcoma)*

leucovorin calcium USP *antianemic; folate replenisher; antidote to folic acid antagonist; methotrexate "rescue" (orphan)* [also: calcium folinate] 5, 15, 25 mg oral; 3 mg/mL injection; 50, 100, 350 mg/vial injection

leukemia inhibitory factor (LIF) *investigational multilineage cytokine for leukemia*

Leukeran tablets ℞ *alkylating antineoplastic for multiple leukemias, lymphomas, and neoplasms* [chlorambucil] 2 mg

Leukine powder for IV infusion ℞ *myeloid reconstitution after autologous bone marrow transplant (orphan); investigational AIDS drug* [sargramostim] 250, 500 μg

leukocyte interferon [now: interferon alfa-n3]

leukocyte protease inhibitor, secretory *(orphan: bronchopulmonary dysplasia)*

leukocyte protease inhibitor, secretory, recombinant *(orphan: congenital alpha₁ antitrypsin deficiency; cystic fibrosis)*

leukocyte typing serum USP *in vitro blood test*

leukopoietin [see: sargramostim]

leukotriene inhibitor *investigational 5-lipoxygenase inhibitor for topical treatment of psoriasis*

leupeptin *(orphan: aid in microsurgical peripheral nerve repair)*

leuprolide acetate USAN *hormonal antineoplastic for various cancers; LHRH agonist; for central precocious puberty (orphan)* [also: leuprorelin]

leuprorelin INN, BAN *antineoplastic; LHRH agonist* [also: leuprolide acetate]

leurocristine (LCR) [see: vincristine]

leurocristine sulfate [see: vincristine sulfate]

Leustatin IV infusion ℞ *antineoplastic (orphan: hairy cell and chronic lymphocytic leukemias; chronic multiple sclerosis)* [cladribine] 1 mg/mL

Leutrol ℞ *investigational 5-lipoxygenase inhibitor for asthma* [zileuton]

levacecarnine (acetyl L-carnitine) *investigational treatment for Alzheimer's disease*

levacetylmethadol INN *narcotic analgesic* [also: levomethadyl acetate]

levallorphan INN, BAN [also: levallorphan tartrate] ⑨ levorphanol

levallorphan tartrate USP [also: levallorphan]

levamfetamine INN *anorectic* [also: levamfetamine succinate; levamphetamine]

levamfetamine succinate USAN *anorectic* [also: levamfetamine; levamphetamine]

levamisole INN, BAN *antineoplastic; veterinary anthelmintic* [also: levamisole HCl]

levamisole HCl USAN *antineoplastic; veterinary anthelmintic; investigational immunomodulator for AIDS* [also: levamisole]

levamphetamine BAN *anorectic* [also: levamfetamine succinate; levamfetamine]

levarterenol [see: norepinephrine bitartrate]

levarterenol bitartrate [now: norepinephrine bitartrate]

Levatol tablets ℞ *antihypertensive; β-blocker* [penbutolol sulfate] 20 mg

Levbid extended-release tablets ℞ *GI anticholinergic; antispasmodic* [hyoscyamine sulfate] 0.375 mg

levcromakalim USAN, INN, BAN *antiasthmatic; antihypertensive*

levcycloserine USAN, INN *enzyme inhibitor; (orphan: Gaucher's disease)*

levdobutamine INN *cardiotonic* [also: levdobutamine lactobionate]

levdobutamine lactobionate USAN *cardiotonic* [also: levdobutamine]

levdropropizine INN

levemopamil INN *investigational treatment for stroke*

levisoprenaline INN

Levlen tablets ℞ *monophasic oral contraceptive* [levonorgestrel; ethinyl estradiol] 0.15 mg•30 μg

levlofexidine INN

levobetaxolol INN *antiadrenergic (β-receptor)* [also: levobetaxolol HCl]

levobetaxolol HCl USAN *antiadrenergic (β-receptor)* [also: levobetaxolol]

levobunolol INN, BAN *antiadrenergic (β-receptor); topical antiglaucoma agent* [also: levobunolol HCl]

levobunolol HCl USAN, USP *antiadrenergic; topical antiglaucoma agent (β-blocker)* [also: levobunolol] 0.25%, 0.5% eye drops

levocabastine INN, BAN *antihistamine* [also: levocabastine HCl]

levocabastine HCl USAN *antihistamine; for vernal keratoconjunctivitis (orphan)* [also: levocabastine]

levocarbinoxamine tartrate [see: rotoxamine tartrate]

levocarnitine USAN, USP, INN *dietary amino acid; (orphan: genetic carnitine deficiency; pediatric cardiomyopathy)* 250 mg oral

levodopa USAN, USP, INN, BAN, JAN *antiparkinsonian* ▷ methyldopa

Levo-Dromoran tablets, subcu or IV injection ℞ *narcotic analgesic; anxiolytic* [levorphanol tartrate] 2 mg; 2 mg/mL

levofacetoperane INN

levofenfluramine INN

levofloxacin INN *investigational antibacterial*

levofuraltadone USAN, INN *antibacterial; antiprotozoal*

levoglutamide INN *nonessential amino acid*

levoleucovorin calcium USAN *antidote to folic acid antagonists*

levomenol INN

levomepate [see: atromepine]

levomepromazine INN *analgesic* [also: methotrimeprazine]

levomethadone INN

levomethadyl acetate USAN *narcotic analgesic* [also: levacetylmethadol]

levomethadyl acetate HCl USAN *narcotic analgesic; narcotic agonist for management of opiate dependence (orphan)*

levomethorphan INN, BAN

levometiomeprazine INN

levomoprolol INN

levomoramide INN, BAN

levonantradol INN, BAN *analgesic* [also: levonantradol HCl]

levonantradol HCl USAN *analgesic* [also: levonantradol]

levonordefrin USP *adrenergic; vasoconstrictor* [also: corbadrine]

levonorgestrel USAN, USP, INN, BAN *progestin; contraceptive implant*

Levophed IV infusion ℞ *vasopressor for acute hypotensive shock* [norepinephrine bitartrate] 1 mg/mL

Levophed Bitartrate IV infusion ℞ *blood pressure control for acute or profound hypotension* [norepinephrine bitartrate]

levophenacylmorphan INN, BAN

Levoprome IM injection ℞ *central analgesic; CNS depressant* [methotrimeprazine HCl] 20 mg/mL

levopropicillin INN *antibacterial* [also: levopropylcillin potassium]

levopropicillin potassium [see: levopropylcillin potassium]

levopropoxyphene INN, BAN *antitussive* [also: levopropoxyphene napsylate]

levopropoxyphene napsylate USAN *antitussive* [also: levopropoxyphene]

levopropylcillin potassium USAN *antibacterial* [also: levopropicillin]

levopropylhexedrine INN

levoprotiline INN

Levora tablets ℞ *monophasic oral contraceptive* [levonorgestrel; ethinyl estradiol] 0.15 mg•30 μg

levorin INN

levorphanol INN, BAN *narcotic analgesic* [also: levorphanol tartrate] ▷ levallorphan

levorphanol tartrate USP *narcotic analgesic* [also: levorphanol]

Levo-T tablets ℞ *thyroid hormone* [levothyroxine sodium] 25, 50, 75, 100, 125, 150, 200, 300 μg

Levothroid tablets, powder for injection ℞ *thyroid hormone* [levothyroxine sodium] 25, 50, 75, 88, 100, 112, 125, 137, 150, 175, 200, 300 μg; 200, 500 μg

levothyroxine sodium (T_4) USP, INN *thyroid hormone* [also: thyroxine] 0.1,

0.15, 0.2, 0.3 mg oral; 200, 500 μg/vial injection ℞ liothyronine

Levovist intracoronary injection ℞ *ultrasound contrast agent* [galactose]

levoxadrol INN *local anesthetic; smooth muscle relaxant* [also: levoxadrol HCl]

levoxadrol HCl USAN *local anesthetic; smooth muscle relaxant* [also: levoxadrol]

Levoxine powder for IV injection (discontinued 1994) ℞ *thyroid hormone* [levothyroxine sodium] 200, 500 μg ℞ Lanoxin

Levoxine tablets (name changed to Levoxyl in 1994)

Levoxyl tablets ℞ *thyroid hormone* [levothyroxine sodium] 25, 50, 75, 88, 100, 112, 125, 137, 150, 175, 200, 300 μg

Levsin tablets, drops, IV, subcu or IM injection, elixir ℞ *GI anticholinergic; antispasmodic* [hyoscyamine sulfate] 0.125 mg; 0.125 mg/mL; 0.5 mg/mL; 0.125 mg/5 mL

Levsin PB drops ℞ *GI anticholinergic; sedative* [hyoscyamine sulfate; phenobarbital; alcohol 5%] 0.125•15 mg/mL

Levsin with Phenobarbital tablets ℞ *GI anticholinergic; sedative* [hyoscyamine sulfate; phenobarbital] 0.125•15 mg

Levsinex Timecaps (timed-release capsules) ℞ *GI anticholinergic; antispasmodic* [hyoscyamine sulfate] 0.375 mg

Levsinex with Phenobarbital Timecaps (timed-release capsules) (discontinued 1992) ℞ *GI anticholinergic; sedative* [hyoscyamine sulfate; phenobarbital] 0.375•45 mg

Levsin-PB drops ℞ *anticholinergic; sedative* [hyoscyamine sulfate; phenobarbital; alcohol 5%] 0.125•15 mg/mL

Levsin/SL sublingual tablets (also may be chewed or swallowed) ℞ *GI anticholinergic; antispasmodic* [hyoscyamine sulfate] 0.125 mg

levulose BAN *nutrient; caloric replacement* [also: fructose]

lexipafant USAN *platelet activating factor (PAF) antagonist*

lexithromycin USAN, INN *antibacterial*

lexofenac INN

LFA3TIP *investigational anti-inflammatory*

LHRF (luteinizing hormone-releasing factor) acetate hydrate [see: gonadorelin acetate]

LHRF diacetate tetrahydrate [now: gonadorelin acetate]

LHRF dihydrochloride [now: gonadorelin HCl]

LHRF HCl [see: gonadorelin HCl]

liarozole INN, BAN *investigational antipsoriatic and antineoplastic for prostatic cancer*

liarozole fumarate USAN *antipsoriatic; aromatase inhibitor*

liarozole HCl USAN *antineoplastic; aromatase inhibitor*

libecillide INN

libenzapril USAN, INN *angiotensin-converting enzyme (ACE) inhibitor*

Librax capsules ℞ *GI anticholinergic; anxiolytic* [clidinium bromide; chlordiazepoxide HCl] 2.5•5 mg

Libritabs film-coated tablets ℞ *anxiolytic* [chlordiazepoxide] 10, 25 mg

Librium capsules, powder for injection ℞ *anxiolytic* [chlordiazepoxide HCl] 5, 10, 25 mg; 100 mg

Lice-Enz foam shampoo OTC *pediculicide* [pyrethrins; piperonyl butoxide] 0.3%•3%

Licetrol 400 liquid (discontinued 1993) OTC *pediculicide* [pyrethrins; piperonyl butoxide; petroleum distillate]

Licoplex DS IM injection (discontinued 1995) ℞ *hematinic* [ferrous gluconate; multiple B vitamins; procaine HCl] 3 mg/mL• ± •2%

licryfilcon A USAN *hydrophilic contact lens material*

licryfilcon B USAN *hydrophilic contact lens material*

Lid Wipes-SPF solution, pads OTC *eyelid cleansing wipes for blepharitis or contact lenses*

Lidakol ℞ *investigational treatment for herpes simplex* [aliphatic alcohol compound]

Lida-Mantle-HC cream ℞ *local anesthetic; topical corticosteroid* [lidocaine; hydrocortisone acetate] 3%•0.5%

lidamidine INN *antiperistaltic* [also: lidamidine HCl]

lidamidine HCl USAN *antiperistaltic* [also: lidamidine]

Lidex cream, gel, ointment, topical solution ℞ *topical corticosteroid* [fluocinonide] 0.05% ⓡ Lasix; Lidox; Wydase

Lidex-E cream ℞ *topical corticosteroid; emollient* [fluocinonide] 0.05%

lidimycin INN *antifungal* [also: lydimycin]

lidocaine USP, INN *topical local anesthetic* [also: lignocaine]

lidocaine benzyl benzoate [see: denatonium benzoate]

lidocaine HCl USP *topical/injectable local anesthetic; antiarrhythmic* [also: lignocaine HCl] 2%, 4%, 5% topical; 1%, 1.5%, 2% injection; 4%, 10%, 20% IV admixture

lidofenin USAN, INN *hepatic function test*

lidofilcon A USAN *hydrophilic contact lens material*

lidofilcon B USAN *hydrophilic contact lens material*

lidoflazine USAN, INN, BAN *coronary vasodilator*

Lidoject-1; Lidoject-2 injection ℞ *injectable local anesthetic* [lidocaine HCl] 1%; 2%

LidoPen auto-injector (automatic IM injection device) ℞ *emergency injection for cardiac arrhythmias* [lidocaine HCl] 10%

Lidox capsules (discontinued 1995) ℞ *GI anticholinergic; anxiolytic* [clidinium bromide; chlordiazepoxide HCl] 2.5•5 mg ⓡ Lidex

Lids-N-Lashes ℞ *investigational eyelid hygiene product*

LIF (leukemia inhibitory factor) [q.v.]

lifarizine USAN *platelet aggregation inhibitor; investigational neural cell protector in stroke*

lifibrate USAN, INN *antihyperlipoproteinemic*

lifibrol USAN, INN *antihyperlipidemic*

Lifoject IM injection (discontinued 1993) ℞ *antianemic; vitamin supplement* [liver extracts; vitamin B$_{12}$; folic acid]

Lifolbex IM injection (discontinued 1994) ℞ *hematinic; vitamin supplement* [liver extracts; folic acid; cyanocobalamin]

Lifomin-R IM injection (discontinued 1994) ℞ *antianemic; vitamin supplement* [liver extracts; vitamin B$_{12}$; folic acid]

light mineral oil [see: mineral oil, light]

lignocaine BAN *topical local anesthetic* [also: lidocaine]

lignocaine HCl BAN *local anesthetic; antiarrhythmic* [also: lidocaine HCl]

lignosulfonic acid, sodium salt [see: polignate sodium]

lilopristone INN

limaprost INN

limarsol [see: acetarsone]

Limbitrol DS 10-25 tablets ℞ *antidepressant; anxiolytic* [chlordiazepoxide; amitryptyline HCl] 10•25 mg

lime USP *pharmaceutic necessity*

lime, sulfurated (calcium polysulfide, calcium thiosulfate) USP *wet dressing/soak for cystic acne and seborrhea*

linarotene USAN, INN *antikeratinizing agent*

Lincocin capsules, pediatric capsules, IV or IM injection ℞ *antibiotic* [lincomycin HCl] 500 mg; 250 mg; 300 mg/mL ⓡ Cleocin; Indocin

lincomycin USAN, INN, BAN *bactericidal antibiotic*

lincomycin HCl USP *bactericidal antibiotic*

Lincorex IV or IM injection ℞ *antibiotic* [lincomycin HCl] 300 mg/mL

lindane USAN, USP, INN, BAN *pediculicide; scabicide* 1% topical

Linguets (trademarked form) *buccal tablets*

linogliride USAN, INN *antidiabetic*

linogliride fumarate USAN *antidiabetic*

linolexamide [see: clinolamide]

Linomide ℞ *investigational (Phase II) immunomodulator for HIV (orphan: bone marrow transplant for leukemia)* [roquinimex]

linopiridine USAN, INN *cognition enhancer for Alzheimer's disease*

linsidomine INN

lintopride INN

Lioresal intrathecal injection ℞ *skeletal muscle relaxant; intractable spasticity treatment (orphan)* [baclofen] 10 mg/20 mL (500 μg/mL), 10 mg/5 mL (2000 μg/mL)

Lioresal tablets ℞ *skeletal muscle relaxant (orphan: spasticity)* [baclofen] 10, 20 mg

liothyronine INN, BAN *radioactive agent* [also: liothyronine I 125] ⑨ levothyroxine

liothyronine I 125 USAN *radioactive agent* [also: liothyronine]

liothyronine I 131 USAN *radioactive agent*

liothyronine sodium (T_3) USP, BAN *thyroid hormone; treatment of myxedema coma or precoma (orphan)* 25 μg oral

liotrix USAN, USP *thyroid hormone* ⑨ Klotrix

Lip Medex ointment OTC *topical antipruritic/counterirritant; mild local anesthetic* [camphor; phenol] 1%•0.54%

lipancreatin [see: pancrelipase]

lipase of pancreas [see: pancrelipase]

lipase triacylglycerol [see: pancrelipase]

Lipidil capsules (discontinued 1994) ℞ *triglyceride-lowering agent* [fenofibrate]

Lipidox ℞ *investigational antineoplastic for breast cancer* [liposomal doxorubicin]

Lipisorb powder OTC *enteral nutritional therapy* [lactose-free formula]

Liple (commercially available in Japan) ℞ *investigational agent for peripheral arterial occlusive disease and diabetic peripheral neuropathy* [liposomal PGE_1]

Lipoflavonoid capsules OTC *dietary lipotropic with vitamin supplementation* [choline; inositol; multiple B vitamins; vitamin C; lemon bioflavonoids] 111.3•111.3•≛•100•100 mg

Lipogen capsules, caplets OTC *dietary lipotropic with vitamin supplementation* [choline; inositol; multiple vitamins] 111•111•≛ mg

Lipomul liquid OTC *dietary fat supplement* [corn oil] 10 g/15 mL

Lipo-Nicin/100 tablets (discontinued 1996) ℞ *peripheral vasodilator* [niacin; niacinamide; multiple vitamins] 100•75•≛ mg

Lipo-Nicin/250 tablets (discontinued 1994) ℞ *peripheral vasodilator* [niacin; niacinamide; multiple vitamins] 250•75•≛ mg

Lipo-Nicin/300 timed-release capsules (discontinued 1996) ℞ *peripheral vasodilator* [niacin; multiple vitamins] 300•≛ mg

Liponol capsules OTC *dietary lipotropic with vitamin supplementation* [choline; inositol; methionine; multiple B vitamins] 115•83•110•≛ mg

Lipo-Plus soft capsules OTC *dietary supplement* [choline; inositol; L-methionine; porcine liver concentrate; lecithin]

liposomal gentamicin [see: gentamicin liposome]

liposome-encapsulated recombinant interleukin-2 [see: interleukin-2, liposome-encapsulated recombinant]

liposome-encapsulated T4 endonuclease V [see: T4 endonuclease V, liposome encapsulated]

Liposyn II 10%; Liposyn III 10% IV infusion (discontinued 1996) ℞ *nutritional therapy* [intravenous fat emulsion]

Liposyn II 20%; Liposyn III 20% IV infusion ℞ *nutritional therapy* [intravenous fat emulsion]

Lipo-Tears eye drops (discontinued 1993) OTC *ocular moisturizer/lubricant*

Lipotriad caplets OTC *dietary lipotropic with vitamin supplementation* [choline; inositol; multiple vitamins] 111•≛•≛ mg

Lipotriad liquid (discontinued 1994) OTC *dietary lipotropic with vitamin supplementation* [choline; inositol; multiple B vitamins] 334•≛•≛ mg/5 mL

Lipovite capsules (discontinued 1995) OTC *vitamin supplement* [multiple B vitamins] ≛

Liquaemin Sodium IV or deep subcu injection ℞ *anticoagulant* [heparin sodium] 1000, 5000, 10,000, 20,000, 40,000 U/mL

liquefied phenol [see: phenol, liquefied]

Liquibid sustained-release tablet ℞ *expectorant* [guaifenesin] 600 mg

Liqui-Cal softgels OTC *calcium supplement* [calcium carbonate]

Liqui-Char oral liquid OTC *adsorbent antidote for poisoning* [activated charcoal] 12.5 g/60 mL, 15 g/75 mL, 25 g/120 mL, 30 g/120 mL, 50 g/240 mL

Liquid Cal-600 soft capsule OTC *calcium supplement* [calcium carbonate]

Liquid Caps (dosage form) *soft liquid-filled capsules*

liquid glucose [see: glucose, liquid]

Liquid Lather body wash (discontinued 1995) OTC *bath emollient*

liquid petrolatum [see: mineral oil]

Liquid Pred syrup ℞ *glucocorticoids* [prednisone; alcohol 5%] 5 mg/5 mL

Liquid Tabs (dosage form) *liquid-filled tablets*

Liqui-Doss emulsion OTC *emollient laxative* [mineral oil]

Liquifilm Tears; Liquifilm Forte eye drops OTC *ocular moisturizer/lubricant* [polyvinyl alcohol] 1.4%; 3%

Liquifilm Wetting solution OTC *wetting solution for hard contact lenses*

Liqui-Histine DM syrup ℞ *antitussive; decongestant; antihistamine* [dextromethorphan hydrobromide; phenylpropanolamine HCl; brompheniramine maleate] 10•12.5•2 mg/5 mL

Liqui-Histine-D elixir ℞ *decongestant; antihistamine* [phenylpropanolamine HCl; phenyltoloxamine citrate; pyrilamine maleate; pheniramine maleate] 12.5•4•4•4 mg/5 mL

Liquimat lotion OTC *antibacterial and exfoliant for acne* [sulfur] 4%

Liquipake suspension ℞ *GI contrast radiopaque agent* [barium sulfate] 100%

Liquiprin elixir, infant's drops OTC *analgesic; antipyretic* [acetaminophen] 160 mg/5 mL; 120 mg/2.5 mL

Liquitab (trademarked dosage form) *chewable tablet*

liquor carbonis detergens (LCD) [see: coal tar]

liroldine INN

lisadimate USAN, INN *sunscreen*

lisinopril USAN, INN, BAN *antihypertensive; angiotensin-converting enzyme (ACE) inhibitor for CHF and acute MI*

lisofylline USAN *immunomodulator*

Listerex Scrub lotion (discontinued 1995) OTC *topical keratolytic for acne* [salicylic acid] 2%

Listerine; Cool-Mint Listerine; FreshBurst Listerine mouthwash/gargle OTC *oral antiseptic* [thymol; eucalyptol; methyl salicylate; menthol; alcohol 22%–26%] 0.06%•0.09%•0.06%•0.04%

Listerine Throat; Listerine Antiseptic lozenges (discontinued 1994) OTC *oral antiseptic* [hexylresorcinol] 2.4 mg; 4 mg

Listermint Arctic Mint mouthwash/gargle OTC

Listermint with Fluoride oral rinse (discontinued 1995) OTC *topical dental caries preventative* [sodium fluoride] 0.02%

lisuride INN [also: lysuride]

Lithane tablets ℞ *antipsychotic* [lithium carbonate] 300 mg

lithium *element (Li)*

lithium benzoate NF

lithium carbonate USAN, USP *antimanic; immunity booster in chemotherapy and AIDS* 150, 300, 600 mg oral

lithium citrate USP *antimanic; immunity booster in chemotherapy and AIDS* 300 mg/5 mL oral

lithium hydroxide USP *antimanic*

lithium hydroxide monohydrate [see: lithium hydroxide]

lithium salicylate NF

Lithobid slow-release tablets ℞ *antipsychotic* [lithium carbonate] 300 mg

Lithonate capsules ℞ *antipsychotic* [lithium carbonate] 300 mg

Lithostat tablets ℞ *adjunctive therapy in urea-splitting urinary tract infections* [acetohydroxamic acid] 250 mg

Lithotabs film-coated tablets ℞ *antipsychotic* [lithium carbonate] 300 mg

litracen INN

Liver Combo No. 5 IM injection ℞ *antianemic; vitamin supplement* [liver extracts; vitamin B_{12}; folic acid] 10 μg•100 μg•0.4 mg per mL

liver derivative complex *claimed to be an anti-inflammatory for various dermatological conditions*

liver extracts *source of vitamin B_{12}*

Livial (commercially available in Europe, Asia, and South America) ℞ *investigational agent for hormone replacement therapy*

lividomycin INN

Livifol IM injection (discontinued 1994) ℞ *antianemic; vitamin supplement* [liver extracts; vitamin B_{12}; folic acid]

Livitamin capsules (discontinued 1995) OTC *hematinic* [ferrous fumarate; desiccated liver; multiple vitamins] 33•150•≟ mg

Livitamin chewable tablets (discontinued 1995) OTC *hematinic* [ferrous fumarate; multiple B vitamins; vitamin C] 16.4•≟•100 mg

Livitamin liquid (discontinued 1995) OTC *hematinic* [peptonized iron; liver fraction 1; multiple B vitamins] 35.5•500•≟ mg/15 mL

Livitamin with Intrinsic Factor capsules (discontinued 1995) ℞ *hematinic* [ferrous fumarate; multiple B vitamins; ascorbic acid; desiccated liver; intrinsic factor concentrate] 33 mg•≟•100 mg•150 mg•0.33 U

Livitrinsic-f capsules ℞ *hematinic* [ferrous fumarate; cyanocobalamin; ascorbic acid; intrinsic factor concentrate; folic acid] 110 mg•15 μg•75 mg•240 mg•0.5 mg

Livostin eye drop suspension ℞ *topical antihistamine for allergic conjunctivitis* [levocarbastine HCl] 0.05%

Livostin nasal spray ℞ *investigational treatment for seasonal allergic rhinitis* [levocarbastine HCl]

Livroben IM injection (discontinued 1993) ℞ *antianemic; vitamin supplement* [liver extracts; vitamin B_{12}; folic acid]

lixazinone sulfate USAN *cardiotonic; phosphodiesterase inhibitor*

LKV Infant Drops powder + liquid OTC *vitamin supplement* [multiple vitamins; biotin] ≟•75 μg/0.6 mL

LLD factor [see: cyanocobalamin]

10% LMD IV injection ℞ *plasma volume expander for shock due to hemorrhage, burns, or surgery* [dextran 40] 10%

LMD (low molecular weight dextran) [see: dextran 40]

LMF (Leukeran, methotrexate, fluorouracil) *chemotherapy protocol*

LMWD (low molecular weight dextran) [see: dextran 40]

Lobac capsules ℞ *skeletal muscle relaxant; analgesic* [salicylamide; phenyltoloxamine; acetaminophen] 200•20•300 mg

Lobana Body lotion OTC *moisturizer; emollient*

Lobana Body Shampoo; Lobana Liquid Lather liquid OTC *soap-free therapeutic skin cleanser* [chloroxylenol]

Lobana Derm-Ade cream OTC *moisturizer; emollient* [vitamins A, D, and E]

Lobana Peri-Garde ointment OTC *moisturizer; emollient; antiseptic* [vitamins A, D, and E; chloroxylenol]

lobeline INN *nicotine withdrawal aid* [also: lobeline HCl]

lobeline HCl JAN *nicotine withdrawal aid* [also: lobeline]

lobendazole USAN, INN *veterinary anthelmintic*

lobenzarit INN *antirheumatic* [also: lobenzarit sodium]

lobenzarit sodium USAN *antirheumatic* [also: lobenzarit]

lobucavir USAN *antiviral; investigational (Phase I) for AIDS-related asymptomatic cytomegalovirus*

lobuprofen INN

Loceryl cream, nail lacquer (commercially available in Europe) ℞ *investigational antifungal* [amorolfine]

locicortolone dicibate INN

locicortone [see: locicortolone dicibate]

Locoid ointment, cream (discontinued 1993) ℞ *topical corticosteroid* [hydrocortisone butyrate]

Locoid solution ℞ *topical corticosteroid* [hydrocortisone butyrate; alcohol 50%] 0.1%

lodaxaprine INN

lodazecar INN

lodelaben USAN, INN *antiarthritic; emphysema therapy adjunct*

Lodine film-coated tablets, capsules ℞ *nonsteroidal anti-inflammatory drug (NSAID); analgesic; antiarthritic* [etodolac] 200, 300, 400, 500 mg

Lodine ER; Lodine SR ℞ *investigational once-daily anti-inflammatory* [etodolac]

lodinixil INN

lodiperone INN

Lodosyn tablets ℞ *antiparkinsonian agent when used with levodopa (no effect when given alone)* [carbidopa] 25 mg

lodoxamide INN, BAN *antiallergic; antiasthmatic* [also: lodoxamide ethyl]

lodoxamide ethyl USAN *antiallergic; antiasthmatic* [also: lodoxamide]

lodoxamide trometamol BAN *antiallergic; antiasthmatic* [also: lodoxamide tromethamine]

lodoxamide tromethamine USAN *antiallergic; antiasthmatic; for vernal keratoconjunctivitis (orphan)* [also: lodoxamide trometamol]

Lodrane LD sustained-release capsules ℞ *decongestant; antihistamine* [pseudoephedrine HCl; brompheniramine maleate] 60•6 mg

Loestrin 21 1/20; Loestrin 21 1.5/30 tablets ℞ *monophasic oral contraceptive* [norethindrone acetate; ethinyl estradiol] 1 mg•20 µg; 1.5 mg•30 µg

Loestrin Fe 1/20; Loestrin Fe 1.5/30 tablets ℞ *monophasic oral contraceptive; iron supplement* [norethindrone acetate; ethinyl estradiol; ferrous fumarate] 1 mg•20 µg•75 mg; 1.5 mg•30 µg•75 mg

lofemizole INN *anti-inflammatory; analgesic; antipyretic* [also: lofemizole HCl]

lofemizole HCl USAN *anti-inflammatory; analgesic; antipyretic* [also: lofemizole]

Lofenalac powder OTC *special diet for infants with phenylketonuria*

lofendazam INN, BAN

Lofene tablets (discontinued 1993) ℞ *antidiarrheal* [diphenoxylate HCl; atropine sulfate]

lofentanil INN, BAN *narcotic analgesic* [also: lofentanil oxalate]

lofentanil oxalate USAN *narcotic analgesic* [also: lofentanil]

lofepramine INN, BAN *antidepressant* [also: lofepramine HCl]

lofepramine HCl USAN *antidepressant* [also: lofepramine]

lofexidine INN, BAN *antihypertensive* [also: lofexidine HCl]

lofexidine HCl USAN *antihypertensive* [also: lofexidine]

loflucarban INN

LoFrin ℞ *5-lipoxygenase inhibitor* [fenleuton]

Logen tablets ℞ *antidiarrheal* [diphenoxylate HCl; atropine sulfate] 2.5•0.025 mg

Logiparin ℞ *investigational antithrombotic for deep vein thrombosis* [low molecular weight heparin]

LOMAC (leucovorin, Oncovin, methotrexate, Adriamycin, cyclophosphamide) *chemotherapy protocol*

Lomanate liquid ℞ *antidiarrheal* [diphenoxylate HCl; atropine sulfate] 2.5•0.025 mg/5 mL

lombazole INN, BAN

lomefloxacin USAN, INN, BAN *antibacterial*

lomefloxacin HCl USAN *broad-spectrum bactericidal antibiotic*

lomefloxacin mesylate USAN *antibacterial*

lometraline INN *antipsychotic; antiparkinsonian* [also: lometraline HCl]

lometraline HCl USAN *antipsychotic; antiparkinsonian* [also: lometraline]

lometrexol INN *antineoplastic* [also: lometrexol sodium]

lometrexol sodium USAN *antineoplastic* [also: lometrexol]

lomevactone INN

lomifylline INN

Lomodix tablets (discontinued 1993) ℞ *antidiarrheal* [diphenoxylate HCl; atropine sulfate]

lomofungin USAN *antifungal*

Lomotil tablets, liquid ℞ *antidiarrheal* [diphenoxylate HCl; atropine sulfate] 2.5•0.025 mg; 2.5•0.025 mg/5 mL

lomustine USAN, INN, BAN *alkylating antineoplastic*

Lonalac powder OTC *enteral nutritional therapy* [milk-based formula]

lonapalene USAN *antipsoriatic*

lonaprofen INN

lonazolac INN

lonidamine INN

Loniten tablets ℞ *antihypertensive; vasodilator* [minoxidil] 2.5, 10 mg ☒ clonidine

Lonox tablets ℞ *antidiarrheal* [diphenoxylate HCl; atropine sulfate] 2.5•0.025 mg

Lo/Ovral tablets ℞ *monophasic oral contraceptive* [norgestrel; ethinyl estradiol] 0.3 mg•30 μg

loperamide INN, BAN *antiperistaltic; antidiarrheal* [also: loperamide HCl]

loperamide HCl USAN, USP, JAN *antiperistaltic; antidiarrheal* [also: loperamide] 2 mg oral; 1 mg/5 mL oral

loperamide oxide INN, BAN *investigational antiperistaltic*

Lopid tablets ℞ *antihyperlipidemic agent (cholesterol-lowering)* [gemfibrozil] 600 mg

Lopid-SR ℞ *investigational cholesterol-lowering agent* [gemfibrozil]

lopirazepam INN

loprazolam INN, BAN

lopremone [now: protirelin]

Lopressor tablets, IV injection ℞ *antianginal; antihypertensive; β-blocker* [metoprolol tartrate] 50, 100 mg; 1 mg/mL

Lopressor HCT 50/25; Lopressor HCT 100/25; Lopressor HCT 100/50 tablets ℞ *antihypertensive* [metoprolol tartrate; hydrochlorothiazide] 50•25 mg; 100•25 mg; 100•50 mg

loprodiol INN

Loprox cream, lotion ℞ *topical antifungal* [ciclopirox olamine] 1%

Lorabid Pulvules (capsules), powder for oral suspension ℞ *carbacephem-type antibiotic* [loracarbef] 200, 400, 500 mg; 100, 200 mg/5 mL

loracarbef USAN, INN *antibacterial*

lorajmine INN *antiarrhythmic* [also: lorajmine HCl]

lorajmine HCl USAN *antiarrhythmic* [also: lorajmine]

lorapride INN

loratadine USAN, INN, BAN *antihistamine*

lorazepam USAN, USP, INN, BAN *anxiolytic; minor tranquilizer* 0.5, 1, 2 mg oral; 2 mg/mL oral; 2, 4 mg/mL injection

lorbamate USAN, INN *muscle relaxant*

lorcainide INN, BAN *antiarrhythmic* [also: lorcainide HCl]

lorcainide HCl USAN *antiarrhythmic* [also: lorcainide]

Lorcet; Lorcet Plus; Lorcet 10/650 tablets ℞ *narcotic analgesic* [hydrocodone bitartrate; acetaminophen] 5•500 mg; 7.5•650 mg; 10•650 mg

Lorcet-HD capsules ℞ *narcotic analgesic* [hydrocodone bitartrate; acetaminophen] 5•500 mg ☒ Fioricet

lorcinadol USAN, INN, BAN *analgesic*

loreclezole USAN, INN, BAN *antiepileptic*

Lorelco tablets (discontinued 1996) ℞ *serum cholesterol reduction* [probucol] 250, 500 mg

lorglumide INN

lormetazepam USAN, INN, BAN *sedative; hypnotic*

lornoxicam USAN, INN, BAN *analgesic; anti-inflammatory*

Lorothidol (available only from the Centers for Disease Control) ℞ *investigational anti-infective for paragonimiasis and fascioliasis* [bithionol]

Loroxide lotion OTC *topical keratolytic for acne* [benzoyl peroxide] 5.5%

lorpiprazole INN

Lortab elixir ℞ *narcotic analgesic* [hydrocodone bitartrate; acetaminophen; alcohol 7%] 2.5•167 mg/5 mL

Lortab 2.5/500; Lortab 5/500; Lortab 7.5/500; Lortab 10/500 tablets ℞ *narcotic analgesic* [hydrocodone bitartrate; acetaminophen] 2.5•500 mg; 5•500 mg; 7.5•500 mg; 10•500 mg

Lortab ASA tablets ℞ *narcotic analgesic* [hydrocodone bitartrate; aspirin] 5•500 mg

lortalamine USAN, INN *antidepressant*

lorzafone USAN, INN *minor tranquilizer*
losartan INN *antihypertensive; angiotensin II antagonist* [also: losartan potassium]
losartan potassium USAN *antihypertensive; angiotensin II antagonist* [also: losartan]
Losec (foreign name for U.S. product Prilosec)
losigamone INN
losindole INN
losmiprofen INN
Losotron Plus liquid (discontinued 1994) OTC *antacid; antiflatulent* [magaldrate; simethicone] 108•4 mg/mL
losoxantrone INN *antineoplastic* [also: losoxantrone HCl]
losoxantrone HCl USAN *antineoplastic* [also: losoxantrone]
losulazine INN *antihypertensive* [also: losulazine HCl]
losulazine HCl USAN *antihypertensive* [also: losulazine]
Lotensin tablets ℞ *antihypertensive; angiotensin-converting enzyme (ACE) inhibitor* [benazepril HCl] 5, 10, 20, 40 mg
Lotensin HCT 5/6.25; Lotensin HCT 10/12.5; Lotensin HCT 20/12.5; Lotensin HCT 20/25 tablets ℞ *antihypertensive* [benazepril; hydrochlorothiazide] 5•6.25 mg; 10•12.5 mg; 20•12.5 mg; 20•25 mg
loteprednol INN *topical anti-inflammatory* [also: loteprednol etabonate]
loteprednol etabonate USAN *topical anti-inflammatory* [also: loteprednol]
lotifazole INN
Lotrel capsules ℞ *antihypertensive* [amlodipine besylate; benazepril HCl] 2.5•10, 5•10, 5•20 mg
lotrifen INN
Lotrimin cream, solution, lotion ℞ *topical antifungal* [clotrimazole] 1% ② Otrivin
Lotrimin AF cream, solution, lotion OTC *topical antifungal* [clotrimazole] 1%
Lotrimin AF powder, spray powder, spray liquid OTC *topical antifungal* [miconazole nitrate] 2%
Lotrisone cream ℞ *topical corticosteroid; antifungal* [betamethasone dipropionate; clotrimazole] 0.05%•1%

lotucaine INN
Lovan ℞ *investigational obesity and bulimia treatment* [fluoxetine]
lovastatin USAN, INN, BAN *antihypercholesterolemic; HMG-CoA reductase inhibitor*
Lovenox subcu injection ℞ *anticoagulant; antithrombotic for deep vein thrombosis following hip replacement* [enoxaparin sodium (low molecular weight heparin)] 30 mg/0.3 mL
loviride INN *investigational treatment for AIDS*
low molecular weight dextran (LMD; LMWD) [see: dextran 40]
Lowila Cake bar OTC *soap-free therapeutic skin cleanser*
Low-Quel tablets (discontinued 1993) ℞ *antidiarrheal* [diphenoxylate HCl; atropine sulfate]
Lowsium chewable tablets, oral suspension (tablets discontinued and suspension renamed Lowsium Plus in 1994)
Lowsium Plus oral suspension OTC *antacid; antiflatulent* [magaldrate; simethicone] 540•40 mg/5 mL
loxanast INN
loxapine USAN, INN, BAN *minor tranquilizer; antipsychotic*
loxapine HCl *minor tranquilizer; antipsychotic*
loxapine succinate USAN *minor tranquilizer; antipsychotic* 5, 10, 25, 50 mg oral
loxiglumide INN
Loxitane capsules ℞ *antipsychotic* [loxapine succinate] 5, 10, 25, 50 mg
Loxitane C oral concentrate ℞ *antipsychotic* [loxapine HCl] 25 mg/mL
Loxitane IM injection ℞ *antipsychotic* [loxapine HCl] 50 mg/mL
loxoprofen INN
loxoribine USAN, INN *immunostimulant; vaccine adjuvant; (orphan: common variable immunodeficiency)*
loxotidine [now: lavoltidine succinate]
loxtidine BAN *antiulcerative; histamine H_2-receptor blocker* [also: lavoltidine succinate; lavoltidine]
lozilurea INN
Lozi-Tabs (trademarked form) *lozenges*

Lozol film-coated tablets ℞ *antihypertensive; diuretic* [indapamide] 1.25, 2.5 mg

L-PAM (L-phenylalanine mustard) [see: melphalan]

LR (lactated Ringer's) solution [see: Ringer's injection, lactated]

LSD (lysergic acid diethylamide) [see: lysergide]

lubeluzole INN *investigational therapy for ischemic stroke*

LubraSol Bath Oil OTC *bath emollient*

Lubricating Gel OTC *vaginal antimicrobial and lubricant* [chlorhexidine gluconate; glycerin]

Lubricating Jelly OTC *vaginal lubricant* [glycerin; propylene glycol]

Lubriderm cream, lotion OTC *moisturizer; emollient*

Lubriderm Bath Oil OTC *bath emollient*

Lubrin vaginal inserts OTC *lubricant for sexual intercourse* [glycerin; caprylic triglyceride] ♀

LubriTears eye drops OTC *ocular moisturizer/lubricant* [hydroxypropyl methylcellulose] 0.3%

LubriTears ophthalmic ointment OTC *ocular moisturizer/lubricant* [white petrolatum; mineral oil; lanolin]

lucanthone INN, BAN *antischistosomal* [also: lucanthone HCl]

lucanthone HCl USAN, USP *antischistosomal* [also: lucanthone]

lucartamide INN

lucensomycin [see: lucimycin]

lucimycin INN

Ludiomil coated tablets ℞ *tetracyclic antidepressant* [maprotiline HCl] 25, 50, 75 mg

lufironil USAN, INN *collagen inhibitor*

lufuradom INN

Lufyllin tablets, elixir, IM injection ℞ *bronchodilator* [dyphylline] 200, 400 mg; 100 mg/15 mL; 250 mg/mL

Lufyllin-EPG tablets, elixir ℞ *antiasthmatic; bronchodilator; decongestant; expectorant; sedative* [dyphylline; ephedrine HCl; guaifenesin; phenobarbital] 100•16•200•16 mg; 150•24•300•24 mg/15 mL

Lufyllin-GG tablets, elixir ℞ *antiasthmatic; bronchodilator; expectorant* [dyphylline; guaifenesin] 200•200 mg; 100•100 mg/15 mL

Lugol solution ℞ *thyroid-blocking therapy; topical antimicrobial* [iodine; potassium iodide] 5%•10%

LumenHance ℞ *investigational GI contrast agent for MRI* [manganese chloride]

Luminal Sodium IV or IM injection ℞ *long-acting barbiturate sedative, hypnotic and anticonvulsant* [phenobarbital sodium] 130 mg/mL ⓢ Tuinal

Lumirem (European name for U.S. product Gastromark)

Lung Check sputum test for professional use (discontinued 1993) *in vitro diagnostic aid for precancerous lung cells*

lung surfactant, synthetic [see: colfosceril palmitate]

2,6-lupetidine [see: nanofin]

lupitidine INN *veterinary antagonist to histamine H_2 receptors* [also: lupitidine HCl]

lupitidine HCl USAN *veterinary antagonist to histamine H_2 receptors* [also: lupitidine]

Lupron subcu injection (daily) ℞ *hormonal chemotherapy for prostatic cancer and central precocious puberty (CPP)* [leuprolide acetate] 5 mg/mL

Lupron Depot microspheres for IM injection (monthly) ℞ *hormonal chemotherapy for prostatic cancer, endometriosis, and uterine fibroids* [leuprolide acetate] 3.75, 7.5 mg

Lupron Depot–3 month microspheres IM injection ℞ *hormonal chemotherapy for prostatic cancer* [leuprolide acetate] 22.5 mg

Lupron Depot-Ped microspheres for IM injection (monthly) ℞ *hormonal chemotherapy for prostatic cancer and central precocious puberty (CPP)* [leuprolide acetate] 7.5, 11.25, 15 mg

luprostiol INN, BAN

Luramide tablets (discontinued 1993) ℞ *loop diuretic* [furosemide]

Luride Lozi-Tabs (chewable tablets), drops, gel ℞ *dental caries preventative* [sodium fluoride] 0.25, 1.1, 2.2 mg; 1.1 mg/mL; 1.2%

Luride SF Lozi-Tabs (lozenges) ℞ *dental caries preventative* [sodium fluoride] 2.2 mg

Lurline PMS tablets OTC *analgesic; antipyretic; diuretic; vitamin* [acetaminophen; pamabrom; pyridoxine] 500•25•50 mg

lurosetron mesylate USAN *antiemetic*

luteinizing hormone-releasing factor acetate hydrate [see: gonadorelin acetate]

luteinizing hormone-releasing factor diacetate tetrahydrate [now: gonadorelin acetate]

luteinizing hormone-releasing factor dihydrochloride [now: gonadorelin HCl]

luteinizing hormone-releasing factor HCl [see: gonadorelin HCl]

lutetium *element* (Lu)

lutrelin INN *luteinizing hormone-releasing hormone (LHRH) agonist* [also: lutrelin acetate]

lutrelin acetate USAN *luteinizing hormone-releasing hormone (LHRH) agonist* [also: lutrelin]

Lutrepulse powder for continuous ambulatory infusion ℞ *gonadotropin-releasing hormone for hypothalamic amenorrhea (orphan)* [gonadorelin acetate] 0.8, 3.2 mg

LuVax ℞ *investigational treatment for small cell lung cancer* [anti-idiotypic antiboby vaccine] ② Luvox

Luvox tablets ℞ *antidepressant; selective serotonin reuptake inhibitor (SSRI) for obsessive-compulsive disorder* [fluvoxamine maleate] 50, 100 mg ② LuVax

luxabendazole INN, BAN

L-VAM (leuprolide acetate, vinblastine, Adriamycin, mitomycin) *chemotherapy protocol*

LY 293111 *investigational antiasthmatic*

lyapolate sodium USAN *anticoagulant* [also: sodium apolate]

lycetamine USAN *topical antimicrobial*

lycine HCl [see: betaine HCl]

Lycolan elixir (discontinued 1993) OTC *oral amino acid supplement* [L-lysine]

lydimycin USAN *antifungal* [also: lidimycin]

lymecycline INN, BAN

Lymphazurin 1% injection ℞ *adjunct radiopaque agent for lymphography* [isosulfan blue] 1%

lymphocyte immune globulin, antithymocyte *passive immunizing agent*

lymphogranuloma venereum antigen USP

lynestrenol USAN, INN *progestin* [also: lynoestrenol]

lynoestrenol BAN *progestin* [also: lynestrenol]

Lyo-Ject (trademarked delivery system) *prefilled dual-chambered syringe with lyophilized powder and diluent*

Lyphazome ℞ *investigational treatment for burns* [liposomal silver sulfadiazine]

Lyphocin powder for IV or IM injection ℞ *glycopeptide-type antibiotic* [vancomycin HCl] 0.5, 1, 5 g

Lypholized Vitamin B Complex & Vitamin C with B_{12} injection ℞ *parenteral vitamin therapy* [multiple B vitamins; vitamin C] ±•50 mg/mL

Lypholyte; Lypholyte II IV admixture ℞ *intravenous electrolyte therapy* [combined electrolyte solution]

lypressin USAN, USP, INN, BAN *posterior pituitary hormone; antidiuretic; vasoconstrictor*

lysergic acid diethylamide (LSD) [see: lysergide]

lysergide INN, BAN

lysine (L-lysine) USAN, INN *essential amino acid; symbols:* Lys, K 312, 500, 1000 mg oral

lysine acetate USP *amino acid*

DL-lysine acetylsalicylate (*orphan status withdrawn 1993*) [see: aspirin DL-lysine]

lysine HCl USAN, USP *amino acid*

L-lysine monoacetate [see: lysine acetate]

L-lysine monohydrochloride [see: lysine HCl]

8-L-lysine vasopressin [see: lypressin]

Lysodren tablets ℞ *antisteroidal antineoplastic for inoperable adrenal cortical carcinoma and Cushing syndrome* [mitotane] 500 mg

lysostaphin USAN *antibacterial enzyme*

LysPro [see: Humalog]

lysuride BAN [also: lisuride]

M2 3 + E tablets OTC *vitamin/mineral supplement* [calcium aspartate; magnesium aspartate; potassium aspartate; vitamin E]

M2 B60 timed-release capsules OTC *vitamin/mineral supplement* [multiple B vitamins; vitamin C; magnesium]

M2 B125 timed-release tablets OTC *vitamin supplement* [multiple B vitamins]

M2 C timed-release capsules OTC *vitamin supplement* [ascorbic acid; rutin]

M-2 protocol (vincristine, carmustine, cyclophosphamide, melphalan, prednisone) *chemotherapy protocol*

MAA (macroaggregated albumin) [see: albumin, aggregated]

Maalox chewable tablets, oral suspension OTC *antacid* [aluminum hydroxide; magnesium hydroxide] 200•200, 350•350 mg; 225•200 mg/5 mL ⑨ Marax

Maalox, Extra Strength oral suspension OTC *antacid; antiflatulent* [aluminum hydroxide; magnesium hydroxide; simethicone] 500•450•40 mg/5 mL

Maalox Antacid caplets OTC *antacid* [calcium carbonate] 1 g

Maalox Anti-Diarrheal caplets OTC *antidiarrheal* [loperamide HCl] 2 mg

Maalox Anti-Gas chewable tablets OTC *antiflatulent* [simethicone] 80 mg

Maalox Daily Fiber Therapy powder OTC *bulk laxative* [psyllium hydrophilic mucilloid] 3.4 g/dose

Maalox HRF (Heartburn Relief Formula) liquid OTC *antacid* [aluminum hydroxide; magnesium carbonate] 140•175 mg/5 mL

Maalox Plus chewable tablets, oral suspension OTC *antacid; antiflatulent* [aluminum hydroxide; magnesium hydroxide; simethicone] 200•200•25 mg; 500•450•40 mg/5 mL

Maalox TC chewable tablets, oral suspension (tablets discontinued 1994; suspension renamed Maalox Therapeutic Concentrate)

Maalox Therapeutic Concentrate oral suspension OTC *antacid* [aluminum hydroxide; magnesium hydroxide] 600•300 mg/5 mL

MAb; MAB (monoclonal antibody)

MABOP (Mustargen, Adriamycin, bleomycin, Oncovin, prednisone) *chemotherapy protocol*

mabuterol INN

MAC (methotrexate, actinomycin D, chlorambucil) *chemotherapy protocol*

MAC; MAC III (methotrexate, actinomycin D, cyclophosphamide) *chemotherapy protocol*

MAC (mitomycin, Adriamycin, cyclophosphamide) *chemotherapy protocol*

MACC (methotrexate, Adriamycin, cyclophosphamide, CCNU) *chemotherapy protocol*

MACHO (methotrexate, asparaginase, cyclophosphamide, hydroxydaunomycin, Oncovin) *chemotherapy protocol*

MACOP-B (methotrexate, Adriamycin, cyclophosphamide, Oncovin, prednisone, bleomycin) *chemotherapy protocol*

macroaggregated albumin (MAA) [see: albumin, aggregated]

macroaggregated iodinated (^{131}I) human albumin [see: macrosalb (^{131}I)]

Macrobid capsules ℞ *urinary bacteriostatic* [nitrofurantoin (macrocrystals); nitrofurantoin monohydrate] 25•75 mg

Macrodantin capsules ℞ *urinary bacteriostatic* [nitrofurantoin (macrocrystals)] 25, 50, 100 mg

Macrodantin MACPAC (box of 7 cards of 4 capsules each) (discontinued 1993) ℞ *urinary antibacterial* [nitrofurantoin (macrocrystals)]

Macrodex IV infusion ℞ *plasma volume expander for shock due to hemorrhage, burns, or surgery* [dextran 70] 6%

macrogol 4000 INN, BAN [also: polyethylene glycol 4000]

macrogol ester 2000 INN *surfactant* [also: polyoxyl 40 stearate]

macrogol ester 400 INN *surfactant* [also: polyoxyl 8 stearate]

Macrolin R *investigational agent for fungal disease and advanced cancer* [macrophage colony-stimulating factor (CSF)]

macrophage colony-stimulating factor (M-CSF) *investigational antiviral for AIDS and various forms of cancer*

macrophage-targeted β-glucocerebrosidase [now: alglucerase]

macrosalb (^{131}I) INN, BAN

macrosalb (^{99m}Tc) INN, BAN [also: technetium (^{99m}Tc) labeled macroaggregated human ...]

Macroscint R *investigational inflammation and infection imaging aid*

Macstim R *investigational antineoplastic for various cancers; investigational antihyperlipidemic* [macrophage colony-stimulating factor]

MAD (MeCCNU, Adriamycin) *chemotherapy protocol*

MADDOC (mechlorethamine, Adriamycin, dacarbazine, DDP, Oncovin, cyclophosphamide) *chemotherapy protocol*

maduramicin USAN, INN *anticoccidal*

mafenide USAN, INN, BAN *bacteriostatic; adjunct to burn therapy*

mafenide acetate USP *bacteriostatic;* (orphan: meshed autograft loss in burns)

mafenide HCl

mafilcon A USAN *hydrophilic contact lens material*

mafoprazine INN

mafosfamide INN

Mag-200 tablets OTC *magnesium supplement* [magnesium oxide] 400 mg

magaldrate USAN, USP, INN *antacid* 540 mg/5 mL oral

Magaldrate Plus oral suspension OTC *antacid; antiflatulent* [magaldrate; simethicone] 540•40 mg/5 mL

Magalox Plus chewable tablets OTC *antacid; antiflatulent* [aluminum hydroxide; magnesium hydroxide; simethicone] 200•200•25 mg

Magan tablets R *analgesic; antirheumatic* [magnesium salicylate] 545 mg

Mag-Cal tablets OTC *dietary supplement* [calcium carbonate; vitamin D; multiple minerals] 416.7 mg•66.7 IU•≛

Mag-Cal Mega tablets OTC *mineral supplement* [magnesium; calcium] 800•400 mg

Magnacal ready-to-use liquid OTC *enteral nutritional therapy* [lactose-free formula]

Magnagel chewable tablets (discontinued 1994) OTC *antacid* [aluminum hydroxide; magnesium carbonate]

Magnalox liquid OTC *antacid* [aluminum hydroxide; magnesium hydroxide] 225•220 mg/5 mL

Magnalox Plus liquid OTC *antacid; antiflatulent* [aluminum hydroxide; magnesium hydroxide; simethicone]

Magnaprin; Magnaprin Arthritis Strength Captabs film-coated tablets OTC *analgesic; antipyretic; anti-inflammatory; antirheumatic* [aspirin, buffered with aluminum hydroxide, magnesium hydroxide, and calcium carbonate] 325 mg

Magnatril chewable tablets (discontinued 1994) OTC *antacid* [aluminum hydroxide; magnesium hydroxide; magnesium trisilicate]

Magnatril oral suspension (discontinued 1994) OTC *antacid* [aluminum hydroxide; calcium carbonate; magnesium trisilicate] 30•16•80 mg/mL

magnesia, milk of USP *antacid; laxative* [also: magnesium hydroxide] 400 mg/5 mL oral

magnesia magma [now: magnesia, milk of]

magnesium *element* (Mg)

magnesium aluminosilicate hydrate [see: almasilate]

magnesium aluminum silicate NF *suspending agent*

magnesium amino acid chelate *dietary magnesium supplement*

magnesium aspartate [see: potassium aspartate & magnesium aspartate]

magnesium carbonate USP *antacid; dietary magnesium supplement*

magnesium carbonate hydrate [see: magnesium carbonate]

magnesium chloride USP *electrolyte replenisher* 1.97 mEq/mL (20%) injection

magnesium chloride hexahydrate [see: magnesium chloride]

magnesium citrate USP *saline laxative*

magnesium clofibrate INN

magnesium D-gluconate dihydrate [see: magnesium gluconate]

magnesium D-gluconate hydrate [see: magnesium gluconate]

magnesium gluconate USP *magnesium replenisher*

magnesium glycinate USAN

magnesium hydroxide USP *antacid; saline laxative* [also: magnesia, milk of]

magnesium oxide USP *antacid; sorbent* 500 mg oral

magnesium phosphate USP *antacid*

magnesium phosphate pentahydrate [see: magnesium phosphate]

magnesium salicylate USP *analgesic; antipyretic; anti-inflammatory; antirheumatic*

magnesium salicylate tetrahydrate [see: magnesium salicylate]

magnesium silicate NF *tablet excipient*

magnesium silicate hydrate [see: magnesium trisilicate]

magnesium stearate NF *tablet and capsule lubricant*

magnesium sulfate USP, JAN *anticonvulsant; saline laxative; electrolyte replenisher* 0.8, 1, 4 mEq/mL (10%, 12.5%, 50%) injection

magnesium sulfate heptahydrate [see: magnesium sulfate]

magnesium trisilicate USP *antacid*

Magnevist injection R *parenteral radiopaque agent for magnetic imaging of the brain and spine* [gadopentetate dimeglumine] 46.9%

Magnox oral suspension OTC *antacid* [aluminum hydroxide; magnesium hydroxide] 225•200 mg/5 mL

Magonate tablets, liquid OTC *magnesium supplement* [magnesium gluconate] 500 mg; 54 mg/5 mL

Mag-Ox 400 tablets OTC *antacid; magnesium supplement* [magnesium oxide] 400 mg

Magsal tablets R *analgesic; antipyretic; anti-inflammatory; antihistamine* [magnesium salicylate; phenyltoloxamine citrate] 600•25 mg

Mag-Tab SR sustained-release caplets OTC *magnesium supplement* [magnesium lactate] 7 mEq (84 mg)

Magtrate tablets OTC *magnesium supplement* [magnesium gluconate] 500 mg

MAID (mesna [rescue], Adriamycin, ifosfamide, dacarbazine) *chemotherapy protocol*

MainStream R *investigational IV system*

maitansine INN *antineoplastic* [also: maytansine]

Major-Con chewable tablets OTC *antiflatulent* [simethicone] 80 mg

Major-gesic tablets OTC *antihistamine; analgesic* [phenyltoloxamine citrate; acetaminophen] 30•325 mg

MAK 195 F *investigational therapy for graft vs. host disease* [monoclonal antibodies]

Malatal tablets R *GI anticholinergic; sedative* [atropine sulfate; scopolamine hydrobromide; hyoscyamine hydrobromide; phenobarbital] 0.0194•0.0065•0.1037•16.2 mg

malathion USP, BAN *pediculicide*

maletamer INN *antiperistaltic* [also: malethamer]

malethamer USAN *antiperistaltic* [also: maletamer]

maleylsulfathiazole INN

malic acid NF *acidifying agent*

malidone [see: aloxidone]

Mallamint chewable tablets OTC *antacid* [calcium carbonate] 420 mg

Mallazine eye drops OTC *topical ocular decongestant/vasoconstrictor* [tetrahydrozoline HCl] 0.05%

Mallergan VC Cough syrup (discontinued 1994) R *narcotic antitussive; decongestant; antihistamine* [codeine phosphate; phenylephrine HCl; promethazine HCl; alcohol]

Mallisol ointment OTC *broad-spectrum antimicrobial* [povidone-iodine]

Mallisol surgical scrub (discontinued 1992) OTC *broad-spectrum antimicrobial* [povidone-iodine]

malonal [see: barbital]

malotilate USAN, INN *liver disorder treatment*

Malotuss syrup (discontinued 1992) OTC *expectorant* [guaifenesin; alcohol 3.5%] 100 mg/5 mL

Maltsupex liquid OTC *bulk laxative* [nondiastatic barley malt extract] 16 g/tbsp.

Maltsupex powder OTC *bulk laxative* [nondiastatic barley malt extract] 8 g/tbsp.

Maltsupex tablets OTC *bulk laxative* [nondiastatic barley malt extract] 750 mg

Mammol ointment OTC *emollient for nipples of nursing mothers* [bismuth subnitrate] 40%

***m*-AMSA (acridinylamine methanesulphon anisidide)** [see: amsacrine]

Mandameth enteric-coated tablets ℞ *urinary bactericidal* [methenamine mandelate] 0.5, 1 g

Mandelamine film-coated tablets (discontinued 1995) ℞ *urinary bactericidal* [methenamine mandelate] 0.5, 1 g

Mandelamine oral suspension, suspension forte, granules (discontinued 1993) ℞ *urinary bactericidal* [methenamine mandelate] 50 mg/mL; 100 mg/mL; 1 g/dose

mandelic acid NF

Mandol powder for IV or IM injection ℞ *cephalosporin-type antibiotic* [cefamandole nafate] 1, 2, 10 g ② nadolol

Manerex tablets (available only in Canada) ℞ *antidepressant* [moclobemide] 100, 150 mg

manganese *element* (Mn)

manganese chloride USP *dietary manganese supplement; investigational GI contrast agent for MRI* 0.1 mg/mL injection

manganese chloride tetrahydrate [see: manganese chloride]

manganese gluconate (manganese D-gluconate) USP *dietary manganese supplement*

manganese glycerophosphate NF

manganese hypophosphite NF

manganese phosphinate [see: manganese hypophosphite]

manganese sulfate USP *dietary manganese supplement* 0.1 mg/mL injection

manganese sulfate monohydrate [see: manganese sulfate]

Manga-Pak IV injection (discontinued 1992) ℞ *intravenous nutritional therapy* [manganese sulfate]

manidipine 6300 INN

manna sugar [see: mannitol]

Mannest tablets (discontinued 1992) ℞ *estrogen hormone replacement* [conjugated estrogens]

mannite [see: mannitol]

mannitol (D-mannitol) USP *renal function test aid; osmotic diuretic; urologic irrigant* 10%, 15%, 20%, 25% injection

mannitol hexanitrate INN

mannityl nitrate [see: mannitol hexanitrate]

mannomustine INN, BAN

mannosulfan INN

Manoplax film-coated tablets (discontinued 1993) ℞ *vasodilator for congestive heart failure* [flosequinan]

manozodil INN

Mantadil cream ℞ *topical corticosteroid; antihistamine* [hydrocortisone acetate; chlorcyclizine HCl] 0.5%•2%

Mantoux test [see: tuberculin]

Maolate tablets ℞ *skeletal muscle relaxant* [chlorphenesin carbamate] 400 mg

Maox tablets (name changed to Maox 420 in 1995)

Maox 420 tablets OTC *antacid* [magnesium oxide] 420 mg

MAP (mitomycin, Adriamycin, Platinol) *chemotherapy protocol*

Mapap tablets OTC *analgesic; antipyretic* [acetaminophen] 325, 500 mg

Mapap, Children's elixir OTC *pediatric analgesic and antipyretic* [acetaminophen (alcohol free)] 160 mg/5 mL

Mapap Cold Formula tablets OTC *antitussive; decongestant; antihistamine; analgesic* [dextromethorphan hydrobromide; pseudoephedrine HCl; chlorpheniramine maleate; acetaminophen] 15•30•2•325 mg

Mapap Infant Drops OTC *pediatric analgesic and antipyretic* [acetaminophen] 100 mg/mL

maprotiline USAN, INN *tetracyclic antidepressant*

maprotiline HCl USP *tetracyclic antidepressant* 25, 50, 75 mg oral

Maranox tablets OTC *analgesic; antipyretic* [acetaminophen] 325 mg

Marax tablets ℞ *antiasthmatic; bronchodilator; decongestant* [theophylline; ephedrine sulfate] 130•25 mg ❷ Atarax; Maalox

Marax-DF pediatric syrup ℞ *antiasthmatic; bronchodilator; decongestant; anxiolytic* [theophylline; ephedrine sulfate; hydroxyzine HCl] 97.5•18.75•7.5 mg/15 mL

Marbaxin 750 tablets (discontinued 1993) ℞ *skeletal muscle relaxant* [methocarbamol]

Marbec tablets (discontinued 1995) OTC *dietary supplement* [multiple B vitamins; vitamin C; brewer's yeast] ±•300•120 mg

Marblen tablets, liquid OTC *antacid* [calcium carbonate; magnesium carbonate] 520•400 mg; 540•400 mg/5 mL

Marcaine HCl injection ℞ *injectable local anesthetic* [bupivacaine HCl] 0.25%, 0.5%, 0.75%

Marcaine HCl injection ℞ *injectable local anesthetic* [bupivacaine HCl; epinephrine bitartrate] 0.25%•1:200,000, 0.5%•1:200,000, 0.75%•1:200,000 ❷ Narcan

Marcaine Spinal injection ℞ *injectable local anesthetic* [bupivacaine HCl] 0.75%

Marcaine with Epinephrine injection ℞ *injectable local anesthetic* [bupivacaine HCl; epinephrine] 0.5%•1:200,000

Marcillin capsules, powder for oral suspension ℞ *penicillin-type antibiotic* [ampicillin trihydrate] 500 mg; 250 mg/100 mL

Marcof Expectorant syrup ℞ *narcotic antitussive; expectorant* [hydrocodone bitartrate; potassium guaiacolsulfonate] 5•300 mg/5 mL

Marezine IM injection (discontinued 1993) ℞ *antiemetic; anticholinergic; antihistamine; motion sickness preventative* [cyclizine lactate] 50 mg/mL

Marezine tablets OTC *antiemetic; anticholinergic; antihistamine; motion sickness preventative* [cyclizine HCl] 50 mg

Marflex tablets (discontinued 1993) ℞ *skeletal muscle relaxant* [orphenadrine citrate]

Margesic capsules ℞ *analgesic; anti-inflammatory; sedative* [acetaminophen; caffeine; butalbital] 325•40•50 mg

Margesic H capsules ℞ *narcotic analgesic* [hydrocodone bitartrate; acetaminophen] 5•500 mg

Margesic No. 3 tablets ℞ *narcotic analgesic* [codeine phosphate; acetaminophen] 30•650 mg

maridomycin INN

Marine Lipid Concentrate softgels OTC *dietary supplement* [omega-3 fatty acids] 1200 mg

Marinol capsules ℞ *antiemetic for chemotherapy; appetite stimulant for AIDS patients (orphan)* [dronabinol] 2.5, 5, 10 mg

mariptiline INN

Marlin Salt System tablets OTC *rinsing/storage solution for soft contact lenses* [sodium chloride for normal saline solution] 250 mg

Marlin Salt System II tablets OTC *rinsing/storage solution for soft contact lenses* [sodium chloride for normal saline solution] 250 mg

Marlipids III capsules (discontinued 1993) OTC *dietary supplement* [omega-3 fatty acids] 1000 mg

Marmine IV or IM injection ℞ *antinauseant; antiemetic; antivertigo; motion sickness preventative* [dimenhydrinate] 50 mg/mL

Marmine tablets OTC *antinauseant; antiemetic; antivertigo; motion sickness preventative* [dimenhydrinate] 50 mg

Marnal tablets, capsules ℞ *analgesic; antipyretic; anti-inflammatory; sedative* [aspirin; caffeine; butalbital] 325•40•50 mg

Marnatal-F film-coated tablets ℞ *vitamin/mineral/calcium/iron supplement* [multiple vitamins & minerals; calcium; iron; folic acid] ±•250•60•1 mg

Marogen ℞ *investigational substitute for blood transfusion (orphan: anemia of end-stage renal disease)* [epoetin beta]

maroxepin INN

Marplan tablets (discontinued 1994) ℞ *antidepressant; monoamine oxidase (MAO) inhibitor* [isocarboxazid] 10 mg

Marpres tablets ℞ *antihypertensive* [hydrochlorothiazide; reserpine; hydralazine HCl] 15•0.1•25 mg

Marthritic tablets ℞ *analgesic; antipyretic; anti-inflammatory; antirheumatic* [salsalate] 750 mg

masoprocol USAN, INN *antineoplastic for actinic keratoses (AK)*

Massé Breast cream OTC *moisturizer and emollient for nipples of nursing women*

Massengill Baking Soda Freshness solution OTC *vaginal cleanser and deodorizer; acidity modifier* [sodium bicarbonate]

Massengill Disposable Douche solution OTC *antiseptic/germicidal; vaginal cleanser and deodorizer; acidity modifier* [cetylpyridinium chloride; lactic acid; sodium lactate]

Massengill Disposable Douche; Massengill Vinegar & Water Extra Mild solution OTC *vaginal cleanser and deodorizer; acidity modifier* [vinegar (acetic acid)]

Massengill Douche powder OTC *astringent; antipruritic/counterirritant; vaginal cleanser and deodorizer* [ammonium alum; phenol; methyl salicylate; menthol; thymol]

Massengill Douche solution concentrate OTC *vaginal cleanser and deodorizer; acidity modifier* [lactic acid; sodium lactate; sodium bicarbonate]

Massengill Feminine Cleansing Wash liquid OTC *for external perivaginal cleansing*

Massengill Medicated towelettes OTC *topical corticosteroidal anti-inflammatory* [hydrocortisone] 0.5%

Massengill Medicated Douche with Cepticin; Massengill Medicated Disposable Douche with Cepticin solution OTC *antiseptic/germicidal; vaginal cleanser and deodorizer* [povidone-iodine] 12%; 10%

Massengill Unscented solution (discontinued 1995) OTC *vaginal cleanser and deodorizer; acidity modifier* [lactic acid]

Massengill Vinegar & Water Extra Cleansing with Puraclean solution OTC *antiseptic/germicidal; vaginal cleanser and deodorizer; acidity modifier* [cetylpyridinium chloride; vinegar (acetic acid)]

Materna tablets ℞ *vitamin/mineral/calcium/iron supplement* [multiple vitamins & minerals; calcium; iron; folic acid; biotin] ≟•250•60•1•0.03 mg

matrix metalloproteinase inhibitor *(orphan: treatment of corneal ulcers)*

Matulane capsules ℞ *antibiotic antineoplastic for Hodgkin's disease; investigational for lymphoma, brain and lung cancer* [procarbazine HCl] 50 mg

Mavik tablets ℞ *antihypertensive; ACE inhibitor* [trandolapril] 1, 2, 4 mg

Maxair Autohaler (breath-activated metered-dose inhaler) ℞ *bronchodilator for bronchospasm* [pirbuterol acetate] 0.2 mg/dose

Maxaquin film-coated tablets ℞ *broad-spectrum fluoroquinolone-type antibiotic* [lomefloxacin HCl] 400 mg

Max-Caro capsules (discontinued 1996) OTC *to reduce photosensitivity reaction* [beta-carotene] 15 mg

MaxEPA soft capsules OTC *dietary supplement* [omega-3 fatty acids; multiple vitamins & minerals] 1000• ≟ mg

Maxicam ℞ *investigational nonsteroidal anti-inflammatory drug (NSAID); antiarthritic; analgesic; antipyretic* [isoxicam]

Maxidex Drop-Tainers (eye drop suspension), ophthalmic ointment ℞ *ophthalmic topical corticosteroidal anti-inflammatory* [dexamethasone] 0.1%; 0.05%

Maxiflor cream, ointment ℞ *topical corticosteroidal anti-inflammatory* [diflorasone diacetate] 0.05%

Maxilube Personal Lubricant jelly (discontinued 1995) OTC *vaginal lubricant*

Maximum Blue Label; Maximum Green Label tablets OTC *vitamin/*

mineral supplement [multiple vitamins & minerals; folic acid; biotin] ≚•130•50 µg

Maximum Red Label tablets OTC *vitamin/mineral/iron supplement* [multiple vitamins & minerals; iron; folic acid; biotin] ≚•3.3 mg•0.13 mg•50 µg

"Maximum Strength" products [see under product name]

Maxipime powder for IV or IM injection ℞ *broad-spectrum cephalosporin antibiotic* [cefepime HCl] 0.5, 1, 2 g

Maxitrol eye drop suspension, ophthalmic ointment ℞ *topical ophthalmic corticosteroidal anti-inflammatory; antibiotic* [dexamethasone; neomycin sulfate; polymyxin B sulfate] 0.1%•0.35%•10,000 U/mL; 0.1%•0.35%•10,000 U/g

Maxivate ointment, cream, lotion ℞ *topical corticosteroid* [betamethasone diproprionate] 0.05%

Maxivent ℞ *investigational antiasthmatic* [doxofylline]

Maxi-Vite tablets OTC *vitamin/mineral/calcium/iron supplement* [multiple vitamins & minerals; calcium; iron; folic acid; biotin] ≚•53.5•1.5•0.4•0.001 mg

Maxolon tablets ℞ *antidopaminergic; antiemetic for chemotherapy; peristaltic* [metoclopramide monohydrochloride monohydrate] 10 mg

Maxovite sustained-release tablets OTC *vitamin/mineral supplement* [multiple vitamins & minerals; folic acid; biotin] ≚•330•11.7 µg

Maxzide tablets ℞ *diuretic; antihypertensive* [triamterene; hydrochlorothiazide] 37.5•25, 75•50 mg

Mayotic ear drop suspension (discontinued 1992) ℞ *topical corticosteroidal anti-inflammatory; antibiotic* [hydrocortisone; neomycin sulfate; polymyxin B sulfate]

maytansine USAN *antineoplastic* [also: maitansine]

May-Vita elixir ℞ *vitamin supplement* [multiple B vitamins; folic acid] ≚•0.1 mg

Mazanor tablets ℞ *anorexiant* [mazindol] 1 mg

mazapertine succinate USAN *antipsychotic; dopamine receptor antagonist*

mazaticol INN

MAZE (m-AMSA, azacitidine, etoposide) *chemotherapy protocol*

Mazicon IV injection (name changed to Romazicon in 1993)

mazindol USAN, USP, INN, BAN *anorexiant (orphan: Duchenne muscular dystrophy)* ② mebendazole

mazipredone INN

MB (methylene blue) [q.v.]

m-BACOD; M-BACOD (methotrexate, bleomycin, Adriamycin, cyclophosphamide, Oncovin, dexamethasone) *chemotherapy protocol* "m" is 200 mg/m^2; "M" is 3 g/m^2

M-BACOS (methotrexate, bleomycin, Adriamycin, cyclophosphamide, Oncovin, Solu-Medrol) *chemotherapy protocol*

MBC (methotrexate, bleomycin, cisplatin) *chemotherapy protocol*

MBD (methotrexate, bleomycin, DDP) *chemotherapy protocol*

MBR (methylene blue, reduced) [see: methylene blue]

MC (mitoxantrone, cytarabine) *chemotherapy protocol*

M-Caps capsules ℞ *urinary acidifier to control ammonia production* [racemethionine] 200 mg

MCBP (melphalan, cyclophosphamide, BCNU, prednisone) *chemotherapy protocol*

MCH (microfibrillar collagen hemostat) [q.v.]

MCP (melphalan, cyclophosphamide, prednisone) *chemotherapy protocol*

M-CSF (macrophage colony-stimulating factor) [q.v.]

MCT oil OTC *dietary fat supplement* [medium chain triglycerides from coconut oil]

MCT (medium chain triglycerides) [q.v.]

MCV (methotrexate, cisplatin, vinblastine) *chemotherapy protocol*

MD-60; MD-76 injection ℞ *parenteral radiopaque agent* [diatrizoate meglumine; diatrizoate sodium] 52%•8%; 66%•10%

MD-Gastroview solution ℞ *GI contrast radiopaque agent* [diatrizoate meglumine; diatrizoate sodium] 66%•10%

MDL 27,192 *investigational anticonvulsant*

MDL 28,314 *investigational antineoplastic for leukemia and solid tumors*

MDL 28,574 *investigational (Phase II) antiviral glucosidase inhibitor for HIV*

MDL 100,240 *investigational treatment for hypertension and congestive heart failure*

MDL 201,404 *investigational agent for adult respiratory disorders*

MDP (methylene diphosphonate) [now: medronate disodium]

MEA (mercaptoethylamine) [see: mercaptamine]

measles, mumps & rubella virus vaccine, live USP *active immunizing agent for measles (rubeola), mumps and rubella*

measles immune globulin USP

measles & rubella virus vaccine, live USP *active immunizing agent for measles (rubeola) and rubella*

measles virus vaccine, live USP *active immunizing agent for measles (rubeola)*

Measurin timed-release tablets (discontinued 1992) OTC *analgesic; antipyretic; anti-inflammatory* [aspirin]

Mebadin (available only from the Centers for Disease Control) ℞ *investigational anti-infective for amebiasis and amebic dysentery* [dehydroemetine]

meballymal [see: secobarbital]

mebamoxine [see: benmoxin]

mebanazine INN, BAN

Mebaral tablets ℞ *long-acting barbiturate sedative, hypnotic and anticonvulsant* [mephobarbital] 32, 50, 100 mg ⓘ Medrol; Mellaril

mebendazole USAN, USP, INN *anthelmintic* 100 mg oral ⓘ mazindol

mebenoside INN

mebeverine INN *smooth muscle relaxant* [also: mebeverine HCl]

mebeverine HCl USAN *smooth muscle relaxant* [also: mebeverine]

mebezonium iodide INN, BAN

mebhydrolin INN, BAN

mebiquine INN

mebolazine INN

mebrofenin USAN, INN *hepatobiliary function test*

mebrophenhydramine HCl [see: embramine HCl]

mebubarbital [see: pentobarbital]

mebumal [see: pentobarbital]

mebutamate USAN, INN *antihypertensive*

mebutizide INN

mecamylamine INN *antihypertensive* [also: mecamylamine HCl]

mecamylamine HCl USP *antihypertensive* [also: mecamylamine]

mecarbinate INN

mecarbine [see: mecarbinate]

MeCCNU (methyl chloroethyl-cyclohexyl-nitrosourea) [see: semustine]

mecetronium ethylsulfate USAN *antiseptic* [also: mecetronium etilsulfate]

mecetronium etilsulfate INN *antiseptic* [also: mecetronium ethylsulfate]

mechlorethamine HCl USP *alkylating antineoplastic* [also: chlormethine; mustine; nitrogen mustard N-oxide HCl]

Mechol tablets (discontinued 1994) OTC *dietary supplement* [multiple B vitamins; vitamin C] ≐•75 mg

meciadanol INN

mecillinam INN, BAN *antibacterial* [also: amdinocillin]

mecinarone INN

Meclan cream ℞ *topical antibiotic for acne* [meclocycline sulfosalicylate] 1% ⓘ Meclomen; Mezlin

meclizine HCl USP *antiemetic; antihistamine; anticholinergic; motion sickness relief* [also: meclozine] 12.5, 25, 50 mg oral

meclocycline USAN, INN, BAN *antibacterial*

meclocycline sulfosalicylate USAN, USP *antibacterial antibiotic*

meclofenamate sodium USAN, USP *analgesic; antiarthritic; nonsteroidal anti-inflammatory drug (NSAID)* 50, 100 mg oral

meclofenamic acid USAN, INN *nonsteroidal anti-inflammatory drug (NSAID)*

meclofenoxate INN, BAN

Meclomen capsules (discontinued 1996) ℞ *nonsteroidal anti-inflammatory drug (NSAID); antiarthritic; analgesic* [meclofenamate sodium] 50, 100 mg ② Meclan

meclonazepam INN

mecloqualone USAN, INN *sedative; hypnotic*

mecloralurea INN

meclorisone INN, BAN *topical anti-inflammatory* [also: meclorisone dibutyrate]

meclorisone dibutyrate USAN *topical anti-inflammatory* [also: meclorisone]

mecloxamine INN

meclozine INN, BAN *antiemetic; antihistamine; anticholinergic; motion sickness relief* [also: meclizine HCl]

mecobalamin USAN, INN *vitamin; hematopoietic*

mecrilate INN *tissue adhesive* [also: mecrylate]

mecrylate USAN *tissue adhesive* [also: mecrilate]

Mectizan ℞ *investigational antiparasitic*

MECY (methotrexate, cyclophosphamide) *chemotherapy protocol*

mecysteine INN

Med Timolol eye drops (available only in Canada) ℞ *antiglaucoma agent (β-blocker)* [timolol maleate] 0.25%, 0.5%

Meda Cap capsules OTC *analgesic; antipyretic* [acetaminophen] 500 mg

Meda Syrup Forte (discontinued 1992) OTC *decongestant; antihistamine; antitussive; expectorant* [phenylephrine HCl; chlorpheniramine maleate; dextromethorphan hydrobromide; guaifenesin]

Meda Tab tablets OTC *analgesic; antipyretic* [acetaminophen] 325 mg

Medacote lotion OTC *topical antihistamine; astringent; antipruritic* [pyrilamine maleate; zinc oxide] 1%•?

Medadyne liquid OTC *topical oral anesthetic; antiseptic; astringent* [benzocaine; methylbenzethonium chloride; tannic acid; camphor; menthol]

Medadyne throat spray OTC *topical anesthetic; oral antiseptic* [lidocaine; cetalkonium chloride]

Medalone 40; Medalone 80 [see: depMedalone 40; depMedalone 80]

Medamint throat lozenges OTC *topical oral anesthetic* [benzocaine]

Medatussin syrup, pediatric syrup (discontinued 1994) OTC *antitussive; expectorant; demulcent* [dextromethorphan hydrobromide; guaifenesin; potassium citrate; citric acid]

Medatussin Plus syrup (discontinued 1994) ℞ *decongestant; antihistamine; antitussive; expectorant* [phenylpropanolamine HCl; chlorpheniramine maleate; phenyltoloxamine citrate; dextromethorphan hydrobromide; guaifenesin]

medazepam INN *minor tranquilizer* [also: medazepam HCl]

medazepam HCl USAN *minor tranquilizer* [also: medazepam]

medazomide INN

medazonamide [see: medazomide]

Medazyme chewable tablets (discontinued 1992) OTC *digestive enzymes; antiflatulent* [amylase; protease; lipase; cellulase; simethicone]

medetomidine INN, BAN *veterinary analgesic; veterinary sedative* [also: medetomidine HCl]

medetomidine HCl USAN *veterinary analgesic; veterinary sedative* [also: medetomidine]

MEDI 488 *investigational HIV vaccine*

Mediatric capsules (discontinued 1993) ℞ *geriatric dietary supplement with hormones* [multiple B vitamins; iron; methyltestosterone; conjugated estrogens; methamphetamine HCl]

medibazine INN

medical air [see: air, medical]

Medicated Acne Cleanser OTC *topical acne treatment* [colloidal sulfur; resorcinol] 4%•2%

medicinal zinc peroxide [see: zinc peroxide, medicinal]

Medicone anorectal ointment OTC *topical local anesthetic* [benzocaine] 20%

Medicone rectal suppositories OTC *topical vasoconstrictor* [phenylephrine HCl] 0.25%

Medicone Derma ointment (discontinued 1992) OTC *topical local anesthetic; antibacterial; counterirritant* [benzocaine; zinc oxide; hydroxyquinoline sulfate; ichthammol; menthol] 2%•13.7%•1.05%•1%•0.18%

Medicone Derma-HC ointment (discontinued 1992) ℞ *topical corticosteroid; anesthetic; antifungal; vasoconstrictor* [hydrocortisone acetate; benzocaine; oxyquinoline sulfate; ephedrine; menthol; ichthammol; zinc oxide]

Medicone Dressing cream (discontinued 1992) OTC *topical local anesthetic; antibacterial; astringent* [benzocaine; hydroxyquinoline sulfate; cod liver oil; zinc oxide; menthol]

Mediconet anorectal wipes (discontinued 1992) OTC *emollient; astringent; antiseptic; antifungal* [witch hazel; glycerin; benzalkonium chloride; ethoxylated lanolin] 50%•10%•0.02%•0.5%

Medi-Flu caplets, liquid (discontinued 1995) OTC *antitussive; decongestant; antihistamine; analgesic* [dextromethorphan hydrobromide; pseudoephedrine HCl; chlorpheniramine maleate; acetaminophen] 15•30•2•500 mg; 5•10•0.67•167 mg/5 mL

medifoxamine INN

Medigesic capsules ℞ *analgesic; antipyretic; sedative* [acetaminophen; caffeine; butalbital] 325•40•50 mg

Medihaler Ergotamine inhaler (discontinued 1992) ℞ *migraine-specific vasoconstrictor* [ergotamine tartrate] 9 mg/mL (0.36 mg/dose)

Medihaler-Epi inhalation aerosol (discontinued 1996) OTC *bronchodilator for bronchial asthma* [epinephrine bitartrate] 0.3 mg/dose

Medihaler-Iso inhalation aerosol ℞ *bronchodilator* [isoproterenol sulfate] 0.2% (80 µg/dose)

Medilax chewable tablets OTC *laxative* [phenolphthalein] 120 mg

medinal [see: barbital sodium]

Medipain 5 capsules ℞ *narcotic analgesic* [hydrocodone bitartrate; acetaminophen] 5•500 mg

Mediplast plaster OTC *topical keratolytic* [salicylic acid] 40%

Mediplex Tabules (tablets) OTC *vitamin/mineral supplement* [multiple vitamins & minerals] ≜

Medipren tablets, caplets (discontinued 1996) OTC *nonsteroidal anti-inflammatory drug (NSAID); antiarthritic; analgesic* [ibuprofen] 200 mg

Medi-Quik aerosol (discontinued 1995) OTC *topical local anesthetic; antiseptic* [lidocaine HCl; benzalkonium chloride]

Medi-Quik ointment OTC *topical antibiotic* [polymyxin B sulfate; neomycin; bacitracin] 5000 U•3.5 mg•400 U per g

Medi-Quik spray OTC *topical local anesthetic; antiseptic* [lidocaine; benzalkonium chloride] 2%•0.13%

medium chain triglycerides (MCT) *dietary lipid supplement*

medorinone USAN, INN *cardiotonic*

medorubicin INN

Medotar ointment OTC *topical antipsoriatic; antiseborrheic; astringent; antiseptic* [coal tar; zinc oxide] 1%•≜

MEDR-640 *investigational agent to prevent reperfusion injury following a heart attack*

Medralone 40; Medralone 80 intralesional, soft tissue, and IM injection ℞ *glucocorticoid; anti-inflammatory; immunosuppressant* [methylprednisolone acetate] 40 mg/mL; 80 mg/mL

medrogestone USAN, INN, BAN *progestin*

Medrol tablets, Dosepak (unit of use package) ℞ *glucocorticoid; anti-inflammatory; immunosuppressant* [methylprednisolone] 2, 4, 8, 16, 24, 32 mg ⧈ Mebaral

Medrol Acetate Topical ointment (discontinued 1993) ℞ *topical corticosteroid* [methylprednisolone acetate] 0.25%, 1%

medronate disodium USAN *pharmaceutic aid*

medronic acid USAN, INN, BAN *pharmaceutic aid*

medroxalol USAN, INN, BAN *antihypertensive*

medroxalol HCl USAN *antihypertensive*

medroxiprogesterone acetate [see: medroxyprogesterone acetate]

medroxyprogesterone INN, BAN *progestin; antineoplastic* [also: medroxyprogesterone acetate]

medroxyprogesterone acetate USP *progestin for secondary amenorrhea or abnormal uterine bleeding; antineoplastic* [also: medroxyprogesterone] 10 mg oral

medrylamine INN

medrysone USAN, USP, INN *glucocorticoid; ophthalmic anti-inflammatory*

mefeclorazine INN

mefenamic acid USAN, USP, INN, BAN *analgesic; nonsteroidal anti-inflammatory drug (NSAID)*

mefenidil USAN, INN *cerebral vasodilator*

mefenidil fumarate USAN *cerebral vasodilator*

mefenidramium metilsulfate INN

mefenorex INN *anorectic* [also: mefenorex HCl]

mefenorex HCl USAN *anorectic* [also: mefenorex]

mefeserpine INN

mefexamide USAN, INN *CNS stimulant*

mefloquine USAN, INN, BAN *antimalarial schizonticide*

mefloquine HCl USAN *antimalarial schizonticide (orphan)*

Mefoxin powder for IV or IM injection ℞ *cephalosporin-type antibiotic* [cefoxitin sodium] 1, 2, 10 g

mefruside USAN, INN *diuretic*

Mega B with C tablets (discontinued 1995) OTC *vitamin supplement* [multiple B vitamins; vitamin C; folic acid; biotin] $\pm$•500 mg•400 μg•100 μg

Mega VM-80 tablets OTC *geriatric vitamin/mineral supplement* [multiple vitamins & minerals; folic acid; biotin] $\pm$•400•80 μg

Mega-B tablets OTC *vitamin supplement* [multiple B vitamins; folic acid; biotin] $\pm$•100•100 μg

Megace oral suspension ℞ *for AIDS-related anorexia and cachexia (orphan); antineoplastic for breast or endometrial cancer* [megestrol acetate] 40 mg/mL

Megace tablets ℞ *antineoplastic for advanced carcinoma of the breast or endometrium* [megestrol acetate] 20, 40 mg

Megadose tablets (discontinued 1995) OTC *geriatric vitamin/mineral supplement* [multiple vitamins & minerals; folic acid; biotin] $\pm$•400•80 μg

megallate INN *combining name for radicals or groups*

megalomicin INN *antibacterial* [also: megalomicin potassium phosphate]

megalomicin potassium phosphate USAN *antibacterial* [also: megalomicin]

Megalone ℞ *investigational quinolone antibiotic* [fleroxacin]

Megaton elixir ℞ *vitamin/mineral supplement* [multiple B vitamins & minerals; folic acid] $\pm$•0.1 mg

megestrol INN, BAN *antineoplastic* [also: megestrol acetate]

megestrol acetate USAN, USP *antineoplastic for breast or endometrial cancer; for AIDS-related anorexia and cachexia (orphan)* [also: megestrol] 20, 40 mg oral

meglitinide INN

meglucycline INN

meglumine USP, INN *radiopaque medium*

meglumine diatrizoate BAN *radiopaque medium* [also: diatrizoate meglumine]

meglumine iocarmate BAN *radiopaque medium* [also: iocarmate meglumine]

meglumine iothalamate BAN *radiopaque medium* [also: iothalamate meglumine]

meglumine ioxaglate BAN *radiopaque medium* [also: ioxaglate meglumine]

meglutol USAN, INN *antihyperlipoproteinemic*

mel B [see: melarsoprol]

mel W [see: melarsonyl potassium]

Melacine ℞ *investigational antineoplastic (orphan: stage III-IV melanoma)* [theraccine]

meladrazine INN, BAN

melafocon A USAN *hydrophobic contact lens material*

Melaine ℞ *investigational oral contraceptive and for use in hormone replacement therapy* [ethinyl estradiol; gestodene]

Melanex solution ℞ *hyperpigmentation bleaching agent* [hydroquinone] 3%

melanoma vaccine *(orphan: stage III-IV melanoma)*

melarsonyl potassium INN, BAN

melarsoprol INN, BAN, DCF *investigational anti-infective for trypanosomiasis*

melatonin *sleep aid (orphan: circadian rhythm sleep disorders in blind people with no light perception)*

melengestrol INN *antineoplastic; progestin* [also: melengestrol acetate]

melengestrol acetate USAN *antineoplastic; progestin* [also: melengestrol]

meletimide INN

melfalan [see: melphalan]

Melfiat-105 Unicelles (sustained-release capsules) ℞ *anorexiant* [phendimetrazine tartrate] 105 mg

Melimmune-1; Melimmune-2 ℞ *investigational treatment for malignant melanoma* [melanoma vaccine]

melinamide INN

melitracen INN *antidepressant* [also: melitracen HCl]

melitracen HCl USAN *antidepressant* [also: melitracen]

melizame USAN, INN *sweetener*

Mellaril tablets, oral concentrate ℞ *antipsychotic* [thioridazine HCl] 10, 15, 25, 50, 100, 150, 200 mg; 30, 100 mg/mL ⓡ Elavil; Mebaral; Moderil

Mellaril-S oral suspension ℞ *antipsychotic* [thioridazine HCl] 25, 100 mg/5 mL

meloxicam INN

Melpaque HP cream ℞ *hyperpigmentation bleaching agent; sunscreen* [hydroquinone in a sunblock base] 4%

melperone INN, BAN

melphalan (MPL) USAN, USP, INN, BAN *alkylating antineoplastic; (orphan: multiple myeloma; metastatic melanoma)*

Melquin HP cream ℞ *hyperpigmentation bleaching agent* [hydroquinone] 4%

MelVax ℞ *investigational treatment for malignant melanoma* [melanoma vaccine]

memantine INN

Memorette (trademarked packaging form) *patient compliance package*

memotine INN *antiviral* [also: memotine HCl]

memotine HCl USAN *antiviral* [also: memotine]

menabitan INN *analgesic* [also: menabitan HCl]

menabitan HCl USAN *analgesic* [also: menabitan]

menadiol BAN *vitamin K_4; prothrombogenic* [also: menadiol sodium diphosphate]

menadiol sodium diphosphate USP *vitamin K_4; prothrombogenic* [also: menadiol]

menadiol sodium sulfate INN

menadione USP *vitamin K_3; prothrombogenic*

menadione sodium bisulfite USP, INN

Menadol tablets OTC *nonsteroidal anti-inflammatory drug (NSAID); antiarthritic; analgesic* [ibuprofen] 200 mg

menaphthene [see: menadione]

menaphthone [see: menadione]

menaphthone sodium bisulfite [see: menadione sodium bisulfite]

menaquinone *vitamin K_2; prothrombogenic*

menatetrenone INN

menbutone INN, BAN

mendelevium *element (Md)*

Menest film-coated tablets ℞ *estrogen replacement therapy; hypogonadism; inoperable prostatic and breast cancer* [esterified estrogens] 0.3, 0.625, 1.25, 2.5 mg

menfegol INN

menglytate INN

menichlopholan [see: niclofolan]

Meni-D capsules ℞ *anticholinergic; antivertigo agent; motion sickness preventative* [meclizine HCl] 25 mg

meningococcal polysaccharide vaccine, group A USP *active bacterin for meningitis (Neisseria meningitidis)*

meningococcal polysaccharide vaccine, group C USP *active bacterin for meningitis (Neisseria meningitidis)*

meningococcal polysaccharide vaccine, group W-135 *active bacterin for meningitis (Neisseria meningitidis)*

meningococcal polysaccharide vaccine, group Y *active bacterin for meningitis (Neisseria meningitidis)*

menitrazepam INN

menoctone USAN, INN *antimalarial*

menogaril USAN, INN *antibiotic antineoplastic*

Menomune-A/C/Y/W-135 powder for subcu injection ℞ *meningitis vaccine* [meningococcal polysaccharide vaccine, groups A, C, Y, and W-135] 200 μg/0.5 mL

Menoplex tablets OTC *analgesic; antipyretic; antihistamine* [acetaminophen; phenyltoloxamine citrate] 325•30 mg

Menorest transdermal patch ℞ *investigational estrogen replacement therapy* [estradiol]

menotropins USAN, USP *gonad-stimulating principle; gonadotropin*

Menrium 5-2; Menrium 5-4; Menrium 10-4 tablets ℞ *estrogen replacement therapy for postmenopausal disorders* [chlordiazepoxide; esterified estrogens] 5•0.2 mg; 5•0.4 mg; 10•0.4 mg

Mentane ℞ *investigational cholinesterase inhibitor for Alzheimer's disease* [velnacrine]

menthol USP *topical antipruritic/antiseptic; mild local anesthetic*

MenthoRub vaporizing ointment OTC *counterirritant* [menthol; camphor; eucalyptus oil; oil of turpentine] 2.6%•4.73%•?•?

meobentine INN *antiarrhythmic* [also: meobentine sulfate]

meobentine sulfate USAN *antiarrhythmic* [also: meobentine]

mepacrine INN *anthelmintic; antimalarial* [also: quinacrine HCl]

mepacrine HCl [see: quinacrine HCl]

meparfynol [see: methylpentynol]

mepartricin USAN, INN *antifungal; antiprotozoal*

mepazine acetate [see: pecazine]

mepenzolate bromide USP, INN *peptic ulcer adjunct*

mepenzolate methylbromide [see: mepenzolate bromide]

mepenzolone bromide [see: mepenzolate bromide]

Mepergan injection ℞ *narcotic analgesic; sedative* [meperidine HCl; promethazine HCl] 25•25 mg/mL

Mepergan Fortis capsules ℞ *narcotic analgesic; sedative* [meperidine HCl; promethazine HCl] 50•25 mg

meperidine HCl USP *narcotic analgesic* [also: pethidine] 50, 100 mg oral; 50 mg/5 mL oral; 10, 25, 50, 75, 100 mg/mL injection ② meprobamate

Mephaquin ℞ *antimalarial; for acute chloroquine-resistant malaria (orphan)* [mefloquine HCl]

mephenesin NF, INN

mephenhydramine [see: moxastine]

mephenoxalone INN

mephentermine INN *adrenergic; vasoconstrictor; vasopressor for hypotensive shock* [also: mephentermine sulfate]

mephentermine sulfate USP *adrenergic; vasoconstrictor; vasopressor for hypotensive shock* [also: mephentermine]

mephenytoin USAN, USP, INN *hydantoin-type anticonvulsant* [also: methoin] ② Mephyton; Mesantoin

mephobarbital USP, JAN *anticonvulsant; sedative* [also: methylphenobarbital; methylphenobarbitone]

Mephyton tablets ℞ *coagulant; correct anticoagulant-induced prothrombin deficiency; vitamin K supplement* [phytonadione] 5 mg ② mephenytoin; methadone

mepicycline [see: pipacycline]

Mepig ℞ *(orphan: pulmonary infections of cystic fibrosis)* [mucoid exopolysaccharide Pseudomonas hyperimmune globulin]

mepindolol INN, BAN

mepiperphenidol bromide

mepiprazole INN, BAN

mepirizole [see: epirizole]

mepiroxol INN

mepitiostane INN

mepivacaine INN *local anesthetic* [also: mepivacaine HCl]
mepivacaine HCl USP *local anesthetic* [also: mepivacaine] 1%, 2% injection
mepixanox INN
mepramidil INN
meprednisone USAN, USP, INN
meprobamate USP, INN *anxiolytic; minor tranquilizer* 200, 400 mg oral 2 meperidine
Meprogesic Q tablets (discontinued 1995) ℞ *analgesic; antipyretic; anti-inflammatory; anxiolytic* [aspirin; meprobamate] 325•200 mg
Mepron film-coated tablets (discontinued 1995) ℞ *antiprotozoal for AIDS-related Pneumocystis carinii pneumonia (PCP)* [atovaquone] 250 mg
Mepron oral suspension ℞ *antiprotozoal for AIDS-related Pneumocystis carinii pneumonia (PCP); (orphan: Toxoplasma gondii)* [atovaquone] 750 mg/5 mL
meproscillarin INN, BAN
Meprospan sustained-release capsules ℞ *anxiolytic* [meprobamate] 200, 400 mg 2 Naprosyn
meprothixol BAN [also: meprotixol]
meprotixol INN [also: meprothixol]
meprylcaine INN *local anesthetic* [also: meprylcaine HCl]
meprylcaine HCl USP *local anesthetic* [also: meprylcaine]
meptazinol INN, BAN *analgesic* [also: meptazinol HCl]
meptazinol HCl USAN *analgesic* [also: meptazinol]
mepyramine INN, BAN *antihistamine* [also: pyrilamine maleate]
mepyramine maleate [see: pyrilamine maleate]
mepyrium [see: amprolium]
mepyrrotazine [see: dimelazine]
mequidox USAN, INN *antibacterial*
mequinol INN
mequitamium iodide INN
mequitazine INN, BAN
mequitazium iodide [see: mequitamium iodide]
meragidone sodium
meralein sodium USAN, INN *topical anti-infective*

meralluride NF, INN
merbaphen USP
merbromin NF, INN *general antiseptic*
mercaptamine INN *antiurolithic* [also: cysteamine]
mercaptoarsenical [see: arsthinol]
mercaptoarsenol [see: arsthinol]
mercaptoethylamine (MEA) [see: mercaptamine]
mercaptomerin (MT6) INN [also: mercaptomerin sodium]
mercaptomerin sodium USP [also: mercaptomerin]
mercaptopurine (6-MP) USP, INN *antimetabolic antineoplastic*
mercuderamide INN
mercufenol chloride USAN *topical anti-infective*
mercumatilin sodium INN
mercuric oxide, yellow NF *ophthalmic antiseptic* (FDA ruled it "not safe and effective" in 1992)
mercuric salicylate NF
mercuric succinimide NF
mercurobutol INN
Mercurochrome solution OTC *antiseptic* [merbromin] 2%
mercurophylline NF, INN
mercurous chloride [see: calomel]
mercury *element (Hg)*
mercury, ammoniated USP *topical anti-infective; antipsoriatic*
mercury amide chloride [see: mercury, ammoniated]
mercury oleate NF
merethoxylline procaine
mergocriptine INN
Meridia ℞ *investigational anorexiant and antidepressant* [sibutramine HCl]
merisoprol acetate Hg 197 USAN *radioactive agent*
merisoprol acetate Hg 203 USAN *radioactive agent*
merisoprol Hg 197 USAN *renal function test; radioactive agent*
Meritene powder OTC *enteral nutritional therapy* [milk-based formula]
Meritene ready-to-use liquid (discontinued 1994) OTC *enteral nutritional therapy* [milk-based formula] 250 mL
Merlenate ointment (discontinued 1992) ℞ *topical antifungal* [zinc

undecylenate; caprylic acid; sodium propionate]

meropenem USAN, INN, BAN *investigational carbapenem antibiotic for intra-abdominal infections and bacterial meningitis*

Merrem powder for IV infusion ℞ *carbapenem antibiotic for intra-abdominal infections and bacterial meningitis* [meropenem] 500, 1000 mg

mersalyl INN

mersalyl sodium [see: mersalyl]

Mersol solution, tincture OTC *antiseptic; antibacterial; antifungal* [thimerosal] 1:1000

Merthiolate solution, tincture (discontinued 1992) OTC *antiseptic; antibacterial; antifungal* [thimerosal]

mertiatide INN

Meruvax II powder for subcu injection ℞ *rubella vaccine* [rubella virus vaccine, live] 0.5 mL

mesabolone INN

mesalamine USAN *anti-inflammatory; treatment of ulcerative colitis and proctitis* [also: mesalazine]

mesalazine INN, BAN *anti-inflammatory; treatment of ulcerative colitis and proctitis* [also: mesalamine]

Mesantoin tablets ℞ *hydantoin-type anticonvulsant* [mephenytoin] 100 mg ⓥ mephenytoin; Mestinon; Metatensin

Mescolor film-coated, sustained-release tablets ℞ *decongestant; antihistamine; anticholinergic* [pseudoephedrine HCl; chlorpheniramine maleate; methscopolamine nitrate] 120•8•2.5 mg

meseclazone USAN, INN *anti-inflammatory*

mesifilcon A USAN *hydrophilic contact lens material*

mesilate INN *combining name for radicals or groups* [also: mesylate]

M-Eslon (Canadian/German name for U.S. product Capros)

mesna USAN, INN, BAN *urotoxic antidote; for hemorrhagic cystitis and cyclophosphamide-induced urotoxicity* (orphan)

Mesnex IV injection ℞ *urotoxic antidote; for hemorrhagic cystitis and cyclophosphamide-induced urotoxicity* (orphan) [mesna] 100 mg/mL

mesocarb INN

meso-inositol [see: inositol]

meso-NDGA (nordihydroguaiaretic acid) [see: masoprocol]

meso-nordihydroguaiaretic acid (NDGA) [see: masoprocol]

mesoridazine USAN, INN *antipsychotic*

mesoridazine besylate USP *antipsychotic*

mespirenone INN

mestanolone INN, BAN

mestenediol [see: methandriol]

mesterolone USAN, INN *androgen*

Mestinon tablets, syrup, Timespan (sustained-release tablets), IM or IV injection ℞ *anticholinesterase muscle stimulant; muscle relaxant reversal* [pyridostigmine bromide] 60 mg; 60 mg/5 mL; 180 mg; 5 mg/mL ⓥ Mesantoin; Metatensin

mestranol USAN, USP, INN *estrogen*

mesudipine INN

mesulergine INN

mesulfamide INN

mesulfen INN [also: mesulphen]

mesulphen BAN [also: mesulfen]

mesuprine INN *vasodilator; smooth muscle relaxant* [also: mesuprine HCl]

mesuprine HCl USAN *vasodilator; smooth muscle relaxant* [also: mesuprine]

mesuximide INN *anticonvulsant* [also: methsuximide]

mesylate USAN, USP, BAN *combining name for radicals or groups* [also: mesilate]

metabromsalan USAN, INN *disinfectant*

metabutethamine HCl NF

metabutoxycaine HCl NF

metacetamol INN, BAN

metaclazepam INN

metacycline INN *antibacterial* [also: methacycline]

metaglycodol INN

metahexamide INN

metahexanamide [see: metahexamide]

Metahydrin tablets ℞ *diuretic; antihypertensive* [trichlormethiazide] 4 mg ⓥ Metandren

metalkonium chloride INN
metallibure INN *anterior pituitary activator for swine* [also: methallibure]
metalol HCl USAN *antiadrenergic (β-receptor)*
metamelfalan INN
metamfazone INN [also: methamphazone]
metamfepramone INN [also: dimepropion]
metamfetamine INN *CNS stimulant* [also: methamphetamine HCl]
metamizole sodium INN *analgesic; antipyretic* [also: dipyrone]
metampicillin INN
Metamucil effervescent powder OTC *bulk laxative; antacid* [psyllium hydrophilic mucilloid; sodium bicarbonate; potassium bicarbonate] 3.4•?•? g/packet
Metamucil powder, wafers OTC *bulk laxative* [psyllium hydrophilic mucilloid] 3.4 g/tsp.; 1.7 g
metandienone INN [also: methandrostenolone; methandienone]
Metandren tablets (discontinued 1992) ℞ *androgen for male hypogonadism, impotence and breast cancer* [methyltestosterone] ② Metahydrin
metanixin INN
metaoxedrine chloride [see: phenylephrine HCl]
metaphosphoric acid, potassium salt [see: potassium metaphosphate]
metaphosphoric acid, trisodium salt [see: sodium trimetaphosphate]
metaphyllin [see: aminophylline]
metapramine INN
Metaprel syrup ℞ *bronchodilator* [metaproterenol sulfate] 10 mg/5 mL
Metaprel tablets, inhalation aerosol powder, solution for inhalation (discontinued 1996) ℞ *bronchodilator* [metaproterenol sulfate] 10, 20 mg; 0.65 mg/dose; 0.4%, 0.6%, 5%
metaproterenol polistirex USAN *bronchodilator* [also: orciprenaline] ② metoprolol
metaproterenol sulfate USAN, USP *bronchodilator* 10, 20 mg oral; 10 mg/5 mL oral; 0.4%, 0.6%, 5% inhalation

metaradrine bitartrate [see: metaraminol bitartrate]
metaraminol INN *adrenergic; vasopressor for acute hypotensive shock, anaphylaxis, or traumatic shock* [also: metaraminol bitartrate]
metaraminol bitartrate USP *adrenergic; vasopressor for acute hypotensive shock, anaphylaxis, or traumatic shock* [also: metaraminol]
Metasep shampoo (discontinued 1992) OTC *antibacterial; antiseborrheic* [parachlorometaxylenol]
Metasome ℞ *investigational antiasthmatic* [liposomal metaproterenol]
Metastron IV injection ℞ *analgesic for metastatic bone pain* [strontium chloride Sr 89] 10.9–22.6 mg/mL (4 mCi)
Metatensin #2; Metatensin #4 tablets ℞ *antihypertensive* [trichlormethiazide; reserpine] 2•0.1 mg; 4•0.1 mg ② Mesantoin; Mestinon
metaterol INN
metaxalone USAN, INN, BAN *skeletal muscle relaxant* ② metolazone
metazamide INN
metazepium iodide [see: buzepide metiodide]
metazide INN
metazocine INN, BAN
metbufen INN
metcaraphen HCl
metembonate INN *combining name for radicals or groups*
meteneprost USAN, INN *oxytocic; prostaglandin*
metenolone INN *anabolic* [also: methenolone acetate]
metenolone acetate [see: methenolone acetate]
metergoline INN, BAN
metergotamine INN
metescufylline INN
metesculetol INN
metethoheptazine INN
metetoin INN *anticonvulsant* [also: methetoin]
metformin USAN, INN, BAN *biguanide-type antidiabetic* [also: metformin HCl]
metformin HCl USAN, JAN *biguanide-type antidiabetic* [also: metformin]
methacholine bromide NF

methacholine chloride USP, INN *cholinergic; bronchoconstrictor for pulmonary challenge tests*

methacrylic acid copolymer NF *tablet-coating agent*

methacycline USAN *antibacterial* [also: metacycline]

methacycline HCl USP *gram-negative and gram-positive bacteriostatic; antirickettsial*

methadol [see: dimepheptanol]

methadone INN *narcotic analgesic* [also: methadone HCl] ② Mephyton

methadone HCl USP *narcotic analgesic* [also: methadone] 5, 10, 40 mg oral; 5, 10 mg/5 mL oral; 10 mg/mL oral

methadonium chloride [see: methadone HCl]

methadyl acetate USAN *narcotic analgesic* [also: acetylmethadol]

methafilcon B USAN *hydrophilic contact lens material*

Methagual OTC *counterirritant* [methyl salicylate; guaiacol] 8%•2%

Methalgen cream OTC *counterirritant* [methyl salicylate; menthol; camphor; mustard oil]

methallenestril INN

methallenestrol [see: methallenestril]

methallibure USAN *anterior pituitary activator for swine* [also: metallibure]

methalthiazide USAN *diuretic; antihypertensive*

methamoctol

methamphazone BAN [also: metamfazone]

methamphetamine HCl USP *CNS stimulant* [also: metamfetamine]

methampyrone [now: dipyrone]

methanabol [see: methandriol]

methandienone BAN [also: methandrostenolone; metandienone]

methandriol

methandrostenolone USP [also: metandienone; methandienone]

methaniazide INN

methanol [see: methyl alcohol]

methantheline bromide USP *peptic ulcer adjunct* [also: methanthelinium bromide]

methanthelinium bromide INN, BAN *anticholinergic* [also: methantheline bromide]

methaphenilene INN, BAN [also: methaphenilene HCl]

methaphenilene HCl NF [also: methaphenilene]

methapyrilene INN [also: methapyrilene fumarate]

methapyrilene fumarate USP [also: methapyrilene]

methapyrilene HCl USP

methaqualone USAN, USP, INN *hypnotic; sedative*

methaqualone HCl USP

metharbital USP, INN, JAN *anticonvulsant* [also: metharbitone]

metharbitone BAN *anticonvulsant* [also: metharbital]

MethaSite ℞ *investigational ophthalmic steroidal anti-inflammatory* [fluorometholone]

methastyridone INN

Methatropic capsules OTC *dietary lipotropic with vitamin supplementation* [choline; inositol; methionine; multiple B vitamins] 115•83•110• ± mg

methazolamide USP, INN *carbonic anhydrase inhibitor* 25, 50 mg oral

Methblue 65 tablets ℞ *urinary anti-infective/antiseptic; antidote to cyanide poisoning* [methylene blue] 65 mg

Meth-Choline caplets (discontinued 1992) OTC *dietary lipotropic with vitamin supplementation* [choline; inositol; methionine; multiple B vitamins; desiccated liver; liver concentrate]

methdilazine USP, INN *antipruritic*

methdilazine HCl USP *antipruritic; antihistamine*

methenamine USP, INN *urinary bactericidal* ② methionine

methenamine hippurate USAN, USP *urinary bactericidal* [also: hexamine hippurate]

methenamine mandelate USP *urinary bactericidal* 0.5, 1 g oral; 0.5 g/5 mL oral

methenolone acetate USAN *anabolic* [also: metenolone]

methenolone enanthate USAN *anabolic*

metheptazine INN

Methergine coated tablets, IV or IM injection ℞ *control postpartum uterine atony; postpartum hemorrhage* [methylergonovine maleate] 0.2 mg; 0.2 mg/mL
methestrol INN
methetharimide [see: bemegride]
methetoin USAN *anticonvulsant* [also: metetoin]
methicillin sodium USAN, USP *bactericidal antibiotic* [also: meticillin]
methimazole USP *thyroid inhibitor* [also: thiamazole]
methindizate BAN [also: metindizate]
methiodal sodium USP, INN
methiomeprazine INN
methiomeprazine HCl [see: methiomeprazine]
methionine (DL-methionine) NF, JAN *urinary acidifier* [also: racemethionine] 500 mg oral
methionine (L-methionine) USAN, USP, INN, JAN *essential amino acid; symbols:* Met, M 2 methenamine
methionine-enkephalin *investigational (Phase I) immunomodulator for AIDS*
methionyl granulocyte CSF, recombinant (*orphan: myelodysplastic syndrome*)
methionyl human granulocyte CSF, recombinant (*orphan: neutropenia in bone marrow transplants*)
methiothepin [see: metitepine]
methisazone USAN *antiviral* [also: metisazone]
methisoprinol [now: inosine pranobex]
methitural INN
methixene HCl USAN *smooth muscle relaxant* [also: metixene] 2 methoxsalen
methocamphone methylsulfate [see: trimethidinium methosulfate]
methocarbamol USP, INN, BAN, JAN *skeletal muscle relaxant* 500, 750 mg oral; 100 mg/mL injection
methocidin INN
methohexital USP, INN *general anesthetic* [also: methohexitone]
methohexital sodium USP *general anesthetic*
methohexitone BAN *general anesthetic* [also: methohexital]

methoin BAN *anticonvulsant* [also: mephenytoin]
methonaphthone [see: menbutone]
methophedrine [see: methoxyphedrine]
methophenazine [see: metofenazate]
methopholine USAN *analgesic* [also: metofoline]
methoprene INN
methopromazine INN
methopromazine maleate [see: methopromazine]
methopyrimazole [see: epirizole]
d-methorphan [see: dextromethorphan]
d-methorphan hydrobromide [see: dextromethorphan hydrobromide]
methoserpidine INN, BAN
methotrexate (MTX) USAN, USP, INN, BAN, JAN *antimetabolic antineoplastic; antirheumatic; antipsoriatic* (*orphan: juvenile rheumatoid arthritis*) 2.5 mg oral; 1 g injection
methotrexate & laurocapram (*orphan: topical mycosis fungoides*)
Methotrexate LPF Sodium preservative-free injection (discontinued 1994) ℞ *antineoplastic for leukemia, psoriasis and rheumatoid arthritis* [methotrexate sodium] 1 g
methotrexate sodium USP *antimetabolic antineoplastic; antirheumatic; for osteogenic sarcoma* (*orphan*) 2.5 mg oral; 20, 1000 mg/vial injection; 2.5, 25 mg/mL injection
Methotrexate/Azone ℞ (*orphan: topical mycosis fungoides*) [methotrexate; laurocapram]
methotrimeprazine USAN, USP *central analgesic; CNS depressant* [also: levomepromazine]
methoxamine INN *adrenergic; vasoconstrictor; vasopressor for hypotensive shock during surgery* [also: methoxamine HCl]
methoxamine HCl USP *adrenergic; vasoconstrictor; vasopressor for hypotensive shock during surgery* [also: methoxamine]
methoxiflurane [see: methoxyflurane]
methoxsalen USP *pigmentation agent for vitiligo; antipsoriatic* (*orphan: pre-*

vent rejection of cardiac allografts) ▣
methixene
methoxy polyethylene glycol [see: polyethylene glycol monomethyl ether]
methoxyfenoserpin [see: mefeserpine]
methoxyflurane USAN, USP, INN, BAN *inhalation general anesthetic*
methoxyphedrine INN
methoxyphenamine INN [also: methoxyphenamine HCl]
methoxyphenamine HCl USP [also: methoxyphenamine]
4-methoxyphenol [see: mequinol]
o-methoxyphenyl salicylate acetate [see: guacetisal]
methoxypromazine maleate [see: methopromazine]
8-methoxypsoralen (8-MOP) [see: methoxsalen]
5-methoxyresorcinol [see: flamenol]
methphenoxydiol [see: guaifenesin]
methscopolamine bromide USP *peptic ulcer adjunct* [also: hyoscine methobromide]
methsuximide USP, BAN *anticonvulsant* [also: mesuximide]
methyclothiazide USAN, USP, INN *diuretic; antihypertensive* 2.5, 5 mg oral
methydromorphine [see: methyldihydromorphine]
methyl alcohol NF *solvent*
methyl benzoquate BAN *coccidiostat for poultry* [also: nequinate]
methyl cresol [see: cresol]
methyl cysteine [see: mecysteine]
methyl p-hydroxybenzoate [see: methylparaben]
methyl isobutyl ketone NF *alcohol denaturant*
methyl nicotinate USAN
methyl palmoxirate USAN *antidiabetic*
methyl phthalate [see: dimethyl phthalate]
methyl salicylate NF *flavoring agent; counterirritant; topical anesthetic*
methyl sulfoxide [see: dimethyl sulfoxide]
methyl violet [see: gentian violet]
l-methylaminoethanolcatechol [see: epinephrine]

methylaminopterin [see: methotrexate]
methylandrostenediol [see: methandriol]
methylatropine nitrate USAN *anticholinergic* [also: atropine methonitrate]
methylbenactyzium bromide INN
methylbenzethonium chloride USP, INN *topical anti-infective/antiseptic*
α-methylbenzylhydrazine [see: mebanazine]
methylcarbamate of salicylanilide [see: anilamate]
methyl-CCNU (chloroethyl-cyclohexyl-nitrosourea) [see: semustine]
methylcellulose USP, INN *suspending and viscosity-increasing agent*
methylcellulose, propylene glycol ether of [see: hydroxypropyl methylcellulose]
methylchromone INN, BAN
methyldesorphine INN, BAN
methyldigoxin [see: metildigoxin]
methyldihydromorphine INN
methyldihydromorphinone HCl [see: metopon]
methyldinitrobenzamide [see: dinitolmide]
methyldioxatrine [see: meletimide]
N-methyldiphenethylamine [see: demelverine]
α-methyl-DL-thyroxine ethyl ester [see: etiroxate]
methyldopa USAN, USP, INN *antihypertensive* 125, 250, 500 mg oral; 250 mg/5 mL oral ▣ levodopa
α-methyldopa [now: methyldopa]
methyldopate HCl USAN, USP *antihypertensive* 250 mg/5 mL injection
6-methylenandrosta-1,4-diene-3,17-dione (*orphan: hormonal therapy for metastatic carcinoma of the breast*)
methylene blue (MB) USP *antimethemoglobinemic; GU antiseptic; antidote to cyanide poisoning* [also: methylthioninium chloride] 65 mg oral; 10 mg/mL injection
methylene chloride NF *solvent*
methylene diphosphonate (MDP) [now: medronate disodium]
6-methyleneoxytetracycline (MOTC) [see: methacycline]

methylenprednisolone [see: prednylidene]
methylergometrine INN *oxytocic* [also: methylergonovine maleate]
methylergometrine maleate [see: methylergonovine maleate]
methylergonovine maleate USP *oxytocic* [also: methylergometrine]
methylergonovinium bimaleate [see: methylergonovine maleate]
methylergotamine [see: metergotamine]
methylestrenolone [see: normethandrone]
methyl-GAG (methylglyoxal-*bis*-guanylhydrazone) [see: mitoguazone]
Methylgesic liquid (discontinued 1992) OTC *counterirritant* [methyl salicylate; menthol; camphor; methyl nicotinate; dipropylene glycol salicylate]
methylglyoxal-*bis*-guanylhydrazone (methyl-GAG; MGBG) [see: mitoguazone]
1-methylhexylamine [see: tuaminoheptane]
1-methylhexylamine sulfate [see: tuaminoheptane sulfate]
N-methylhydrazine [see: procarbazine]
methylmorphine [see: codeine]
methyl-nitro-imidazole [see: carnidazole]
methylnortestosterone [see: normethandrone]
methylparaben USAN, NF *antifungal agent; preservative*
methylparaben sodium USAN, NF *antimicrobial preservative*
methylparafynol [see: meparfynol]
methylpentynol INN, BAN
methylperidol [see: moperone]
(+)-methylphenethylamine [see: dextroamphetamine]
(−)-methylphenethylamine [see: levamphetamine]
methylphenethylamine HCl [see: amphetamine HCl]
methylphenethylamine phosphate [see: amphetamine phosphate]
(−)-methylphenethylamine succinate [see: levamfetamine succinate]
methylphenethylamine sulfate [see: amphetamine sulfate]
(+)-methylphenethylamine sulfate [see: dextroamphetamine sulfate]
methylphenidate INN, BAN *CNS stimulant for attention deficit hyperactivity disorders (ADHD) and narcolepsy* [also: methylphenidate HCl]
methylphenidate HCl USP, JAN *CNS stimulant for attention deficit hyperactivity disorders (ADHD) and narcolepsy* [also: methylphenidate] 5, 10, 20 mg oral
methylphenobarbital INN *anticonvulsant; sedative* [also: mephobarbital; methylphenobarbitone]
methylphenobarbitone BAN *anticonvulsant; sedative* [also: mephobarbital; methylphenobarbital]
d-methylphenylamine sulfate [see: dextroamphetamine sulfate]
methylphytyl napthoquinone [see: phytonadione]
methylprednisolone USP, INN, BAN, JAN *corticosteroid; anti-inflammatory; immunosuppressant* 4, 16 mg oral
methylprednisolone aceponate INN
methylprednisolone acetate USP, JAN *corticosteroid; anti-inflammatory; immunosuppressant* 20, 40, 80 mg/mL injection
methylprednisolone hemisuccinate USP *corticosteroid*
methylprednisolone sodium phosphate USAN *corticosteroid* 40, 125, 500, 1000 mg/vial injection
methylprednisolone sodium succinate USP, JAN *corticosteroid; anti-inflammatory; immunosuppressant*
methylprednisolone suleptanate USAN, INN *anti-inflammatory*
methylpromazine
4-methylpyrazole (4-MP) [see: fomepizole]
methylrosaniline chloride [now: gentian violet]
methylrosanilinium chloride INN *topical anti-infective* [also: gentian violet]
methylscopolamine bromide [see: methscopolamine bromide]
methylsulfate USP *combining name for radicals or groups* [also: metilsulfate]

methyltestosterone USP, INN, BAN *oral androgen* 10, 25 mg oral
methyltheobromine [see: caffeine]
methylthionine chloride [see: methylene blue]
methylthionine HCl [see: methylene blue]
methylthioninium chloride INN *antimethemoglobinemic; antidote to cyanide poisoning* [also: methylene blue]
methylthiouracil USP, INN
methyltrienolone [see: metribolone]
methynodiol diacetate USAN *progestin* [also: metynodiol]
methyprylon USP, INN *sedative; hypnotic* [also: methprylone]
methyprylone BAN *sedative* [also: methyprylon]
methyridene BAN [also: metyridine]
methysergide USAN, INN, BAN *migraine-specific vasoconstrictor*
methysergide maleate USP *migraine-specific vasoconstrictor*
metiamide USAN, INN *antagonist to histamine H$_2$ receptors*
metiapine USAN, INN *antipsychotic*
metiazinic acid INN
metibride INN
meticillin INN *antibacterial* [also: methicillin sodium]
meticillin sodium [see: methicillin sodium]
Meticorten tablets ℞ *glucocorticoid; anti-inflammatory; immunosuppressant* [prednisone] 1 mg
meticrane INN
metildigoxin INN
metilsulfate INN *combining name for radicals or groups* [also: methylsulfate]
Metimyd eye drop suspension, ophthalmic ointment ℞ *ophthalmic topical corticosteroidal anti-inflammatory; bacteriostatic* [prednisolone acetate; sulfacetamide sodium] 0.5%•10%
metindizate INN [also: methindizate]
metioprim USAN, INN, BAN *antibacterial*
metioxate INN
metipirox INN
metipranolol USAN, INN, BAN *ophthalmic antihypertensive (β-blocker)*

metipranolol HCl *topical antiglaucoma agent (β-blocker)*
metiprenaline INN
metirosine INN *antihypertensive* [also: metyrosine]
metisazone INN *antiviral* [also: methisazone]
metitepine INN
metixene INN *smooth muscle relaxant* [also: methixene HCl]
metixene HCl [see: methixene HCl]
metizoline INN *adrenergic; vasoconstrictor* [also: metizoline HCl]
metizoline HCl USAN *adrenergic; vasoconstrictor* [also: metizoline]
metkefamide INN *analgesic* [also: metkephamid acetate]
metkefamide acetate [see: metkephamid acetate]
metkephamid acetate USAN *analgesic* [also: metkefamide]
metochalcone INN
metocinium iodide INN
metoclopramide INN *antiemetic for chemotherapy; GI stimulant; antidopaminergic* [also: metoclopramide HCl]
metoclopramide HCl USAN, USP *antiemetic for chemotherapy; GI stimulant; antidopaminergic* [also: metoclopramide] 5, 10 mg oral; 5, 10 mg/5 mL oral; 5 mg/mL injection
metoclopramide monohydrochloride monohydrate *antiemetic for chemotherapy; GI stimulant; antidopaminergic* 5, 10 mg oral; 5, 10 mg/5 mL oral; 5 mg/mL injection
metocurine iodide USAN, USP *neuromuscular blocker; muscle relaxant* 2 mg/mL injection
metofenazate INN
metofoline INN *analgesic* [also: methopholine]
metogest USAN, INN *hormone*
metolazone USAN, INN *diuretic; antihypertensive* ⑨ metaxalone
metomidate INN, BAN
metopimazine USAN, INN *antiemetic*
Metopirone tablets (discontinued 1994) ℞ *pituitary function test* [metyrapone] 250 mg ⑨ metyrapone
metopon INN
metopon HCl [see: metopon]

metoprine USAN *antineoplastic*

metoprolol USAN, INN, BAN *antiadrenergic (β-receptor)* ② metaproterenol

metoprolol fumarate USAN *antihypertensive*

metoprolol succinate USAN *antianginal; antihypertensive*

metoprolol tartrate USAN, USP *antiadrenergic (β-receptor)* 50, 100 mg oral; 1 mg/mL injection

metoquizine USAN, INN *anticholinergic*

metoserpate INN *veterinary sedative* [also: metoserpate HCl]

metoserpate HCl USAN *veterinary sedative* [also: metoserpate]

metostilenol INN

metoxepin INN

metoxiestrol [see: moxestrol]

Metra tablets (discontinued 1994) ℞ *anorexiant* [phendimetrazine tartrate] 35 mg

metrafazoline INN

metralindole INN

metrazifone INN

metrenperone USAN, INN, BAN *veterinary myopathic*

Metreton Ophthalmic eye drops (discontinued 1993) ℞ *ophthalmic topical corticosteroidal anti-inflammatory* [prednisolone sodium phosphate]

metribolone INN

Metric 21 tablets (discontinued 1995) ℞ *antibiotic; antiprotozoal; amebicide* [metronidazole]

metrifonate INN *investigational treatment for Alzheimer's disease* [also: metriphonate]

metrifudil INN

metriphonate BAN *investigational treatment for Alzheimer's disease* [also: metrifonate]

metrizamide USAN, INN *radiopaque medium*

metrizoate sodium USAN *radiopaque medium* [also: sodium metrizoate]

Metro I.V. ready-to-use injection ℞ *antibiotic; antiprotozoal; amebicide* [metronidazole] 500 mg/100 mL

MetroCream ℞ *topical antibiotic, antiprotozoal, and amebicide for rosacea* [metronidazole] 0.75%

Metrodin powder for IM injection ℞ *ovulation stimulant in polycystic ovarian disease (orphan)* [urofollitropin] 0.83, 1.66 mg/ampule

Metrodin HP ℞ *investigational infertility treatment* [urofollitropin]

MetroGel ℞ *antibacterial; antiprotozoal; (orphan: decubitus ulcers; acne rosacea; perioral dermatitis)* [metronidazole] 0.75%

MetroGel Vaginal gel ℞ *antibacterial; antiprotozoal* [metronidazole] 0.75%

metronidazole USAN, USP, INN, BAN *antibiotic; antiprotozoal; amebicide; (orphan: decubitus ulcers; acne rosacea; perioral dermatitis)* 250, 500 mg oral; 500 mg/100 mL injection

metronidazole benzoate *antiprotozoal (Trichomonas)*

metronidazole HCl USAN *antibiotic; antiprotozoal; amebicide*

metronidazole phosphate USAN *antibacterial; antiprotozoal*

Metryl tablets (discontinued 1992) ℞ *antibiotic; antiprotozoal; amebicide* [metronidazole]

Metubine Iodide IV injection ℞ *anesthesia adjunct* [metocurine iodide] 2 mg/mL

metuclazepam [see: metaclazepam]

meturedepa USAN, INN *antineoplastic*

metynodiol INN *progestin* [also: methynodiol diacetate]

metynodiol diacetate [see: methynodiol diacetate]

metyrapone USAN, USP, INN *pituitary function test* ② Metopirone; metyrosine

metyrapone tartrate USAN *pituitary function test*

metyridine INN [also: methyridene]

metyrosine USAN, USP *antihypertensive; pheochromocytomic agent* ② metyrapone

Mevacor tablets ℞ *cholesterol-lowering antihyperlipidemic; antiatherosclerotic* [lovastatin] 10, 20, 40 mg

Mevanin-C capsules (discontinued 1992) OTC *vitamin/mineral/iron supplement* [multiple vitamins & minerals; iron; folic acid; hesperidin complex]

mevastatin INN

mevinolin [now: lovastatin]

mexafylline INN
mexazolam INN
mexenone INN, BAN
mexiletine INN, BAN *antiarrhythmic* [also: mexiletine HCl]
mexiletine HCl USAN, USP *antiarrhythmic* [also: mexiletine] 150, 200, 250 mg oral
mexiprostil
Mexitil capsules ℞ *antiarrhythmic* [mexiletine HCl] 150, 200, 250 mg
mexoprofen INN
mexrenoate potassium USAN, INN *aldosterone antagonist*
Mexsana Medicated powder OTC *topical diaper rash treatment* [kaolin; zinc oxide; eucalyptus oil; camphor; corn starch]
mezacopride INN
mezepine INN
mezilamine INN
Mezlin powder for IV or IM injection ℞ *extended-spectrum penicillin-type antibiotic* [mezlocillin sodium] 1, 2, 3, 4, 20 g ② Meclan
mezlocillin USAN, INN *antibacterial*
mezlocillin sodium USP *bactericidal antibiotic*
MF (methotrexate [with leucovorin rescue], fluorouracil) *chemotherapy protocol*
MF (mitomycin, fluorouracil) *chemotherapy protocol*
MFP (melphalan, fluorouracil, medroxyprogesterone acetate) *chemotherapy protocol*
MG Cold Sore Formula solution OTC *topical oral anesthetic; antipruritic/counterirritant* [lidocaine; menthol] 2•1%
MG217 Dual Treatment lotion OTC *topical antipsoriatic; antiseborrheic* [coal tar solution] 5%
MG217 Medicated conditioner OTC *topical antipsoriatic; antiseborrheic* [coal tar solution] 2%
MG217 Medicated ointment, shampoo OTC *topical antipsoriatic; antiseborrheic; antifungal; keratolytic* [coal tar solution; colloidal sulfur; salicylic acid] 2%•1.1%•1.5%; 5%•1.5%•2%
MG400 shampoo OTC *antiseborrheic; keratolytic* [salicylic acid; sulfur] 3%•5%

MGA (melengestrol acetate) [q.v.]
MGBG (methylglyoxal-*bis*-guanyl-hydrazone) [see: mitoguazone]
MGW (magnesium sulfate + glycerin + water) enema [q.v.]
Miacalcin nasal spray ℞ *calcium regulator for postmenopausal osteoporosis (only)* [calcitonin (salmon)] 200 IU/0.09 mL
Miacalcin subcu or IM injection ℞ *calcium regulator for hypercalcemia, Paget's disease, and postmenopausal osteoporosis* [calcitonin (salmon)] 200 IU/mL
Mi-Acid gelcaps OTC *antacid* [calcium carbonate; magnesium carbonate] 311•232 mg
Mi-Acid; Mi-Acid II liquid OTC *antacid; antiflatulent* [aluminum hydroxide; magnesium hydroxide; simethicone] 200•200•20 mg/5 mL; 400•400•40 mg/5 mL
mianserin INN *serotonin inhibitor; antihistamine; investigational antidepressant* [also: mianserin HCl]
mianserin HCl USAN *serotonin inhibitor; antihistamine; investigational antidepressant* [also: mianserin]
mibefradil *investigational calcium channel blocker for hypertension, angina, and congestive heart failure*
mibefradil dihydrochloride USAN *vasodilator; anti-ischemic; calcium modulator*
MIBG-I-123 [see: iobenguane sulfate I 123]
mibolerone USAN, INN *anabolic; androgen*
Micatin cream, powder, aerosol powder, liquid spray OTC *topical antifungal* [miconazole nitrate] 2%
MICE (mesna [rescue], ifosfamide, carboplatin, etoposide) *chemotherapy protocol* [also: ICE]
Mi-Cebrin; Mi-Cebrin T tablets (discontinued 1993) OTC *vitamin/mineral/iron supplement* [multiple vitamins & minerals; iron]
micinicate INN
miconazole USP, INN, BAN, JAN *fungicidal*

miconazole nitrate USAN, USP, JAN *antifungal* 2% topical

Micrainin tablets ℞ *analgesic; antipyretic; anti-inflammatory; anxiolytic* [aspirin; meprobamate] 325•200 mg

MICRhoGAM IM injection ℞ *obstetric Rh factor immunity suppressant* [Rh$_0$(D) immune globulin] 50 μg ② microgram

microbubble contrast agent *(orphan: diagnostic aid for intracranial tumors)*

microcrystalline cellulose [see: cellulose, microcrystalline]

microcrystalline wax [see: wax, microcrystalline]

microfibrillar collagen hemostat (MCH) *topical local hemostatic*

Micro-K; Micro-K 10 Extencaps (controlled-release capsules) ℞ *potassium supplement* [potassium chloride] 600 mg (8 mEq); 750 mg (10 mEq)

Micro-K LS extended-release powder ℞ *potassium supplement* [potassium chloride] 20 mEq/packet

Microlipid emulsion OTC *dietary fat supplement* [safflower oil] 50%

Micronase tablets ℞ *sulfonylurea antidiabetic* [glyburide] 1.25, 2.5, 5 mg

microNefrin solution for inhalation OTC *bronchodilator for bronchial asthma and COPD* [racepinephrine] 2.25%

micronized aluminum *astringent*

micronomicin INN

Micronor tablets ℞ *oral contraceptive (progestin only)* [norethindrone] 0.35 mg

Microstix-3 reagent strips for professional use *in vitro diagnostic aid for nitrate, uropathogens, or bacteria in the urine*

MicroTrak Chlamydia trachomatis slide test for professional use *in vitro diagnostic aid for Chlamydia trachomatis*

MicroTrak HSV 1/HSV 2 Culture Identification/Typing Test culture test for professional use *in vitro diagnostic aid for herpes simplex virus in tissue cultures*

MicroTrak HSV 1/HSV 2 Direct Specimen Identification/Typing Test slide test for professional use *in vitro diagnostic aid for herpes simplex virus in external lesions*

MicroTrak Neisseria gonorrhoeae Culture Confirmation Test reagent kit for professional use *in vitro diagnostic aid for Neisseria gonorrhoeae*

mictine [see: aminometradine]

Micturin ℞ *investigational agent for urinary incontinence (clinical trials discontinued in 1994)* [terodiline HCl]

midaflur USAN, INN *sedative*

midaglizole INN

midalcipran [see: milnacipran]

midamaline INN

Midamine ℞ *(orphan: idiopathic orthostatic hypotension)* [midodrine HCl]

Midamor tablets ℞ *potassium-sparing diuretic* [amiloride HCl] 5 mg

midazogrel INN

midazolam INN, BAN, JAN *general anesthetic* [also: midazolam HCl]

midazolam HCl USAN *general anesthetic* [also: midazolam]

midazolam maleate USAN *intravenous anesthetic*

Midchlor capsules ℞ *vasoconstrictor; sedative; analgesic (for migraine)* [isometheptene mucate; dichloralphenazone; acetaminophen] 65•100•325 mg

midecamycin INN

midkine factor *investigational protectant for nerve cells*

midodrine INN, BAN *antihypertensive; vasoconstrictor* [also: midodrine HCl]

midodrine HCl USAN, JAN *antihypertensive; vasoconstrictor; (orphan: idiopathic orthostatic hypotension)* [also: midodrine]

Midol; Midol for Cramps caplets (discontinued 1995) OTC *analgesic; antipyretic; anti-inflammatory; muscle relaxant* [aspirin; caffeine; cinnamedrine HCl] 545•32.4•14.9 mg; 500•32.4•14.9 mg

Midol, Teen caplets OTC *analgesic; anti-inflammatory; diuretic* [acetaminophen; pamabrom] 400•25 mg

Midol 200 tablets (discontinued 1996) OTC *nonsteroidal anti-inflammatory drug (NSAID); antiarthritic; analgesic* [ibuprofen] 200 mg

Midol IB tablets OTC *nonsteroidal anti-inflammatory drug (NSAID); antiarthritic; analgesic* [ibuprofen] 200 mg

Midol Multi-Symptom Formula caplets OTC *analgesic; anti-inflammatory; antihistaminic sleep aid* [acetaminophen; pyrilamine maleate] 325•12.5 mg

Midol Multi-Symptom Menstrual caplets OTC *analgesic; anti-inflammatory; antihistaminic sleep aid* [acetaminophen; caffeine; pyrilamine maleate] 500•60•15 mg

Midol PM caplets OTC *analgesic; antipyretic; antihistaminic sleep aid* [acetaminophen; diphenhydramine] 500•25 mg

Midol PMS caplets, gelcaps OTC *analgesic; anti-inflammatory; diuretic; antihistaminic sleep aid* [acetaminophen; pamabrom; pyrilamine maleate] 500•25•15 mg

Midon R *investigational treatment for orthostatic hypotension* [midodrine]

Midrin capsules R *vasoconstrictor; sedative; analgesic (for migraine)* [isometheptene mucate; dichloralphenazone; acetaminophen] 65•100•325 mg ② Mydfrin

MIFA (mitomycin, fluorouracil, Adriamycin) *chemotherapy protocol*

mifarmonab [see: imciromab pentetate]

Mifegyne (available in France, Sweden, and the U.K.) R *abortifacient; investigational glucocorticosteroid antagonist for Cushing syndrome* [mifepristone]

mifentidine INN

mifepristone INN, BAN *progesterone antagonist; abortifacient; investigational (Phase III) for unresectable meningioma*

mifobate USAN, INN *antiatherosclerotic*

Mighty Vite T tablets OTC *vitamin/ mineral supplement* [multiple vitamins & minerals]

miglitol USAN, INN, BAN *α-glucosidase inhibitor; investigational antidiabetic agent*

Migranal nasal spray R *investigational antimigraine agent* [dihydroergotamine]

Migrastat intranasal R *investigational antimigraine agent* [propranolol HCl]

Migratine capsules R *vasoconstrictor; sedative; analgesic (for migraine)* [isometheptene mucate; dichloralphenazone; acetaminophen] 65•100•325 mg

mikamycin INN, BAN

Mil Adrene; Mil Adrene Forte tablets OTC *dietary supplement* [raw adrenal concentrate]

milacemide INN *anticonvulsant; antidepressant* [also: milacemide HCl]

milacemide HCl USAN *anticonvulsant; antidepressant* [also: milacemide]

Mil-Adregen tablets OTC *dietary supplement* [multiple glandular concentrates; multiple vitamins; zinc]

Mil-A-Mulsion drops OTC *vitamin supplement* [vitamin A palmitate; vitamin E]

Milco B tablets OTC *vitamin supplement* [multiple B vitamins]

Milco-B-Forte tablets OTC *vitamin/ mineral supplement* [multiple B vitamins; vitamin C; zinc]

Milco-Zyme timed-release tablets OTC *dietary supplement* [multiple enzymes]

mild silver protein [see: silver protein, mild]

Mild-C chewable tablets, capsules, timed-release caplets OTC *vitamin supplement* [calcium ascorbate]

milenperone USAN, INN, BAN *antipsychotic*

Miles Nervine caplets OTC *antihistaminic sleep aid* [diphenhydramine HCl] 25 mg

milipertine USAN, INN *antipsychotic*

milk of bismuth [see: bismuth, milk of]

milk of magnesia [see: magnesia, milk of]

Milk of Magnesia-Cascara, Concentrated oral suspension OTC *antacid; laxative* [milk of magnesia; aromatic cascara fluidextract; alcohol 7%] 30•5 mL/15 mL

Milkinol emulsion OTC *emollient laxative* [mineral oil]

milnacipran INN *investigational antidepressant*

Milontin Kapseals (capsules) R *anticonvulsant* [phensuximide] 500 mg ② Miltown; Mylanta

Milophene tablets ℞ *ovulation stimulant* [clomiphene citrate] 50 mg

miloxacin INN

milrinone USAN, INN, BAN *cardiotonic*

milrinone lactate *vasodilator for congestive heart failure*

Miltab #1 tablets OTC *dietary supplement* [multiple vitamins; levoglutamide; magnesium aspartate]

miltefosine INN

Miltown; Miltown-600 tablets ℞ *anxiolytic* [meprobamate] 200, 400 mg; 600 mg ⓓ Milontin

milverine INN

Mil-V-Zyme capsules OTC *dietary supplement* [multiple enzymes]

mimbane INN *analgesic* [also: mimbane HCl]

mimbane HCl USAN *analgesic* [also: mimbane]

minaprine USAN, INN, BAN *psychotropic*

minaprine HCl USAN *antidepressant*

minaxolone USAN, INN *anesthetic*

mindodilol INN

mindolic acid [see: clometacin]

mindoperone INN

MINE (mesna [rescue], ifosfamide, Novantrone, etoposide) *chemotherapy protocol*

MINE-ESHAP (alternating cycles of MINE and ESHAP) *chemotherapy protocol*

minepentate INN, BAN

Mineral Compleet caplets OTC *mineral supplement* [multiple minerals; kelp]

Mineral Ice [see: Therapeutic Mineral Ice]

mineral oil USP *emollient/protectant; laxative; solvent*

mineral oil, light NF *tablet and capsule lubricant; vehicle*

Mini Thin Asthma Relief tablets OTC *decongestant; expectorant* [ephedrine HCl; guaifenesin] 25•100, 25•200 mg

Mini Thin Pseudo tablets OTC *nasal decongestant* [pseudoephedrine HCl] 60 mg

mini-BEAM (BCNU, etoposide, ara-C, melphalan) *chemotherapy protocol*

mini-COAP (cyclophosphamide, Oncovin, ara-C, prednisone) *chemotherapy protocol*

Minidyne solution OTC *broad-spectrum antimicrobial* [povidone-iodine] 10%

Mini-Gamulin Rh IM injection ℞ *obstetric Rh factor immunity suppressant* [$Rh_0(D)$ immune globulin] 50 μg

Miniguard disposable pads *adhesive foam pad to seal urethral opening for stress urinary incontinence in women*

Min-I-Mix (delivery system) *dual-chambered prefilled syringe*

Minipress capsules ℞ *antihypertensive; antiadrenergic* [prazosin HCl] 1, 2, 5 mg

Minipress XL extended-release tablets ℞ *antihypertensive* [prazosin HCl]

Minitran transdermal patch ℞ *antianginal* [nitroglycerin] 9, 18, 36, 54 mg

Minit-Rub OTC *counterirritant* [methyl salicylate; menthol; camphor] 15%•3.5%•2.3%

Minizide 1; Minizide 2; Minizide 5 capsules ℞ *antihypertensive* [prazosin HCl; polythiazide] 1•0.5 mg; 2•0.5 mg; 5•0.5 mg

Minocin pellet-filled capsules, oral suspension, powder for IV injection ℞ *tetracycline-type antibiotic; (orphan: chronic malignant pleural effusion)* [minocycline HCl] 50, 100 mg; 50 mg/5 mL; 100 mg ⓓ Indocin; Mithracin; niacin

minocromil USAN, INN, BAN *prophylactic antiallergic*

minocycline USAN, INN, BAN *gram-negative and gram-positive bacteriostatic; antirickettsial*

minocycline HCl USP *antibacterial; (orphan: chronic malignant pleural effusion)* 50, 100 mg oral

Minodyl tablets (discontinued 1993) ℞ *antihypertensive; vasodilator* [minoxidil]

minoxidil USAN, USP, INN, BAN *antihypertensive; peripheral vasodilator; hair growth stimulant* 2.5, 10 mg oral

Minoxidil for Men topical solution OTC *hair growth stimulant* [minoxidil] 2%

Mintezol chewable tablets, oral suspension ℞ *anthelmintic* [thiabendazole] 500 mg; 500 mg/5 mL

Mintox chewable tablets, oral suspension OTC *antacid* [aluminum hydroxide; magnesium hydroxide] 200•200 mg; 225•200 mg/5 mL

Mintox Plus liquid OTC *antacid; antiflatulent* [aluminum hydroxide; magnesium hydroxide; simethicone] 500•450•40 mg/5 mL

Minulet ℞ *investigational monophasic oral contraceptive* [gestodene]

Minute-Gel ℞ *topical dental caries preventative* [acidulated phosphate fluoride] 1.23%

Miochol solution (discontinued 1996) ℞ *direct-acting miotic for ophthalmic surgery* [acetylcholine chloride] 1:100

Miochol-E solution ℞ *direct-acting miotic for ophthalmic surgery* [acetylcholine chloride] 1:100

mioflazine INN, BAN *coronary vasodilator* [also: mioflazine HCl]

mioflazine HCl USAN *coronary vasodilator* [also: mioflazine]

Mio-Rel injection ℞ *muscle relaxant* [orphenadrine citrate]

Miostat solution ℞ *direct-acting miotic for ophthalmic surgery* [carbachol] 0.01%

MIP-1 alpha *investigational antineoplastic*

mipafilcon A USAN *hydrophilic contact lens material*

mipimazole INN

Mirac [see: Tilarin]

Miradon tablets ℞ *anticoagulant* [anisindione] 50 mg

MiraFlow solution OTC *cleaning solution for hard or soft contact lenses*

MiraSept System solutions OTC *two-step chemical disinfecting system for soft contact lenses* [hydrogen peroxide based] 3%

mirfentanil INN *analgesic* [also: mirfentanil HCl]

mirfentanil HCl USAN *analgesic* [also: mirfentanil]

mirincamycin INN *antibacterial; antimalarial* [also: mirincamycin HCl]

mirincamycin HCl USAN *antibacterial; antimalarial* [also: mirincamycin]

mirisetron maleate USAN *anxiolytic*

miristalkonium chloride INN

miroprofen INN

mirosamicin INN

mirtazapine USAN, INN *investigational antidepressant; 5HT-1A agonist*

misonidazole USAN, INN *antiprotozoal (Trichomonas)*

misoprostol USAN, INN, BAN *prevention of NSAID-induced gastric ulcers*

Mission Prenatal; Mission Prenatal F.A.; Mission Prenatal H.P. tablets OTC *vitamin/iron supplement* [multiple vitamins; ferrous gluconate; folic acid] ±•30•0.4 mg; ±•30•0.8 mg; ±•30•0.8 mg

Mission Prenatal Rx tablets ℞ *vitamin/calcium/iron supplement* [multiple vitamins; calcium; iron; folic acid] ±•175•60•1 mg

Mission Surgical Supplement tablets OTC *vitamin/iron supplement* [multiple vitamins; ferrous gluconate] ±•27 mg

Mistometer (trademarked form) *metered-dose inhalation aerosol*

Mithracin powder for IV infusion ℞ *antineoplastic for testicular cancer* [plicamycin] 2.5 mg ⚠ Minocin

mithramycin [now: plicamycin] ⚠ mitomycin

mitindomide USAN, INN *antineoplastic*

mitobronitol INN, BAN

mitocarcin USAN, INN *antineoplastic*

mitoclomine INN, BAN

mitocromin USAN *antineoplastic*

mitoflaxone INN

mitogillin USAN, INN *antineoplastic*

mitoguazone INN *investigational antineoplastic for lymphomas, multiple myeloma, head, esophagus, and prostate cancer*

mitolactol INN *investigational antineoplastic (orphan: cervical squamous carcinoma)*

mitomalcin USAN, INN *antineoplastic*

mitomycin USAN, USP, INN, BAN *antibiotic antineoplastic; (orphan: refractory glaucoma; glaucoma surgery)* ⚠ mithramycin; Mutamycin

mitomycin C (MTC) [see: mitomycin]

mitonafide INN

mitopodozide INN, BAN

mitoquidone INN, BAN

mitosper USAN, INN *antineoplastic*

mitotane USAN, USP, INN *antineoplastic; adrenal cytotoxic agent*

mitotenamine INN, BAN

mitoxantrone INN *antibiotic antineoplastic* [also: mitoxantrone HCl; mitozantrone]

mitoxantrone HCl USAN *antibiotic antineoplastic; for acute myelogenous (nonlymphocytic) leukemia (orphan)* [also: mitoxantrone; mitozantrone]

mitozantrone BAN *antineoplastic* [also: mitoxantrone HCl; mitoxantrone]

mitozolomide INN, BAN

Mitran capsules ℞ *anxiolytic* [chlordiazepoxide HCl] 10 mg

Mitrolan chewable tablets OTC *bulk laxative; antidiarrheal* [calcium polycarbophil] 500 mg

mitronal [see: cinnarizine]

MIV (mitoxantrone, ifosfamide, VePesid) *chemotherapy protocol*

Mivacron IV infusion ℞ *muscle relaxant; adjunct to anesthesia* [mivacurium chloride] 0.5, 2 mg/mL

mivacurium chloride USAN, INN, BAN *neuromuscular blocking agent*

mixed respiratory vaccine (MRV) *active bacterin for respiratory tract infections*

mixed tocopherols [see: vitamin E]

mixidine USAN, INN *coronary vasodilator*

Mix-O-Vial (trademarked packaging form) *two-compartment vial*

Mixtard 70/30 subcu injection (discontinued 1994) OTC *antidiabetic* [isophane insulin (pork); insulin (pork)]

Mixtard Human 70/30 subcu injection (discontinued 1994) OTC *antidiabetic* [isophane insulin (human semisynthetic); human insulin (semisynthetic)]

mizoribine INN

MK-383 *investigational fibrinogen receptor antagonist for cardiac platelet aggregation disorders*

MK-462 *investigational serotonin reuptake receptor inhibitor for migraine*

MK-499 *investigational calcium channel blocker for atrial and ventricular arrhythmias*

M-KYA capsules (discontinued 1996) OTC *prevention and treatment of nocturnal leg cramps* [quinine sulfate] 64.8 mg

MM (mercaptopurine, methotrexate) *chemotherapy protocol*

MMOPP (methotrexate, mechlorethamine, Oncovin, procarbazine, prednisone) *chemotherapy protocol*

MMP injection ℞ *diagnosis and treatment of allergies* [mold allergenic extracts]

MMR (measles, mumps & rubella vaccines) [q.v.]

M-M-R II powder for subcu injection ℞ *measles, mumps and rubella vaccine* [measles, mumps & rubella virus vaccine, live] 0.5 mL

MM-Zyme tablets OTC *dietary supplement* [multiple enzymes]

MOB (mechlorethamine, Oncovin, bleomycin) *chemotherapy protocol*

MOB-III (mitomycin, Oncovin, bleomycin, cisplatin) *chemotherapy protocol*

Moban tablets, oral concentrate ℞ *antipsychotic* [molindone HCl] 5, 10, 25, 50, 100 mg; 20 mg/mL ② Mobidin; Modane

mobecarb INN

mobenzoxamine INN

Mobidin tablets ℞ *analgesic; antipyretic; anti-inflammatory; antirheumatic* [magnesium salicylate] 600 mg ② Moban

Mobigesic tablets OTC *analgesic; antipyretic; anti-inflammatory; antihistamine* [magnesium salicylate; phenyltoloxamine citrate] 325•30 mg

Mobisyl Creme OTC *topical analgesic* [trolamine salicylate] 10%

moccasin snake antivenin [see: antivenin (Crotalidae) polyvalent]

mocimycin INN

mociprazine INN

moclobemide USAN, INN, BAN *antidepressant; investigational treatment for panic disorder and social phobia*

moctamide INN

Moctanin biliary infusion ℞ *anticholelithogenic; for dissolution of cholesterol gallstones (orphan)* [monoctanoin]

modafinil USAN, INN *analeptic (orphan: excessive daytime sleepiness)*

modaline INN *antidepressant* [also: modaline sulfate]

modaline sulfate USAN *antidepressant* [also: modaline]
Modane tablets OTC *laxative* [white phenolphthalein] 130 mg ② Moban; Mudrane
Modane Bulk liquid OTC *bulk laxative* [psyllium hydrophilic mucilloid] 50%
Modane Plus tablets OTC *laxative; stool softener* [white phenolphthalein; docusate sodium] 65•100 mg
Modane Soft capsules OTC *stool softener* [docusate sodium] 100 mg
modecainide USAN, INN *antiarrhythmic*
Moderil tablets (discontinued 1995) ℞ *antihypertensive* [rescinnamine] 0.25, 0.5 mg ② Mellaril
Modicon tablets ℞ *monophasic oral contraceptive* [norethindrone; ethinyl estradiol] 0.5 mg•35 μg ② Mylicon
modified bovine lung surfactant extract [see: beractant]
modified Burow solution [see: aluminum acetate solution]
modified cellulose gum [now: croscarmellose sodium]
modified Shohl solution (sodium citrate & citric acid) *urinary alkalinizer; compounding agent*
Modiodal (commercially available in France) ℞ *investigational analeptic for narcolepsy and hypersomnia* [modafinil]
Modivid ℞ *investigational cephalosporin antibiotic* [cefodizime]
Modrastane capsules (discontinued 1995) ℞ *adrenal steroid inhibitor; antisteroidal antineoplastic for Cushing syndrome* [trilostane] 30, 60 mg
Modual powder OTC *carbohydrate caloric supplement* [glucose polymers]
Moduretic tablets ℞ *diuretic; antihypertensive* [amiloride HCl; hydrochlorothiazide] 5•50 mg
moexipril INN, BAN *antihypertensive*
moexipril HCl USAN *antihypertensive; angiotensin-converting enzyme (ACE) inhibitor*
moexiprilat INN
MOF (MeCCNU, Oncovin, fluorouracil) *chemotherapy protocol*
mofebutazone INN
mofedione [see: oxazidione]

mofegiline INN *antiparkinsonian; investigational Alzheimer's treatment; investigational antiasthmatic* [also: mofegiline HCl]
mofegiline HCl USAN *antiparkinsonian; investigational Alzheimer's treatment; investigational antiasthmatic* [also: mofegiline]
mofetil USAN, INN *combining name for radicals or groups*
mofloverine INN
mofoxime INN
MOF-STREP; MOF-Strep (MeCCNU, Oncovin, fluorouracil, streptozocin) *chemotherapy protocol*
Mogadon ℞ *investigational benzodiazepine-type tranquilizer; anxiolytic; anticonvulsant; hypnotic* [nitrazepam]
moguisteine INN
Moist Again vaginal gel OTC *lubricant* [glycerin; aloe vera]
Moi-Stir oral spray, Swabsticks OTC *saliva substitute* ② moisture
Moi-Stir 10 oral spray (name changed to Entertainer's Secret Throat Relief in 1994)
Moisture Derm lotion OTC *emollient* [mineral oil; stearic acid; petrolatum; lanolin; lanolin alcohol; trolamine; cetyl alcohol]
Moisture Drops eye drops OTC *ocular moisturizer/lubricant* [hydroxypropyl methylcellulose] 0.5%
Moisturel lotion OTC *moisturizer; emollient* [dimethicone] 3%
molecusol & carbamazepine *(orphan: emergency rescue of grand mal status epilepticus)*
molfarnate INN
molgramostim USAN, INN, BAN *antineutropenic; hematopoietic stimulant; investigational cytokine to AIDS (orphan: aplastic anemia)*
molinazone USAN, INN *analgesic*
molindone INN *antipsychotic* [also: molindone HCl]
molindone HCl USAN *antipsychotic* [also: molindone]
Mol-Iron tablets OTC *hematinic* [ferrous sulfate] 195 mg

Mol-Iron with Vitamin C tablets OTC *hematinic* [ferrous sulfate; ascorbic acid] 39•75 mg

Mollifene Ear Wax Removing Formula drops OTC *agent to emulsify and disperse ear wax* [carbamide peroxide] 6.5%

molracetam INN

molsidomine USAN, INN *antianginal; coronary vasodilator*

Moly-B capsule OTC *dietary supplement* [molybdenum]

molybdenum *element (Mo)*

Moly-Pak IV injection (discontinued 1992) ℞ *intravenous nutritional therapy* [ammonium molybdate tetrahydrate]

Molypen IV injection ℞ *intravenous nutritional therapy* [ammonium molybdate tetrahydrate] 25 µg/mL

Momentum caplets OTC *analgesic; antipyretic; anti-inflammatory; antihistamine* [aspirin; phenyltoloxamine citrate] 500•15 mg

Momentum Muscular Backache Formula caplets OTC *analgesic; antipyretic; anti-inflammatory* [magnesium salicylate tetrahydrate] 580 mg

mometasone INN, BAN *topical corticosteroid* [also: mometasone furoate]

mometasone furoate USAN *topical corticosteroid; investigational agent for allergic rhinitis in nasal spray form* [also: mometasone]

MOMP (mechlorethamine, Oncovin, methotrexate, prednisone) *chemotherapy protocol*

monalazone disodium INN

monalium hydrate [see: magaldrate]

monatepil INN *antianginal; antihypertensive* [also: monatepil maleate]

monatepil maleate USAN *antianginal; antihypertensive* [also: monatepil]

monensin USAN, INN *antiprotozoal; antibacterial; antifungal*

Monistat 3 vaginal suppositories + cream OTC *antifungal* [miconazole nitrate] 200 mg; 2%

Monistat 5 tampons (discontinued 1994; previously available only in California) ℞ *antifungal* [miconazole nitrate] 100 mg

Monistat 7 vaginal suppositories, vaginal cream OTC *antifungal* [miconazole nitrate] 100 mg; 2%

Monistat 7 Combination Pack vaginal suppositories + cream OTC *antifungal* [miconazole nitrate] 100 mg; 2%

Monistat Dual-Pak vaginal suppositories + cream ℞ *antifungal* [miconazole nitrate] 200 mg; 2%

Monistat i.v. intrathecal or IV injection ℞ *systemic antifungal* [miconazole] 10 mg/mL

Monistat-Derm cream ℞ *topical antifungal* [miconazole nitrate] 2%

mono- & di-acetylated monoglycerides NF *plasticizer*

mono- & di-glycerides NF *emulsifying agent*

monobasic potassium phosphate [see: potassium phosphate, monobasic]

monobasic sodium phosphate [see: sodium phosphate, monobasic]

monobenzone USP, INN *depigmenting agent for vitiligo*

monobenzyl ether of hydroquinone [see: monobenzone]

monobromated camphor [see: camphor, monobromated]

monocalcium phosphate [see: calcium phosphate, dibasic] 2]

Monocaps tablets OTC *vitamin/mineral/ iron supplement* [multiple vitamins & minerals; ferrous fumarate; folic acid; biotin] ≛•14 mg•0.1 mg•15 µg

Monocete liquid (discontinued 1995) ℞ *cauterant; keratolytic* [monochloroacetic acid] 80% 2 Monoket

Mono-Chlor liquid ℞ *cauterant; keratolytic* [monochloroacetic acid] 80% 2 Monocor

monochloroacetic acid *strong keratolytic/cauterant*

monochlorothymol [see: chlorothymol]

monochlorphenamide [see: clofenamide]

Monocid powder for IV or IM injection ℞ *cephalosporin-type antibiotic* [cefonicid sodium] 0.5, 1, 10 g

Monoclate powder for IV injection (discontinued 1996) ℞ *antihemophilic to correct coagulation deficiency*

[antihemophilic factor VIII:C, heat treated] ☑

Monoclate P powder for IV injection ℞ *antihemophilic to correct coagulation deficiency* [antihemophilic factor VIII:C] ☑

monoclonal antibody (human) to hepatitis B virus (*orphan: hepatitis B prophylaxis for liver transplant*)

monoclonal antibody (murine) anti-idiotype melanoma assorted antigen (*orphan: invasive cutaneous melanoma*)

monoclonal antibody (murine or human) to B-cell lymphoma (*orphan: B-cell lymphoma*)

monoclonal antibody 17-1A (*orphan: pancreatic cancer*)

monoclonal antibody 7E3 [see: abciximab]

monoclonal antibody E5 *investigational treatment for sepsis*

monoclonal antibody IgG *investigational treatment for multiple sclerosis*

monoclonal antibody PM-81 (*orphan: acute myelogenous leukemia*)

monoclonal antibody PM-81 & AML-2-23 (*orphan: bone marrow transplant for acute myelogenous leukemia*)

monoclonal antibody r24 *investigational treatment for Hodgkin's disease*

monoclonal antibody to CD4, 5a8 (*orphan: prophylaxis for occupational exposure to HIV*)

monoclonal antibody to lupus nephritis (*orphan: immunization against lupus nephritis*)

monoclonal antiendotoxin antibody XMMEN-OE5 (*orphan: gram-negative sepsis*)

monoclonal factor IX [see: factor IX complex]

Monocor (name changed to Probeta in 1992) ☑ Mono-Chlor

monoctanoin USAN, BAN *anticholelithogenic; for dissolution of cholesterol gallstones* (*orphan*)

monoctanoin component A
monoctanoin component B
monoctanoin component C
monoctanoin component D

Mono-Diff reagent kit for professional use *in vitro diagnostic aid for mononucleosis*

Monodox capsules ℞ *antibiotic* [doxycycline monohydrate] 50, 100 mg

Mono-Drop (trademarked delivery system) *prefilled eye drop dispenser*

monoethanolamine NF *surfactant*

monoethanolamine oleate INN *sclerosing agent* [also: ethanolamine oleate]

Monogen ℞ *investigational treatment for T-cell leukemia* [monoclonal antibodies]

Mono-Gesic film-coated tablets ℞ *analgesic; antipyretic; anti-inflammatory; antirheumatic* [salsalate] 750 mg

Mono-IX ℞ *investigational treatment for hemophilia B* [factor IX complex]

Monoket tablets ℞ *angina preventative* [isosorbide mononitrate] 10, 20 mg ☑ Monocete

Mono-Latex reagent kit for professional use *in vitro diagnostic aid for mononucleosis*

monolaurin (*orphan: congenital primary ichthyosis*)

Mono-Lisa reagent kit for professional use (discontinued 1992) *in vitro diagnostic aid for mononucleosis*

monomercaptoundecahydro-closo-DO decaborate sodium (*orphan: boron neutron capture therapy for glioblastoma multiforme*)

monometacrine INN

N-monomethyl arginine (NMA) *investigational treatment for septic shock and hypotension following chemotherapy*

Mononine powder for IV infusion ℞ *antihemophilic for factor IX deficiency; coagulant for hemophilia B* (*orphan*) [factor IX complex] 100 IU/mL

monooctanoin [see: monoctanoin]

monophenylbutazone [see: mofebutazone]

monophosphoryl lipid A (MPL-A) *investigational (Phase I) vaccine for AIDS; investigational for septic shock in surgical patients*

monophosphoryl lipid C (MPL-C) *investigational agent to prevent cardiac reperfusion injury*

monophosphoryl lipid S (MPL-S) *investigational immunostimulant for sepsis*

monophosphothiamine INN

Mono-Plus reagent kit for professional use *in vitro diagnostic aid for mononucleosis*

monopotassium 4-aminosalicylate [see: aminosalicylate potassium]

monopotassium carbonate [see: potassium bicarbonate]

monopotassium D-gluconate [see: potassium gluconate]

monopotassium monosodium tartrate tetrahydrate [see: potassium sodium tartrate]

monopotassium phosphate [see: potassium phosphate, monobasic]

Monopril tablets ℞ *antihypertensive; angiotensin-converting enzyme (ACE) inhibitor* [fosinopril sodium] 10, 20 mg

monosodium *p*-aminohippurate [see: aminohippurate sodium]

monosodium 4-aminosalicylate dihydrate [see: aminosalicylate sodium]

monosodium carbonate [see: sodium bicarbonate]

monosodium D-gluconate [see: sodium gluconate]

monosodium D-thyroxine hydrate [see: dextrothyroxine sodium]

monosodium glutamate NF *flavoring agent; perfume*

monosodium L-ascorbate [see: sodium ascorbate]

monosodium L-thyroxine hydrate [see: levothyroxine sodium]

monosodium phosphate dihydrate [see: sodium phosphate, monobasic]

monosodium phosphate monohydrate [see: sodium phosphate, monobasic]

monosodium salicylate [see: sodium salicylate]

monosodium sulfite [see: sodium bisulfite]

Monospot slide test for professional use *in vitro diagnostic aid for mononucleosis*

monostearin [see: glyceryl monostearate]

Monosticon Dri-Dot slide test for professional use *in vitro diagnostic aid for mononucleosis*

monosulfiram BAN [also: sulfiram]

Mono-Sure slide test for professional use *in vitro diagnostic aid for mononucleosis*

Mono-Test slide test for professional use *in vitro diagnostic aid for mononucleosis*

Mono-Test (FTB) test kit for professional use (discontinued 1994) *in vitro diagnostic aid for mononucleosis*

monothioglycerol NF *preservative*

Mono-Vacc Test (O.T.) single-use intradermal puncture test device ℞ *tuberculosis skin test* [old tuberculin] 5 U

monoxerutin INN

montelukast sodium USAN *antiasthmatic; leukotriene D_4 antagonist*

monteplase INN

montirelin INN

Monuril (commercially available in 11 countries) ℞ *investigational antibiotic for urinary tract infection* [fosfomycin trometanol]

Monurol [see: Monuril]

8-MOP capsules ℞ *to increase tolerance to sunlight and enhance pigmentation* [methoxsalen] 10 mg

MOP (mechlorethamine, Oncovin, prednisone) *chemotherapy protocol*

MOP (mechlorethamine, Oncovin, procarbazine) *chemotherapy protocol*

8-MOP (8-methoxypsoralen) [see: methoxsalen]

MOP-BAP (mechlorethamine, Oncovin, procarbazine, bleomycin, Adriamycin, prednisone) *chemotherapy protocol*

moperone INN

mopidamol INN

mopidralazine INN

MOPP (mechlorethamine, Oncovin, procarbazine, prednisone) *chemotherapy protocol*

MOPP (mustine HCl, Oncovin, procarbazine, prednisone) *chemotherapy protocol*

**MOPP/ABV (mechlorethamine, Oncovin, procarbazine, predni-

sone, Adriamycin, bleomycin, vinblastine) *chemotherapy protocol*

MOPP/ABVD (alternating cycles of MOPP and ABVD) *chemotherapy protocol*

MOPP-BLEO; MOPP-Bleo (mechlorethamine, Oncovin, procarbazine, prednisone, bleomycin) *chemotherapy protocol*

MOPPHDB (mechlorethamine, Oncovin, procarbazine, prednisone, high-dose bleomycin) *chemotherapy protocol*

MOPPLDB (mechlorethamine, Oncovin, procarbazine, prednisone, low-dose bleomycin) *chemotherapy protocol*

MOPr (mechlorethamine, Oncovin, procarbazine) *chemotherapy protocol*

moprolol INN

moquizone INN

moracizine INN, BAN *antiarrhythmic* [also: moricizine]

morantel INN *anthelmintic* [also: morantel tartrate]

morantel tartrate USAN *anthelmintic* [also: morantel]

Moranyl (available only from the Centers for Disease Control) ℞ *investigational anti-infective for trypanosomiasis and onchocerciasis* [suramin sodium]

morazone INN, BAN

morclofone INN

More-Dophilus powder OTC *dietary supplement; fever blister treatment; not generally regarded as safe and effective as an antidiarrheal* [Lactobacillus acidophilus] 4 billion U/g

morforex INN

moricizine USAN *antiarrhythmic* [also: moracizine]

moricizine HCl *antiarrhythmic*

morinamide INN

morniflumate USAN, INN *anti-inflammatory*

morocromen INN

moroxydine INN, BAN

morphazinamide [see: morinamide]

morpheridine INN, BAN

morphine BAN *narcotic analgesic* [also: morphine sulfate]

morphine dinicotinate ester [see: nicomorphine]

morphine HCl USP

morphine sulfate (MS) USP *narcotic analgesic; intraspinal microinfusion for intractable chronic pain (orphan)* [also: morphine] 25, 50 mg/mL injection

4-morpholinecarboximidoylguanidine [see: moroxydine]

2-morpholinoethylrutin [see: ethoxazorutoside]

3-morpholinosydnoneimine [see: linsidomine]

morpholinyl succinimide [see: morsuximide]

morpholinylethyl morphine [see: pholcodine]

morrhuate sodium USP *sclerosing agent* [also: sodium morrhuate] 50 mg/mL injection

morsuximide INN

morsydomine [see: molsidomine]

Morton Salt Substitute; Morton Seasoned Salt Substitute OTC *salt substitute* [potassium chloride] 64 mEq/5 g; 56 mEq/5 g

Mosco liquid OTC *topical keratolytic* [salicylic acid in flexible collodion] 17.6%

Mostarinia ℞ *investigational antineoplastic for leukemia, lymphoma, ovarian, breast, and prostatic cancers* [prednimustine]

motapizone INN

MOTC (methyleneoxytetracycline) [see: methacycline]

Motilium ℞ *investigational antiemetic for diabetic gastroparesis* [domperidone]

Motofen tablets ℞ *antidiarrheal* [difenoxin HCl; atropine sulfate] 1 • 0.025 mg

motrazepam INN

motretinide USAN, INN *keratolytic*

Motrin tablets, chewable tablets, oral suspension ℞ *nonsteroidal anti-inflammatory drug (NSAID); antiarthritic; analgesic* [ibuprofen] 300, 400, 600, 800 mg; 50, 100 mg; 100 mg/5 mL

Motrin, Children's drops OTC *nonsteroidal anti-inflammatory drug*

(NSAID); *analgesic; antipyretic* [ibuprofen] 40 mg/mL
Motrin, Children's oral suspension OTC *nonsteroidal anti-inflammatory drug (NSAID); analgesic; antipyretic* [ibuprofen] 100 mg/5 mL
Motrin, Junior film-coated caplets OTC *nonsteroidal anti-inflammatory drug (NSAID); antiarthritic; analgesic* [ibuprofen] 100 mg
Motrin IB caplets, tablets, gelcaps OTC *nonsteroidal anti-inflammatory drug (NSAID); antiarthritic; analgesic* [ibuprofen] 200 mg
Motrin IB Sinus caplets OTC *decongestant; analgesic* [pseudoephedrine HCl; ibuprofen] 30•200 mg
MouthKote oral spray OTC *saliva substitute*
MouthKote F/R oral rinse OTC *topical dental caries preventative* [sodium fluoride] 0.04%
MouthKote O/R mouthwash OTC *anesthetic and antimicrobial throat irrigation* [benzyl alcohol; menthol]
MouthKote O/R oral solution OTC *topical antihistamine* [diphenhydramine] 1.25%
MouthKote P/R oral solution, ointment OTC *topical antihistamine* [diphenhydramine HCl] 1.25%; 25%
moveltipril INN
moxadolen INN
moxalactam disodium USAN, USP *bactericidal antibiotic* [also: latamoxef]
Moxam powder for IV or IM injection (discontinued 1992) ℞ *cephalosporin-type antibiotic* [moxalactam disodium]
moxantrazole [now: teloxantrone HCl]
moxaprindine INN
moxastine INN
moxaverine INN, BAN
moxazocine USAN, INN *analgesic; antitussive*
moxestrol INN
moxicoumone INN
moxidectin USAN, INN *veterinary antiparasitic*
moxipraquine INN, BAN
moxiraprine INN
moxisylyte INN [also: thymoxamine]

moxnidazole USAN, INN *antiprotozoal (Trichomonas)*
moxonidine INN *investigational antihypertensive*
Moxy Compound tablets (discontinued 1993) ℞ *antiasthmatic; bronchodilator; decongestant; anxiolytic* [theophylline; ephedrine sulfate; hydroxyzine HCl]
MP (melphalan, prednisone) *chemotherapy protocol*
4-MP (4-methylpyrazole) [see: fomepizole]
6-MP (6-mercaptopurine) [see: mercaptopurine]
MPF [see: Mucoprotective Factor]
m-PFL (methotrexate, Platinol, fluorouracil, leucovorin [rescue]) *chemotherapy protocol*
MPL (melphalan) [q.v.]
MPL + PRED (melphalan, prednisone) *chemotherapy protocol*
MPL-A (monophosphoryl lipid A) [q.v.]
MPL-C (monophosphoryl lipid C) [q.v.]
MPL-S (monophosphoryl lipid S) [q.v.]
M-Prednisol-40; M-Prednisol-80 intralesional, soft tissue, and IM injection ℞ *glucocorticoid; antiinflammatory; immunosuppressant* [methylprednisolone acetate] 40 mg/mL; 80 mg/mL
MRV subcu injection ℞ *active respiratory bacteria immunizing agent* [mixed respiratory vaccine]
MRV (mixed respiratory vaccine) [q.v.]
M-R-Vax II powder for subcu injection ℞ *measles and rubella vaccine* [measles & rubella virus vaccine, live] 0.5 mL
MS (magnesium salicylate) [q.v.]
MS (morphine sulfate) [q.v.]
MS Contin controlled-release tablets ℞ *narcotic analgesic; preoperative sedative and anxiolytic* [morphine sulfate] 15, 100, 200 mg
MSI-78 *investigational broad-spectrum anti-infective for impetigo*

MSIR immediate-release tablets, oral solution, oral concentrate ℞ *narcotic analgesic; preoperative sedative and anxiolytic* [morphine sulfate] 15, 30 mg; 10, 20 mg/5 mL; 20 mg/mL

MS/L; MS/L Concentrate oral liquid ℞ *narcotic analgesic; preoperative sedative and anxiolytic* [morphine sulfate] 10 mg/5 mL; 100 mg/5 mL

MS/S suppositories ℞ *narcotic analgesic; preoperative sedative and anxiolytic* [morphine sulfate] 5, 10, 20, 30 mg

MSTA (Mumps Skin Test Antigen) intradermal injection ℞ *diagnostic aid to assess immune system competency (not effective in testing immunity to mumps virus)* [mumps skin test antigen] 0.1 mL (4 U/0.1 mL)

MT6 (mercaptomerin) [q.v.]

MTC (mitomycin C) [see: mitomycin]

M.T.E.-4; M.T.E.-5; M.T.E.-6; M.T.E.-7; M.T.E.-4 Concentrated; M.T.E.-5 Concentrated; M.T.E.-6 Concentrated IV injection ℞ *intravenous nutritional therapy* [multiple trace elements (metals)]

mTHPC [see: temoporfin]

MTX (methotrexate) [q.v.]

MTX + MP (methotrexate, mercaptopurine) *chemotherapy protocol*

MTX + MP + CTX (methotrexate, mercaptopurine, cyclophosphamide) *chemotherapy protocol*

MTXCP-PDAdr (methotrexate [with leucovorin rescue], cisplatin, doxorubicin) *chemotherapy protocol*

Muco-Fen-DM timed-release tablets ℞ *antitussive; expectorant* [dextromethorphan hydrobromide; guaifenesin] 30•600 mg

Muco-Fen-LA timed-release tablets ℞ *expectorant* [guaifenesin] 600 mg

mucoid exopolysaccharide Pseudomonas hyperimmune globulin *(orphan: pulmonary infections of cystic fibrosis)*

Mucomyst solution for nebulization or intratracheal instillation ℞ *mucolytic; (orphan: severe acetaminophen overdose)* [acetylcysteine sodium] 10%, 20%

Mucomyst 10 IV ℞ *(orphan: moderate to severe acetaminophen overdose)* [acetylcysteine]

Mucoplex tablets (discontinued 1995) OTC *dietary supplement* [vitamins B_2 and B_{12}; liver fraction] 1.5 mg•5 µg•750 mg

Mucoprotective Factor (MPF) (trademarked ingredient) *aromatic flavored syrup* [eriodictyon]

Mucosil-10; Mucosil-20 solution for nebulization or intratracheal instillation ℞ *mucolytic* [acetylcysteine sodium] 10%; 20%

Mudrane tablets ℞ *antiasthmatic; bronchodilator; decongestant; expectorant; sedative* [aminophylline; ephedrine HCl; potassium iodide; phenobarbital] 111•16•195•8 mg ⓘ Modane

Mudrane GG elixir (discontinued 1995) ℞ *antiasthmatic; decongestant; expectorant; sedative* [theophylline; ephedrine HCl; guaifenesin; phenobarbital] 4•0.8•5.2•0.5 mg/mL

Mudrane GG tablets ℞ *antiasthmatic; decongestant; expectorant; sedative* [theophylline; ephedrine HCl; guaifenesin; phenobarbital] 111•16•100•8 mg

Mudrane GG-2 tablets ℞ *antiasthmatic; bronchodilator; expectorant* [theophylline; guaifenesin] 111•100 mg

Mudrane-2 tablets (discontinued 1995) ℞ *antiasthmatic; expectorant* [aminophylline; potassium iodide] 111•195 mg

Multa-Gen 12+E capsules (discontinued 1992) OTC *vitamin supplement* [multiple vitamins; folic acid]

MulTE-Pak-4; MulTE-Pak-5 IV injection ℞ *intravenous nutritional therapy* [multiple trace elements (metals)] ≜

Multi 75 timed-release tablets OTC *vitamin/mineral supplement* [multiple vitamins & minerals; folic acid; biotin] ≜•0.4•≟ mg

Multi Vit drops (discontinued 1993) OTC *vitamin supplement* [multiple vitamins]

Multi Vit with Fluoride drops *vitamin supplement; dental caries prophylaxis* [multiple vitamins; fluoride]

Multi Vit with Iron drops OTC *vitamin/iron supplement* [multiple vitamins; iron] ± •10 mg/mL

Multi Vitamin Concentrate injection ℞ *parenteral vitamin supplement* [multiple vitamins] ±

Multibret-500 Hematinic timed-release tablets (discontinued 1995) ℞ *hematinic* [ferrous sulfate; multiple B vitamins; sodium ascorbate] 105• ± •500 mg

Multibret-Folic-500 timed-release tablets (discontinued 1995) ℞ *hematinic* [ferrous sulfate; multiple B vitamins; sodium ascorbate; folic acid] 105• ± •500•0.8 mg

Multi-Day tablets OTC *vitamin supplement* [multiple vitamins; folic acid] ± •0.4 mg

Multi-Day Plus Iron tablets OTC *vitamin/iron supplement* [multiple vitamins; iron; folic acid] ± •18•0.4 mg

Multi-Day Plus Minerals tablets OTC *vitamin/mineral/iron supplement* [multiple vitamins & minerals; iron; folic acid; biotin] ± •18 mg•0.4 mg•30 μg

Multi-Day with Calcium and Extra Iron tablets OTC *vitamin/calcium/iron supplement* [multiple vitamins; calcium; iron; folic acid] ± • ± •27•0.4 mg

Multi-Gel soft capsules OTC *vitamin/mineral supplement* [multiple vitamins & minerals; papaya concentrate; bioflavonoids; lecithin]

Multi-Glan tablets OTC *dietary supplement* [multiple glandular concentrates]

Multilex; Multilex-T & M tablets OTC *vitamin/mineral/iron supplement* [multiple vitamins & minerals; iron] ± •15 mg

Multilyte effervescent tablets (discontinued 1993) OTC *vitamin/mineral supplement* [multiple vitamins & minerals; folic acid; biotin; phenylalanine]

Multilyte-20; Multilyte-40 IV admixture ℞ *intravenous electrolyte therapy* [combined electrolyte solution]

Multi-Mineral tablets OTC *mineral supplement* [multiple minerals]

Multiple Trace Element; Multiple Trace Element Concentrated; Multiple Trace Element Neonatal; Multiple Trace Element Pediatric IV injection ℞ *intravenous nutritional therapy* [multiple trace elements (metals)]

Multiple Trace Element with Selenium; Multiple Trace Element with Selenium Concentrated IV injection ℞ *intravenous nutritional therapy* [multiple trace elements (metals)]

Multistix; Multistix 2; Multistix 7; Multistix 8 SG; Multistix 9; Multistix 9 SG; Multistix 10 SG; Multistix SG reagent strips *in vitro diagnostic aid for multiple urine products*

Multitest CMI single-use intradermal skin test device ℞ *skin test for multiple allergen sensitivity* [skin test antigens (seven different); glycerin (one for test control)]

Multitrace-5 Concentrate IV injection ℞ *intravenous nutritional therapy* [multiple trace elements (metals)] ±

Multi-Vita-Drops (discontinued 1993) OTC *vitamin supplement* [multiple vitamins]

Multi-Vita-Drops with Fluoride (discontinued 1993) ℞ *pediatric vitamin supplement and dental caries preventative* [multiple vitamins; fluoride]

Multi-Vita-Drops with Iron (discontinued 1993) OTC *vitamin/iron supplement* [multiple vitamins; iron]

multivitamin infusion (neonatal formula) *(orphan: total parenteral nutrition for very low birthweight infants)*

Multi-Vitamin Mineral with Beta-Carotene tablets OTC *vitamin/mineral/iron supplement* [multiple vitamins & minerals; ferrous fumarate; folic acid; biotin] ± •27•0.4•0.45 mg

Multivitamin with Fluoride drops ℞ *pediatric vitamin supplement and dental caries preventative* [multiple vitamins; fluoride] ± •0.25, ± •0.5 mg/mL

Multivitamins capsules OTC *vitamin supplement* [multiple vitamins] ≐

Mulvidren-F Softabs (chewable tablets) ℞ *pediatric vitamin supplement and dental caries preventative* [multiple vitamins; fluoride] ≐•1 mg

Mumps Skin Test Antigen [see: MSTA]

mumps skin test antigen (MSTA) USP *diagnostic aid to assess immune system competency*

mumps vaccine [see: mumps virus vaccine, inactivated]

mumps virus vaccine, inactivated NF

mumps virus vaccine, live USP *active immunizing agent for mumps*

Mumpsvax powder for subcu injection ℞ *mumps vaccine* [mumps virus vaccine, live] 0.5 mL

mupirocin USAN, INN, BAN *topical antibacterial antibiotic*

mupirocin calcium USAN *topical antibacterial antibiotic*

murabutide INN

muramyl-tripeptide *investigational immunomodulator for AIDS (clinical trials discontinued 1994)*

Murine eye drops OTC *ocular moisturizer/lubricant* [polyvinyl alcohol] 0.5%

Murine Contact Lens Cleaner solution (discontinued 1992) OTC *surfactant cleaning solution for soft contact lenses*

Murine Ear Drops OTC *agent to emulsify and disperse ear wax* [carbamide peroxide; alcohol] 6.5%•6.3%

murine monoclonal antibody [see: muromonab-CD3]

Murine Plus eye drops OTC *topical ocular decongestant/vasoconstrictor* [tetrahydrozoline HCl] 0.05%

Murine Preserved All-Purpose Saline solution (discontinued 1992) OTC *rinsing/storage solution for soft contact lenses* [preserved saline solution]

Murine Regular Formula ophthalmic solution (discontinued 1993) OTC *extraocular irrigating solution* [balanced saline solution]

Murine Sterile Lubricating and Rewetting Drops (discontinued 1992) OTC *rewetting solution for soft or hard contact lenses*

Muro 128 eye drops, ophthalmic ointment OTC *corneal edema-reducing agent* [hypertonic saline solution] 2%, 5%; 5%

Muro Tears eye drops (discontinued 1993) OTC *ocular moisturizer/lubricant*

murocainide INN

Murocel eye drops OTC *ocular moisturizer/lubricant* [methylcellulose] 1%

Murocoll-2 eye drops ℞ *cycloplegic; mydriatic* [scopolamine hydrobromide; phenylephrine HCl] 0.3%•10%

murodermin INN

muromonab-CD3 USAN, INN *monoclonal antibody immunosuppressive for renal, hepatic, and cardiac transplants*

Muroptic-5 eye drops OTC *corneal edema-reducing agent* [hypertonic saline solution] 5%

Muro's Opcon eye drops (discontinued 1995) ℞ *topical ocular decongestant/vasoconstrictor* [naphazoline HCl] 0.1%

muscarinic agonists *investigational analgesic*

MuscleRub ointment OTC *counterirritant* [methyl salicylate; menthol] 15%•10%

Mus-Lax capsules (discontinued 1996) ℞ *skeletal muscle relaxant; analgesic* [chlorzoxazone; acetaminophen] 250•300 mg

mustaral oil [see: allyl isothiocyanate]

mustard oil [see: allyl isothiocyanate]

Mustargen powder for IV or intracavitary injection ℞ *antineoplastic for multiple myelomas, lymphomas and leukemias, and breast, lung, and ovarian cancers* [mechlorethamine HCl] 10 mg

Musterole Deep Strength Rub OTC *counterirritant* [methyl salicylate; methyl nicotinate; menthol] 30%•0.5%•3%

Musterole Extra Strength OTC *counterirritant* [camphor; menthol] 5%•3%

mustine BAN *alkylating antineoplastic* [also: mechlorethamine HCl; chlormethine; nitrogen mustard N-oxide HCl]

mustine HCl [see: mechlorethamine HCl]

Mutamycin powder for IV injection ℞ *antibiotic antineoplastic for stomach, pancreatic, breast, colon, head, neck, and lung cancers* [mitomycin] 5, 20, 40 mg ② mitomycin

muzolimine USAN, INN *diuretic; antihypertensive*

MV (mitomycin, vinblastine) *chemotherapy protocol*

MV (mitoxantrone, VePesid) *chemotherapy protocol*

MVAC; M-VAC (methotrexate, vinblastine, Adriamycin, cisplatin) *chemotherapy protocol*

M.V.C. 9+3 injection (discontinued 1995) ℞ *parenteral vitamin supplement* [multiple vitamins; folic acid; biotin] ± •0.4 mg•60 μg per 5 mL

M.V.C. 9+4 Pediatric powder for injection ℞ *vitamin therapy* [multiple vitamins; folic acid; biotin]

MVF (mitoxantrone, vincristine, fluorouracil) *chemotherapy protocol*

M.V.I. Neonatal IV infusion ℞ *(orphan: total parenteral nutrition for very low birthweight infants)* [multiple vitamins]

M.V.I. Pediatric injection ℞ *parenteral vitamin supplement* [multiple vitamins; folic acid; biotin] ± •140• 20 μg/5 mL

M.V.I.-12 injection ℞ *parenteral vitamin supplement* [multiple vitamins; folic acid; biotin] ± •400•60 μg/5 mL

M.V.M. capsules OTC *vitamin/mineral/iron supplement* [multiple vitamins & minerals; iron; folic acid; biotin] ± • 3.6 mg•0.08 mg•160 μg

MVP (mitomycin, vinblastine, Platinol) *chemotherapy protocol*

MVPP (mechlorethamine, vinblastine, procarbazine, prednisone) *chemotherapy protocol*

MVT (mitoxantrone, VePesid, thiotepa) *chemotherapy protocol*

MVVPP (mechlorethamine, vincristine, vinblastine, procarbazine, prednisone) *chemotherapy protocol*

Myadec tablets OTC *vitamin/mineral/iron supplement* [multiple vitamins & minerals; iron; folic acid; biotin] ± • 18 mg•0.4 mg•30 μg

Myambutol film-coated tablets ℞ *tuberculostatic* [ethambutol HCl] 100, 400 mg ② Nembutal

Myapap drops ℞ *analgesic; antipyretic* [acetaminophen] 100 mg/mL

Mycelex cream, solution ℞ *topical antifungal* [clotrimazole] 1%

Mycelex troches ℞ *antifungal; oral candidiasis prophylaxis or treatment* [clotrimazole] 10 mg

Mycelex OTC cream, solution OTC *topical antifungal* [clotrimazole] 1%

Mycelex Twin Pack vaginal tablets + cream ℞ *antifungal* [clotrimazole] 500 mg; 1%

Mycelex-7 vaginal cream, vaginal tablets, combination pack (cream + vaginal suppositories) OTC *antifungal* [clotrimazole] 1%; 100 mg

Mycelex-G vaginal cream (discontinued 1994) ℞ *antifungal* [clotrimazole] 500 mg

Mycelex-G vaginal tablets ℞ *antifungal* [clotrimazole] 500 mg

Mycifradin Sulfate oral solution ℞ *aminoglycoside-type antibiotic* [neomycin sulfate] 125 mg/5 mL

Myciguent ointment, cream OTC *topical antibiotic* [neomycin sulfate] 3.5 mg/g

Mycinette throat spray OTC *topical anesthetic; oral antiseptic; astringent* [phenol; alum] 1.4%•0.3%

Mycinettes lozenges OTC *topical oral anesthetic* [benzocaine] 15 mg

Myci-Spray nasal spray OTC *nasal decongestant; antihistamine* [phenylephrine HCl; pyrilamine maleate] 0.25%•0.15%

Mycitracin Plus ointment OTC *topical antibiotic; local anesthetic* [polymyxin B sulfate; neomycin sulfate; bacitracin; lidocaine] 5000 U•3.5 mg•500 U•40 mg per g

Mycitracin Triple Antibiotic ointment OTC *topical antibiotic* [polymyxin B sulfate; neomycin sulfate; bacitracin] 5000 U•3.5 mg•500 U per g

Mycobax ℞ *investigational immunizing agent for high-risk tuberculosis populations* [BCG vaccine]

Myco-Biotic II cream ℞ *topical corticosteroid; antifungal* [triamcinolone acetonide; neomycin sulfate; nystatin] 0.1%•0.5%•100,000 U per g

Mycobutin capsules ℞ *prevention of Mycobacterium avium complex (MAC) in advanced HIV patients (orphan)* [rifabutin] 150 mg

Mycocide NS solution OTC *topical antiseptic* [benzalkonium chloride] ?

Mycogen II cream, ointment ℞ *topical corticosteroid; antifungal* [triamcinolone acetonide; nystatin] 0.1%•100,000 U per g

Mycolog-II cream, ointment ℞ *topical corticosteroid; antifungal* [triamcinolone acetonide; nystatin] 0.1%•100,000 U per g

Myconel cream ℞ *topical corticosteroid; antifungal* [triamcinolone acetonide; nystatin] 0.1%•100,000 U per g

mycophenolate mofetil USAN *immunomodulator; purine biosynthesis inhibitor; kidney transplant rejection preventative*

mycophenolic acid USAN, INN *antineoplastic*

Mycostatin cream, ointment, powder, vaginal tablets ℞ *topical antifungal* [nystatin] 100,000 U/g; 100,000 U/g; 100,000 U/g; 100,000 U

Mycostatin film-coated tablets ℞ *systemic antifungal* [nystatin] 500,000 U

Mycostatin oral suspension, Pastilles (troches) ℞ *antifungal; oral candidiasis treatment* [nystatin] 100,000 U/mL; 200,000 U

Myco-Triacet II cream, ointment ℞ *topical corticosteroid; antifungal* [triamcinolone acetonide; nystatin] 0.1%•100,000 U per g

mydeton [see: tolperisone]

Mydfrin 2.5% eye drops ℞ *ophthalmic decongestant/vasoconstrictor; mydriatic* [phenylephrine HCl] 2.5% ⑨ Midrin; Myfedrine

Mydrapred Drop-Tainers (eye drop suspension) (discontinued 1994) ℞ *ophthalmic topical corticosteroidal antiinflammatory; cycloplegic; mydriatic* [prednisolone acetate; atropine sulfate] 0.25%•1%

Mydriacyl Drop-Tainers (eye drops) ℞ *cycloplegic; mydriatic* [tropicamide] 0.5%, 1%

myelin *(orphan: multiple sclerosis)*

myelosan [see: busulfan]

myfadol INN

Myfedrine liquid (discontinued 1993) OTC *nasal decongestant* [pseudoephedrine HCl] ⑨ Mydfrin

Myfedrine Plus liquid (discontinued 1993) OTC *decongestant; antihistamine* [pseudoephedrine HCl; chlorpheniramine maleate]

Mygel; Mygel II oral suspension OTC *antacid; antiflatulent* [aluminum hydroxide; magnesium hydroxide; simethicone] 200•200•20 mg/5 mL; 400•400•40 mg/5 mL

Myidone tablets (discontinued 1992) ℞ *anticonvulsant* [primidone]

Myidyl syrup ℞ *antihistamine* [triprolidine HCl] 1.25 mg/5 mL

My-K Elixir (discontinued 1992) ℞ *potassium supplement* [potassium gluconate]

Mykinac cream ℞ *topical antifungal* [nystatin]

Mykrox tablets ℞ *diuretic; antihypertensive* [metolazone] 0.5 mg

Mylagen gelcaps OTC *antacid* [calcium carbonate; magnesium carbonate] 311•232 mg

Mylagen; Mylagen II liquid OTC *antacid; antiflatulent* [aluminum hydroxide; magnesium hydroxide; simethicone] 200•200•20 mg/5 mL; 400•400•40 mg/5 mL

Mylanta chewable tablets, liquid OTC *antacid; antiflatulent* [aluminum hydroxide; magnesium hydroxide; simethicone] 200•200•20, 400•400•40 mg; 200•200•20, 400•400•40 mg/5 mL ⑨ Milontin

Mylanta gelcaps OTC *antacid* [calcium carbonate; magnesium carbonate] 311•232 mg

Mylanta lozenges OTC *antacid* [calcium carbonate] 600 mg

Mylanta, Children's oral liquid, chewable tablets OTC *antacid* [calcium carbonate] 400 mg/5 mL; 400 mg

Mylanta Gas chewable tablets OTC *antiflatulent* [simethicone] 40, 80, 125 mg

Mylanta Natural Fiber Supplement powder OTC *laxative* [psyllium hydrophilic mucilloid] 3.4 g/tsp.

Myleran tablets ℞ *alkylating antineoplastic for palliation in chronic myelogenous leukemia* [busulfan] 2 mg ⚠ Mylicon

Mylicon drops OTC *antiflatulent* [simethicone] 40 mg/0.6 mL ⚠ Modicon; Myleran

Mylicon; Mylicon-80; Mylicon-125 chewable tablets (name changed to Mylanta Gas in 1992)

Myloral ℞ *investigational oral treatment for multiple sclerosis* [bovine myelin]

Myminic syrup (discontinued 1993) OTC *antihistamine; decongestant* [phenylpropanolamine HCl; chlorpheniramine maleate]

Myminic Expectorant liquid OTC *decongestant; expectorant* [phenylpropanolamine HCl; guaifenesin; alcohol 5%] 12.5•100 mg/5 mL

Myminicol liquid OTC *antitussive; decongestant; antihistamine* [dextromethorphan hydrobromide; phenylpropanolamine HCl; chlorpheniramine maleate] 10•12.5•2 mg/5 mL

Mynatal capsules ℞ *vitamin/mineral/calcium/iron supplement* [multiple vitamins & minerals; calcium; iron; folic acid; biotin] ±•300•65•1•0.03 mg

Mynatal FC caplets ℞ *vitamin/mineral/calcium/iron supplement* [multiple vitamins & minerals; calcium; iron; folic acid; biotin] ±•250•60•1•0.03 mg

Mynatal P.N. captabs ℞ *vitamin/calcium/iron supplement* [multiple vitamins; calcium; iron; folic acid] ±•125•60•1 mg

Mynatal P.N. Forte caplets ℞ *vitamin/mineral/calcium/iron supplement* [multiple vitamins & minerals; calcium; iron; folic acid] ±•250•60•1 mg

Mynatal Rx caplets ℞ *vitamin/mineral/calcium/iron supplement* [multiple vitamins & minerals; calcium; iron; folic acid; biotin] ±•200•60•1•0.03 mg

Mynate 90 Plus delayed-release caplets ℞ *vitamin/calcium/iron supplement* [multiple vitamins; calcium; iron; folic acid] ±•250•90•1 mg

Myochrysine IM injection (discontinued 1996) ℞ *antirheumatic* [gold sodium thiomalate] 25, 50 mg/mL

Myocide NS solution OTC *topical antiseptic* [benzalkonium chloride] ±

Myoflex Creme OTC *topical analgesic* [trolamine salicylate] 10%

Myolin IV or IM injection ℞ *skeletal muscle relaxant* [orphenadrine citrate] 30 mg/mL

Myoscint (commercially available in Europe) ℞ *investigational imaging agent for cardiac necrosis and myocarditis (orphan)* [indium In 111 murine monoclonal antibody Fab to myosin; imciromab pentetate]

Myotonachol tablets ℞ *postsurgical cholinergic bladder muscle stimulant* [bethanechol chloride] 10, 25 mg

Myotrophin ℞ *investigational adjunct to chemotherapy (orphan: amyotrophic lateral sclerosis)* [insulin-like growth factor-1, recombinant]

Myoview ℞ *investigational cardiovascular imaging aid* [technetium Tc 99m tetrofosmin]

Myphetane DC Cough syrup ℞ *narcotic antitussive; decongestant; antihistamine* [codeine phosphate; phenylpropanolamine HCl; brompheniramine maleate; alcohol 1.2%] 10•12.5•2 mg/5 mL

Myphetane DX Cough syrup ℞ *antitussive; decongestant; antihistamine* [dextromethorphan hydrobromide; pseudoephedrine HCl; brompheniramine maleate; alcohol 1%] 10•30•2 mg/5 mL

Myphetapp elixir (discontinued 1993) OTC *decongestant; antihistamine* [phenylpropanolamine HCl; brompheniramine maleate]

myralact INN, BAN

myricodine [see: myrophine]

myristica oil [see: nutmeg oil]

myristyl alcohol NF *stiffening agent*

myristyltrimethylammonium bromide *antiseborrheic*

myrophine INN, BAN
myrtecaine INN
Mysoline tablets, oral suspension ℞ *anticonvulsant* [primidone] 50, 250 mg; 250 mg/5 mL
myspamol [see: proquamezine]
Mytelase caplets ℞ *anticholinesterase muscle stimulant; myasthenia gravis treatment* [ambenonium chloride] 10 mg
Mytrex cream, ointment ℞ *topical corticosteroid; antifungal* [triamcinolone acetonide; nystatin] 0.1% • 100,000 U/g
Mytussin syrup OTC *expectorant* [guaifenesin; alcohol 3.5%] 100 mg/5 mL
Mytussin AC Cough syrup ℞ *narcotic antitussive; expectorant* [codeine phosphate; guaifenesin; alcohol 3.5%] 10 • 100 mg/5 mL
Mytussin DAC syrup ℞ *narcotic antitussive; decongestant; expectorant* [codeine phosphate; pseudoephedrine HCl; guaifenesin; alcohol 1.7%] 10 • 30 • 100 mg/5 mL
Mytussin DM liquid OTC *antitussive; expectorant* [dextromethorphan hydrobromide; guaifenesin; alcohol 1.6%] 10 • 100 mg/5 mL
myuizone [see: thioacetazone; thiacetazone]
My-Vitalife capsules OTC *vitamin/mineral/calcium/iron supplement* [multiple vitamins & minerals; calcium; iron; folic acid; biotin] ± • 130 • 27 • 0.4 • 0.03 mg
MZM tablets ℞ *carbonic anhydrase inhibitor; diuretic* [methazolamide] 25, 50 mg
MZM (methazolamide) [q.v.]

N₂ (nitrogen) [q.v.]
N-3 polyunsaturated fatty acids [see: doconexent; icosapent; omega-3 marine triglycerides]
N901-blocked ricin *investigational antineoplastic for small cell lung cancer*
²²Na [see: sodium chloride Na 22]
nabazenil USAN, INN *anticonvulsant*
nabilone USAN, INN, BAN *minor tranquilizer*
nabitan INN *analgesic* [also: nabitan HCl]
nabitan HCl USAN *analgesic* [also: nabitan]
naboctate INN *antiglaucoma agent; antinauseant* [also: naboctate HCl]
naboctate HCl USAN *antiglaucoma agent; antinauseant* [also: naboctate]
nabumetone USAN, INN, BAN *nonsteroidal anti-inflammatory drug (NSAID); antiarthritic*
nabutan HCl [now: nabitan HCl]
NAC (nitrogen mustard, Adriamycin, CCNU) *chemotherapy protocol*
nacartocin INN
NaCl (sodium chloride) [q.v.]
NAD (nicotinamide-adenine dinucleotide) [see: nadide]
nadide USAN, INN *antagonist to alcohol and narcotics*
nadisan [see: carbutamide]
nadolol USAN, USP, INN, BAN *antianginal; antihypertensive; antiadrenergic (β-receptor)* 20, 40, 80, 120, 160 mg oral ⑨ Nandol
nadoxolol INN
naepaine HCl NF
nafamostat INN *anticoagulant; antifibrinolytic* [also: nafamostat mesylate; nafamostat mesilate]
nafamostat mesilate JAN *anticoagulant; antifibrinolytic* [also: nafamostat mesylate; nafamostat]
nafamostat mesylate USAN *anticoagulant; antifibrinolytic* [also: nafamostat mesilate]
nafarelin INN, BAN *luteinizing hormone-releasing hormone (LHRH) agonist* [also: nafarelin acetate]
nafarelin acetate USAN *luteinizing hormone-releasing hormone (LHRH) ago-*

nist; *for central precocious puberty (orphan)* [also: nafarelin]

Nafazair eye drops ℞ *topical ocular decongestant/vasoconstrictor* [naphazoline HCl] 0.1%

Nafazair A eye drops (discontinued 1995) ℞ *topical ocular decongestant and antihistamine* [naphazoline HCl; pheniramine maleate] 0.025%•0.3%

nafazatrom INN, BAN

nafcaproic acid INN

Nafcil powder for IV or IM injection ℞ *bactericidal antibiotic (penicillinase-resistant penicillin)* [nafcillin sodium] 0.5, 1, 2, 10 g

nafcillin INN *antibacterial* [also: nafcillin sodium]

nafcillin sodium USAN, USP *bactericidal antibiotic* [also: nafcillin] 0.5, 1, 2, 10 g/vial injection

nafenodone INN

nafenopin USAN, INN *antihyperlipoproteinemic*

nafetolol INN

nafimidone INN *anticonvulsant* [also: nafimidone HCl]

nafimidone HCl USAN *anticonvulsant* [also: nafimidone]

nafiverine INN

naflocort USAN, INN *topical adrenocortical steroid*

nafomine INN *muscle relaxant* [also: nafomine malate]

nafomine malate USAN *muscle relaxant* [also: nafomine]

nafoxadol INN

nafoxidine HCl USAN, INN *antiestrogen*

nafronyl oxalate USAN *vasodilator* [also: naftidrofuryl]

naftalofos USAN, INN *veterinary anthelmintic*

naftazone INN, BAN

naftidrofuryl INN *vasodilator* [also: nafronyl oxalate]

naftifine INN, BAN *broad-spectrum antifungal* [also: naftifine HCl]

naftifine HCl USAN *broad-spectrum antifungal* [also: naftifine]

Naftin cream, gel ℞ *topical antifungal* [naftifine HCl] 1%

naftopidil INN

naftoxate INN

naftypramide INN

Naganol (available only from the Centers for Disease Control) ℞ *investigational anti-infective for trypanosomiasis and onchocerciasis* [suramin sodium]

naganol [see: suramin sodium]

nalazosulfamide [see: salazosulfamide]

nalbuphine INN, BAN *narcotic agonist-antagonist analgesic; narcotic antagonist* [also: nalbuphine HCl]

nalbuphine HCl USAN *narcotic agonist-antagonist analgesic; narcotic antagonist* [also: nalbuphine] 10, 20 mg/mL injection

Naldec Pediatric syrup ℞ *decongestant; antihistamine* [phenylpropanolamine HCl; phenylephrine HCl; phenyltoloxamine citrate; chlorpheniramine maleate]

Naldecon sustained-release tablets, syrup, pediatric syrup, pediatric drops ℞ *decongestant; antihistamine* [phenylpropanolamine HCl; phenylephrine HCl; chlorpheniramine maleate; phenyltoloxamine citrate] 40•10•5•15 mg; 20•5•2.5•7.5 mg/5 mL; 5•1.25•0.5•2 mg/5 mL; 5•1.25•0.5•2 mg/mL ② Nalfon

Naldecon CX Adult liquid ℞ *narcotic antitussive; decongestant; expectorant* [codeine phosphate; phenylpropanolamine HCl; guaifenesin] 10•12.5•200 mg/5 mL

Naldecon DX children's syrup, pediatric drops OTC *pediatric antitussive, decongestant, and expectorant* [dextromethorphan hydrobromide; phenylpropanolamine HCl; guaifenesin] 5•6.25•100 mg/5 mL; 5•6.25•50 mg/mL

Naldecon DX Adult liquid OTC *antitussive; decongestant; expectorant* [dextromethorphan hydrobromide; phenylpropanolamine HCl; guaifenesin] 10•12.5•200 mg/5 mL

Naldecon EX children's syrup, pediatric drops OTC *pediatric decongestant and expectorant* [phenylpropanolamine HCl; guaifenesin] 6.25•100 mg/5 mL; 6.25•50 mg/mL

Naldecon Senior DX liquid OTC *antitussive; expectorant* [dextromethorphan hydrobromide; guaifenesin] 10•200 mg/5 mL

Naldecon Senior EX liquid OTC *expectorant* [guaifenesin] 200 mg/5 mL

Naldegesic tablets OTC *decongestant; analgesic* [pseudoephedrine HCl; acetaminophen]

Naldelate syrup, pediatric syrup ℞ *decongestant; antihistamine* [phenylpropanolamine HCl; phenylephrine HCl; chlorpheniramine maleate; phenyltoloxamine citrate] 20•5•2.5•7.5 mg/5 mL; 5•1.25•0.5•2 mg/5 mL

Naldelate DX Adult liquid OTC *antitussive; decongestant; expectorant* [dextromethorphan hydrobromide; phenylpropanolamine HCl; guaifenesin] 10•12.5•200 mg/5 mL

Nalfon Pulvules (capsules) ℞ *nonsteroidal anti-inflammatory drug (NSAID); antiarthritic; analgesic* [fenoprofen calcium] 200, 300 mg ② Naldecon

Nalfon tablets (discontinued 1994) ℞ *nonsteroidal anti-inflammatory drug (NSAID); antiarthritic; analgesic* [fenoprofen calcium] 600 mg

Nalgest sustained-release tablets, syrup, pediatric syrup, pediatric drops ℞ *decongestant; antihistamine* [phenylpropanolamine HCl; phenylephrine HCl; chlorpheniramine maleate; phenyltoloxamine citrate] 40•10•5•15 mg; 20•5•2.5•7.5 mg/5 mL; 5•1.25•0.5•2 mg/5 mL; 5•1.25•0.5•2 mg/mL

nalidixane [see: nalidixic acid]

nalidixate sodium USAN *antibacterial*

nalidixic acid USAN, USP, INN *urinary bactericidal*

Nallpen IV or IM injection ℞ *bactericidal antibiotic (penicillinase-resistant penicillin)* [nafcillin sodium] 0.5, 1, 2, 10 g

nalmefene USAN, INN, BAN *narcotic antagonist; investigational treatment for stroke, interstitial cystitis, and pruritus*

nalmefene HCl *narcotic antagonist*

nalmetrene [now: nalmefene]

nalmexone INN *analgesic; narcotic antagonist* [also: nalmexone HCl]

nalmexone HCl USAN *analgesic; narcotic antagonist* [also: nalmexone]

nalorphine INN [also: nalorphine HCl]

nalorphine HCl USP [also: nalorphine]

naloxiphane tartrate [see: levallorphan tartrate]

naloxone INN *narcotic antagonist; investigational treatment for constipation* [also: naloxone HCl]

naloxone HCl USAN, USP *narcotic antagonist; investigational treatment for constipation* [also: naloxone] 0.02, 0.4 mg/mL injection

Nalspan syrup (discontinued 1993) ℞ *decongestant; antihistamine* [phenylpropanolamine HCL; phenylephrine HCl; chlorpheniramine maleate; phenyltoloxamine citrate]

naltrexone USAN, INN, BAN *narcotic antagonist*

naltrexone HCl *opiate blockage and maintenance in formerly opiate-dependent individuals (orphan)*

naminterol INN

[^{13}N]ammonia [see: ammonia N 13]

namoxyrate USAN, INN *analgesic*

namuron [see: cyclobarbitone]

nanafrocin INN

Nandrobolic IM injection (discontinued 1994) ℞ *anabolic steroid for metastatic breast cancer in women* [nandrolone phenpropionate] 25 mg/mL

nandrolone BAN *anabolic* [also: nandrolone cyclotate]

nandrolone cyclotate USAN *anabolic* [also: nandrolone]

nandrolone decanoate USAN, USP *androgen; anabolic steroid* 50, 100, 200 mg/mL injection (in oil)

nandrolone phenpropionate USP *androgen; anabolic steroid* 25, 50 mg/mL injection (in oil)

naniopine [see: nanofin]

nanofin INN

nanterinone INN, BAN

nantradol INN *analgesic* [also: nantradol HCl]

nantradol HCl USAN *analgesic* [also: nantradol]

Napa ℞ *investigational antiarrhythmic* [acecainide HCl]

NAPA (N-acetyl-p-aminophenol) [see: acetaminophen]

NAPA (N-acetylprocainamide) [q.v.]

napactadine INN *antidepressant* [also: napactadine HCl]

napactadine HCl USAN *antidepressant* [also: napactadine]

napadisilate INN *combining name for radicals or groups* [also: napadisylate]

napadisylate BAN *combining name for radicals or groups* [also: napadisilate]

napamezole INN *antidepressant* [also: napamezole HCl]

napamezole HCl USAN *antidepressant* [also: napamezole]

Napamide capsules ℞ *antiarrhythmic* [disopyramide phosphate]

Naphazole-A eye drops (discontinued 1995) ℞ *topical ocular decongestant and antihistamine* [naphazoline HCl; pheniramine maleate] 0.025%•0.3%

naphazoline INN, BAN *topical ocular vasoconstrictor; nasal decongestant* [also: naphazoline HCl]

naphazoline HCl USP *topical ocular vasoconstrictor; nasal decongestant* [also: naphazoline] 0.1% eye drops

Naphazoline Plus eye drops OTC *topical ocular decongestant and antihistamine* [naphazoline HCl; pheniramine maleate] 0.025%•0.3%

Naphazoline-A eye drops (name changed to Naphazoline Plus in 1993)

Naphcon eye drops OTC *topical ocular decongestant/vasoconstrictor* [naphazoline HCl] 0.012%

Naphcon Forte Drop-Tainers (eye drops) ℞ *topical ocular decongestant/vasoconstrictor* [naphazoline HCl] 0.1%

Naphcon-A Drop-Tainers (eye drops) OTC *topical ocular decongestant and antihistamine* [naphazoline HCl; pheniramine maleate] 0.025%•0.3%

Naphoptic-A eye drops ℞ *topical ocular decongestant and antihistamine* [naphazoline HCl; pheniramine maleate] 0.025%•0.3%

2-naphthol [see: betanaphthol]

naphthonone INN

naphthypramide [see: naftypramide]

Naphuride (available only from the Centers for Disease Control) ℞ *investigational anti-infective for trypanosomiasis and onchocerciasis* [suramin sodium]

napirimus INN

Naprelan controlled-release tablets ℞ *once-daily nonsteroidal anti-inflammatory drug (NSAID); antiarthritic; analgesic* [naproxen (from naproxen sodium)] 375 (412.5), 500 (550) mg

Napril tablets (discontinued 1994) OTC *decongestant; antihistamine* [pseudoephedrine HCl; chlorpheniramine maleate] 60•4 mg

naprodoxime INN

Napron X tablets ℞ *nonsteroidal anti-inflammatory drug (NSAID); antiarthritic; analgesic* [naproxen] 500 mg

Naprosyn tablets, oral suspension ℞ *nonsteroidal anti-inflammatory drug (NSAID); antiarthritic; analgesic* [naproxen] 250, 375, 500 mg; 125 mg/5 mL ℞ Meprospan; naproxen; Natacyn

Naprosyn EC [see: EC-Naprosyn]

Naprosyn SR ℞ *investigational nonsteroidal anti-inflammatory drug (NSAID); antiarthritic; analgesic* [naproxen]

naproxen USAN, USP, INN, BAN, JAN *analgesic; antiarthritic; nonsteroidal anti-inflammatory drug (NSAID); antipyretic* 250, 375, 500 mg oral; 125 mg/5 mL oral ℞ Naprosyn

naproxen sodium USAN, USP *analgesic; antiarthritic; nonsteroidal anti-inflammatory drug (NSAID); antipyretic* 250, 500 mg oral

naproxol USAN, INN *anti-inflammatory; analgesic; antipyretic*

napsagatran USAN, INN *antithrombotic*

napsilate INN *combining name for radicals or groups* [also: napsylate]

napsylate USAN, BAN *combining name for radicals or groups* [also: napsilate]

Naqua tablets ℞ *diuretic; antihypertensive* [trichlormethiazide] 2, 4 mg

naranol INN *antipsychotic* [also: naranol HCl]

naranol HCl USAN *antipsychotic* [also: naranol]

narasin USAN, INN, BAN *coccidiostat; veterinary growth stimulant*

naratriptan HCl USAN *antimigraine agent*

Narcan IV, IM, or subcu injection, neonatal injection ℞ *narcotic antagonist for opiate dependence or overdose; hypotension treatment* [naloxone HCl] 0.4, 1 mg/mL; 0.02 mg/mL ⚠ Marcaine

narcotine [see: noscapine]

narcotine HCl [see: noscapine HCl]

Nardil sugar-coated tablets ℞ *antidepressant; antipsychotic; monoamine oxidase (MAO) inhibitor* [phenelzine sulfate] 15 mg ⚠ Norinyl

Nasabid prolonged-action capsules ℞ *decongestant; expectorant* [pseudoephedrine HCl; guaifenesin] 90•250 mg

Nasacort nasal spray ℞ *intranasal steroidal anti-inflammatory* [triamcinolone acetonide] 55 μg/spray

Nasacort AQ metered-dose aerosol ℞ *once-daily aqueous intranasal corticosteroidal anti-inflammatory* [triamcinolone acetonide] 55 μg/spray

Nasahist sustained-release capsules (discontinued 1993) ℞ *decongestant; antihistamine* [phenylpropanolamine HCl; phenylephrine HCl; chlorpheniramine maleate]

Nasahist B subcu or IM injection ℞ *antihistamine; anaphylaxis* [brompheniramine maleate] 10 mg/mL

NāSal nasal spray, nose drops OTC *nasal moisturizer* [sodium chloride (saline)] 0.65%

Nasal Decongestant spray OTC *nasal decongestant* [oxymetazoline HCl] 0.05%

Nasal Moist nasal spray OTC *nasal moisturizer* [sodium chloride (saline)] 0.65%

Nasal Relief nasal spray OTC *nasal decongestant* [oxymetazoline HCl] 0.05%

Nasalcrom nasal spray ℞ *bronchodilator for bronchial asthma and bronchospasm* [cromolyn sodium] 40 mg/mL (5.2 mg/dose)

Nasalide nasal spray ℞ *intranasal steroidal anti-inflammatory* [flunisolide] 25 μg/dose

Nasarel metered dose nasal spray ℞ *intranasal steroidal anti-inflammatory* [flunisolide] 0.025% (25 μg/dose)

Nasatab LA long-acting film-coated tablets ℞ *decongestant; expectorant* [pseudoephedrine HCl; guaifenesin] 120•500 mg

Nashville rabbit antithymocyte serum *(orphan: prevent allograft rejection)* [see: lymphocyte immune globulin, antithymocyte]

Natabec Kapseals (capsules) (discontinued 1992) OTC *vitamin/mineral/iron supplement* [multiple vitamins & minerals; iron]

Natabec FA Kapseals (capsules) (discontinued 1992) OTC *vitamin/mineral/iron supplement* [multiple vitamins & minerals; iron; folic acid]

Natabec Rx Kapseals (capsules) (discontinued 1995) ℞ *vitamin/calcium/iron supplement* [multiple vitamins; calcium; iron; folic acid] ≛•240•30•1 mg

Natabec with Fluoride capsules (discontinued 1992) ℞ *pediatric vitamin deficiency and dental caries prevention* [multiple vitamins; fluoride; iron]

Natacomp-FA film-coated tablets (discontinued 1993) ℞ *vitamin/mineral/iron supplement* [multiple vitamins & minerals; iron; folic acid]

Natacyn eye drop suspension ℞ *ophthalmic antifungal agent* [natamycin] 5% ⚠ Naprosyn

Natafort Filmseal (film-coated tablets) (discontinued 1995) ℞ *vitamin/calcium/iron supplement* [multiple vitamins; calcium; iron; folic acid] ≛•350•65•1 mg

Nata-Key coated caplets OTC *vitamin/mineral supplement* [multiple vitamins & minerals; bioflavonoids]

Natalins tablets OTC *vitamin/calcium/iron supplement* [multiple vitamins; calcium; iron; folic acid] ≛•200•30•0.5 mg

Natalins Rx tablets ℞ *vitamin/calcium/iron supplement* [multiple vitamins; calcium; iron; folic acid; biotin] ≛•200•60•1•0.03 mg

natamycin USAN, USP, INN, BAN *ophthalmic fungicidal antibiotic* [also: pimaricin]

Natarex Prenatal tablets ℞ *vitamin/calcium/iron supplement* [multiple vitamins; calcium; iron; folic acid; biotin] ± •200•60•1•0.03 mg

natural killer cell stimulatory factor [see: interleukin-12]

Natural Vegetable powder OTC *bulk laxative* [psyllium hydrophilic mucilloid] 3.4 g/tsp.

Naturalyte oral solution OTC *electrolyte replacement* [sodium, potassium, and chloride electrolytes] 240 mL, 1 L

Nature's Bounty 1 timed-release tablets (discontinued 1995) OTC *vitamin/mineral/calcium/iron supplement* [multiple vitamins & minerals; calcium; iron; folic acid; biotin] ± • 50•10•0.4•0.05 mg

Nature's Remedy tablets OTC *laxative* [cascara sagrada] 150 mg

Nature's Tears eye drops OTC *ocular moisturizer/lubricant* [hydroxypropyl methylcellulose] 0.4%

Naturetin tablets ℞ *diuretic; antihypertensive* [bendroflumethiazide] 5, 10 mg

Naus-A-Way solution OTC *antinauseant; antiemetic* [phosphorated carbohydrate solution]

Nausetrol solution OTC *antinauseant; antiemetic* [phosphorated carbohydrate solution]

Navane capsules ℞ *antipsychotic* [thiothixene] 1, 2, 5, 10, 20 mg

Navane oral concentrate, IM solution, powder for IM injection ℞ *antipsychotic* [thiothixene HCl] 5 mg/mL; 2 mg/mL; 5 mg/mL

Navelbine IV injection ℞ *antineoplastic for Hodgkin's disease and lung, breast and ovarian cancer* [vinorelbine tartrate] 10 mg/mL

Navoban ℞ *investigational treatment for nausea and vomiting related to chemotherapy* [tropisetron]

naxagolide INN *antiparkinsonian; dopamine agonist* [also: naxagolide HCl]

naxagolide HCl USAN *antiparkinsonian; dopamine agonist* [also: naxagolide]

naxaprostene INN

N-B-P ointment (discontinued 1994) OTC *topical antibiotic* [polymyxin B sulfate; neomycin sulfate; bacitracin] 5000 U•3.5 mg•400 U per g

ND Clear sustained-release capsules ℞ *decongestant; antihistamine* [pseudoephedrine HCl; chlorpheniramine maleate] 120•8 mg

ND Stat subcu or IM injection ℞ *antihistamine; anaphylaxis* [brompheniramine maleate] 10 mg/mL

ND-Gesic tablets OTC *decongestant; antihistamine; analgesic* [phenylephrine HCl; chlorpheniramine maleate; pyrilamine maleate; acetaminophen] 5•2•12.5•300 mg

nealbarbital INN [also: nealbarbitone]

nealbarbitone BAN [also: nealbarbital]

nebacumab USAN, INN, BAN *antiendotoxin monoclonal antibody; (orphan: gram-negative bacteremia in endotoxin shock)*

Nebcin IV or IM injection, pediatric injection, powder for injection ℞ *aminoglycoside-type antibiotic* [tobramycin sulfate] 10, 40 mg/mL; 10 mg/mL; 30 mg/mL

nebidrazine INN

nebivolol USAN, INN *antihypertensive (β-blocker)*

nebracetam INN

nebramycin USAN, INN *antibacterial*

nebramycin factor 6 [see: tobramycin]

NebuPent inhalation aerosol ℞ *antiprotozoal; treatment and prophylaxis of Pneumocystis carinii pneumonia (orphan)* [pentamidine isethionate] 300 mg

nedocromil USAN, INN, BAN *prophylactic antiallergic*

nedocromil calcium USAN *prophylactic antiallergic*

nedocromil sodium USAN *prophylactic antiallergic; antiasthmatic*

N.E.E. 1/35 tablets ℞ *monophasic oral contraceptive* [norethindrone; ethinyl estradiol] 1 mg•35 μg

nefazodone INN *antidepressant* [also: nefazodone HCl]

nefazodone HCl USAN *antidepressant* [also: nefazodone]

neflumozide INN *antipsychotic* [also: neflumozide HCl]

neflumozide HCl USAN *antipsychotic* [also: neflumozide]

nefocon A USAN *hydrophobic contact lens material*

nefopam INN *analgesic* [also: nefopam HCl]

nefopam HCl USAN *analgesic* [also: nefopam]

nefrolan [see: clorexolone]

NegGram caplets, oral suspension ℞ *urinary bactericidal* [nalidixic acid] 250, 500, 1000 mg; 250 mg/5 mL

neldazosin INN

nelezaprine INN *muscle relaxant* [also: nelezaprine maleate]

nelezaprine maleate USAN *muscle relaxant* [also: nelezaprine]

nelfinavir *investigational protease inhibitor for HIV*

Nelova 1/35E; Nelova 0.5/35E tablets ℞ *monophasic oral contraceptive* [norethindrone; ethinyl estradiol] 1 mg•35 μg; 0.5 mg•35 μg

Nelova 1/50M tablets ℞ *monophasic oral contraceptive* [norethindrone; mestranol] 1 mg•50 μg

Nelova 10/11 tablets ℞ *biphasic oral contraceptive* [norethindrone; ethinyl estradiol] Phase 1: 0.5 mg•35 μg; Phase 2: 1 mg•35 μg

Nelulen 1/35E; Nelulen 1/50E tablets (discontinued 1994) ℞ *oral contraceptive* [ethynodiol diacetate; ethinyl estradiol] 1 mg•35 μg; 1 mg•50 μg

nemadectin USAN, INN *veterinary antiparasitic*

nemazoline INN *nasal decongestant* [also: nemazoline HCl]

nemazoline HCl USAN *nasal decongestant* [also: nemazoline]

Nembutal elixir (discontinued 1993) ℞ *sedative; hypnotic* [pentobarbital] ② Myambutal

Nembutal Sodium capsules, IV, IM injection, suppositories ℞ *sedative; hypnotic* [pentobarbital sodium] 50, 100 mg; 50 mg/mL; 30, 60, 120, 200 mg

neoarsphenamine NF, INN

Neocaf ℞ *(orphan: apnea of prematurity)* [caffeine]

Neo-Calglucon syrup OTC *calcium supplement* [calcium glubionate] 1.8 g/5 mL

neocarzinostatin [now: zinostatin]

Neo-Castaderm liquid (discontinued 1995) OTC *topical antifungal; astringent; antiseptic* [resorcinol; boric acid; acetone; sodium bisulfite; phenol; alcohol]

Neocate One + ready-to-use liquid OTC *pediatric enteral nutritional therapy* [lactose-free formula] 237 mL

Neocera (trademarked ingredient) *suppository base* [PEG 400, 1450, 8000; polysorbate 60]

neocid [see: chlorophenothane]

Neocidin eye drops (discontinued 1993) ℞ *ophthalmic antibiotic* [polymyxin B sulfate; neomycin sulfate; gramicidin]

neocinchophen NF, INN

NeoCitran DM Coughs & Colds powder for oral solution (available only in Canada) OTC *antitussive; decongestant; antihistamine* [dextromethorphan hydrobromide; phenylephrine HCl; pheniramine maleate] 30•10•20 mg/dose

Neo-Cortef cream (discontinued 1993) ℞ *topical corticosteroid; antibiotic* [hydrocortisone; neomycin sulfate] 1%•0.5%

Neo-Cortef ointment ℞ *topical corticosteroid; antibiotic* [hydrocortisone; neomycin sulfate] 0.5%•0.5%, 1%•0.5%

Neo-Cultol jelly OTC *emollient laxative* [mineral oil]

Neocyten IV or IM injection (discontinued 1993) ℞ *skeletal muscle relaxant* [orphenadrine citrate]

NeoDecadron cream ℞ *topical corticosteroid; antibiotic* [dexamethasone phosphate; neomycin sulfate] 0.1%•0.5%

NeoDecadron Ocumeter (eye drops), ophthalmic ointment ℞ *topical ophthalmic corticosteroidal anti-inflammatory; antibiotic* [dexamethasone sodium phosphate; neomycin sulfate] 0.1%•0.35%; 0.05%•0.35%

Neo-Dexair eye drops ℞ *topical ophthalmic corticosteroidal anti-inflammatory; antibiotic* [dexamethasone sodium phosphate; neomycin sulfate] 0.1%•0.35%

Neo-Dexameth eye drops ℞ *topical ophthalmic corticosteroidal anti-inflammatory; antibiotic* [dexamethasone sodium phosphate; neomycin sulfate] 0.1%•0.35%

Neo-Diaral capsules OTC *antidiarrheal* [loperamide] 2 mg

Neo-Durabolic IM injection ℞ *anabolic steroid for anemia of renal insufficiency* [nandrolone decanoate] 50, 200 mg/mL

neodymium *element (Nd)*

Neo-fradin oral solution ℞ *aminoglycoside-type antibiotic* [neomycin sulfate] 125 mg/5 mL

Neoloid oil OTC *stimulant laxative* [castor oil] 36.4%

Neomac ointment OTC *topical antibiotic* [polymyxin B sulfate; neomycin sulfate; bacitracin]

Neo-Medrol Acetate liquid (discontinued 1993) ℞ *topical corticosteroid; antibiotic* [methylprednisolone acetate; neomycin sulfate] 0.25%•0.5%, 1%•0.5%

neo-mercazole [see: carbimazole]

Neomixin ointment OTC *topical antibiotic* [polymyxin B sulfate; neomycin sulfate; bacitracin zinc] 5000 U•3.5 mg•400 U per g ⑨ neomycin

neomycin INN, BAN *antibacterial* [also: neomycin palmitate] ⑨ Neomixin

neomycin B [see: framycetin]

neomycin palmitate USAN *antibacterial* [also: neomycin]

neomycin sulfate USP *aminoglycoside antibacterial antibiotic* 500 mg oral; 3.5 mg/g topical

neomycin undecenoate [see: neomycin undecylenate]

neomycin undecylenate USAN *antibacterial; antifungal*

Neomycin-Dex ophthalmic solution ℞ *topical corticosteroid; antibiotic* [neomycin sulfate; dexamethasone sodium phosphate]

neon *element (Ne)*

Neopap suppositories OTC *analgesic; antipyretic* [acetaminophen] 125 mg

neopenyl [see: clemizole penicillin]

neoquate [see: nequinate]

Neoquess IM injection (discontinued 1994) ℞ *gastrointestinal antispasmodic* [dicyclomine HCl] 10 mg/mL

Neoquess tablets (discontinued 1994) ℞ *gastrointestinal antispasmodic* [hyoscyamine sulfate] 0.125 mg

Neoral soft gelatin capsules for microemulsion, oral solution for microemulsion ℞ *immunosuppressant for allogenic kidney, liver, and heart transplants* [cyclosporine] 25, 100 mg; 100 mg/mL

NeoRespin timed-release capsules OTC *bronchodilator for bronchial asthma and bronchospasm* [ephedrine HCl]

Neosar powder for IV injection ℞ *alkylating antineoplastic for multiple leukemias, lymphomas, blastomas, sarcomas and organ cancers* [cyclophosphamide] 100, 200, 500, 1000, 2000 mg

Neosporin cream OTC *topical antibiotic* [polymyxin B sulfate; neomycin sulfate] 10,000 U•3.5 mg per g

Neosporin Drop Dose (eye drops) ℞ *ophthalmic antibiotic* [polymyxin B sulfate; neomycin sulfate; gramicidin] 10,000 U•1.75 mg•0.025 mg per mL

Neosporin ointment OTC *topical antibiotic* [polymyxin B sulfate; neomycin sulfate; bacitracin] 5000 U•3.5 mg•400 U, 10,000 U•3.5 mg•500 U per g

Neosporin ophthalmic ointment ℞ *ophthalmic antibiotic* [polymyxin B sulfate; neomycin sulfate; bacitracin zinc] 10,000 U•3.5 mg•400 U per g

Neosporin G.U. Irrigant solution ℞ *bactericidal* [neomycin sulfate; polymyxin B sulfate] 40 mg•200,000 U per mL

Neosporin Plus cream OTC *topical antibiotic; anesthetic* [polymyxin B sulfate; neomycin; lidocaine] 10,000 U•3.5 mg•40 mg per g

Neosporin Plus ointment OTC *topical antibiotic; anesthetic* [polymyxin B sulfate; bacitracin zinc; neomycin; lidocaine] 10,000 U•500 U•3.5 mg•40 mg per g

neostigmine BAN *cholinergic muscle stimulant* [also: neostigmine bromide]

neostigmine bromide USP, INN, BAN *cholinergic muscle stimulant* [also: neostigmine] 15 mg oral

neostigmine methylsulfate USP *cholinergic muscle stimulant* 1:1000, 1:2000, 1:4000 (1, 0.5, 0.25 mg/mL) injection

Neostrata AHA for Age Spots and Skin Lightening gel OTC *hyperpigmentation bleaching agent; sunscreen* [hydroquinone; glycolic acid] 2% • 2

Neo-Synalar cream (discontinued 1995) ℞ *topical corticosteroid; antibacterial* [fluocinolone acetonide; neomycin sulfate] 0.025% • 0.5%

Neo-Synephrine eye drops, viscous solution ℞ *ophthalmic decongestant/vasoconstrictor; mydriatic* [phenylephrine HCl] 2.5%, 10%; 10%

Neo-Synephrine jelly (discontinued 1992) OTC *nasal decongestant* [phenylephrine HCl]

Neo-Synephrine nasal spray, nose drops OTC *nasal decongestant* [phenylephrine HCl] 0.25%, 0.5%, 1%; 0.125%, 0.25%, 0.5%, 1%

Neo-Synephrine 12 Hour nasal spray OTC *nasal decongestant* [oxymetazoline HCl] 0.05%

Neo-Synephrine 12 Hour nose drops (discontinued 1992) OTC *nasal decongestant* [oxymetazoline HCl]

Neo-Synephrine HCl IV, IM, or subcu injection ℞ *vasopressor for hypotensive or cardiac shock* [phenylephrine HCl] 1% (10 mg/mL)

Neo-Tabs tablets ℞ *aminoglycoside-type antibiotic* [neomycin sulfate] 500 mg

Neotal ophthalmic ointment (discontinued 1995) ℞ *ophthalmic antibiotic* [polymyxin B sulfate; neomycin sulfate; bacitracin zinc] 5000 U • 5 mg • 400 U per g

Neothylline tablets ℞ *bronchodilator* [dyphylline] 200, 400 mg

Neothylline-GG tablets (discontinued 1995) ℞ *antiasthmatic; bronchodilator; expectorant* [dyphylline; guaifenesin] 200 • 200 mg

Neotrace-4 IV injection ℞ *intravenous nutritional therapy* [multiple trace elements (metals)]

Neotricin ointment, eye drops (name changed to Ocutricin in 1992)

Neotricin HC ophthalmic ointment ℞ *ophthalmic topical corticosteroidal anti-inflammatory; antibiotic* [hydrocortisone acetate; neomycin sulfate; bacitracin zinc; polymyxin B sulfate] 1% • 3.5% • 400 U/g • 10,000 U/g

NeoVadrin B Complex "50"; NeoVadrin B Complex "100" tablets (discontinued 1992) OTC *vitamin B supplement* [multiple B vitamins; folic acid; biotin; inositol; choline bitartrate]

NeoVadrin Children's Chewable Tablets (discontinued 1992) OTC *vitamin supplement* [multiple vitamins; folic acid]

NeoVadrin Oystershell Calcium with Vitamin D tablets (discontinued 1992) OTC *dietary supplement* [calcium carbonate; vitamin D]

NeoVadrin Therapeutic M tablets (discontinued 1992) OTC *vitamin/mineral/iron supplement* [multiple vitamins & minerals; iron; biotin; folic acid]

Nephplex Rx tablets ℞ *vitamin supplement* [multiple B vitamins; ascorbic acid; folic acid; biotin] ± • 60 • 1 • 0.3 mg

NephrAmine 5.4% IV infusion ℞ *nutritional therapy for renal failure* [multiple essential amino acids; electrolytes]

Nephrobiss ℞ *investigational atrial natriuretic peptide to prevent renal failure after heart transplant* [urodilatin]

Nephro-Calci tablets OTC *calcium supplement* [calcium carbonate] 1.5 g

Nephrocaps capsules ℞ *vitamin supplement* [multiple B vitamins; vitamin C; folic acid; biotin] ± • 100 mg • 1 mg • 150 μg

Nephro-Derm cream OTC *moisturizer; emollient; antipruritic; counterirritant* [camphor; menthol]

Nephro-Fer tablets OTC *hematinic* [ferrous fumarate] 350 mg

Nephro-Fer Rx film-coated tablets ℞ *hematinic* [ferrous fumarate; folic acid] 106.9•1 mg

Nephron solution for inhalation OTC *bronchodilator for bronchial asthma* [racepinephrine] 2.25%

Nephron FA tablets (name changed to Nephplex Rx in 1995; reintroduced with a different formulation in 1996—see below)

Nephron FA tablets ℞ *hematinic* [ferrous fumarate; multiple B vitamins; ascorbic acid; folic acid; biotin; docusate sodium] 66.6•±•40•1•0.3•75 mg

Nephro-Vite tablets OTC *vitamin supplement* [multiple B vitamins; vitamin C]

Nephro-Vite Rx film-coated tablets ℞ *vitamin supplement* [multiple B vitamins; vitamin C; folic acid; biotin] ±•60 mg•1 mg•300 μg

Nephro-Vite Rx + Fe film-coated tablets ℞ *hematinic* [ferrous fumarate; multiple B vitamins; ascorbic acid; folic acid; biotin] 100•±•60•1•0.3 mg

Nephro-Vite Vitamin B Complex and C Supplement tablets OTC *vitamin supplement* [multiple B vitamins; vitamin C; folic acid; biotin] ±•60•0.8•0.3 mg

Nephrox oral suspension OTC *antacid; laxative* [aluminum hydroxide; mineral oil 10%] 320 mg/5 mL

Nepro oral liquid OTC *enteral nutritional therapy for acute or chronic renal failure* [lactose-free formula] 240 mL

neptamustine INN *antineoplastic* [also: pentamustine]

Neptazane tablets ℞ *carbonic anhydrase inhibitor; diuretic* [methazolamide] 25, 50 mg

neptunium *element (Np)*

nequinate USAN, INN *coccidiostat for poultry* [also: methyl benzoquate]

neraminol INN

nerbacadol INN

neridronic acid INN

nerve growth factor (NGF) *investigational agent for chemotherapy-induced peripheral neuropathy*

nerve growth factor receptor antagonist *investigational treatment for degenerative CNS disorders*

Nervine Nighttime Sleep-Aid tablets (name changed to Miles Nervine in 1993)

Nervocaine 1% injection ℞ *injectable local anesthetic* [lidocaine HCl] 1%

Nervocaine 2% injection (discontinued 1995) ℞ *injectable local anesthetic* [lidocaine HCl] 2%

Nesacaine; Nesacaine MPF injection ℞ *injectable local anesthetic* [chloroprocaine HCl] 1%, 2%; 2%, 3%

nesapidil INN

nesosteine INN

Nestabs tablets OTC *vitamin/calcium/iron supplement* [multiple vitamins; calcium; ferrous fumarate; folic acid] ±•200•36•0.8 mg

Nestabs FA tablets ℞ *vitamin/calcium/iron supplement* [multiple vitamins; calcium; ferrous fumarate; folic acid] ±•200•36•1 mg

Nestrex tablets OTC *vitamin supplement* [pyridoxine HCl] 25 mg

nethalide [see: pronetalol]

netilmicin INN, BAN *aminoglycoside bactericidal antibiotic* [also: netilmicin sulfate]

netilmicin sulfate USAN, USP *aminoglycoside bactericidal antibiotic* [also: netilmicin]

netobimin USAN, INN, BAN *veterinary anthelmintic*

netrafilcon A USAN *hydrophilic contact lens material*

Netromicina (Mexican name for U.S. product Netromycin)

Netromycin IV or IM injection ℞ *aminoglycoside-type antibiotic* [netilmicin sulfate] 100 mg/mL

NEU differentiation factor *investigational treatment for breast cancer*

Neucef ℞ *investigational cephalosporin antibiotic* [cefodizime]

Neumega; Numega ℞ *investigational treatment for thrombocytopenia related to chemotherapy or radiation* [interleukin-11, recombinant human]

Neupogen IV or subcu injection ℞ *severe chronic neutropenia (orphan);*

myelodysplastic syndrome; investigational cytokine for AIDS [filgrastim] 300 μg/mL

Neuprex ℞ *investigational agent for sepsis, hemorrhagic shock, gram-negative pneumonia, ARDS, cystic fibrosis*

Neuralgon ℞ *muscle relaxant for intractable spasticity of spinal cord injury or multiple sclerosis (orphan)* [baclofen]

Neuramate tablets ℞ *anxiolytic* [meprobamate] 400 mg

NeuRecover-DA; NeuRecover-LT; NeuRecover-SA capsules OTC *dietary supplement* [multiple vitamins, minerals, and amino acids; folic acid] ± • 0.067 mg; ± • 0.03 mg; ± • 0.067 mg

NeuroCRIB ℞ *investigational treatment for Alzheimer's and Parkinson's diseases* [cellular implants]

Neurodep injection OTC *parenteral vitamin therapy* [multiple B vitamins; vitamin C] ± • 50 mg/mL

Neurodep-Caps capsules OTC *vitamin supplement* [vitamins B_1, B_6, and B_{12}] 125 • 125 • 1 mg

Neuroforte-R injection ℞ *vitamin B_{12} therapy* [cyanocobalamin]

Neuroforte-Six injection ℞ *vitamin therapy* [multiple B vitamins; vitamin C]

Neurogard ℞ *investigational stroke treatment* [dizocilpine]

Neurolite injection ℞ *imaging aid for SPECT brain scans* [technetium Tc 99m bicisate]

Neuromax ℞ *investigational muscle relaxant* [doxacurium]

Neurontin capsules ℞ *anticonvulsant* [gabapentin] 100, 300, 400 mg

neurosin [see: calcium glycerophosphate]

NeuroSlim capsules OTC *dietary supplement* [multiple vitamins, minerals, and amino acids; folic acid; biotin] ± • 0.066 • 0.05 mg

neurotrophic growth factor *investigational treatment for neurologic conditions*

neurotrophin-1 *(orphan: motor neuron disease; amyotrophic lateral sclerosis)*

neurotrophin-2 *investigational treatment for amyotrophic lateral sclerosis*

neurotrophin-3 *investigational agent for treating peripheral neuropathies*

neustab [see: thioacetazone; thiacetazone]

Neut IV or subcu injection ℞ *pH buffer for metabolic acidosis; urinary alkalinizer* [sodium bicarbonate] 4% (0.48 mEq/mL)

neutral acriflavine [see: acriflavine]

neutral insulin INN, BAN *antidiabetic* [also: insulin, neutral]

neutramycin USAN, INN *antibacterial*

Neutra-Phos capsules (discontinued 1994) OTC *phosphorus supplement* [monobasic sodium phosphate; monobasic potassium phosphate; dibasic sodium phosphate; dibasic potassium phosphate] 250 mg (P)

Neutra-Phos powder OTC *phosphorus supplement* [monobasic sodium phosphate; monobasic potassium phosphate; dibasic sodium phosphate; dibasic potassium phosphate] 250 mg/packet (P)

Neutra-Phos-K capsules (discontinued 1994) OTC *phosphorus supplement* [monobasic potassium phosphate; dibasic potassium phosphate] 250 mg (P)

Neutra-Phos-K powder OTC *phosphorus supplement* [monobasic potassium phosphate; dibasic potassium phosphate] 250 mg/packet (P)

NeuTrexin powder for IV injection ℞ *antineoplastic for AIDS-related Pneumocystis carinii pneumonia (PCP); folate antagonist* [trimetrexate glucuronate] 25 mg

neutroflavine [see: acriflavine]

Neutrogena Acne Mask OTC *topical keratolytic cleansing mask for acne* [benzoyl peroxide] 5%

Neutrogena Antiseptic Cleanser for Acne-Prone Skin liquid OTC *topical cleanser for acne* [benzethonium chloride]

Neutrogena Body lotion, oil OTC *moisturizer; emollient*

Neutrogena Drying gel OTC *topical astringent and antiseptic for acne* [hamamelis water; isopropyl alcohol]

Neutrogena Moisture lotion OTC *moisturizer; emollient*

Neutrogena Non-Drying Cleansing lotion OTC *soap-free therapeutic skin cleanser*

Neutrogena Norwegian Formula Hand cream OTC *moisturizer; emollient*

Neutrogena Oil-Free Acne Wash liquid OTC *topical keratolytic cleanser for acne* [salicylic acid] 2%

Neutrogena Soap; Neutrogena Cleansing for Acne-Prone Skin; Neutrogena Baby Cleansing Formula Soap; Neutrogena Dry Skin Soap; Neutrogena Oily Skin Soap bar OTC *therapeutic skin cleanser*

Neutrogena T/Derm oil OTC *topical antipsoriatic; antiseborrheic* [coal tar] 5%

Neutrogena T/Gel shampoo, conditioner OTC *antiseborrheic; antipsoriatic; antipruritic; antibacterial* [coal tar] 2%; 1.5%

Neutrogena T/Gel Scalp Solution gel (discontinued 1992) OTC *antiseborrheic; antipsoriatic* [coal tar]

Neutrogena T/Sal shampoo OTC *antiseborrheic; antipsoriatic; antipruritic; antibacterial* [salicylic acid; coal tar] 2% • 2%

nevirapine USAN, INN *antiviral; nonnucleoside reverse transcriptase inhibitor (NNRTI) for HIV-1*

New Decongest syrup (discontinued 1993) ℞ *decongestant; antihistamine* [phenylpropanolamine HCl; phenylephrine HCl; chlorpheniramine maleate; phenyltoloxamine citrate]

New Decongest Pediatric syrup, drops (name changed to Tri-Phen-Mine in 1995)

New Decongestant sustained-release tablets (discontinued 1993) ℞ *decongestant; antihistamine* [phenylpropanolamine HCl; phenylephrine HCl; chlorpheniramine maleate; phenyltoloxamine citrate]

new-estranol 1 [see: diethylstilbestrol]

new-oestranol 1 [see: diethylstilbestrol]

new-oestranol 11 [see: diethylstilbestrol dipropionate]

NewPaks (trademarked delivery form) *ready-to-use closed system containers*

New-Skin liquid, spray OTC *skin protectant; antiseptic* [hydroxyquinoline]

nexeridine INN *analgesic* [also: nexeridine HCl]

nexeridine HCl USAN *analgesic* [also: nexeridine]

NFL (Novantrone, fluorouracil, leucovorin [rescue]) *chemotherapy protocol*

NG-29 (orphan: *diagnostic aid for pituitary release of growth hormone*)

NGD 91-1 *investigational anxiolytic*

NGF (nerve growth factor) [q.v.]

N.G.T. cream ℞ *topical corticosteroid; antifungal* [triamcinolone acetonide; nystatin] 0.1% • 100,000 U per g

Nia-Bid sustained-action capsules OTC *vitamin supplement* [niacin] 400 mg

Niac timed-release capsules (discontinued 1994) OTC *vitamin supplement* [niacin] 300 mg

Niacels timed-release capsules OTC *vitamin supplement* [niacin] 400 mg

niacin USP *vitamin B₃; vasodilator; antihyperlipidemic* [also: nicotinic acid] 25, 50, 100, 125, 250, 500 mg oral; 100 mg/mL injection ☒ Minocin

niacinamide USP *vitamin B₃; enzyme cofactor* [also: nicotinamide] 50, 100, 125, 250, 500 mg oral

niacinamide hydroiodide *expectorant*

Niacin-Time time-release wax-matrix tablet OTC *vitamin supplement* [niacin]

Niacor immediate-release tablets ℞ *antihyperlipidemic* [niacin] 500 mg

nialamide NF, INN

niaprazine INN

Niazide tablets (discontinued 1993) ℞ *diuretic; antihypertensive* [trichlormethiazide]

nibroxane USAN, INN *topical antimicrobial*

Nicabate (European name for U.S. product Nicoderm)

nicafenine INN

nicainoprol INN

nicametate INN, BAN

nicaraven INN

nicarbazin BAN
nicardipine INN, BAN *vasodilator; calcium channel blocker* [also: nicardipine HCl]
nicardipine HCl USAN *vasodilator; calcium channel blocker* [also: nicardipine] 20, 30 mg oral
N'Ice throat spray OTC *topical antipruritic/counterirritant; mild local anesthetic* [menthol] 0.12%
N'Ice; N'Ice 'n Clear lozenges OTC *topical antipruritic/counterirritant; mild local anesthetic* [menthol] 5 mg
N'Ice Vitamin C Drops (lozenges) OTC *vitamin supplement* [ascorbic acid; menthol; sorbitol] 60 mg
NicErase-IA injection ℞ *investigational treatment for nicotine withdrawal* [lobeline]
nicergoline USAN, INN *vasodilator*
niceritrol INN, BAN
nicethamide BAN [also: nikethamide]
niceverine INN
nickel *element (Ni)*
Niclocide chewable tablets (discontinued 1995) ℞ *anthelmintic (tapeworm)* [niclosamide] 500 mg
niclofolan INN, BAN
niclosamide USAN, INN *anthelmintic*
Nico-400 timed-release capsules OTC *vitamin supplement* [niacin] 400 mg
Nicobid Tempules (timed-release capsules) OTC *niacin therapy* [niacin] 125, 250, 500 mg ② Nitro-Bid
nicoboxil INN
nicoclonate INN
nicocodine INN, BAN
nicocortonide INN
Nicoderm transdermal patch ℞ *smoking deterrent; nicotine withdrawal aid* [nicotine] 36, 78, 114 mg
Nicoderm CQ transdermal patch OTC *smoking deterrent; nicotine withdrawal aid* [nicotine] 7, 14, 21 mg/day
Nicoderm HP transdermal patch ℞ *investigational high-potency form* [nicotine]
nicodicodine INN, BAN
nicoduozide (isoniazid + nicothiazone)
nicofibrate INN
nicofuranose INN
nicofurate INN
nicogrelate INN
Nicolar tablets ℞ *niacin therapy; antihyperlipidemic* [niacin] 500 mg
nicomol INN
nicomorphine INN, BAN
nicopholine INN
nicorandil USAN, INN *coronary vasodilator*
Nicorette chewing pieces OTC *smoking deterrent; nicotine withdrawal aid* [nicotine polacrilex] 2 mg
Nicorette nasal spray, inhaler, throat pastilles *investigational delivery forms* [nicotine]
Nicorette DS chewing pieces ℞ *smoking deterrent; nicotine withdrawal aid* [nicotine polacrilex] 4 mg
nicothiazone INN
nicotinaldehyde thiosemicarbazone [see: nicothiazone]
nicotinamide INN, BAN, JAN *vitamin B_3; enzyme cofactor* [also: niacinamide]
nicotinamide-adenine dinucleotide (NAD) [now: nadide]
nicotine polacrilex USAN *smoking deterrent; nicotine withdrawal aid*
nicotine resin complex [see: nicotine polacrilex]
Nicotinex elixir OTC *vitamin supplement* [niacin] 50 mg/5 mL
nicotinic acid INN, BAN, JAN *vitamin B_3; vasodilator; antihyperlipidemic* [also: niacin]
nicotinic acid amide [see: niacinamide]
nicotinic acid 1-oxide [see: oxiniacic acid]
nicotinohydroxamic acid [see: nicoxamat]
6-nicotinoyl dihydrocodeine [see: nicodicodine]
6-nicotinoylcodeine [see: nicocodine]
4-nicotinoylmorpholine [see: nicopholine]
nicotinyl alcohol USAN, BAN *peripheral vasodilator*
nicotinyl tartrate
Nicotrol transdermal patch OTC *smoking deterrent; nicotine withdrawal aid* [nicotine] 15 mg
Nicotrol transdermal patch ℞ *smoking deterrent; nicotine withdrawal aid;*

investigational treatment for ulcerative colitis [nicotine] 8.3, 16.6, 24.9 mg

Nicotrol NS nasal spray ℞ *smoking deterrent; nicotine withdrawal aid* [nicotine] 0.5 mg/spray

nicotylamide [see: niacinamide]

nicoumalone BAN [also: acenocoumarol]

Nico-Vert capsules (discontinued 1995) ℞ *anticholinergic; antiemetic; antivertigo agent; motion sickness preventative* [meclizine] 30, 50 mg

nicoxamat INN

nictiazem INN

nictindole INN

nidroxyzone INN

Nidryl elixir (discontinued 1996) OTC *antihistamine; antitussive* [diphenhydramine HCl] 12.5 mg/5 mL

nifedipine USAN, USP, INN, BAN *coronary vasodilator; calcium channel blocker; (orphan: interstitial cystitis)* 10, 20 mg oral

nifenalol INN

nifenazone INN, BAN

Niferex film-coated tablets, elixir OTC *hematinic* [polysaccharide-iron complex] 50 mg; 100 mg/5 mL

Niferex Daily tablets OTC *vitamin/mineral supplement* [multiple vitamins & minerals]

Niferex Forte elixir ℞ *hematinic* [polysaccharide-iron complex; cyanocobalamin; folic acid] 300 mg•75 μg•3 mg per 15 mL

Niferex with Vitamin C chewable tablets OTC *hematinic* [polysaccharide-iron complex; ascorbic acid; sodium ascorbate] 50•100•169 mg

Niferex-150 capsules OTC *hematinic* [polysaccharide-iron complex] 150 mg

Niferex-150 Forte capsules ℞ *hematinic* [polysaccharide-iron complex; cyanocobalamin; folic acid] 150 mg•25 μg•1 mg

Niferex-PN film-coated tablets ℞ *prenatal vitamin/iron supplement* [polysaccharide-iron complex; multiple vitamins and minerals; folic acid] 60• ± •1 mg

Niferex-PN Forte film-coated tablets ℞ *prenatal vitamin/mineral/calcium/iron supplement* [multiple vitamins & minerals; calcium; polysaccharide-iron complex; folic acid] ± •250•60•1 mg

niflumic acid INN

nifluridide USAN *ectoparasiticide*

nifungin USAN, INN

nifuradene USAN, INN *antibacterial*

nifuralazine [see: furalazine]

nifuraldezone USAN, INN *antibacterial*

nifuralide INN

nifuramizone [see: nifurethazone]

nifuratel USAN, INN *antibacterial; antifungal; antiprotozoal (Trichomonas)*

nifuratrone USAN, INN *antibacterial*

nifurazolidone [see: furazolidone]

nifurdazil USAN, INN *antibacterial*

nifurethazone INN

nifurfoline INN

nifurhydrazone [see: nihydrazone]

nifurimide USAN, INN *antibacterial*

nifurizone INN

nifurmazole INN

nifurmerone USAN, INN *antifungal*

nifuroquine INN

nifuroxazide INN

nifuroxime NF, INN

nifurpipone (NP) INN

nifurpirinol USAN, INN *antibacterial*

nifurprazine INN

nifurquinazol USAN, INN *antibacterial*

nifursemizone USAN, INN *antiprotozoal for poultry (Histomonas)*

nifursol USAN, INN *antiprotozoal for poultry (Histomonas)*

nifurthiazole USAN, INN *antibacterial*

nifurthiline [see: thiofuradene]

nifurtimox INN, BAN *investigational anti-infective for Chagas disease (available only from Centers for Disease Control)*

nifurtoinol INN

nifurvidine INN

nifurzide INN

Night-Time Effervescent Cold tablets for oral solution OTC *decongestant; antihistamine; analgesic; antipyretic* [phenylpropanolamine HCl; diphenhydramine citrate; aspirin] 15•38.33•325 mg

niguldipine INN

nihydrazone INN

nikethamide NF, INN [also: nicethamide]

Nil vaginal cream (discontinued 1992) ℞ *bacteriostatic antibiotic; antiseptic; vulnerary* [sulfanilamide; aminacrine HCl; allantoin] 15%•0.2%•1.5%

Nilandron (marketed in Europe, Canada, and Latin America as Anandron) ℞ *investigational antiandrogen antineoplastic for prostate cancer* [nilutamide]

nileprost INN

nilestriol INN *estrogen* [also: nylestriol]

nilprazole INN

Nilstat cream, ointment ℞ *topical antifungal* [nystatin] 100,000 U/g ⊇ Nitrostat; nystatin

Nilstat film-coated tablets ℞ *systemic antifungal* [nystatin] 500,000 U

Nilstat oral suspension, powder for oral suspension ℞ *antifungal; oral candidiasis treatment* [nystatin] 100,000 U/mL; 150 million, 500 million, 1 billion, 2 billion U

Nilstat vaginal tablets (discontinued 1993) ℞ *topical antifungal* [nystatin]

niludipine INN

nilutamide USAN, INN, BAN *antiandrogen antineoplastic for prostate cancer*

nilvadipine USAN, INN, JAN *calcium channel antagonist*

nimazone USAN, INN *anti-inflammatory*

Nimbex IV infusion ℞ *nondepolarizing neuromuscular blocking agent for anesthesia* [cisatracurium besylate] 2, 10 mg/mL

Nimbus; Nimbus Quick Strip test kit for home use OTC *in vitro diagnostic aid for urine pregnancy test* [monoclonal antibody-based enzyme immunoassay]

Nimbus II test kit for professional use (discontinued 1992) *in vitro diagnostic aid for urine pregnancy test* [monoclonal antibody-based enzyme immunoassay]

Nimbus Plus test kit for professional use *in vitro diagnostic aid for urine pregnancy test*

nimesulide INN, BAN

nimetazepam INN

nimidane USAN, INN *veterinary acaricide*

nimodipine USAN, INN, BAN *vasodilator; calcium channel blocker; investigational Alzheimer's treatment*

nimorazole INN, BAN

Nimotop soft liquid-filled capsules ℞ *calcium channel blocker for subarachnoid hemorrhage; investigational Alzheimer's treatment* [nimodipine] 30 mg

nimustine INN

935U *investigational treatment for HIV*

niobium *element (Nb)*

niometacin INN

Nion B Plus C caplets OTC *vitamin supplement* [multiple B vitamins; vitamin C] ≛•300 mg

Nipent powder for IV injection ℞ *antibiotic antineoplastic; for hairy cell and chronic lymphocytic leukemias (orphan)* [pentostatin] 10 mg

niperotidine INN

nipradilol INN

Nipride powder for IV infusion (discontinued 1992) ℞ *antihypertensive for hypertensive crisis* [sodium nitroprusside] 50 mg

niprofazone INN

niridazole USAN, INN *antischistosomal*

Nisaval tablets (discontinued 1992) ℞ *antihistamine* [pyrilamine maleate] 25 mg

nisbuterol INN *bronchodilator* [also: nisbuterol mesylate]

nisbuterol mesylate USAN *bronchodilator* [also: nisbuterol]

nisobamate USAN, INN *minor tranquilizer*

nisoldipine USAN, INN, BAN, JAN *coronary vasodilator; calcium channel blocker for hypertension*

nisoxetine USAN, INN *antidepressant*

nisterime INN *androgen* [also: nisterime acetate]

nisterime acetate USAN *androgen* [also: nisterime]

nitarsone USAN, INN *antiprotozoal (Histomonas)*

nitazoxanide (NTZ) INN *investigational (Phase II) anti-infective for AIDS-related cryptosporidiosis*

Nite Time Cold Formula liquid OTC *antitussive; decongestant; antihistamine; analgesic* [dextromethorphan hydrobromide; pseudoephedrine

HCl; doxylamine succinate; acetaminophen; alcohol 25%] 5•10•1.25•167 mg/5 mL

NiteLite OTC *investigational cough/cold medication*

nithiamide USAN *veterinary antibacterial* [also: aminitrozole; acinitrazole]

nitracrine INN

nitrafudam INN *antidepressant* [also: nitrafudam HCl]

nitrafudam HCl USAN *antidepressant* [also: nitrafudam]

nitralamine HCl USAN *antifungal*

nitramisole INN *anthelmintic* [also: nitramisole HCl]

nitramisole HCl USAN *anthelmintic* [also: nitramisole]

nitraquazone INN

nitratophenylmercury [see: phenylmercuric nitrate]

nitrazepam USAN, INN, BAN, JAN *anticonvulsant; hypnotic*

Nitrazine paper for professional use *in vitro diagnostic aid for urine pH determination*

nitre, sweet spirit of [see: ethyl nitrite]

nitrefazole INN, BAN

nitrendipine USAN, INN, BAN, JAN *antihypertensive; calcium channel blocker*

nitric acid NF *acidifying agent*

nitric oxide (orphan: *neonatal primary pulmonary hypertension*)

nitricholine perchlorate INN

***p*-nitrobenzenearsonic acid** [see: nitarsone]

Nitro-Bid Plateau Caps (controlled-release capsules), ointment ℞ *antianginal* [nitroglycerin] 2.5, 6.5, 9 mg; 2% (15 mg/inch) ② Nicobid

Nitro-Bid IV infusion ℞ *antianginal; perioperative antihypertensive; for congestive heart failure with myocardial infarction* [nitroglycerin] 5 mg/mL

Nitrocine Timecaps (timed-release capsules) ℞ *antianginal* [nitroglycerin] 2.5, 6.5, 9 mg

Nitrocine transdermal patch (discontinued 1995) ℞ *antianginal* [nitroglycerin] 187.5 mg

nitroclofene INN

nitrocycline USAN, INN *antibacterial*

nitrodan USAN, INN *anthelmintic*

Nitro-Derm transdermal patch ℞ *antianginal* [nitroglycerin] 160 mg

Nitrodisc transdermal patch ℞ *antianginal* [nitroglycerin] 16, 24, 32 mg

Nitro-Dur transdermal patch ℞ *antianginal* [nitroglycerin] 20, 40, 60, 80, 120, 160 mg

nitroethanolamine [see: aminoethyl nitrate]

Nitrofan capsules ℞ *urinary bacteriostatic* [nitrofurantoin] 50, 100 mg

nitrofuradoxadone [see: furmethoxadone]

nitrofural INN *broad-spectrum bactericidal; adjunct to burn treatment* [also: nitrofurazone]

nitrofurantoin USP, INN *urinary bacteriostatic* 50, 100 mg oral

nitrofurantoin sodium

nitrofurazone USP, BAN *broad-spectrum bactericidal; adjunct to burn treatment* [also: nitrofural] 0.2% topical

nitrofurmethone [see: furaltadone]

nitrofuroxizone [see: nidroxyzone]

Nitrogard transmucosal extended-release tablets *antianginal* [nitroglycerin] 1, 2, 3 mg

nitrogen (N_2) NF *air displacement agent; element (N)*

nitrogen monoxide [see: nitrous oxide]

nitrogen mustard N-oxide HCl JAN *alkylating antineoplastic* [also: mechlorethamine HCl; chlormethine; mustine]

nitrogen oxide (N_2O) [see: nitrous oxide]

nitroglycerin USP *coronary vasodilator; antianginal* [also: glyceryl trinitrate] 2.5, 6.5, 9 mg oral; 5 mg/mL injection; 16–187.5 mg transdermal; 2% topical ② Nitroglyn

Nitroglyn extended-release capsules ℞ *antianginal* [nitroglycerin] 2.5, 6.5, 9, 13 mg ② nitroglycerin

nitrohydroxyquinoline [see: nitroxoline]

Nitrol ointment, Appli-Kit (ointment & adhesive dosage covers) ℞ *antianginal* [nitroglycerin] 2% (15 mg/inch)

Nitrolan liquid OTC *enteral nutritional therapy* [lactose-free formula]

Nitrolingual Spray lingual aerosol ℞ *antianginal* [nitroglycerin] 0.4 mg/spray

nitromannitol [see: mannitol hexanitrate]

nitromersol USP *topical anti-infective*

nitromide USAN *coccidiostat for poultry; antibacterial*

nitromifene INN

nitromifene citrate USAN *antiestrogen*

Nitrong sustained-release tablets ℞ *antianginal* [nitroglycerin] 2.6, 6.5, 9 mg

Nitropress powder for IV injection, fliptop vials ℞ *emergency antihypertensive* [sodium nitroprusside] 50 mg/dose

nitroprusside sodium [see: sodium nitroprusside]

nitroscanate USAN, INN *veterinary anthelmintic*

Nitrostat IV infusion (discontinued 1992) ℞ *antianginal* [nitroglycerin] ② Hyperstat; Nilstat; nystatin

Nitrostat sublingual tablets ℞ *antianginal* [nitroglycerin] 0.3, 0.4, 0.6 mg

nitrosulfathiazole INN [also: paranitrosulfathiazole]

Nitro-Time extended-release capsules ℞ *antianginal* [nitroglycerin] 2.5, 6.5, 9 mg

nitrous acid, sodium salt [see: sodium nitrite]

nitrous oxide (N_2O) USP *inhalation general anesthetic*

nitroxinil INN

nitroxoline INN, BAN

nivacortol INN *glucocorticoid* [also: nivazol]

nivadipine [see: nilvadipine]

nivaquine [see: chloroquine phosphate]

nivazol USAN *glucocorticoid* [also: nivacortol]

Nivea After Tan; Nivea Moisturizing; Nivea Moisturizing Extra Enriched lotion OTC *moisturizer; emollient*

Nivea Moisturizing; Nivea Skin oil OTC *moisturizer; emollient*

Nivea Moisturizing Creme Soap bar OTC *therapeutic skin cleanser*

Nivea Ultra Moisturizing Creme OTC *moisturizer; emollient*

nivimedone sodium USAN *antiallergic*

Nix creme rinse (discontinued 1993) OTC *pediculicide; scabicide* [permethrin; alcohol 20%] 1%

nixylic acid INN

nizatidine USAN, USP, INN, BAN, JAN *treatment of gastric and duodenal ulcers; histamine H_2 antagonist*

nizofenone INN

Nizoral cream, shampoo ℞ *topical antifungal* [ketoconazole] 2%

Nizoral tablets ℞ *systemic antifungal (orphan: diminish cyclosporine-induced nephrotoxicity of transplants)* [ketoconazole] 200 mg

NMA (N-monomethyl arginine) [q.v.]

N-Multistix; N-Multistix SG reagent strips *in vitro diagnostic aid for multiple urine products*

no more burn; no more ouchies spray (discontinued 1995) OTC *topical local anesthetic; antiseptic* [lidocaine HCl; benzethonium chloride] 2.3%•0.13%

no more germies soap (discontinued 1995) OTC *antiseptic; disinfectant* [triclosan] 0.25%

no more germies towelettes (discontinued 1995) OTC *antiseptic wipes* [benzalkonium chloride]

no more itchies spray (discontinued 1995) OTC *topical corticosteroid* [hydrocortisone] 1%

No Pain-HP roll-on OTC *topical analgesic* [capsaicin] 0.075%

nobelium *element (No)*

noberastine USAN, INN, BAN *antihistamine*

nocloprost INN

nocodazole USAN, INN *antineoplastic*

Noctec capsules, syrup (discontinued 1992) ℞ *sedative; hypnotic* [chloral hydrate] 250, 500 mg; 500 mg/5 mL

N'Odor softgels OTC *urinary and fecal odor control* [chlorophyllin copper complex]

NōDōz chewable tablets OTC *CNS stimulant; analeptic* [caffeine] 100 mg

nofecainide INN

nofetumomab merpentan *monoclonal antibody imaging agent for small cell lung cancer*

nogalamycin USAN, INN *antineoplastic*

noggin *investigational neurotrophic factor for neurologic diseases*

No-Hist capsules ℞ *nasal decongestant* [phenylephrine HCl; phenylpropanolamine HCl; pseudoephedrine HCl] 5•40•40 mg

Nolahist tablets OTC *antihistamine* [phenindamine tartrate] 25 mg

Nolamine timed-release tablets ℞ *decongestant; antihistamine* [phenylpropanolamine HCl; chlorpheniramine maleate; phenindamine tartrate] 50•4•24 mg

Nolex LA long-acting tablets (name changed to Exgest LA in 1994)

nolinium bromide USAN, INN *antisecretory; antiulcerative*

Noludar 300 capsules (discontinued 1993) ℞ *sedative; hypnotic* [methyprylon] 300 mg

Nolvadex tablets ℞ *antiestrogen antineoplastic for advanced postmenopausal breast cancer* [tamoxifen citrate] 10, 20 mg

nomegestrol INN

nomelidine INN

nomifensine INN *antidepressant* [also: nomifensine maleate]

nomifensine maleate USAN *antidepressant* [also: nomifensine]

nonabine INN, BAN

nonabsorbable surgical suture [see: suture, nonabsorbable surgical]

nonachlazine [now: azaclorzine HCl]

nonaperone INN

nonapyrimine INN

nonathymulin INN

nondestearinated cod liver oil [see: cod liver oil, nondestearinated]

nonivamide INN

non-nucleoside reverse transcriptase inhibitor *investigational (Phase II) antiviral for HIV*

nonoxinol 4 INN *surfactant* [also: nonoxynol 4]

nonoxinol 9 INN *wetting and solubilizing agent; spermaticide* [also: nonoxynol 9]

nonoxinol 15 INN *surfactant* [also: nonoxynol 15]

nonoxinol 30 INN *surfactant* [also: nonoxynol 30]

nonoxynol 4 USAN *surfactant* [also: nonoxinol 4]

nonoxynol 9 USAN, USP *wetting and solubilizing agent; spermicide* [also: nonoxinol 9]

nonoxynol 10 NF *surfactant*

nonoxynol 15 USAN *surfactant* [also: nonoxinol 15]

nonoxynol 30 USAN *surfactant* [also: nonoxinol 30]

nonylphenoxypolyethoxyethanol [see: nonoxynol 4, 9, 15, & 30]

Nootropic ℞ *investigational treatment for Alzheimer's disease* [oxiracetam]

Nootropil ℞ *cognition adjuvant; (orphan: myoclonus)* [piracetam]

noracymethadol INN *analgesic* [also: noracymethadol HCl]

noracymethadol HCl USAN *analgesic* [also: noracymethadol]

Noradex tablets (discontinued 1993) ℞ *skeletal muscle relaxant* [orphenadrine citrate]

noradrenaline bitartrate [see: norepinephrine bitartrate]

Noralac chewable tablets OTC *antacid* [calcium carbonate; magnesium carbonate; bismuth subnitrate]

noramidopyrine methanesulfonate sodium [see: dipyrone]

norandrostenolone phenylpropionate [see: nandrolone phenpropionate]

norbolethone USAN *anabolic* [also: norboletone]

norboletone INN *anabolic* [also: norbolethone]

norbudrine INN [also: norbutrine]

norbutrine BAN [also: norbudrine]

Norcept-E 1/35 tablets (discontinued 1994) ℞ *monophasic oral contraceptive* [norethindrone; ethinyl estradiol] 1 mg•35 μg

Norcet capsules (discontinued 1995) ℞ *narcotic analgesic* [hydrocodone bitartrate; acetaminophen] 5•500 mg

norclostebol INN

norcodeine INN, BAN

Norcuron powder for IV injection ℞ *nondepolarizing neuromuscular blocker; adjunct to anesthesia* [vecuronium bromide] 10, 20 mg/vial

norcycline [see: sancycline]
nordazepam INN
nordefrin HCl NF
Nordette tablets ℞ *monophasic oral contraceptive* [levonorgestrel; ethinyl estradiol] 0.15 mg•30 μg
Nordiate ℞ *investigational treatment for hemophilia* [antihemophilic factor]
Nordimmun ℞ *investigational antibody replacement therapy for immunologic thrombocytic disorders* [immunoglobulin]
nordinone INN
Norditropin powder for subcu injection ℞ *human growth hormone (orphan: growth failure; Turner syndrome; anovulation; burns)* [somatropin] 4 mg (12 IU), 8 mg (24 IU)
Nordryl capsules, elixir, cough syrup, injection (discontinued 1992) ℞ *antihistamine; motion sickness preventative; sleep aid; antiparkinsonian* [diphenhydramine HCl] 25, 50 mg; 12.5 mg/5 mL; 12.5 mg/5 mL; 10, 50 mg/mL
Norel Plus capsules ℞ *decongestant; antihistamine; analgesic* [phenylpropanolamine HCl; chlorpheniramine maleate; phenyltoloxamine dihydrogen citrate; acetaminophen] 25•4•25•325 mg
norephedrine HCl [see: phenylpropanolamine HCl]
norepinephrine INN *adrenergic; vasoconstrictor; vasopressor for shock* [also: norepinephrine bitartrate]
norepinephrine bitartrate USAN, USP *adrenergic; vasoconstrictor; vasopressor for acute hypotensive shock* [also: norepinephrine]
norethandrolone NF, INN
Norethin 1/35E tablets ℞ *monophasic oral contraceptive* [norethindrone; ethinyl estradiol] 1 mg•35 μg
Norethin 1/50M tablets ℞ *monophasic oral contraceptive* [norethindrone; mestranol] 1 mg•50 μg
norethindrone USP *progestin for amenorrhea, abnormal uterine bleeding, and endometriosis* [also: norethisterone]
norethindrone acetate USP *progestin for amenorrhea, abnormal uterine bleeding, and endometriosis*

norethisterone INN, BAN, JAN *progestin* [also: norethindrone]
norethynodrel USAN, USP *progestin* [also: noretynodrel]
noretynodrel INN *progestin* [also: norethynodrel]
noreximide INN
norfenefrine INN
Nor-Feran IM, IV injection (discontinued 1992) ℞ *antianemic* [iron dextran]
Norflex sustained-release tablets, IV or IM injection ℞ *skeletal muscle relaxant* [orphenadrine citrate] 100 mg; 30 mg/mL
norfloxacin USAN, USP, INN, BAN, JAN *broad-spectrum bactericidal antibiotic*
norfloxacin succinil INN
norflurane USAN, INN *inhalation anesthetic*
Norforms powder OTC *absorbs vaginal moisture; astringent* [cornstarch; zinc oxide]
Norforms vaginal suppositories OTC *feminine deodorant*
Norgesic; Norgesic Forte tablets ℞ *skeletal muscle relaxant; analgesic* [orphenadrine citrate; aspirin; caffeine] 25•385•30 mg; 50•770•60 mg
norgesterone INN
norgestimate USAN, INN, BAN *progestin*
Norgestimate/EE ℞ *investigational cyclophasic oral contraceptive*
norgestomet USAN, INN *progestin*
norgestrel USAN, USP, INN *progestin*
d-norgestrel (incorrect enantiomer designation) [now: levonorgestrel]
D-norgestrel [see: levonorgestrel]
norgestrienone INN
Norinyl 1 + 35 tablets ℞ *monophasic oral contraceptive* [norethindrone; ethinyl estradiol] 1 mg•35 μg ② Nardil
Norinyl 1 + 50 tablets ℞ *monophasic oral contraceptive* [norethindrone; mestranol] 1 mg•50 μg
Norisodrine Aerotrol (inhalation aerosol) ℞ *bronchodilator* [isoproterenol HCl]
Norisodrine with Calcium Iodide syrup ℞ *bronchodilator; expectorant* [isoproterenol sulfate; calcium iodide; alcohol 6%] 3•150 mg

Norlac Rx tablets (discontinued 1995) ℞ *vitamin/mineral/calcium/iron supplement* [multiple vitamins & minerals; calcium; iron; folic acid] ± •200•60•1 mg

Norlestrin 1/50 tablets (discontinued 1993) ℞ *monophasic oral contraceptive* [norethindrone acetate; ethinyl estradiol] 1 mg•50 μg

Norlestrin 21 2.5/50 tablets (discontinued 1994) ℞ *monophasic oral contraceptive* [norethindrone acetate; ethinyl estradiol] 2.5 mg•50 μg

Norlestrin Fe 1/50; Norlestrin Fe 2.5/50 tablets (discontinued 1994) ℞ *monophasic oral contraceptive* [norethindrone acetate; ethinyl estradiol; ferrous fumarate] 1 mg•50 μg•75 mg

norletimol INN

norleusactide INN [also: pentacosactride]

norlevorphanol INN, BAN

Norlutate tablets (discontinued 1995) ℞ *progestin for amenorrhea, abnormal uterine bleeding, or endometriosis* [norethindrone acetate] 5 mg ⊇ Norlutin

Norlutin tablets (discontinued 1995) ℞ *progestin for amenorrhea, abnormal uterine bleeding, or endometriosis* [norethindrone] 5 mg ⊇ Norlutate

½ normal saline (½ NS; 0.45% sodium chloride) *electrolyte replacement*

normal saline (NS; 0.9% sodium chloride) *electrolyte replacement* [also: saline solution]

normal serum albumin [see: albumin, human]

normethadone INN, BAN

normethandrolone [see: normethandrone]

normethandrone

normethisterone [see: normethandrone]

Normiflo; Normiflow tablets ℞ *investigational anticoagulant for hip and knee surgery* [ardeparin sodium]

Normodyne tablets, IV ℞ *antihypertensive; alpha- and beta-adrenergic blocking agent* [labetalol HCl] 100, 200, 300 mg; 5 mg/mL

normorphine INN, BAN

Normosang ℞ *(orphan: acute symptomatic porphyria; myelodysplastic syndromes)* [heme arginate]

Normosol-M and 5% Dextrose; Normosol-R and 5% Dextrose IV infusion ℞ *intravenous nutritional/electrolyte therapy* [combined electrolyte solution; dextrose]

Normosol-R; Normosol-R pH 7.4 IV infusion ℞ *intravenous electrolyte therapy* [combined electrolyte solution]

Normozide film-coated tablets (discontinued 1994) ℞ *antihypertensive* [labetalol HCl; hydrochlorothiazide] 100•25, 200•25, 300•25 mg

Normylin ℞ *investigational antidiabetic* [AC 137 (code name—generic name not yet approved)]

Noroxin film-coated tablets ℞ *broad-spectrum fluoroquinolone-type antibiotic* [norfloxacin] 400 mg

Norpace capsules ℞ *antiarrhythmic* [disopyramide phosphate] 100, 150 mg

Norpace CR controlled-release capsules ℞ *antiarrhythmic* [disopyramide phosphate] 100, 500 mg

norpipanone INN, BAN

Norplant implantable Silastic capsules ℞ *implant contraceptive system* [levonorgestrel] 36 mg

Norplant II ℞ *investigational implant contraceptive system* [levonorgestrel]

Norpramin film-coated tablets ℞ *tricyclic antidepressant* [desipramine HCl] 10, 25, 50, 75, 100, 150 mg ⊇ imipramine

norpseudoephedrine [see: cathine]

Nor-Q.D. tablets ℞ *oral contraceptive (progestin only)* [norethindrone] 0.35 mg

nortestosterone phenylpropionate [see: nandrolone phenpropionate]

Nor-Tet capsules ℞ *broad-spectrum antibiotic* [tetracycline HCl] 250, 500 mg

nortetrazepam INN

nortriptyline HCl USAN, USP, INN *tricyclic antidepressant* [10, 25, 50, 75 mg oral] ⊇ amitriptyline

Norvasc tablets ℞ *antianginal; antihypertensive; calcium channel blocker* [amlodipine] 2.5, 5, 10 mg

norvinisterone INN

norvinodrel [see: norgesterone]

Norvir capsules, oral solution ℞ *antiviral protease inhibitor for HIV* [ritonavir] 100 mg; 80 mg/mL

Norwich tablets OTC *analgesic; antipyretic; anti-inflammatory; antirheumatic* [aspirin] 325, 500 mg

Norzine IM injection, suppositories, tablets ℞ *antiemetic* [thiethylperazine maleate] 5 mg/mL; 10 mg; 10 mg

NoSalt; NoSalt Seasoned OTC *salt substitute* [potassium chloride] 64 mEq/5 g; 34 mEq/5 g

nosantine INN, BAN

noscapine USP, INN *antitussive*

noscapine HCl NF

nosiheptide USAN, INN *veterinary growth stimulant*

Nōstril; Children's Nōstril nasal spray OTC *nasal decongestant* [phenylephrine HCl] 0.5%; 0.25%

Nōstrilla nasal spray OTC *nasal decongestant* [oxymetazoline HCl] 0.05%

notensil maleate [see: acepromazine]

Novacet lotion ℞ *topical acne treatment* [sodium sulfacetamide; sulfur] 10%•5%

Nova-Dec tablets OTC *vitamin/mineral/iron supplement* [multiple vitamins & minerals; iron; folic acid; biotin] ±• 30 mg•0.4 mg•30 µg

Novafed timed-release capsules (discontinued 1996) ℞ *nasal decongestant* [pseudoephedrine HCl] 120 mg

Novafed A sustained-release capsules ℞ *decongestant; antihistamine* [pseudoephedrine HCl; chlorpheniramine maleate] 120•8 mg

Novagest Expectorant with Codeine liquid ℞ *narcotic antitussive; decongestant; expectorant* [codeine phosphate; pseudoephedrine HCl; guaifenesin; alcohol 1.4%] 10•30•100 mg/5 mL

Novahistine elixir OTC *decongestant; antihistamine* [phenylephrine HCl; chlorpheniramine maleate] 5•2 mg/5 mL

Novahistine DH liquid ℞ *narcotic antitussive; decongestant; antihistamine* [codeine phosphate; pseudoephedrine HCl; chlorpheniramine maleate; alcohol 5%] 10•30•2 mg/5 mL

Novahistine DMX liquid OTC *antitussive; decongestant; expectorant* [dextromethorphan hydrobromide; pseudoephedrine HCl; guaifenesin; alcohol 10%] 10•30•100 mg/5 mL

Novahistine Expectorant liquid ℞ *narcotic antitussive; decongestant; expectorant* [codeine phosphate; pseudoephedrine HCl; guaifenesin; alcohol 7.5%] 10•30•100 mg/5 mL

novamidon [see: aminopyrine]

Novamine; Novamine 15% IV infusion ℞ *total parenteral nutrition; peripheral parenteral nutrition* [multiple essential and nonessential amino acids]

Novantrone IV injection ℞ *antibiotic antineoplastic; for acute myelogenous (nonlymphocytic) leukemia (orphan)* [mitoxantrone HCl] 2 mg/mL

Novapren ℞ *investigational (Phase I) antiviral for HIV*

novel plasminogen activator (NPA) *investigational treatment for heart attack and blood clotting disorders; modified tPA*

novobiocin INN, BAN *bacteriostatic antibiotic* [also: novobiocin calcium]

novobiocin calcium USP *bacteriostatic antibiotic* [also: novobiocin]

novobiocin sodium USP *bacteriostatic antibiotic*

Novocain injection ℞ *injectable local anesthetic* [procaine HCl] 1%, 2%, 10%

Novolin 70/30 subcu injection OTC *antidiabetic* [isophane insulin (human semisynthetic); human insulin (semisynthetic)] 100 U/mL

Novolin 70/30 PenFill NovoPen cartridge OTC *antidiabetic* [isophane insulin (human semisynthetic); human insulin (semisynthetic)] 100 U/mL

Novolin L subcu injection OTC *antidiabetic* [insulin zinc (human semisynthetic)] 100 U/mL

Novolin N subcu injection OTC *antidiabetic* [isophane insulin (human semisynthetic)] 100 U/mL

Novolin N PenFill NovoPen cartridge OTC *antidiabetic* [isophane insulin (human semisynthetic)] 100 U/mL

Novolin R subcu injection OTC *antidiabetic* [human insulin (semisynthetic)] 100 U/mL

Novolin R PenFill NovoPen cartridges OTC *antidiabetic* [human insulin (semisynthetic)] 100 U/mL

NovoNorm ℞ *investigational antidiabetic agent; stimulates pancreatic insulin production*

NovoPen 1.5 prefilled reusable syringe *uses Novolin PenFill cartridges and NovoFine 30-gauge disposable needles* [insulin (several types available)] 1–40 U/injection

NovoSeven ℞ *investigational antihemophilic* [recombinant factor VIIa]

Novo-Timol eye drops (available only in Canada) ℞ *antiglaucoma agent (β-blocker)* [timolol maleate] 0.25%, 0.5%

NOVP (Novantrone, Oncovin, vinblastine, prednisone) *chemotherapy protocol*

noxiptiline INN [also: noxiptyline]

noxiptyline BAN [also: noxiptiline]

noxythiolin BAN [also: noxytiolin]

noxytiolin INN [also: noxythiolin]

NP (nifurpipone) [q.v.]

NP-27 solution, powder, spray powder, cream OTC *topical antifungal* [tolnaftate] 1%

NPA (novel plasminogen activator) [q.v.]

NPH (neutral protamine Hagedorn) insulin [see: insulin, isophane]

NPH Iletin I subcu injection OTC *antidiabetic* [isophane insulin (beef-pork)] 100 U/mL

NPH Iletin I (beef) subcu injection (discontinued 1994) OTC *antidiabetic* [isophane insulin]

NPH Iletin I (pork) subcu injection (discontinued 1994) OTC *antidiabetic* [isophane insulin]

NPH Iletin II (beef) subcu injection (discontinued 1994) OTC *antidiabetic* [isophane insulin]

NPH Iletin II (pork) subcu injection OTC *antidiabetic* [isophane insulin] 100 U/mL

NPH Insulin subcu injection OTC *antidiabetic* [isophane insulin (beef)] 100 U/mL

NPH Purified Pork Isophane Insulin subcu injection (name changed to NPH-N in 1994)

NPH-N subcu injection OTC *antidiabetic* [isophane insulin (pork)] 100 U/mL

NR-LU-10-PE *investigational diagnostic aid for small cell lung cancer*

NS (normal saline) [q.v.]

NTS transdermal patches ℞ *antianginal* [nitroglycerin]

NTZ (nitazoxanide) [q.v.]

NTZ Long Acting nasal spray, nose drops OTC *nasal decongestant* [oxymetazoline HCl] 0.05%

Nubain IV, subcu or IM injection ℞ *narcotic agonist-antagonist analgesic* [nalbuphine HCl] 10, 20 mg/mL

nuclomedone INN

nuclotixene INN

Nucofed capsules, syrup ℞ *narcotic antitussive; decongestant* [codeine phosphate; pseudoephedrine HCl] 20•60 mg; 20•60 mg/5 mL

Nucofed Expectorant; Nucofed Pediatric Expectorant syrup ℞ *narcotic antitussive; decongestant; expectorant* [codeine phosphate; pseudoephedrine HCl; guaifenesin; alcohol 12.5%•6%] 20•60•200 mg/5 mL; 10•30•100 mg/5 mL

Nucotuss Expectorant; Nucotuss Pediatric Expectorant liquid *narcotic antitussive; decongestant; expectorant* [codeine phosphate; pseudoephedrine HCl; guaifenesin; alcohol 12.5%•6%] 20•60•200 mg/5 mL; 10•30•100 mg/5 mL

nufenoxole USAN, INN *antiperistaltic*

Nu-Iron elixir OTC *hematinic* [polysaccharide-iron complex] 100 mg/5 mL

Nu-Iron 150 capsules OTC *hematinic* [polysaccharide-iron complex] 150 mg

Nu-Iron Plus elixir ℞ *hematinic* [polysaccharide iron complex; cyanocobalamin; folic acid] 300 mg•75 μg•3 mg per 15 mL

Nu-Iron V film-coated tablets ℞ *vitamin/iron supplement* [polysaccharide iron complex; multiple vitamins; folic acid] 60•≛•1 mg

Nu-knit (trademarked form) *oxidized cellulose hemostatic pad*

Nulicaine injection (discontinued 1995) ℞ *injectable local anesthetic* [lidocaine HCl] 1%, 2%

Nullo tablets (discontinued 1996) OTC *vulnerary; fecal and urinary odor control* [chlorophyllin copper complex] 33.3 mg

NuLytely powder for oral solution ℞ *pre-procedure bowel cleansing* [polyethylene glycol-electrolyte solution] 105 g/L

Numorphan IV, IM, or subcu injection, suppositories ℞ *narcotic analgesic; preoperative support of anesthesia (orphan: intractable narcotic-tolerant pain)* [oxymorphone HCl] 1, 1.5 mg/mL; 5 mg

Numzident gel OTC *topical oral anesthetic* [benzocaine] 10%

Numzit Teething gel OTC *topical oral anesthetic* [benzocaine] 7.5%

Numzit Teething lotion OTC *topical oral anesthetic* [benzocaine; alcohol 12.1%] 0.2%

Nupercainal ointment, cream OTC *topical local anesthetic* [dibucaine] 1%; 0.5%

Nupercainal rectal suppositories OTC *emollient; astringent* [cocoa butter; zinc oxide] 2.1•0.25 g

Nuprin tablets, caplets OTC *nonsteroidal anti-inflammatory drug (NSAID); antiarthritic; analgesic* [ibuprofen] 200 mg

Nuquin HP cream, gel ℞ *hyperpigmentation bleaching agent; sunscreen* [hydroquinone; dioxybenzone] 4%•30 mg

Nuromax IV injection ℞ *nondepolarizing neuromuscular blocker; adjunct to anesthesia* [doxacurium chloride] 1 mg/mL

Nursette (trademarked form) *prefilled disposable bottle*

Nursoy liquid, powder (discontinued 1996) OTC *hypoallergenic infant food* [soy protein formula]

Nu-Salt OTC *salt substitute* [potassium chloride] 68 mEq/5 g

Nu-Tears eye drops OTC *ocular moisturizer/lubricant* [polyvinyl alcohol] 1.4%

Nu-Tears II eye drops OTC *ocular moisturizer/lubricant* [polyvinyl alcohol; polyethylene glycol 400] 1%•1%

Nu-Timolol eye drops (available only in Canada) ℞ *antiglaucoma agent (β-blocker)* [timolol maleate] 0.25%, 0.5%

nutmeg oil NF

Nutracort cream, lotion ℞ *topical corticosteroid* [hydrocortisone] 1%

Nutraderm cream, lotion OTC *moisturizer; emollient*

Nutraderm OTC *lotion base*

Nutraderm Bath Oil OTC *bath emollient*

Nutraloric powder OTC *enteral nutritional therapy* [milk-based formula]

Nutramigen liquid, powder OTC *hypoallergenic infant food* [enzymatically hydrolyzed protein formula]

Nutra-Plex liquid (discontinued 1995) OTC *vitamin/mineral supplement* [multiple B vitamins & minerals; alcohol 13.5%]

Nutraplus cream, lotion OTC *moisturizer; emollient; keratolytic* [urea] 10%

Nutra-Soothe bath oil OTC *bath emollient* [colloidal oatmeal; light mineral oil]

Nutra-Support capsules OTC *dietary supplement* [multiple vitamins & minerals]

NutraTear eye drops (discontinued 1994) OTC *ocular moisturizer/lubricant*

Nutren 1.0 liquid OTC *enteral nutritional therapy* [lactose-free formula]

Nutren 1.5 liquid OTC *enteral nutritional therapy* [lactose-free formula]

Nutren 2.0 ready-to-use liquid OTC *enteral nutritional therapy* [lactose-free formula]

Nutrex tablets (discontinued 1992) OTC *vitamin/mineral/iron supplement* [multiple vitamins & minerals; iron; biotin]

Nutricon tablets OTC *vitamin/mineral/calcium/iron supplement* [multiple vitamins & minerals; calcium; iron; folic acid; biotin] ≛•200•20•0.4•0.15 mg

Nutrilan ready-to-use liquid OTC *enteral nutritional therapy* [lactose-free formula]

NutriLipid 10%; NutriLipid 20% IV infusion (discontinued 1992) ℞ *nutritional therapy* [intravenous fat emulsion]

Nutrilyte; Nutrilyte II IV admixture ℞ *intravenous electrolyte therapy* [combined elecrolyte solution]

Nutrineal PD-2 Peritoneal Dialysis Solution with 1.1% Amino Acid (discontinued 1994) ℞ *(orphan: malnourishment of continuous ambulatory peritoneal dialysis)*

Nutropin powder for subcu injection ℞ *(orphan: growth failure; Turner syndrome; anovulation; severe burns); investigational AIDS cytokine* [somatropin] 5, 10 mg (13, 26 IU)

Nutropin AQ subcu injection ℞ *(orphan: growth failure; Turner syndrome; anovulation; severe burns); investigational AIDS cytokine* [somatropin] 10 mg (30 IU)/vial

Nutrox capsules OTC *dietary supplement* [multiple vitamins, minerals, and amino acids] ≛

nuvenzepine INN

nyctal [see: carbromal]

nydrane [see: benzchlorpropamid]

Nydrazid IM injection ℞ *tuberculostatic* [isoniazid] 100 mg/mL

nylestriol USAN *estrogen* [also: nilestriol]

nylidrin HCl USP *peripheral vasodilator* [also: buphenine] 6, 12 mg oral

NyQuil Allergy/Head Cold, Children's liquid (discontinued 1995) OTC *pediatric decongestant and antihistamine* [pseudoephedrine HCl; chlorpheniramine maleate] 10•0.67 mg/5 mL

NyQuil Hot Therapy powder for oral solution OTC *antitussive; decongestant; antihistamine; analgesic* [dextromethorphan hydrobromide; pseudoephedrine HCl; doxylamine succinate; acetaminophen] 30•60•12.5•1000 mg/packet

NyQuil LiquiCaps (liquid-filled capsules) OTC *antitussive; decongestant; antihistamine; analgesic* [dextromethorphan hydrobromide; pseudoephedrine HCl; doxylamine succinate; acetaminophen] 10•30•6.25•250 mg

NyQuil Multisymptom Cold Flu Relief; NyQuilNighttime Cold/Flu Medicine liquid OTC *antitussive; decongestant; antihistamine; analgesic* [dextromethorphan hydrobromide; pseudoephedrine HCl; doxylamine succinate; acetaminophen; alcohol 10%•25%] 5•10•2.1•167 mg/5 mL; 5•10•1.25•167 mg/5 mL

NyQuil Nighttime Cough/Cold, Children's liquid OTC *pediatric antitussive, decongestant, and antihistamine* [dextromethorphan hydrobromide; pseudoephedrine HCl; chlorpheniramine maleate] 5•10•0.67 mg/5 mL

nystatin USP, INN, BAN, JAN *antifungal* 100,000, 500,000 U/mL oral; 100,000 mg vaginal; 100,000 U/g topical ▣ Nilstat; Nitrostat

Nystatin-LF (liposomal formulation) IV injection ℞ *investigational (Phase II) antiviral for HIV* [AR-121 (code name—generic name not yet approved)]

Nystex cream, ointment ℞ *topical antifungal* [nystatin] 100,000 U/g

Nystex oral suspension ℞ *antifungal; oral candidiasis treatment* [nystatin] 100,000 U/mL

Nytcold Medicine liquid OTC *antitussive; decongestant; antihistamine; analgesic* [dextromethorphan hydrobromide; pseudoephedrine HCl; doxylamine succinate; acetaminophen; alcohol 25%] 5•10•1.25•167 mg/5 mL

NyteTime liquid OTC *analgesic; antipyretic; antitussive; antihistamine; decongestant* [acetaminophen; dextromethorphan hydrobromide; doxylamine succinate; pseudoephedrine HCl]

Nytol tablets OTC *antihistaminic sleep aid* [diphenhydramine HCl] 25, 50 mg

Nytyme liquid OTC *analgesic; decongestant; antihistamine; antitussive* [acetaminophen; doxylamine succinate; pseudoephedrine HCl; dextromethorphan hydrobromide; alcohol]

O₂ (oxygen) [q.v.]
OAP (Oncovin, ara-C, prednisone) *chemotherapy protocol*
oatmeal, colloidal *demulcent*
Obalan tablets (discontinued 1996) ℞ *anorexiant* [phendimetrazine tartrate] 35 mg
obecalp *placebo (spelled backward)*
Obe-nix capsules ℞ *appetite suppressant* [phentermine HCl] 37.5 mg
Obephen capsules ℞ *anorexiant* [phentermine HCl] 30 mg
Obermine capsules (discontinued 1992) ℞ *anorexiant* [phentermine HCl] 30 mg
Obestin-30 capsules (discontinued 1992) ℞ *anorexiant* [phentermine HCl] 30 mg
Obetrol tablets (name changed to Adderall in 1994)
obidoxime chloride USAN, INN *cholinesterase reactivator*
Obtundia topical spray, swab pads, liquid, cream (discontinued 1992) OTC *germicide; fungicide; topical anesthetic* [camphor; metacresol]
Obtundia Calamine cream (discontinued 1992) OTC *astringent; antiseptic; topical anesthetic* [camphor; metacresol; zinc oxide; calamine]
Oby-Cap capsules ℞ *anorexiant* [phentermine HCl] 30 mg
O-Cal f.a. tablets ℞ *vitamin/mineral/calcium/iron supplement and dental caries preventative* [multiple vitamins & minerals; calcium; iron; folic acid; sodium fluoride] ± •200•66•1•1.1 mg
ocaperidone USAN, INN, BAN *antipsychotic*
Occlusal liquid (discontinued 1994) OTC *topical keratolytic* [salicylic acid in polyacrylic vehicle] 17%
Occlusal-HP liquid OTC *topical keratolytic* [salicylic acid in polyacrylic vehicle] 17%
Occucoat ophthalmic solution ℞ *ophthalmic surgical aid* [hydroxypropyl methylcellulose] 2%

Ocean Mist nasal spray OTC *nasal moisturizer* [sodium chloride (saline)] 0.65%
ocfentanil INN *narcotic analgesic* [also: ocfentanil HCl]
ocfentanil HCl USAN *narcotic analgesic* [also: ocfentanil]
ociltide INN
ocinaplon USAN *anxiolytic*
OCL oral solution ℞ *pre-procedure bowel evacuant* [polyethylene glycol-electrolyte solution]
ocrase INN
ocrilate INN *tissue adhesive* [also: ocrylate]
ocrylate USAN *tissue adhesive* [also: ocrilate]
octabenzone USAN, INN *ultraviolet screen*
octacaine INN
octacosactrin BAN [also: tosactide]
octadecafluorodecehydronaphthalene [see: perflunafene]
octadecanoic acid, calcium salt [see: calcium stearate]
octadecanoic acid, sodium salt [see: sodium stearate]
octadecanoic acid, zinc salt [see: zinc stearate]
1-octadecanol [see: stearyl alcohol]
9-octadecenylamine hydrofluoride [see: dectaflur]
octafonium chloride INN
Octamide tablets (discontinued 1992) ℞ *antidopaminergic; antiemetic; peristaltic* [metoclopramide HCl] 10 mg
Octamide PFS IV or IM injection ℞ *antiemetic for chemotherapy; GI stimulant; peristaltic* [metoclopramide monohydrochloride monohydrate] 5 mg/mL
octamoxin INN
octamylamine INN
octanoic acid USAN, INN *antifungal*
octapinol INN
octastine INN
octatropine methylbromide INN, BAN *anticholinergic; peptic ulcer adjunct* [also: anisotropine methylbromide]
octatropone bromide [see: anisotropine methylbromide]

octaverine INN, BAN
octazamide USAN, INN *analgesic*
octenidine INN, BAN *topical anti-infective* [also: octenidine HCl]
octenidine HCl USAN *topical anti-infective* [also: octenidine]
octenidine saccharin USAN *dental plaque inhibitor*
Octicare ear drops, ear drop suspension ℞ *topical corticosteroidal anti-inflammatory; antibiotic* [hydrocortisone; neomycin sulfate; polymyxin B sulfate] 1%•5 mg•10,000 U per mL
octicizer USAN *plasticizer*
octil INN *combining name for radicals or groups*
octimibate INN
octisamyl [see: octamylamine]
Octocaine HCl injection ℞ *injectable local anesthetic* [lidocaine HCl; epinephrine] 2%•1:50,000, 2%•1:100,000
octoclothepine [see: clorotepine]
octocrilene INN *ultraviolet screen* [also: octocrylene]
octocrylene USAN *ultraviolet screen* [also: octocrilene]
octodecactide [see: codactide]
octodrine USAN, INN *adrenergic; vasoconstrictor; local anesthetic*
octopamine INN
octotiamine INN
octoxinol INN *surfactant/wetting agent* [also: octoxynol 9]
octoxynol 9 USAN, NF *surfactant/wetting agent; spermicide* [also: octoxinol]
OctreoScan powder for injection ℞ *parenteral radiopaque agent* [oxidronate sodium] 2 mg
OctreoScan 111 ℞ *investigational tumor imaging agent for SPECT scans* [indium In 111 pentetreotide]
octreotide USAN, INN, BAN *gastric antisecretory*
octreotide acetate USAN *gastric antisecretory*
octriptyline INN *antidepressant* [also: octriptyline phosphate]
octriptyline phosphate USAN *antidepressant* [also: octriptyline]
octrizole USAN, INN *ultraviolet screen*
S-octyl thiobenzoate [see: tioctilate]

octyl-2-cyanoacrylate [see: ocrylate]
octyldodecanol NF *oleaginous vehicle*
Ocu-Bath Eye Lotion ophthalmic solution (discontinued 1992) OTC *extraocular irrigating solution* [balanced saline solution]
OcuCaps caplets OTC *vitamin/mineral supplement* [vitamins A, C, and E; multiple minerals] 5000 IU•400 mg•182 mg• ≐
Ocu-Carpine eye drops (discontinued 1995) ℞ *antiglaucoma agent; direct-acting miotic* [pilocarpine HCl] 0.5%, 1%, 2%, 3%, 4%, 6%
OcuClear eye drops OTC *topical ocular decongestant/vasoconstrictor* [oxymetazoline HCl] 0.025%
OcuClenz solution, pads (discontinued 1996) OTC *eyelid cleanser for blepharitis or contact lenses*
OcuCoat prefilled syringe OTC *ophthalmic surgical aid* [hydroxypropyl methylcellulose] 2%
OcuCoat; OcuCoat PF eye drops OTC *ocular moisturizer/lubricant* [hydroxypropyl methylcellulose] 0.8%
Ocudose (trademarked delivery device) *single-use eye drop dispenser*
Ocu-Drop ophthalmic solution (discontinued 1992) OTC *extraocular irrigating solution* [balanced saline solution]
Ocufen eye drops ℞ *ocular nonsteroidal anti-inflammatory drug (NSAID); intraoperative miosis inhibitor* [flurbiprofen sodium] 0.03%
ocufilcon A USAN *hydrophilic contact lens material*
ocufilcon B USAN *hydrophilic contact lens material*
ocufilcon C USAN *hydrophilic contact lens material*
ocufilcon D USAN *hydrophilic contact lens material*
Ocuflox eye drops ℞ *ophthalmic quinolone-type antibiotic for corneal ulcers* [ofloxacin] 3 mg/mL
Oculinum powder (name changed to Botox in 1993)
Ocumeter (trademarked delivery device) *prefilled eye drop dispenser*

Ocupress eye drops ℞ *topical antiglaucoma agent (β-blocker)* [carteolol HCl] 1%

Ocusert Pilo-20; Ocusert Pilo-40 continuous-release ocular wafer ℞ *antiglaucoma agent; direct-acting miotic* [pilocarpine] 20 μg/hour; 40 μg/hour

OCuSOFT solution, pads OTC *eyelid cleanser for blepharitis or contact lenses*

OCuSoft VMS film-coated tablets OTC *vitamin/mineral supplement* [vitamins A, C, and E; multiple minerals] 5000 IU•60 mg•30 mg• ±

Ocusulf-10 eye drops ℞ *ophthalmic bacteriostatic* [sulfacetamide sodium] 10%

Ocutears eye drops (available only in Canada) OTC *ocular moisturizer/lubricant* [hydroxypropyl methylcellulose] 0.5%

Ocutricin eye drops (discontinued 1995) ℞ *ophthalmic antibiotic* [polymyxin B sulfate; neomycin sulfate; gramicidin] 10,000 U•1.75 mg•0.025 mg per mL

Ocutricin ophthalmic ointment ℞ *ophthalmic antibiotic* [polymyxin B sulfate; neomycin sulfate; bacitracin zinc] 10,000 U•3.5 mg•400 U per g

Ocuvite film-coated tablets OTC *vitamin/mineral supplement* [vitamins A, C, and E; multiple minerals] 5000 IU•60 mg•30 IU• ±

Ocuvite Extra tablets OTC *vitamin/mineral supplement* [vitamins A, C, and E; multiple minerals] 6000 IU•200 mg•50 IU• ±

OCuZIN tablets OTC *vitamin/mineral supplement* [vitamins A, C, and E; zinc; copper; selenium]

Odor Free ArthriCare [see: ArthriCare, Odor Free]

Oesto-Mins powder OTC *vitamin/mineral supplement* [vitamins C and D; calcium; magnesium; potassium] 500 mg•100 IU•250 mg•250 mg•45 mg per 4.5 g

oestradiol BAN *estrogen* [also: estradiol]

oestradiol benzoate BAN [also: estradiol benzoate]

oestradiol valerate BAN *estrogen* [also: estradiol valerate]

Oestring (Swedish name for U.S. product Estring)

oestriol succinate BAN *estrogen* [also: estriol; estriol succinate]

oestrogenine [see: diethylstilbestrol]

oestromenin [see: diethylstilbestrol]

oestrone BAN *estrogen* [also: estrone]

Off-Ezy Corn & Callus Remover kit (liquid + cushion pads) OTC *topical keratolytic* [salicylic acid in a collodion-like vehicle] 17%

Off-Ezy Wart Remover liquid OTC *topical keratolytic* [salicylic acid in a collodion-like vehicle] 17%

O-Flex IV or IM injection (discontinued 1993) ℞ *skeletal muscle relaxant* [orphenadrine citrate]

ofloxacin USAN, INN, BAN, JAN *broad-spectrum quinolone-type bactericidal antibiotic; for corneal ulcers (orphan)*

ofornine USAN, INN *antihypertensive*

oftasceine INN

Ogen tablets ℞ *hormone replacement therapy for postmenopausal disorders* [estrogen (from estropipate)] 0.625 (0.75), 1.25 (1.5), 2.5 (3) mg

Ogen vaginal cream ℞ *topical estrogen replacement for postmenopausal disorders* [estropipate] 1.5 mg/g

oidiomycin *diagnostic aid for cell-mediated immunity; extract of the Oidiomycetes fungus family*

oil of mustard [see: allyl isothiocyanate]

Oil of Olay Foaming Face Wash liquid OTC *topical cleanser for acne*

oil ricini [see: castor oil]

Oilatum Soap bar OTC *therapeutic skin cleanser*

ointment, hydrophilic USP *ointment base; oil-in-water emulsion*

ointment, white USP *oleaginous ointment base*

ointment, yellow USP *ointment base*

OK-B7 *investigational monoclonal antibody used for the treatment of lymphoma*

olaflur USAN, INN, BAN *dental caries prophylactic*

olamine USAN, INN *combining name for radicals or groups*

olanzapine USAN *antipsychotic*

olaquindox INN, BAN

old tuberculin (OT) [see: tuberculin]

oleandomycin INN [also: oleandomycin phosphate]
oleandomycin, triacetate ester [see: troleandomycin]
oleandomycin phosphate NF [also: oleandomycin]
oleic acid NF *emulsion adjunct*
oleic acid I 125 USAN *radioactive agent*
oleic acid I 131 USAN *radioactive agent*
oleovitamin A [now: vitamin A]
oleovitamin A & D USP *source of vitamins A and D*
oleovitamin D, synthetic [now: ergocalciferol]
olethytan 20 [see: polysorbate 80]
oletimol INN
oleum caryophylii [see: clove oil]
oleum gossypii seminis [see: cottonseed oil]
oleum maydis [see: corn oil]
oleum ricini [see: castor oil]
oleyl alcohol NF *emulsifying agent; emollient*
oligomycin D [see: rutamycin]
olive oil NF *pharmaceutic aid*
olivomycin INN
olmidine INN
olopatadine INN *antiallergic; antiasthmatic*
olopatadine HCl USAN *antiallergic; antiasthmatic*
olpimedone INN
olsalazine INN, BAN *GI anti-inflammatory* [also: olsalazine sodium]
olsalazine sodium USAN *GI anti-inflammatory; treatment of ulcerative colitis* [also: olsalazine]
oltipraz INN
olvanil USAN, INN *analgesic*
OLX-102 *investigational adjuvant to chemotherapy in small-cell lung cancer*
OM 401 (*orphan: sickle cell disease*)
OMAD (**O**ncovin, **m**ethotrexate/ citrovorum factor, **A**driamycin, **d**actinomycin) *chemotherapy protocol*
Omega Oil (discontinued 1992) OTC *counterirritant; topical antiseptic* [methyl salicylate; methyl nicotinate; capsicum oleoresin; histamine dihydrochloride; alcohol]

omega-3 fatty acids [see: doconexent; icosapent; omega-3 marine triglycerides]
omega-3 marine triglycerides BAN [12% doconexent (q.v.) + 18% icosapent (q.v.)]
omeprazole USAN, INN, BAN, JAN *gastric acid antisecretory; proton pump inhibitor*
omeprazole sodium USAN *gastric antisecretory*
omidoline INN
Omnicef ℞ *investigational broad-spectrum cephalosporin antibiotic* [cefdinir]
Omniflox film-sealed tablets (discontinued 1992) ℞ *broad-spectrum fluoroquinolone-type antibiotic* [temafloxacin HCl]
OmniHIB powder for IM injection, prefilled syringes ℞ *Haemophilus influenzae type b (HIB) vaccine* [Hemophilus b conjugate vaccine; tetanus toxoid] 10•24 µg/0.5 mL
OMNIhist L.A. long-acting tablets ℞ *decongestant; antihistamine; anticholinergic* [phenylephrine HCl; chlorpheniramine maleate; methscopolamine nitrate] 20•8•2.5 mg
Omnipaque injection ℞ *parenteral radiopaque agent* [iohexol] 140, 180, 210, 240, 300, 350 mg/mL
Omnipen capsules ℞ *penicillin-type antibiotic* [ampicillin, anhydrous] 250, 500 mg ② Unipen
Omnipen powder for oral suspension ℞ *penicillin-type antibiotic* [ampicillin trihydrate] 125, 250 mg/5 mL
Omnipen-N powder for IV or IM injection ℞ *penicillin-type antibiotic* [ampicillin sodium] 0.125, 0.25, 0.5, 1, 2, 10 g
Omniscan IV injection ℞ *magnetic resonance imaging agent for the central nervous system* [gadodiamide] 287 mg/mL
omoconazole INN
omonasteine INN
OMS Concentrate drops ℞ *narcotic analgesic* [morphine sulfate] 20 mg/mL
onapristone INN *investigational antineoplastic for hormone-dependent cancers*
Oncaspar IV or IM injection ℞ *antineoplastic for acute lymphoblastic leu-*

kemia; and acute lymphocytic leukemia (orphan) [pegaspargase] 750 IU/mL

Oncet capsules ℞ *narcotic antitussive; analgesic* [hydrocodone bitartrate; acetaminophen] 5•500 mg

Oncoject ℞ *investigational antineoplastic*

Oncolym ℞ *investigational treatment for non-Hodgkin's B-cell lymphoma* [iodine I 131 Lym-1 monoclonal antibody]

Oncolysin B ℞ *investigational antineoplastic for B-cell lymphoma, leukemia, AIDS lymphoma, and myeloma* [CD19 anti-B4-blocked ricin monoclonal antibodies]

Oncolysin CD6 ℞ *investigational treatment for cutaneous T-cell lymphoma* [CD6-blocked ricin]

Oncolysin M ℞ *investigational treatment for myeloid leukemias* [anti-My9-blocked ricin]

Oncolysin S ℞ *investigational antineoplastic for small cell lung cancer* [N901-blocked ricin]

Onconase ℞ *investigational treatment for pancreatic, breast, colorectal, prostate, and small cell lung cancers* [p30 protein; tamoxifen]

OncoPurge ℞ *investigational antineoplastic for breast cancer* [Pseudomonas exotoxin monoclonal antibody]

OncoRad GI103 ℞ *investigational antineoplastic for gastrointestinal cancer* [CYT-103-Y-90 (code name—generic name not yet approved)]

OncoRad OV103 ℞ *investigational antineoplastic for colorectal cancer (orphan: ovarian cancer)* [CYT-103-Y-90 (code name—generic name not yet approved)]

OncoRad-Prostate ℞ *investigational antineoplastic for prostatic cancer* [CYT-356-Y-90 (code name—generic name not yet approved)]

OncoScint CR372 ℞ *investigational imaging aid for colorectal cancer detection and staging* [CYT-372-In-111 (code name—generic name not yet approved)]

OncoScint CR/OV ℞ *investigational imaging aid for colorectal cancer; imaging aid for ovarian cancer (orphan)* [satumomab pendetide]

OncoScint OV103 ℞ *(orphan: diagnostic aid in ovarian carcinoma)* [indium In 111 murine monoclonal antibody B72.3]

OncoScint PR356 ℞ *investigational imaging aid for prostatic cancer detection and staging* [CYT-356-In-111 (code name—generic name not yet approved)]

OncoScint-Breast ℞ *investigational imaging aid for breast cancer detection and staging* [TC-CYT-380 (code name—generic name not yet approved)]

OncoScint-NSC Lung ℞ *investigational imaging aid for non-small cell lung cancer detection and staging* [TC-CYT-380 fragment (code name—generic name not yet approved)]

OncoSpect ℞ *investigational imaging aid for colon cancer* [monoclonal antibodies]

Oncostate ℞ *(orphan: renal cell carcinoma)* [coumarin]

OncoTher 130 ℞ *investigational treatment for breast and ovarian cancer* [aminopterin sodium]

OncoTICE (foreign name for U.S. product Tice BCG)

OncoTrac ℞ *(orphan: diagnostic imaging agent for metastasis of malignant melanoma and small cell lung cancer)* [technetium Tc 99m antimelanoma murine monoclonal antibody]

Oncovin IV injection, Hyporets (prefilled syringes) ℞ *antineoplastic for lung and breast cancers, various leukemias, lymphomas, and sarcomas* [vincristine sulfate] 1 mg/mL ▣ Ancobon

Oncozole ℞ *investigational antineoplastic* [3-deazaguanine]

ondansetron INN, BAN *antiemetic for chemotherapy; antischizophrenic; anxiolytic; investigational Alzheimer's treatment* [also: ondansetron HCl]

ondansetron HCl USAN *antiemetic for chemotherapy; antischizophrenic; anxiolytic; investigational Alzheimer's treatment* [also: ondansetron]

Ondrox sustained-release tablets OTC *vitamin/mineral/calcium/iron supplement* [multiple vitamins, minerals and amino acids; calcium; iron; folic acid; biotin] ±•25•3•0.67•0.005 mg

1 + 1-F Creme ℞ *topical corticosteroid; antifungal; antibacterial; local anesthetic* [hydrocortisone; clioquinol; pramoxine] 1%•3%•1%

1% HC ointment ℞ *topical corticosteroid* [hydrocortisone] 1%

One Step Midstream Pregnancy Test stick for home use OTC *in vitro diagnostic aid for urine pregnancy test*

One Touch reagent strips for home use OTC *in vitro diagnostic aid for blood glucose*

1069C *investigational antineoplastic*

1370U *investigational antidepressant*

141W94 *investigational (Phase I) antiviral protease inhibitor for HIV*

142780 *investigational antiestrogen steroid for advanced breast cancer*

1592U89 *investigational (Phase I/II) antiviral for HIV*

One-A-Day 55 Plus tablets OTC *geriatric vitamin/mineral supplement* [multiple vitamins and minerals; folic acid; biotin] ±•400•30 µg

One-A-Day Essential tablets OTC *vitamin supplement* [multiple vitamins; folic acid] ±•0.4 mg

One-A-Day Extras Antioxidant softgel capsules OTC *vitamin/mineral supplement* [vitamins A, C, and E; multiple minerals] 5000 IU•250 mg•200 IU•±

One-A-Day Extras Vitamin C tablets OTC *vitamin supplement* [vitamin C] 500 mg

One-A-Day Extras Vitamin E soft gel capsules OTC *vitamin supplement* [vitamin E] 400 IU

One-A-Day Maximum Formula tablets OTC *vitamin/mineral/iron supplement* [multiple vitamins & minerals; iron; folic acid; biotin] ±•18 mg•0.4 mg•30 µg

One-A-Day Men's Vitamins tablets OTC *vitamin supplement* [multiple vitamins; folic acid] ±•0.4 mg

One-A-Day Plus Extra C tablets (discontinued 1994) OTC *vitamin supplement* [multiple vitamins; folic acid] ±•0.4 mg

One-A-Day Stressgard tablets (discontinued 1994) OTC *vitamin/mineral/iron supplement* [multiple vitamins & minerals; iron; folic acid] ±•18•0.4 mg

One-A-Day Within (name changed to One-A-Day Women's Formula in 1993)

One-A-Day Women's Formula tablets OTC *vitamin/calcium/iron supplement* [multiple vitamins; calcium; iron; folic acid] ±•450•27•0.4 mg

One-Tablet-Daily OTC *vitamin supplement* [multiple vitamins; folic acid] ±•0.4 mg

One-Tablet-Daily with Iron OTC *vitamin/iron supplement* [multiple vitamins; iron; folic acid] ±•18•0.4 mg

One-Tablet-Daily with Minerals OTC *vitamin/mineral/iron supplement* [multiple vitamins & minerals; iron; folic acid; biotin] ±•18 mg•0.4 mg•30 µg

ONO-1078 *investigational leukotriene antagonist for asthma*

ontazolast USAN *antiasthmatic; leukotriene biosynthesis inhibitor*

ontianil INN

Ontosein ℞ *investigational treatment for osteoarthritis* [orgotein]

Ony-Clear aerosol spray ℞ *topical antifungal* [miconazole nitrate] 2%

Ony-Clear Nail (name changed to Ony-Clear in 1996)

Onysin liquid OTC *vitamin supplement* [multiple vitamins]

OPA (Oncovin, prednisone, Adriamycin) *chemotherapy protocol*

OPAL (Oncovin, prednisone, L-asparaginase) *chemotherapy protocol*

OPC-14117 *investigational vitamin E-like antioxidant for cognitive impairment and HIV-related nerve damage*

Opcon eye drops (name changed to Muro's Opcon in 1993)

Opcon-A eye drops OTC *topical ocular decongestant and antihistamine* [naphazoline HCl; pheniramine maleate] 0.027%•0.315%

OPEN (Oncovin, prednisone, etoposide, Novantrone) *chemotherapy protocol*

Operand solution, prep pads, swab sticks, surgical scrub, perineal wash concentrate, aerosol, Iofoam skin cleanser, ointment OTC *broad-spectrum antimicrobial* [povidone-iodine] 1%; 1%; 1%; 7.5%; 1%; 0.5%; 1%; 1%

Operand Douche concentrate OTC *antiseptic/germicidal; vaginal cleanser and deodorizer* [povidone-iodine]

Ophtha P/S Ophthalmic eye drop suspension (discontinued 1992) ℞ *topical ophthalmic corticosteroidal anti-inflammatory; bacteriostatic* [prednisolone acetate; sulfacetamide sodium]

Ophthacet eye drops (discontinued 1993) ℞ *ophthalmic bacteriostatic* [sodium sulfacetamide]

Ophthaine eye drops ℞ *topical ophthalmic anesthetic* [proparacaine HCl] 0.5%

Ophthalgan eye drops ℞ *corneal edema-reducing and clearing agent* [glycerin]

Ophthetic eye drops ℞ *topical ophthalmic anesthetic* [proparacaine HCl] 0.5%

Ophthifluor IV injection ℞ *corneal disclosing agent* [fluorescein sodium] 10%

Ophthochlor eye drops (discontinued 1992) ℞ *ophthalmic antibiotic* [chloramphenicol] ⓘ Ophthocort

Ophthocort ophthalmic ointment (discontinued 1996) ℞ *ophthalmic topical corticosteroidal anti-inflammatory; antibiotic* [hydrocortisone acetate; chloramphenicol; polymyxin B sulfate] 0.5%•1%•10,000 U/g ⓘ Ophthochlor

opiniazide INN

opipramol INN *antidepressant; antipsychotic* [also: opipramol HCl]

opipramol HCl USAN *antidepressant; antipsychotic* [also: opipramol]

opium USP *narcotic analgesic* 10% oral

opium, powdered USP *narcotic analgesic*

OPOL ℞ *investigational oral polio vaccine*

OPP (Oncovin, procarbazine, prednisone) *chemotherapy protocol*

OPPA (Oncovin, prednisone, procarbazine, Adriamycin) *chemotherapy protocol*

Opticare PMS tablets OTC *vitamin/mineral supplement; digestive enzymes* [multiple vitamins & minerals; iron; folic acid; biotin; amylase; protease; lipase] ±•2.5 mg•0.033 mg•10.4 μg•2500 U•2500 U•200 U

Opti-Clean solution OTC *cleaning solution for hard, soft, or rigid gas permeable contact lenses*

Opti-Clean II solution OTC *cleaning solution for hard or soft contact lenses*

Opti-Clean II Especially for Sensitive Eyes solution OTC *cleaning solution for rigid gas permeable contact lenses*

Opticrom 4% eye drops (discontinued 1993) ℞ *ocular antiallergic; for vernal keratoconjunctivitis (orphan)* [cromolyn sodium]

Opticyl eye drops ℞ *cycloplegic; mydriatic* [tropicamide] 0.5%, 1%

Opti-Free solution OTC *chemical disinfecting solution for soft contact lenses* [note: one of four different products with the same name]

Opti-Free solution OTC *rewetting solution for soft contact lenses* [note: one of four different products with the same name]

Opti-Free solution OTC *surfactant cleaning solution for soft contact lenses* [note: one of four different products with the same name]

Opti-Free tablets OTC *enzymatic cleaner for soft contact lenses* [pork pancreatin; note: one of four different products with the same name]

Optigene ophthalmic solution OTC *extraocular irrigating solution* [sterile isotonic solution]

Optigene 3 eye drops OTC *topical ocular decongestant/vasoconstrictor* [tetrahydrozoline HCl] 0.05%

Optilets-500 Filmtabs (film-coated tablets) OTC *vitamin supplement* [multiple vitamins] ±

Optilets-M-500 Filmtabs (film-coated tablets) OTC *vitamin/mineral/iron supplement* [multiple vitamins & minerals; iron] ±•20 mg

Optimine tablets ℞ *antihistamine* [azatadine maleate] 1 mg

Optimmune ℞ *(orphan: keratoconjunctivitis sicca in Sjögren syndrome)* [cyclosporine]

Optimoist oral spray OTC *saliva substitute*

Optimox Prenatal tablets OTC *vitamin/mineral/calcium/iron supplement* [multiple vitamins & minerals; calcium; iron; folic acid] ± • 100 • 5 • 0.133 mg

Optimyd eye drops (discontinued 1995) ℞ *topical ophthalmic corticosteroidal anti-inflammatory; bacteriostatic* [prednisolone sodium phosphate; sulfacetamide sodium] 0.5% • 10%

Opti-One solution OTC *rewetting solution for soft contact lenses*

Opti-One Multi-Purpose solution OTC *chemical disinfecting solution for soft contact lenses*

OptiPranolol eye drops ℞ *topical antiglaucoma agent (β-blocker)* [metipranolol HCl] 0.3%

Opti-Pure aerosol solution (discontinued 1993) OTC *rinsing/storage solution for soft contact lenses*

Optiray 160; Optiray 240; Optiray 320; Optiray 350 injection ℞ *parenteral radiopaque agent* [ioversol (source of iodine)] 34% (16%); 51% (24%); 68% (32%); 74% (35%)

Optised eye drops (discontinued 1993) OTC *topical ocular decongestant; astringent; antiseptic* [phenylephrine HCl; zinc sulfate]

Opti-Soft Especially for Sensitive Eyes solution OTC *rinsing/storage solution for soft contact lenses* [preserved saline solution]

Opti-Tears solution OTC *rewetting solution for hard or soft contact lenses*

Optivite P.M.T. tablets OTC *geriatric vitamin/mineral supplement* [multiple vitamins & minerals; folic acid; biotin] ± • 30 • ? μg

Opti-Zyme Enzymatic Cleaner Especially for Sensitive Eyes tablets OTC *enzymatic cleaner for soft or rigid gas permeable contact lenses* [pork pancreatin]

OPV (oral poliovirus vaccine) [see: poliovirus vaccine, live oral]

ORA5 liquid OTC *oral anti-infective* [copper sulfate; iodine; potassium iodide] ? • ? • ?

Orabase gel OTC *mucous membrane anesthetic* [benzocaine] 15%

Orabase Baby gel OTC *topical oral anesthetic* [benzocaine] 7.5%

Orabase HCA oral paste ℞ *topical corticosteroid* [hydrocortisone acetate] 0.5%

Orabase Lip Healer cream OTC *topical oral anesthetic; antipruritic/counterirritant; vulnerary* [benzocaine; menthol; allantoin] 5% • 0.5% • 1.5%

Orabase-B oral paste OTC *topical oral anesthetic* [benzocaine] 20% ⓘ Orinase

Orabase-O orthodontic gel (discontinued 1994) OTC *topical oral anesthetic* [benzocaine] 20%

Orabase-Plain oral paste OTC *relief from minor oral irritations* [plasticized hydrocarbon gel]

Oracin lozenges (discontinued 1994) OTC *topical oral anesthetic; antipruritic/counterirritant* [benzocaine; menthol] 6.25 mg • 0.1% ⓘ orarsan; Orasone

Oracit solution ℞ *urinary alkalinizing agent* [sodium citrate; citric acid] 490 • 640 mg/5 mL

Oradex-C lozenges (discontinued 1995) OTC *topical anesthetic; counterirritant* [dyclonine HCl] 3 mg

Oradex-C troches (discontinued 1994) OTC *topical oral anesthetic; antiseptic* [benzocaine; cetylpyridinium chloride] 10 • 2.5 mg

Ora-Fresh mouthwash (discontinued 1994) OTC *oral antiseptic/antifungal* [methylparaben; zinc chloride]

Oragest SR sustained-release capsules (discontinued 1993) ℞ *decongestant; antihistamine* [phenylpropanolamine HCl; chlorpheniramine maleate]

Oragrafin Calcium granules for oral suspension ℞ *oral cholecystographic radiopaque agent* [ipodate calcium] 3 g/packet

Oragrafin Sodium capsules ℞ *oral cholecystographic radiopaque agent* [ipodate sodium] 500 mg

Orajel liquid OTC *topical oral anesthetic* [benzocaine; alcohol 44.2%] 20%

Orajel; Orajel Brace-aid; Orajel/d; Denture Orajel; Baby Orajel; Baby Orajel Nighttime Formula gel OTC *topical oral anesthetic* [benzocaine] 20%; 20%; 10%; 10%; 7.5%; 10%

Orajel Brace-aid rinse (discontinued 1993) OTC *topical oral anti-inflammatory/anti-infective for braces* [carbamide peroxide] 10%

Orajel Mouth-Aid liquid, gel OTC *mucous membrane anesthetic* [benzocaine] 20%

Orajel Perioseptic liquid OTC *topical oral anti-inflammatory/anti-infective for braces* [carbamide peroxide] 15%

Orajel Tooth & Gum Cleanser, Baby gel OTC *removes plaque-like film* [poloxamer 407; simethicone] 2%•0.12%

Oralet (trademarked dosage form) *oral lozenge/lollipop*

Oralone Dental paste ℞ *topical corticosteroid* [triamcinolone acetonide] 0.1%

Oramide tablets ℞ *antidiabetic* [tolbutamide]

Oraminic II subcu or IM injection ℞ *antihistamine; anaphylaxis* [brompheniramine maleate] 10 mg/mL

Oramorph SR sustained-release tablets ℞ *narcotic analgesic* [morphine sulfate] 15, 30, 60, 100 mg

orange flower oil NF *flavoring agent; perfume*

orange flower water NF
orange oil NF
orange peel tincture, sweet NF
orange spirit, compound NF
orange syrup NF

Oranyl tablets OTC *decongestant* [pseudoephedrine HCl]

Oranyl Plus tablets OTC *decongestant; analgesic; antipyretic* [pseudoephedrine HCl; acetaminophen]

Orap tablets ℞ *antipsychotic* [pimozide] 2 mg

Oraphen-PD elixir OTC *analgesic; antipyretic* [acetaminophen] 120 mg/5 mL

orarsan [see: acetarsone] ② Oracin; Orasone

OraScan ℞ *investigational diagnostic aid for oral cancers*

Orasept liquid OTC *oral astringent; antiseptic* [tannic acid; methylbenzethonium chloride; alcohol 53.31%] 12.16%•1.53%

Orasept throat spray OTC *topical oral anesthetic; antiseptic* [benzocaine; methylbenzethonium chloride] 0.996%•1.037%

Orasol liquid OTC *topical oral anesthetic; antipruritic/counterirritant; antiseptic* [benzocaine; phenol; alcohol 70%] 6.3%•0.5%

Orasone tablets ℞ *glucocorticoid; anti-inflammatory; immunosuppressant* [prednisone] 1, 5, 10, 20, 50 mg ② Oracin; orarsan

Ora-stetic liquid OTC *topical anesthetic; antiseptic; antipruritic* [phenol; phenolate sodium]

OraSure reagent kit for home use OTC *in vitro diagnostic aid for HIV antibodies*

OraSure HIV-1 reagent kit for professional use ℞ *in vitro diagnostic aid for HIV antibodies*

Oratect gel (discontinued 1995) OTC *topical oral anesthetic* [benzocaine; alcohol 65.8%] 15%

Oratrast powder for oral suspension ℞ *GI contrast medium* [barium sulfate]

orazamide INN

Orazinc capsules, tablets OTC *zinc supplement* [zinc sulfate] 220 mg; 110 mg

orbutopril INN

orciprenaline INN, BAN *bronchodilator* [also: metaproterenol polistirex]

orciprenaline polistirex [see: metaproterenol polistirex]

orconazole INN *antifungal* [also: orconazole nitrate]

orconazole nitrate USAN *antifungal* [also: orconazole]

Ordrine AT extended-release capsules ℞ *antitussive; decongestant* [caramiphen edisylate; phenylpropanolamine HCl] 40•75 mg

Ordrine S.R. sustained-release capsules ℞ *decongestant; antihistamine* [phenylpropanolamine HCl; chlorpheniramine maleate]

orestrate INN

orestrol [see: diethylstilbestrol dipropionate]

Oretic tablets ℞ *diuretic; antihypertensive* [hydrochlorothiazide] 25, 50 mg ② Oreton

Oreticyl 25; Oreticyl 50; Oreticyl Forte tablets (discontinued 1994) ℞ *antihypertensive* [hydrochlorothiazide; deserpidine] 25•0.125 mg; 50•0.125 mg; 25•0.25 mg

Oreton Methyl tablets, buccal tablets ℞ *androgen for male hypogonadism, impotence and breast cancer* [methyltestosterone] 10 mg ② Oretic

Orex oral solution (discontinued 1994) OTC *saliva substitute* ② Ornex

Orexin chewable tablets OTC *vitamin supplement* [vitamins B_1, B_6, and B_{12}] 8.1 mg•4.1 mg•25 µg

Org 32489 *investigational recombinant follicle-stimulating hormone for infertility*

Organidin tablets, elixir, drops (discontinued 1993; Organidin NR ["Newly Reformulated"] replaced it in 1994) ℞ *expectorant* [iodinated glycerol] 30 mg; 60 mg/5 mL; 50 mg/mL

Organidin NR tablets, oral liquid ℞ *expectorant* [guaifenesin] 200 mg; 100 mg/5 mL

Orgaran ℞ *investigational therapy for stroke and deep venous thrombosis* [danaproid]

orgotein USAN, INN, BAN *anti-inflammatory; antirheumatic (orphan: protection of organ donor tissue; familial ALS)*

Orimune oral suspension ℞ *poliomyelitis vaccine* [poliovirus vaccine, live oral trivalent] 0.5 mL

Orinase tablets ℞ *sulfonylurea-type antidiabetic* [tolbutamide] 500 mg ② Orabase; Ornade; Ornex; Tolinase

Orinase Diagnostic powder for IV injection ℞ *in vivo pancreas function test* [tolbutamide sodium] 1 g

Orlaam IV injection ℞ *narcotic agonist for management of opiate dependence (orphan)* [levomethadyl acetate HCl] 10 mg/mL

orlipastat [see: orlistat]

orlistat USAN, INN *pancreatic lipase inhibitor; investigational adjunct to weight loss*

ormaplatin USAN *antineoplastic*

Ormazine IV or IM injection ℞ *antipsychotic* [chlorpromazine HCl] 25 mg/mL

ormetroprim USAN, INN *antibacterial*

Ornade Spansules (sustained-release capsules) ℞ *decongestant; antihistamine* [phenylpropanolamine HCl; chlorpheniramine maleate] 75•12 mg ② Orinase; Ornex

Ornex caplets (name changed to Ornex No Drowsiness in 1995) ② Orex; Orinase; Ornade

Ornex No Drowsiness caplets OTC *decongestant; analgesic; antipyretic* [pseudoephedrine HCl; acetaminophen] 30•325 mg

Ornex Severe Cold No Drowsiness caplets (discontinued 1995) OTC *antitussive; decongestant; analgesic* [dextromethorphan hydrobromide; pseudoephedrine HCl; acetaminophen] 15•30•500 mg

ornidazole USAN, INN *anti-infective*

Ornidyl IV injection concentrate ℞ *antiprotozoal; (orphan: sleeping sickness; Pneumocystis carinii pneumonia)* [eflornithine HCl] 200 mg/mL

ornipressin INN

ornithine (L-ornithine) INN

ornithine vasopressin [see: ornipressin]

ornoprostil INN

orotic acid INN

orotirelin INN

orpanoxin USAN, INN *anti-inflammatory*

orphenadrine citrate [see: orphenadrine citrate]

orphenadrine INN, BAN *skeletal muscle relaxant; antihistamine* [also: orphenadrine citrate]

orphenadrine citrate USP *skeletal muscle relaxant; antihistamine* [also: orphenadrine] 100 mg oral; 30 mg/mL injection

Orphenate IV or IM injection (discontinued 1993) ℞ *skeletal muscle relaxant* [orphenadrine citrate]

Orphengesic; Orphengesic Forte tablets (discontinued 1996) ℞ *skeletal muscle relaxant; analgesic; CNS stimulant* [orphenadrine citrate; aspirin; caffeine] 25•385•30 mg; 50•770•60 mg

orpressin [see: ornipressin]

Ortega Otic M ear drops (discontinued 1992) ℞ *topical corticosteroidal anti-inflammatory; antibiotic* [hydrocortisone; neomycin sulfate; polymyxin B sulfate]

ortetamine INN

orthesin [see: benzocaine]

Ortho Dienestrol vaginal cream ℞ *estrogen replacement for postmenopausal disorders* [dienestrol] 0.01%

Ortho Drops eye drop suspension (discontinued 1993) ℞ *topical ophthalmic corticosteroidal anti-inflammatory; antibiotic* [hydrocortisone acetate; neomycin sulfate]

Ortho Tri-Cept ℞ *investigational triphasic oral contraceptive* [ethinyl estradiol; desogestrel]

Ortho Tri-Cyclen tablets ℞ *triphasic oral contraceptive* [norgestimate; ethinyl estradiol] Phase 1: 0.18 mg•35 µg; Phase 2: 0.215 mg•35 µg; Phase 3: 0.25 mg•35 µg

Ortho-Cept tablets ℞ *monophasic oral contraceptive* [desogestrel; ethinyl estradiol] 0.15 mg•30 µg

Orthoclone OKT3 IV injection ℞ *immunosuppressant for renal, cardiac, and hepatic transplants* [muromonab-CD3] 5 mg/5 mL ⑨ Ortho-Creme

Orthoclone OKT4A ℞ *investigational immunosuppressant for cardiac and hepatic transplantation* ⑨ Ortho-Creme

Ortho-Creme vaginal cream (discontinued 1994) OTC *spermicidal contraceptive* [nonoxynol 9] 2% ⑨ Orthoclone

orthocresol NF

Ortho-Cyclen tablets ℞ *monophasic oral contraceptive* [norgestimate; ethinyl estradiol] 0.25 mg•35 µg

Ortho-Est tablets ℞ *hormone replacement therapy for postmenopausal disorders* [estropipate] 0.75, 1.5 mg

Ortho-Est Plus ℞ *investigational hormone for menopause*

Ortho-Gynol vaginal gel OTC *spermicidal contraceptive (for use with a diaphragm)* [octoxynol 9] 1%

Ortholinum ℞ *(orphan: spasmodic torticollis)* [botulinum toxin]

Ortho-Novum 1/35 tablets ℞ *monophasic oral contraceptive* [norethindrone; ethinyl estradiol] 1 mg•35 µg

Ortho-Novum 1/50 tablets ℞ *monophasic oral contraceptive* [norethindrone; mestranol] 1 mg•50 µg

Ortho-Novum 7/7/7 tablets ℞ *triphasic oral contraceptive* [norethindrone; ethinyl estradiol] Phase 1: 0.5 mg•35 µg; Phase 2: 0.75 mg•35 µg; Phase 3: 1 mg•35 µg

Ortho-Novum 10/11 tablets ℞ *biphasic oral contraceptive* [norethindrone; ethinyl estradiol] Phase 1: 0.5 mg•35 µg; Phase 2: 1 mg•35 µg

orthotolidine

Orthovisc ℞ *investigational treatment for temporomandibular joint syndrome* [hyaluronic acid]

Orthoxicol Cough syrup OTC *antitussive; decongestant; antihistamine* [dextromethorphan hydrobromide; phenylpropanolamine HCl; chlorpheniramine maleate; alcohol 8%] 6.7•8.3•1.3 mg/5 mL

Orthozyme-CD5+ ℞ *investigational graft vs. host disease preventative* [zolimomab aritox]

Or-Toptic M eye drop suspension (discontinued 1992) ℞ *topical ophthalmic corticosteroidal anti-inflammatory; bacteriostatic* [prednisolone acetate; sulfacetamide sodium]

Or-Tyl IM injection (discontinued 1992) ℞ *gastrointestinal antispasmodic* [dicyclomine HCl] 10 mg/mL

Orudis capsules ℞ *nonsteroidal anti-inflammatory drug (NSAID); antiarthritic; analgesic* [ketoprofen] 25, 50, 75 mg

Orudis KT tablets OTC *nonsteroidal anti-inflammatory drug (NSAID); analgesic; antiarthritic* [ketoprofen] 12.5 mg

Orudis SR ℞ *investigational once-daily anti-inflammatory* [ketoprofen]

Oruvail sustained-release pellets in capsules ℞ *once-daily nonsteroidal anti-inflammatory drug (NSAID); antiarthritic; analgesic* [ketoprofen] 100, 150, 200 mg

osalmid INN
osarsal [see: acetarsone]
Os-Cal 250+D; Os-Cal 500+D film-coated tablets OTC *dietary supplement* [calcium carbonate; vitamin D] 250 mg•125 IU; 500 mg•125 IU
Os-Cal 500 tablets, chewable tablets OTC *calcium supplement* [calcium carbonate] 1.25 g
Os-Cal Fortified tablets OTC *vitamin/calcium/iron supplement* [multiple vitamins; calcium carbonate; iron] ≟•250•5 mg
Os-Cal Fortified Multivitamin & Minerals tablets OTC *vitamin/mineral/calcium/iron supplement* [multiple vitamins & minerals; calcium carbonate; iron] ≟•250•5 mg
Os-Cal Plus tablets (discontinued 1995) OTC *vitamin/calcium/iron supplement* [multiple vitamins; calcium carbonate; iron] ≟•250•16.6 mg
osmadizone INN
Osmitrol IV infusion ℞ *osmotic diuretic* [mannitol] 5%, 10%, 15%, 20%
osmium *element (Os)*
Osmoglyn solution ℞ *osmotic diuretic* [glycerin] 50%
Osmolite; Osmolite HN liquid OTC *enteral nutritional therapy* [lactose-free formula]
Osmovist injection ℞ *parenteral radiopaque agent* [iotrolan]
Ossirene ℞ *investigational bone marrow protectant for chemotherapy*
Osteocalcin subcu or IM injection ℞ *calcium regulator for hypercalcemia, Paget's disease, and postmenopausal osteoporosis* [calcitonin (salmon)] 200 IU/mL
Osteo-D ℞ *calcium regulator (orphan: familial hypophosphatemic rickets)* [secalciferol]
Osteomark ℞ *investigational enzyme-linked immunoassay for monitoring breakdown of bone mass* [monoclonal antibodies]
Osteo-Mins powder OTC *dietary supplement* [multiple minerals; vitamins C and D] ≟•500 mg•100 IU

Osteon-D tablets (discontinued 1992) OTC *calcium supplement* [calcium; vitamin D; phosphorus; magnesium]
Ostiderm lotion OTC *for hyperhidrosis and bromhidrosis* [aluminum sulfate; zinc oxide] 14.5•≟ mg/g
Ostiderm roll-on OTC *for hyperhidrosis and bromhidrosis* [aluminum chlorohydrate; camphor; alcohol] ≟•≟•≟
Osto-K chewable tablets (discontinued 1992) OTC *potassium supplement* [potassium gluconate; potassium chloride; potassium citrate; vitamin C]
ostreogrycin INN, BAN
osvarsan [see: acetarsone]
OT (old tuberculin) [see: tuberculin]
Otic Domeboro ear drops ℞ *antibacterial/antifungal* [acetic acid; aluminum acetate] 2%•≟
Otic Tridesilon ear drops (discontinued 1995) ℞ *topical corticosteroidal anti-inflammatory; antibacterial/antifungal* [desonide; acetic acid] 0.05%•2%
Otic-Care ear drops, otic suspension ℞ *topical corticosteroidal anti-inflammatory; antibiotic* [hydrocortisone; neomycin sulfate; polymyxin B sulfate] 1%•5 mg•10,000 U per mL
Otic-HC ear drops (discontinued 1992) ℞ *topical corticosteroid; antibacterial/antifungal; anesthetic* [hydrocortisone; pramoxine; chloroxylenol; acetic acid]
Otic-Plain ear drops (discontinued 1992) ℞ *anesthetic; antibacterial/antifungal; anesthetic* [pramoxine HCl; acetic acid; parachlorometaxylenol]
otilonium bromide INN, BAN
Oti-Med ear drops ℞ *topical corticosteroidal anti-inflammatory; antibacterial; topical local anesthetic* [hydrocortisone; chloroxylenol; pramoxine HCl] 10•1•10 mg/mL
otimerate sodium INN
OtiTricin otic suspension ℞ *topical corticosteroidal anti-inflammatory; antibiotic* [hydrocortisone; neomycin sulfate; polymyxin B sulfate] 1%•5 mg•10,000 U per mL

Oto Ear Drops (discontinued 1992) ℞ *topical local anesthetic; analgesic* [benzocaine; antipyrine; glycerin]

Otobiotic Otic ear drops ℞ *topical corticosteroidal anti-inflammatory; antibiotic* [hydrocortisone; polymyxin B sulfate] 0.5%•10,000 U per mL ⓓ Urobiotic

Otocain ear drops ℞ *topical local anesthetic* [benzocaine] 20%

Otocalm ear drops ℞ *topical local anesthetic; analgesic* [benzocaine; antipyrine] 1.4%•5.4%

Otocort ear drops, otic suspension ℞ *topical corticosteroidal anti-inflammatory; antibiotic* [hydrocortisone; neomycin sulfate; polymyxin B sulfate] 1%•5 mg•10,000 U per mL

Otomycet-HC ear drops ℞ *topical corticosteroidal anti-inflammatory; antibacterial/antifungal* [hydrocortisone; acetic acid] 1%•2%

Otomycin-HPN Otic ear drops ℞ *topical corticosteroidal anti-inflammatory; antibiotic* [hydrocortisone; neomycin sulfate; polymyxin B sulfate] 1%•5 mg•10,000 U per mL

Otosporin ear drops ℞ *topical corticosteroidal anti-inflammatory; antibiotic* [hydrocortisone; neomycin sulfate; polymyxin B sulfate] 1%•5 mg•10,000 U per mL

Otrivin nasal spray, nose drops, pediatric drops OTC *nasal decongestant* [xylometazoline HCl] 0.1%; 0.1%; 0.05% ⓓ Lotrimin

ouabain USP

Outgro solution OTC *pain relief for ingrown toenails* [tannic acid; chlorobutanol; isopropyl alcohol 83%] 25%•5%

O-V Statin package with both oral tablets & vaginal tablets (discontinued 1992) ℞ *antifungal* [nystatin]

ovandrotone albumin INN, BAN

Ovastat ℞ *(orphan: ovarian cancer)* [treosulfan]

Ovcon-35; Ovcon-50 tablets ℞ *monophasic oral contraceptive* [norethindrone; ethinyl estradiol] 1 mg•35 μg; 1 mg•50 μg

Ovide lotion ℞ *pediculicide* [malathion; isopropyl alcohol 78%] 0.5%

ovine corticotropin-releasing hormone [see: corticorelin ovine triflutate]

Ovoid (trademarked dosage form) *sugar-coated tablet*

Ovral tablets ℞ *monophasic oral contraceptive* [norgestrel; ethinyl estradiol] 0.5 mg•50 μg

Ovrette tablets ℞ *oral contraceptive (progestin only)* [norgestrel] 0.075 mg

OvuGen test kit OTC *in vitro diagnostic aid to predict ovulation time*

OvuKIT Self-Test kit for home use OTC *in vitro diagnostic aid to predict ovulation time*

OvuQuick Self-Test kit for home use OTC *in vitro diagnostic aid to predict ovulation time*

[^{15}O]**water** [see: water O 15]

ox bile extract [see: bile salts]

oxabolone cipionate INN

oxabrexine INN

oxaceprol INN

oxacillin INN *antibacterial* [also: oxacillin sodium]

oxacillin sodium USAN, USP *bactericidal antibiotic* [also: oxacillin] 250, 500 mg oral; 0.25, 0.5, 1, 2, 4, 10 g/vial injection

oxadimedine INN

oxadimedine HCl [see: oxadimedine]

oxaflozane INN

oxaflumazine INN

oxafuradene [see: nifuradene]

oxagrelate USAN, INN *platelet antiaggregatory agent*

oxalinast INN

oxaliplatin INN *(orphan: ovarian cancer)*

oxamarin INN *hemostatic* [also: oxamarin HCl]

oxamarin HCl USAN *hemostatic* [also: oxamarin]

oxametacin INN

oxamisole INN *immunoregulator* [also: oxamisole HCl]

oxamisole HCl USAN *immunoregulator* [also: oxamisole]

oxamniquine USAN, USP, INN *antischistosomal; anthelmintic*

oxamphetamine hydrobromide [see: hydroxyamphetamine hydrobromide]
oxamycin [see: cycloserine]
oxanamide INN
Oxandrin tablets ℞ *anabolic steroid for weight gain; (orphan: Turner syndrome; growth and puberty delay; AIDS)* [oxandrolone] 2.5 mg
oxandrolone USAN, USP, INN, BAN, JAN *androgen; anabolic steroid (orphan: Turner syndrome; growth and puberty delay; AIDS; hepatitis)*
oxantel INN *anthelmintic* [also: oxantel pamoate]
oxantel pamoate USAN *anthelmintic* [also: oxantel]
oxantrazole HCl [see: piroxantrone HCl]
oxapadol INN
oxapium iodide INN
oxaprazine
oxapropanium iodide INN
oxaprotiline INN *antidepressant* [also: oxaprotiline HCl]
oxaprotiline HCl USAN *antidepressant* [also: oxaprotiline]
oxaprozin USAN, INN, BAN *nonsteroidal anti-inflammatory drug (NSAID)*
oxarbazole USAN, INN *antiasthmatic*
oxarutine [see: ethoxazorutoside]
oxatomide USAN, INN *antiallergic; antiasthmatic*
oxazafone INN
oxazepam USAN, USP, INN *anxiolytic; minor tranquilizer; alcohol withdrawal therapy* 10, 15, 30 mg oral
oxazidione INN
oxazolam INN
oxazolidin [see: oxyphenbutazone]
oxazorone INN
oxcarbazepine INN *antiepileptic*
oxdralazine INN
oxeladin INN, BAN
oxendolone USAN, INN *antiandrogen for benign prostatic hypertrophy*
oxepinac INN
oxerutins BAN
oxetacaine INN *topical anesthetic* [also: oxethazaine]
oxetacillin INN
2-oxetanone [see: propiolactone]

oxethazaine USAN, BAN *topical anesthetic* [also: oxetacaine]
oxetorone INN *migraine-specific analgesic* [also: oxetorone fumarate]
oxetorone fumarate USAN *migraine-specific analgesic* [also: oxetorone]
oxfenamide [see: oxiramide]
oxfendazole USAN, INN *anthelmintic*
oxfenicine USAN, INN, BAN *vasodilator*
oxibendazole USAN, INN *anthelmintic*
oxibetaine INN
oxibuprocaine chloride [see: benoxinate HCl]
oxichlorochine sulfate [see: hydroxychloroquine sulfate]
oxicinchophen [see: oxycinchophen]
oxiconazole INN, BAN *antifungal* [also: oxiconazole nitrate]
oxiconazole nitrate USAN *antifungal* [also: oxiconazole]
oxicone [see: oxycodone]
oxidized cellulose [see: cellulose, oxidized]
oxidized cholic acid [see: dehydrocholic acid]
oxidized regenerated cellulose [see: cellulose, oxidized regenerated]
oxidopamine USAN, INN *ophthalmic adrenergic*
oxidronic acid USAN, INN, BAN *calcium regulator*
oxifenamate [see: hydroxyphenamate]
oxifentorex INN
Oxi-Freeda tablets OTC *dietary supplement* [multiple vitamins, minerals, and amino acids] ≛
oxifungin INN *antifungal* [also: oxifungin HCl]
oxifungin HCl USAN *antifungal* [also: oxifungin]
oxilorphan USAN, INN *narcotic antagonist*
oximetazoline HCl [see: oxymetazoline HCl]
oximetholone [see: oxymetholone]
oximonam USAN, INN *antibacterial*
oximonam sodium USAN *antibacterial*
oxindanac INN
oxiniacic acid INN
oxiperomide USAN, INN *antipsychotic*
oxipertine [see: oxypertine]
oxipethidine [see: hydroxypethidine]

oxiphenbutazone [see: oxyphenbutazone]

oxiphencyclimine chloride [see: oxyphencyclimine HCl]

Oxipor VHC lotion OTC *topical antipsoriatic; antiseborrheic; keratolytic* [coal tar solution; alcohol 79%] 25%

oxiprocaine [see: hydroxyprocaine]

oxiprogesterone caproate [see: hydroxyprogesterone caproate]

oxipurinol INN *xanthine oxidase inhibitor* [also: oxypurinol]

oxiracetam INN, BAN *investigational treatment for Alzheimer's disease*

oxiramide USAN, INN *antiarrhythmic*

oxisopred INN

Oxistat cream, lotion ℞ *topical antifungal* [oxiconazole nitrate] 1%

oxistilbamidine isethionate [see: hydroxystilbamidine isethionate]

oxisuran USAN, INN *antineoplastic*

oxitefonium bromide INN

oxitetracaine [see: hydroxytetracaine]

oxitetracycline [see: oxytetracycline]

oxitriptan INN

oxitriptyline INN

oxitropium bromide INN, BAN

oxmetidine INN, BAN *antagonist to histamine H_2 receptors* [also: oxmetidine HCl]

oxmetidine HCl USAN *antagonist to histamine H_2 receptors* [also: oxmetidine]

oxmetidine mesylate USAN *antagonist to histamine H_2 receptors*

oxodipine INN

oxogestone INN *progestin* [also: oxogestone phenpropionate]

oxogestone phenpropionate USAN *progestin* [also: oxogestone]

oxoglurate INN *combining name for radicals or groups*

oxolamine INN

oxolinic acid USAN, INN *antibacterial*

oxomemazine INN

oxonazine INN

4-oxopentanoic acid, calcium salt [see: calcium levulinate]

oxophenarsine INN [also: oxophenarsine HCl]

oxophenarsine HCl USP [also: oxophenarsine]

5-oxoproline [see: pidolic acid]

oxoprostol INN, BAN

oxothiazolidine carboxylate (L-2-oxothiazolidine-4-carboxylic acid) *investigational (Phase II) immunomodulator for AIDS (orphan: adult respiratory distress syndrome)*

oxozepam [see: oxazepam]

oxpentifylline BAN *vasodilator; hemorheologic agent* [also: pentoxifylline]

oxpheneridine INN

oxprenoate potassium INN

oxprenolol INN *coronary vasodilator* [also: oxprenolol HCl]

oxprenolol HCl USAN, USP *coronary vasodilator* [also: oxprenolol]

Oxsoralen capsules (discontinued 1993) ℞ *antipsoriatic* [methoxsalen] 10 mg

Oxsoralen lotion ℞ *repigmenting adjunct with ultraviolet A for vitiligo; investigational treatment for scleroderma* [methoxsalen] 1%

Oxsoralen-Ultra capsules ℞ *antipsoriatic* [methoxsalen] 10 mg

oxtriphylline USP *bronchodilator* [also: choline theophyllinate] 100, 200 mg oral; 50, 100 mg/5 mL oral

Oxy 5 lotion (discontinued 1994) OTC *topical keratolytic for acne* [benzoyl peroxide] 5%

Oxy 5 Advanced Formula for Sensitive Skin gel (name changed to Advanced Formula Oxy 5 for Sensitive Skin in 1995)

Oxy 5 for Sensitive Skin, Advanced Formula; Oxy for Sensitive Skin, Advanced Formula gel OTC *topical keratolytic for acne* [benzoyl peroxide] 5%; 2.5%

Oxy 5 Tinted lotion OTC *topical keratolytic for acne* [benzoyl peroxide] 5%

Oxy 10 lotion, cover cream (discontinued 1994) OTC *topical keratolytic for acne* [benzoyl peroxide] 10%

Oxy 10 Advanced Formula gel OTC *topical keratolytic for acne* [benzoyl peroxide] 10%

Oxy 10 Wash liquid OTC *topical keratolytic for acne* [benzoyl peroxide] 10%

Oxy Clean Lathering Facial scrub (discontinued 1994) OTC *abrasive cleanser for acne* [sodium tetraborate decahydrate dissolving particles]

Oxy Clean Soap bar (discontinued 1994) OTC *medicated cleanser for acne* [salicylic acid] 3.5%

Oxy Medicated Cleanser & Pads OTC *topical keratolytic cleanser for acne* [salicylic acid; alcohol] 0.5%•22%, 0.5%•40%, 2%•50%

Oxy Medicated Soap bar OTC *medicated cleanser for acne* [triclosan] 1%

Oxy Night Watch; Oxy Night Watch for Sensitive Skin lotion OTC *topical keratolytic for acne* [salicylic acid] 2%; 1%

Oxy ResiDon't Medicated Face Wash liquid OTC *topical cleanser for acne* [triclosan] 0.6%

oxybenzone USAN, USP, INN *ultraviolet screen*

oxybuprocaine INN, BAN *topical anesthetic* [also: benoxinate HCl; oxybuprocaine HCl]

oxybuprocaine HCl JAN *topical anesthetic* [also: benoxinate HCl; oxybuprocaine]

oxybutynin INN, BAN *anticholinergic; urinary antispasmodic* [also: oxybutynin chloride]

oxybutynin chloride USAN, USP *anticholinergic; urinary antispasmodic* [also: oxybutynin] 5 mg oral; 1 mg/mL oral

Oxycel pads, pledgets, strips ℞ *topical local hemostat for surgery* [oxidized cellulose]

oxychlorosene USAN *topical anti-infective*

oxychlorosene sodium USAN *topical anti-infective*

oxycinchophen INN, BAN

oxyclipine INN *anticholinergic* [also: propenzolate HCl]

oxyclipine HCl [see: propenzolate HCl]

oxyclozanide INN, BAN

oxycodone USAN, INN, BAN *narcotic analgesic*

oxycodone HCl USAN, USP *narcotic analgesic*

oxycodone terephthalate USP *narcotic analgesic*

OxyContin controlled-release tablets ℞ *narcotic analgesic* [oxycodone HCl] 10, 20, 40 mg

Oxydess II tablets ℞ *CNS stimulant; amphetamine* [dextroamphetamine sulfate] 10 mg

oxydimethylquinazine [see: antipyrine]

oxydipentonium chloride INN

oxyethyltheophylline [see: etofylline]

oxyfedrine INN, BAN

oxyfenamate INN *minor tranquilizer* [also: hydroxyphenamate]

oxyfilcon A USAN *hydrophilic contact lens material*

oxygen (O_2) USP *medicinal gas; element (O)*

oxygen, polymeric (orphan: sickle cell anemia)

oxygen 93 percent USP *medicinal gas*

Oxygent ℞ *investigational blood substitute* [perflubron]

OxyIR capsules ℞ *narcotic analgesic* [oxycodone HCl] 5 mg

oxymesterone INN, BAN

Oxymeta 12 nasal spray OTC *decongestant* [oxymetazoline HCl]

oxymetazoline INN, BAN *topical ocular vasoconstrictor; nasal decongestant* [also: oxymetazoline HCl] ⊘ oxymetholone

oxymetazoline HCl USAN, USP *topical ocular vasoconstrictor; nasal decongestant* [also: oxymetazoline] 0.05% nose drops or spray

oxymetholone USAN, USP, INN, BAN *androgen; anabolic steroid* ⊘ oxymetazoline; oxymorphone

oxymethylene urea [see: polynoxylin]

oxymorphone INN, BAN *narcotic analgesic* [also: oxymorphone HCl] ⊘ oxymetholone

oxymorphone HCl USP *narcotic analgesic; (orphan: intractable narcotic-tolerant pain)* [also: oxymorphone]

oxypendyl INN

oxypertine USAN, INN *antidepressant*

oxyphenbutazone USP, INN *anti-inflammatory; antirheumatic; antipyretic; analgesic*

oxyphencyclimine INN *anticholinergic* [also: oxyphencyclimine HCl]

oxyphencyclimine HCl USP *peptic ulcer adjunct* [also: oxyphencyclimine]

oxyphenhydrazine [see: carsalam]

oxyphenisatin BAN *laxative* [also: oxyphenisatin acetate; oxyphenisatine]

oxyphenisatin acetate USAN *laxative* [also: oxyphenisatine; oxyphenisatin]

oxyphenisatine INN *laxative* [also: oxyphenisatin acetate; oxyphenisatin]

oxyphenonium bromide

oxyphylline [see: etofylline]

oxypurinol USAN *xanthine oxidase inhibitor* [also: oxipurinol]

oxypyrronium bromide INN

oxyquinoline USAN *disinfectant/antiseptic*

oxyquinoline benzoate [see: benzoxiquine]

oxyquinoline sulfate USAN, NF *complexing agent*

oxyridazine INN

Oxysept solution + tablets OTC *two-step chemical disinfecting system for soft contact lenses* [hydrogen peroxide-based] 3%

Oxysept 2 solution OTC *rinsing/storage solution for soft contact lenses* [preservative-free saline solution]

oxysonium iodide INN

oxytetracycline USP, INN *bacteriostatic antibiotic; antirickettsial*

oxytetracycline calcium USP *antibacterial*

oxytetracycline HCl USP *bacteriostatic antibiotic; antirickettsial* 250 mg oral

oxytocin USP, INN *oxytocic; posterior pituitary hormone* 10 U/mL injection

Oxyzal Wet Dressing liquid OTC *antiseptic dressing for minor infections* [oxyquinoline sulfate; benzalkonium chloride]

Oysco 500 chewable tablets OTC *calcium supplement* [calcium carbonate] 1.25 g

Oysco D tablets (discontinued 1993) OTC *dietary supplement* [calcium carbonate; vitamin D] 250 mg•125 IU

Oyst-Cal 500 film-coated tablets OTC *calcium supplement* [calcium carbonate] 1.25 g

Oyst-Cal-D film-coated tablets OTC *dietary supplement* [calcium carbonate; vitamin D] 250 mg•125 IU

Oyster Calcium tablets OTC *dietary supplement* [calcium carbonate; vitamins A and D] 375 mg•800 IU•200 IU

Oyster Calcium 500 + D tablets OTC *dietary supplement* [calcium carbonate; vitamin D] 500 mg•125 IU

Oyster Calcium with Vitamin D tablets OTC *dietary supplement* [calcium carbonate; vitamin D] 250 mg•125 IU

Oyster Shell Calcium with Vitamin D tablets OTC *calcium supplement* [calcium carbonate; vitamin D] 250 mg•125 IU

Oyster Shell Calcium-500 tablets OTC *calcium supplement* [calcium carbonate] 1.25 g

Oystercal 500 tablets OTC *calcium supplement* [calcium carbonate] 1.25 g

Oystercal-D 250 tablets OTC *dietary supplement* [calcium carbonate; vitamin D] 250 mg•125 IU

ozagrel INN *investigational antiasthmatic*

ozolinone USAN, INN *diuretic*

P & S liquid OTC *antimicrobial hair dressing* [phenol]

P & S shampoo OTC *antiseborrheic; keratolytic* [salicylic acid] 2%

P & S Plus gel OTC *topical antipsoriatic; antiseborrheic; keratolytic* [coal tar solution; salicylic acid] 8%•2%

P_1E_1; P_2E_1; P_3E_1; P_4E_1; P_6E_1 Drop-Tainers (eye drops) ℞ *antiglaucoma agent* [pilocarpine HCl; epinephrine bitartrate] 1%•1%; 2%•1%; 3%•1%; 4%•1%; 6%•1%

p30 protein *investigational adjunct to chemotherapy*

^{32}P [see: chromic phosphate P 32]

^{32}P [see: polymetaphosphate P 32]

^{32}P [see: sodium phosphate P 32]

PAB (para-aminobenzoate) [see: aminobenzoic acid]

PABA (para-aminobenzoic acid) [now: aminobenzoic acid]

PABA sodium [see: aminobenzoate sodium]

Pabalate enteric-coated tablets OTC *analgesic; antipyretic; anti-inflammatory* [sodium salicylate; aminobenzoate sodium] 300•300 mg

Pabalate-SF enteric-coated tablets (discontinued 1995) ℞ *analgesic; antipyretic; anti-inflammatory* [potassium salicylate; potassium aminobenzoate] 300•300 mg

PAB-Esc-C (Platinol, Adriamycin, bleomycin, escalating doses of cyclophosphamide) *chemotherapy protocol*

pabestrol D [see: diethylstilbestrol dipropionate]

P-A-C tablets (discontinued 1995) OTC *analgesic; antipyretic; anti-inflammatory* [aspirin; caffeine] 400•32 mg

PAC; PAC-I (Platinol, Adriamycin, cyclophosphamide) *chemotherapy protocol*

PACE (Platinol, Adriamycin, cyclophosphamide, etoposide) *chemotherapy protocol*

PACIS injection (available only in Canada) ℞ *immunizing agent* [BCG vaccine, Montreal strain] 2–10×10^6 CFU (colony-forming units)

Packer's Pine Tar shampoo, soap OTC *antiseborrheic; antipsoriatic; antipruritic; antibacterial* [pine tar]

paclitaxel USAN, INN, BAN *antineoplastic*

pacrinolol INN

padimate INN *ultraviolet screen* [also: padimate A]

padimate A USAN *ultraviolet screen* [also: padimate]

padimate O USAN *ultraviolet screen*

pafenolol INN

pagoclone USAN *anxiolytic*

PAH (para-aminohippurate) [see: aminohippuric acid]

PAHA (para-aminohippuric acid) [see: aminohippuric acid]

Pain Bust-R II cream OTC *topical local anesthetic; counterirritant* [methyl salicylate; menthol] 17%•12%

Pain Doctor cream OTC *topical analgesic; topical anesthetic; antipruritic* [capsaicin; methyl salicylate; menthol] 0.025%•25%•10%

Pain Gel Plus OTC *counterirritant* [menthol] 4%

Pain Reliever tablets OTC *analgesic; antipyretic; anti-inflammatory* [acetaminophen; aspirin; caffeine] 250•250•65 mg

PALA disodium [see: sparfosate sodium]

palatrigine INN, BAN

paldimycin USAN, INN *antibacterial*

paldimycin A [see: paldimycin]

paldimycin B [see: paldimycin]

palestrol [see: diethylstilbestrol]

palinavir USAN *antiviral; HIV-1 protease inhibitor*

palinum [see: cyclobarbitone]

palladium *element (Pd)*

palmidrol INN

Palmitate-A 5000 tablets OTC *vitamin supplement* [vitamin A] 5000 IU

palmoxirate sodium USAN *antidiabetic* [also: palmoxiric acid]

palmoxiric acid INN *antidiabetic* [also: palmoxirate sodium]

PALS coated tablets OTC *systemic deodorant for ostomy, breath, and body odors* [chlorophyllin copper complex] 100 mg

PAM; L-PAM (phenylalanine mustard) [see: melphalan]

2-PAM (2-pyridine aldoxime methylchloride) [see: pralidoxime chloride]

pamabrom USAN *nonprescription diuretic*

pamaquine naphthoate NF

pamatolol INN *antiadrenergic (β-receptor)* [also: pamatolol sulfate]

pamatolol sulfate USAN *antiadrenergic (β-receptor)* [also: pamatolol]

Pamelor capsules, oral solution ℞ *tricyclic antidepressant* [nortriptyline HCl] 10, 25, 50, 75 mg; 10 mg/5 mL ⓓ Dymelor

pamidronate disodium USAN *bone resorption suppressant*

pamidronic acid INN, BAN

Pamine tablets ℞ *anticholinergic; peptic ulcer treatment* [methscopolamine bromide] 2.5 mg

Pamisyl ℞ *(orphan: ulcerative colitis)* [aminosalicylic acid]

pamoate USAN, USP *combining name for radicals or groups* [also: embonate]

Pamprin caplets (name changed to Multi-Symptom Pamprin in 1994)

Pamprin, Multi-Symptom caplets, tablets OTC *analgesic; antipyretic; diuretic; antihistaminic sleep aid* [acetaminophen; pamabrom; pyrilamine maleate] 500•25•15 mg

Pamprin, Nighttime powder OTC *antihistaminic sleep aid; analgesic* [diphenhydramine HCl; acetaminophen] 50•650 mg

Pamprin Maximum Cramp Relief caplets (name changed to Multi-Symptom Pamprin in 1994)

Pamprin Maximum Cramp Relief capsules (discontinued 1992) OTC *analgesic; antipyretic; diuretic; antihistaminic sleep aid* [acetaminophen; pamabrom; pyrilamine maleate]

Pamprin Maximum Pain Relief caplets OTC *analgesic; antipyretic; diuretic* [acetaminophen; magnesium salicylate; pamabrom] 250•250•25 mg

Pamprin-IB coated tablets (discontinued 1993) OTC *nonsteroidal anti-inflammatory drug (NSAID); antiarthritic; analgesic* [ibuprofen] 200 mg

Pan C-500 tablets OTC *dietary supplement* [vitamin C; citrus bioflavonoids & hesperidin] 1000•250 mg

Panacet 5/500 tablets ℞ *narcotic analgesic* [hydrocodone bitartrate; acetaminophen] 5•500 mg

panadiplon USAN, INN *anxiolytic*

Panadol tablets, caplets OTC *analgesic; antipyretic* [acetaminophen] 500 mg

Panadol, Children's chewable tablets, liquid OTC *analgesic; antipyretic* [acetaminophen] 80 mg; 160 mg/5 mL

Panadol, Infants' drops OTC *analgesic; antipyretic* [acetaminophen] 100 mg/mL

Panadol, Junior caplets OTC *analgesic; antipyretic* [acetaminophen] 160 mg

Panadyl sustained-release tablets (discontinued 1992) ℞ *decongestant; antihistamine* [phenylpropanolamine HCl; pyrilamine maleate; pheniramine maleate]

Panadyl Forte sustained-release tablets (discontinued 1993) ℞ *decongestant; antihistamine* [phenylpropanolamine HCl; phenylephrine HCl; chlorpheniramine maleate]

Panafil ointment ℞ *topical enzyme for wound debridement; vulnerary; wound deodorant* [papain; urea; chlorophyllin copper complex] 10%•10%•0.5%

Panafil White ointment ℞ *topical enzyme for wound debridement; vulnerary* [papain; urea] 10%•10%

Panalgesic cream OTC *counterirritant* [methyl salicylate; menthol] 35%•4%

Panalgesic Gold liniment OTC *counterirritant; topical antiseptic* [methyl salicylate; camphor; menthol; alcohol 22%] 55%•3.1%•1.25%

Panasal 5/500 tablets ℞ *narcotic analgesic* [hydrocodone bitartrate; aspirin] 5•500 mg

Panasol-S tablets ℞ *glucocorticoid; anti-inflammatory; immunosuppressant* [prednisone] 1 mg ② Panscol

pancopride USAN, INN *antiemetic; anxiolytic; peristaltic stimulant*

Pancrease; Pancrease MT 4; Pancrease MT 10; Pancrease MT 16; Pancrease MT 20 capsules containing enteric-coated microtablets ℞ *digestive enzymes* [lipase; protease; amylase] 4.5•25•20; 4.5•12•12; 10•30•30; 16•48•48; 20•44•56 thousand USP units

Pancrease MT 25; Pancrease MT 32 capsules containing enteric-coated microtablets (discontinued 1994) ℞ *digestive enzymes* [lipase; protease; amylase] 25,000•70,000•55,000 U; 32,000•90,000•70,000 U

pancreatin USP *digestive enzyme*

Pancreatin, 4X; Pancreatin, 8X tablets OTC *digestive enzymes* [pancreatin; lipase; protease; amylase] 2400 mg•12,000 U•60,000 U•60,000 U;

7200 mg•22,500 U•180,000 U•180,000 U

pancrelipase USAN, USP *digestive enzyme*

Pancrezyme 4X tablets OTC *digestive enzymes* [pancreatin; lipase; protease; amylase] 2400 mg•12,000 U•60,000 U•60,000 U

pancuronium bromide USAN, INN *nondepolarizing neuromuscular blocker; muscle relaxant; adjunct to anesthesia* 1, 2 mg/mL injection

Panex; Panex 500 tablets OTC *analgesic; antipyretic* [acetaminophen] 325 mg; 500 mg

Panhematin powder for IV injection ℞ *enzyme inhibitor; for acute intermittent porphyria and hereditary coproporphyria (orphan)* [hemin] 7 mg/mL

panidazole INN, BAN

Panmycin capsules ℞ *broad-spectrum antibiotic* [tetracycline HCl] 250 mg

panomifene INN

Panorex ℞ *investigational antineoplastic for colorectal cancer; (orphan: pancreatic cancer)* [monoclonal antibody 17-1A] ⓓ Panarex

Panoxyl cleansing bar ℞ *topical keratolytic for acne* [benzoyl peroxide] 5%, 10% ⓓ Benoxyl

Panoxyl AQ 2½; Panoxyl 5; Panoxyl AQ 5; Panoxyl 10; Panoxyl AQ 10 gel ℞ *topical keratolytic for acne* [benzoyl peroxide] 2.5%; 5%; 5%; 10%; 10%

Panscol lotion, ointment OTC *topical keratolytic* [salicylic acid] 3% ⓓ Panasol

pantenicate INN

panthenol USAN, USP, INN *B complex vitamin*

D-panthenol [see: dexpanthenol]

Panthoderm cream OTC *antipruritic; vulnerary; emollient* [dexpanthenol] 2%

Pantopon injection (discontinued 1993) ℞ *narcotic analgesic; sedative; hypnotic* [opium alkaloids HCl] 20 mg/mL ⓓ Parafon

pantoprazole USAN, INN, BAN *antiulcerative*

pantothenic acid BAN *vitamin B_5; enzyme cofactor* [also: calcium pantothenate]

DL-pantothenic acid [see: calcium pantothenate, racemic]

pantothenol [see: dexpanthenol]

pantothenyl alcohol [see: panthenol]

D-pantothenyl alcohol [see: dexpanthenol]

panuramine INN, BAN

Panwarfin tablets (discontinued 1993) ℞ *anticoagulant* [warfarin sodium] 2, 2.5, 5, 7.5, 10 mg

Papadeine #3 tablets ℞ *narcotic analgesic* [codeine phosphate; acetaminophen]

papain USP *topical proteolytic enzyme for necrotic tissue debridement*

papaverine BAN *smooth muscle relaxant; peripheral vasodilator; (orphan: sexual dysfunction in spinal cord injuries)* [also: papaverine HCl]

papaverine HCl USP *smooth muscle relaxant; peripheral vasodilator* [also: papaverine] 30, 60, 100, 150, 200, 300 mg oral; 30 mg/mL injection

papaveroline INN, BAN

Papaya Enzyme chewable tablets OTC *digestive enzymes* [papain; amylase] 60•60 mg

Paplex solution (discontinued 1994) ℞ *topical keratolytic* [salicylic acid in flexible collodion; lactic acid] 17%•17%

Paplex Ultra solution ℞ *topical keratolytic* [salicylic acid in flexible collodion] 26%

Par Decon sustained-action tablets (discontinued 1993) ℞ *decongestant; antihistamine* [phenylpropanolamine HCl; phenylephrine HCl; phenyltoloxamine citrate; chlorpheniramine maleate]

Par Glycerol elixir ℞ *expectorant* [iodinated glycerol] 60 mg/5 mL

Par Glycerol C liquid (discontinued 1993) ℞ *narcotic antitussive; expectorant* [codeine phosphate; iodinated glycerol]

Par Glycerol DM liquid (discontinued 1993) ℞ *expectorant; antitussive* [iodinated glycerol; dextromethorphan hydrobromide]

para-aminobenzoate (PAB) [see: aminobenzoic acid]

Para-Aminobenzoic Acid tablets, powder OTC *"possibly effective" for scleroderma and other skin diseases, and Peyronie's disease* [aminobenzoic acid] 100, 500 mg; 120 g

para-aminobenzoic acid (PABA) [now: aminobenzoic acid]

para-aminohippurate (PAH) [see: aminohippuric acid]

para-aminohippurate sodium [see: aminohippurate sodium]

para-aminohippuric acid (PAHA) [see: aminohippuric acid]

para-aminosalicylate (PAS) [see: aminosalicylic acid]

para-aminosalicylic acid (PASA) [see: aminosalicylic acid]

parabromdylamine maleate [see: brompheniramine maleate]

paracetaldehyde [see: paraldehyde]

paracetamol INN, BAN *analgesic; antipyretic* [also: acetaminophen]

parachlorometaxylenol (PCMX) *topical antiseptic; broad-spectrum antibacterial*

parachlorophenol (PCP) USP *topical antibacterial*

parachlorophenol, camphorated USP *topical dental anti-infective*

paracodin [see: dihydrocodeine]

Paradione capsules, oral solution (discontinued 1994) ℞ *anticonvulsant* [paramethadione] 150, 300 mg

paraffin NF *stiffening agent*

paraffin, liquid [see: mineral oil]

paraffin, synthetic NF *stiffening agent*

Paraflex caplets ℞ *skeletal muscle relaxant* [chlorzoxazone] 250 mg

paraflutizide INN

Parafon Forte DSC caplets ℞ *skeletal muscle relaxant* [chlorzoxazone] 500 mg ② Pantopon

paraformaldehyde USP

ParaGard IUD ℞ *contraceptive* [copper]

Para-Hist AT syrup (discontinued 1994) ℞ *narcotic antitussive; decongestant; antihistamine* [codeine phosphate; phenylephrine HCl; promethazine HCl; alcohol] 10•5•6.25 mg/5 mL

Para-Hist HD liquid ℞ *narcotic antitussive; decongestant; antihistamine* [hydrocodone bitartrate; phenylephrine HCl; chlorpheniramine maleate] 1.67•5•2 mg/5 mL

parahydrecin [now: isomerol]

Paral oral liquid, rectal liquid ℞ *sedative; hypnotic* [paraldehyde]

paraldehyde USP *hypnotic; sedative; anticonvulsant* 1 g/mL oral or rectal

paramethadione USP, INN, BAN *anticonvulsant* ② paramethasone

paramethasone INN *glucocorticoid* [also: paramethasone acetate] ② paramethadione

paramethasone acetate USAN, USP *glucocorticoid* [also: paramethasone]

para-nitrosulfathiazole NF [also: nitrosulfathiazole]

paranyline HCl USAN *anti-inflammatory* [also: renytoline]

parapenzolate bromide USAN, INN *anticholinergic*

Paraplatin powder for IV injection ℞ *alkylating antineoplastic for ovarian cancer* [carboplatin] 50, 150, 450 mg

parapropamol INN

pararosaniline embonate INN *antischistosomal* [also: pararosaniline pamoate]

pararosaniline pamoate USAN *antischistosomal* [also: pararosaniline embonate]

Parathar powder for IV injection ℞ *in vivo diagnostic aid for parathyroid-induced hypocalcemia (orphan)* [teriparatide acetate] 200 U

parathesin [see: benzocaine]

parathiazine INN

parathyroid USP *hormone*

paraxazone INN

parbendazole USAN, INN *anthelmintic*

parconazole INN *antifungal* [also: parconazole HCl]

parconazole HCl USAN *antifungal* [also: parconazole]

Par-Drix sustained-release tablets (discontinued 1994) ℞ *decongestant; antihistamine* [pseudoephedrine sulfate; dexbrompheniramine maleate] 120•6 mg

Paredrine eye drops ℞ *mydriatic* [hydroxyamphetamine hydrobromide] 1%

paregoric (PG) (a preparation of opium, anise oil, benzoic acid, camphor, alcohol, and glycerin) USP *antiperistaltic; narcotic analgesic* 2 mg/5 mL oral

Paremyd eye drops ℞ *mydriatic; weak cycloplegic* [hydroxyamphetamine hydrobromide; tropicamide] 1%•0.25%

parenabol [see: boldenone undecylenate]

Parepectolin concentrated liquid OTC *GI adsorbent; antidiarrheal* [attapulgite] 600 mg/15 mL

pareptide INN *antiparkinsonian* [also: pareptide sulfate]

pareptide sulfate USAN *antiparkinsonian* [also: pareptide]

parethoxycaine INN

parethoxycaine HCl [see: parethoxycaine]

Par-F tablets ℞ *vitamin/mineral/calcium/iron supplement* [multiple vitamins & minerals; calcium; iron; folic acid] ±•250•60•1 mg

pargeverine INN

pargolol INN

pargyline INN *antihypertensive* [also: pargyline HCl]

pargyline HCl USAN, USP *antihypertensive* [also: pargyline]

Parhist SR sustained-release capsules (discontinued 1995) ℞ *decongestant; antihistamine* [phenylpropanolamine HCl; chlorpheniramine maleate] 75•12 mg

paridocaine INN

Parlodel SnapTabs (scored tablets), capsules ℞ *antiparkinsonian; lactation preventative; treats acromegaly, infertility, and hypogonadism* [bromocriptine mesylate] 2.5 mg; 5 mg

Par-Natal Plus 1 Improved tablets ℞ *vitamin/calcium/iron supplement* [multiple vitamins; calcium; iron; folic acid] ±•200•65•1 mg

Parnate film-coated tablets ℞ *antidepressant; monoamine oxidase (MAO) inhibitor* [tranylcypromine sulfate] 10 mg

parodilol INN

parodyne [see: antipyrine]

paroleine [see: mineral oil]

Paromomycin ℞ *(orphan: visceral leishmaniasis)* [aminosidine]

paromomycin INN, BAN *aminoglycoside bactericidal antibiotic; amebicide* [also: paromomycin sulfate]

paromomycin sulfate USP *aminoglycoside bactericidal antibiotic; amebicide* [also: paromomycin]

paroxetine USAN, INN, BAN *antidepressant; selective serotonin reuptake inhibitor*

paroxetine HCl *antidepressant*

paroxyl [see: acetarsone]

paroxypropione INN

parpanit HCl [see: caramiphen HCl]

parsalmide INN

Parsidol tablets ℞ *anticholinergic; antiparkinsonian* [ethopropazine HCl] 10, 50 mg

Partapp elixir (discontinued 1994) OTC *decongestant; antihistamine* [phenylpropanolamine HCl; brompheniramine maleate] 12.5•2 mg/5 mL

Partapp TD timed-release tablets (discontinued 1995) ℞ *decongestant; antihistamine* [phenylpropanolamine HCl; phenylephrine HCl; brompheniramine maleate] 15•15•12 mg

partricin USAN, INN *antifungal; antiprotozoal*

Partuss LA long-acting tablets ℞ *decongestant; expectorant* [phenylpropanolamine HCl; guaifenesin] 75•400 mg

parvaquone INN, BAN

Parvlex tablets OTC *hematinic* [ferrous fumarate; multiple B vitamins and minerals; vitamin C; folic acid] 100•±•50•0.1 mg

PAS (para-aminosalicylate) [see: aminosalicylic acid]

PASA (para-aminosalicylic acid) [see: aminosalicylic acid]

Paser granules ℞ *tuberculostatic* [aminosalicylic acid] 4 g/packet

pasiniazid INN

PassHIV ℞ *investigational immunotherapy for HIV and AIDS*

Pastilles (dosage form) *troches*

PATCO (prednisone, ara-C, thioguanine, cyclophosphamide, Oncovin) *chemotherapy protocol*

Pathilon film-coated tablets ℞ *peptic ulcer treatment adjunct* [tridihexethyl chloride] 25 mg ☒ Pathocil

Pathocil capsules, powder for oral suspension ℞ *bactericidal antibiotic (penicillinase-resistant penicillin)* [dicloxacillin sodium monohydrate] 250, 500 mg; 62.5 mg/5 mL ☒ Bactocill; Pathilon; Placidyl

paulomycin USAN, INN *antibacterial*

Pavabid Plateau Caps (controlled-release capsules) ℞ *cerebral and peripheral vasodilator* [papaverine HCl] 150 mg ☒ Pavased; Pavabid

Pavabid HP capsulets (tablets) (discontinued 1995) ℞ *cerebral and peripheral vasodilator* [papaverine HCl] 300 mg

Pavarine Spancaps (timed-release capsules) ℞ *cerebral and peripheral vasodilator* [papaverine HCl] 150 mg

Pavased timed-release capsules (discontinued 1996) ℞ *peripheral vasodilators* [papaverine HCl] 150 mg

Pavatine timed-release capsules ℞ *peripheral vasodilators* [papaverine HCl] 150 mg ☒ Pavatym

Pavatym timed-release capsules (discontinued 1992) ℞ *muscle relaxant* [papaverine HCl] 150 mg ☒ Pavatine

PAVe (procarbazine, Alkeran, Velban) *chemotherapy protocol*

Paverolan Lanacaps (timed-release capsules) ℞ *peripheral vasodilators* [papaverine HCl] 150 mg ☒ Pavulon

Pavulon IM injection ℞ *nondepolarizing neuromuscular blocker; adjunct to anesthesia* [pancuronium bromide] 1, 2 mg/mL ☒ Paverolan

paxamate INN

Paxarel tablets ℞ *anxiolytic; sedative* [acetylcarbromal] 250 mg

Paxil film-coated tablets ℞ *antidepressant; selective serotonin reuptake inhibitor for panic disorder and OCD* [paroxetine HCl] 20, 30 mg

Paxipam tablets (discontinued 1995) ℞ *anxiolytic* [halazepam] 20, 40 mg

pazelliptine INN

pazinaclone USAN *anxiolytic*

Pazo Hemorrhoid ointment OTC *temporary relief of hemorrhoidal symptoms; topical vasoconstrictor; counterirritant; astringent* [ephedrine sulfate; camphor; zinc oxide] 0.2%•2%•5%

Pazo Hemorrhoid suppositories OTC *temporary relief of hemorrhoidal symptoms; topical vasoconstrictor; astringent* [ephedrine sulfate; zinc oxide] 3.8•96.5 mg

pazoxide USAN, INN *antihypertensive*

PBV (Platinol, bleomycin, vinblastine) *chemotherapy protocol*

PBZ tablets, elixir ℞ *antihistamine* [tripelennamine HCl] 25, 50 mg; 37.5 mg/5 mL

PBZ (pyribenzamine) [see: tripelennamine]

PBZ-SR sustained-release tablets ℞ *antihistamine* [tripelennamine HCl] 100 mg

PC (paclitaxel, carboplatin) *chemotherapy protocol*

PC (phosphatidylcholine) [see: lecithin]

PCE Dispertabs (delayed-release tablets) ℞ *macrolide antibiotic* [erythromycin] 333, 500 mg

PCE (Platinol, cyclophosphamide, etoposide) *chemotherapy protocol*

PCE (polymer-coated erythromycin) [see: erythromycin]

PCMX (parachlorometaxylenol) [q.v.]

PCP (parachlorophenol) [q.v.]

PCP (phenylcyclohexyl piperidine) [see: phencyclidine HCl]

PCV (procarbazine, CCNU, vincristine) *chemotherapy protocol*

PDA-641 *investigational anti-inflammatory and bronchodilator for asthma*

PDGA (pteroyldiglutamic acid)

PDLA (phosphinicodilactic acid) [see: foscolic acid]

PDP Liquid Protein OTC *dietary supplement* [hydrolyzed protein; L-tryptophan] 15•$\underline{2}$ g/30 mL

PE (phenylephrine) [q.v.]

PE (polyethylene) [q.v.]

peanut oil NF *solvent*

PEB (Platinol, etoposide, bleomycin) *chemotherapy protocol*

pecazine INN, BAN

pecazine acetate [see: pecazine]

pecilocin INN, BAN
pecocycline INN
pectin USP *suspending agent; protectant; GI adsorbent*
Pedameth capsules, liquid ℞ *urinary acidifier to control ammonia production* [racemethionine] 200 mg; 75 mg/5 mL
PediaCare Allergy Formula liquid OTC *antihistamine* [chlorpheniramine maleate] 1 mg/5 mL
PediaCare Cold-Allergy chewable tablets OTC *pediatric decongestant and antihistamine* [pseudoephedrine HCl; chlorpheniramine maleate] 15•1 mg
PediaCare Cough-Cold Formula chewable tablets, liquid OTC *pediatric antitussive, decongestant, and antihistamine* [dextromethorphan hydrobromide; pseudoephedrine HCl; chlorpheniramine maleate] 5•15•1 mg; 5•15•1 mg/5 mL
PediaCare Infant's Decongestant drops OTC *nasal decongestant* [pseudoephedrine HCl] 7.5 mg/0.8 mL
PediaCare NightRest Cough-Cold liquid OTC *pediatric antitussive, decongestant, and antihistamine* [dextromethorphan hydrobromide; pseudoephedrine HCl; chlorpheniramine maleate] 7.5•15•1 mg/5 mL
Pediacof syrup ℞ *pediatric narcotic antitussive, decongestant, antihistamine, and expectorant* [codeine phosphate; phenylephrine HCl; chlorpheniramine maleate; potassium iodide; alcohol 5%] 5•2.5•0.75•75 mg/5 mL
Pediacon DX children's syrup, pediatric drops OTC *pediatric antitussive, decongestant, and expectorant* [dextromethorphan hydrobromide; phenylpropanolamine HCl; guaifenesin] 5•6.25•100 mg/5 mL; 5•6.25•50 mg/mL
Pediacon EX pediatric drops OTC *pediatric decongestant and expectorant* [phenylpropanolamine HCl; guaifenesin] 6.25•50 mg/mL
Pediaflor drops ℞ *dental caries preventative* [sodium fluoride] 1.1 mg/mL
Pedialyte oral solution OTC *electrolyte replacement* [sodium, potassium, and chloride electrolytes]
PediaPatch transdermal patch (name changed to Trans-Ver-Sal Pedia-Patch in 1995)
Pediapred oral liquid ℞ *glucocorticoids* [prednisolone sodium phosphate] 5 mg/5 mL
PediaProfen oral suspension (name changed to Children's Motrin in 1993)
PediaSure ready-to-use liquid OTC *total or supplementary infant feeding*
Pediatric Electrolyte oral solution OTC *electrolyte replacement* [dextrose; multiple electrolytes] 1 L
Pediatric Maintenance Solution (discontinued 1992) ℞ *electrolyte replacement* [sodium chloride; dextrose; sodium lactate]
Pediazole oral suspension ℞ *antibiotic* [erythromycin ethylsuccinate; sulfisoxazole acetyl] 200•600 mg/5 mL
Pedi-Bath Salts OTC *bath emollient*
Pedi-Boro Soak Paks powder packets OTC *astringent wet dressing (modified Burow solution)* [aluminum sulfate; calcium acetate]
Pedi-Cort V Creme ℞ *topical corticosteroid; antifungal; antibacterial* [hydrocortisone; clioquinol] 1%•3%
Pedi-Dri powder ℞ *topical antifungal* [nystatin] 100,000 U/g
Pediotic ear drop suspension ℞ *topical corticosteroidal anti-inflammatory; antibiotic* [hydrocortisone; neomycin sulfate; polymyxin B sulfate] 1%•5 mg•10,000 U per mL
Pedi-Pro foot powder OTC *topical antifungal; anhidrotic* [zinc undecylenate; aluminum chlorhydroxide; menthol; chloroxylenol]
Pedituss Cough syrup ℞ *pediatric narcotic antitussive, decongestant, antihistamine, and expectorant* [codeine phosphate; phenylephrine HCl; chlorpheniramine maleate; potassium iodide] 5•2.5•0.75•75 mg/5 mL
Pedi-Vit-A Creme OTC *moisturizer; emollient* [vitamin A] 100,000 U/30 g
Pedotic otic suspension ℞ *topical corticosteroidal anti-inflammatory; antibiotic* [hydrocortisone; neomycin sul-

fate; polymyxin B sulfate] 1%•5 mg•10,000 U per mL

PedTE-Pak-4 IV injection ℞ *intravenous nutritional therapy* [multiple trace elements (metals)] ≛

Pedtrace-4 IV injection ℞ *intravenous nutritional therapy* [multiple trace elements (metals)]

PedvaxHIB powder for IM injection ℞ *Haemophilus influenzae type b (HIB) vaccine* [Hemophilus b conjugate vaccine]

PeeWee's Children's Vitamins chewable tablets (discontinued 1995) OTC *vitamin/iron supplement* [multiple vitamins; iron; folic acid] ≛•15•0.3 mg

pefloxacin USAN, INN, BAN *antibacterial*

pefloxacin mesylate USAN *antibacterial*

PEG (polyethylene glycol) [q.v.]

P.E.G. Ointment OTC *ointment base* [polyethylene glycol 400; polyethylene glycol 3350]

PEG-ADA (polyethylene glycol-adenosine deaminase) [see: pegademase bovine]

pegademase INN *adenosine deaminase replacement* [also: pegademase bovine]

pegademase bovine USAN *adenosine deaminase replacement; (orphan: severe combined immunodeficiency disease)* [also: pegademase]

PEG-adenosine deaminase (PEG-ADA) [see: pegademase bovine]

Peganone tablets ℞ *hydantoin-type anticonvulsant* [ethotoin] 250, 500 mg

pegaspargase (PEG-L-asparaginase) USAN, INN *antineoplastic for acute lymphoblastic leukemia (ALL); acute lymphocytic leukemia (orphan)*

PEG-ES (polyethylene glycol-electrolyte solution) [q.v.]

PEG-glucocerebrosidase (polyethylene glycol-glucocerebrosidase) *(orphan: enzyme replacement in Gaucher's disease)*

PEG-hemoglobin (polyethylene glycol-hemoglobin) *investigational blood replacement*

PEG-interleukin-2 (polyethylene glycol-interleukin-2) *investigational (Phase II) cytokine for AIDS; (orphan: primary immunodeficiencies)*

PEG-intron A (polyethylene glycol-intron A) *investigational*

PEG-L-asparaginase [see: pegaspargase]

peglicol 5 oleate USAN *emulsifying agent*

pegorgotein USAN *investigational free-radical scavenger to prevent irreversible brain damage after head trauma*

pegoterate USAN, INN *suspending agent*

pegoxol 7 stearate USAN *emulsifying agent*

PEG-SOD (polyethylene glycol-superoxide dismutase) [see: pegorgotein]

Pelamine tablets ℞ *antihistamine* [tripelennamine HCl] 50 mg

pelanserin INN *antihypertensive; vasodilator; serotonin adrenergic blocker* [also: pelanserin HCl]

pelanserin HCl USAN *antihypertensive; vasodilator; serotonin adrenergic blocker* [also: pelanserin]

peliomycin USAN, INN *antineoplastic*

pelretin USAN, INN *antikeratinizing agent*

pelrinone INN *cardiotonic* [also: pelrinone HCl]

pelrinone HCl USAN *cardiotonic* [also: pelrinone]

PEM-420 *investigational oral analgesic*

pemedolac USAN, INN *analgesic*

pemerid INN *antitussive* [also: pemerid nitrate]

pemerid nitrate USAN *antitussive* [also: pemerid]

pemirolast INN *antiallergic; mediator release inhibitor* [also: pemirolast potassium]

pemirolast potassium USAN *antiallergic; mediator release inhibitor* [also: pemirolast]

pemoline USAN, INN, BAN, JAN *CNS stimulant for attention deficit hyperactivity disorders (ADHD) and narcolepsy*

pempidine INN, BAN

penamecillin USAN, INN, BAN *antibacterial*

penbutolol INN, BAN *antiadrenergic (β-receptor)* [also: penbutolol sulfate]

penbutolol sulfate USAN *antiadrenergic (β-receptor)* [also: penbutolol]

penciclovir USAN, INN, BAN *antiviral for herpes*
pendecamaine INN, BAN
pendiomide [see: azamethonium bromide]
Penecare cream, lotion OTC *moisturizer; emollient*
Penecort cream, solution ℞ *topical corticosteroid* [hydrocortisone] 1%
penem antibiotics *a class of broad-spectrum anti-infectives*
Penetrex film-coated tablets ℞ *broad-spectrum fluoroquinolone-type antibiotic* [enoxacin] 200, 400 mg
PenFill (trademarked form) *insulin injector refill cartridge*
penfluridol USAN, INN *antipsychotic*
penflutizide INN
pengitoxin INN
penicillamine USAN, USP, INN *metal chelating agent; antirheumatic* ⑨ penicillin
penicillin aluminum
penicillin benzathine phenoxymethyl [now: penicillin V benzathine]
penicillin calcium USP
penicillin G benzathine USP *bactericidal antibiotic* [also: benzathine benzylpenicillin; benzathine penicillin; benzylpenicillin benzathine]
penicillin G hydrabamine
penicillin G potassium USP *bactericidal antibiotic* [also: benzylpenicillin potassium] 200, 250, 400, 500 thousand U oral; 1, 2, 3, 5, 10, 20 million U/vial injection
penicillin G procaine USP *bactericidal antibiotic* [also: procaine penicillin]
penicillin G redox [see: redox-penicillin G]
penicillin G sodium USP *bactericidal antibiotic* [also: benzylpenicillin sodium]
penicillin hydrabamine phenoxymethyl [now: penicillin V hydrabamine]
penicillin N [see: adicillin]
penicillin O [see: almecillin]
penicillin O chloroprocaine
penicillin O potassium
penicillin O sodium
penicillin phenoxymethyl [now: penicillin V]
penicillin potassium G [see: penicillin G potassium]
penicillin potassium phenoxymethyl [now: penicillin V potassium]
penicillin V USAN, USP *bactericidal antibiotic* [also: phenoxymethylpenicillin]
penicillin V benzathine USAN, USP *antibacterial*
penicillin V hydrabamine USAN, USP *antibacterial*
penicillin V potassium USAN, USP *bactericidal antibiotic*
penicillin-152 potassium [see: phenethicillin potassium] ⑨ penicillamine; Polycillin
penicillinase INN, BAN
penicillinphenyrazine [see: phenyracillin]
Penicillin-VK tablets, oral solution ℞ *bactericidal antibiotic* [penicillin V potassium] 250, 500 mg; 125, 250 mg/5 mL
penidural [see: benzathine penicillin]
penimepicycline INN
penimocycline INN
penirolol INN
Pen-Kera cream OTC *moisturizer; emollient*
penmesterol INN
penoctonium bromide INN
penprostene INN
pentabamate USAN, INN *minor tranquilizer*
Pentacarinat IV or IM injection ℞ *antiprotozoal; treatment and prophylaxis of Pneumocystis carinii pneumonia (orphan)* [pentamidine isethionate] 300 mg
Pentacef powder for IV or IM injection ℞ *cephalosporin-type antibiotic* [ceftazidime]
pentacosactride BAN [also: norleusactide]
pentacynium chloride INN
pentacyone chloride [see: pentacynium chloride]
pentaerithritol tetranicotinate [see: niceritrol]
pentaerithrityl tetranitrate INN *vasodilator* [also: pentaerythritol tetranitrate]

pentaerythritol tetranitrate (PETN) USP *vasodilator; "possibly effective" antianginal* [also: pentaerithrityl tetranitrate]
pentaerythritol trinitrate [see: pentrinitrol]
pentafilcon A USAN *hydrophilic contact lens material*
pentafluranol INN
pentagastrin USAN, INN *gastric secretion indicator*
pentagestrone INN
pentalamide INN, BAN
pentalyte USAN, USP, NF *electrolyte combination*
Pentam 300 IV or IM injection ℞ *antiprotozoal; treatment and prophylaxis of Pneumocystis carinii pneumonia (orphan)* [pentamidine isethionate] 300 mg
pentamethazene [see: azamethonium bromide]
pentamethonium bromide INN, BAN
pentamethylenetetrazol [see: pentylenetetrazol]
pentamidine INN, BAN
pentamidine isethionate *antiprotozoal; treatment and prophylaxis of Pneumocystis carinii pneumonia (orphan)* 300 mg injection
pentamin [see: azamethonium bromide]
pentamorphone USAN, INN *narcotic analgesic*
pentamoxane INN
pentamoxane HCl [see: pentamoxane]
pentamustine USAN *antineoplastic* [also: neptamustine]
pentanedial [see: glutaral]
pentanitrol [see: pentaerythritol tetranitrate]
pentaphonate
pentapiperide INN
pentapiperium methylsulfate USAN *anticholinergic* [also: pentapiperium metilsulfate]
pentapiperium metilsulfate INN *anticholinergic* [also: pentapiperium methylsulfate]
pentaquine INN [also: pentaquine phosphate]
pentaquine phosphate USP [also: pentaquine]

Pentasa controlled-release capsules ℞ *for ulcerative colitis, proctosigmoiditis, and proctitis; investigational for Crohn's disease* [mesalamine] 250 mg
pentasodium colistinmethanesulfonate [see: colistimethate sodium]
Pentaspan ℞ *leukapheresis adjunct to improve leukocyte yield (orphan)* [pentastarch]
pentastarch USAN, BAN *leukapheresis adjunct; red cell sedimenting agent; centrifugal leukocyte harvesting aid (orphan)*
pentavalent gas gangrene antitoxin
Pentazine injection ℞ *antihistamine; motion sickness; sleep aid; antiemetic; sedative* [promethazine HCl] 50 mg/mL ⚠ Phenazine
Pentazine VC with Codeine liquid ℞ *narcotic antitussive; antihistamine* [codeine phosphate; promethazine HCl] 10•6.25 mg/5 mL
pentazocine USAN, USP, INN, BAN *narcotic agonist-antagonist analgesic*
pentazocine HCl USAN, USP *analgesic*
pentazocine lactate USAN, USP *analgesic*
pentetate calcium trisodium USAN *plutonium chelating agent* [also: calcium trisodium pentetate]
pentetate calcium trisodium Yb 169 USAN *radioactive agent*
pentetate disodium [see: pentetic acid, sodium salts]
pentetate indium disodium In 111 USAN *diagnostic aid; radioactive agent*
pentetate monosodium [see: pentetic acid, sodium salts]
pentetate pentasodium [see: pentetic acid, sodium salts]
pentetate tetrasodium [see: pentetic acid, sodium salts]
pentetate trisodium [see: pentetic acid, sodium salts]
pentetate trisodium calcium [see: pentetate calcium trisodium]
pentethylcyclanone [see: cyclexanone]
pentetic acid USAN, BAN *diagnostic aid*
pentetic acid, sodium salts *diagnostic aid*
pentetrazol INN [also: pentylenetetrazol]

penthanil diethylenetriamine pentaacetic acid (DTPA) [see: pentetic acid]

penthienate bromide NF

Penthrane liquid for vaporization ℞ *inhalation general anesthetic* [methoxyflurane]

penthrichloral INN, BAN

pentiapine INN *antipsychotic* [also: pentiapine maleate]

pentiapine maleate USAN *antipsychotic* [also: pentiapine]

penticide [see: chlorophenothane]

Pentids '400'; Pentids '800' tablets (discontinued 1993) ℞ *bactericidal antibiotic* [penicillin G potassium] 400,000 U; 800,000 U

Pentids '400' for Syrup powder for oral solution (discontinued 1993) ℞ *bactericidal antibiotic* [penicillin G potassium] 400,000 U/5 mL

pentifylline INN, BAN

pentigetide USAN, INN *antiallergic*

pentisomicin USAN, INN *anti-infective*

pentisomide INN

pentizidone INN *antibacterial* [also: pentizidone sodium]

pentizidone sodium USAN *antibacterial* [also: pentizidone]

pentobarbital USP, INN *sedative; hypnotic* [also: pentobarbitone; pentobarbital calcium] ② phenobarbital

pentobarbital calcium JAN *sedative; hypnotic* [also: pentobarbital; pentobarbitone]

pentobarbital sodium USP, JAN *sedative; hypnotic* [also: pentobarbitone sodium] 100 mg oral; 50 mg/mL injection

pentobarbitone BAN *sedative; hypnotic* [also: pentobarbital]

pentobarbitone sodium BAN *sedative; hypnotic* [also: pentobarbital sodium]

Pentolair eye drops ℞ *mydriatic; cycloplegic* [cyclopentolate HCl] 1%

pentolinium tartrate NF [also: pentolonium tartrate]

pentolonium tartrate INN [also: pentolinium tartrate]

pentolonum bitartrate [see: pentolinium tartrate]

pentomone USAN, INN *prostate growth inhibitor*

pentopril USAN, INN *angiotensin-converting enzyme (ACE) inhibitor*

pentorex INN

pentosalen BAN

pentosan polysulfate sodium USAN, INN *anti-inflammatory* (orphan: interstitial cystitis)

Pentostam (available only from the Centers for Disease Control) ℞ *investigational anti-infective for leishmaniasis* [sodium stibogluconate]

pentostatin USAN, INN *potentiator; antibiotic antineoplastic for hairy cell and chronic lymphocytic leukemias* (orphan)

Pentothal powder for IV injection, rectal suspension ℞ *general anesthetic* [thiopental sodium] 2%, 2.5%; 400 mg/g ② pentrinitrol;

pentoxifylline USAN, INN *vasodilator; hemorheologic agent* [also: oxpentifylline]

pentoxiverine citrate [see: carbetapentane citrate]

pentoxyverine INN [also: carbetapentane citrate]

pentoxyverine citrate [see: carbetapentane citrate]

Pentrax; Pentrax Gold shampoo OTC *antiseborrheic; antipsoriatic; antipruritic; antibacterial* [coal tar] 4.3%; 4%

pentrinitrol USAN, INN *coronary vasodilator* ② Pentothal

***tert*-pentyl alcohol** [see: amylene hydrate]

Pentylan tablets (discontinued 1995) ℞ *antianginal* [pentaerythritol tetranitrate] 10, 20 mg

6-pentyl-*m*-cresol [see: amylmetacresol]

pentylenetetrazol NF [also: pentetrazol]

pentymal [see: amobarbital]

Pen-V tablets ℞ *bactericidal antibiotic* [penicillin V potassium] 250, 500 mg

Pen-Vee K tablets, powder for oral solution ℞ *bactericidal antibiotic* [penicillin V potassium] 250, 500 mg; 125, 250 mg/5 mL

Pepcid film-coated tablets, powder for oral suspension, IV injection, preloaded syringes for IV ℞ *gastric and*

duodenal ulcer treatment; histamine H_2 *antagonist* [famotidine] 20, 40 mg; 40 mg/5 mL; 10 mg/mL; 20 mg

Pepcid AC tablets OTC *"acid controller" for heartburn and acid indigestion* [famotidine] 10 mg

pepleomycin [see: peplomycin sulfate]

peplomycin INN *antineoplastic* [also: peplomycin sulfate]

peplomycin sulfate USAN *antineoplastic* [also: peplomycin]

peppermint NF *flavoring agent; perfume*

peppermint oil NF *flavoring agent*

peppermint spirit USP *flavoring agent; perfume*

peppermint water NF *flavored vehicle*

pepsin *digestive aid*

pepstatin USAN, INN *pepsin enzyme inhibitor*

Peptamen ready-to-use liquid OTC *enteral nutritional therapy for GI impairment*

Peptavlon subcu injection ℞ *in vivo gastrointestinal function test* [pentagastrin] 250 µg/mL

peptide copper compound *investigational treatment for peptic ulcers, surgical wound repair, and bone healing*

peptide metal compound *investigational hair growth enhancer*

peptide T *investigational antiviral for AIDS (clinical trials discontinued 1994)*

Pepto Diarrhea Control oral solution OTC *antidiarrheal* [loperamide HCl] 1 mg/5 mL

Pepto-Bismol chewable tablets, caplets, liquid OTC *antidiarrheal; antinauseant* [bismuth subsalicylate] 262 mg; 262 mg; 262, 524 mg/15 mL

peraclopone INN

peradoxime INN

perafensine INN

peralopride INN

peraquinsin INN

perastine INN

peratizole INN, BAN

perbufylline INN

Perchloracap capsules ℞ *pertechnetate Tc 99m accumulation blocker; for hyperthyroidism* [potassium perchlorate] 200 mg

Percocet tablets ℞ *narcotic analgesic* [oxycodone HCl; acetaminophen] 5•325 mg

Percodan; Percodan-Demi tablets ℞ *narcotic analgesic* [oxycodone HCl; oxycodone terephthalate; aspirin] 4.5•0.38•325 mg; 2.25•0.19•325 mg ⑨ Decadron

Percogesic tablets OTC *antihistamine; analgesic* [phenyltoloxamine citrate; acetaminophen] 30•325 mg

Perdiem granules OTC *laxative* [psyllium husks; senna extract] 3.25•0.74 g/tsp. ⑨ Pyridium

Perdiem Fiber granules OTC *laxative* [psyllium] 4.03 g/tsp.

Perfectoderm gel OTC *topical keratolytic for acne* [benzoyl peroxide] 5%

perfilcon A USAN *hydrophilic contact lens material*

perfluamine INN, BAN

perflubron USAN, INN *blood substitute; MRI imaging agent*

perflunafene INN, BAN

perfluorochemical (PFC) emulsion (discontinued 1995) *synthetic blood oxygen carrier for PTCA*

perfomedil INN

perfosfamide USAN *antineoplastic; (orphan: ex vivo treatment of autologous bone marrow for leukemia)*

Pergamid ℞ *investigational antineoplastic (orphan: ex vivo treatment of autologous bone marrow in leukemia)* [perfosfamide]

pergolide INN, BAN *dopamine agonist* [also: pergolide mesylate]

pergolide mesylate USAN *dopamine agonist; antiparkinsonian* [also: pergolide]

Pergonal powder for IM injection ℞ *ovulation stimulant for women; spermatogenesis stimulant for men* [menotropins] 75, 150 IU/ampule

perhexiline INN *coronary vasodilator* [also: perhexiline maleate]

perhexiline maleate USAN *coronary vasodilator* [also: perhexiline]

Periactin tablets, syrup ℞ *antihistamine; cold urticaria; anticholinergic* [cyproheptadine HCl] 4 mg; 2 mg/5 mL ⑨ Taractan

periciazine INN [also: pericyazine]

Peri-Colace capsules, syrup OTC *laxative; stool softener* [casanthranol; docusate sodium] 30•100 mg; 30•60 mg/15 mL

pericyazine BAN [also: periciazine]

Peridex mouth rinse ℞ *antimicrobial; gingivitis treatment; (orphan: oral mucositis)* [chlorhexidine gluconate; alcohol 11.6%] 0.12%

Peridin-C tablets OTC *vitamin supplement* [ascorbic acid; hesperidin complex; hesperidin methyl chalcone bioflavonoids] 200•150•50 mg

Peri-Dos softgels OTC *laxative; stool softener* [casanthranol; docusate sodium] 30•100 mg

Perimed oral rinse (discontinued 1994) OTC *oral antibacterial* [hydrogen peroxide; povidone-iodine] 1.5%•5%

perimetazine INN

perindopril USAN, INN, BAN *angiotensin-converting enzyme (ACE) inhibitor*

perindopril erbumine USAN *antihypertensive*

perindoprilat INN, BAN

PerioGard mouth rinse ℞ *antimicrobial; gingivitis treatment* [chlorhexidine gluconate; alcohol 11.6%] 0.12%

perisoxal INN

Peritrate tablets (discontinued 1995) ℞ *antianginal* [pentaerythritol tetranitrate] 10, 20, 40 mg

Peritrate SA sustained-action tablets (discontinued 1995) ℞ *antianginal* [pentaerythritol tetranitrate] 80 mg

perlapine USAN, INN *hypnotic*

Perle (dosage form) *soft gelatin capsule*

permanganic acid, potassium salt [see: potassium permanganate]

Permapen Isoject (unit dose syringe) ℞ *bactericidal antibiotic* [penicillin G benzathine] 1,200,000 U

Permax tablets ℞ *antiparkinsonian agent* [pergolide mesylate] 0.05, 0.25, 1 mg

permethrin USAN, INN, BAN *ectoparasiticide*

Permitil tablets, oral concentrate ℞ *antipsychotic* [fluphenazine HCl] 2.5, 5, 10 mg; 5 mg/mL

Pernivit-R injection ℞ *vitamin therapy* [liver concentrate; folic acid; cyanocobalamin]

Pernox Scrub; Pernox Lathering Lotion OTC *abrasive cleanser for acne* [sulfur; salicylic acid]

peroxide, dibenzoyl [see: benzoyl peroxide]

Peroxin A 5; Peroxin A 10 gel ℞ *topical keratolytic for acne* [benzoyl peroxide] 5%; 10%

Peroxyl mouth rinse, oral gel OTC *cleansing of oral wounds* [hydrogen peroxide] 1.5%

perphenazine USP, INN *antipsychotic; antiemetic; antidopaminergic; intractable hiccough relief* 2, 4, 8, 16 mg oral

Persa-Gel; Persa-Gel W 5%; Persa-Gel W 10% gel ℞ *topical keratolytic for acne* [benzoyl peroxide] 5%, 10%; 5%; 10%

Persantine sugar-coated tablets ℞ *antiplatelet agent* [dipyridamole] 25, 50, 75 mg ☒ Pertofrane

Persantine IV injection ℞ *in vivo coronary artery function test* [dipyridamole] 10 mg

persic oil NF *vehicle*

persilic acid INN

Personal Lubricant vaginal gel (discontinued 1992) OTC *lubricant* [glycerin; propylene glycol]

Pertofrane capsules ℞ *tricyclic antidepressant* [desipramine HCl] 25, 50 mg ☒ Persantine

Pertropin capsules OTC *dietary lipotropic agent* [linolenic acid; multiple essential fatty acids] 7 mins.

Pertussin All-Night PM liquid (discontinued 1994) OTC *decongestant; antihistamine; antitussive; analgesic* [pseudoephedrine HCl; doxylamine succinate; dextromethorphan hydrobromide; acetaminophen; alcohol 25%] 2•0.25•1•33.4 mg/mL

Pertussin AM liquid (discontinued 1994) OTC *decongestant; antitussive; expectorant* [pseudoephedrine HCl; dextromethorphan hydrobromide; guaifenesin; alcohol]

Pertussin CS; Pertussin ES syrup OTC *antitussive* [dextromethorphan hydrobromide] 3.5 mg/5 mL; 15 mg/5 mL

Pertussin PM liquid (discontinued 1994) OTC *decongestant; antihistamine; antitussive; analgesic* [pseudoephedrine HCl; doxylamine succinate; dextromethorphan hydrobromide; acetaminophen; alcohol]

pertussis immune globulin USP *passive immunizing agent*

pertussis immune human globulin [now: pertussis immune globulin]

pertussis vaccine USP *active immunizing agent*

pertussis vaccine adsorbed USP *active immunizing agent*

peruvian balsam NF *topical local protectant; rubefacient*

pethidine INN, BAN *narcotic analgesic* [also: meperidine HCl]

pethidine HCl [see: meperidine HCl]

PETN (pentaerythritol tetranitrate) [q.v.]

petrichloral INN

petrolatum USP *ointment base; emollient/protectant* [also: yellow petrolatum]

petrolatum, hydrophilic USP *absorbent ointment base; topical protectant*

petrolatum, liquid [see: mineral oil]

petrolatum, liquid emulsion [see: mineral oil emulsion]

petrolatum, white USP, JAN *oleaginous ointment base; topical protectant*

petrolatum gauze [see: gauze, petrolatum]

petroleum benzin [see: benzin, petroleum]

petroleum jelly [see: petrolatum]

pexantel INN

PFA (phosphonoformic acid) [see: foscarnet sodium]

PFC (perfluorochemical) emulsion [q.v.]

Pfeiffer's Allergy tablets OTC *antihistamine* [chlorpheniramine maleate] 4 mg

Pfeiffer's Cold Sore lotion OTC *topical oral anesthetic; antipruritic/counterirritant* [gum benzoin; camphor; menthol; eucalyptol; alcohol 85%] 7%•$\underline{?}$•$\underline{?}$•$\underline{?}$

Pfizerpen powder for injection ℞ *bactericidal antibiotic* [penicillin G potassium] 1, 5, 20 million units

Pfizerpen-AS IM injection ℞ *bactericidal antibiotic* [penicillin G procaine] 300,000 U/mL

PFL (Platinol, fluorouracil, leucovorin [rescue]) *chemotherapy protocol*

PFT (L-phenylalanine mustard, fluorouracil, tamoxifen) *chemotherapy protocol*

PG (paregoric) [q.v.]

PG (prostaglandin) [q.v.]

PGA (pteroylglutamic acid) [see: folic acid]

PGE$_1$ (prostaglandin E$_1$) [now: alprostadil]

PGE$_2$ (prostaglandin E$_2$) [now: dinoprostone]

PGF$_{2\alpha}$ (prostaglandin F$_{2\alpha}$) [see: dinoprost]

PGF$_{2\alpha}$ (prostaglandin F$_{2\alpha}$) THAM [see: dinoprost tromethamine]

PGI$_2$ (prostaglandin I$_2$) [now: epoprostenol]

PGX (prostaglandin X) [now: epoprostenol]

Phacotron Gold ℞ *investigational phacoemulsification system for cataract surgery*

Phanacōl Cough syrup (discontinued 1995) OTC *decongestant; antitussive; expectorant; analgesic; antipyretic* [phenylpropanolamine HCl; dextromethorphan hydrobromide; guaifenesin; acetaminophen] 25•10•100•325 mg/5 mL

Phanadex Cough syrup OTC *antitussive; decongestant; antihistamine; expectorant* [dextromethorphan hydrobromide; phenylpropanolamine HCl; pyrilamine maleate; guaifenesin] 15•25•40•100 mg/5 mL

Phanatuss Cough syrup OTC *antitussive; expectorant* [dextromethorphan hydrobromide; guaifenesin] 10•85 mg/5 mL

phanchinone [see: phanquinone; phanquone]

phanquinone INN [also: phanquone]

phanquone BAN [also: phanquinone]

pharmaceutical glaze [see: glaze, pharmaceutical]

Pharmadine ointment, perineal wash, skin cleanser, solution, swabs, swab sticks, spray, surgical scrub, whirlpool solution (discontinued 1992) OTC *broad-spectrum antimicrobial* [povidone-iodine]

Pharmaflur; Pharmaflur df; Pharmaflur 1.1 chewable tablets ℞ *dental caries preventative* [sodium fluoride] 2.2 mg; 2.2 mg; 1.1 mg

Pharmalgen subcu or IM injection ℞ *venom sensitivity testing (subcu); venom desensitization therapy (IM)* [extracts of honeybee, yellow jacket, yellow hornet, white-faced hornet, mixed vespid, and wasp venom]

Pharmorubicin PFS; Pharmorubicin RDF injection (available only in Canada) ℞ *antibiotic antineoplastic* [epirubicin HCl] 2 mg/mL; 10, 20, 50, 150 mg

Phazyme tablets, drops OTC *antiflatulent* [simethicone] 60 mg; 40 mg/0.6 mL ❷ Pherazine

Phazyme 95 tablets OTC *antiflatulent* [simethicone] 95 mg

Phazyme 125 softgels OTC *antiflatulent* [simethicone] 125 mg

phebutazine [see: febuverine]
phebutyrazine [see: febuverine]
phemfilcon A USAN *hydrophilic contact lens material*
phenacaine INN [also: phenacaine HCl]
phenacaine HCl USP [also: phenacaine]

PhenaCal capsules (discontinued 1993) OTC *dietary supplement* [multiple amino acids, vitamins, and minerals]

phenacemide USP, INN, BAN *anticonvulsant*

phenacetin USP, INN (*withdrawn from market*) ❷ phenazocine

phenacon [see: fenaclon]
phenactropinium chloride INN, BAN
phenacyl 4-morpholineacetate [see: mobecarb]
N-phenacylhomatropinium chloride [see: phenactropinium chloride]
phenacylpivalate [see: pibecarb]

Phenadex Children's Cough/Cold syrup OTC *pediatric antitussive, decongestant, and expectorant* [dextromethorphan hydrobromide; phenylpropanolamine HCl; guaifenesin; alcohol 5%] 5•6.25•100 mg/5 mL

Phenadex Pediatric Cough/Cold drops OTC *pediatric antitussive, decongestant, and expectorant* [dextromethorphan hydrobromide; phenylpropanolamine HCl; guaifenesin] 5•6.25•50 mg/mL

Phenadex Senior liquid OTC *antitussive; expectorant* [dextromethorphan hydrobromide; guaifenesin] 10•200 mg/5 mL

phenadoxone INN, BAN
phenaglycodol INN

Phenahist-TR sustained-release tablets ℞ *decongestant; antihistamine; anticholinergic* [phenylpropanolamine HCl; phenylephrine HCl; chlorpheniramine maleate; hyoscyamine sulfate; atropine sulfate; scopolamine hydrobromide] 50•25•8•0.19•0.04•0.01 mg

phenamazoline INN
phenamazoline HCl [see: phenamazoline]

Phenameth tablets ℞ *antihistamine; motion sickness; sleep aid; antiemetic; sedative* [promethazine HCl] 25 mg

Phenameth DM syrup ℞ *antitussive; antihistamine* [dextromethorphan hydrobromide; promethazine HCl; alcohol] 15•6.25 mg/5 mL

phenampromide INN

Phenapap Sinus Headache & Congestion tablets OTC *decongestant; antihistamine; analgesic* [pseudoephedrine HCl; chlorpheniramine maleate; acetaminophen] 30•2•325 mg

Phenaphen caplets (discontinued 1993) OTC *analgesic; antipyretic* [acetaminophen] 325 mg ❷ Betapen; Phenergan

Phenaphen with Codeine No. 2 capsules (discontinued 1993) ℞ *narcotic analgesic* [codeine phosphate; acetaminophen] 15•325 mg

Phenaphen with Codeine No. 3 & No. 4 capsules ℞ *narcotic analgesic* [codeine phosphate; acetaminophen] 30•325 mg; 60•325 mg

Phenaphen-650 with Codeine tablets (discontinued 1995) ℞ *narcotic*

analgesic [codeine phosphate; acetaminophen] 30•650 mg
phenaphthazine
phenarbutal [see: phetharbital]
phenarsone sulfoxylate INN
Phenaseptic mouthwash/gargle (discontinued 1995) OTC *topical antipruritic/counterirritant; mild local anesthetic* [phenol] 1.4%
Phenate timed-release tablets ℞ *decongestant; antihistamine; analgesic* [phenylpropanolamine HCl; chlorpheniramine maleate; acetaminophen] 40•4•325 mg
Phenazine 25 injection (discontinued 1996) ℞ *antihistamine; motion sickness; sleep aid; antiemetic; sedative* [promethazine HCl] 25 mg/mL ⓓ Pentazine; phenelzine; Phenoxine; Pherazine
Phenazine 50 injection ℞ *antihistamine; motion sickness; sleep aid; antiemetic; sedative* [promethazine HCl] 50 mg/mL ⓓ Pentazine; phenelzine; Phenoxine; Pherazine
phenazocine INN ⓓ phenacetin
phenazocine hydrobromide [see: phenazocine]
Phenazodine tablets (discontinued 1996) ℞ *urinary analgesic* [phenazopyridine HCl] 100, 200 mg
phenazone INN, BAN *analgesic* [also: antipyrine]
phenazopyridine INN, BAN *urinary tract analgesic* [also: phenazopyridine HCl]
phenazopyridine HCl USAN, USP *urinary tract analgesic* [also: phenazopyridine] 100, 200 mg oral
phenbenicillin BAN [also: fenbenicillin]
phenbutazone sodium glycerate USAN *anti-inflammatory*
phenbutrazate BAN [also: fenbutrazate]
phencarbamide USAN *anticholinergic* [also: fencarbamide]
Phencen-50 injection (discontinued 1994) ℞ *sedative; antihistamine* [promethazine HCl] 50 mg/mL
Phenchlor S.H.A. sustained-release tablets ℞ *decongestant; antihistamine; anticholinergic* [phenylpropanolamine HCl; phenylephrine HCl; chlorpheniramine maleate; hyoscyamine sulfate; atropine sulfate; scopolamine hydrobromide] 50•25•8•0.19•0.04•0.01 mg

phencyclidine INN *anesthetic* [also: phencyclidine HCl]
phencyclidine HCl USAN *anesthetic* [also: phencyclidine]
phendimetrazine INN *anorexiant* [also: phendimetrazine tartrate] 35 mg oral
phendimetrazine tartrate USP *anorexiant; CNS stimulant* [also: phendimetrazine] 35, 105 mg oral
Phendry; Phendry Children's Allergy Medicine elixir OTC *antihistamine* [diphenhydramine HCl] 12.5 mg/5 mL
phenelzine INN *antidepressant; MAO inhibitor* [also: phenelzine sulfate] ⓓ Phenazine; Phenylzin
phenelzine sulfate USP *antidepressant; MAO inhibitor* [also: phenelzine]
phenemal [see: phenobarbital]
Phenerbel-S tablets ℞ *GI anticholinergic; sedative; analgesic* [belladonna alkaloids; phenobarbital; ergotamine tartrate] 0.2•40•0.6 mg
Phenergan tablets, suppositories, injection ℞ *antihistamine; motion sickness; sleep aid; antiemetic; sedative* [promethazine HCl] 12.5, 25 mg; 12.5, 25, 50 mg; 25, 50 mg/mL ⓓ Phenaphen; Theragran
Phenergan Fortis syrup ℞ *antihistamine; motion sickness; sleep aid; antiemetic; sedative* [promethazine HCl; alcohol 1.5%] 25 mg/5 mL
Phenergan Plain syrup ℞ *antihistamine; motion sickness; sleep aid; antiemetic; sedative* [promethazine HCl] 6.25 mg/5 mL
Phenergan VC syrup ℞ *decongestant; antihistamine* [phenylephrine HCl; promethazine HCl; alcohol 7%] 5•6.25 mg/5 mL
Phenergan VC with Codeine syrup ℞ *narcotic antitussive; decongestant; antihistamine* [codeine phosphate; phenylephrine HCl; promethazine HCl; alcohol 7%] 10•5•6.25 mg/5 mL
Phenergan with Codeine syrup ℞ *narcotic antitussive; antihistamine*

[codeine phosphate; promethazine HCl; alcohol 7%] 10•6.25 mg/5 mL

Phenergan with Dextromethorphan syrup ℞ *antitussive; antihistamine* [dextromethorphan hydrobromide; promethazine HCl; alcohol 7%] 15•6.25 mg/5 mL

Phenergan-D tablets ℞ *antihistamine; decongestant* [promethazine HCl; pseudoephedrine HCl]

pheneridine INN

phenethanol [see: phenylethyl alcohol]

phenethazine [see: fenethazine]

phenethicillin potassium USP [also: pheneticillin]

phenethyl alcohol BAN *antimicrobial agent* [also: phenylethyl alcohol]

N-phenethylanthranilic acid [see: enfenamic acid]

phenethylazocine bromide [see: phenazocine hydrobromide]

phenethylhydrazine sulfate [see: phenelzine sulfate]

pheneticillin INN [also: phenethicillin potassium]

pheneticillin potassium [see: phenethicillin potassium]

Phenetron tablets, syrup ℞ *antihistamine; antitussive* [chlorpheniramine maleate] 4 mg; 2 mg/5 mL

Phenetron Compound sugar-coated tablets (discontinued 1993) OTC *antihistamine; analgesic* [chlorpheniramine maleate; aspirin; caffeine]

phenetsal [see: acetaminosalol]

pheneturide INN, BAN [also: acetylpheneturide]

Phenex-1 powder OTC *formula for infants with phenylketonuria*

Phenex-2 powder OTC *enteral nutritional therapy for phenylketonuria*

phenformin INN, BAN *hypoglycemic agent* [also: phenformin HCl]

phenformin HCl USP *hypoglycemic agent (removed from market by FDA in 1977, now available as an investigational drug)* [also: phenformin]

phenglutarimide INN, BAN

Phenhist DH with Codeine liquid ℞ *narcotic antitussive; decongestant; antihistamine* [codeine phosphate; pseudoephedrine HCl; chlorpheniramine maleate; alcohol 5%] 10•30•2 mg/5 mL

Phenhist Expectorant liquid ℞ *narcotic antitussive; decongestant; expectorant* [codeine phosphate; pseudoephedrine HCl; guaifenesin; alcohol 7.5%] 10•30•100 mg/5 mL

phenicarbazide INN

phenidiemal [see: phetharbital]

phenindamine INN *antihistamine* [also: phenindamine tartrate]

phenindamine tartrate USAN *antihistamine* [also: phenindamine]

phenindione USP, INN *anticoagulant*

pheniodol sodium INN [also: iodoalphionic acid]

pheniprazine INN, BAN

pheniprazine HCl [see: pheniprazine]

pheniramine INN [also: pheniramine maleate]

pheniramine maleate USAN [also: pheniramine]

phenisonone hydrobromide

Phenistix reagent strips for professional use (discontinued 1994) *in vitro diagnostic aid for phenylketonuria*

phenmetraline HCl [see: phenmetrazine HCl]

phenmetrazine INN *anorexiant* [also: phenmetrazine HCl]

phenmetrazine HCl USP *anorexiant; CNS stimulant* [also: phenmetrazine]

phenobamate [see: febarbamate]

phenobarbital USP, INN, JAN *anticonvulsant; hypnotic; sedative* [also: phenobarbitone] 15, 30, 60, 100 mg oral; 15, 20 mg/5 mL oral ▽ pentobarbital

phenobarbital sodium USP, INN, JAN *anticonvulsant; hypnotic; sedative* 30, 60, 65, 130 mg/mL injection

phenobarbitone BAN *anticonvulsant; hypnotic; sedative* [also: phenobarbital]

phenobutiodil INN

phenododecinium bromide [see: domiphen bromide]

Phenoject-50 injection ℞ *antihistamine; motion sickness; sleep aid; antiemetic; sedative* [promethazine HCl] 50 mg/mL

phenol USP *topical antiseptic/antipruritic; local anesthetic; preservative*

phenol, liquefied USP *topical antipruritic*

phenol, sodium salt [see: phenolate sodium]

phenol red [see: phenolsulfonphthalein]

phenolate sodium USAN *disinfectant*

Phenolated Calamine lotion OTC *topical poison ivy treatment* [calamine; zinc oxide; phenol] 8%•8%•1%

Phenolax wafers OTC *laxative* [phenolphthalein] 64.8 mg

phenolphthalein USP, INN *stimulant laxative*

phenolphthalein, white [see: phenolphthalein]

phenolphthalein, yellow USP *stimulant laxative*

phenolsulfonphthalein USP

phenolsulphonate sodium USP

phenomorphan INN, BAN

phenomycilline [see: penicillin V]

phenoperidine INN, BAN

phenopryldiasulfone sodium [see: solasulfone]

Phenoptic eye drops ℞ *ophthalmic decongestant/vasoconstrictor; mydriatic* [phenylephrine HCl] 2.5%

phenosulfophthalein [see: phenolsulfonphthalein]

phenothiazine NF, INN *antipsychotic*

phenothrin INN, BAN

phenoxazoline HCl [see: fenoxazoline HCl]

Phenoxine tablets OTC *diet aid* [phenylpropanolamine HCl] 25 mg ⊡ Phenazine

phenoxybenzamine INN *antihypertensive* [also: phenoxybenzamine HCl]

phenoxybenzamine HCl USP *antihypertensive; pheochromocytomic agent* [also: phenoxybenzamine]

phenoxymethylpenicillin INN *bactericidal antibiotic* [also: penicillin V]

phenoxypropazine BAN [also: fenoxypropazine]

phenoxypropylpenicillin [see: propicillin]

phenozolone [see: fenozolone]

phenprobamate INN, BAN

phenprocoumon USAN, USP, INN *anticoagulant*

phenprocumone [see: phenprocoumon]

phenpromethadrine [see: phenpromethamine]

phenpromethamine INN

phenpropamine citrate [see: alverine citrate]

phensuximide USP, INN, BAN *anticonvulsant*

phentermine USAN, INN *anorexiant* ⊡ phentolamine

phentermine HCl USP *anorexiant; CNS stimulant* 8, 15, 18.75, 30, 37.5 mg oral

phenthiazine [see: phenothiazine]

phentolamine INN, BAN *antihypertensive; pheochromocytomic agent* [also: phentolamine HCl] ⊡ phentermine; Ventolin

phentolamine HCl USP *antihypertensive; pheochromocytomic agent* [also: phentolamine]

phentolamine mesilate INN, JAN *antiadrenergic; antihypertensive; pheochromocytomic agent* [also: phentolamine mesylate]

phentolamine mesylate USP *antiadrenergic; antihypertensive; pheochromocytomic agent* [also: phentolamine mesilate]

phentolamine methanesulfonate [now: phentolamine mesylate]

Phentrol tablets ℞ *anorexiant* [phentermine HCl] 8 mg

Phentrol 2; Phentrol 4; Phentrol 5 capsules ℞ *anorexiant* [phentermine HCl] 30 mg

phentydrone

Phenurone tablets ℞ *anticonvulsant* [phenacemide] 500 mg

phenyl aminosalicylate USAN, BAN *antibacterial; tuberculostatic* [also: fenamisal]

phenyl salicylate NF *analgesic; not generally regarded as safe and effective as an antidiarrheal*

phenylalanine (L-phenylalanine) USAN, USP, INN *essential amino acid; symbols:* Phe, F

phenylalanine mustard (PAM) [see: melphalan]

L-phenylalanine mustard (L-PAM) [see: melphalan]

phenylazo diamino pyridine HCl [see: phenazopyridine HCl]

phenylbenzyl atropine [see: xenytropium bromide]

phenylbutazone USP, INN *antirheumatic; anti-inflammatory; antipyretic; analgesic*

phenylbutyrate sodium *(orphan: sickling disorders; S-S, S-C and S-thalassemia hemoglobinopathy)*

2-phenylbutyrylurea [see: pheneturide; acetylpheneturide]

phenylcarbinol [see: benzyl alcohol]

phenylcinchoninic acid [now: cinchophen]

α-phenyl-*p*-cresol carbamate [see: diphenan]

2-phenylcyclopentylamine HCl [see: cypenamine HCl]

phenyldimazone [see: normethadone]

Phenyldrine timed-release tablets OTC *diet aid* [phenylpropanolamine HCl] 75 mg

phenylephrine (PE) INN, BAN *nasal decongestant; ocular vasoconstrictor; vasopressor for hypotensive or cardiac shock* [also: phenylephrine HCl]

phenylephrine bitartrate *bronchodilator; vasoconstrictor*

phenylephrine HCl USP *nasal decongestant; ocular vasoconstrictor; vasopressor for hypotensive or cardiac shock* [also: phenylephrine] 0.25%, 0.5%, 1% nose drops or spray; 2.5%, 10% eye drops; 1% injection

phenylephrine tannate

phenylethanol [see: phenylethyl alcohol]

phenylethyl alcohol USP *antimicrobial agent; preservative* [also: phenethyl alcohol]

phenylethylmalonylurea [see: phenobarbital]

Phenylfenesin L.A. long-acting tablets ℞ *decongestant; expectorant* [phenylpropanolamine HCl; guaifenesin] 75•400 mg

Phenyl-Free liquid OTC *special diet for infants with phenylketonuria (PKU)*

Phenylgesic tablets OTC *antihistamine; analgesic* [phenyltoloxamine citrate; acetaminophen] 30•325 mg

phenylindanedione [see: phenindione]

phenylmercuric acetate NF *antimicrobial agent; preservative*

phenylmercuric borate INN

phenylmercuric chloride NF

phenylmercuric nitrate NF *antimicrobial agent; preservative; topical antiseptic*

phenylone [see: antipyrine]

phenylpropanolamine (PPA) INN, BAN *vasoconstrictor; nasal decongestant; nonprescription diet aid* [also: phenylpropanolamine HCl]

phenylpropanolamine HCl USP *vasoconstrictor; nasal decongestant; nonprescription diet aid* [also: phenylpropanolamine] 25, 50, 75 mg oral

phenylpropanolamine polistirex USAN *adrenergic; vasoconstrictor*

1-phenylsemicarbazide [see: phenicarbazide]

phenylthilone [see: phenythilone]

phenyltoloxamine INN

phenyltoloxamine citrate *antihistamine*

Phenylzin eye drops (discontinued 1993) OTC *topical ocular decongestant; astringent; antiseptic* [phenylephrine HCl; zinc sulfate] ⓖ phenelzine

phenyracillin INN

phenyramidol HCl USAN *analgesic; skeletal muscle relaxant* [also: fenyramidol]

phenythilone INN

phenytoin USAN, USP, INN, BAN *hydantoin-type anticonvulsant*

phenytoin redox [see: redox-phenytoin]

phenytoin sodium USP *hydantoin-type anticonvulsant* 100 mg oral; 50 mg/mL injection

Pherazine syrup ℞ *antihistamine* [promethazine HCl] ⓖ Phazyme; Phenazine

Pherazine DM syrup ℞ *antitussive; antihistamine* [dextromethorphan hydrobromide; promethazine HCl; alcohol 7%] 15•6.25 mg/5 mL

Pherazine VC syrup (name changed to Promethazine VC Plain in 1995)

Pherazine VC with Codeine syrup ℞ *narcotic antitussive; decongestant; antihistamine* [codeine phosphate; phenylephrine HCl; promethazine HCl; alcohol 7%] 10•5•6.25 mg/5 mL

Pherazine with Codeine syrup ℞ *narcotic antitussive; antihistamine* [codeine phosphate; promethazine HCl; alcohol 7%] 10•6.25 mg/5 mL

Pheryl E 400 tablets OTC *vitamin supplement* [vitamin E]

phetharbital INN

phezathion [see: fezatione]

Phicon cream OTC *topical anesthetic; emollient* [pramoxine HCl; vitamins A and E] 0.5%•7500 IU•2000 IU

Phicon F cream OTC *topical anesthetic; antifungal* [pramoxine HCl; undecylenic acid] 0.05%•8%

Phillips' Chewable tablets OTC *antacid* [magnesium hydroxide] 311 mg

Phillips' Laxative gelcaps OTC *laxative; stool softener* [phenolphthalein; docusate sodium] 90•83 mg

Phillips' LaxCaps capsules OTC *laxative; stool softener* [phenolphthalein; docusate sodium] 90•83 mg

Phillips' Milk of Magnesia; Concentrated Phillips' Milk of Magnesia liquid OTC *antacid; laxative* [magnesium hydroxide] 400 mg/5 mL; 800 mg/5 mL

pHisoAc BP cream (discontinued 1992) OTC *topical keratolytic for acne* [benzoyl peroxide] 10%

pHisoDerm; pHisoDerm for Baby liquid OTC *soap-free therapeutic skin cleanser*

pHisoDerm Cleansing Bar OTC *therapeutic skin cleanser*

pHisoHex liquid ℞ *bacteriostatic skin cleanser* [hexachlorophene] 3% 2 Fostex

phloropropiophenone [see: flopropione]

pholcodine INN

pholedrine INN, BAN

pholescutol [see: folescutol]

PhosChol softgels, liquid concentrate OTC *neurotransmitter; lipotropic* [phosphatidylcholine] 565, 900 mg; 3 g/5 mL

phoscolic acid [see: foscolic acid]

Phos-Ex 62.5 Mini-Tabs; Phos-Ex 167; Phos-Ex 250 tablets (discontinued 1994) OTC *calcium supplement* [calcium acetate] 250 mg; 668 mg; 1000 mg

Phos-Ex 125 capsules (discontinued 1994) OTC *calcium supplement* [calcium acetate] 500 mg

Phos-Flur oral rinse ℞ *dental caries preventative* [acidulated phosphate fluoride] 0.44 mg/mL

PhosLo tablets ℞ *buffering agent; for hyperphosphatemia in end-stage renal failure (orphan)* [calcium acetate] 667 mg

pHos-pHaid E.C. enteric-coated tablets (discontinued 1993) ℞ *urinary acidifier* [ammonium biphosphate; sodium biphosphate; sodium acid pyrophosphate] 95•100•55, 190•200•110 mg

Phosphaljel oral suspension (discontinued 1994) OTC *no longer labeled for use as an antacid* [aluminum phosphate gel] 44.6 mg/mL

phosphate salt of tricyclic nucleoside [now: triciribine phosphate]

phosphatidylcholine (PC) [see: lecithin]

phosphinic acid [see: hypophosphorous acid]

2,2′-phosphinicodilactic acid (PDLA) [see: foscolic acid]

Phosphocol P 32 suspension for intracavitary instillation, interstitial injection ℞ *radiopharmaceutical antineoplastic* [chromic phosphate P 32] 10, 15 mCi

phosphocysteamine *(orphan: cystinosis)*

Phospholine Iodide powder for eye drops ℞ *antiglaucoma agent; irreversible cholinesterase inhibitor miotic* [echothiophate iodide] 0.03%, 0.06%, 0.125%, 0.25%

phosphonoformic acid (PFA) [see: foscarnet sodium]

phosphorated carbohydrate solution (fructose, dextrose & orthophosphoric acid) *antinauseant; antiemetic*

phosphoric acid NF *solvent; acidifying agent*

phosphoric acid, aluminum salt [see: aluminum phosphate gel]

phosphoric acid, calcium salt [see: calcium phosphate, dibasic]

phosphoric acid, chromium salt [see: chromic phosphate Cr 51 & P 32]
phosphoric acid, diammonium salt [see: ammonium phosphate]
phosphoric acid, dipotassium salt [see: potassium phosphate, dibasic]
phosphoric acid, disodium salt heptahydrate [see: sodium phosphate, dibasic]
phosphoric acid, disodium salt hydrate [see: sodium phosphate, dibasic]
phosphoric acid, magnesium salt [see: magnesium phosphate]
phosphoric acid, monopotassium salt [see: potassium phosphate, monobasic]
phosphoric acid, monosodium salt dihydrate [see: sodium phosphate, monobasic]
phosphoric acid, monosodium salt monohydrate [see: sodium phosphate, monobasic]
phosphorofluoridic acid, disodium salt [see: sodium monofluorophosphate]
phosphorus *element (P)*
Phospho-Soda [see: Fleet Phospho-Soda]
phosphothiamine [see: monophosphothiamine]
Photofrin powder for IV injection *laser light-activated antineoplastic for photodynamic therapy (PDT) of esophageal cancer* [porfimer sodium] 75 mg
Photoplex lotion OTC *broad-spectrum sunscreen* [avobenzone; padimate O]
phoxim INN, BAN
Phrenilin tablets ℞ *analgesic; antipyretic; sedative* [acetaminophen; butalbital] 325•50
Phrenilin Forte capsules ℞ *analgesic; antipyretic; sedative* [acetaminophen; butalbital] 650•50 mg
PHRT (procarbazine, hydroxyurea, radiotherapy) *chemotherapy protocol*
phthalofyne USAN *veterinary anthelmintic* [also: ftalofyne]
phthalylsulfacetamide NF
phthalylsulfamethizole INN
phthalylsulfathiazole USP, INN

phylcardin [see: aminophylline]
phyllindon [see: aminophylline]
Phyllocontin controlled-release tablets ℞ *bronchodilator* [aminophylline] 225 mg
phylloquinone [see: phytonadione]
Phylorinol liquid OTC *topical antipruritic/counterirritant; mild local anesthetic; antiseptic; astringent; oral deodorant* [phenol; boric acid; strong iodine solution; chlorophyllin copper complex] 0.6%•?•?•?
Phylorinol mouthwash/gargle OTC *topical antipruritic/counterirritant; mild local anesthetic* [phenol] 0.6%
physiological irrigating solution *for general irrigating, washing and rinsing; not for injection*
Physiolyte liquid ℞ *sterile irrigant* [physiological irrigating solution]
PhysioSol liquid ℞ *sterile irrigant* [physiological irrigating solution]
Physiotens ℞ *investigational antihypertensive* [monoxidine]
physostigmine USP, BAN *antiglaucoma agent; reversible cholinesterase inhibitor miotic* ⓘ pyridostigmine; Prostigmin
physostigmine salicylate USP *cholinergic to reverse anticholinergic overdose; (orphan: Friedreich's and other ataxias)*
physostigmine sulfate USP *ophthalmic cholinergic*
phytate persodium USAN *pharmaceutic aid*
phytate sodium USAN *calcium-chelating agent*
phytic acid [see: fytic acid]
phytomenadione INN, BAN *vitamin K_1; prothrombogenic* [also: phytonadione]
phytonadiol sodium diphosphate INN
phytonadione USP *vitamin K_1; prothrombogenic* [also: phytomenadione] 2 mg/mL injection
PIA (Platinol, ifosfamide, Adriamycin) *chemotherapy protocol*
pibecarb INN
piberaline INN
picafibrate INN
picartamide INN
picenadol INN *analgesic* [also: picenadol HCl]

picenadol HCl USAN *analgesic* [also: picenadol]
picilorex INN
piclonidine INN
piclopastine INN
picloxydine INN, BAN
picobenzide INN
picodralazine INN
picolamine INN
piconol INN
picoperine INN
picoprazole INN
picotrin INN *keratolytic* [also: picotrin diolamine]
picotrin diolamine USAN *keratolytic* [also: picotrin]
picric acid [see: trinitrophenol]
picrotoxin NF
picumast INN, BAN
picumeterol INN, BAN *bronchodilator* [also: picumeterol fumarate]
picumeterol fumarate USAN *bronchodilator* [also: picumeterol]
pidolacetamol INN
pidolic acid INN
pifarnine USAN, INN *gastric antiulcerative*
pifenate INN, BAN
pifexole INN
piflutixol INN
pifoxime INN
piketoprofen INN
Pilagan eye drops ℞ *antiglaucoma agent; direct-acting miotic* [pilocarpine nitrate] 1%, 2%, 4%
pildralazine INN
Pilocar eye drops ℞ *antiglaucoma agent; direct-acting miotic* [pilocarpine HCl] 0.5%, 1%, 2%, 3%, 4%, 6%
pilocarpine USP, BAN *antiglaucoma agent; ophthalmic cholinergic*
pilocarpine HCl USP *ophthalmic cholinergic; antiglaucoma miotic; (orphan: xerostomia; keratoconjunctivitis sicca)* 0.5%, 1%, 2%, 4%, 6%, 8% eye drops
pilocarpine nitrate USP *ophthalmic cholinergic; antiglaucoma agent; miotic*
Pilocarpine SME ℞ *investigational glaucoma treatment* [pilocarpine]
Pilopine HS ophthalmic gel ℞ *antiglaucoma agent; direct-acting miotic* [pilocarpine HCl] 4%

Piloptic-½; Piloptic-1; Piloptic-2; Piloptic-3; Piloptic-4; Piloptic-6 eye drops ℞ *antiglaucoma agent; direct-acting miotic* [pilocarpine HCl] 0.5%; 1%; 2%; 3%; 4%; 6%
Pilopto-Carpine eye drops ℞ *antiglaucoma agent; direct-acting miotic* [pilocarpine HCl] 4%
Pilostat eye drops ℞ *antiglaucoma agent; direct-acting miotic* [pilocarpine HCl] 0.5%, 1%, 2%, 3%, 4%, 6%
Pilpak (trademarked packaging form) *patient compliance package*
Pima syrup ℞ *expectorant* [potassium iodide] 325 mg/5 mL
pimagedine HCl USAN *advanced glycosylation end-product formation inhibitor for diabetes*
pimaricin JAN *ophthalmic antibacterial/antifungal antibiotic* [also: natamycin]
pimeclone INN
pimefylline INN
pimelautide INN
pimetacin INN
pimethixene INN
pimetine INN *antihyperlipoproteinemic* [also: pimetine HCl]
pimetine HCl USAN *antihyperlipoproteinemic* [also: pimetine]
pimetixene [see: pimethixene]
pimetremide INN
pimeverine [see: pimetremide]
piminodine INN [also: piminodine esylate]
piminodine esylate NF [also: piminodine]
piminodine ethanesulfonate [see: piminodine esylate]
pimobendan USAN, INN *cardiotonic*
pimonidazole INN, BAN
pimozide USAN, USP, INN, BAN, JAN *antipsychotic; neuroleptic; suppresses symptoms of Tourette syndrome*
pinacidil USAN, INN *antihypertensive*
pinadoline USAN, INN *analgesic*
pinafide INN
pinaverium bromide INN
pinazepam INN
pincainide INN
Pindac ℞ *investigational antihypertensive* [pinacidil]

pindolol USAN, USP, INN, BAN *vasodilator; antiadrenergic (β-receptor)* 5, 10 mg oral
pine needle oil NF
pine tar USP
Pink Bismuth liquid OTC *antidiarrheal; antinauseant* [bismuth subsalicylate] 130, 262 mg/15 mL
pinolcaine INN
pinoxepin INN *antipsychotic* [also: pinoxepin HCl]
pinoxepin HCl USAN *antipsychotic* [also: pinoxepin]
Pin-Rid soft gel capsules, liquid OTC *anthelmintic* [pyrantel pamoate] 180 mg; 144 mg/mL
Pin-X liquid OTC *anthelmintic* [pyrantel pamoate] 50 mg/mL
pioglitazone INN *antidiabetic* [also: pioglitazone HCl]
pioglitazone HCl USAN *antidiabetic* [also: pioglitazone]
pipacycline INN
pipamazine INN
pipamperone USAN, INN *antipsychotic*
pipaneperone [see: pipamperone]
pipazetate INN *antitussive* [also: pipazethate]
pipazethate USAN *antitussive* [also: pipazetate]
pipebuzone INN
pipecuronium bromide USAN, INN, BAN *muscle relaxant; nondepolarizing neuromuscular blocker; adjunct to anesthesia*
pipemidic acid INN
pipenzolate bromide INN
pipenzolate methylbromide [see: pipenzolate bromide]
pipenzolone bromide [see: pipenzolate bromide]
pipequaline INN
piperacetazine USAN, USP, INN *antipsychotic* ⑨ piperazine
piperacillin INN, BAN *bactericidal antibiotic* [also: piperacillin sodium]
piperacillin sodium USAN, USP, JAN *bactericidal antibiotic* [also: piperacillin]
piperamide INN *anthelmintic* [also: piperamide maleate]
piperamide maleate USAN *anthelmintic* [also: piperamide]

piperamine [see: bamipine]
piperazine USP *anthelmintic* ⑨ piperacetazine
piperazine calcium edetate INN *anthelmintic* [also: piperazine edetate calcium]
piperazine citrate USP *anthelmintic* 250 mg oral; 500 mg/mL oral
piperazine citrate hydrate [see: piperazine citrate]
piperazine edetate calcium USAN *anthelmintic* [also: piperazine calcium edetate]
piperazine estrone sulfate [now: estropipate]
piperazine hexahydrate [see: piperazine citrate]
piperazine phosphate
piperazine phosphate monohydrate [see: piperazine phosphate]
piperazine theophylline ethanoate [see: acefylline piperazine]
piperidine phosphate
piperidolate INN [also: piperidolate HCl]
piperidolate HCl USP [also: piperidolate]
piperilate [see: pipethanate]
piperine USP
piperocaine INN [also: piperocaine HCl]
piperocaine HCl USP [also: piperocaine]
piperonyl butoxide *pediculicide*
piperoxan
piperphenidol HCl
piperylone INN
pipethanate INN
pipobroman USAN, USP, INN *alkylating antineoplastic*
pipoctanone INN
pipofezine INN
piposulfan USAN, INN *antineoplastic*
pipotiazine INN *antipsychotic* [also: pipotiazine palmitate]
pipotiazine palmitate USAN *antipsychotic* [also: pipotiazine]
pipoxizine
pipoxolan INN *muscle relaxant* [also: pipoxolan HCl]
pipoxolan HCl USAN *muscle relaxant* [also: pipoxolan]

Pipracil powder for IV or IM injection ℞ *extended-spectrum penicillin-type antibiotic* [piperacillin sodium] 2, 3, 4, 20 g
pipradimadol INN
pipradrol INN [also: pipradrol HCl]
pipradrol HCl NF [also: pipradrol]
pipramadol INN
pipratecol INN
piprinhydrinate INN, BAN
piprocurarium iodide INN
piprofurol INN
piprozolin USAN, INN *choleretic*
piquindone INN *antipsychotic* [also: piquindone HCl]
piquindone HCl USAN *antipsychotic* [also: piquindone]
piquizil INN *bronchodilator* [also: piquizil HCl]
piquizil HCl USAN *bronchodilator* [also: piquizil]
piracetam USAN, INN, BAN *cognition adjuvant; (orphan: myoclonus)* ② piroxicam
pirandamine INN *antidepressant* [also: pirandamine HCl]
pirandamine HCl USAN *antidepressant* [also: pirandamine]
pirarubicin INN
piraxelate INN
pirazmonam INN *antimicrobial* [also: pirazmonam sodium]
pirazmonam sodium USAN *antimicrobial* [also: pirazmonam]
pirazofurin INN *antineoplastic* [also: pyrazofurin]
pirazolac USAN, INN, BAN *antirheumatic*
pirbenicillin INN *antibacterial* [also: pirbenicillin sodium]
pirbenicillin sodium USAN *antibacterial* [also: pirbenicillin]
pirbuterol INN *bronchodilator* [also: pirbuterol acetate]
pirbuterol acetate USAN *bronchodilator* [also: pirbuterol]
pirbuterol HCl USAN *bronchodilator*
pirdonium bromide INN
pirenoxine INN
pirenperone USAN, INN, BAN *tranquilizer*
pirenzepine INN, BAN *antiulcerative* [also: pirenzepine HCl]
pirenzepine HCl USAN, JAN *antiulcerative* [also: pirenzepine]

pirepolol INN
piretanide USAN, INN *diuretic*
pirfenidone USAN, INN *analgesic; antiinflammatory; antipyretic*
piribedil INN
piribenzyl methylsulfate [see: bevonium metilsulfate]
piridicillin INN *antibacterial* [also: piridicillin sodium]
piridicillin sodium USAN *antibacterial* [also: piridicillin]
piridocaine INN
piridocaine HCl [see: piridocaine]
piridoxilate INN, BAN
piridronate sodium USAN *calcium regulator*
piridronic acid INN
pirifibrate INN
pirinidazole INN
pirinitramide [see: piritramide]
pirinixic acid INN
pirinixil INN
piriprost USAN *antiasthmatic*
piriprost potassium USAN *antiasthmatic*
piriqualone INN
pirisudanol INN
piritramide INN, BAN
piritrexim INN *antiproliferative agent* [also: piritrexim isethionate]
piritrexim isethionate USAN *antiproliferative; (orphan: Pneumocystis carinii; Mycobacterium avium complex; Toxoplasma gondii)* [also: piritrexim]
pirlimycin HCl USAN *antibacterial*
pirlindole INN
pirmagrel USAN, INN *thromboxane synthetase inhibitor*
pirmenol INN *antiarrhythmic* [also: pirmenol HCl]
pirmenol HCl USAN *antiarrhythmic* [also: pirmenol]
pirnabin INN *antiglaucoma agent* [also: pirnabine]
pirnabine USAN *antiglaucoma agent* [also: pirnabin]
piroctone USAN, INN *antiseborrheic*
piroctone olamine USAN *antiseborrheic*
pirodavir USAN, INN, BAN *antiviral*
pirogliride INN *antidiabetic* [also: pirogliride tartrate]
pirogliride tartrate USAN *antidiabetic* [also: pirogliride]

piroheptine INN
pirolate USAN, INN *antiasthmatic*
pirolazamide USAN, INN *antiarrhythmic*
piromidic acid INN
piroxantrone INN *antineoplastic* [also: piroxantrone HCl]
piroxantrone HCl USAN *antineoplastic* [also: piroxantrone]
piroxicam USAN, USP, INN, BAN, JAN *antiarthritic; nonsteroidal anti-inflammatory drug (NSAID); analgesic; antiarthritic* 10, 20 mg oral ⊠ piracetam
piroxicam cinnamate USAN *anti-inflammatory*
piroxicam olamine USAN *analgesic; anti-inflammatory*
piroxicillin INN
piroximone USAN, INN, BAN *cardiotonic*
pirozadil INN
pirprofen USAN, INN, BAN *anti-inflammatory*
pirquinozol USAN, INN *antiallergic*
pirralkonium bromide INN
pirroksan [now: proroxan HCl]
pirsidomine USAN, INN *vasodilator*
pirtenidine INN
pitenodil INN
Pitocin IV, IM injection ℞ *induction of labor; postpartum bleeding; incomplete abortion* [oxytocin] 10 U/mL ⊠ Pitressin
pitofenone INN
Pitressin Synthetic IM or subcu injection ℞ *pituitary antidiuretic hormone for diabetes insipidus or prevention of abdominal distention* [vasopressin] 20 U/mL ⊠ Pitocin
pituitary, anterior
pituitary, posterior USP *antidiuretic hormone*
pituxate INN
pivalate USAN, INN, BAN *combining name for radicals or groups*
pivampicillin INN *antibacterial* [also: pivampicillin HCl]
pivampicillin HCl USAN *antibacterial* [also: pivampicillin]
pivampicillin pamoate USAN *antibacterial*
pivampicillin probenate USAN *antibacterial*
pivenfrine INN

pivmecillinam INN, BAN *antibacterial* [also: amdinocillin pivoxil; pivmecillinam HCl]
pivmecillinam HCl JAN *antibacterial* [also: amdinocillin pivoxil; pivmecillinam]
pivopril USAN *antihypertensive*
pivoxazepam INN
pivoxetil USAN, INN *combining name for radicals or groups*
pivoxil USAN, INN *combining name for radicals or groups*
pivsulbactam BAN *β-lactamase inhibitor; penicillin/cephalosporin synergist* [also: sulbactam pivoxil]
pix pini [see: pine tar]
PIXY-321 (GM-CSF + IL-3) *investigational treatment for non-Hodgkin's lymphoma*
Pixykine ℞ *investigational second-generation colony stimulating factor for neutropenia and thrombocytopenia* [PIXY-321 (granulocyte macrophage-colony stimulating factor + interleukin-3)]
pizotifen INN, BAN *anabolic; antidepressant; serotonin inhibitor (migraine specific)* [also: pizotyline]
pizotyline USAN *anabolic; antidepressant; serotonin inhibitor (migraine specific)* [also: pizotifen]
placebo *no medicinal value* [also: obecalp]
Placidyl capsules ℞ *hypnotic* [ethchlorvynol] 200, 500, 750 mg ⊠ Pathocil
plafibride INN
plague vaccine USP *active bacterin for plague (Yersinia pestis)* $1.8–2.2 \times 10^8$ bacilli/mL IM injection
planadalin [see: carbromal]
plantago seed USP *laxative*
plantain seed [see: plantago seed]
Plaquenil Sulfate tablets ℞ *antimalarial; antirheumatic* [hydroxychloroquine sulfate] 200 mg
Plasbumin-5; Plasbumin-25 IV infusion ℞ *blood volume expander for shock, burns, and hypoproteinemia* [human albumin] 5%; 25%
plasma, antihemophilic human USP
plasma concentrate factor IX [see: factor IX complex]

plasma protein fraction USP *blood volume supporter*

plasma protein fraction, human [now: plasma protein fraction]

plasma thromboplastin component (PTC) [see: factor IX]

Plasma-Lyte A pH 7.4; Plasma-Lyte R; Plasma-Lyte 56; Plasma-Lyte 148 IV infusion ℞ *intravenous electrolyte therapy* [combined electrolyte solution]

Plasma-Lyte M (R; 56; 148) and 5% Dextrose IV infusion ℞ *intravenous nutritional/electrolyte therapy* [combined electrolyte solution; dextrose]

Plasmanate IV infusion ℞ *blood volume expander for shock due to burns, trauma and surgery* [plasma protein fraction] 5%

Plasma-Plex IV infusion ℞ *blood volume expander for shock due to burns, trauma and surgery* [plasma protein fraction] 5%

Plasmatein IV infusion ℞ *blood volume expander for shock due to burns, trauma and surgery* [plasma protein fraction] 5%

plasmin BAN [also: fibrinolysin, human]

Plateau Cap (trademarked dosage form) *controlled-release capsule*

platelet cofactor II [see: factor IX]

platelet concentrate USP *platelet replenisher*

platelet factor 4, recombinant (rPF4) *investigational antineoplastic for various cancers and heparin neutralizer*

platelet-derived growth factor *investigational treatment for diabetic skin ulcers and pressure ulcers*

Platinol powder for IV injection ℞ *alkylating antineoplastic for testicular, ovarian, bladder, lung, head, neck, and esophageal cancers* [cisplatin] 10, 50 mg

Platinol-AQ IV injection ℞ *alkylating antineoplastic for testicular, ovarian, bladder, lung, head, neck, and esophageal cancers* [cisplatin] 1 mg/mL

platinum *element (Pt)*

cis-**platinum** [now: cisplatin]

cis-**platinum II** [now: cisplatin]

platinum diamminodichloride [see: cisplatin]

plaunotol INN

plauracin USAN, INN *veterinary growth stimulant*

Plax, Advanced Formula mouthwash/gargle OTC [sodium pyrophosphate]

Plegine tablets ℞ *anorexiant* [phendimetrazine tartrate] 35 mg

Plegisol solution ℞ *cardioplegic solution* [calcium chloride; magnesium chloride; potassium chloride; sodium chloride] 17.6•325.3•119.3•643 mg/100 mL

Plendil extended-release tablets ℞ *antihypertensive; investigational antianginal* [felodipine] 2.5, 5, 10 mg

pleuromulin INN

Pliagel solution OTC *surfactant cleaning solution for soft contact lenses*

plicamycin USAN, USP, INN *antibiotic antineoplastic*

plomestane USAN *antineoplastic; aromatase inhibitor*

plutonium *element (Pu)*

PMB 200; PMB 400 tablets ℞ *estrogen replacement therapy for postmenopausal disorders* [conjugated estrogens; meprobamate] 0.45•200 mg; 0.45•400 mg

PMEA *investigational (Phase I/II) antiviral nucleoside analog for HIV and various herpesvirus types*

PMMA (polymethylmethacrylate) [q.v.]

P-MVAC (Platinol, methotrexate, vinblastine, Adriamycin, carboplatin) *chemotherapy protocol*

pneumococcal vaccine, polyvalent *active bacterin for pneumococcal pneumonia (23 types)*

Pneumomist sustained-release tablets ℞ *expectorant* [guaifenesin] 600 mg

Pneumopent for inhalation ℞ *(orphan: Pneumocystis carinii pneumonia)* [pentamidine isethionate]

Pneumotussin HC syrup ℞ *narcotic antitussive; expectorant* [hydrocodone bitartrate; guaifenesin] 5•100 mg/5 mL

Pneumovax 23 subcu or IM injection ℞ *pneumonia vaccine* [pneumococcal vaccine, polyvalent] 0.5 mL

Pnu-Imune 23 subcu or IM injection ℞ *pneumonia vaccine* [pneumococcal vaccine, polyvalent] 0.5 mL
pobilukast edamine USAN *antiasthmatic*
POC (procarbazine, Oncovin, CCNU) *chemotherapy protocol*
POCA (prednisone, Oncovin, cytarabine, Adriamycin) *chemotherapy protocol*
POCC (procarbazine, Oncovin, cyclophosphamide, CCNU) *chemotherapy protocol*
Pockethaler (trademarked delivery device) *nasal inhalation aerosol*
Pod-Ben-25 liquid (discontinued 1994) ℞ *topical keratolytic* [podophyllum resin] 25%
podilfen INN
Podocon-25 liquid ℞ *topical keratolytic for genital warts* [podophyllum resin] 25%
podofilox USAN *antimitotic* [also: podophyllotoxin]
Podofin liquid ℞ *topical keratolytic for genital warts* [podophyllum resin] 25% ⑨ podophyllin
podophyllin [see: podophyllum resin] ⑨ Podofin
podophyllotoxin BAN *antimitotic* [also: podofilox]
podophyllum USP *pharmaceutic necessity*
podophyllum resin USP *caustic; cytotoxic agent for genital warts*
Point-Two oral rinse ℞ *topical dental caries preventative* [sodium fluoride; alcohol 6%] 0.2%
Poison Antidote Kit OTC *emergency treatment for various poisons* [syrup of ipecac; charcoal suspension] 30•60 mL
poison ivy extract, alum precipitated USAN *ivy poisoning counteractant*
poison oak extract USAN *antiallergic*
Poison Oak-N-Ivy Armor lotion OTC *topical poison ivy protectant*
polacrilin USAN, INN *pharmaceutic aid*
polacrilin potassium USAN, NF *tablet disintegrant*
Poladex timed-release tablets ℞ *antihistamine* [dexchlorpheniramine maleate] 4, 6 mg

Polaramine tablets, Repetabs (repeat-action tablets), syrup ℞ *antihistamine* [dexchlorpheniramine maleate] 2 mg; 6 mg; 2 mg/5 mL
Polaramine Expectorant liquid ℞ *decongestant; antihistamine; expectorant* [pseudoephedrine sulfate; dexchlorpheniramine maleate; guaifenesin; alcohol 7.2%] 20•2•100 mg/5 mL
poldine methylsulfate USAN, USP *anticholinergic* [also: poldine metilsulfate]
poldine metilsulfate INN *anticholinergic* [also: poldine methylsulfate]
policapram USAN, INN *tablet binder*
policresulen INN
polidexide sulfate INN
polidocanol
polifeprosan INN *pharmaceutic aid* [also: polifeprosan 20]
polifeprosan 20 USAN *pharmaceutic aid* [also: polifeprosan]
poligeenan USAN, INN *dispersing agent*
poliglecaprone 25 USAN *absorbable surgical suture material*
poliglecaprone 90 USAN *absorbable surgical suture coating*
poliglusam USAN *antihemorrhagic*
polignate sodium USAN *pepsin enzyme inhibitor*
polihexanide INN [also: polyhexanide]
poliomyelitis vaccine [now: poliovirus vaccine, inactivated]
Poliovax subcu injection (discontinued 1993) ℞ *poliomyelitis vaccine* [poliovirus vaccine, inactivated] 0.5 mL
poliovirus vaccine, inactivated (IPV) USP *active immunizing agent for poliomyelitis*
poliovirus vaccine, live oral (OPV) USP *active immunizing agent for poliomyelitis*
polipropene 25 USAN *tablet excipient*
polisaponin INN
politef INN *prosthetic aid* [also: polytef]
polixetonium chloride USAN, INN *preservative*
Polocaine injection ℞ *injectable local anesthetic* [mepivacaine HCl] 1%, 2%, 3%
Polocaine injection ℞ *injectable local anesthetic* [mepivacaine HCl; levonordefrin] 2%•1:20,000

Polocaine MPF injection ℞ *injectable local anesthetic* [mepivacaine HCl] 1%, 1.5%, 2%

polonium *element (Po)*

Poloris Dental Poultice (discontinued 1994) OTC *topical oral anesthetic; antipruritic/counterirritant* [benzocaine; capsicum] 7.5•4.6 mg

poloxalene USAN, INN, BAN *surfactant*

poloxamer USAN, NF, INN, BAN *ointment and suppository base; tablet binder*

poloxamer 124 USAN *surfactant; emulsifier; solubilizer; stabilizer*

poloxamer 188 USAN *surfactant; emulsifier; solubilizer; (orphan: sickle cell crisis; severe burns)*

poloxamer 237 USAN *surfactant; emulsifier; solubilizer; stabilizer*

poloxamer 331 *(orphan: toxoplasmosis of AIDS)*

poloxamer 338 USAN *surfactant; emulsifier; solubilizer; stabilizer*

poloxamer 407 USAN *surfactant; emulsifier; solubilizer; stabilizer*

poly I: poly C12U *investigational antiviral/immunomodulator; (orphan: AIDS; renal cell carcinoma; chronic fatigue)*

polyamine resin [see: polyamine-methylene resin]

polyamine-methylene resin

polyanhydroglucose [see: dextran]

polyanhydroglucuronic acid [see: dextran]

polybenzarsol INN

polybutester USAN *surgical suture material*

polybutilate USAN *surgical suture coating*

polycarbokane [see: polycarbophil]

polycarbophil USP, INN, BAN *bulk laxative*

Polycillin capsules, powder for oral suspension, pediatric drops ℞ *penicillin-type antibiotic* [ampicillin trihydrate] 250, 500 mg; 125, 250, 500 mg/5 mL; 100 mg/mL ⌘ penicillin

Polycillin-N powder for IV or IM injection ℞ *penicillin-type antibiotic* [ampicillin sodium] 0.125, 0.25, 0.5, 1, 2, 10 g

Polycillin-PRB powder for oral suspension ℞ *antibiotic for Neisseria gonorrhoeae* [ampicillin trihydrate; probenecid] 3.5•1 g

Polycitra syrup ℞ *urinary alkalinizing agent* [potassium citrate; sodium citrate; citric acid] 550•500•334 mg/5 mL

Polycitra-K solution, crystals ℞ *urinary alkalizing agent; (orphan: dissolution of uric acid and cysteine calculi)* [potassium citrate; citric acid] 1100• 334 mg/5 mL; 3300•1002 mg/packet

Polycitra-LC solution ℞ *urinary alkalizing agent; (orphan: dissolution of urinary stones)* [potassium citrate; sodium citrate; citric acid] 550• 500•334 mg/5 mL

Polycose liquid, powder OTC *carbohydrate caloric supplement* [glucose polymers]

polydextrose USAN *food additive*

polydimethylsiloxane *surgical aid (retinal tamponade) for retinal detachment*

Polydine ointment, scrub, solution OTC *broad-spectrum antimicrobial* [povidone-iodine]

polydioxanone USAN *absorbable surgical suture material*

polyelectrolyte 211 [see: sodium alginate]

polyestradiol phosphate INN, BAN *antineoplastic; estrogen*

polyetadene INN *antacid* [also: polyethadene]

polyethadene USAN *antacid* [also: polyetadene]

polyethylene excipient NF *stiffening agent*

polyethylene glycol (PEG) NF *ointment and suppository base; solvent*

polyethylene glycol n [n refers to the molecular weight: 300, 400, 1000, etc.]

polyethylene glycol n dioleate [n refers to the molecular weight: 300, 400, 1000, etc.]

polyethylene glycol 8 monostearate [see: polyoxyl 8 stearate]

polyethylene glycol 1000 monocetyl ether [see: cetomacrogol 1000]

polyethylene glycol 1540 NF

polyethylene glycol 4000 USP [also: macrogol 4000]

polyethylene glycol 6000 USP
polyethylene glycol monoleyl ether [see: polyoxyl 10 oleyl ether]
polyethylene glycol monomethyl ether NF *excipient*
polyethylene glycol monostearate [see: polyoxyl 40 & 50 stearate]
polyethylene glycol-electrolyte solution (PEG-ES) *pre-procedure bowel evacuant* [contains PEG 3350]
polyethylene glycol-superoxide dismutase (PEG-SOD) [see: pegorgotein]
polyethylene oxide NF *suspending and viscosity agent; tablet binder*
polyferose USAN *hematinic*
Polygam (name changed to Polygam S/D in 1994)
Polygam S/D freeze-dried powder for IV infusion ℞ *passive immunizing agent; immunomodulator for AIDS/ARC* [immune globulin, solvent/detergent treated] 50 mg/mL
polygeline INN, BAN
polyglactin 370 USAN *absorbable surgical suture coating*
polyglactin 910 USAN *absorbable surgical suture material*
polyglycolic acid USAN, INN *surgical suture material*
polyglyconate USAN, BAN *absorbable surgical suture material*
polyhexanide BAN [also: polihexanide]
Poly-Histine elixir ℞ *antihistamine* [pheniramine maleate; pyrilamine maleate; phenyltoloxamine citrate] 4•4•4 mg/5 mL
Poly-Histine CS syrup ℞ *narcotic antitussive; decongestant; antihistamine* [codeine phosphate; phenylpropanolamine HCl; brompheniramine maleate] 10•12.5•2 mg/5 mL
Poly-Histine DM syrup ℞ *antitussive; decongestant; antihistamine* [dextromethorphan hydrobromide; phenylpropanolamine HCl; brompheniramine maleate] 10•12.5•2 mg/5 mL
Poly-Histine-D sustained-release capsules, elixir ℞ *decongestant; antihistamine* [phenylpropanolamine HCl; phenyltoloxamine citrate; pyrilamine maleate; pheniramine maleate] 50•16•16•16 mg; 12.5•4•4•4 mg/5 mL
Poly-Histine-D Ped Caps sustained-release capsules ℞ *pediatric decongestant and antihistamine* [phenylpropanolamine HCl; phenyltoloxamine citrate; pyrilamine maleate; pheniramine maleate] 25•8•8•8 mg
polyloxyl 8 stearate USAN *surfactant*
polymacon USAN *hydrophilic contact lens material*
polymanoacetate [now: acemannan]
polymeric oxygen [see: oxygen, polymeric]
polymetaphosphate P 32 USAN *radioactive agent*
polymethyl methacrylate (PMMA) *rigid hydrophobic polymer used for hard contact lenses*
polymixin E [see: colistin sulfate]
polymonine
Polymox capsules, powder for oral suspension, pediatric drops ℞ *penicillin-type antibiotic* [amoxicillin trihydrate] 250, 500 mg; 125, 250 mg/5 mL; 50 mg/mL
polymyxin BAN *bactericidal antibiotic* [also: polymyxin B sulfate; polymyxin B]
polymyxin B INN *bactericidal antibiotic* [also: polymyxin B sulfate; polymyxin]
polymyxin B sulfate USP *bactericidal antibiotic* [also: polymyxin B; polymyxin] 500,000 U/vial eye drops or injection
polymyxin B_1 [see: polymyxin B]
polymyxin B_2 [see: polymyxin B]
polymyxin B_3 [see: polymyxin B]
polymyxin E [see: colistin sulfate]
polynoxylin INN, BAN
polyoxyethylene 20 sorbitan monolaurate [see: polysorbate 20]
polyoxyethylene 20 sorbitan monooleate [see: polysorbate 80]
polyoxyethylene 20 sorbitan monopalmitate [see: polysorbate 40]
polyoxyethylene 20 sorbitan monostearate [see: polysorbate 60]
polyoxyethylene 20 sorbitan trioleate [see: polysorbate 85]
polyoxyethylene 20 sorbitan tristearate [see: polysorbate 65]

polyoxyethylene 50 stearate [now: polyoxyl 50 stearate]

polyoxyethylene glycol 1000 monocetyl ether [see: cetomacrogol 1000]

polyoxyethylene nonyl phenol *surfactant/wetting agent*

polyoxyl 10 oleyl ether NF *surfactant*

polyoxyl 20 cetostearyl ether NF *surfactant*

polyoxyl 35 castor oil NF *emulsifying agent; surfactant*

polyoxyl 40 hydrogenated castor oil NF *emulsifying agent; surfactant*

polyoxyl 40 stearate USAN, NF *surfactant*

polyoxyl 50 stearate NF *surfactant; emulsifying agent*

polyoxypropylene 15 stearyl ether USAN *solvent*

polyphosphoric acid, sodium salt [see: sodium polyphosphate]

Poly-Pred eye drop suspension ℞ *topical ophthalmic corticosteroidal anti-inflammatory; antibiotic* [prednisolone acetate; neomycin sulfate; polymyxin B sulfate] 0.5%•0.35%•10,000 U per mL

polypropylene glycol NF

polyribonucleotide [see: poly I: poly C12U]

polysaccharide-iron complex *hematinic* 150 mg oral

Polysorb Hydrate cream OTC *moisturizer; emollient*

polysorbate 20 USAN, NF, INN *surfactant/wetting agent*

polysorbate 40 USAN, NF, INN *surfactant*

polysorbate 60 USAN, NF, INN *surfactant*

polysorbate 65 USAN, INN *surfactant*

polysorbate 80 USAN, NF, INN *surfactant/wetting agent; viscosity-increasing agent*

polysorbate 85 USAN, INN *surfactant*

Polysporin aerosol spray (discontinued 1993) OTC *topical/ophthalmic antibiotic* [polymyxin B sulfate; bacitracin zinc] 2222•111 U/mL

Polysporin ointment, powder OTC *topical antibiotic* [polymyxin B sulfate; bacitracin zinc] 10,000•500 U/g

Polysporin ophthalmic ointment OTC *ophthalmic antibiotic* [polymyxin B sulfate; bacitracin zinc] 10,000•500 U/g

Polytabs-F chewable tablets ℞ *pediatric vitamin supplement and dental caries preventative* [multiple vitamins; fluoride; folic acid] ±•1•0.3 mg

Polytar shampoo, soap OTC *antiseborrheic; antipsoriatic; antipruritic; antibacterial* [coal tar, pine tar, and juniper tar solution] 2.5%; 1%

Polytar Bath oil OTC *antipsoriatic; antiseborrheic; antipruritic; emollient* [coal tar, pine tar, and juniper tar solution] 25%

polytef USAN *prosthetic aid* [also: politef]

polytetrafluoroethylene (PTFE) [see: polytef]

polythiazide USAN, USP, INN *diuretic; antihypertensive*

Polytrim eye drops ℞ *ophthalmic antibiotic* [polymyxin B sulfate; trimethoprim] 10,000 U•1 mg per mL

polyurethane foam USAN *internal bone splint*

polyvalent Crotaline antivenin [see: antivenin (Crotalidae) polyvalent]

polyvalent gas gangrene antitoxin [see: gas gangrene antitoxin, pentavalent]

polyvidone INN *dispersing, suspending and viscosity-increasing agent* [also: povidone]

Poly-Vi-Flor chewable tablets ℞ *pediatric vitamin supplement and dental caries preventative* [multiple vitamins; sodium fluoride; folic acid] ±•0.25•0.3, ±•0.5•0.3, ±•1•0.3 mg

Poly-Vi-Flor drops ℞ *pediatric vitamin supplement and dental caries preventative* [multiple vitamins; sodium fluoride] ±•0.25, ±•0.5 mg/mL

Poly-Vi-Flor with Iron chewable tablets ℞ *pediatric vitamin/iron supplement and dental caries preventative* [multiple vitamins & minerals; sodium fluoride; iron; folic acid] ±•0.25•12•0.3, ±•0.5•12•0.3, ±•1•12•0.3 mg

Poly-Vi-Flor with Iron drops ℞ *pediatric vitamin/iron supplement and dental caries preventative* [multiple vitamins & minerals; sodium fluoride; iron] ≛•0.25•10, ≛•0.5•10 mg/mL

polyvinyl acetate phthalate NF *coating agent*

polyvinyl alcohol (PVA) USP *viscosity-increasing agent*

polyvinylpyrrolidone [now: povidone]

Poly-Vi-Sol chewable tablets OTC *vitamin supplement* [multiple vitamins; folic acid] ≛•0.3 mg

Poly-Vi-Sol drops OTC *vitamin supplement* [multiple vitamins] ≛

Poly-Vi-Sol with Iron chewable tablets OTC *vitamin/iron supplement* [multiple vitamins; iron; folic acid] ≛•12•0.3 mg

Poly-Vi-Sol with Iron drops OTC *vitamin/iron supplement* [multiple vitamins; iron] ≛•10 mg/mL

Poly-Vitamin drops OTC *vitamin supplement* [multiple vitamins] ≛

Polyvitamin Fluoride chewable tablets ℞ *pediatric vitamin supplement and dental caries preventative* [multiple vitamins; fluoride; folic acid] ≛•0.5•0.3, ≛•1•0.3 mg

Polyvitamin Fluoride drops ℞ *pediatric vitamin supplement and dental caries preventative* [multiple vitamins; fluoride] ≛•0.25, ≛•0.5 mg/mL

Polyvitamin Fluoride with Iron chewable tablets ℞ *pediatric vitamin/iron supplement and dental caries preventative* [multiple vitamins & minerals; fluoride; iron; folic acid] ≛•1•12•0.3 mg

Poly-Vitamin with Iron drops OTC *vitamin/iron supplement* [multiple vitamins; iron] ≛•10 mg/mL

Polyvitamin with Iron and Fluoride drops ℞ *pediatric vitamin/iron supplement and dental caries preventative* [multiple vitamins; iron; fluoride] ≛•10•0.25 mg/mL

Polyvitamins with Fluoride and Iron chewable tablets ℞ *pediatric vitamin/iron supplement and dental caries preventative* [multiple vitamins; fluoride; iron; folic acid] ≛•0.5•12•0.3 mg

Polyvite with Fluoride drops (discontinued 1993) ℞ *pediatric vitamin deficiency and dental caries prevention* [multiple vitamins; fluoride]

POMP (prednisone, Oncovin, methotrexate, Purinethol) *chemotherapy protocol*

ponalrestat USAN, INN, BAN *aldose reductase inhibitor*

Pondimin tablets ℞ *anorexiant; CNS depressant* [fenfluramine HCl] 20 mg

ponfibrate INN

Ponstel capsules ℞ *nonsteroidal anti-inflammatory drug (NSAID); analgesic; for primary dysmenorrhea* [mefenamic acid] 250 mg ⓘ Pronestyl

Pontocaine cream OTC *topical local anesthetic* [tetracaine HCl] 1%

Pontocaine ointment OTC *topical local anesthetic* [tetracaine; menthol] 0.5%•0.5%

Pontocaine HCl Mono-Drop (eye drops) ℞ *topical ophthalmic anesthetic* [tetracaine HCl] 0.5%

Pontocaine HCl ophthalmic ointment (discontinued 1995) ℞ *topical ophthalmic anesthetic* [tetracaine HCl] 0.5%

Pontocaine HCl solution ℞ *nose/throat anesthetic to abolish laryngeal and esophageal reflex* [tetracaine HCl; chlorobutanol] 2%•0.4%

Pontocaine HCl spinal injection, powder for reconstitution ℞ *injectable local anesthetic* [tetracaine HCl] 0.2%, 0.3%, 1%

Po-Pon-S sugar-coated tablets OTC *vitamin/mineral supplement* [multiple vitamins & minerals] ≛

Porcelana cream OTC *hyperpigmentation bleaching agent* [hydroquinone] 2%

Porcelana with Sunscreen cream OTC *hyperpigmentation bleaching agent; sunscreen* [hydroquinone; padimate O] 2%•2.5%

porfimer sodium USAN, INN *antineoplastic; photosensitizing agent for photodynamic therapy (PDT)*

porfiromycin USAN, INN *antibacterial; antineoplastic*

porofocon A USAN *hydrophobic contact lens material*

porofocon B USAN *hydrophobic contact lens material*

Portagen powder OTC *enteral nutritional therapy* [lactose-free formula]
porton asparaginase [see: Erwinia L-asparaginase]
posatirelin INN
posedrine [see: benzchlorpropamid]
poskine INN, BAN
posterior pituitary [see: pituitary, posterior]
Posture tablets OTC *calcium supplement* [calcium phosphate, tribasic] 1565.2 mg
Posture-D film-coated tablets OTC *dietary supplement* [calcium phosphate, tribasic; vitamin D] 600 mg•125 IU
Potaba tablets, capsules, Envules (powder for reconstitution), powder ℞ *"possibly effective" for scleroderma and other skin diseases, and Peyronie's disease* [aminobenzoate potassium] 500 mg; 500 mg; 2 g; 100 g, 1 lb.
Potable Aqua tablets OTC *emergency disinfectant for drinking water* [tetraglycine hydroperiodide (source of iodine)] 16.7% (6.68%)
Potachlor 10%; Potachlor 20% liquid (discontinued 1992) ℞ *potassium supplement* [potassium chloride]
Potasalan liquid ℞ *potassium supplement* [potassium chloride; alcohol 4%] 20 mEq/15 mL
potash, sulfurated USP *source of sulfides*
potassic saline, lactated NF
potassium *element (K)*
potassium acetate USP *electrolyte replenisher* 2, 4 mEq/mL injection
potassium acid phosphate *urinary acidifier*
potassium alpha-phenoxyethyl penicillin [see: phenethicillin potassium]
potassium alum [see: alum, potassium]
potassium aspartate [see: L-aspartate potassium]
potassium aspartate & magnesium aspartate USAN *nutrient*
potassium benzoate NF *preservative*
potassium benzyl penicillin [see: penicillin G potassium]
potassium bitartrate USAN
potassium borate *pH buffer*

potassium canrenoate JAN *aldosterone antagonist* [also: canrenoate potassium; canrenoic acid]
potassium carbonate USP *alkalizing agent*
potassium chloride (KCl) USP *electrolyte replenisher* 600, 750 mg oral; 20, 40 mEq/15 mL oral; 20 mEq/pkt oral; 2, 10, 20, 30, 40, 60, 90 mEq/mL injection
potassium chloride K 42 USAN *radioactive agent*
potassium citrate USP *alkalizer; electrolyte replacement; nephrolithiasis and hypocitraturia prevention (orphan)*
potassium citrate & citric acid *(orphan: dissolution of uric acid and cysteine calculi)*
Potassium Cl enteric-coated tablets (discontinued 1992) ℞ *potassium supplement* [potassium chloride]
potassium clavulanate & amoxicillin [see: amoxicillin]
potassium clavulanate & ticarcillin [see: ticarcillin disodium]
potassium dichloroisocyanurate [see: troclosene potassium]
potassium glucaldrate USAN, INN *antacid*
potassium gluconate USP *electrolyte replenisher* 500, 595 mg oral; 20 mEq/15 mL oral
potassium guaiacolsulfonate USP *expectorant* [also: sulfogaiacol]
potassium hydroxide (KOH) NF *alkalizing agent*
potassium hydroxymethoxybenzenesulfonate hemihydrate [see: potassium guaiacolsulfonate]
potassium iodide USP *antifungal; expectorant; iodine supplement* 1 g/mL oral
potassium mercuric iodide NF
potassium metabisulfite NF *antioxidant*
potassium metaphosphate NF *buffering agent*
potassium nitrate *tooth desensitizer*
potassium nitrazepate INN
potassium para-aminobenzoate (PAB) [see: aminobenzoate potassium]
potassium penicillin G [see: penicillin G potassium]

potassium perchlorate *adjunct in radioimaging*

potassium permanganate USP *topical anti-infective*

potassium phosphate, dibasic USP *calcium regulator; phosphorus replacement; pH buffer*

potassium phosphate, monobasic NF *pH buffer; phosphorus replacement*

potassium sodium tartrate USP *laxative*

potassium sorbate NF *antimicrobial agent*

potassium tetraborate *pH buffer*

potassium thiocyanate NF

potasssium bicarbonate USP *pH buffer; electrolyte replacement*

Povadyne ointment, scrub, solution, swabsticks, wipes, whirlpool concentrate (discontinued 1992) OTC *broad-spectrum antimicrobial* [povidone-iodine]

Povidine ointment, scrub, solution OTC *broad-spectrum antimicrobial* [povidone-iodine] 10%, 5%, 10%

povidone USAN, USP *dispersing, suspending and viscosity-increasing agent* [also: polyvidone]

povidone I 125 USAN *radioactive agent*

povidone I 131 USAN *radioactive agent*

povidone-iodine USP, BAN *broad-spectrum antimicrobial* 10% topical

powdered cellulose [see: cellulose, powdered]

powdered ipecac [see: ipecac, powdered]

powdered opium [see: opium, powdered]

PowerMate tablets OTC *vitamin/mineral supplement* [multiple vitamins & minerals] ≛

PowerVites tablets OTC *vitamin/mineral supplement* [multiple vitamins and minerals; folic acid; biotin] ≛•150•25 μg

PPA (phenylpropanolamine) [q.v.]

PPA/Guaifenesin tablets (discontinued 1992) ℞ *decongestant; expectorant* [phenylpropanolamine HCl; guaifenesin]

PPD (purified protein derivative [of tuberculin]) [see: tuberculin]

PPG-15 stearyl ether [now: polyoxypropylene 15 stearyl ether]

PPI-002 (*orphan: malignant mesothelioma*)

PR-122 (redox-phenytoin) (*orphan: emergency rescue of status epilepticus*)

PR-225 (redox-acyclovir) (*orphan: herpes simplex encephalitis in AIDS*)

PR-239 (redox penicillin G) (*orphan: AIDS-associated neurosyphilis*)

PR-320 (molecusol & carbamazepine) (*orphan: emergency rescue of status epilepticus*)

practolol USAN, INN *antiadrenergic (β-receptor)*

prajmalium bitartrate INN, BAN

pralidoxime chloride USAN, USP *cholinesterase reactivator for organophosphate poisoning and anticholinesterase overdose* 600 mg injection ② pyridoxine; pramoxine

pralidoxime iodide USAN, INN *cholinesterase reactivator* ② pyridoxine; pramoxine

pralidoxime mesylate USAN *cholinesterase reactivator* ② pyridoxine; pramoxine

PrameGel gel OTC *topical local anesthetic* [pramoxine HCl; menthol] 1%•0.5%

Pramet FA controlled-release Filmtabs (film-coated tablets) (discontinued 1995) ℞ *prenatal vitamin/calcium/iron supplement* [multiple vitamins; calcium; iron; folic acid] ≛•250•60•1 mg

Pramilet FA Filmtabs (film-coated tablets) ℞ *prenatal vitamin/mineral/calcium/iron supplement* [multiple vitamins & minerals; calcium; iron; folic acid] ≛•250•40•1 mg

pramipexole USAN, INN *investigational dopamine agonist for Parkinson's disease, depression, and schizophrenia*

pramiracetam INN *cognition adjuvant* [also: pramiracetam HCl]

pramiracetam HCl USAN *cognition adjuvant* [also: pramiracetam]

pramiracetam sulfate USAN *cognition adjuvant*; (*orphan: adjunct to electroconvulsive therapy*)

pramiverine INN, BAN

pramocaine INN *topical anesthetic* [also: pramoxine HCl; pramoxine]

pramocaine HCl [see: pramoxine HCl]

Pramosone cream, lotion, ointment ℞ *topical corticosteroid; local anesthetic* [hydrocortisone acetate; pramoxine] 1%•1%, 2.5%•1%; 2.5%•1%; 2.5%•1% ℞ pramoxine

pramoxine BAN *topical local anesthetic* [also: pramoxine HCl; pramocaine] ℞ pralidoxime; Pramosone

Pramoxine HC anorectal aerosol foam ℞ *topical corticosteroidal anti-inflammatory; local anesthetic* [hydrocortisone acetate; pramoxine HCl] 1%•1%

pramoxine HCl USP *topical local anesthetic* [also: pramocaine; pramoxine]

prampine INN, BAN

pranidipine INN

pranlukast INN *investigational treatment for asthma*

pranolium chloride USAN, INN *antiarrhythmic*

pranoprofen INN

pranosal INN

praseodymium *element (Pr)*

prasterone INN

Pravachol tablets ℞ *cholesterol-lowering antihyperlipidemic* [pravastatin sodium] 10, 20, 40 mg

pravadoline INN *analgesic* [also: pravadoline maleate]

pravadoline maleate USAN *analgesic* [also: pravadoline]

pravastatin INN, BAN *antihyperlipidemic* [also: pravastatin sodium]

pravastatin sodium USAN, JAN *antihyperlipidemic* [also: pravastatin]

Prax lotion, cream OTC *topical local anesthetic* [pramoxine HCl] 1%

praxadine INN

prazepam USAN, USP, INN *sedative* 5 mg oral ℞ prazepine; prazosin

prazepine INN ℞ prazepam

praziquantel USAN, USP, INN, BAN *anthelmintic; (orphan: neurocysticercosis)*

prazitone INN, BAN

prazocillin INN

prazosin INN, BAN *antihypertensive; α_1-adrenergic blocker* [also: prazosin HCl] 1, 2, 5 mg oral ℞ prazepam

prazosin HCl USAN, USP, JAN *antihypertensive; α_1-adrenergic blocker* [also: prazosin]

Pre-Attain liquid OTC *enteral nutritional therapy* [lactose-free formula]

Precef powder for IV or IM injection, StrapKap vials (discontinued 1993) ℞ *cephalosporin-type antibiotic* [ceforanide]

precipitated calcium carbonate JAN *antacid; calcium replenisher* [also: calcium carbonate]

precipitated chalk [see: calcium carbonate]

precipitated sulfur [see: sulfur, precipitated]

Precision High Nitrogen Diet powder OTC *enteral nutritional therapy* [lactose-free formula]

Precision Isotonic Diet powder (discontinued 1994) OTC *oral nutritional supplement* 58.4 g/packet

Precision LR Diet powder OTC *enteral nutritional therapy* [lactose-free formula]

preclamol INN

Precose tablets ℞ *alpha-glucosidase inhibitor for type II diabetes mellitus* [acarbose] 50, 100 mg

Pred Mild; Pred Forte eye drop suspension ℞ *ophthalmic topical corticosteroidal anti-inflammatory* [prednisolone acetate] 0.12%; 1%

Predaject-50 IM injection (discontinued 1996) ℞ *glucocorticoid* [prednisolone acetate] 50 mg/mL

Predalone 50 IM injection ℞ *glucocorticoids* [prednisolone acetate] 50 mg/mL

Predalone T.B.A. intra-articular, intralesional, or soft tissue injection (discontinued 1994) ℞ *glucocorticoids* [prednisolone tebutate] 20 mg/mL

Predamide eye drop suspension (discontinued 1992) ℞ *topical ophthalmic corticosteroidal anti-inflammatory; bacteriostatic* [prednisolone acetate; sulfacetamide sodium]

Predcor-25 IM injection (discontinued 1994) ℞ *glucocorticoids* [prednisolone acetate] 25 mg/mL

Predcor-50 IM injection ℞ *glucocorticoids* [prednisolone acetate] 50 mg/mL

Pred-G eye drop suspension ℞ *topical ophthalmic corticosteroidal anti-inflam-*

matory; antibiotic [prednisolone acetate; gentamicin sulfate] 1%•0.3%

Pred-G S.O.P. ophthalmic ointment ℞ ophthalmic topical corticosteroidal anti-inflammatory; antibiotic [prednisolone acetate; gentamicin sulfate; chlorobutanol] 0.6%•0.3%•0.5%

prednazate USAN, INN anti-inflammatory

prednazoline INN

prednicarbate USAN, INN glucocorticoid

Prednicen-M tablets ℞ glucocorticoid; anti-inflammatory; immunosuppressant [prednisone] 5 mg

prednimustine USAN, INN antineoplastic; (orphan: malignant non-Hodgkin's lymphomas)

Prednisol TBA intra-articular, intralesional, or soft tissue injection ℞ glucocorticoids [prednisolone tebutate] 20 mg/mL

prednisolamate INN, BAN

prednisolone USP, INN glucocorticoid 5 mg oral ⑨ prednisone

prednisolone acetate USP, BAN glucocorticoid; ophthalmic anti-inflammatory 1% eye drops; 25, 50 mg/mL injection

prednisolone hemisuccinate USP glucocorticoid

prednisolone sodium phosphate USP glucocorticoid; ophthalmic anti-inflammatory 0.125%, 1% eye drops

prednisolone sodium succinate USP glucocorticoid

prednisolone steaglate INN, BAN

prednisolone tebutate USP glucocorticoid 20 mg/mL injection

prednisone USP, INN glucocorticoid; anti-inflammatory; immunosuppressant 1 mg oral ⑨ prednisolone

prednival USAN glucocorticoid

prednylidene INN, BAN

Predsulfair eye drop suspension, ophthalmic ointment (discontinued 1993) ℞ topical ophthalmic corticosteroidal anti-inflammatory; bacteriostatic [prednisolone acetate; sulfacetamide sodium]

prefenamate INN

Prefill (dosage form) prefilled applicator

Preflex Daily Cleaner Especially for Sensitive Eyes solution OTC surfactant cleaning solution for soft contact lenses

Prefrin Liquifilm eye drops OTC topical ocular decongestant [phenylephrine HCl] 0.12%

Prefrin-A eye drops (discontinued 1993) ℞ topical ocular decongestant and antihistamine; local anesthetic [phenylephrine HCl; pyrilamine maleate; antipyrine]

pregelatinized starch [see: starch, pregelatinized]

Pregestimil powder OTC hypoallergenic infant food for severe malabsorption disorders [enzymatically hydrolyzed protein formula]

pregnandiol JAN

pregneninolone [see: ethisterone]

pregnenolone INN non-hormonal sterol derivative [also: pregnenolone succinate]

pregnenolone succinate USAN non-hormonal sterol derivative [also: pregnenolone]

Pregnosis slide test for home use OTC in vitro diagnostic aid for urine pregnancy test [latex agglutination test]

Pregnyl powder for IM injection ℞ hormone for prepubertal cryptorchidism and hypogonadism; ovulation stimulant [chorionic gonadotropin] 1000 U/mL

Pre-H Cal tablets (discontinued 1995) ℞ vitamin/calcium/iron supplement [multiple vitamins; calcium; iron; folic acid] ±•47.5•51.7•0.5 mg

Prehist sustained-release capsules ℞ decongestant; antihistamine [phenylephrine HCl; chlorpheniramine maleate] 20•8 mg

Prehist D sustained-release tablets, sustained-release capsules ℞ decongestant; antihistamine; anticholinergic [phenylephrine HCl; chlorpheniramine maleate; methscopolamine nitrate] 20•8•2.5 mg

Prelone syrup ℞ glucocorticoids [prednisolone; alcohol 5%] 15 mg/5 mL

Prelu-2 timed-release capsules ℞ anorexiant [phendimetrazine tartrate] 105 mg

Preludin sustained-release tablets (discontinued 1992) ℞ *anorexiant* [phenmetrazine HCl] 75 mg

premafloxacin USAN, INN *veterinary antibacterial*

Premarin tablets ℞ *estrogen replacement therapy; palliative therapy for prostatic and breast cancer* [conjugated estrogens] 0.3, 0.625, 0.9, 1.25, 2.5 mg

Premarin vaginal cream ℞ *estrogen replacement therapy for postmenopausal disorders* [conjugated estrogens] 0.625 mg/g

Premarin Intravenous IV or IM injection ℞ *treatment of abnormal uterine bleeding due to hormonal imbalance* [conjugated estrogens] 25 mg

Premarin MPA ℞ *investigational osteoporosis treatment* [conjugated estrogens; medroxyprogesterone acetate]

Premarin with Methyltestosterone tablets ℞ *estrogen/androgen for menopausal vasomotor symptoms* [conjugated estrogens; methyltestosterone] 0.625•5, 1.25•10 mg

premazepam INN, BAN

Premphase tablets (28 per package, 14 of each phase) ℞ *treatment of menopausal symptoms including osteoporosis* [Phase 1: conjugated estrogens; Phase 2: medroxyprogesterone acetate] 0.625 mg; 5 mg

Prempro tablets (the single-phase product replaced the two-phase product in 1996) [Phase 1: conjugated estrogens; Phase 2: medroxyprogesterone acetate] 0.625 mg; 2.5 mg

Prempro tablets ℞ *treatment of menopausal symptoms including osteoporosis* [conjugated estrogens; medroxyprogesterone acetate] 0.625•2.5 mg

Prēmsyn PMS caplets OTC *analgesic; antipyretic; diuretic; antihistaminic sleep aid* [acetaminophen; pamabrom; pyrilamine maleate] 500•25•15 mg

Prēmsyn PMS capsules (discontinued 1992) OTC *analgesic; antipyretic; diuretic; antihistaminic sleep aid* [acetaminophen; pamabrom; pyrilamine maleate]

prenalterol INN, BAN *adrenergic* [also: prenalterol HCl]

prenalterol HCl USAN *adrenergic* [also: prenalterol]

Pre-Natal cellulose-coated caplets OTC *vitamin/mineral supplement for pregnant and lactating women* [multiple vitamins & minerals]

Prenatal 1/1 tablets ℞ *vitamin/mineral supplement* [multiple vitamins & minerals]

Prenatal FA tablets ℞ *prenatal vitamin/mineral supplement* [multiple vitamins & minerals]

Prenatal Maternal tablets ℞ *vitamin/mineral/calcium/iron supplement* [multiple vitamins & minerals; calcium; iron; folic acid; biotin] ≟•250•60•1•0.03 mg

Prenatal MR 90 film-coated delayed-release tablets ℞ *vitamin/calcium/iron supplement* [multiple vitamins; calcium; iron; folic acid] ≟•250•90•1 mg

Prenatal One film-coated tablets (discontinued 1995) ℞ *vitamin/calcium/iron supplement* [multiple vitamins; calcium; iron; folic acid] ≟•200•65•1 mg

Prenatal Plus tablets ℞ *vitamin/calcium/iron supplement* [multiple vitamins; calcium; iron; folic acid] ≟•200•65•1 mg

Prenatal Plus Improved tablets ℞ *vitamin/calcium/iron supplement* [multiple vitamins; calcium; iron; folic acid] ≟•200•65•1 mg

Prenatal Plus with Betacarotene tablets ℞ *vitamin/calcium/iron supplement* [multiple vitamins; calcium; iron; folic acid] ≟•200•65•1 mg

Prenatal Rx tablets (name changed to Prenatal Rx with Betacarotene in 1995)

Prenatal Rx with Betacarotene tablets ℞ *vitamin/calcium/iron supplement* [multiple vitamins; calcium; iron; folic acid; biotin] ≟•200•60•1•0.03 mg

Prenatal with Folic Acid tablets OTC *vitamin/calcium/iron supplement* [multiple vitamins; calcium; iron; folic acid] ±•200•60•0.8 mg

Prenatal Z film-coated delayed-release tablets ℞ *vitamin/calcium/iron supplement* [multiple vitamins; calcium; iron; folic acid] ±•300•65•1 mg

Prenatal-1 + Iron tablets ℞ *vitamin/calcium/iron supplement* [multiple vitamins; calcium; iron; folic acid] ±•200•65•1 mg

Prenatal-S tablets OTC *vitamin/calcium/iron supplement* [multiple vitamins; calcium; iron; folic acid] ±•200•60•0.8 mg

Prenate 90 film-coated delayed-release tablets ℞ *vitamin/calcium/iron supplement* [multiple vitamins; calcium; iron; folic acid] ±•250•90•1 mg

Prenavite tablets OTC *vitamin/calcium/iron supplement* [multiple vitamins; calcium; iron; folic acid] ±•200•60•0.8 mg

prenisteine INN

prenoverine INN

prenoxdiazine INN

prenylamine USAN, INN *coronary vasodilator*

Preparation H anorectal cream, anorectal ointment OTC *temporary relief of hemorrhoidal symptoms* [shark liver oil; phenylephrine HCl] 3%•0.25%

Preparation H cleansing pads (discontinued 1992) OTC *moisturizer and cleanser for external rectal/vaginal areas; astringent; antiseptic; antifungal* [witch hazel; alcohol] 50%•7.4%

Preparation H cleansing tissues OTC *moisturizer and cleanser for external rectal/vaginal areas* [propylene glycol]

Preparation H rectal suppositories OTC *temporary relief of hemorrhoidal symptoms* [shark liver oil] 3%

prepared chalk [see: calcium carbonate]

Prepcat suspension ℞ *GI contrast radiopaque agent* [barium sulfate] 1.5%

Pre-Pen solution for dermal scratch test ℞ *penicillin hypersensitivity assessment* [benzylpenicilloyl polylysine] 0.25 mL

Pre-Pen/MDM solution for dermal scratch test ℞ *(orphan: penicillin hypersensitivity assessment)* [benzylpenicillin

Prepidil gel ℞ *prostaglandin for cervical ripening at term* [dinoprostone] 0.5 mg

Prepulsid (Canadian name for U.S. product Propulsid)

Presalin tablets (discontinued 1995) OTC *analgesic; antipyretic; anti-inflammatory; antacid* [acetaminophen; aspirin; salicylamide; aluminum hydroxide] 120•260•120•100 mg

Presaril (name changed to Demadex in 1993)

pretamazium iodide INN, BAN

prethcamide

prethrombin [see: prothrombin complex, activated]

pretiadil INN

Pretts Diet-Aid chewable tablets OTC *diet aid* [sodium carboxymethylcellulose; alginic acid; sodium bicarbonate] 100•200•70 mg

Pretty Feet & Hands cream OTC *moisturizer; emollient*

Pretz solution OTC *nasal moisturizer* [sodium chloride (saline)] 0.6%

Pretz Irrigating solution OTC *for postoperative irrigation* [sodium chloride (saline); glycerin; eriodictyon] 0.75%

Pretz Moisturizing nose drops OTC *nasal moisturizer* [sodium chloride (saline); glycerin; eriodictyon] 0.75%

Pretz-D nasal spray OTC *nasal decongestant and moisturizer* [ephedrine sulfate] 0.25%

PretzPak ointment OTC *antimicrobial postoperative nasal pack* [benzyl alcohol; PEG; carboxymethylcellulose; urea; allantoin]

Prevacid enteric-coated granules in delayed-release capsules ℞ *proton pump inhibitor; antiulcerative/antisecretory for duodenal ulcer and erosive esophagitis* [lansoprazole] 15, 30 mg

Prevalite powder for oral suspension ℞ *cholesterol-lowering antihyperlipidemic* [cholestyramine resin; phenylalanine] 4000•14.1 mg/dose

PreviDent topical gel (for self-application) ℞ *dental caries preventative* [sodium fluoride] 1.1%

PreviDent Plus topical gel (for professional application) ℞ *dental caries preventative* [sodium fluoride]

PreviDent Rinse oral solution ℞ dental caries preventative [sodium fluoride] 0.2%

prezatide copper acetate USAN, INN immunomodulator

pribecaine INN

pridefine INN antidepressant [also: pridefine HCl]

pridefine HCl USAN antidepressant [also: pridefine]

prideperone INN

pridinol INN

prifelone USAN, INN dermatologic anti-inflammatory

prifinium bromide INN

prifuroline INN

prilocaine INN local anesthetic [also: prilocaine HCl]

prilocaine HCl USAN, USP local anesthetic [also: prilocaine]

Prilosec delayed-release capsules ℞ proton pump inhibitor for gastric and duodenal ulcers and gastroesophageal reflux disease [omeprazole] 10, 20 mg

primachine phosphate [see: primaquine phosphate]

Primacor IV infusion ℞ vasodilator for congestive heart failure [milrinone lactate] 0.2, 1 mg/mL

Primacor in 5% Dextrose IV infusion ℞ vasodilator for congestive heart failure [milrinone lactate; dextrose] 200 μg/mL; 5%

Primaderm ointment (discontinued 1992) OTC moisturizer; emollient; astringent; antiseptic [cod liver oil concentrate; zinc oxide]

Primaderm-B anorectal ointment (discontinued 1995) OTC topical anesthetic; astringent [benzocaine; zinc oxide; cod liver oil]

primaperone INN

primaquine INN antimalarial [also: primaquine phosphate]

primaquine phosphate USP cure for malaria; prevention of malarial relapse [also: primaquine] 26.3 mg oral

primaquine phosphate & clindamycin (orphan: AIDS-associated Pneumocystis carinii pneumonia)

Primatene tablets OTC antiasthmatic; bronchodilator; decongestant; sedative [theophylline; ephedrine HCl; phenobarbital] 130•24•7.5 mg

Primatene Dual Action tablets OTC antiasthmatic; bronchodilator; decongestant; expectorant [theophylline; ephedrine HCl; guaifenesin] 60•12.5•100 mg

Primatene Mist inhalation aerosol OTC bronchodilator for bronchial asthma [epinephrine] 0.2 mg/dose

Primatene Mist Suspension inhalation aerosol OTC bronchodilator for bronchial asthma [epinephrine bitartrate] 0.3 mg/dose

Primatuss Cough Mixture 4 liquid OTC antitussive; antihistamine [dextromethorphan hydrobromide; chlorpheniramine maleate; alcohol 10%] 15•2 mg/5 mL

Primatuss Cough Mixture 4D liquid OTC antitussive; decongestant; expectorant [dextromethorphan hydrobromide; pseudoephedrine HCl; guaifenesin; alcohol 10%] 10•20•67 mg/5 mL

Primaxin I.M. powder for injection ℞ thienamycin-type bactericidal antibiotic [imipenem; cilastatin sodium] 500•500, 750•750 mg

Primaxin I.V. powder for injection ℞ thienamycin-type bactericidal antibiotic [imipenem; cilastatin sodium] 250•250, 500•500 mg

primidolol USAN, INN antihypertensive; antianginal; antiarrhythmic

primidone USP, INN, BAN anticonvulsant 250 mg oral

primycin INN

Principen capsules, powder for oral suspension ℞ penicillin-type antibiotic [ampicillin trihydrate] 250, 500 mg; 125, 250 mg/5 mL

Principen with Probenecid capsules ℞ antibiotic for Neisseria gonorrhoeae [ampicillin trihydrate; probenecid]

Prinivil tablets ℞ antihypertensive; angiotensin-converting enzyme (ACE) inhibitor for CHF and acute MI [lisinopril] 2.5, 5, 10, 20, 40 mg

prinodolol [see: pindolol]

prinomide INN antirheumatic [also: prinomide tromethamine]

prinomide tromethamine USAN *antirheumatic* [also: prinomide]

prinoxodan USAN, INN *cardiotonic*

Prinzide tablets ℞ *antihypertensive* [hydrochlorothiazide; lisinopril] 12.5•10 mg

Prinzide 12.5; Prinzide 25 tablets ℞ *antihypertensive* [hydrochlorothiazide; lisinopril] 12.5•20 mg; 25•20 mg

Priscoline HCl IV injection ℞ *antihypertensive* [tolazoline HCl] 25 mg/mL ② Apresoline

pristinamycin INN, BAN

Privine nasal spray, nose drops OTC *nasal decongestant* [naphazoline HCl] 0.05%

prizidilol INN, BAN *antihypertensive* [also: prizidilol HCl]

prizidilol HCl USAN *antihypertensive* [also: prizidilol]

Pro Skin capsules OTC *vitamin/zinc supplement* [vitamins A, B_5, C, and E; zinc] 6250 IU•10 mg•100 mg•100 IU•10 mg

Pro-50 injection ℞ *antihistamine; motion sickness; sleep aid; antiemetic; sedative* [promethazine HCl] 50 mg/mL

proadifen INN *non-specific synergist* [also: proadifen HCl]

proadifen HCl USAN *non-specific synergist* [also: proadifen]

Pro-Air ℞ *investigational antiasthmatic* [procaterol]

Probalan tablets ℞ *uricosuric for gout* [probenecid] 500 mg

Probampacin powder for oral suspension ℞ *antibiotic for Neisseria gonorrhoeae* [ampicillin trihydrate; probenecid] 3.5•1 g

Pro-Banthīne tablets ℞ *peptic ulcer treatment adjunct; antispasmodic; antisecretory* [propantheline bromide] 7.5, 15 mg

probarbital sodium NF, INN

Probax gel OTC *relief from minor oral irritations* [propolis] 2%

Probec-T tablets OTC *vitamin supplement* [multiple B vitamins; vitamin C] ±•600 mg

Proben-C tablets ℞ *uricosuric for gout* [probenecid; colchicine] 500•0.5 mg

probenecid USP, INN, BAN *uricosuric* 500 mg oral

Probeta ℞ *investigational antihypertensive (β-blocker)* [bisoprolol]

probicromil calcium USAN *prophylactic antiallergic* [also: ambicromil]

Pro-Bionate capsules, powder OTC *dietary supplement; fever blister treatment; not generally regarded as safe and effective as an antidiarrheal* [Lactobacillus acidophilus] 2 billion U; 2 billion U/g

probucol USAN, USP, INN *antihyperlipoproteinemic*

procainamide INN *antiarrhythmic* [also: procainamide HCl]

procainamide HCl USP *antiarrhythmic* [also: procainamide] 250, 375, 500, 750 mg oral; 100, 500 mg/mL injection

procaine INN [also: procaine borate] ② Procan

procaine borate NF [also: procaine]

procaine HCl USP *injectable local anesthetic* 1%, 2%

procaine penicillin BAN *bactericidal antibiotic* [also: penicillin G procaine]

ProcalAmine IV infusion ℞ *peripheral parenteral nutrition* [multiple essential and nonessential amino acids; electrolytes]

Pro-Cal-Sof capsules OTC *stool softener* [docusate calcium] 240 mg

Procan SR sustained-release tablets (replaced by Procanbid in 1996) ℞ *antiarrhythmic* [procainamide HCl] 250, 500, 750, 1000 mg ② procaine

Procanbid extended-release film-coated tablets ℞ *twice-daily antiarrhythmic* [procainamide HCl] 500, 1000 mg

procarbazine INN *antibiotic antineoplastic* [also: procarbazine HCl] ② dacarbazine

procarbazine HCl USAN, USP *antibiotic antineoplastic for Hodgkin's disease* [also: procarbazine]

Procardia capsules ℞ *antianginal* [nifedipine] 10, 20 mg

Procardia XL film-coated sustained-release tablets ℞ *antianginal; antihypertensive* [nifedipine] 30, 60, 90 mg

procaterol INN, BAN *bronchodilator* [also: procaterol HCl]

procaterol HCl USAN *bronchodilator* [also: procaterol]

prochlorperazine USP, INN *antiemetic; antipsychotic; antidopaminergic* 25 mg suppositories

prochlorperazine edisylate USP *antiemetic; antipsychotic* 5 mg/mL injection

prochlorperazine ethanedisulfonate [see: prochlorperazine edisylate]

prochlorperazine maleate USP *antiemetic; antipsychotic* 5, 10, 25 mg oral

procinolol INN

procinonide USAN, INN *adrenocortical steroid*

proclonol USAN, INN *anthelmintic; antifungal*

procodazole INN

proconvertin [see: factor VII]

Procort cream, spray OTC *topical corticosteroid* [hydrocortisone] 1%

Procrit IV or subcu injection ℞ *stimulates RBC production; (orphan: anemia of end-stage renal disease, HIV, or chemotherapy)* [epoetin alfa] 2000, 3000, 4000, 10,000 U/mL

Proctocort anorectal cream ℞ *topical corticosteroidal anti-inflammatory* [hydrocortisone] 1%

ProctoCream-HC anorectal cream ℞ *topical corticosteroidal anti-inflammatory* [hydrocortisone acetate] 2.5%

ProctoCream-HC anorectal cream ℞ *topical corticosteroidal anti-inflammatory; local anesthetic* [hydrocortisone acetate; pramoxine HCl] 1%•1%

ProctoFoam NS anorectal aerosol foam OTC *topical local anesthetic* [pramoxine HCl] 1%

Proctofoam-HC anorectal aerosol foam ℞ *topical corticosteroidal anti-inflammatory; local anesthetic* [hydrocortisone acetate; pramoxine HCl] 1%•1%

Pro-Cute lotion OTC *moisturizer; emollient*

ProCycle Gold tablets OTC *vitamin/mineral/iron supplement* [multiple vitamins & minerals; iron; folic acid; biotin] ≚•3•0.067•≚ mg

procyclidine INN *antiparkinsonian; skeletal muscle relaxant; anticholinergic* [also: procyclidine HCl]

procyclidine HCl USP *antiparkinsonian; skeletal muscle relaxant; anticholinergic* [also: procyclidine]

procymate INN

Procysteine ℞ *investigational (Phase II) immunomodulator for AIDS (orphan: adult respiratory distress syndrome)* [oxothiazolidine carboxylate]

prodeconium bromide INN

Pro-Depo IM injection (discontinued 1993) ℞ *progestin for amenorrhea and dysfunctional uterine bleeding* [hydroxyprogesterone caproate in oil]

Proderm Topical dressing OTC *dressing for decubitus ulcers* [castor oil; balsam Peru] 650•72.5 mg/0.82 mL

prodilidine INN *analgesic* [also: prodilidine HCl]

prodilidine HCl USAN *analgesic* [also: prodilidine]

prodipine INN

Prodium tablets OTC *urinary analgesic* [phenazopyridine HCl] 95 mg

prodolic acid USAN, INN *anti-inflammatory*

profadol INN *analgesic* [also: profadol HCl]

profadol HCl USAN *analgesic* [also: profadol]

Profasi powder for IM injection ℞ *hormone for prepubertal cryptorchidism and hypogonadism; ovulation stimulant* [chorionic gonadotropin] 500, 1000 U/mL

Profasi HP powder for IM injection (name changed to Profasi in 1994)

Profen LA; Profen II timed-release tablets ℞ *decongestant; expectorant* [phenylpropanolamine HCl; guaifenesin] 75•600 mg; 37.5•600 mg

Profenal Drop-Tainers (eye drops) ℞ *ocular nonsteroidal anti-inflammatory drug (NSAID); intraoperative miosis inhibitor* [suprofen] 1%

profenamine INN *antiparkinsonian* [also: ethopropazine HCl; ethopropazine]

profenamine HCl [see: ethopropazine HCl]

profexalone INN

Profiber liquid OTC *enteral nutritional therapy* [lactose-free formula]

Profilate HP IV injection ℞ *antihemophilic to correct coagulation deficiency* [antihemophilic factor VIII:C in heptane] 2

Profilate OSD IV injection (discontinued 1996) ℞ *antihemophilic to correct coagulation deficiency* [antihemophilic factor VIII:C] 2

Profilnine Heat-Treated IV suspension (discontinued 1995) ℞ *anticoagulant to correct factor IX deficiency* [factor IX complex, heat treated] 2

Profilnine SD powder for IV injection ℞ *antihemophilic to correct factor IX deficiency* [factor IX complex, solvent/detergent treated] 2

proflavine INN [also: proflavine dihydrochloride]

proflavine dihydrochloride NF [also: proflavine]

proflavine sulfate NF

proflazepam INN

ProFree/GP Weekly Enzymatic Cleaner tablets OTC *enzymatic cleaner for rigid gas permeable contact lenses* [papain]

progabide USAN, INN *anticonvulsant; muscle relaxant*

Pro-gesic liquid (discontinued 1995) OTC *topical analgesic* [trolamine salicylate] 10%

Progestasert IUD ℞ *intrauterine contraceptive* [progesterone] 38 mg

progesterone USP, INN *progestin; intrauterine contraceptive (orphan: in vitro fertilization and embryo transfer)* 50 mg/mL IM injection (in oil); also available as powder for compounding

proglumetacin INN

proglumide USAN, INN *anticholinergic; investigational antiulcerative*

Proglycem capsules, oral suspension ℞ *glucose-elevating agent* [diazoxide] 50 mg; 50 mg/mL

Prograf capsules ℞ *liver transplant rejection preventative; investigational preventative for other transplant rejection* [tacrolimus] 1, 5 mg

Prograf IV infusion ℞ *liver transplant rejection preventative* [tacrolimus] 5 mg/mL

proguanil INN, BAN [also: chloroguanide HCl]

proguanil HCl [see: chloroguanide HCl]

ProHance injection ℞ *contrast media for magnetic imaging of the brain and spine* [gadoteridol] 279.3 mg/mL

proheptazine INN

ProHIBiT IM injection ℞ *Haemophilus influenzae type b (HIB) vaccine* [Hemophilus b conjugate vaccine] 0.5 mL

proinsulin human USAN *antidiabetic*

Prokine powder for IV infusion (discontinued 1993) ℞ *myeloid reconstitution after autologous bone marrow transplant* [sargramostim] 250, 500 μg

prolactin *investigational immune stimulator for burns and chemotherapy*

Prolamine capsules (discontinued 1992) OTC *diet aid* [phenylpropanolamine HCl] 37.5 mg

Prolastin IV injection ℞ *replacement therapy for alpha$_1$-proteinase inhibitor deficiency (orphan)* [alpha$_1$-proteinase inhibitor] 20 mg/mL

Proleukin powder for IV infusion ℞ *antineoplastic (orphan: metastatic renal cell carcinoma; immunodeficiency diseases)* [aldesleukin] 18 million IU/mL

Proleukin-PEG ℞ *investigational immune enhancer for AIDS and human papillomavirus* [aldesleukin; polyethylene glycol]

proligestone INN

proline (L-proline) USAN, USP, INN *nonessential amino acid; symbols: Pro, P* ⑨ Prolene

prolintane INN *antidepressant* [also: prolintane HCl]

prolintane HCl USAN *antidepressant* [also: prolintane]

Prolixin tablets, elixir, oral concentrate, IM injection ℞ *antipsychotic* [fluphenazine HCl] 1, 2.5, 5, 10 mg; 2.5 mg/5 mL; 5 mg/mL; 2.5 mg/mL

Prolixin Decanoate subcu or IM injection, Unimatic (prefilled) syringe ℞ *antipsychotic* [fluphenazine decanoate] 25 mg/mL

Prolixin Enanthate subcu or IM injection ℞ *antipsychotic* [fluphenazine enanthate] 25 mg/mL

Proloid tablets (discontinued 1992) ℞ *hypothyroidism; thyroid cancer* [thyroglobulin] 30, 60, 90, 120, 180 mg
prolonium iodide INN
Proloprim tablets ℞ *anti-infective; antibacterial* [trimethoprim] 100, 200 mg
ProMACE (prednisone, methotrexate [with leucovorin rescue], Adriamycin, cyclophosphamide, etoposide) *chemotherapy protocol*
ProMACE/cytaBOM (ProMACE [above], cytarabine, bleomycin, Oncovin, mitoxantrone) *chemotherapy protocol*
ProMACE/MOPP (full course of ProMACE, followed by MOPP) *chemotherapy protocol*
promazine INN *antipsychotic* [also: promazine HCl] 🔁 Promethazine
promazine HCl USP *antipsychotic* [also: promazine] 25, 50 mg/mL injection
Promedrol ℞ *investigational treatment for asthma, shock, and kidney transplant rejection* [methylprednisolone suleptanate]
Promega Pearls (softgels) OTC *dietary supplement* [omega-3 fatty acids; multiple vitamins & minerals] 600•≛, 1000•≛ mg
promegestone INN
promelase INN
promestriene INN
Prometa syrup (discontinued 1995) ℞ *bronchodilator* [metaproterenol sulfate] 10 mg/5 mL
Prometh syrup (discontinued 1996) ℞ *antihistamine* [promethazine HCl; alcohol]
Prometh VC Plain liquid ℞ *decongestant; antihistamine* [phenylephrine HCl; promethazine HCl] 5•6.25 mg/5 mL
Prometh VC with Codeine syrup ℞ *narcotic antitussive; decongestant; antihistamine* [codeine phosphate; phenylephrine HCl; promethazine HCl; alcohol] 10•5•6.25 mg/5 mL
Prometh with Codeine syrup ℞ *narcotic antitussive; antihistamine* [codeine phosphate; promethazine HCl] 10•6.25 mg/5 mL
Prometh with Dextromethorphan syrup ℞ *antitussive; antihistamine* [dextromethorphan hydrobromide; promethazine HCl; alcohol 7%] 15•6.25 mg/5 mL
Prometh-50 injection ℞ *antihistamine; motion sickness; sleep aid; antiemetic; sedative* [promethazine HCl] 50 mg/mL
promethazine INN *antiemetic; antihistamine; antidopaminergic; motion sickness relief* [also: promethazine HCl]
Promethazine DC Plain syrup (discontinued 1993) ℞ *decongestant; antihistamine* [promethazine HCl; phenylephrine HCl; alcohol] 🔁 promazine
Promethazine DM syrup ℞ *antitussive; antihistamine* [dextromethorphan hydrobromide; promethazine HCl; alcohol] 15•6.25 mg/5 mL
promethazine HCl USP *antiemetic; antihistamine; antidopaminergic* [also: promethazine] 12.5, 25, 50 mg oral; 6.25, 25 mg/5 mL oral; 50 mg suppositories; 25, 50 mg/mL injection
promethazine teoclate INN
Promethazine VC syrup ℞ *decongestant; antihistamine* [phenylephrine HCl; promethazine HCl] 5•6.25 mg/5 mL
Promethazine VC Plain syrup ℞ *decongestant; antihistamine* [phenylephrine HCl; promethazine HCl; alcohol 7%] 5•6.25 mg/5 mL
Promethazine VC with Codeine syrup ℞ *narcotic antitussive; decongestant; antihistamine* [codeine phosphate; phenylephrine HCl; promethazine HCl; alcohol] 10•5•6.25 mg/5 mL
promethestrol [see: methestrol]
Promethist with Codeine syrup ℞ *narcotic antitussive; decongestant; antihistamine* [codeine phosphate; phenylephrine HCl; promethazine HCl; alcohol] 10•5•6.25 mg/5 mL
promethium *element (Pm)*
Prometrium ℞ *investigational oral progesterone for secondary amenorrhea and abnormal uterine bleeding*
Promine capsules ℞ *antiarrhythmic* [procainamide HCl]

Prominol tablets ℞ *analgesic; antipyretic; sedative* [acetaminophen; butalbital] 650•50 mg

Promise with Fluoride toothpaste (discontinued 1994) OTC *tooth desensitizer; dental caries preventative* [potassium nitrate; sodium monofluorophosphate]

Promit IV injection ℞ *monovalent hapten for prophylaxis of dextran-induced anaphylactic reactions* [dextran 1] 150 mg/mL

ProMod powder OTC *oral protein supplement* [D-whey protein concentrate; soy lecithin]

promolate INN

promoxolane INN

prompt insulin zinc [see: insulin zinc, prompt]

Pronemia Hematinic capsules ℞ *hematinic* [ferrous fumarate; cyanocobalamin; ascorbic acid; intrinsic factor concentrate; folic acid] 115 mg•15 μg•150 mg•75 mg•1 mg

Pronestyl capsules, tablets, IV or IM injection ℞ *antiarrhythmic* [procainamide HCl] 250, 375, 500 mg; 250, 375, 500 mg; 100, 500 mg/mL ⓘ Ponstel

Pronestyl-SR sustained-release tablets ℞ *antiarrhythmic* [procainamide HCl] 500 mg

pronetalol INN [also: pronethalol]

pronethalol BAN [also: pronetalol]

Pronto shampoo + creme rinse OTC *pediculicide* [pyrethrins; piperonyl butoxide] 0.33%•4%

Pronto-Gel (discontinued 1992) OTC *counterirritant* [methyl salicylate; methyl nicotinate; camphor; menthol; isopropanol]

Propa P.H. liquid soap (discontinued 1992) OTC *topical keratolytic for acne* [benzoyl peroxide] 10%

Propa P.H. with Aloe cleansing pads (discontinued 1994) OTC *topical acne treatment* [salicylic acid; alcohol] 0.5%•25%

Propa P.H. with Aloe cream (discontinued 1993) OTC *topical acne treatment* [salicylic acid] 2%

Propa P.H. with Aloe stick (discontinued 1992) OTC *topical acne treatment* [salicylic acid] 2%

Propac powder OTC *oral protein supplement* [whey protein; lactose]

Propacet 100 film-coated tablets ℞ *narcotic analgesic* [propoxyphene napsylate; acetaminophen] 100•650 mg

propacetamol INN

propafenone INN, BAN *antiarrhythmic* [also: propafenone HCl]

propafenone HCl USAN *antiarrhythmic* [also: propafenone]

Propagest tablets OTC *nasal decongestant; diet aid* [phenylpropanolamine HCl] 25 mg

propamidine INN, BAN

propamidine isethionate (orphan: *Acanthamoeba keratitis*)

propaminodiphen [see: pramiverine]

propane NF *aerosol propellant*

1,2-propanediol [see: propylene glycol]

propanidid USAN, INN *intravenous anesthetic*

propanocaine INN

propanoic acid, sodium salt hydrate [see: sodium propionate]

2-propanol [see: isopropyl alcohol]

2-propanone [see: acetone]

propantheline bromide USP, INN *peptic ulcer adjunct* 15 mg oral

PROPApH Acne cream OTC *topical keratolytic for acne* [salicylic acid] 2%

PROPApH Cleansing; PROPApH Cleansing for Sensitive Skin; PROPApH Cleansing Maximum Strength pads OTC *topical keratolytic for acne* [salicylic acid] 0.5%; 0.5%; 2%

PROPApH Cleansing for Normal/Combination Skin; PROPApH Cleansing for Oily Skin lotion OTC *topical keratolytic for acne* [salicylic acid] 0.5%

PROPApH Foaming Face Wash liquid ℞ *topical keratolytic cleanser for acne* [salicylic acid] 2%

PROPApH Peel-Off Acne Mask OTC *topical keratolytic for acne* [salicylic acid] 2%

proparacaine HCl USP *topical ophthalmic anesthetic* [also: proxymetacaine] 0.5% eye drops

propatyl nitrate USAN *coronary vasodilator* [also: propatylnitrate]

propatylnitrate INN *coronary vasodilator* [also: propatyl nitrate]

propazolamide INN

1-propene homopolymer [see: polipropene 25]

propenidazole INN

propentofylline INN

p-**propenylanisole** [see: anethole]

propenzolate HCl USAN *anticholinergic* [also: oxyclipine]

propericiazine [see: periciazine]

properidine INN, BAN

propetamide INN

propetandrol INN

prophenamine HCl [see: ethopropazine HCl]

Pro-Phree powder OTC *supplement to breast milk* [protein-free formula with vitamins & minerals]

Prophyllin ointment OTC *topical antifungal; vulnerary; wound deodorant* [sodium propionate; chlorophyll derivatives] 5%•0.0125%

Prophyllin powder (discontinued 1994) OTC *topical antifungal; vulnerary; wound deodorant* [sodium propionate; chlorophyll derivatives] 1%•0.0025%

propicillin INN, BAN

propikacin USAN, INN *antibacterial*

Propimex-1 powder OTC *formula for infants with propionic or methylmalonicacidemia*

Propimex-2 powder OTC *enteral nutritional therapy for propionic or methylmalonicacidemia*

Propine eye drops ℞ *antiglaucoma agent* [dipivefrin HCl] 0.1%

propinetidine INN

propiodal [see: prolonium iodide]

propiolactone (β-propiolactone) USAN, INN *disinfectant*

propiomazine USAN, INN *preanesthetic sedative*

propiomazine HCl USP *sedative; analgesic adjunct*

propionic acid NF *antimicrobial; acidifying agent*

propionyl erythromycin lauryl sulfate [see: erythromycin estolate]

propipocaine INN

propiram INN *narcotic analgesic* [also: propiram fumarate]

propiram fumarate USAN *narcotic analgesic* [also: propiram]

propisergide INN

propitocaine HCl [now: prilocaine HCl]

propiverine INN

propizepine INN

Proplex T IV infusion ℞ *antihemophilic to correct factor IX deficiency and control bleeding in factor VII deficiency* [factor IX complex, heat treated] 30 mL

propofol USAN, INN, BAN *general anesthetic*

propoxate INN

propoxycaine INN *local anesthetic* [also: propoxycaine HCl]

propoxycaine HCl USP *local anesthetic* [also: propoxycaine]

propoxyphene HCl USAN, USP *narcotic analgesic* [also: dextropropoxyphene HCl] 65 mg oral

propoxyphene napsylate USAN, USP *narcotic analgesic*

propranolol INN, BAN *antiarrhythmic; migraine preventative; antiadrenergic (β-receptor)* [also: propranolol HCl]

propranolol HCl USAN, USP *antiarrhythmic; migraine preventative; antiadrenergic (β-receptor)* [also: propranolol] 10, 20, 40, 60, 80, 90, 120, 160 mg oral; 4, 8, 80 mg/mL oral; 1 mg/mL injection

Propulsid tablets, oral suspension ℞ *treatment for nocturnal heartburn due to gastroesophageal reflux disease (GERD)* [cisapride] 10, 20 mg; 1 mg/mL

propyl *p*-aminobenzoate [see: risocaine]

propyl docetrizoate INN, BAN

propyl gallate NF *antioxidant*

propyl *p*-hydroxybenzoate [see: propylparaben]

propyl *p*-hydroxybenzoate, sodium salt [see: propylparaben sodium]

N-propylajmalinium tartrate [see: prajmalinum bitartrate]

propylene carbonate NF *gelling agent*

propylene glycol USP *humectant; solvent; suspending and viscosity-increasing agent*

propylene glycol alginate NF *suspending agent; viscosity-increasing agent*

propylene glycol diacetate NF *solvent*

propylene glycol ether of methylcellulose [see: hydroxypropyl methylcellulose]

propylene glycol monostearate NF *emulsifying agent*

propylhexedrine USP, INN, BAN *vasoconstrictor; nasal decongestant*

propyliodone USP, INN *radiopaque medium*

propylorvinol [see: etorphine]

propylparaben USAN, NF *antifungal agent; preservative*

propylparaben sodium USAN, NF *antimicrobial preservative*

2-propylpentanoic acid [see: valproic acid]

propylthiouracil (PTU) USP, INN *thyroid inhibitor*

2-propylvaleramide [see: valpromide]

propylvaleric acid [see: valproic acid]

5-propynylarabinofuranosyluracil *investigational treatment for varicella-zoster virus*

propyperone INN

propyphenazone INN, BAN

propyromazine bromide INN

proquamezine BAN [also: aminopromazine]

proquazone USAN, INN *anti-inflammatory*

proquinolate USAN, INN *coccidiostat for poultry*

prorenoate potassium USAN, INN *aldosterone antagonist*

Prorex-25; Prorex-50 injection ℞ *antihistamine; motion sickness; sleep aid; antiemetic; sedative* [promethazine HCl] 25 mg/mL; 50 mg/mL

proroxan INN *antiadrenergic (α-receptor)* [also: proroxan HCl]

proroxan HCl USAN *antiadrenergic (α-receptor)* [also: proroxan]

Proscar film-coated tablets ℞ *androgen hormone inhibitor for benign prostatic hyperplasia (BPH)* [finasteride] 5 mg

proscillaridin USAN, INN *cardiotonic*

proscillaridin A [see: proscillaridin]

Prosed/DS sugar-coated tablets ℞ *urinary anti-infective; antiseptic; analgesic; antispasmodic* [methenamine; phenyl salicylate; methylene blue; benzoic acid; atropine sulfate; hyoscyamine sulfate] 81.6•36.2•10.8•9•0.06•0.06 mg

ProSobee liquid, powder OTC *hypoallergenic infant food* [soy protein formula]

Pro-Sof capsules, syrup (discontinued 1992) OTC *stool softener* [docusate sodium] 100, 250 mg; 60 mg/15 mL

Pro-Sof Plus capsules OTC *laxative; stool softener* [casanthranol; docusate sodium] 30•100 mg

ProSom tablets ℞ *sedative; hypnotic* [estazolam] 1, 2 mg

prospidium chloride INN

prostacyclin [now: epoprostenol]

prostaglandin E_1 (PGE_1) [now: alprostadil]

prostaglandin E_1 alphacyclodextrin *(orphan: severe peripheral arterial occlusive disease)*

prostaglandin E_2 (PGE_2) [see: dinoprostone]

prostaglandin $F_{2\alpha}$ ($PGF_{2\alpha}$) [see: dinoprost]

prostaglandin I_2 (PGI_2) [now: epoprostenol]

prostaglandin X (PGX) [now: epoprostenol]

prostalene USAN, INN *prostaglandin*

Prostaphlin capsules, powder for oral solution, powder for IV or IM injection ℞ *bactericidal antibiotic (penicillinase-resistant penicillin)* [oxacillin sodium] 250, 500 mg; 250 mg/5 mL; 0.5, 1, 2, 4, 10 g

ProStep transdermal patch ℞ *smoking deterrent; nicotine withdrawal aid* [nicotine] 15, 30 mg

Prostigmin subcu or IM injection ℞ *postsurgical cholinergic bladder muscle stimulant* [neostigmine methylsulfate] 1:1000 (1 mg/mL), 1:2000 (0.5 mg/mL), 1:4000 (0.25 mg/mL) ⑨ physostigmine

Prostigmin tablets ℞ *myasthenia gravis treatment; antidote for neuromuscular blockers* [neostigmine bromide] 15 mg

Prostin E2 vaginal suppository ℞ *prostaglandin-type abortifacient* [dinoprostone] 20 mg

Prostin VR Pediatric IV injection ℞ *vasodilator; platelet aggregate inhibitor* [alprostadil] 500 µg/mL

prosulpride INN

prosultiamine INN

Protac troches (discontinued 1994) OTC *topical oral anesthetic; antiseptic* [benzocaine; cetylpyridinium chloride] 10•2.5 mg

protactinium *element (Pa)*

protamine sulfate USP, INN *antidote to heparin* [also: protamine sulphate] 10 mg/mL injection

protamine sulphate BAN *antidote to heparin* [also: protamine sulfate]

Protamine Zinc Iletin I subcu injection (discontinued 1992) OTC *antidiabetic* [protamine zinc insulin (beef-pork)] ▷ Protopam

Protamine Zinc Iletin II (beef) subcu injection (discontinued 1992) OTC *antidiabetic* [protamine zinc insulin]

Protamine Zinc Iletin II (pork) subcu injection (discontinued 1992) OTC *antidiabetic* [protamine zinc insulin]

protamine zinc insulin (PZI) INN *antidiabetic* [also: insulin, protamine zinc]

Protar Protein shampoo OTC *antiseborrheic; antipsoriatic; antipruritic; antibacterial* [coal tar] 5%

protargin, mild [see: silver protein, mild]

protease inhibitors *a class of investigational (Phase II) antivirals for HIV*

ProTec ℞ *investigational immunomodulator* [lisofylline]

ProTech First Aid Stick liquid OTC *topical antiseptic; analgesic* [lidocaine; povidone-iodine] 2.5%•10%

Protectol Medicated powder OTC *topical antifungal* [calcium undecylenate] 15%

Protegra softgels OTC *vitamin/mineral supplement* [multiple vitamins & minerals] ±

protein C concentrate *investigational anticoagulant (orphan: protein C deficiency)*

protein hydrolysate USP *fluid and nutrient replenisher*

α₁-proteinase inhibitor [see: alpha₁-proteinase inhibitor]

Protenate IV infusion ℞ *blood volume expander for shock due to burns, trauma and surgery* [plasma protein fraction] 5%

proterguride INN

Prothazine subcu or IM injection ℞ *antihistamine; motion sickness; sleep aid; antiemetic; sedative* [promethazine HCl] 25, 50 mg/mL

Prothazine Plain syrup ℞ *antihistamine; motion sickness; sleep aid; antiemetic; sedative* [promethazine HCl] 6.25 mg/5 mL

protheobromine INN

Prothera liquid (discontinued 1995) OTC *soap-free therapeutic skin cleanser*

Prothiaden ℞ *investigational tricyclic antidepressant* [dothiepin HCl]

prothionamide BAN [also: protionamide]

prothipendyl INN

prothipendyl HCl [see: prothipendyl]

prothixene INN

prothrombin complex, activated BAN

Protilase capsules containing enteric-coated spheres ℞ *digestive enzymes* [lipase; protease; amylase] 4000•25,000•20,000 U

protiofate INN

protionamide INN [also: prothionamide]

protirelin USAN, INN, BAN *prothyrotropin; (orphan: infant respiratory distress syndrome of prematurity)*

protizinic acid INN

protokylol HCl

proton pump inhibitor [see: reversible proton pump inhibitor]

Protopam Chloride IV injection ℞ *antidote for organophosphate poisoning and anticholinesterase overdose* [pralidoxime chloride] 1 g ▷ Protamine

Protopam Chloride tablets (discontinued 1995) ℞ *antidote for organophosphate and anticholinesterase chemicals* [pralidoxime chloride] 500 mg ② Protamine

Protostat tablets ℞ *antibiotic; antiprotozoal; amebicide* [metronidazole] 250, 500 mg

protoveratrine A

Protovir ℞ *investigational antiviral for cytomegalovirus* [sevirumab]

Protox ℞ *(orphan: toxoplasmosis of AIDS)* [poloxamer 331]

protriptyline INN *tricyclic antidepressant* [also: protriptyline HCl]

protriptyline HCl USAN, USP *tricyclic antidepressant* [also: protriptyline]

Protropin powder for IM or subcu injection ℞ *growth hormone (orphan: growth failure; Turner syndrome)* [somatrem] 5, 10 mg (13, 26 IU)

Protropin II ℞ *(orphan: growth failure; Turner syndrome; anovulation; severe burns)* [somatropin]

Protuss liquid ℞ *narcotic antitussive; expectorant* [hydrocodone bitartrate; potassium guaiacolsulfonate] 5•300 mg/5 mL

Protuss-D liquid ℞ *narcotic antitussive; decongestant; expectorant* [hydrocodone bitartrate; pseudoephedrine HCl; potassium guaiacolsulfonate] 5•30•300 mg/5 mL

prourokinase [see: saruplase]

Provatene soft gel perles (discontinued 1996) OTC *to reduce photosensitivity reaction* [beta-carotene] 15 mg

Proventil inhalation aerosol ℞ *bronchodilator* [albuterol] 90 μg/dose

Proventil tablets, Repetabs (extended-release tablets), syrup, solution for inhalation ℞ *bronchodilator* [albuterol sulfate] 2, 4 mg; 4 mg; 2 mg/5 mL; 0.083%

Provera tablets ℞ *progestin for secondary amenorrhea or abnormal uterine bleeding* [medroxyprogesterone acetate] 2.5, 5, 10 mg

Provir ℞ *investigational antiviral for respiratory viruses*

Provisc ℞ *investigational ophthalmic agent*

provitamin A [see: beta carotene]

Provocholine powder for reconstitution for inhalation ℞ *bronchoconstrictor for in vivo pulmonary function challenge test* [methacholine chloride] 100 mg/5 mL

proxazole USAN, INN *smooth muscle relaxant; analgesic; anti-inflammatory*

proxazole citrate USAN *smooth muscle relaxant; analgesic; anti-inflammatory*

proxetil INN *combining name for radicals or groups*

proxibarbal INN

proxibutene INN

proxicromil USAN, INN *antiallergic*

proxifezone INN

Proxigel OTC *topical oral anti-inflammatory/anti-infective for braces* [carbamide peroxide] 10%

proxorphan INN *analgesic; antitussive* [also: proxorphan tartrate]

proxorphan tartrate USAN *analgesic; antitussive* [also: proxorphan]

Proxy 65 tablets ℞ *analgesic* [propoxyphene HCl; acetaminophen]

proxymetacaine INN, BAN *topical ophthalmic anesthetic* [also: proparacaine HCl]

proxymetacaine HCl [see: proparacaine HCl]

proxyphylline INN, BAN

Prozac Pulvules (capsules), liquid ℞ *antidepressant; selective serotonin reuptake inhibitor; treatment for obsessive-compulsive disorder* [fluoxetine HCl] 10, 20 mg; 20 mg/5 mL

prozapine INN

Prozine-50 IM injection ℞ *antipsychotic* [promazine HCl] 50 mg/mL

Prulet tablets OTC *laxative* [white phenolphthalein] 60 mg

Pryme ℞ *investigational vaccine for Lyme disease*

PSC-833 *investigational adjunct to chemotherapy for multi–drug-resistant tumors*

Pseudo liquid OTC *nasal decongestant* [pseudoephedrine HCl] 30 mg/5 mL

Pseudo-Car DM syrup ℞ *antitussive; decongestant; antihistamine* [dextromethorphan hydrobromide; pseudoephedrine HCl; carbinoxamine maleate] 15•60•4 mg/5 mL

Pseudo-Chlor sustained-release capsules ℞ *decongestant; antihistamine* [pseudoephedrine HCl; chlorpheniramine maleate] 120•8 mg

pseudoephedrine INN, BAN *vasoconstrictor; nasal decongestant* [also: pseudoephedrine HCl]

pseudoephedrine HCl USAN, USP *vasoconstrictor; nasal decongestant* [also: pseudoephedrine] 30, 60 mg oral; 30 mg/5 mL oral

pseudoephedrine polistirex USAN *nasal decongestant*

pseudoephedrine sulfate USAN, USP *bronchodilator; nasal decongestant*

Pseudo-Gest tablets OTC *nasal decongestant* [pseudoephedrine HCl] 30, 60 mg

Pseudo-Gest Plus tablets OTC *decongestant; antihistamine* [pseudoephedrine HCl; chlorpheniramine maleate] 60•4 mg

pseudomonas hyperimmune globulin [see: mucoid exopolysaccharide pseudomonas hyperimmune globulin]

pseudomonic acid A [see: mupirocin]

psilocybine INN, BAN

Psor-a-set bar OTC *therapeutic skin cleanser; topical keratolytic* [salicylic acid] 2%

Psorcon cream, ointment ℞ *topical corticosteroidal anti-inflammatory* [diflorasone diacetate] 0.05%

PsoriGel OTC *topical antipsoriatic; antiseborrheic; antiseptic* [coal tar solution; alcohol 33%] 7.5%

PsoriNail liquid (discontinued 1994) OTC *topical antipsoriatic; antiseborrheic; antiseptic* [coal tar solution] 2.5%

Psorion cream (discontinued 1995) ℞ *topical corticosteroid* [betamethasone dipropionate] 0.05%

psyllium husk USP *bulk laxative*

psyllium hydrocolloid *bulk laxative*

psyllium hydrophilic mucilloid *bulk laxative*

psyllium seed [see: plantago seed]

PTC (plasma thromboplastin component) [see: factor IX]

P.T.E.-4; P.T.E.-5 IV injection ℞ *intravenous nutritional therapy* [multiple trace elements (metals)]

pteroyldiglutamic acid (PDGA)

pteroylglutamic acid (PGA) [see: folic acid]

PTFE (polytetrafluoroethylene) [see: polytef]

PTU (propylthiouracil) [q.v.]

Pulmicort Turbuhaler ℞ *investigational steroidal inhalant for asthma and chronic bronchitis* [budesonide]

Pulmocare ready-to-use liquid OTC *enteral nutritional therapy for pulmonary problems*

pulmonary surfactant replacement (*orphan: infant respiratory distress syndrome*)

Pulmozyme solution for nebulization ℞ *treatment for the respiratory effects of cystic fibrosis* (*orphan*) [dornase alfa] 1 mg/mL

pulse VAC (vincristine, actinomycin D, cyclophosphamide) *chemotherapy protocol* [also: VAC]

pulse VAC (vincristine, Adriamycin, cyclophosphamide) *chemotherapy protocol* [also: VAC]

Pulvule (trademarked dosage form) *bullet-shaped capsule*

pumice USP *dental abrasive*

pumitepa INN

Punctum Plug ℞ *blocks the puncta and canaliculus to eliminate tear loss in keratitis sicca* [silicone plug]

Puralube ophthalmic ointment OTC *ocular moisturizer/lubricant* [white petrolatum; mineral oil]

Puralube Tears eye drops OTC *ocular moisturizer/lubricant* [polyvinyl alcohol; polyethylene glycol 400] 1%•1%

Pure Sept solutions (discontinued 1992) OTC *two-step chemical disinfecting system for soft contact lenses*

Purge liquid OTC *stimulant laxative* [castor oil] 95%

purified cotton [see: cotton, purified]

purified protein derivative (PPD) of tuberculin [see: tuberculin]

purified rayon [see: rayon, purified]

purified siliceous earth [see: siliceous earth, purified]

purified water [see: water, purified]

H-purin-6-amine [see: adenine]

Purinethol tablets ℞ *antimetabolic antineoplastic for multiple leukemias* [mercaptopurine] 50 mg

Purisol 4 solution (discontinued 1992) OTC *rinsing/storage solution for soft contact lenses* [saline solution]

puromycin USAN, INN *antineoplastic; antiprotozoal (Trypanosoma)*

puromycin HCl USAN *antineoplastic; antiprotozoal (Trypanosoma)*

Purpose Dry Skin cream OTC *moisturizer; emollient*

Purpose Soap bar OTC *therapeutic skin cleanser*

PVA (polyvinyl alcohol) [q.v.]

PVB (Platinol, vinblastine, bleomycin) *chemotherapy protocol*

PVDA (prednisone, vincristine, daunorubicin, asparaginase) *chemotherapy protocol*

PVP; PVP-16 (Platinol, VP-16) *chemotherapy protocol*

P-V-Tussin syrup ℞ *narcotic antitussive; decongestant; antihistamine* [hydrocodone bitartrate; pseudoephedrine HCl; chlorpheniramine maleate; alcohol 5%] 2.5•30•2 mg/5 mL

P-V-Tussin tablets ℞ *narcotic antitussive; antihistamine; expectorant* [hydrocodone bitartrate; phenindamine tartrate; guaifenesin] 5•25•200 mg

9-[3-pydidylmethyl]-9-deazaguanine (*orphan: cutaneous T-cell lymphoma*)

Pyloriset reagent kit for professional use *in vitro diagnostic aid for GI disorders*

Pyocidin-Otic ear drops (discontinued 1992) ℞ *topical corticosteroidal anti-inflammatory; antibiotic* [hydrocortisone; polymyxin B sulfate]

pyrabrom USAN *antihistamine*

pyradone [see: aminopyrine]

pyrantel INN *anthelmintic* [also: pyrantel pamoate]

pyrantel pamoate USAN, USP *anthelmintic* [also: pyrantel]

pyrantel tartrate USAN *anthelmintic*

pyrathiazine HCl [see: parathiazine]

pyrazinamide (PZA) USP, INN, BAN *bactericidal; primary tuberculostatic* 500 mg oral

pyrazinecarboxamide [see: pyrazinamide]

pyrazofurin USAN *antineoplastic* [also: pirazofurin]

pyrazoline [see: antipyrine]

pyrbenzindole [see: benzindopyrine HCl]

pyrbuterol HCl [see: pirbuterol HCl]

pyrethrins

pyribenzamine (PBZ) [see: tripelennamine]

pyricarbate INN

pyridarone INN

Pyridiate tablets ℞ *urinary analgesic* [phenazopyridine HCl] 100 mg

4-pyridinamine [see: fampridine]

2-pyridine aldoxime methylchloride (2-PAM) [see: pralidoxime chloride]

3-pyridinecarboxamide [see: niacinamide]

3-pyridinecarboxylic acid [see: niacin]

4-pyridinecarboxylic acid hydrazide [see: isoniazid]

3-pyridinecarboxylic acid methyl ester [see: methyl nicotinate]

3-pyridinemethanol [see: nicotinyl alcohol]

2-pyridinemethanol [see: piconol]

3-pyridinemethanol tartrate [see: nicotinyl tartrate]

Pyridium tablets ℞ *urinary analgesic* [phenazopyridine HCl] 100, 200 mg ℞ Dyrenium; pyridoxine; pyrithione; pyritidium

Pyridium Plus tablets (discontinued 1993) ℞ *urinary analgesic; antispasmodic; sedative* [phenazopyridine HCl; hyoscyamine hydrobromide; butabarbital] 150•0.3•15 mg

pyridofylline INN

pyridostigmine bromide USP, INN *cholinergic; anticholinesterase muscle stimulant* ℞ physostigmine

pyridoxal [see: pyridoxine HCl]

pyridoxamine [see: pyridoxine HCl]

pyridoxine INN *vitamin B_6; enzyme cofactor* [also: pyridoxine HCl] ℞ pralidoxime; Pyridium

pyridoxine HCl USP *vitamin B_6; enzyme cofactor* [also: pyridoxine] 25, 50, 100 mg oral; 100 mg/mL injection ℞ pralidoxime; Pyridium

β-pyridylcarbinol [see: nicotinyl alcohol]

pyridylmethanol *me+* [see: nicotinyl alcohol]

pyrilamine maleate USP *anticholinergic; antihistamine; sleep aid* [also: mepyramine]

pyrilamine tannate

pyrimethamine USP, INN *malaria suppression and transmission control; folic acid antagonist*

pyrimitate INN, BAN

Pyrinex Pediculicide shampoo OTC *pediculicide* [pyrethrins; piperonyl butoxide; deodorized kerosene] 0.2%•2%•0.8%

pyrinoline USAN, INN *antiarrhythmic*

Pyrinyl liquid OTC *pediculicide* [pyrethrins; piperonyl butoxide; deodorized kerosene] 0.2%•2%•0.8%

Pyrinyl II liquid OTC *pediculicide* [pyrethrins; piperonyl butoxide] 0.3%•3%

Pyrinyl Plus shampoo OTC *pediculicide* [pyrethrins; piperonyl butoxide] 0.3%•3%

pyrithen [see: chlorothen citrate]

pyrithione sodium USAN *topical antimicrobial* ② Pyridium

pyrithione zinc USAN, INN, BAN *antibacterial; antifungal; antiseborrheic*

pyrithyldione INN

pyritidium bromide INN ② Pyridium

pyritinol INN, BAN

pyrodifenium bromide [see: prifinium bromide]

pyrogallic acid [see: pyrogallol]

pyrogallol NF

pyrophendane INN

pyrophenindane [see: pyrophendane]

pyrovalerone INN *CNS stimulant* [also: pyrovalerone HCl]

pyrovalerone HCl USAN *CNS stimulant* [also: pyrovalerone]

pyroxamine INN *antihistamine* [also: pyroxamine maleate]

pyroxamine maleate USAN *antihistamine* [also: pyroxamine]

pyroxylin USP, INN *pharmaceutic necessity for collodion*

pyrrobutamine phosphate USP

pyrrocaine USAN, INN *local anesthetic*

pyrrocaine HCl NF

pyrrolifene INN *analgesic* [also: pyrroliphene HCl]

pyrrolifene HCl [see: pyrroliphene HCl]

pyrroliphene HCl USAN *analgesic* [also: pyrrolifene]

pyrrolnitrin USAN, INN *antifungal*

pyrroxane [now: proroxan HCl]

Pyrroxate capsules OTC *decongestant; antihistamine; analgesic* [phenylpropanolamine HCl; chlorpheniramine maleate; acetaminophen] 25•4•650 mg

pyrvinium chloride INN

pyrvinium embonate [see: pyrvinium pamoate]

pyrvinium pamoate USP *anthelmintic* [also: viprynium embonate]

pytamine INN

PZA (pyrazinamide) [q.v.]

PZI (protamine zinc insulin) [q.v.]

Q.B. liquid (discontinued 1993) ℞ *antiasthmatic; bronchodilator; expectorant* [theophylline; guaifenesin]

Q-Pam tablets (discontinued 1993) ℞ *skeletal muscle relaxant* [diazepam]

QTest test stick for home use OTC *in vitro diagnostic aid for urine pregnancy test*

QTest Ovulation test kit for professional use *in vitro diagnostic aid to predict ovulation time*

quadazocine INN, BAN *opioid antagonist* [also: quadazocine mesylate]

quadazocine mesylate USAN *opioid antagonist* [also: quadazocine]

Quadra-Hist extended-release tablets (discontinued 1995) ℞ *decongestant;*

antihistamine [phenylpropanolamine HCl; phenylephrine HCl; chlorpheniramine maleate; phenyltoloxamine citrate] 40•10•5•15 mg

Quadra-Hist ER syrup (discontinued 1993) ℞ *decongestant; antihistamine* [phenylpropanolamine HCl; phenylephrine HCl; phenyltoloxamine citrate; chlorpheniramine maleate]

Quadra-Hist Pediatric syrup (discontinued 1995) ℞ *pediatric decongestant and antihistamine* [phenylpropanolamine HCl; phenylephrine HCl; chlorpheniramine maleate; phenyltoloxamine citrate] 5•1.25•0.5•2 mg/5 mL

Quadrinal tablets ℞ *antiasthmatic; bronchodilator; decongestant; expectorant; sedative* [theophylline; ephedrine HCl; potassium iodide; phenobarbital] 65•24•320•24 mg

quadrosilan INN

Quantaffirm reagent kit for professional use *in vitro diagnostic aid for mononucleosis*

Quarzan capsules ℞ *anticholinergic; peptic ulcer treatment* [clidinium bromide] 2.5, 5 mg ⓘ Questran

quatacaine INN

quazepam USAN, INN *sedative; hypnotic*

quazinone USAN, INN *cardiotonic*

quazodine USAN, INN *cardiotonic; bronchodilator*

quazolast USAN, INN *antiasthmatic; mediator release inhibitor*

Quelan liquid ℞ *bronchodilator; expectorant* [theophylline; guaifenesin]

Quelicin IV or IM injection ℞ *neuromuscular blocker* [succinylcholine chloride] 20, 50, 100 mg/mL

Quelidrine Cough syrup OTC *antitussive; decongestant; antihistamine; expectorant* [dextromethorphan hydrobromide; ephedrine HCl; phenylephrine HCl; chlorpheniramine maleate; ammonium chloride; ipecac; alcohol 2%] 10 mg•5 mg•5 mg•2 mg•40 mg•0.005 mL per 5 mL

Queltuss tablets (discontinued 1993) OTC *antitussive; expectorant* [dextromethorphan hydrobromide; guaifenesin]

Quercetin tablets OTC *dietary supplement* [eucalyptus bioflavonoids] 50, 250 mg

Questran wax-coated tablets (discontinued 1994) ℞ *cholesterol-lowering antihyperlipidemic* [cholestyramine resin] 1 g ⓘ Quarzan

Questran; Questran Light powder for oral suspension ℞ *cholesterol-lowering antihyperlipidemic* [cholestyramine resin] 4 g/dose

Quibron liquid (discontinued 1992) ℞ *antiasthmatic; bronchodilator; expectorant* [theophylline; guaifenesin]

Quibron; Quibron-300 capsules ℞ *antiasthmatic; bronchodilator; expectorant* [theophylline; guaifenesin] 150•90 mg; 300•180 mg

Quibron Plus capsules (discontinued 1992) ℞ *antiasthmatic; bronchodilator; decongestant; expectorant; sedative* [theophylline; ephedrine HCl; guaifenesin; butabarbital]

Quibron Plus elixir (discontinued 1993) ℞ *antiasthmatic; bronchodilator; decongestant; expectorant; sedative* [theophylline; ephedrine HCl; guaifenesin; butabarbital]

Quibron-T Dividose (multiple-scored tablets) ℞ *bronchodilator* [theophylline] 300 mg

Quibron-T/SR sustained-release Dividose (multiple-scored tablets) ℞ *bronchodilator* [theophylline] 300 mg

Quick Care solutions OTC *two-step chemical disinfecting system for soft contact lenses* [hydrogen peroxide-based]

Quick Pep tablets OTC *CNS stimulant; analeptic* [caffeine] 150 mg

QuickVue test cassettes for professional use *in vitro diagnostic aid for urine pregnancy test*

Quiess IM injection ℞ *anxiolytic* [hydroxyzine HCl] 50 mg/mL

Quiet World tablets (discontinued 1992) OTC *antihistaminic sleep aid; analgesic* [pyrilamine maleate; acetaminophen; aspirin]

quifenadine INN

quiflapon sodium USAN *leukotriene biosynthesis inhibitor for asthma and inflammatory bowel disease*

quillifoline INN

quinacainol INN
quinacillin INN, BAN
quinacrine HCl USP *anthelmintic; antimalarial* [also: mepacrine] ▣ quinidine
Quinaglute Dura-Tabs (sustained-release tablets) ℞ *antiarrhythmic* [quinidine gluconate] 324 mg
Quinalan sustained-release tablets ℞ *antiarrhythmic* [quinidine gluconate] 324 mg
quinalbarbitone sodium BAN *hypnotic; sedative* [also: secobarbital sodium]
quinaldine blue USAN *obstetric diagnostic aid*
quinambicide [see: clioquinol]
Quinamm tablets (discontinued 1996) ℞ *prevention and treatment of nocturnal leg cramps* [quinine sulfate] 260 mg
quinapril INN, BAN *antihypertensive; angiotensin-converting enzyme (ACE) inhibitor* [also: quinapril HCl]
quinapril HCl USAN *antihypertensive; angiotensin-converting enzyme (ACE) inhibitor* [also: quinapril]
quinaprilat USAN, INN *antihypertensive; angiotensin-converting enzyme (ACE) inhibitor*
Quinatime sustained-release tablets (discontinued 1992) ℞ *antiarrhythmic* [quinidine gluconate] ▣ quinidine
quinazosin INN *antihypertensive* [also: quinazosin HCl]
quinazosin HCl USAN *antihypertensive* [also: quinazosin]
quinbolone USAN, INN *anabolic*
quincarbate INN
quindecamine INN *antibacterial* [also: quindecamine acetate]
quindecamine acetate USAN *antibacterial* [also: quindecamine]
quindonium bromide USAN, INN *antiarrhythmic*
quindoxin INN, BAN
quinelorane INN *antihypertensive; antiparkinsonian* [also: quinelorane HCl]
quinelorane HCl USAN *antihypertensive; antiparkinsonian* [also: quinelorane]
quinestradol INN, BAN
quinestrol USAN, USP, INN, BAN *estrogen*
quinetalate INN *smooth muscle relaxant* [also: quinetolate]

quinethazone USP, INN *diuretic; antihypertensive*
quinetolate USAN *smooth muscle relaxant* [also: quinetalate]
quinezamide INN
quinfamide USAN, INN *antiamebic*
quingestanol INN *progestin* [also: quingestanol acetate]
quingestanol acetate USAN *progestin* [also: quingestanol]
quingestrone USAN, INN *progestin*
Quinidex Extentabs (extended-release tablets) ℞ *antiarrhythmic* [quinidine sulfate] 300 mg
quinidine NF, BAN *antiarrhythmic* ▣ clonidine; quinacrine; Quinatime; quinine
quinidine gluconate USP *antiarrhythmic* 324 mg oral; 80 mg/mL injection
quinidine polygalacturonate *antiarrhythmic*
quinidine sulfate USP *antiarrhythmic* 300 mg oral
quinine NF, BAN ▣ quinidine
quinine ascorbate USAN *smoking deterrent*
quinine biascorbate [now: quinine ascorbate]
quinine bisulfate NF
quinine dihydrochloride NF *investigational anti-infective for pernicious malaria*
quinine ethylcarbonate NF
quinine glycerophosphate NF
quinine HCl NF
quinine hydrobromide NF
quinine hypophosphite NF
quinine monohydrobromide [see: quinine hydrobromide]
quinine monohydrochloride [see: quinine HCl]
quinine monosalicylate [see: quinine salicylate]
quinine phosphate NF
quinine phosphinate [see: quinine hypophosphite]
quinine salicylate NF
quinine sulfate USP *antimalarial schizonticide; treatment of nocturnal leg cramps* 200, 260, 325 mg oral
quinine sulfate dihydrate [see: quinine sulfate]
quinine tannate USP

quinisocaine INN [also: dimethisoquin HCl; dimethisoquin]
quinocide INN
8-quinolinol [see: oxyquinoline]
8-quinolinol benzoate [see: benzoxiquine]
Quinora tablets ℞ *antiarrhythmic* [quinidine sulfate] 300 mg
quinotolast *investigational antiallergic/antiasthmatic agent*
quinoxyl [see: chiniofon]
quinpirole INN *antihypertensive* [also: quinpirole HCl]
quinpirole HCl USAN *antihypertensive* [also: quinpirole]
quinprenaline INN *bronchodilator* [also: quinterenol sulfate]
quinprenaline sulfate [see: quinterenol sulfate]
Quin-Release sustained-release tablets ℞ *antiarrhythmic* [quinidine gluconate]
Quinsana Plus powder OTC *topical antifungal* [tolnaftate] 1%
Quintabs tablets OTC *vitamin supplement* [multiple vitamins; folic acid] ≟•0.1 mg

Quintabs-M tablets OTC *vitamin/mineral/iron supplement* [multiple vitamins & minerals; iron; folic acid] ≟•18•0.4 mg
quinterenol sulfate USAN *bronchodilator* [also: quinprenaline]
quintiofos INN, BAN
3-quinuclidinol benzoate [see: benzoclidine]
quinuclium bromide USAN, INN *antihypertensive*
quinupramine INN
quinupristin USAN, INN *antibacterial*
quipazine INN *antidepressant; oxytocic* [also: quipazine maleate]
quipazine maleate USAN *antidepressant; oxytocic* [also: quipazine]
Quiphile tablets (discontinued 1996) ℞ *prevention and treatment of nocturnal leg cramps* [quinine sulfate] 260 mg
quisultazine INN
quisultidine [see: quisultazine]
Q-Vel soft caplets (discontinued 1996) OTC *prevention and treatment of nocturnal leg cramps* [quinine sulfate] 64.8 mg

R

r24 antibody [see: monoclonal antibody r24]
R 87,926 *investigational treatment for stroke*
R 89,439 *investigational agent for HIV*
R 91,274 *investigational antimigraine agent in clinical trials as a patch, injection, and nasal spray*
R 93,777 *investigational treatment for irritable bowel syndrome*
R 93,877 *investigational therapy for chronic constipation*
R & C shampoo OTC *pediculicide* [pyrethrins; piperonyl butoxide] 0.3%•3%
R & D Calcium Carbonate/600 ℞ (*orphan: hyperphosphatemia of end-stage renal disease*) [calcium carbonate]
RA Lotion OTC *topical acne treatment* [resorcinol; alcohol 43%] 3%

rabeprazole INN *antiulcerative; proton pump inhibitor* [also: rabeprazole sodium]
rabeprazole sodium USAN *antiulcerative; proton pump inhibitor* [also: rabeprazole]
rabies immune globulin (RIG) USP *passive immunizing agent*
rabies vaccine USP *active immunizing agent* Challenge Virus Standard (CVS)
rabies vaccine, adsorbed (RVA) [see: rabies vaccine]
rabies vaccine, HDCV (human diploid cell vaccine) [see: rabies vaccine]
racefemine INN
racefenicol INN *antibacterial* [also: racephenicol]
racemethadol [see: dimepheptanol]

racemethionine USAN, USP *urinary acidifier* [also: methionine (the DL- form)]
racemethorphan INN, BAN
racemetirosine INN
racemic amphetamine phosphate
racemic amphetamine sulfate [see: amphetamine sulfate]
racemic calcium pantothenate [see: calcium pantothenate, racemic]
racemoramide INN, BAN
racemorphan INN
racephedrine HCl USAN
racephenicol USAN *antibacterial* [also: racefenicol]
racepinefrine INN *bronchodilator* [also: racepinephrine]
racepinephrine USP *bronchodilator* [also: racepinefrine]
racepinephrine HCl USP *bronchodilator*
raclopride INN, BAN
ractopamine INN *veterinary growth stimulant* [also: ractopamine HCl]
ractopamine HCl USAN *veterinary growth stimulant* [also: ractopamine]
Radinyl ℞ *investigational antineoplastic for breast cancer* [etanidazole]
radio-chromated serum albumin [see: albumin, chromated]
radio-iodinated I 125 serum albumin [see: albumin, iodinated]
radio-iodinated I 131 serum albumin [see: albumin, iodinated]
radiomerisoprol ^{197}Hg [see: merisoprol Hg 197]
radioselenomethionine ^{75}Se [see: selenomethionine Se 75]
radiotolpovidone I 131 INN *hypoalbuminemia test; radioactive agent* [also: tolpovidone I 131]
radium *element (Ra)*
radon *element (Rn)*
rafoxanide USAN, INN *anthelmintic*
Ragus tablets OTC *dietary supplement* [multiple vitamins, minerals, and amino acids]
ralitoline USAN, INN *anticonvulsant*
raloxifene INN *antiestrogen; investigational treatment for osteoporosis* [also: raloxifene HCl]
raloxifene HCl USAN *antiestrogen; investigational treatment for osteoporosis* [also: raloxifene]

rambufaside [see: meproscillarin]
ramciclane INN
ramifenazone INN
ramipril USAN, INN, BAN *antihypertensive; angiotensin-converting enzyme (ACE) inhibitor*
ramiprilat INN
ramixotidine INN
ramnodigin INN
ramoplanin USAN, INN *antibacterial antibiotic; investigational decontaminant for bowel surgery and wound infections*
RAMP Urine hCG Assay test kit for professional use (discontinued 1994) *in vitro diagnostic aid for urine pregnancy test* [monoclonal antibody-based enzyme immunoassay]
Ramses vaginal jelly OTC *spermicidal contraceptive* [nonoxynol 9] 5%
Ramses Extra premedicated condom OTC *spermicidal/barrier contraceptive* [nonoxynol 9] 15%
ranimustine INN
ranimycin USAN, INN *antibacterial*
ranitidine USAN, INN, BAN *treatment of GI ulcers; histamine H$_2$ antagonist*
ranitidine bismuth citrate USAN *treatment of GI ulcers; histamine H$_2$ blocker* [also: ranitidine bismutrex]
ranitidine bismutrex BAN *treatment of GI ulcers; histamine H$_2$ blocker* [also: ranitidine bismuth citrate]
ranitidine HCl USP, JAN *treatment of GI ulcers; histamine H$_2$ antagonist* 15 mg/mL oral
ranolazine INN *antianginal* [also: ranolazine HCl]
ranolazine HCl USAN *antianginal; investigational treatment for peripheral artery disease* [also: ranolazine]
Rapamune ℞ *investigational adjunct for organ transplant and treatment for autoimmune diseases* [sirolimus]
rapamycin [now: sirolimus]
RapidTest Strep test kit for professional use (discontinued 1995) *in vitro diagnostic test for streptococcal antigens in throat swabs*
RapidVue test kit for home use OTC *in vitro diagnostic aid for urine pregnancy test*

rasagiline INN
rasagiline mesylate USAN *antiparkinsonian; monoamine oxidase B (MAO-B) inhibitor*
raspberry [syrup] USP
rathyronine INN
rattlesnake antivenin [see: antivenin (Crotalidae) polyvalent]
Raudixin tablets (discontinued 1995) ℞ *antihypertensive; antipsychotic* [rauwolfia serpentina (whole root)] 50, 100 mg
Rauverid tablets (discontinued 1995) ℞ *antihypertensive; antipsychotic* [rauwolfia serpentina (whole root)] 50 mg
rauwolfia derivatives *all rauwolfia derivatives except reserpine were discontinued 1991–1995*
rauwolfia serpentina USP *antihypertensive; peripheral antiadrenergic*
Rauzide tablets ℞ *antihypertensive* [bendroflumethiazide; rauwolfia serpentina] 4•50 mg
Ravocaine & Novocaine with Levophed injection ℞ *injectable local anesthetic for dental procedures* [proproxycaine HCl; procaine; norepinephrine] 7.2•36•0.12 mg/1.8 mL
Ravocaine & Novocaine with Neo-Cobefrin injection (discontinued 1995) ℞ *injectable local anesthetic for dental procedures* [proproxycaine HCl; procaine; levonordefrin] 7.2•36•0.09 mg/1.8 mL
rayon, purified USAN, USP *surgical aid*
razinodil INN
razobazam INN
razoxane INN, BAN
[86]Rb [see: rubidium chloride Rb 86]
RBC-CD4 *investigational (Phase I/II) antiviral for HIV*
rCD4 (recombinant soluble human CD4) [see: CD4, recombinant soluble human]
RCF liquid OTC *hypoallergenic infant formula* [soy protein formula, carbohydrate free]
Reabilan; Reabilan HN ready-to-use liquid OTC *enteral nutritional therapy* [lactose-free formula]
Reactine (Canadian name for U.S. product Zyrtec)
reactrol [see: clemizole HCl]

Rea-Lo cream, lotion (discontinued 1992) OTC *moisturizer; emollient; keratolytic* [urea]
rebamipide INN
Rebif (commercially available in Italy) ℞ *investigational treatment for multiple sclerosis, hepatitis C, genital warts, and malignant gliomas* [interferon beta, recombinant]
reboxetine INN *investigational fast-acting antidepressant*
recainam INN, BAN *antiarrhythmic* [also: recainam HCl]
recainam HCl USAN *antiarrhythmic* [also: recainam]
recainam tosylate USAN *antiarrhythmic*
recanescin [see: deserpidine]
Receptin ℞ *(orphan: AIDS)* [CD4, recombinant soluble human]
reclazepam USAN, INN *sedative*
Reclomide tablets ℞ *antidopaminergic; antiemetic for chemotherapy; peristaltic* [metoclopramide monohydrochloride monohydrate] 10 mg
Recombigen HIV-1 LA Test reagent kit for professional use *in vitro diagnostic aid for HIV-1 antibodies in blood, serum, or plasma* [latex agglutination test]
recombinant alpha$_1$ antitrypsin [see: alpha$_1$ antitrypsin, recombinant]
recombinant antihemophilic factor [see: antihemophilic factor, recombinant]
recombinant factor VIIa [see: factor VIIa, recombinant]
recombinant factor VIII [see: antihemophilic factor, recombinant]
recombinant human CD4 immunoglobulin G [CD4 immunoglobulin G, recombinant human]
recombinant human deoxyribonuclease (rhDNase) [see: deoxyribonuclease, recombinant human]
recombinant human erythropoietin [see: erythropoietin, recombinant human]
recombinant human growth hormone (rhGH) [see: somatropin]
recombinant human interferon beta [see: interferon beta, recombinant human]

recombinant human interleukin-1 receptor (rhIL-1R; rhu IL-1R) [see: interleukin-1 receptor]
recombinant human nerve growth factor (rhNGF) [see: nerve growth factor]
recombinant human serum albumin (rHSA)
recombinant human superoxide dismutase (SOD) [see: superoxide dismutase, recombinant human]
recombinant interferon alfa-2a [see: interferon alfa-2a, recombinant]
recombinant interferon alfa-2b [see: interferon alfa-2b, recombinant]
recombinant interferon beta [see: interferon beta, recombinant]
recombinant interleukin-2 [see: interleukin-2, recombinant]
recombinant methionyl granulocyte CSF [see: methionyl granulocyte CSF, recombinant]
recombinant methionyl human granulocyte CSF [see: methionyl human granulocyte CSF, recombinant]
recombinant soluble human CD4 (rCD4) [see: CD4, recombinant soluble human]
recombinant tissue plasminogen activator (rtPA; rt-PA) [see: alteplase]
recombinant TNF receptor fusion protein *investigational treatment for rheumatoid arthritis and septic shock*
recombinant vaccinia (human papillomavirus) *(orphan: cervical cancer)*
Recombinate powder for IV injection ℞ *antihemophilic to correct coagulation deficiency* [antihemophilic factor VIII, recombinant] 250, 500, 1000 IU
Recombivax HB adult IM injection, pediatric IM injection, adolescent/high-risk infant IM injection, dialysis formulation ℞ *hepatitis B vaccine* [hepatitis B virus vaccine, recombinant] 10 μg/mL; 2.5 μg/0.5 mL; 5 μg/0.5 mL; 40 μg/mL
Recormon ℞ *investigational blood cell growth factor* [erythropoietin]
Rectacort rectal suppositories ℞ *topical corticosteroidal anti-inflammatory* [hydrocortisone acetate] 10%
Rectagene rectal suppositories OTC *temporary relief of hemorrhoidal symptoms* [live yeast cell derivative; shark liver oil] 2000 SRF U/oz.
Rectagene II rectal suppositories OTC *temporary relief of hemorrhoidal symptoms* [bismuth subgallate; bismuth resorcin compound; benzyl benzoate; peruvian balsam; zinc oxide] 2.25%•1.75%•1.2%•1.8%•11%
Rectagene Medicated Rectal Balm ointment OTC *temporary relief of hemorrhoidal symptoms* [shark liver oil; phenyl mercuric nitrate; live yeast cell derivative] 3%•1:10,000•66.67 U/g
Rectolax suppositories OTC *laxative* [bisacodyl] 10 mg
red blood cells [see: blood cells, red]
Red Cross Toothache liquid OTC *topical oral analgesic* [eugenol] 85%
red ferric oxide [see: ferric oxide, red]
red veterinarian petrolatum (RVP) [see: petrolatum]
Redi Vial (trademarked packaging form) *dual-compartment vial*
Redi Vial (trademarked packaging form) *two-compartment vial*
Rediject (trademarked delivery system) *prefilled disposable syringe*
Redipak (trademarked packaging form) *unit dose or unit-of-issue package*
redox-acyclovir *(orphan: herpes simplex encephalitis in AIDS)*
redox-penicillin G *(orphan: AIDS-associated neurosyphilis)*
redox-phenytoin *(orphan: emergency rescue of grand mal status epilepticus)*
Reducin ℞ *(orphan: nonoperative management of cutaneous fistulas of the GI tract)* [somatostatin]
Redutemp tablets OTC *analgesic; antipyretic* [acetaminophen] 500 mg
Redux capsules ℞ *anorexiant and appetite suppressant for long-term dieting* [dexfenfluramine HCl] 15 mg
Reese's Pinworm liquid OTC *anthelmintic* [pyrantel pamoate] 50 mg/mL
Refresh eye drops OTC *ocular moisturizer/lubricant* [polyvinyl alcohol] 1.4%

Refresh Plus eye drops OTC *ocular moisturizer/lubricant* [carboxymethylcellulose] 0.5%

Refresh P.M. ophthalmic ointment OTC *ocular moisturizer/lubricant* [white petrolatum; mineral oil; lanolin]

Rēgain snack bar OTC *enteral nutritional therapy for impaired renal function* [essential amino acids] ⓧ Rogaine

Regitine IV or IM injection ℞ *antihypertensive for pheochromocytoma* [phentolamine mesylate] 5 mg/mL

Reglan tablets, syrup, IV infusion ℞ *antidopaminergic; antiemetic for chemotherapy; peristaltic* [metoclopramide monohydrochloride monohydrate] 5, 10 mg; 5 mg/5 mL; 5 mg/mL ⓧ Regonol

Regonol IM or IV injection ℞ *anticholinesterase muscle stimulant; muscle relaxant reversal* [pyridostigmine bromide] 5 mg/mL ⓧ Reglan

regramostim USAN, INN *antineutropenic; hematopoietic stimulant; biologic response modifier; bone marrow stimulant*

Regranex *investigational recombinant platelet-derived growth factor B for chronic dermal ulcers* [becaplermin]

Regroton tablets ℞ *antihypertensive* [chlorthalidone; reserpine] 50•0.25 mg ⓧ Hygroton

Regulace capsules OTC *laxative; stool softener* [casanthranol; docusate sodium] 30•100 mg

Regular Iletin I subcu injection OTC *antidiabetic* [insulin (beef-pork)] 100 U/mL

Regular Iletin II (beef) subcu injection (discontinued 1994) OTC *antidiabetic* [insulin]

Regular Iletin II (pork) subcu injection OTC *antidiabetic* [insulin] 100 U/mL

Regular Iletin II U-500 (concentrated) subcu or IM injection ℞ *antidiabetic* [insulin (pork)] 500 U/mL

Regular Insulin subcu injection OTC *antidiabetic* [insulin (pork)] 100 U/mL

Regular Purified Pork Insulin subcu injection OTC *antidiabetic* [insulin] 100 U/mL

Regulax SS capsules OTC *stool softener* [docusate sodium] 100, 250 mg

Reguloid powder OTC *bulk laxative* [psyllium hydrophilic mucilloid] 3.4 g/tsp.

Regutol tablets OTC *stool softener* [docusate sodium] 100 mg

Rehydralyte oral solution OTC *electrolyte replacement* [sodium, potassium, and chloride electrolytes]

Rela sugar-coated tablets (discontinued 1993) ℞ *skeletal muscle relaxant* [carisoprodol]

Relafen film-coated tablets ℞ *antiarthritic; nonsteroidal anti-inflammatory drug (NSAID)* [nabumetone] 500, 750 mg

Relaxadon tablets (discontinued 1995) ℞ *GI anticholinergic; sedative* [atropine sulfate; scopolamine hydrobromide; hyoscyamine hydrobromide; phenobarbital] 0.0194•0.0065•0.1037•16.2 mg

relaxin *investigational agent to facilitate childbirth (clinical trials discontinued 1994)*

Release-Tabs (dosage form) *timed-release tablets*

Relefact TRH IV injection (name changed to Thyrel-TRH in 1995)

Relief eye drops OTC *topical ocular decongestant* [phenylephrine HCl] 0.12%

relomycin USAN, INN *antibacterial*

remacemide INN *neuroprotective anticonvulsant; investigational treatment for stroke and Huntington's disease* [also: remacemide HCl]

remacemide HCl USAN *neuroprotective anticonvulsant; investigational treatment for stroke and Huntington's disease* [also: remacemide]

Remcol Cold capsules (discontinued 1995) OTC *decongestant; antihistamine; analgesic* [phenylpropanolamine HCl; chlorpheniramine maleate; acetaminophen] 25•2•300 mg

Remcol-C capsules (discontinued 1995) OTC *antitussive; antihistamine; analgesic* [dextromethorphan hydrobromide; chlorpheniramine maleate; acetaminophen] 15•2•300 mg

Remeron tablets ℞ *tetracyclic antidepressant* [mirtazapine] 15, 30 mg

remifentanil INN, BAN *short-acting opioid analgesic* [also: remifentanil HCl]

remifentanil HCl USAN *short-acting opioid analgesic* [also: remifentanil]

remikiren INN

remiprostol USAN, INN *antiulcerative*

Remisar ℞ *investigational oncolytic and immunomodulator for bladder cancer and lymphoma* [bropirimine]

remoxipride USAN, INN, BAN *antipsychotic*

remoxipride HCl USAN *antipsychotic*

Remular-S tablets ℞ *skeletal muscle relaxant* [chlorzoxazone] 250 mg

Renacidin powder for solution ℞ *bladder and catheter irrigant for calcifications* [citric acid; d-gluconic acid lactone; magnesium hydroxycarbonate] 6.602•0.198•3.177 g/100 mL

Renacidin Irrigation solution ℞ *bladder and catheter irrigant for calcifications (orphan)* [citric acid; gluconodelta-lactone; magnesium carbonate]

RenAmin IV infusion ℞ *nutritional therapy for renal failure* [multiple essential and nonessential amino acids; electrolytes]

renanolone INN

Renese tablets ℞ *diuretic; antihypertensive* [polythiazide] 1, 2, 4 mg

Renese-R tablets ℞ *antihypertensive* [polythiazide; reserpine] 2•0.25 mg

Renografin-60; Renografin-76 injection ℞ *parenteral radiopaque agent* [diatrizoate meglumine; diatrizoate sodium] 52%•8%; 66%•10%

Reno-M-30; Reno-M-60; Reno-M-Dip intracavitary instillation ℞ *urologic radiopaque agent* [diatrizoate meglumine] 30%; 60%; 30%

Renoquid tablets ℞ *broad-spectrum bacteriostatic* [sulfacytine] 250 mg

Renormax tablets (discontinued 1995) ℞ *antihypertensive; ACE inhibitor* [spirapril] 3, 6, 12, 24 mg

Renova cream ℞ *retinoid for photodamage, fine wrinkles, mottled hyperpigmentation, and roughness of facial skin* [tretinoin] 0.05%

Renovist; Renovist II injection ℞ *parenteral radiopaque agent* [diatrizoate meglumine; diatrizoate sodium] 34.3%•35%; 28.5%•29.1%

Renovue-Dip; Renovue-65 injection ℞ *parenteral renal radiopaque agent* [iodamide meglumine] 24%; 65%

Rentamine Pediatric oral suspension ℞ *pediatric antitussive, decongestant, and antihistamine* [carbetapentane tannate; phenylephrine tannate; ephedrine tannate; chlorpheniramine tannate] 30•5•5•4 mg/5 mL

rentiapril INN

ReNu solution OTC *rinsing/storage solution for soft contact lenses* [preserved saline solution]

ReNu Effervescent Enzymatic Cleaner; ReNu Thermal Enzymatic Cleaner tablets OTC *enzymatic cleaner for soft contact lenses* [subtilisin]

ReNu Multi-Purpose solution OTC *chemical disinfecting solution for soft contact lenses*

renytoline INN *anti-inflammatory* [also: paranyline HCl]

renytoline HCl [see: paranyline HCl]

renzapride INN, BAN

ReoPro IV injection ℞ *antiplatelet agent for acute arterial occlusive disorders (antianginal trials discontinued 1995)* [abciximab] 2 mg/mL

Repan tablets, capsules ℞ *analgesic; antipyretic; sedative* [acetaminophen; caffeine; butalbital] 325•40•50 mg
Ⓡ Riopan

Repan CF tablets ℞ *analgesic; antipyretic; sedative* [acetaminophen; butalbital] 650•50 mg

Repetab (trademarked dosage form) *extended-release tablet*

repirinast USAN, INN *antiallergic; antiasthmatic*

Replena (name changed to Suplena in 1992)

Replens vaginal gel OTC *lubricant* [glycerin; mineral oil]

Replete ready-to-use liquid OTC *enteral nutritional therapy* [lactose-free formula]

Replistatin ℞ *investigational antineoplastic and postsurgery coagulation restorer (heparin reversal)* [platelet factor 4, recombinant]

rEPO (recombinant erythropoietin) [see: epoetin alfa; epoetin beta]

Reposans-10 capsules ℞ *anxiolytic* [chlordiazepoxide HCl] 10 mg

repository corticotropin [see: corticotropin, repository]

Rep-Pred 40; Rep-Pred 80 injection (discontinued 1994) ℞ *glucocorticoid; anti-inflammatory; immunosuppressant* [methylprednisolone acetate] 40 mg/mL; 80 mg/mL

repromicin USAN, INN *antibacterial*

reproterol INN, BAN *bronchodilator* [also: reproterol HCl]

reproterol HCl USAN *bronchodilator* [also: reproterol]

Resaid sustained-release capsules ℞ *decongestant; antihistamine* [phenylpropanolamine HCl; chlorpheniramine maleate] 75•12 mg

Rescaps-D S.R. sustained-release capsules ℞ *antitussive; decongestant* [caramiphen edisylate; phenylpropanolamine HCl] 40•75 mg

rescimetol INN

rescinnamine NF, INN, BAN *antihypertensive; rauwolfia derivative*

Rescon liquid OTC *decongestant; antihistamine* [phenylpropanolamine HCl; chlorpheniramine maleate] 12.5•2 mg/5 mL

Rescon sustained-release capsules ℞ *decongestant; antihistamine* [pseudoephedrine HCl; chlorpheniramine maleate] 120•12 mg

Rescon JR controlled-release capsules ℞ *pediatric decongestant and antihistamine* [pseudoephedrine HCl; chlorpheniramine maleate] 60•4 mg

Rescon-DM liquid OTC *antitussive; decongestant; antihistamine* [dextromethorphan hydrobromide; pseudoephedrine HCl; chlorpheniramine maleate] 10•30•2 mg/5 mL

Rescon-ED controlled-release capsules ℞ *decongestant; antihistamine* [pseudoephedrine HCl; chlorpheniramine maleate] 120•8 mg

Rescon-GG liquid OTC *decongestant; expectorant* [phenylephrine HCl; guaifenesin] 5•100 mg/5 mL

Rescriptor ℞ *investigational (Phase III) reverse transcriptase inhibitor for HIV and AIDS* [delvaridine mesylate]

Rescue Pak (trademarked dosage form) *unit dose package*

Resectisol solution ℞ *genitourinary irrigant* [mannitol] 5 g/100 mL

reserpine USP, INN *antihypertensive; peripheral antiadrenergic; rauwolfia derivative* 0.1, 0.25 mg oral

resibufogenin [see: bufogenin]

Resinol ointment OTC *topical poison ivy treatment* [calamine; zinc oxide; resorcinol] 6%•12%•2%

resocortol butyrate USAN *topical anti-inflammatory*

Resol oral solution OTC *electrolyte replacement* [sodium, potassium, chloride, calcium, magnesium, and phosphate electrolytes]

Resolve/GP solution OTC *cleaning solution for hard or rigid gas permeable contact lenses*

resorantel INN

resorcin [see: resorcinol]

resorcin acetate [see: resorcinol monoacetate]

resorcin brown NF

resorcinol USP *keratolytic; antifungal*

resorcinol monoacetate USP *antiseborrheic; keratolytic*

Resource; Resource Plus ready-to-use liquid OTC *enteral nutritional therapy* [lactose-free formula]

Respa-1st sustained-release tablets ℞ *decongestant; expectorant* [pseudoephedrine HCl; guaifenesin] 60•600 mg

Respa-DM sustained-release tablets ℞ *antitussive; expectorant* [dextromethorphan hydrobromide; guaifenesin] 30•600 mg

Respa-GF sustained-release tablets ℞ *expectorant* [guaifenesin] 600 mg

Respahist sustained-release capsules ℞ *decongestant; antihistamine* [pseudoephedrine HCl; brompheniramine maleate] 60•6 mg

Respaire-60; Respaire-120 extended-release capsules ℞ *decongestant; expectorant* [pseudoephedrine HCl; guaifenesin] 60•200 mg; 120•250 mg

Respalor ready-to-use liquid OTC *enteral nutritional therapy for pulmonary problems*

Respbid sustained-release tablets ℞ *bronchodilator* [theophylline] 250, 500 mg

RespiGam IV infusion ℞ *preventative for respiratory syncytial virus (RSV) infections in high-risk infants* [respiratory syncytial virus immune globulin (RSV-IG)] 2500 mg/dose (50 mg/mL)

Respihaler (trademarked delivery system) *oral inhalation aerosol*

Respinol-G film-coated tablets (discontinued 1994) ℞ *decongestant; expectorant* [phenylpropanolamine HCl; phenylephrine HCl; guaifenesin]

Respiracult-Strep culture paddles for professional use *in vitro diagnostic test for Group A streptococci from throat and nasopharyngeal sources*

Respiralex test kit for professional use *in vitro diagnostic test for Group A streptococcal antigens in throat and pharynx* [latex agglutination test]

respiratory syncytial virus (RSV) immune globulin, human *respiratory syncytial virus preventative (orphan)*

Respirgard II (trademarked delivery system) *nebulizer*

Respivir (name changed to RespiGam in 1994)

Respond tablets OTC *dietary supplement* [multiple vitamins; levoglutamide; bovine brain concentrate]

Resporal sustained-release tablets (discontinued 1993) OTC *decongestant; antihistamine* [pseudoephedrine sulfate; dexbrompheniramine maleate]

Res-Q powder (discontinued 1996) OTC *universal antidote* [activated charcoal; magnesium hydroxide; tannic acid] 50% • 25% • ?

Restore powder OTC *bulk laxative* [psyllium hydrophilic mucilloid] 3.4 g/dose

Restoril capsules ℞ *sedative; hypnotic* [temazepam] 7.5, 15, 30 mg ② Vistaril

retelliptine INN

Retin-A cream, gel, liquid ℞ *topical keratolytic for acne* [tretinoin] 0.025%, 0.5%, 1%; 0.025%, 0.1%; 0.05%

retinoic acid (all-*trans*-retinoic acid) [see: tretinoin]

9-*cis*-retinoic acid *investigational (Phase I/III) for AIDS-related Kaposi sarcoma (orphan: acute promyelocytic leukemia)*

13-*cis*-retinoic acid [see: isotretinoin]

Retinol cream OTC *moisturizer; emollient* [vitamin A] 100,000 IU

retinol INN, BAN *vitamin A_1*

Retinol-A cream OTC *moisturizer; emollient* [vitamin A palmitate] 10,000 IU/g

Retrovector ℞ *investigational (Phase II) gene therapy for asymptomatic HIV infection* [HIV immunotherapeutic (HIV-IT)]

Retrovir capsules, syrup, IV injection ℞ *antiviral for HIV, AIDS and AIDS-related complex (orphan)* [zidovudine] 100 mg; 50 mg/5 mL; 10 mg/mL

revenast INN

reversible proton pump inhibitor *investigational treatment for peptic ulcers*

Reversol IV or IM injection ℞ *myasthenia gravis treatment; antidote to curare-type overdose* [edrophonium chloride] 10 mg/mL

Revex IV, IM, or subcu injection ℞ *opioid antagonist for narcotic overdose* [nalmefene] 100 μg/mL, 1 mg/mL

Rēv-Eyes powder for eye drops ℞ *miotic to reverse iatrogenic mydriasis* [dapiprazole HCl] 0.5%

ReVia tablets ℞ *narcotic antagonist for alcoholism, opiate dependence or overdose (orphan)* [naltrexone HCl] 50 mg

revospirone INN, BAN

Rexigen Forte sustained-release capsules ℞ *anorexiant* [phendimetrazine tartrate] 105 mg

Rexolate IM injection ℞ *analgesic; antipyretic; anti-inflammatory; antirheumatic* [sodium thiosalicylate] 50 mg/mL

Rezamid lotion OTC *topical acne treatment* [sulfur; resorcinol; alcohol] 5% • 2% • 28%

Rezine tablets (discontinued 1995) ℞ *anxiolytic* [hydroxyzine HCl] 10, 25 ml

Rezipas ℞ *(orphan: ulcerative colitis)* [aminosalicylic acid]

R-Frone ℞ *(orphan: metastatic renal cell carcinoma; T-cell lymphoma; malignant melanoma; Kaposi sarcoma)* [interferon beta, recombinant]

RG 12525 *investigational leukotriene D4 antagonist for asthma*

RG 12915 *investigational antiemetic for chemotherapy (clinical trials discontinued 1994)*

RG 12986 *investigational antithrombotic* [recombinant human von Willebrand factor]

RG 201 *investigational (Phase I) anti-infective for AIDS-related Pneumocystis carinii pneumonia (PCP)*

rGCR (recombinant glucocerebrosidase) *(orphan: Gaucher's disease)*

rG-CSF (recombinant granulocyte colony-stimulating factor) [see: lenograstim]

R-Gel OTC *topical analgesic* [capsaicin] 0.025%

R-Gen elixir ℞ *expectorant* [iodinated glycerol] 60 mg/5 mL

R-gene 10 IV injection ℞ *pituitary (growth hormone) function diagnostic aid* [arginine HCl] 10% (950 mOsm/L)

rGM-CSF; rhGM-CSF; rhuGM-CSF (granulocyte-macrophage colony-stimulating factor) [q.v.]

rgp160; rgp160 IIIB; rgp160 MN (recombinant glycoprotein) *investigational (Phase I/II) antiviral (treatment) and vaccine (preventative) for HIV* [also: AIDS vaccine]

$Rh_0(D)$ immune globulin USP *passive immunizing agent; (orphan: immune thrombocytopenic purpura)*

$Rh_0(D)$ immune human globulin [now: $Rh_0(D)$ immune globulin]

rhamnus purshiana [see: cascara sagrada]

rhDNase (recombinant human deoxyribonuclease) [see: dornase alfa]

Rheaban caplets OTC *antidiarrheal; GI adsorbent* [activated attapulgite] 750 mg

rhenium *element (Re)*

Rheomacrodex IV infusion ℞ *plasma volume expander for shock due to hemorrhage, burns, or surgery* [dextran 40] 10%

RheothRx Copolymer ℞ *investigational therapy for heart attack and malaria; (orphan: sickle cell crisis; severe burns)* [poloxamer 188]

rheotran (45) [see: dextran 45]

Rhesonativ IM injection (discontinued 1995) ℞ *obstetric Rh factor immunity suppressant* [$Rh_0(D)$ immune globulin]

rhetinic acid [see: enoxolone]

Rheumatex slide tests for professional use *in vitro diagnostic aid for rheumatoid factor in the blood* ⓓ Rheumatrex

Rheumaton slide tests for professional use *in vitro diagnostic aid for rheumatoid factor in serum or synovial fluid*

Rheumatrex Dose Pack (tablets) ℞ *antirheumatic; antipsoriatic; antineoplastic for leukemia (orphan: juvenile rheumatoid arthritis)* [methotrexate sodium] 2.5 mg ⓓ Rheumatex

Rheumox ℞ *investigational nonsteroidal anti-inflammatory drug (NSAID)* [azapropazone]

rhFSH (recombinant human follicle-stimulating hormone) [see: menotropins]

rhGH (recombinant human growth hormone) [see: somatropin]

rhIL-1R; rhu IL-1R (recombinant human interleukin-1 receptor) [see: interleukin-1 receptor]

rhIL-11 (recombinant human interleukin-11) [see: interleukin-11, recombinant human]

rhIL-12 (recombinant human interleukin-12) [see: interleukin-12]

Rhinall nasal spray, nose drops OTC *nasal decongestant* [phenylephrine HCl] 0.25%

Rhinall-10 solution (discontinued 1992) OTC *nasal decongestant* [phenylephrine HCl]

Rhinatate tablets ℞ *decongestant; antihistamine* [phenylephrine tannate; chlorpheniramine tannate; pyrilamine tannate] 25•8•25 mg

Rhindecon timed-release capsules (discontinued 1993) ℞ *nasal decon-*

gestant; diet aid [phenylpropanolamine HCl] 75 mg

Rhinocaps capsules OTC *decongestant; analgesic; antipyretic* [phenylpropanolamine HCl; acetaminophen; aspirin] 20•162•162 mg

Rhinocort nasal inhalation aerosol ℞ *intranasal steroidal anti-inflammatory* [budesonide] 32 μg/dose

Rhinocort Aqua nasal spray (available only in Canada) ℞ *intranasal steroidal anti-inflammatory* [budesonide] 100 μg/spray

Rhinocort Turbuhaler powder for nasal inhalation (available only in Canada) ℞ *intranasal steroidal anti-inflammatory* [budesonide] 100 μg/dose

Rhinogesic tablets (discontinued 1995) OTC *decongestant; antihistamine; analgesic* [phenylephrine HCl; chlorpheniramine maleate; acetaminophen; salicylamide] 5•2•150•250 mg

Rhinolar sustained-release capsules (discontinued 1995) ℞ *decongestant; antihistamine; anticholinergic* [phenylpropanolamine HCl; chlorpheniramine maleate; methscopolamine nitrate] 75•8•2.5 mg

Rhinolar-EX; Rhinolar-EX 12 sustained-release capsules ℞ *decongestant; antihistamine* [phenylpropanolamine HCl; chlorpheniramine maleate] 75•8 mg; 75•12 mg

Rhinosyn; Rhinosyn-PD liquid OTC *decongestant; antihistamine* [pseudoephedrine HCl; chlorpheniramine maleate; alcohol] 60•4 mg/5 mL; 30•2 mg/5 mL

Rhinosyn-DM liquid OTC *antitussive; decongestant; antihistamine* [dextromethorphan hydrobromide; pseudoephedrine HCl; chlorpheniramine maleate; alcohol 1.4%] 15•30•2 mg/5 mL

Rhinosyn-DMX syrup OTC *antitussive; expectorant* [dextromethorphan hydrobromide; guaifenesin] 15•100 mg/5 mL

Rhinosyn-X liquid OTC *antitussive; decongestant; expectorant* [dextromethorphan hydrobromide; pseudoephedrine HCl; guaifenesin; alcohol 7.5%] 10•30•100 mg/5 mL

rhNGF (recombinant human nerve growth factor) [see: nerve growth factor]

rhodine [see: aspirin]

rhodium *element (Rh)*

RhoGAM IM injection ℞ *obstetric Rh factor immunity suppressant* [Rh$_0$(D) immune globulin] 300 μg

rHSA (recombinant human serum albumin)

Rhuli cream (discontinued 1994) OTC *topical poison ivy treatment* [benzocaine; calamine; camphor] 5%•3%•0.3%

Rhuli gel OTC *topical poison ivy treatment* [benzyl alcohol; menthol; camphor] 2%•0.3%•0.3%

Rhuli spray OTC *topical poison ivy treatment* [benzocaine; calamine; camphor] 5%•13.8%•0.7%

Rhythmin sustained-release tablets ℞ *antiarrhythmic* [procainamide HCl]

ribaminol USAN, INN *memory adjuvant*

ribavirin USP, INN *antiviral; investigational (Phase II/III) for HIV; (orphan: hemorrhagic fever with renal syndrome)* [also: tribavirin]

riboflavin USP, INN *vitamin B$_2$; vitamin G; enzyme cofactor* 25, 50, 100 mg oral

riboflavin 5′-phosphate sodium USP *vitamin*

riboflavine [see: riboflavin]

riboprine USAN, INN *antineoplastic*

ribostamycin INN, BAN

riboxamide [see: tiazofurin]

ricainide [see: indecainide HCl]

Ricelyte oral solution (name changed to Infalyte in 1994)

ricin (blocked) conjugated murine monoclonal antibody (anti-B4) *(orphan: B-cell leukemia and lymphoma; ex vivo treatment of autologous bone marrow in leukemia)*

ricin (blocked) conjugated murine monoclonal antibody (anti-MY9) *(orphan: myeloid leukemia; ex vivo treatment of autologous bone marrow in leukemia)*

ricin (blocked) conjugated murine monoclonal antibody (CD6)

(orphan: T-cell leukemias, lymphomas, and other T-cell malignancies)
ricin (blocked) conjugated murine monoclonal antibody (N901) *(orphan: small cell lung cancer)*
RID liquid OTC *pediculicide* [pyrethrins; piperonyl butoxide; petroleum distillate] 0.3%•3•1.2%
Rid-A-Pain drops (discontinued 1994) OTC *topical oral anesthetic; antiseptic* [benzocaine; cetalkonium chloride; alcohol 20%] 2.5•0.02%
Rid-A-Pain gel OTC *topical oral anesthetic* [benzocaine] 10%
Rid-A-Pain ointment (discontinued 1992) OTC *counterirritant* [methyl salicylate; methyl nicotinate; menthol; camphor]
Rid-A-Pain with Codeine tablets (discontinued 1995) ℞ *narcotic analgesic* [codeine phosphate; acetaminophen; aspirin; caffeine; salicylamide] 1•97.2•226.8•32.4•32.4 mg
Ridaura capsules ℞ *antirheumatic; investigational antiasthmatic* [auranofin] 3 mg
ridazolol INN
RIDD (recombinant interleukin-2, dacarbazine, DDP) *chemotherapy protocol*
Ridenol elixir OTC *analgesic; antipyretic* [acetaminophen] 80 mg/5 mL
ridogrel USAN, INN, BAN *thromboxane synthetase inhibitor; investigational treatment for ulcerative colitis*
rifabutin USAN, INN *antiviral; antibacterial; (orphan: Mycobacterium avium complex disease in HIV)*
Rifadin capsules, powder for IV injection ℞ *tuberculostatic; (orphan: IV where oral use is not feasible)* [rifampin] 150, 300 mg; 600 mg ⑨ rifampin; Ritalin
Rifamate capsules ℞ *tuberculostatic* [rifampin; isoniazid] 300•150 mg
rifametane USAN, INN *antibacterial*
rifamexil USAN *antibacterial*
rifamide USAN, INN *antibacterial*
rifampicin INN, BAN, JAN *antibacterial* [also: rifampin]
rifampin USAN, USP *antibacterial; antituberculosis treatment (orphan)* [also: rifampicin] ⑨ Rifadin
rifampin, isoniazid & pyrazinamide *(orphan: short-course treatment of tuberculosis)*
rifamycin INN, BAN
rifamycin diethylamide [see: rifamide]
rifamycin M-14 [see: rifamide]
rifapentine USAN, INN, BAN *antibacterial; investigational treatment for Mycobacterium avium complex and tuberculosis*
Rifater tablets ℞ *(orphan: short course treatment of tuberculosis)* [rifampin; isoniazid; pyrazinamide] 120•50•300 mg
rifaxidin [see: rifaximin]
rifaximin USAN, INN *antibacterial*
rIFN-A (recombinant interferon alfa) [see: interferon alfa-2a, recombinant]
rIFN-α2 (recombinant interferon alfa-2) [see: interferon alfa-2b, recombinant]
rIFN-B (recombinant interferon beta) [see: interferon beta-1b, recombinant]
r-IFN-beta ℞ *(orphan: metastatic renal cell carcinoma; T-cell lymphoma; malignant melanoma; Kaposi sarcoma)* [interferon beta, recombinant]
rifomycin [see: rifamycin]
RIG (rabies immune globulin) [q.v.]
rilapine INN
rilmazafone INN
rilmenidine INN
rilopirox INN
rilozarone INN
Rilutek film-coated tablets ℞ *treatment for amyotrophic lateral sclerosis (ALS)* [riluzole] 50 mg
riluzole USAN, INN *(orphan: amyotrophic lateral sclerosis)*
Rimactane capsules ℞ *tuberculostatic* [rifampin] 300 mg
Rimactane/INH Dual Pack (two-product package) ℞ *tuberculostatic* [rifampin (2 capsules); isoniazid (1 tablet)] 300 mg; 300 mg

Rimadyl ℞ *investigational nonsteroidal anti-inflammatory drug (NSAID); analgesic; antipyretic* [carprofen]

rimantadine INN *antiviral* [also: rimantadine HCl]

rimantadine HCl USAN *antiviral* [also: rimantadine]

rimazolium metilsulfate INN

rimcazole INN *antipsychotic* [also: rimcazole HCl]

rimcazole HCl USAN *antipsychotic* [also: rimcazole]

rimexolone USAN, INN, BAN *ophthalmic corticosteroidal anti-inflammatory*

rimiterol INN *bronchodilator* [also: rimiterol hydrobromide]

rimiterol hydrobromide USAN *bronchodilator* [also: rimiterol]

rimoprogin INN

Rimso-50 solution for bladder instillation ℞ *for symptomatic relief of cystitis* [dimethyl sulfoxide (DMSO)] 50%

Rinade B.I.D. sustained-release capsules ℞ *decongestant; antihistamine* [pseudoephedrine HCl; chlorpheniramine maleate] 120•8 mg

Ringer's injection USP *fluid and electrolyte replenisher* [also: compound solution of sodium chloride]

Ringer's injection, lactated USP *fluid and electrolyte replenisher; systemic alkalizer* [also: compound solution of sodium lactate]

Ringer's irrigation USP *irrigation solution*

Ringer's solution [now: Ringer's irrigation]

riodipine INN

Riopan suspension OTC *antacid* [magaldrate] 540 mg/5 mL

Riopan tablets, chewable tablets (discontinued 1994) OTC *antacid* [magaldrate] 480 mg; 480 mg ② Repan

Riopan Plus chewable tablets, oral suspension OTC *antacid; antiflatulent* [magaldrate; simethicone] 480•20, 1080•20 mg; 540•40, 1080•40 mg/5 mL

Riopan Plus 2 chewable tablets, oral suspension (discontinued 1994) OTC *antacid; antiflatulent* [magaldrate; simethicone] 1080•30 mg; 216•6 mg/mL

rioprostil USAN, INN *gastric antisecretory*

ripazepam USAN, INN *minor tranquilizer*

risedronate sodium USAN *biphosphonate calcium regulator*

rismorelin porcine USAN *growth stimulant for growth hormone deficiencies*

risocaine USAN, INN *local anesthetic*

risotilide HCl USAN *antiarrhythmic*

Risperdal tablets, oral solution ℞ *antipsychotic for schizophrenia; serotonin-dopamine antagonist* [risperidone] 1, 2, 3, 4 mg; 1 mg/mL

risperidone USAN, INN, BAN *neuroleptic; antipsychotic*

ristianol INN, BAN *immunoregulator* [also: ristianol phosphate]

ristianol phosphate USAN *immunoregulator* [also: ristianol]

ristocetin USP, INN, BAN

Ritalin tablets ℞ *CNS stimulant for attention deficit hyperactivity disorders (ADHD); analeptic* [methylphenidate HCl] 5, 10, 20 mg ② Ismelin; Rifadin

Ritalin-SR sustained-release tablets ℞ *CNS stimulant for attention deficit hyperactivity disorders (ADHD); analeptic* [methylphenidate HCl] 20 mg

ritanserin USAN, INN, BAN *serotonin antagonist; investigational agent for various psychiatric illnesses and substance abuse* 10 mg oral

ritiometan INN

ritodrine USAN, INN *smooth muscle relaxant*

ritodrine HCl USAN, USP *smooth muscle relaxant; uterine relaxant* 0.3, 10, 15 mg/mL injection

ritolukast USAN, INN *antiasthmatic; leukotriene antagonist*

ritonavir USAN *antiviral; investigational (Phase III) HIV-1 and HIV-2 protease inhibitor*

ritropirronium bromide INN

ritrosulfan INN

rizolipase INN

RMP-7 *investigational drug for AIDS; carries medications across the blood-brain barrier*

RMS suppositories ℞ *narcotic analgesic; preoperative sedative and anxiolytic* [morphine sulfate] 10, 20, 30 mg

rNPA (recombinant novel plasminogen activator) [see: novel plasminogen activator]

Ro 24-7429 *investigational antiviral for AIDS (clinical trials discontinued 1994)*

Roaccutane gel (French name for U.S. product Isotrex)

Robafen AC Cough syrup ℞ *narcotic antitussive; expectorant* [codeine phosphate; guaifenesin; alcohol 3.5%] 10•100 mg/5 mL

Robafen CF liquid OTC *antitussive; decongestant; expectorant* [dextromethorphan hydrobromide; phenylpropanolamine HCl; guaifenesin] 10•12.5•100 mg/5 mL

Robafen DAC syrup ℞ *narcotic antitussive; decongestant; expectorant* [codeine phosphate; pseudoephedrine HCl; guaifenesin; alcohol 1.4%] 10•30•100 mg/5 mL

Robafen DM syrup OTC *antitussive; expectorant* [dextromethorphan hydrobromide; guaifenesin; alcohol 1.4%] 10•100 mg/5 mL

RoBathol Bath Oil OTC *bath emollient*

Robaxacet ℞ *investigational adjunct for musculoskeletal pain* [methocarbamol; acetaminophen] ☒ Robaxisal

Robaxin tablets, IV or IM injection ℞ *skeletal muscle relaxant* [methocarbamol] 500, 750 mg; 100 mg/mL

Robaxisal tablets ℞ *skeletal muscle relaxant; analgesic* [methocarbamol; aspirin] 400•325 mg ☒ Robaxacet

robenidine INN *coccidiostat for poultry* [also: robenidine HCl]

robenidine HCl USAN *coccidiostat for poultry* [also: robenidine]

Robicap (trademarked dosage form) *capsule*

Robicillin VK tablets ℞ *bactericidal antibiotic* [penicillin V potassium] 250, 500 mg

Robimycin Robitabs (enteric-coated tablets) ℞ *macrolide antibiotic* [erythromycin] 250 mg

Robinul tablets, IV or IM injection ℞ *anticholinergic; peptic ulcer treatment adjunct; antisecretory* [glycopyrrolate] 1 mg; 0.2 mg/5 mL

Robinul Forte tablets ℞ *anticholinergic; peptic ulcer treatment adjunct; antisecretory* [glycopyrrolate] 2 mg

Robitab (trademarked dosage form) *tablet*

Robitet Robicaps (capsules) ℞ *broad-spectrum antibiotic* [tetracycline HCl] 250, 500 mg

Robitussin syrup OTC *expectorant* [guaifenesin; alcohol 3.5%] 100 mg/5 mL

Robitussin A-C syrup ℞ *narcotic antitussive; expectorant* [codeine phosphate; guaifenesin; alcohol 3.5%] 10•100 mg/5 mL

Robitussin Cold & Cough Liqui-Gels (capsules) OTC *antitussive; decongestant; expectorant* [dextromethorphan hydrobromide; pseudoephedrine HCl; guaifenesin] 10•30•200 mg

Robitussin Cough Calmers lozenge OTC *antitussive* [dextromethorphan hydrobromide] 5 mg

Robitussin Cough & Cold; Robitussin Pediatric Cough & Cold liquid OTC *antitussive; decongestant* [dextromethorphan hydrobromide; pseudoephedrine HCl] 15•30 mg/5 mL; 7.5•15 mg/5 mL

Robitussin Cough Drops lozenge OTC *mild topical anesthetic* [menthol] 7.4, 10 mg

Robitussin Liquid Center Cough Drops lozenges OTC *topical antipruritic/counterirritant; mild local anesthetic* [menthol] 10 mg

Robitussin Night Relief liquid OTC *antitussive; decongestant; antihistamine; analgesic* [dextromethorphan hydrobromide; pseudoephedrine HCl; pyrilamine maleate; acetaminophen] 5•10•8.3•108.3 mg/5 mL

Robitussin Pediatric liquid OTC *antitussive* [dextromethorphan hydrobromide] 7.5 mg/5 mL

Robitussin Severe Congestion Liqui-Gels (capsules) OTC *expectorant; decongestant* [guaifenesin; pseudoephedrine HCl] 200•30 mg

Robitussin-CF liquid OTC *antitussive; decongestant; expectorant* [dextromethorphan hydrobromide; phenylpropanolamine HCl; guaifenesin; alcohol 4.75%] 10•12.5•100 mg/5 mL

Robitussin-DAC syrup ℞ *narcotic antitussive; decongestant; expectorant* [codeine phosphate; pseudoephedrine HCl; guaifenesin; alcohol 1.9%] 10•30•100 mg/5 mL

Robitussin-DM liquid OTC *antitussive; expectorant* [dextromethorphan hydrobromide; guaifenesin] 10•100 mg/5 mL

Robitussin-PE syrup OTC *decongestant; expectorant* [pseudoephedrine HCl; guaifenesin; alcohol 1.4%] 30•100 mg/5 mL

Robomol-500; Robomol-750 tablets (discontinued 1993) ℞ *skeletal muscle relaxant* [methocarbamol]

Rocaltrol capsules ℞ *treatment of hypocalcemia in dialysis patients; decreases severity of psoriatic lesions* [calcitriol] 0.25, 0.5 μg

rocastine INN *antihistamine* [also: rocastine HCl]

rocastine HCl USAN *antihistamine* [also: rocastine]

Rocephin powder for IV or IM injection, ADD-vantage vials ℞ *cephalosporin-type antibiotic* [ceftriaxone sodium] 0.25, 0.5, 1, 2, 10 g

rochelle salt [see: potassium sodium tartrate]

rociverine INN

Rocky Mountain spotted fever vaccine USP

rocuronium bromide INN, BAN *neuromuscular blocking agent*

R.O.-Dexsone eye drops (available only in Canada) ℞ *ophthalmic topical corticosteroidal anti-inflammatory* [dexamethasone sodium phosphate] 0.1%

rodocaine USAN, INN *local anesthetic*

rodorubicin INN

rofelodine INN

Roferon-A subcu or IM injection ℞ *antineoplastic for hairy cell leukemia, chronic myelogenous leukemia, and Kaposi sarcoma (orphan)* [interferon alfa-2a] 3, 6, 9, 36 million IU/mL

roflurane USAN, INN *inhalation anesthetic*

Rogaine for Men; Rogaine for Women topical solution OTC *hair growth stimulant* [minoxidil] 2% ☑ Regain

Rogenic IM injection (discontinued 1994) ℞ *hematinic* [peptonized iron; vitamin B$_{12}$] 20•500 mg/mL

Rogenic slow-release tablets (discontinued 1994) OTC *hematinic* [ferrous fumarate, ferrous gluconate & ferrous sulfate; desiccated liver; multiple vitamins] 60•25• ≟ mg

rogletimide USAN, INN, BAN *antineoplastic; aromatase inhibitor*

rokitamycin INN

Rolaids, Calcium Rich chewable tablets OTC *antacid* [magnesium hydroxide; calcium carbonate] 80•412 mg

Rolaids Antacid chewable tablets (discontinued 1994) OTC *antacid* [dihydroxyaluminum sodium carbonate] 334 mg

Rolaids Sodium Free chewable tablets (discontinued 1994) OTC *antacid* [magnesium hydroxide; calcium carbonate]

Rolatuss Expectorant liquid ℞ *narcotic antitussive; decongestant; antihistamine; expectorant* [codeine phosphate; phenylephrine HCl; chlorpheniramine maleate; ammonium chloride; alcohol 5%] 9.85•5•2•33.3 mg/5 mL

Rolatuss Plain liquid OTC *decongestant; antihistamine* [phenylephrine HCl; chlorpheniramine maleate; alcohol 5%] 5•2 mg/5 mL

Rolatuss with Hydrocodone liquid ℞ *narcotic antitussive; decongestant; antihistamine* [hydrocodone bitartrate; phenylpropanolamine HCl; phenylephrine HCl; pyrilamine maleate; pheniramine maleate] 1.7•3.3•5•3.3•3.3 mg/5 mL

roletamide USAN, INN *hypnotic*

rolgamidine USAN, INN, BAN *antidiarrheal*

rolicton [see: amisometradine]

rolicyclidine INN

rolicypram BAN *antidepressant* [also: rolicyprine]

rolicyprine USAN, INN *antidepressant* [also: rolicypram]

rolipram USAN, INN *tranquilizer*

rolitetracycline USAN, USP, INN *antibacterial*
rolitetracycline nitrate USAN *antibacterial*
rolodine USAN, INN *skeletal muscle relaxant*
rolziracetam INN, BAN
romazarit USAN, INN, BAN *anti-inflammatory; antirheumatic*
Romazicon IV injection ℞ *benzodiazepine antagonist to reverse anesthesia or treat overdose* [flumazenil] 0.1 mg/mL
rometin [see: clioquinol]
romifenone INN
romifidine INN
romurtide INN
Romycin topical solution (discontinued 1995) ℞ *topical antibiotic for acne* [erythromycin] 2%
ronactolol INN
Rondamine-DM pediatric drops ℞ *pediatric antitussive, decongestant, and antihistamine* [dextromethorphan hydrobromide; pseudoephedrine HCl; carbinoxamine maleate] 4•25•2 mg/5 mL
Rondec film-coated tablets, chewable tablets, syrup, pediatric drops ℞ *decongestant; antihistamine* [pseudoephedrine HCl; carbinoxamine maleate] 60•4 mg; 60•4 mg; 60•4 mg/5 mL; 25•2 mg/mL
Rondec-DM syrup, pediatric drops ℞ *antitussive; decongestant; antihistamine* [dextromethorphan hydrobromide; pseudoephedrine HCl; carbinoxamine maleate] 15•60•4 mg/5 mL; 4•25•2 mg/mL
Rondec-TR timed-release Filmtabs (film-coated tablets) ℞ *decongestant; antihistamine* [pseudoephedrine HCl; carbinoxamine maleate] 120•8 mg
ronidazole USAN, INN *antiprotozoal*
ronifibrate INN
ronipamil INN
ronnel USAN *systemic insecticide* [also: fenclofos; fenchlorphos]
ropinirole INN, BAN *antiparkinsonian* [also: ropinirole HCl]
ropinirole HCl USAN *antiparkinsonian* [also: ropinirole]

ropitoin INN *antiarrhythmic* [also: ropitoin HCl]
ropitoin HCl USAN *antiarrhythmic* [also: ropitoin]
ropivacaine INN *investigational anti-inflammatory and local anesthetic for pain relief in the spinal canal*
ropizine USAN, INN *anticonvulsant*
roquinimex USAN, INN *investigational (Phase II) immunomodulator for HIV (orphan: bone marrow transplant for leukemia)*
rosamicin [now: rosaramicin]
rosamicin butyrate [now: rosaramicin butyrate]
rosamicin propionate [now: rosaramicin propionate]
rosamicin sodium phosphate [now: rosaramicin sodium phosphate]
rosamicin stearate [now: rosaramicin stearate]
rosaprostol INN
rosaramicin USAN, INN *antibacterial*
rosaramicin butyrate USAN *antibacterial*
rosaramicin propionate USAN *antibacterial*
rosaramicin sodium phosphate USAN *antibacterial*
rosaramicin stearate USAN *antibacterial*
rose bengal *corneal injury and pathology diagnostic aid* 1.3 mg/strip
rose bengal sodium (^{131}I) INN *hepatic function test; radioactive agent* [also: rose bengal sodium I 131]
rose bengal sodium I 125 USAN *radioactive agent*
rose bengal sodium I 131 USAN, USP *hepatic function test; radioactive agent* [also: rose bengal sodium (^{131}I)]
rose oil NF *perfume*
rose petal aqueous infusion *ocular emollient*
rose water, stronger NF *perfume*
rose water ointment USP *emollient; ointment base*
Rosets ophthalmic strips OTC *corneal disclosing agent* [rose bengal] 1.3 mg
rosin USP
rosoxacin USAN, INN *antibacterial* [also: acrosoxacin]
Ross SLD powder for oral solution (discontinued 1994) OTC *oral nutri-*

tional supplement for patients on clear liquid diets

rosterolone INN

Rotacaps (trademarked form) *encapsulated powder for inhalation*

Rotalex test kit for professional use (discontinued 1995) *in vitro diagnostic aid for fecal rotavirus* [latex agglutination test]

rotamicillin INN

rotavirus vaccine *investigational immunization against diarrhea*

rotoxamine USAN, INN *antihistamine*

rotoxamine tartrate NF

rotraxate INN

Rovamycine ℞ *(orphan status withdrawn 1994)* [spiramycin]

Rowasa suppositories, rectal suspension enema ℞ *treatment of active ulcerative colitis, proctosigmoiditis and proctitis* [mesalamine] 500 mg; 4 g/60 mL

roxadimate USAN, INN *sunscreen*

Roxanol suppositories ℞ *narcotic analgesic* [morphine sulfate] 5, 10, 20, 30 mg

Roxanol; Roxanol 100; Roxanol Rescudose; Roxanol UD oral solution ℞ *narcotic analgesic* [morphine sulfate] 20 mg/mL; 100 mg/5 mL; 10 mg/2.5 mL; 20 mg/mL

Roxanol SR sustained-release tablets (name changed to Oramorph SR in 1994)

roxarsone USAN, INN *antibacterial*

roxatidine INN, BAN *antiulcerative* [also: roxatidine acetate HCl]

roxatidine acetate HCl USAN *antiulcerative for duodenal and gastric ulcers; histamine H_2 receptor antagonist* [also: roxatidine]

Roxiam (commercially available in the UK, Denmark, and Luxembourg) ℞ *investigational antipsychotic for schizophrenia (clinical trials discontinued 1994)* [remoxipride]

roxibolone INN

Roxicet tablets, oral solution ℞ *narcotic analgesic* [oxycodone HCl; acetaminophen] 5•325 mg; 5•325 mg/5 mL

Roxicet 5/500 caplets ℞ *narcotic analgesic* [oxycodone HCl; acetaminophen] 5•500 mg

Roxicodone tablets, oral solution, Intensol (concentrated oral solution) ℞ *narcotic analgesic* [oxycodone HCl] 5 mg; 5 mg/5 mL; 20 mg/mL

Roxilox capsules ℞ *narcotic analgesic* [oxycodone HCl; acetaminophen] 5•500 mg

Roxin ℞ *investigational treatment for duodenal and gastric ulcers* [roxatidine acetate HCl]

roxindole INN

Roxiprin tablets ℞ *narcotic analgesic* [oxycodone HCl; oxycodone terephthalate; aspirin] 4.5•0.38•325 mg

roxithromycin USAN, INN *antibacterial*

roxolonium metilsulfate INN

roxoperone INN

RP 60180 *investigational kappa agonist for severe pain*

RP 64477 *investigational intestinal ACAT inhibitor for hypercholesterolemia*

RP 73401 *investigational phosphodiesterase type IV inhibitor for asthma*

rp24 *investigational antiviral for AIDS* [also: AIDS vaccine]

rPF4 (recombinant platelet factor 4) [see: platelet factor 4, recombinant]

R/S lotion OTC *topical acne treatment* [sulfur; resorcinol; alcohol] 5%•2%•28%

RS 15385 *investigational alpha$_2$ adrenoreceptor antagonist for male sexual dysfunction*

RS 25259 *investigational 5-HT3 antagonist for postoperative and postchemotherapy nausea and vomiting*

RS 66271 *investigational osteoporosis treatment and preventative*

R-Tannamine tablets, pediatric oral suspension ℞ *decongestant; antihistamine* [phenylephrine tannate; chlorpheniramine tannate; pyrilamine tannate] 25•8•25 mg; 5•2•12.5 mg/5 mL

R-Tannate tablets, pediatric oral suspension ℞ *decongestant; antihistamine* [phenylephrine tannate; chlorpheniramine tannate; pyrilamine tannate] 25•8•25 mg; 5•2•12.5 mg/5 mL

rtPA; rt-PA (recombinant tissue plasminogen activator) [see: alteplase]

Rubacell II test for professional use (discontinued 1995) *in vitro diagnostic aid for rubella virus antibodies in serum or plasma* [passive hemagglutination (PHA) test]

Rubazyme reagent kit for professional use *in vitro diagnostic aid for rubella virus IgG antibodies in serum* [enzyme immunoassay (EIA)]

rubbing alcohol [see: alcohol, rubbing]

rubbing isopropyl alcohol [see: isopropyl alcohol, rubbing]

rubella & mumps virus vaccine, live *active immunizing agent for rubella and mumps*

rubella virus vaccine, live USP *active immunizing agent for rubella*

rubeola vaccine [see: measles virus vaccine, live]

Rubesol-1000 IM or subcu injection ℞ *antianemic; vitamin B_{12} supplement* [cyanocobalamin] 1000 μg/mL

Rubex powder for IV injection ℞ *antineoplastic antibiotic* [doxorubicin HCl] 10, 50, 100 mg

rubidium *element (Rb)*

rubidium chloride Rb 82 USAN *radioactive diagnostic aid for cardiac disease*

rubidium chloride Rb 86 USAN *radioactive agent*

Rubramin PC IM or subcu injection ℞ *antianemic; vitamin B_{12} supplement* [cyanocobalamin] 100, 1000 μg/mL

Rufen film-coated tablets (discontinued 1995) ℞ *nonsteroidal anti-inflammatory drug (NSAID); antiarthritic; analgesic* [ibuprofen] 400, 600, 800 mg

rufloxacin INN

rufocromomycin INN, BAN *antineoplastic* [also: streptonigrin]

Ru-lets 500 film-coated tablets (discontinued 1995) OTC *vitamin/mineral supplement* [multiple vitamins and minerals] ⁑

Ru-lets M 500 film-coated tablets OTC *vitamin/mineral supplement* [multiple vitamins & minerals] ⁑

Rulid ℞ *investigational macrolide antibiotic* [roxithromycin]

RuLox oral suspension OTC *antacid* [aluminum hydroxide; magnesium hydroxide] 225•200 mg/5 mL

RuLox #1; RuLox #2 chewable tablets OTC *antacid* [aluminum hydroxide; magnesium hydroxide] 200•200 mg; 400•400 mg

RuLox Plus chewable tablets, oral suspension OTC *antacid; antiflatulent* [aluminum hydroxide; magnesium hydroxide; simethicone] 200•200•25 mg; 500•450•40 mg/5 mL

Rum-K liquid ℞ *potassium supplement* [potassium chloride] 30 mEq/15 mL

rutamycin USAN, INN *antifungal*

ruthenium *element (Ru)*

rutin NF [also: rutoside]

rutoside INN [also: rutin]

Ru-Tuss liquid OTC *decongestant; antihistamine* [phenylephrine HCl; chlorpheniramine maleate; alcohol 5%] 5•2 mg/5 mL

Ru-Tuss sustained-release tablets (discontinued 1995) ℞ *decongestant; antihistamine; anticholinergic* [phenylpropanolamine HCl; phenylephrine HCl; chlorpheniramine maleate; hyoscyamine sulfate; atropine sulfate; scopolamine hydrobromide] 50•25•8•0.19•0.04•0.01 mg

Ru-Tuss II slow-release capsules (discontinued 1995) ℞ *decongestant; antihistamine* [phenylpropanolamine HCl; chlorpheniramine maleate] 75•12 mg

Ru-Tuss DE prolonged-action film-coated tablets ℞ *decongestant; expectorant* [pseudoephedrine HCl; guaifenesin] 120•600 mg

Ru-Tuss Expectorant liquid OTC *antitussive; decongestant; expectorant* [dextromethorphan hydrobromide; pseudoephedrine HCl; guaifenesin; alcohol 10%] 10•30•100 mg/5 mL

Ru-Tuss with Hydrocodone liquid ℞ *narcotic antitussive; decongestant; antihistamine* [hydrocodone bitartrate; phenylpropanolamine HCl; phenylephrine HCl; pyrilamine maleate; pheniramine maleate; alcohol 5%] 1.7•3.3•5•3.3•3.3 mg/5 mL

ruvazone INN

Ru-Vert-M film-coated tablets ℞ *anticholinergic; antivertigo agent;*

motion sickness preventative [meclizine HCl] 25 mg

RVA (rabies vaccine, adsorbed) [see: rabies vaccine]

r-VIII SQ ℞ *investigational antihemophilic* [recombinant factor VIII]

RVP (red veterinarian petrolatum) [see: petrolatum]

RWJ 23989 *investigational retinoid for acne*

RWJ 26091 *investigational retinoid for acne*

RWJ 26127 *investigational treatment for osteoporosis*

RxPak; ℞Pak (trademarked form) *prescription package*

Rymed capsules ℞ *decongestant; expectorant* [pseudoephedrine HCl; guaifenesin] 30•250 mg

Rymed liquid OTC *decongestant; expectorant* [pseudoephedrine HCl; guaifenesin; alcohol 1.4%] 30•100 mg/5 mL

Rymed-TR long-acting caplets ℞ *decongestant; expectorant* [phenylpropanolamine HCl; guaifenesin] 75•400 mg

Ryna liquid OTC *decongestant; antihistamine* [pseudoephedrine HCl; chlorpheniramine maleate] 30•2 mg/5 mL

Ryna-C liquid ℞ *narcotic antitussive; decongestant; antihistamine* [codeine phosphate; pseudoephedrine HCl; chlorpheniramine maleate] 10•30•2 mg/5 mL

Ryna-CX liquid ℞ *narcotic antitussive; decongestant; expectorant* [codeine phosphate; pseudoephedrine HCl; guaifenesin] 10•30•100 mg/5 mL

Rynatan tablets, pediatric oral suspension ℞ *decongestant; antihistamine* [phenylephrine tannate; chlorpheniramine tannate; pyrilamine tannate] 25•8•25 mg; 5•2•12.5 mg/5 mL

Rynatan-S oral suspension ℞ *pediatric decongestant and antihistamine* [phenylephrine tannate; chlorpheniramine tannate; pyrilamine tannate] 5•2•12.5 mg/5 mL

Rynatuss tablets, pediatric suspension ℞ *antitussive; decongestant; antihistamine* [carbetapentane tannate; phenylephrine tannate; ephedrine tannate; chlorpheniramine tannate] 60•10•10•5 mg; 30•5•5•4 mg/5 mL

Rythmol film-coated tablets ℞ *antiarrhythmic* [propafenone HCl] 150, 225, 300 mg

S

S-2 solution for inhalation OTC *bronchodilator for bronchial asthma* [racepinephrine] 2.25%

^{35}S [see: sodium sulfate S 35]

SA (salicylic acid) [q.v.]

SA (serum albumin) [see: albumin, human]

Saave + capsules (discontinued 1993) OTC *dietary supplement* [multiple amino acids, vitamins, and minerals]

sabeluzole USAN, INN, BAN *anticonvulsant; antihypoxic; investigational treatment for Alzheimer's disease*

Sabin vaccine [see: poliovirus vaccine, live oral]

Sabril (commercially available in 40 foreign countries) ℞ *investigational anticonvulsant* [vigabatrin]

S-A-C tablets (discontinued 1995) OTC *analgesic; antipyretic; anti-inflammatory* [acetaminophen; salicylamide; caffeine] 150•230•30 mg

Sacarase ℞ (*orphan: congenital sucrase-isomaltase deficiency*) [sucrase]

saccharin NF *flavoring agent*

saccharin calcium USP *non-nutritive sweetener*

saccharin sodium USP *non-nutritive sweetener*

Saf-Clens spray OTC *wound cleanser*

Safe Tussin 30 liquid OTC *antitussive; expectorant* [dextromethorphan

hydrobromide; guaifenesin] 15•100 mg/5 mL
safflower oil USP *oleaginous vehicle; essential fatty acid supplement*
safingol USAN *antipsoriatic; antineoplastic adjunct*
safingol HCl USAN *antipsoriatic; antineoplastic adjunct*
safrole USP
Saizen ℞ *(orphan: growth failure; Turner syndrome; anovulation; severe burns)* [somatropin]
SalAc liquid OTC *topical keratolytic cleanser for acne* [salicylic acid] 2%
salacetamide INN
salacetin [see: aspirin]
Sal-Acid plaster OTC *topical keratolytic* [salicylic acid in a collodion-like vehicle] 40%
Salacid 25%; Salacid 60% ointment (discontinued 1994) ℞ *topical keratolytic* [salicylic acid in a petroleum base] 25%; 60%
Salactic Film liquid OTC *topical keratolytic* [salicylic acid in a collodion-like vehicle] 17%
salafibrate INN
Salagen film-coated tablets ℞ *treatment for radiation-induced xerostomia (orphan)* [pilocarpine HCl] 5 mg
salantel USAN, INN *veterinary anthelmintic*
Salazide; Salazide-Demi tablets ℞ *antihypertensive* [hydroflumethiazide; reserpine]
salazodine INN
Salazopyrin (European name for U.S. product Azulfidine)
salazosulfadimidine INN [also: salazosulphadimidine]
salazosulfamide INN
salazosulfapyridine [see: sulfasalazine]
salazosulfathiazole INN
salazosulphadimidine BAN [also: salazosulfadimidine]
salbutamol INN, BAN *bronchodilator* [also: albuterol]
salbutamol sulfate JAN *bronchodilator* [also: albuterol sulfate]
salcatonin BAN *synthetic analog of calcitonin (salmon); calcium regulator; investigational osteoporosis treatment* [also: calcitonin salmon (synthesis)]

salcetogen [see: aspirin]
Sal-Clens Acne Cleanser gel OTC *topical keratolytic for acne* [salicylic acid] 2%
salcolex USAN, INN *analgesic; anti-inflammatory; antipyretic*
saletamide INN *analgesic* [also: salethamide maleate]
saletamide maleate [see: salethamide maleate]
salethamide maleate USAN *analgesic* [also: saletamide]
saletin [see: aspirin]
Saleto tablets OTC *analgesic; antipyretic; anti-inflammatory* [acetaminophen; aspirin; salicylamide; caffeine] 115•210•65•16 mg
Saleto CF tablets OTC *antitussive; decongestant; analgesic* [dextromethorphan hydrobromide; phenylpropanolamine; acetaminophen] 10•12.5•325 mg
Saleto-200 tablets OTC *nonsteroidal anti-inflammatory drug (NSAID); antiarthritic; analgesic* [ibuprofen] 200 mg
Saleto-400; Saleto-600; Saleto-800 tablets ℞ *nonsteroidal anti-inflammatory drug (NSAID); antiarthritic; analgesic* [ibuprofen] 400 mg; 600 mg; 800 mg
Saleto-D capsules OTC *decongestant; analgesic; antipyretic* [phenylpropanolamine HCl; acetaminophen; salicylamide; caffeine] 18•240•120•16 mg
Salflex film-coated tablets OTC *analgesic; antipyretic; anti-inflammatory; antirheumatic* [salsalate] 500, 750 mg
salfluverine INN
salicain [now: salicyl alcohol]
salicin USP
salicyl alcohol USAN *local anesthetic*
salicylamide USP *analgesic*
salicylanilide NF
salicylate meglumine USAN *antirheumatic; analgesic*
salicylazosulfapyridine [now: sulfasalazine]
salicylic acid (SA) USP *keratolytic; antiseborrheic; antipsoriatic*
salicylic acid, bimolecular ester [see: salsalate]
salicylic acid acetate [see: aspirin]

Salicylic Acid Acne Treatment bar (discontinued 1995) OTC *medicated cleanser for acne* [salicylic acid] 2%

Salicylic Acid and Sulfur Soap bar OTC *medicated cleanser for acne* [salicylic acid; precipitated sulfur] 3%•10%

Salicylic Acid Cleansing bar OTC *medicated cleanser for acne* [salicylic acid] 2%

salicylic acid dihydrogen phosphate [see: fosfosal]

salicylsalicylic acid [see: salsalate]

Saligel gel (discontinued 1994) OTC *topical keratolytic for acne* [salicylic acid; alcohol] 5%•14%

saligenin [now: salicyl alcohol]

saligenol [now: salicyl alcohol]

salinazid INN, BAN

saline, lactated potassic [see: potassic saline, lactated]

saline solution (SS) [also: normal saline]

SalineX nasal mist, nose drops OTC *nasal moisturizer* [sodium chloride (saline)] 0.4%

saliniazid [see: salinazid]

salinomycin INN, BAN

Saliva Substitute oral solution OTC *saliva substitute*

Salivart oral spray OTC *saliva substitute*

Salix lozenges OTC *saliva substitute*

salmaterol [see: salmeterol]

salmefamol INN, BAN

salmeterol USAN, INN, BAN *bronchodilator*

salmeterol xinafoate USAN *adrenergic; bronchodilator*

salmisteine INN

salmon calcitonin [see: salcatonin]

Salmonine subcu or IM injection ℞ *calcium regulator for hypercalcemia, Paget's disease, and postmenopausal osteoporosis* [calcitonin (salmon)] 200 IU/mL

salmotin [see: adicillin]

salnacedin USAN *anti-inflammatory*

Salocol tablets (discontinued 1995) OTC *analgesic; antipyretic; anti-inflammatory* [acetaminophen; aspirin; salicylamide; caffeine] 115•210•65•16 mg

Sal-Oil-T hair dressing ℞ *antipsoriatic; antiseborrheic; keratolytic* [coal tar; salicylic acid] 10%•6%

salol [see: phenyl salicylate]

Salonil ointment (discontinued 1992) ℞ *topical keratolytic* [salicylic acid]

Salphenyl capsules (discontinued 1995) OTC *decongestant; antihistamine; analgesic* [phenylephrine HCl; chlorpheniramine maleate; acetaminophen; salicylamide] 10•2•130•200 mg

Sal-Plant gel OTC *topical keratolytic* [salicylic acid in a collodion-like vehicle] 17%

salprotoside INN

salsalate USAN, USP, INN, BAN *analgesic; antipyretic; anti-inflammatory; antirheumatic* 500, 750 mg oral

Salsitab film-coated tablets ℞ *analgesic; antipyretic; anti-inflammatory; antirheumatic* [salsalate] 500, 750 mg

Sal-Tropine tablets ℞ *GI anticholinergic and antispasmodic* [atropine sulfate] 0.4 mg

Saluron tablets ℞ *diuretic; antihypertensive* [hydroflumethiazide] 50 mg

Salutensin tablets ℞ *antihypertensive* [hydroflumethiazide; reserpine] 50•0.125 mg ▣ Diutensen

Salutensin-Demi tablets (discontinued 1995) ℞ *antihypertensive* [hydroflumethiazide; reserpine] 25•0.125 mg

saluzide [see: opiniazide]

salvarsan [see: arsphenamine]

salverine INN

Salzen ℞ *investigational treatment for growth hormone deficiency and chronic renal insufficiency* [human growth hormone]

samarium *element (Sm)*

samarium EDTMP *investigational analgesic for metastatic bone pain*

samarium Sm 153 lexidronam pentasodium USAN *radiopharmaceutical for treatment of bone pain in bone metastases*

Sanchia Silicone cream OTC *skin protectant* [silicone; lanolin]

sancycline USAN, INN *antibacterial*

Sandimmune gel capsules, oral solution, IV injection ℞ *immunosuppressant for allogenic kidney, liver, and heart transplants; investigational for many uses* [cyclosporine] 25, 50, 100 mg; 100 mg/mL; 50 mg/mL

Sandimmune ophthalmic ointment ℞ *(orphan: keratoplasty graft rejection; corneal melting syndrome); investigational antipsoriatic* [cyclosporine] 2%

Sandoglobulin powder for IV infusion ℞ *passive immunizing agent; immunomodulator for AIDS/ARC* [immune globulin] 1, 3, 6, 12 g

SandoPak (trademarked packaging form) *unit dose blister package*

Sandostatin subcu or IV injection ℞ *acromegaly; carcinoid tumors; vasoactive intestinal peptide tumors (VIPomas)* [octreotide acetate] 0.05, 0.1, 0.2, 0.5, 1 mg/mL

Sandostatin LAR ℞ *investigational antineoplastic for breast and colon cancer* [octreotide acetate]

sanfetrinem INN, BAN *antibacterial* [also: sanfetrinem sodium]

sanfetrinem cilexetil USAN *antibacterial*

sanfetrinem sodium USAN *antibacterial* [also: sanfetrinem]

sanguinarine chloride [now: sanguinarium chloride]

sanguinarium chloride USAN, INN *antifungal; antimicrobial; anti-inflammatory*

Sani-Pak (trademarked packaging form) *sanitary dispensing box*

Sani-Supp suppositories OTC *hyperosmolar laxative* [glycerin]

Sanitube ointment (discontinued 1996) OTC *venereal prophylactic* [calomel; benzoxiquine; trolamine] 30% • 2 • 2

Sanorex tablets ℞ *anorexiant (orphan: Duchenne muscular dystrophy)* [mazindol] 1, 2 mg

Sansert tablets ℞ *agent for migraine and vascular headaches* [methysergide maleate] 2 mg

santonin NF

Santyl ointment ℞ *topical enzyme for biochemical debridement* [collagenase] 250 U/g

saperconazole USAN, INN, BAN *antifungal*

saprisartan INN, BAN *antihypertensive* [also: saprisartan potassium]

saprisartan potassium USAN *antihypertensive* [also: saprisartan]

sapropterin INN

saquinavir INN, BAN *antiviral; HIV protease inhibitor* [also: saquinavir mesylate]

saquinavir mesylate USAN *antiviral; HIV protease inhibitor* [also: saquinavir]

sarafloxacin INN, BAN *anti-infective; DNA gyrase inhibitor* [also: sarafloxacin HCl]

sarafloxacin HCl USAN *anti-infective; DNA gyrase inhibitor* [also: sarafloxacin]

saralasin INN *antihypertensive* [also: saralasin acetate]

saralasin acetate USAN *antihypertensive* [also: saralasin]

Saratoga ointment OTC *astringent; antiseptic; wound protectant* [zinc oxide; boric acid; eucalyptol]

sarcolysin INN

L-sarcolysin [see: melphalan]

Sardo Bath & Shower oil OTC *bath emollient*

Sardoettes towelettes OTC *moisturizer; emollient*

sargramostim USAN, INN, BAN *antineutropenic for bone marrow transplant and graft delay (orphan); investigational AIDS cytokine*

Sarisol No. 2 tablets (discontinued 1993) ℞ *sedative; hypnotic* [butabarbital sodium]

sarmazenil INN

sarmoxicillin USAN, INN *antibacterial*

Sarna Anti-Itch foam, lotion OTC *counterirritant* [camphor; menthol] 0.5% • 0.5%

saroten [see: amitriptyline]

sarpicillin USAN, INN *antibacterial*

saruplase INN

Sastid cream OTC *keratolytic for acne* [precipitated sulfur; salicylic acid]

Sastid (AL) Scrub cream (discontinued 1994) OTC *abrasive cleanser for* *acne* [aluminum oxide; sulfur; salicylic acid] 20%•1.6%•1.6%

Sastid Plain Therapeutic Shampoo & Acne Wash (discontinued 1994) OTC *topical acne cleanser* [sulfur; salicylic acid] 1.6%•1.6%

SAStid Soap bar OTC *medicated cleanser for acne* [precipitated sulfur] 10%

saterinone INN

satranidazole INN

satumomab pendetide *(orphan: imaging aid for detection of ovarian carcinoma)*

savoxepin INN

SC (succinylcholine) [see: succinylcholine chloride]

SC-49483 *investigational pro-drug that prevents the clumping of HIV cells which leads to drug resistance*

SCA proteins (single-chain antigen-binding proteins) *investigational class of antineoplastics*

Scabene lotion, shampoo ℞ *scabicide; pediculicide* [lindane] 1%

Scadan scalp lotion OTC *antiseptic; antiseborrheic* [myristyltrimethylammonium bromide; stearyl dimethyl benzyl ammonium chloride] 1%•0.1%

Scalpicin liquid OTC *topical corticosteroid* [hydrocortisone] 1%

scandium *element (Sc)*

scarlet fever streptococcus toxin

scarlet red NF *promotes wound healing*

Scarlet Red Ointment Dressings medication-impregnated gauze ℞ *wound dressings* [scarlet red] 5%

sCD4-PE40 [see: alvircept sudotox]

Schamberg lotion OTC *antiseptic; astringent; antifungal; counterirritant* [zinc oxide; menthol; phenol] 8.25%•0.25%•1.5%

Schick test [see: diphtheria toxin for Schick test]

Schick test control USP *dermal reactivity indicator*

Schirmer Tear Test ophthalmic strips OTC *diagnostic tear flow test aid*

Sclavo PPD Solution intradermal injection (discontinued 1995) ℞ *tuberculosis skin test* [tuberculin purified protein derivative] 5 U/0.1 mL

Sclavo Test-PPD single-use intradermal puncture test device (discontinued 1995) ℞ *tuberculosis skin test* [tuberculin purified protein derivative] 5 U

Sclerex tablets OTC *vitamin/mineral supplement* [multiple vitamins & minerals]

Scleromate IV injection ℞ *sclerosing agent for varicose veins* [morrhuate sodium] 50 mg/mL

Sclerosol ℞ *(orphan: scleroderma)* [dimethyl sulfoxide (DMSO)]

Scooby-Doo Children's Chewable Plus Iron tablets (discontinued 1992) OTC *vitamin/iron supplement* [multiple vitamins; iron; folic acid]

Scooby-Doo Children's Chewable Tablets (discontinued 1992) OTC *vitamin supplement* [multiple vitamins; folic acid]

Scooby-Doo Children's Complete Formula chewable tablets (discontinued 1992) OTC *vitamin/mineral/iron supplement* [multiple vitamins & minerals; iron; folic acid; biotin]

Scooter Rabbit chewable tablets OTC *vitamin/mineral supplement* [multiple vitamins & minerals; bioflavonoids]

scopafungin USAN *antibacterial; antifungal*

Scope mouthwash OTC *oral antiseptic* [cetylpyridinium chloride]

scopolamine *transdermal motion sickness preventative*

scopolamine hydrobromide USP *GI antispasmodic; anticholinergic; motion sickness preventative; cycloplegic; mydriatic* [also: hyoscine hydrobromide] 0.3, 0.4, 0.86, 1 mg/mL injection

scopolamine methyl nitrate [see: methscopolamine nitrate]

scopolamine methylbromide [see: methscopolamine bromide]

Scorbex/12 injection (discontinued 1992) ℞ *vitamin therapy* [multiple B vitamins; vitamin C]

Scott's Emulsion OTC *vitamin supplement* [vitamins A and D] 1250•100 IU/5 mL

Scot-Tussin Allergy liquid OTC *antihistamine* [diphenhydramine HCl] 12.5 mg/5 mL

Scot-Tussin DM liquid OTC *antitussive; antihistamine* [dextromethorphan hydrobromide; chlorpheniramine maleate] 15•2 mg/5 mL

Scot-Tussin DM 2 syrup (discontinued 1992) OTC *antitussive; expectorant* [dextromethorphan hydrobromide; guaifenesin; alcohol]

Scot-Tussin DM Cough Chasers lozenges OTC *antitussive* [dextromethorphan hydrobromide] 2.5 mg

Scot-Tussin Expectorant sugar-free liquid OTC *expectorant* [guaifenesin; alcohol 3.5%] 100 mg/5 mL

Scot-Tussin Original 5-Action Cold Formula syrup, sugar-free liquid OTC *decongestant; antihistamine; analgesic* [phenylephrine HCl; pheniramine maleate; sodium citrate; sodium salicylate; caffeine citrate] 4.2•13.3•83.3•83.3•25 mg

Scot-Tussin Senior Clear liquid OTC *antitussive; expectorant* [dextromethorphan hydrobromide; guaifenesin] 15•200 mg/5 mL

sCR1 (soluble complement receptor 1) *investigational complement inhibitor for severe burns and adult respiratory distress syndrome*

Scriptene ℞ *investigational (Phase I) antiviral for AIDS* [zidovudine; didanosine]

scuroforme [see: butyl aminobenzoate]

SD (streptodornase) [q.v.]

SD Polygam (name changed to Polygam S/D in 1994)

⁷⁵Se [see: selenomethionine Se 75]

Sea Mist nasal spray OTC *nasal moisturizer* [sodium chloride (saline)] 0.65%

Seale's Lotion Modified OTC *topical acne treatment* [sulfur] 6.4%

Sea-Omega 30; Sea-Omega 50 softgels OTC *dietary supplement* [omega-3 fatty acids] 1200 mg; 1000 mg

SEB-324 *investigational anxiolytic and antidepressant*

Sebacide Cleanser liquid (discontinued 1994) OTC *topical acne cleanser* [parachlorometaxylenol] 0.35%

Seba-Nil Cleansing Mask scrub OTC *abrasive cleanser for acne*

Seba-Nil Oily Skin Cleanser liquid OTC *topical cleanser for acne* [alcohol; acetone]

Sebaquin shampoo (discontinued 1994) OTC *antiseborrheic; antimicrobial* [iodoquinol] 3%

Sebasorb liquid (discontinued 1994) OTC *topical acne treatment* [colloidal sulfur; salicylic acid; attapulgite] 2%•2%•10%

Sebasorb lotion OTC *topical keratolytic for acne* [salicylic acid; attapulgite] 2%•10%

Sebex shampoo OTC *antiseborrheic; keratolytic* [sulfur; salicylic acid] 2%•2%

Sebex-T shampoo OTC *antiseborrheic; antipsoriatic; keratolytic* [sulfur; salicylic acid; coal tar] 2%•2%•5%

Sebizon lotion ℞ *bacteriostatic; antiseborrheic* [sulfacetamide sodium] 10%

Sebucare hair lotion OTC *antiseborrheic; keratolytic* [salicylic acid; alcohol 61%] 1.8%

Sebulex; Sebulex with Conditioners shampoo OTC *antiseborrheic; keratolytic* [sulfur; salicylic acid] 2%•2%

Sebulon shampoo OTC *antiseborrheic; antibacterial; antifungal* [pyrithione zinc] 2%

Sebutone cream shampoo, liquid shampoo OTC *antiseborrheic; antipsoriatic; keratolytic* [coal tar; sulfur; salicylic acid] 0.5%•2%•2%

SEC-579 *investigational anxiolytic and 5-HT3 antagonist*

secalciferol USAN, BAN *calcium regulator (orphan: familial hypophosphatemic rickets)*

secbutabarbital sodium INN *sedative; hypnotic* [also: butabarbital sodium]

secbutobarbitone BAN *sedative; hypnotic* [also: butabarbital]

seclazone USAN, INN *anti-inflammatory; uricosuric*

secnidazole INN, BAN

secobarbital USP, INN *hypnotic; sedative*

secobarbital sodium USP, JAN *hypnotic; sedative* [also: quinalbarbitone sodium] 100 mg oral; 50 mg/mL injection

Seconal Sodium IV, IM or rectal injection (discontinued 1992) ℞ *sedative; hypnotic* [secobarbital sodium]

Seconal Sodium Pulvules (capsules) ℞ *sedative; hypnotic* [secobarbital sodium] 100 mg

secoverine INN

Secran liquid OTC *vitamin supplement* [vitamins B_1, B_3, and B_{12}; alcohol 17%] 10 mg•10 mg•25 μg per 5 mL

Secran Prenatal tablets (discontinued 1995) ℞ *vitamin/calcium/iron supplement* [multiple vitamins; calcium; iron; folic acid] ≟•250•60•1 mg

secretin INN, BAN *pancreatic function diagnostic aid*

Secretin Ferring powder for IV injection ℞ *in vivo pancreatic function test* [secretin] 10 CU/mL

Sectral capsules ℞ *antihypertensive; antiarrhythmic; β-blocker* [acebutolol HCl] 200, 400 mg

Secule (trademarked packaging form) *single-dose vial*

securinine INN

sedaform [see: chlorobutanol]

Sedapap-10 tablets ℞ *analgesic; antipyretic; sedative* [acetaminophen; butalbital] 650•50 mg

sedatine [see: antipyrine]

sedecamycin USAN, INN *veterinary antibacterial*

sedeval [see: barbital]

seganserin INN, BAN

seglitide INN *antidiabetic* [also: seglitide acetate]

seglitide acetate USAN *antidiabetic* [also: seglitide]

Seldane tablets ℞ *nonsedating antihistamine* [terfenadine] 60 mg

Seldane-D sustained-release tablets ℞ *decongestant; antihistamine* [pseudoephedrine HCl; terfenadine] 120•60 mg

Selecor tablets ℞ *investigational antihypertensive; antianginal; β-blocker* [celiprolol HCl]

Select-A-Jet (trademarked delivery system) *syringe system*

selegiline INN, BAN *antiparkinsonian; investigational treatment for Alzheimer's disease* [also: selegiline HCl]

selegiline HCl USAN *antiparkinsonian (orphan); investigational treatment for Alzheimer's disease* [also: selegiline]

selenious acid USP *dietary selenium supplement* 65.4 μg/mL injection

selenium *element (Se)*

selenium dioxide, monohydrated [see: selenious acid]

selenium sulfide USP *antifungal; antiseborrheic* 1%, 2.5% topical

selenomethionine (^{75}Se) INN *pancreas function test; radioactive agent* [also: selenomethionine Se 75]

selenomethionine Se 75 USAN, USP *pancreas function test; radioactive agent* [also: selenomethionine (^{75}Se)]

Sele-Pak IV injection ℞ *intravenous nutritional therapy* [selenious acid] 65.4 μg/mL

Selepen IV injection ℞ *intravenous nutritional therapy* [selenious acid] 65.4 μg/mL

Selestoject IV, IM injection (discontinued 1996) ℞ *glucocorticoid* [betamethasone sodium phosphate] 4 mg/mL

selfotel USAN *N-methyl-D-aspartate (NMDA) antagonist for treatment of stroke-induced impairment*

Seloken (foreign name for U.S. product Lopressor)

Seloken ZOC (foreign name for U.S. product Toprol XL)

selprazine INN

Selsun lotion/shampoo ℞ *antiseborrheic; antifungal* [selenium sulfide] 2.5%

Selsun Blue; Selsun Gold for Women lotion/shampoo OTC *antiseborrheic* [selenium sulfide] 1%

sematilide INN *antiarrhythmic* [also: sematilide HCl]

sematilide HCl USAN *antiarrhythmic* [also: sematilide]

semduramicin USAN, INN *coccidiostat*

semduramicin sodium USAN *coccidiostat*

Semicid vaginal suppositories OTC *spermicidal contraceptive* [nonoxynol 9] 100 mg

Semilente Iletin I subcu injection (discontinued 1994) OTC *antidiabetic* [insulin zinc (beef-pork)]

Semilente Insulin subcu injection (discontinued 1994) OTC *antidiabetic* [insulin zinc, prompt (beef)]

semisodium valproate BAN *anticonvulsant* [also: divalproex sodium; valproate semisodium]

Semprex-D capsules ℞ *decongestant; antihistamine* [pseudoephedrine HCl; acrivastine] 60•8 mg

semustine USAN, INN *antineoplastic*

Senexon tablets OTC *laxative* [senna concentrate] 187 mg

Senilezol elixir ℞ *vitamin/iron supplement* [multiple B vitamins; ferric pyrophosphate] ≟•3.3 mg

senna USP *stimulant laxative*

Senna-Gen tablets OTC *laxative* [senna concentrate] 187 mg

sennosides USP *stimulant laxative*

Senokot tablets, granules, suppositories, syrup OTC *laxative* [senna concentrate] 187 mg; 326 mg/tsp.; 652 mg; 218 mg/5 mL

Senokot-S tablets OTC *laxative; stool softener* [docusate sodium; senna concentrate] 50•187 mg

Senokotxtra tablets OTC *laxative* [senna concentrate] 374 mg

Senolax tablets OTC *laxative* [senna concentrate] 187 mg

Sensitive Eyes; Sensitive Eyes Plus solution OTC *rinsing/storage solution for soft contact lenses* [preserved saline solution]

Sensitive Eyes Daily Cleaner; Sensitive Eyes Saline/Cleaning Solution OTC *surfactant cleaning solution for soft contact lenses*

Sensitive Eyes Drops OTC *rewetting solution for soft contact lenses*

Sensitivity Protection Crest toothpaste OTC *tooth desensitizer; dental caries preventative* [potassium nitrate; sodium fluoride]

Sensodyne, Original toothpaste (name changed to Sensodyne-SC in 1994)

Sensodyne Cool Gel toothpaste OTC *tooth desensitizer; dental caries preventative* [potassium nitrate; sodium fluoride]

Sensodyne Fresh Mint toothpaste OTC *tooth desensitizer; dental caries preventative* [potassium nitrate; sodium monofluorophosphate] ≟

Sensodyne-F toothpaste (name changed to Sensodyne Fresh Mint in 1994)

Sensodyne-SC toothpaste OTC *tooth desensitizer* [strontium chloride hexahydrate] 10%

SensoGARD gel OTC *topical oral anesthetic* [benzocaine] 20%

Sensorcaine injection ℞ *injectable local anesthetic* [bupivacaine HCl] 0.25%, 0.5%, 0.75%

Sensorcaine injection ℞ *injectable local anesthetic* [bupivacaine HCl; epinephrine] 0.25%•1:200,000; 0.5%•1:200,000

Sensorcaine MPF injection ℞ *injectable local anesthetic* [bupivacaine HCl] 0.25%, 0.5%, 0.75%

Sensorcaine MPF injection ℞ *injectable local anesthetic* [bupivacaine HCl; epinephrine] 0.25%•1:200,000, 0.5%•1:200,000, 0.75%•1:200,000

Sensorcaine MPF Spinal injection ℞ *injectable local anesthetic* [bupivacaine HCl] 0.75%

sepazonium chloride USAN, INN *topical anti-infective*

seperidol HCl USAN *antipsychotic* [also: clofluperol]

Sepo throat lozenges OTC *topical oral anesthetic; demulcent* [benzocaine; sugar] ⓘ Septa

Seprafilm hydrated gel film *to reduce the incidence, extent, and severity of postoperative adhesions* [sodium hyaluronate; carboxymethylcellulose]

seprilose USAN *antirheumatic*

seproxetine HCl USAN *antidepressant*

Septa ointment OTC *topical antibiotic* [polymyxin B sulfate; neomycin sulfate; bacitracin] 5000 U•3.5 mg•400 U per g ⓘ Sepo; Septra

SeptiGAM ℞ *investigational antibacterial for Staphylococcus aureus-induced sepsis*

Septi-Soft solution ℞ *antiseptic; disinfectant* [triclosan] 0.25%

Septisol foam ℞ *bacteriostatic skin cleanser* [hexachlorophene; alcohol 56%] 0.23%

Septisol solution ℞ *antiseptic; disinfectant* [triclosan] 0.25%

septomonab [see: nebacumab]

Septopal polymethyl methacrylate (PMMA) beads on surgical wire ℞ *(orphan: chronic osteomyelitis)* [gentamicin]

Septra tablets, oral suspension ℞ *anti-infective; antibacterial* [trimethoprim; sulfamethoxazole] 80•400 mg; 40•200 mg/5 mL ② Septa

Septra DS tablets ℞ *anti-infective; antibacterial* [trimethoprim; sulfamethoxazole] 160•800 mg

Septra IV infusion ℞ *anti-infective; antibacterial* [trimethoprim; sulfamethoxazole] 80•400 mg/5 mL

Sequels (trademarked dosage form) *sustained-release capsule or tablet*

sequifenadine INN

seractide INN *adrenocorticotropic hormone* [also: seractide acetate]

seractide acetate USAN *adrenocorticotropic hormone* [also: seractide]

Ser-A-Gen tablets (discontinued 1993) ℞ *antihypertensive* [hydrochlorothiazide; reserpine; hydralazine HCl]

Seralazide tablets (discontinued 1992) ℞ *antihypertensive* [hydrochlorothiazide; reserpine; hydralazine HCl]

Ser-Ap-Es tablets ℞ *antihypertensive* [hydrochlorothiazide; reserpine; hydralazine HCl] 15•0.1•25 mg ② Catapres

seratrodast USAN, INN *anti-inflammatory; antiasthmatic; thromboxane receptor antagonist*

Serax capsules, tablets ℞ *anxiolytic* [oxazepam] 10, 15, 30 mg; 15 mg ② Eurax; Urex; Xerac

serazapine HCl USAN *anxiolytic*

Serc-16 tablets ℞ *treatment for vertigo due to Meniere syndrome* [betahistine]

Sereine solution OTC *cleaning solution for hard contact lenses* [note: one of three different products with the same name]

Sereine solution OTC *wetting solution for hard contact lenses* [note: one of three different products with the same name]

Sereine solution OTC *wetting/soaking solution for hard contact lenses* [note: one of three different products with the same name]

Serentil tablets, oral concentrate, IM injection ℞ *antipsychotic* [mesoridazine besylate] 10, 25, 50, 100 mg; 25 mg/mL; 25 mg/mL ② Surital

Serevent oral metered dose inhaler ℞ *twice-daily bronchodilator for asthma and bronchospasm* [salmeterol xinafoate] 25 μg/dose

serfibrate INN

sergolexole INN *antimigraine* [also: sergolexole maleate]

sergolexole maleate USAN *antimigraine* [also: sergolexole]

serine (L-serine) USAN, USP, INN *nonessential amino acid; symbols: Ser, S*

L-serine diazoacetate [see: azaserine]

84-L-serineplasminogen activator [see: monteplase]

sermetacin USAN, INN *anti-inflammatory*

sermorelin INN, BAN *growth hormone deficiency diagnosis and treatment* [also: sermorelin acetate]

sermorelin acetate USAN *pituitary diagnostic aid; (orphan: growth hormone deficiency; anovulation; AIDS-related weight loss)* [also: sermorelin]

Seromycin Pulvules (capsules) ℞ *tuberculostatic* [cycloserine] 250 mg

Serophene tablets ℞ *ovulation stimulant* [clomiphene citrate] 50 mg

Seroquel ℞ *investigational dopamine and serotonin antagonist for schizophrenia*

Serostim ℞ *treatment for AIDS-related catabolism (wasting syndrome) and cachexia* [somatropin]

Seroxat (European name for U.S. product Paxil)

Serpalan tablets (discontinued 1995) ℞ *antihypertensive; antipsychotic* [reserpine] 0.1, 0.25 mg

Serpasil tablets (discontinued 1992) ℞ *antihypertensive; antipsychotic* [reserpine] 0.1, 0.25 mg

Serpasil-Apresoline #1; Serpasil-Apresoline #2 tablets (discontinued 1992) ℞ *antihypertensive* [reserpine; hydralazine HCl]

Serpasil-Esidrix #1; Serpasil-Esidrex #2 tablets (discontinued 1992) ℞ *antihypertensive* [reserpine; hydrochlorothiazide]

Serpazide tablets ℞ *antihypertensive* [hydrochlorothiazide; reserpine; hydralazine HCl]

serrapeptase INN

Serratia marcescens extract (polyribosomes) *(orphan: primary brain malignancies)*

sertaconazole INN

sertindole USAN, INN *antipsychotic; neuroleptic*

sertraline INN, BAN *antidepressant; selective serotonin reuptake inhibitor* [also: sertraline HCl]

sertraline HCl USAN *antidepressant; selective serotonin reuptake inhibitor* [also: sertraline]

serum albumin (SA) [see: albumin, human]

serum albumin, iodinated (^{125}I) human [see: albumin, iodinated I 125 serum]

serum albumin, iodinated (^{131}I) human [see: albumin, iodinated I 131 serum]

serum fibrinogen (SF) [see: fibrinogen, human]

serum globulin (SG) [see: globulin, immune]

serum gonadotrophin [see: gonadotrophin, serum]

serum gonadotropin [see: gonadotrophin, serum]

serum prothrombin conversion accelerator (SPCA) factor [see: factor VII]

Serutan powder, granules OTC *bulk laxative* [psyllium] 3.4 g/tsp.; 2.5 g/tsp.

Serzone tablets ℞ *antidepressant* [nefazodone HCl] 100, 150, 200, 250 mg

sesame oil NF *solvent; oleaginous vehicle*

Sesame Street Complete chewable tablets OTC *vitamin/mineral/calcium/iron supplement* [multiple vitamins and minerals; calcium; iron; folic acid; biotin] ≛•80•10•0.2•0.015 mg

Sesame Street Plus Extra C chewable tablets OTC *vitamin supplement* [multiple vitamins; folic acid] ≛•0.2 mg

Sesame Street Plus Iron chewable tablets OTC *vitamin/iron supplement* [multiple vitamins; iron; folic acid] ≛•10•0.2 mg

Sesame Street Vitamins chewable tablets (discontinued 1993) OTC *vitamin supplement* [multiple vitamins; folic acid] ≛•0.4 mg

Sesame Street Vitamins and Minerals (name changed to Sesame Street Complete in 1993)

setastine INN

setazindol INN

setiptiline INN

setoperone USAN, INN *antipsychotic*

Seudotabs tablets OTC *nasal decongestant* [pseudoephedrine HCl] 30 mg

7 + 3 protocol (cytarabine, daunorubicin) *chemotherapy protocol*

7 + 3 protocol (cytarabine, idarubicin) *chemotherapy protocol*

7 + 3 protocol (cytarabine, mitoxantrone) *chemotherapy protocol*

7E3 monoclonal antibody [see: abciximab]

7U85 *investigational antineoplastic*

sevirumab USAN, INN *investigational antiviral monoclonal antibody (orphan: cytomegalovirus of organ transplants & AIDS)*

sevitropium mesilate INN

sevoflurane USAN, INN *inhalation general anesthetic*

sevopramide INN

sezolamide HCl USAN *carbonic anhydrase inhibitor*

SF (serum fibrinogen) [see: fibrinogen, human]

SFC lotion OTC *soap-free therapeutic skin cleanser*

sfericase INN

SG (serum globulin) [see: globulin, immune]

SG (soluble gelatin) [see: gelatin]

SH 570 *investigational treatment for acne*

shark liver oil *emollient/protectant*

Sheik Elite premedicated condom OTC *spermicidal/barrier contraceptive* [nonoxynol 9] 8%

shellac NF *tablet coating agent*

Shepard's Cream Lotion; Shepard's Skin Cream OTC *moisturizer; emollient*

Shepard's Moisturizing Soap bar (discontinued 1992) OTC *therapeutic skin cleanser*

Shohl solution, modified (sodium citrate & citric acid) *urinary alkalizer; compounding agent*

short chain fatty acids *(orphan: left-sided ulcerative colitis)*

Shur-Clens solution OTC *wound cleanser* [poloxamer 188] 20%

Shur-Seal vaginal gel OTC *spermicidal contraceptive (for use with a diaphragm)* [nonoxynol 9] 2%

siagoside INN

Sibelium ℞ *vasodilator (orphan: alternating hemiplegia)* [flunarizine HCl]

Siblin granules OTC *bulk laxative* [blond psyllium seed coatings] 2.5 g/tsp.

sibopirdine USAN *cognition enhancer for Alzheimer's disease; nootropic*

sibutramine INN, BAN *anorectic; antidepressant; investigational treatment for obesity* [also: sibutramine HCl]

sibutramine HCl USAN *anorectic; antidepressant; investigational treatment for obesity* [also: sibutramine]

siccanin INN

Sickledex test kit for professional use *in vitro diagnostic aid for hemoglobin S (sickle cell)*

Sigosix ℞ *investigational treatment for radiation- or chemotherapy-induced thrombocytopenia* [recombinant human interleukin-6]

SigPak (trademarked packaging form) *unit-of-use package*

Sigtab tablets OTC *vitamin supplement* [multiple vitamins; folic acid] ≐•0.4 mg

Sigtab-M tablets OTC *vitamin/mineral/calcium/iron supplement* [multiple vitamins & minerals; calcium; iron; folic acid; biotin] ≐•200•18•0.4•0.045 mg

siguazodan INN, BAN

Silace syrup OTC *stool softener* [docusate sodium] 20 mg/5 mL

Silace-C syrup OTC *stimulant laxative; stool softener* [casanthranol; docusate sodium; alcohol 10%] 30•60 mg/15 mL

SilaClean 20/20 solution (discontinued 1995) OTC *cleaning solution for hard contact lenses*

Siladryl elixir OTC *antihistamine* [diphenhydramine HCl] 12.5 mg/5 mL

Silafed syrup OTC *decongestant; antihistamine* [pseudoephedrine HCl; triprolidine HCl] 30•1.25 mg/5 mL

silafilcon A USAN *hydrophilic contact lens material*

silafocon A USAN *hydrophobic contact lens material*

Silaminic Cold syrup OTC *decongestant; antihistamine* [phenylpropanolamine HCl; chlorpheniramine maleate] 12.5•2 mg/5 mL

Silaminic Expectorant syrup OTC *decongestant; expectorant* [phenylpropanolamine HCl; guaifenesin; alcohol 5%] 12.5•100 mg/5 mL

silandrone USAN, INN *androgen*

Silapap, Children's elixir OTC *analgesic; antipyretic* [acetaminophen (alcohol free)] 80 mg/2.5 mL

Silapap, Infant's pediatric drops OTC *analgesic; antipyretic* [acetaminophen] 80 mg/0.8 mL

Sildec-DM syrup, pediatric drops ℞ *antitussive; decongestant; antihistamine* [dextromethorphan hydrobromide; pseudoephedrine HCl; carbinoxamine maleate] 15•60•4 mg/5 mL; 4•25•2 mg/mL

Sildicon-E pediatric drops OTC *pediatric decongestant and expectorant* [phenylpropanolamine HCl; guaifenesin] 6.25•30 mg/mL

Silexin syrup OTC *antitussive; expectorant* [dextromethorphan hydrobromide; guaifenesin]

Silexin tablets OTC *antitussive; topical oral anesthetic* [dextromethorphan hydrobromide; benzocaine]

Silfedrine, Children's liquid OTC *nasal decongestant* [pseudoephedrine HCl] 30 mg/5 mL

silibinin INN

silica, dental-type NF *pharmaceutic aid*

silica gel [now: silicon dioxide]

siliceous earth, purified NF *filtering medium*

silicic acid, magnesium salt [see: magnesium trisilicate]

silicon *element (Si)*

silicon dioxide NF *dispersing and suspending agent*

silicon dioxide, colloidal NF *suspending agent; tablet and capsule diluent*

silicone

Silicone No. 2 ointment OTC *skin protectant* [silicone; hydrophobic starch derivative] 10%•?

silicone oil [see: polydimethylsiloxane]

silicristin INN

silidianin INN

silodrate USAN *antacid* [also: simaldrate]

Silphen Cough syrup OTC *antihistamine; antitussive* [diphenhydramine HCl; alcohol 5%] 12.5 mg/5 mL

Silphen DM syrup OTC *antitussive* [dextromethorphan hydrobromide; alcohol 5%] 10 mg/5 mL

Siltapp with Dextromethorphan HBr Cold & Cough elixir ℞ *antitussive; decongestant; antihistamine* [dextromethorphan hydrobromide; phenylpropanolamine HCl; brompheniramine maleate] 10•12.5•2 mg/5 mL

Sil-Tex liquid ℞ *decongestant; expectorant* [phenylpropanolamine HCl; phenylephrine HCl; guaifenesin; alcohol 5%] 20•5•100 mg/5 mL

Siltussin syrup OTC *expectorant* [guaifenesin; alcohol 3.5%] 100 mg/5 mL

Siltussin DM syrup OTC *antitussive; expectorant* [dextromethorphan hydrobromide; guaifenesin] 10•100 mg/5 mL

Siltussin-CF liquid OTC *antitussive; decongestant; expectorant* [dextromethorphan hydrobromide; phenylpropanolamine HCl; guaifenesin; alcohol 4.75%] 10•12.5•100 mg/5 mL

Silvadene cream ℞ *broad-spectrum bactericidal for adjunctive burn treatment* [silver sulfadiazine] 10 mg/g

silver *element (Ag)*

silver nitrate USP *ophthalmic neonatal anti-infective; strong caustic* 1% eye drops; 10%, 25%, 50%, 75% topical

silver nitrate, toughened USP *caustic*

silver protein, mild NF *ophthalmic antiseptic; ophthalmic surgical aid*

silver sulfadiazine (SSD) USAN, USP *broad-spectrum bactericidal; adjunct to burn therapy* [also: sulfadiazine silver]

Simaal; Simaal II gel (renamed Simaal Gel; Simaal Gel 2 in 1994)

Simaal Gel; Simaal Gel 2 liquid OTC *antacid; antiflatulent* [aluminum hydroxide; magnesium hydroxide; simethicone] 200•200•20 mg/5 mL; 500•400•40 mg/5 mL

simaldrate INN *antacid* [also: silodrate]

simethicone USAN, USP *antiflatulent* 80 mg oral; 40 mg/0.6 mL oral

simetride INN

simfibrate INN

Similac Low Iron liquid, powder OTC *total or supplementary infant feeding*

Similac PM 60/40 Low-Iron liquid OTC *formula for infants predisposed to hypocalcemia* [whey formula with lowered mineral levels]

Similac with Iron liquid, powder OTC *total or supplementary infant feeding*

simple syrup [see: syrup]

Simplet tablets OTC *decongestant; antihistamine; analgesic* [pseudoephedrine HCl; chlorpheniramine maleate; acetaminophen] 60•4•650 mg ② Singlet

Simron soft gelatin capsules OTC *hematinic* [ferrous gluconate] 86 mg

Simron Plus capsules OTC *vitamin/iron supplement* [multiple vitamins; ferrous gluconate; folic acid] ±•10•0.1 mg

simtrazene USAN, INN *antineoplastic*

simvastatin USAN, INN, BAN *antihyperlipidemic*

Sinapils tablets OTC *decongestant; antihistamine; analgesic* [phenylpropanolamine HCl; chlorpheniramine maleate; acetaminophen; caffeine] 12.5•2•325•32.5 mg

Sinarest; Sinarest Sinus tablets OTC *decongestant; antihistamine; analgesic* [pseudoephedrine HCl; chlorpheniramine maleate; acetaminophen] 30•2•500 mg; 30•2•325 mg

Sinarest, No Drowsiness tablets OTC *decongestant; analgesic; antipyretic* [pseudoephedrine HCl; acetaminophen] 30•500 mg

Sinarest 12 Hour nasal spray OTC *nasal decongestant* [oxymetazoline HCl] 0.05%

sincalide USAN, INN *choleretic*

Sine-Aid tablets, caplets, gelcaps OTC *decongestant; analgesic; antipyretic* [pseudoephedrine HCl; acetaminophen] 30•500 mg

Sine-Aid IB caplets OTC *decongestant; analgesic* [pseudoephedrine HCl; ibuprofen] 30•200 mg

sinefungin USAN, INN *antifungal*

Sinemet 10/100; Sinemet 25/100; Sinemet 25/250 tablets ℞ *antiparkinsonian* [carbidopa; levodopa] 10•100 mg; 25•100 mg; 25•250 mg

Sinemet CR sustained-release tablets ℞ *antiparkinsonian* [carbidopa; levodopa] 25•100, 50•200 mg

Sine-Off Allergy/Sinus caplets (name changed to Sine-Off Sinus Medicine in 1995)

Sine-Off No Drowsiness Formula caplets OTC *decongestant; analgesic; antipyretic* [pseudoephedrine HCl; acetaminophen] 30•500 mg

Sine-Off Sinus Medicine caplets OTC *decongestant; antihistamine; analgesic* [pseudoephedrine HCl; chlorpheniramine maleate; acetaminophen] 30•2•500 mg

Sine-Off Sinus Medicine tablets (discontinued 1995) OTC *decongestant; antihistamine; analgesic; antipyretic* [phenylpropanolamine HCl; chlorpheniramine maleate; aspirin] 12.5•2•325 mg

Sinequan capsules, oral concentrate ℞ *anxiolytic; antidepressant* [doxepin HCl] 10, 25, 50, 75, 100, 150 mg; 10 mg/mL

Sinex nasal spray OTC *nasal decongestant* [phenylephrine HCl] 0.5%

Sinex 12-Hour nasal spray OTC *nasal decongestant* [oxymetazoline HCl] 0.05%

Sinex Long-Acting nasal spray (name changed to Sinex 12-Hour in 1994)

single-chain antigen-binding proteins (SCA proteins) *investigational class of antineoplastics*

Singlet for Adults tablets OTC *decongestant; antihistamine; analgesic* [pseudoephedrine HCl; chlorpheniramine maleate; acetaminophen] 60•4•650 mg ⓢ Simplet

Sinografin intracavitary instillation ℞ *radiopaque agent* [diatrizoate meglumine; iodipamide meglumine] 52.7%•26.8%

sinorphan [now: ecadotril]

sintropium bromide INN

Sinubid sustained-release tablets (discontinued 1993) ℞ *decongestant; antihistamine; analgesic* [phenylpropanolamine HCl; phenyltoloxamine citrate; acetaminophen]

Sinufed Timecelles (sustained-release capsules) ℞ *decongestant; expectorant* [pseudoephedrine HCl; guaifenesin] 60•300 mg

Sinulin tablets OTC *decongestant; antihistamine; analgesic* [phenylpropanolamine HCl; chlorpheniramine maleate; acetaminophen] 25•4•650 mg

Sinumist-SR sustained-release Capsulets (capsule-shaped tablet) ℞ *expectorant* [guaifenesin] 600 mg

Sinupan controlled-release capsules ℞ *decongestant; expectorant* [phenylephrine HCl; guaifenesin] 40•200 mg

Sinus Headache & Congestion tablets OTC *decongestant; antihistamine; analgesic* [pseudoephedrine HCl; chlorpheniramine maleate; acetaminophen] 30•2•500 mg

Sinus Relief tablets OTC *decongestant; analgesic* [pseudoephedrine HCl; acetaminophen] 30•325 mg

Sinusol-B subcu or IM injection ℞ *antihistamine; anaphylaxis* [brompheniramine maleate] 10 mg/mL

SinuStat capsules OTC *decongestant* [pseudoephedrine HCl]

Sinustop Pro capsules OTC *nasal decongestant* [pseudoephedrine HCl] 60 mg

Sinutab, Allergy Formula sustained-release tablets (discontinued 1992) OTC *decongestant; antihistamine* [pseudoephedrine sulfate; dexbrompheniramine maleate]

Sinutab Non-Drying liquid capsules OTC *decongestant; expectorant* [pseudoephedrine HCl; guaifenesin] 30•200 mg

Sinutab Sinus Allergy caplets, tablets OTC *decongestant; antihistamine; analgesic* [pseudoephedrine HCl; chlorpheniramine maleate; acetaminophen] 30•2•500 mg

Sinutab Without Drowsiness caplets OTC *decongestant; analgesic; antipyretic* [pseudoephedrine HCl; acetaminophen] 30•500 mg

Sinutab Without Drowsiness tablets OTC *decongestant; analgesic; antipyretic* [pseudoephedrine HCl; acetaminophen] 30•325 mg; 30•500 mg

Sinutrex tablets (discontinued 1995) OTC *decongestant; antihistamine; analgesic* [pseudoephedrine HCl; chlorpheniramine maleate; acetaminophen] 30•2•500 mg

SinuVent long-acting tablets ℞ *decongestant; expectorant* [phenylpropanolamine HCl; guaifenesin] 75•600 mg

Sirdalud (foreign name for U.S. product Zanaflex)

sirolimus USAN *immunosuppressant*

sisomicin USAN, INN *antibacterial* [also: sissomicin]

sisomicin sulfate USAN, USP *antibacterial*

sissomicin BAN *antibacterial* [also: sisomicin]

sitalidone INN

sitofibrate INN

sitogluside USAN, INN *antiprostatic hypertrophy*

sitosterols NF

Sitzmarks capsules ℞ *GI contrast radiopaque agent* [radiopaque polyvinyl chloride] 20 rings

619C *investigational treatment for stroke*

sizofiran INN

SK (streptokinase) [q.v.]

Skeeter Stik liquid OTC *topical local anesthetic; counterirritant* [lidocaine; menthol] 4%•1%

Skelaxin tablets ℞ *skeletal muscle relaxant* [metaxalone] 400 mg

SK&F 97426 *investigational antihyperlipidemic*

SK&F 106203 *investigational leukotriene antagonist for asthma*

SK&F 110679 (orphan: *growth failure due to lack of endogenous growth hormone*)

skin respiratory factor (SRF) claimed to *promote wound healing*

Skin Shield liquid OTC *skin protectant; topical local anesthetic* [dyclonine HCl; benzethonium chloride] 0.75%•0.2%

SL (sodium lactate) [q.v.]

SLC solution (discontinued 1992) OTC *cleaning solution for hard contact lenses*

Sleep-Eze 3 tablets OTC *antihistaminic sleep aid* [diphenhydramine HCl] 25 mg

Sleepinal capsules, soft gels OTC *antihistaminic sleep aid* [diphenhydramine HCl] 50 mg

Sleepwell 2-nite tablets OTC *antihistaminic sleep aid* [diphenhydramine HCl] 25 mg

Slim-Mint gum OTC *decrease taste perception of sweetness* [benzocaine] 6 mg

Sloan's Liniment (discontinued 1992) OTC *counterirritant* [methyl salicylate; oil of camphor; capsicum oleoresin; turpentine oil; oil of pine]

Slo-bid Gyrocaps (extended-release capsules) ℞ *antiasthmatic; bronchodilator* [theophylline] 50, 75, 100, 125, 200, 300 mg

Slocaps (trademarked form) *sustained-release capsules*

Slo-Niacin controlled-release tablets OTC *nutritional supplement* [niacin] 250, 500, 750 mg

Slo-phyllin tablets, syrup, Gyrocaps (extended-release capsules) ℞ *antiasthmatic; bronchodilator* [theophylline] 100, 200 mg; 80 mg/15 mL; 60, 125, 250 mg

Slo-phyllin GG capsules, syrup ℞ *antiasthmatic; bronchodilator; expectorant* [theophylline; guaifenesin] 150•90 mg; 150•90 mg/15 mL

Slo-Salt slow-release tablets (discontinued 1993) OTC *sodium chloride replacement; dehydration preventative* [sodium chloride] 600 mg

Slo-Salt-K slow-release tablets OTC *sodium chloride/potassium replacement;*

dehydration preventative [sodium chloride; potassium chloride] 410•150 mg

Slow Fe slow-release tablets OTC *hematinic* [ferrous sulfate, dried] 160 mg

Slow Fe with Folic Acid slow-release tablets OTC *hematinic* [ferrous sulfate; folic acid] 50•0.4 mg

Slow-K controlled-release tablets ℞ *potassium supplement* [potassium chloride] 600 mg (8 mEq)

Slow-Mag delayed-release enteric-coated tablets OTC *magnesium supplement* [magnesium chloride] 535 mg

SLT hair lotion OTC *antiseborrheic; antipsoriatic; keratolytic; antiseptic* [coal tar; salicylic acid; lactic acid; alcohol 65%] 2%•3%•5%

Slyn-LL sustained-release capsules (discontinued 1993) ℞ *anorexiant* [phendimetrazine tartrate] 105 mg

SMA Iron Fortified liquid, powder (discontinued 1996) OTC *total or supplementary infant feeding*

SMA Lo-Iron liquid, powder (discontinued 1996) OTC *total or supplementary infant feeding*

SMA with Whey liquid (discontinued 1994) OTC *total or supplementary infant feeding* [whey protein formula]

smallpox vaccine USP *active immunizing agent*

SMF (streptozocin, mitomycin, fluorouracil) *chemotherapy protocol*

SMX; SMZ (sulfamethoxazole) [q.v.]

SMZ-TMP (sulfamethoxazole & trimethoprim) [q.v.]

SN (streptonigrin) [q.v.]

snakebite antivenin [see: antivenin, Crotalidae & Micrurus fulvius]

Snaplets-D granules (discontinued 1995) OTC *pediatric decongestant and antihistamine* [phenylpropanolamine HCl; chlorpheniramine maleate] 6.25•1 mg/packet

Snaplets-DM granules OTC *pediatric antitussive and decongestant* [dextromethorphan hydrobromide; phenylpropanolamine HCl] 5•6.25 mg/packet

Snaplets-EX granules OTC *pediatric decongestant and expectorant* [phenylpropanolamine HCl; guaifenesin] 6.25•50 mg/packet

Snaplets-FR granules OTC *analgesic; antipyretic* [acetaminophen] 80 mg/packet

Snaplets-Multi granules OTC *pediatric antitussive, decongestant, and antihistamine* [dextromethorphan hydrobromide; phenylpropanolamine HCl; chlorpheniramine maleate] 5•6.25•1 mg/packet

SnapTab (trademarked dosage form) *scored tablet*

Sno-Strips ophthalmic strips OTC *diagnostic tear flow test aid*

SNX-111 *investigational calcium-channel blocker for neurologic disorders*

Soac-Lens solution OTC *wetting/soaking solution for hard contact lenses*

Soakare solution (discontinued 1992) OTC *storage/soaking solution for hard contact lenses*

soap, green USP *detergent*

SOD (superoxide dismutase) [see: orgotein]

soda lime NF *carbon dioxide absorbent*

Soda Mint tablets OTC *antacid* [sodium bicarbonate]

sodium *element (Na)*

sodium acetate USP *dialysis aid; electrolyte replenisher; pH buffer* 2, 4 mEq/mL (16.4%, 32.8%) injection

sodium acetate trihydrate [see: sodium acetate]

sodium acetrizoate INN, BAN [also: acetrizoate sodium]

sodium acetylsalicylate *analgesic*

sodium acid phosphate *urinary acidifier*

sodium acid pyrophosphate *urinary acidifier*

sodium alginate NF *suspending agent*

sodium amidotrizoate INN *radiopaque medium* [also: diatrizoate sodium; sodium diatrizoate]

sodium aminobenzoate [see: aminobenzoate sodium]

sodium amylopectin sulfate [see: sodium amylosulfate]

sodium amylosulfate USAN *enzyme inhibitor*

sodium anoxynaphthonate BAN *blood volume and cardiac output test* [also: anazolene sodium]

sodium antimony gluconate [see: sodium stibogluconate]

sodium antimonylgluconate BAN

sodium apolate INN, BAN *anticoagulant* [also: lyapolate sodium]

sodium arsenate, exsiccated NF

sodium arsenate As 74 USAN *radioactive agent*

sodium ascorbate USP, INN *vitamin C; antiscorbutic* 500 mg oral; 1800 mg/½ tsp. oral; 222, 500 mg/mL injection

sodium aurothiomalate INN *antirheumatic* [also: gold sodium thiomalate]

sodium aurotiosulfate INN [also: gold sodium thiosulfate]

sodium azodisalicylate [now: olsalazine sodium]

sodium benzoate USAN, NF, JAN *antihyperammonemic; antifungal agent; preservative*

sodium benzoate and sodium phenylacetate (*orphan: urea cycle disorders*)

sodium benzyl penicillin [see: penicillin G sodium]

sodium bicarbonate USP *electrolyte replenisher; systemic alkalizer; antacid* 325, 600, 650 mg oral; 0.5, 0.6, 0.9, 1 mEq/mL (4.2%, 5%, 7.5%, 8.4%) injection

sodium biphosphate *urinary acidifier; pH buffer*

sodium bisulfite NF *antioxidant*

sodium bitionolate INN *topical antiinfective* [also: bithionolate sodium]

sodium borate NF *alkalizing agent; antipruritic*

sodium borocaptate (^{10}B) INN *antineoplastic; radioactive agent* [also: borocaptate sodium B 10]

sodium cacodylate NF

sodium calcium edetate INN *heavy metal chelating agent* [also: edetate calcium disodium; sodium calciumedetate; calcium disodium edetate]

sodium calciumedetate BAN *heavy metal chelating agent* [also: edetate calcium disodium; sodium calcium edetate; calcium disodium edetate]

sodium caprylate *antifungal*

sodium carbonate NF *alkalizing agent*

sodium chloride (NaCl) USP *ophthalmic hypertonic; electrolyte replacement; abortifacient* [sterile isotonic solution] 650, 1000, 2250 mg oral; 0.45%, 0.9%, 3%, 5%, 14.6%, 23.4% injection

0.45% sodium chloride (½ normal saline; ½ NS) *electrolyte replacement*

0.9% sodium chloride (normal saline; NS) *electrolyte replacement* [also: saline solution]

sodium chloride, compound solution of INN *fluid and electrolyte replenisher* [also: Ringer's injection]

sodium chloride Na 22 USAN *radioactive agent*

sodium chondroitin sulfate [see: chondroitin sulfate sodium]

sodium chromate (^{51}Cr) INN *blood volume test; radioactive agent* [also: sodium chromate Cr 51]

sodium chromate Cr 51 USAN *blood volume test; radioactive agent* [also: sodium chromate (^{51}Cr)]

sodium citrate USP *systemic alkalizer; pH buffer; antacid*

sodium colistin methanesulfonate [see: colistimethate sodium]

sodium cyclamate NF, INN

sodium cyclohexanesulfamate [see: sodium cyclamate]

sodium dehydroacetate NF *antimicrobial preservative*

sodium dehydrocholate INN [also: dehydrocholate sodium]

sodium denyl [see: phenytoin sodium]

sodium diatrizoate BAN *radiopaque medium* [also: diatrizoate sodium; sodium amidotrizoate]

sodium dibunate INN, BAN

sodium dicloroacetate (*orphan: lactic acidosis; homozygous hypercholesterolemia*)

sodium diethyldithiocarbamate [see: ditiocarb sodium]

sodium diiodomethanesulfonate [see: dimethiodal sodium]

sodium dioctyl sulfosuccinate INN *stool softener; surfactant* [also: docusate sodium]

sodium diphenylhydantoin [see: phenytoin sodium]
sodium diprotrizoate INN, BAN [also: diprotrizoate sodium]
Sodium Diuril powder for IV injection ℞ *diuretic* [chlorothiazide] 500 mg
Sodium Edecrin powder for IV injection ℞ *loop diuretic* [ethacrynate sodium]
sodium edetate [see: edetate sodium]
sodium etasulfate INN *detergent* [also: sodium ethasulfate]
sodium ethasulfate USAN *detergent* [also: sodium etasulfate]
sodium feredetate INN [also: sodium ironedetate]
sodium fluoride USP *dental caries preventative* 1.1, 2.2 mg oral; 0.125 mg/drop oral
sodium fluoride F 18 USP
sodium fluoride & phosphoric acid USP *dental caries prophylactic*
sodium formaldehyde sulfoxylate NF *preservative*
sodium gammahydroxyburate [see: sodium oxybate]
sodium gentisate INN
sodium glucaspaldrate INN, BAN
sodium gluconate USP *electrolyte replenisher*
sodium glucosulfone USP
sodium glutamate
sodium glycerophosphate NF
sodium glycocholate [see: bile salts]
sodium gualenate INN [also: azulene sulfonate sodium]
sodium hyaluronate [see: hyaluronate sodium]
sodium hydroxide NF *alkalizing agent*
sodium hydroxybenzenesulfonate [see: phenolsulphonate sodium]
sodium 4-hydroxybutyrate [see: sodium oxybate]
sodium hypochlorite USP, JAN *disinfectant; bleach; used for utensils and equipment*
sodium hypochlorite, diluted NF [also: antiformin, dental]
sodium hypophosphite NF
sodium iodide USP *dietary iodine supplement*

sodium iodide (^{125}I) INN *thyroid function test; radioactive agent* [also: sodium iodide I 125]
sodium iodide I 123 USP *thyroid function test; radioactive agent* 3.7, 7.4 MBq oral
sodium iodide I 125 USAN, USP *thyroid function test; radioactive agent* [also: sodium iodide (^{125}I)]
sodium iodide I 131 USAN, USP *antineoplastic for thyroid carcinoma; radioactive agent for hyperthyroidism* 0.75–100 mCi, 3.5–150 mCi oral
sodium iodohippurate (^{131}I) INN *renal function test; radioactive agent* [also: iodohippurate sodium I 131]
sodium iodomethanesulfonate [see: methiodal sodium]
sodium iopodate INN, BAN *radiopaque medium* [also: ipodate sodium]
sodium iotalamate (^{125}I) INN *radioactive agent* [also: iothalamate sodium I 125]
sodium iotalamate (^{131}I) INN *radioactive agent* [also: iothalamate sodium I 131]
sodium iothalamate BAN *radiopaque medium* [also: iothalamate sodium]
sodium ioxaglate BAN *radiopaque medium* [also: ioxaglate sodium]
sodium ironedetate BAN [also: sodium feredetate]
sodium lactate (SL) USP *electrolyte replenisher* 167 mEq/L (1/6 molar) injection
sodium lactate, compound solution of INN *electrolyte and fluid replenisher; systemic alkalizer* [also: Ringer's injection, lactated]
sodium lauryl sulfate NF *surfactant/wetting agent* [also: laurilsulfate]
sodium lignosulfonate [see: polignate sodium]
sodium metabisulfite NF *antioxidant*
sodium metrizoate INN *radiopaque medium* [also: metrizoate sodium]
sodium monododecyl sulfate [see: sodium lauryl sulfate]
sodium monofluorophosphate USP *dental caries prophylactic*
sodium morrhuate INN *sclerosing agent* [also: morrhuate sodium]

sodium nitrite USP *antidote to cyanide poisoning*

sodium nitroferricyanide [see: sodium nitroprusside]

sodium nitroferricyanide dihydrate [see: sodium nitroprusside]

sodium nitroprusside USP *emergency antihypertensive* 50 mg/dose injection

sodium noramidopyrine methanesulfonate [see: dipyrone]

sodium oxybate USAN *adjunct to anesthesia (orphan: narcolepsy; cataplexy; sleep paralysis; hypnagogic hallucinations)*

sodium oxychlorosene [see: oxychlorosene sodium]

sodium paratoluenesulfan chloramide [see: chloramine-T]

Sodium P.A.S. tablets ℞ *tuberculostatic* [aminosalicylate sodium] 500 mg

sodium penicillin G [see: penicillin G sodium]

sodium pentosan polysulfate [see: pentosan polysulfate sodium]

sodium perborate *topical antiseptic/germicidal*

sodium perborate monohydrate USAN

sodium pertechnetate Tc 99m USAN, USP *radioactive agent*

sodium phenolate [see: phenolate sodium]

sodium phenylacetate USAN *antihyperammonemic*

sodium phenylbutyrate USAN *antihyperammonemic for urea cycle disorders (orphan)*

sodium phosphate (^{32}P) INN *antineoplastic; antipolycythemic; neoplasm test* [also: sodium phosphate P 32]

sodium phosphate, dibasic USP *saline laxative; phosphorus replacement; pH buffer*

sodium phosphate, monobasic USP *phosphorus replacement; pH buffer*

sodium phosphate P 32 USAN, USP *antipolycythemic; antineoplastic for various leukemias and skeletal metastases* [also: sodium phosphate (^{32}P)] 0.67 mCi/mL

sodium picofosfate INN

sodium picosulfate INN

sodium polyphosphate USAN *pharmaceutic aid*

sodium polystyrene sulfonate USP *potassium-removing ion-exchange resin* 15 g/60 mL oral

sodium propionate NF *preservative; antifungal*

sodium propionate hydrate [see: sodium propionate]

sodium 2-propylvalerate [see: valproate sodium]

sodium psylliate NF

sodium pyrophosphate USAN *pharmaceutic aid*

sodium radiochromate [see: sodium chromate Cr 51]

sodium rhodanate [see: thiocyanate sodium]

sodium salicylate (SS) USP *analgesic; antipyretic; anti-inflammatory; antirheumatic* 325, 650 mg oral

sodium starch glycolate NF *tablet excipient*

sodium stearate NF *emulsifying and stiffening agent*

sodium stearyl fumarate NF *tablet and capsule lubricant*

sodium stibocaptate INN [also: stibocaptate]

sodium stibogluconate INN, BAN, DCF *investigational anti-infective for leishmaniasis*

Sodium Sulamyd eye drops, ophthalmic ointment ℞ *ophthalmic bacteriostatic* [sulfacetamide sodium] 10%, 30%; 10%

sodium sulfacetamide [see: sulfacetamide sodium]

sodium sulfate USP *calcium regulator*

sodium sulfate S 35 USAN *radioactive agent*

sodium sulfocyanate [see: thiocyanate sodium]

sodium taurocholate [see: bile salts]

sodium tetradecyl (STD) sulfate INN *sclerosing agent; (orphan: bleeding esophageal varices)*

sodium thiomalate, gold [see: gold sodium thiomalate]

sodium thiosalicylate *analgesic; antipyretic; anti-inflammatory; antirheumatic* 50 mg/mL injection

sodium thiosulfate USP *antidote to cyanide poisoning; antiseptic; antifungal* 25% (250 mg/mL) IV injection

sodium thiosulfate, gold [see: gold sodium thiosulfate]

sodium timerfonate INN *topical anti-infective* [also: thimerfonate sodium]

sodium trimetaphosphate USAN *pharmaceutic aid*

sodium tyropanoate INN *cholecystographic radiopaque medium* [also: tyropanoate sodium]

sodium valproate [see: valproate sodium]

Sodol tablets ℞ *skeletal muscle relaxant* [carisoprodol]

Sodol Compound tablets ℞ *skeletal muscle relaxant; analgesic* [carisoprodol; aspirin] 200•325 mg

sofalcone INN

Sofarin tablets (discontinued 1995) ℞ *anticoagulant* [warfarin sodium] 2, 2.5, 5 mg

Sofenol 5 lotion OTC *moisturizer; emollient*

Sof/Pro-Clean; Sof/Pro-Clean (s.a.) solution (discontinued 1995) OTC *surfactant cleaning solution for soft contact lenses*

Soft Mate Comfort Drops for Sensitive Eyes OTC *rewetting solution for soft contact lenses*

Soft Mate Consept solution + aerosol spray OTC *two-step chemical disinfecting system for soft contact lenses* [hydrogen peroxide based] 3%

Soft Mate Daily Cleaning for Sensitive Eyes solution (discontinued 1995) OTC *surfactant cleaning solution for soft contact lenses*

Soft Mate Disinfecting for Sensitive Eyes solution OTC *chemical disinfecting solution for soft contact lenses*

Soft Mate Enzyme Plus Cleaner tablets (discontinued 1995) OTC *enzymatic cleaner for soft contact lenses*

Soft Mate Hands Off Daily Cleaner solution OTC *surfactant cleaning solution for soft contact lenses*

Soft Mate Lens Drops (discontinued 1992) OTC *rewetting solution for soft contact lenses*

Soft Mate Protein Remover solution (discontinued 1993) OTC *surfactant cleaning solution for soft contact lenses*

Soft Mate Saline for Sensitive Eyes solution (discontinued 1995) OTC *rinsing/storage solution for soft contact lenses* [preserved saline solution]

Soft Mate Saline Preservative-Free solution (discontinued 1992) OTC *rinsing/storage solution for soft contact lenses* [saline solution]

Soft Rinse 135 tablets (discontinued 1993) OTC *rinsing/storage solution for soft contact lenses* [sodium chloride for normal saline solution] 135 mg

Soft Rinse 250 tablets (discontinued 1995) OTC *rinsing/storage solution for soft contact lenses* [sodium chloride for normal saline solution] 250 mg

Soft Sense lotion OTC *moisturizer; emollient*

Softabs (trademarked dosage form) *chewable tablets*

softgels (dosage form) *soft gelatin capsules*

Soft-Stress capsules (discontinued 1995) OTC *vitamin/mineral/calcium/iron supplement* [multiple vitamins & minerals; calcium; iron; folic acid; biotin] ≛•50•4.5•0.05•≟ mg

SoftWear solution OTC *rinsing/storage solution for soft contact lenses* [preserved saline solution]

sol particle immunoassay (SPIA) *detects hCG in urine for pregnancy testing*

solapsone BAN [also: solasulfone]

Solaquin cream OTC *hyperpigmentation bleaching agent in a sunscreen base* [hydroquinone] 2%

Solaquin Forte cream, gel ℞ *hyperpigmentation bleaching agent; sunscreen* [hydroquinone; ethyl dihydroxypropyl PABA; dioxybenzone; oxybenzone] 4%•5%•3%•2%

Solarcaine aerosol spray, lotion OTC *topical local anesthetic; antiseptic* [benzocaine; triclosan] 20%•0.13%

Solarcaine cream (name changed to Solarcaine Aloe Extra Burn Relief in 1995)

Solarcaine Aloe Extra Burn Relief spray, gel, cream OTC *topical local anesthetic* [lidocaine] 0.5%

solasulfone INN [also: solapsone]

Solatene capsules (discontinued 1996) ℞ *to reduce photosensitivity reaction* [beta-carotene] 30 mg

Solfoton tablets, capsules ℞ *long-acting barbiturate sedative, hypnotic and anticonvulsant* [phenobarbital] 16 mg

Solganal IM injection ℞ *antirheumatic* [aurothioglucose] 50 mg/mL

solpecainol INN

Soltice Quick-Rub OTC *counterirritant* [methyl salicylate; camphor; menthol; eucalyptus oil]

soluble ferric pyrophosphate [see: ferric pyrophosphate, soluble]

soluble gelatin (SG) [see: gelatin]

Soluble T4 ℞ (orphan: AIDS) [CD4, human truncated 369 AA polypeptide]

Solu-Cortef powder for IV or IM injection ℞ *glucocorticoids* [hydrocortisone sodium succinate] 100, 250, 500, 1000 mg/vial

Solu-Medrol powder for IV or IM injection ℞ *glucocorticoid; anti-inflammatory; immunosuppressant* [methylprednisolone sodium succinate] 40, 125, 500, 1000, 2000 mg/vial

Solumol OTC *ointment base*

Solurex intra-articular, intralesional, soft tissue, or IM injection ℞ *glucocorticoids* [dexamethasone sodium phosphate] 4 mg/mL

Solurex LA intralesional, intra-articular, soft tissue, or IM injection ℞ *glucocorticoids* [dexamethasone acetate] 8 mg/mL

Soluspan (trademarked form) *injectable suspension*

Soluvite C.T. chewable tablets ℞ *pediatric vitamin supplement and dental caries preventative* [multiple vitamins; fluoride; folic acid] ±•1•0.3 mg

Soluvite-f drops ℞ *pediatric vitamin supplement and dental caries preventative* [vitamins A, C, and D; fluoride] 1500 IU•35 mg•400 IU•0.25 mg per 0.6 mL

Solvent-G OTC *liquid base*

Solvet (trademarked dosage form) *soluble tablet*

solypertine INN *antiadrenergic* [also: solypertine tartrate]

solypertine tartrate USAN *antiadrenergic* [also: solypertine]

Soma tablets ℞ *skeletal muscle relaxant* [carisoprodol] 350 mg

Soma Compound tablets ℞ *skeletal muscle relaxant; analgesic* [carisoprodol; aspirin] 200•325 mg

Soma Compound with Codeine tablets ℞ *skeletal muscle relaxant; analgesic* [carisoprodol; aspirin; codeine phosphate] 200•325•16 mg

Somagard ℞ *investigational LHRH agonist (orphan: central precocious puberty)* [deslorelin]

somagrebove USAN *veterinary galactopoietic agent*

somalapor USAN, INN, BAN *porcine growth hormone*

somantadine INN *antiviral* [also: somantadine HCl]

somantadine HCl USAN *antiviral* [also: somantadine]

somatomedin-C [see: insulin-like growth factor-1]

somatorelin INN *growth hormone-releasing factor (GH-RF)*

somatostatin (SS) INN, BAN *growth hormone-release inhibiting factor (orphan: cutaneous gastrointestinal fistulas)*

somatotropin, human [see: somatropin]

Somatrel ℞ (orphan: diagnostic aid for pituitary release of growth hormone) [NG-29 (code name—generic name not yet approved)]

somatrem USAN, INN, BAN *human growth hormone; (orphan: Turner syndrome; growth delay)*

somatropin USAN, INN, BAN, JAN *growth hormone; (orphan: Turner syndrome; growth delay; severe burns; anovulation; AIDS)* [also: human growth hormone]

somavubove USAN, INN *veterinary galactopoietic agent*

somenopor USAN *porcine growth hormone*

sometribove USAN, INN, BAN *veterinary growth stimulant*

sometripor USAN, INN, BAN *veterinary growth stimulant*

somfasepor USAN *veterinary growth stimulant*

somidobove USAN, INN *synthetic bovine growth hormone*

Sominex tablets, caplets OTC *antihistaminic sleep aid* [diphenhydramine HCl] 25 mg; 50 mg

Sominex 2 tablets (name changed to Sominex in 1993)

Sominex Pain Relief tablets OTC *antihistaminic sleep aid; analgesic* [diphenhydramine HCl; acetaminophen] 25•500 mg

SonoRx ℞ *investigational ultrasound contrast agent* [cellulose]

Soothaderm lotion OTC *topical anesthetic; topical antihistamine; emollient* [pyrilamine maleate; benzocaine; zinc oxide] 2.07•2.08•41.35 mg/mL

Soothe eye drops (discontinued 1995) OTC *topical ocular decongestant/vasoconstrictor* [tetrahydrozoline HCl] 0.05%

Soothers Throat Drops lozenges (discontinued 1995) OTC *topical antipruritic/counterirritant; mild local anesthetic* [menthol] 2 mg

sopecainol [see: solpecainol]

sopitazine INN

Soprodol tablets (discontinued 1993) ℞ *skeletal muscle relaxant* [carisoprodol]

sopromidine INN

Soquette solution (discontinued 1992) OTC *storage/soaking solution for hard contact lenses*

soquinolol INN

sorbic acid NF *antimicrobial agent; preservative*

sorbide nitrate [see: isosorbide dinitrate]

sorbimacrogol laurate 300 [see: polysorbate 20]

sorbimacrogol oleate 300 [see: polysorbate 80]

sorbimacrogol palmitate 300 [see: polysorbate 40]

sorbimacrogol stearate [see: polysorbate 60]

sorbimacrogol tristearate 300 [see: polysorbate 65]

sorbinicate INN

sorbinil USAN, INN, BAN *aldose reductase enzyme inhibitor*

sorbitan laurate INN *surfactant* [also: sorbitan monolaurate]

sorbitan monolaurate USAN, NF *surfactant* [also: sorbitan laurate]

sorbitan monooleate USAN, NF *surfactant* [also: sorbitan oleate]

sorbitan monopalmitate USAN, NF *surfactant* [also: sorbitan palmitate]

sorbitan monostearate USAN, NF *surfactant* [also: sorbitan stearate]

sorbitan oleate INN *surfactant* [also: sorbitan monooleate]

sorbitan palmitate INN *surfactant* [also: sorbitan monopalmitate]

sorbitan sesquioleate USAN, INN *surfactant*

sorbitan stearate INN *surfactant* [also: sorbitan monostearate]

sorbitan trioleate USAN, INN *surfactant*

sorbitan tristearate USAN, INN *surfactant*

Sorbi-Tinic-F liquid (discontinued 1992) ℞ *vitamin supplement* [multiple B vitamins; lysine HCl]

sorbitol NF *flavoring agent; tablet excipient; urologic irrigant* 3%, 3.3%

sorbitol (solution) USP *flavoring agent; tablet excipient*

Sorbitrate tablets, sublingual tablets, chewable tablets ℞ *antianginal* [isosorbide dinitrate] 5, 10, 20, 30, 40 mg; 2.5, 5 mg; 5, 10 mg

Sorbitrate SA sustained-action tablets (discontinued 1995) ℞ *antianginal* [isosorbide dinitrate]

Sorbsan pads, wound packing ℞ *wound dressing* [calcium alginate fiber]

Soretts lozenges (discontinued 1993) OTC *topical oral anesthetic; antipruritic/counterirritant* [benzocaine; menthol] 32•0.5 mg

Soriatane capsules (commercially available in Canada) ℞ *investigational antipsoriatic* [acitretin] 10, 25 mg

sorivudine USAN, INN, BAN *antiviral for varicella zoster and herpes zoster in immunocompromised patients*

sornidipine INN

SOSS-10 eye drops (discontinued 1993) ℞ *ophthalmic bacteriostatic* [sodium sulfacetamide]

sotalol INN, BAN *antiadrenergic (β-receptor)* [also: sotalol HCl]

sotalol HCl USAN *antiadrenergic (β-receptor); for ventricular arrhythmias (orphan)* [also: sotalol]

soterenol INN *adrenergic; bronchodilator* [also: soterenol HCl]

soterenol HCl USAN *adrenergic; bronchodilator* [also: soterenol]

Sotradecol IV injection, Dosette (unit-of-use injection) ℞ *sclerosing agent; (orphan: bleeding esophageal varices)* [sodium tetradecyl sulfate] 1%, 3%

Soviet gramicidin [see: gramicidin S]

Soyalac; I-Soyalac liquid, powder OTC *hypoallergenic infant food* [soy protein formula]

soybean oil USP *pharmaceutic necessity*

S/P Cola oral liquid ℞ *glucose tolerance test beverage* [glucose]

spaglumic acid INN

Span C tablets OTC *dietary supplement* [vitamin C; citrus & rose hips bioflavonoids] 200•300 mg

Spancap No. 1 sustained-release capsules ℞ *CNS stimulant* [dextroamphetamine sulfate] 15 mg

Spancaps (dosage form) *timed-release capsules*

Span-FF controlled-release capsules OTC *hematinic* [ferrous fumarate] 325 mg

Spansule (trademarked dosage form) *sustained-release capsule*

sparfloxacin USAN, INN, BAN *antibacterial*

sparfosate sodium USAN *antineoplastic* [also: sparfosic acid]

sparfosic acid INN *antineoplastic* [also: sparfosate sodium]

Sparine tablets, Tubex (cartridge-needle unit for IM injection) ℞ *antipsychotic* [promazine HCl] 25, 50, 100 mg; 50 mg/mL

Sparkles effervescent granules OTC *antacid; aid in endoscopic examination* [sodium bicarbonate; citric acid; simethicone] 2000•1500•≟ mg/dose

sparsomycin USAN, INN *antineoplastic*

sparteine INN *oxytocic* [also: sparteine sulfate]

sparteine sulfate USAN *oxytocic* [also: sparteine]

Spasmoject IM injection (discontinued 1996) ℞ *gastrointestinal antispasmodic* [dicyclomine HCl] 10 mg/mL

Spasmolin capsules (discontinued 1995) ℞ *GI anticholinergic; sedative* [atropine sulfate; scopolamine hydrobromide; hyoscyamine hydrobromide; phenobarbital] 0.0194•0.0065•0.1037•16.2 mg

Spasmolin tablets ℞ *GI anticholinergic; sedative* [atropine sulfate; scopolamine hydrobromide; hyoscyamine hydrobromide; phenobarbital] 0.0194•0.0065•0.1037•16.2 mg

Spasmophen tablets, elixir (discontinued 1995) ℞ *GI anticholinergic; sedative* [atropine sulfate; scopolamine hydrobromide; hyoscyamine hydrobromide; phenobarbital] 0.0194•0.0065•0.1037•15 mg; 0.0194•0.0065•0.1037•16.2 mg/5 mL

Spasquid elixir (discontinued 1995) ℞ *GI anticholinergic; sedative* [atropine sulfate; scopolamine hydrobromide; hyoscyamine hydrobromide; phenobarbital] 0.0194•0.0065•0.1037•16.2 mg/5 mL

Spastosed chewable tablets OTC *antacid* [calcium carbonate; magnesium carbonate]

SPCA (serum prothrombin conversion accelerator) factor [see: factor VII]

spearmint NF

spearmint oil NF

Specifid ℞ *investigational antineoplastic for various B-cell lymphomas (clinical trials discontinued 1994)* [monoclonal antibodies]

Spec-T lozenges OTC *topical oral anesthetic* [benzocaine] 10 mg

Spec-T Sore Throat/Cough Suppressant lozenges OTC *topical oral anesthetic; antitussive* [benzocaine; dextromethorphan hydrobromide] 10•10 mg

Spec-T Sore Throat/Decongestant lozenges OTC *decongestant; topical oral*

anesthetic [phenylpropanolamine HCl; phenylephrine HCl; benzocaine] 10.5•5•10 mg

Spectazole cream ℞ *topical antifungal* [econazole nitrate] 1%

spectinomycin INN *bactericidal antibiotic* [also: spectinomycin HCl]

spectinomycin HCl USAN, USP *bactericidal antibiotic* [also: spectinomycin]

Spectrobid film-coated tablets, powder for oral suspension ℞ *penicillin-type antibiotic* [bacampicillin HCl] 400 mg; 125 mg/5 mL

Spectrocin Plus ointment OTC *topical antibiotic; local anesthetic* [neomycin sulfate; polymyxin B sulfate; bacitracin; lidocaine] 5000 U•3.5 mg•400 U•5 mg per g

Spectro-Jel liquid OTC *soap-free therapeutic skin cleanser*

spenbolic [see: methandriol]

spermaceti, synthetic [see: cetyl esters wax]

Spersadex eye drops (available only in Canada) ℞ *ophthalmic topical corticosteroidal anti-inflammatory* [dexamethasone sodium phosphate] 0.1%

Sperti ointment (discontinued 1992) OTC *treatment for burns, scalds, cuts and abrasions* [live yeast cell derivative; shark liver oil; phenylmercuric nitrate]

Spexil ℞ *investigational broad-spectrum antibiotic for respiratory, gynecologic, and abdominal infections* [trospectomycin]

Spherex ℞ *investigational antineoplastic for liver metastases*

Spherulin intradermal injection ℞ *diagnostic aid for coccidioidomycosis* [coccidioidin] 1:100, 1:10

SPIA (sol particle immunoassay) [q.v.]

spiclamine INN

spiclomazine INN

spider bite antivenin [see: antivenin (Latrodectus mactans)]

Spider-Man Children's Chewable Vitamin Tablets (discontinued 1993) OTC *vitamin supplement* [multiple vitamins; folic acid]

spiperone USAN, INN *antipsychotic*

spiradoline INN *analgesic* [also: spiradoline mesylate]

spiradoline mesylate USAN *analgesic* [also: spiradoline]

spiramide INN

spiramycin USAN, INN, BAN *antibacterial (orphan status withdrawn 1994)* [also: acetylspiramycin]

spirapril INN, BAN *angiotensin-converting enzyme (ACE) inhibitor* [also: spirapril HCl]

spirapril HCl USAN *angiotensin-converting enzyme (ACE) inhibitor* [also: spirapril]

spiraprilat USAN, INN *angiotensin-converting enzyme (ACE) inhibitor*

spirazine INN

spirazine HCl [see: spirazine]

spirendolol INN

spirgetine INN

spirilene INN, BAN

spirit of nitrous ether [see: ethyl nitrite]

Spiro-32 ℞ *investigational antineoplastic for colorectal cancer and rheumatoid arthritis* [spirogermanium]

spirobarbital sodium

spirofylline INN

spirogermanium INN, BAN *antineoplastic* [also: spirogermanium HCl]

spirogermanium HCl USAN *antineoplastic* [also: spirogermanium]

spirohydantoin mustard [now: spiromustine]

spiromustine USAN, INN *antineoplastic*

Spironazide tablets (discontinued 1993) ℞ *diuretic* [spironolactone; hydrochlorothiazide]

spironolactone USP, INN, BAN, JAN *potassium-sparing diuretic; aldosterone antagonist* 25 mg oral

spiroplatin USAN, INN, BAN *antineoplastic*

spirorenone INN

spirotriazine HCl [see: spirazine]

spiroxamide [see: spiroxatrine]

spiroxasone USAN, INN *diuretic*

spiroxatrine INN

spiroxepin INN

Spirozide tablets (discontinued 1994) ℞ *diuretic; antihypertensive* [spironolactone; hydrochlorothiazide] 25•25 mg

spizofurone INN

SPL (staphage lysate) [q.v.]
SPL-Serologic types I and III solution for subcu injection, nasal aerosol, nasal drop, oral, or topical irrigation ℞ *staphylococcal or polymicrobial vaccine* [staphage lysate (Staphylococcus aureus; Staphylococcus bacteriophage plaque-forming units)]

Sporanox capsules ℞ *systemic antifungal* [itraconazole] 100 mg

Sporanox oral solution ℞ *investigational (Phase III) systemic antifungal for esophageal and oropharyngeal candidiasis* [itraconazole]

Sporidin-G ℞ *(orphan: treatment of Cryptosporidium parvum infections in immunocompromised patients)* [bovine immunoglobulin concentrate, Cryptosporidium parvum]

Sports Spray OTC *counterirritant; topical antiseptic* [methyl salicylate; menthol; camphor; alcohol 58%] 3.5%•10%•5%

Sportscreme OTC *topical analgesic* [trolamine salicylate] 10%

Sportscreme Ice gel OTC *topical analgesic; counterirritant* [trolamine; menthol] 2•2%

SPPG (sulfated polysaccharide peptidoglycan) [see: tecogalan sodium]

Spray-U-Thin oral spray OTC *diet aid* [phenylpropanolamine HCl] 6.58 mg

Sprinkle Caps (trademarked form) *powder*

sprodiamide USAN *heart and CNS imaging aid for MRI*

SPS oral suspension ℞ *potassium-removing agent for hyperkalemia* [sodium polystyrene sulfonate] 15 g/60 mL

S-P-T "liquid" capsules ℞ *hypothyroidism; thyroid cancer* [pork thyroid, desiccated] 60, 120, 180, 300 mg

squalane NF *oleaginous vehicle*

^{85}**Sr** [see: strontium chloride Sr 85]

^{85}**Sr** [see: strontium nitrate Sr 85]

^{85}**Sr** [see: strontium Sr 85]

SRC Expectorant liquid ℞ *narcotic antitussive; decongestant; expectorant* [hydrocodone bitartrate; pseudoephedrine HCl; guaifenesin; alcohol 12.5%] 5•60•200 mg/5 mL

SRF (skin respiratory factor) [q.v.]
SS (saline solution)
SS (sodium salicylate) [q.v.]
SS (somatostatin) [q.v.]
SSD (silver sulfadiazine) [q.v.]
SSD; SSD AF cream ℞ *broad-spectrum bactericidal for adjunctive burn treatment* [silver sulfadiazine] 10 mg/g

SSKI oral solution ℞ *expectorant* [potassium iodide] 1 g/mL

S.T. 37 solution OTC *topical antiseptic* [hexylresorcinol] 0.1%

S-T Cort cream (discontinued 1992) ℞ *topical corticosteroid* [hydrocortisone]

S-T Cort lotion ℞ *topical corticosteroid* [hydrocortisone] 0.5%

S-T Forte syrup, liquid ℞ *narcotic antitussive; decongestant; antihistamine; expectorant* [hydrocodone bitartrate; phenylephrine HCl; phenylpropanolamine HCl; pheniramine maleate; guaifenesin; alcohol 5%] 2.5•5•5•13.33•80 mg/5 mL

S-T Forte 2 liquid ℞ *narcotic antitussive; antihistamine* [hydrocodone bitartrate; chlorpheniramine maleate] 2.5•2 mg/5 mL

St. Joseph Adult Chewable Aspirin chewable tablets OTC *analgesic; antipyretic; anti-inflammatory* [aspirin] 81 mg

St. Joseph Anti-Diarrheal for Children liquid OTC *antidiarrheal; GI adsorbent* [attapulgite]

St. Joseph Aspirin-Free Fever Reducer for Children liquid OTC *analgesic; antipyretic* [acetaminophen] 160 mg/5 mL

St. Joseph Aspirin-Free for Children chewable tablets OTC *analgesic; antipyretic* [acetaminophen] 80 mg

St. Joseph Aspirin-Free Infant Drops OTC *analgesic; antipyretic* [acetaminophen] 100 mg/mL

St. Joseph Cold Tablets for Children chewable tablets OTC *pediatric decongestant and analgesic* [phenylpropanolamine HCl; acetaminophen] 3.125•80 mg

St. Joseph Complete Nighttime Cold Relief, Aspirin Free liquid (discontinued 1993) OTC *pediatric decongestant, antihistamine, antitussive*

and analgesic [pseudoephedrine HCl; chlorpheniramine maleate; dextromethorphan hydrobromide; acetaminophen]

St. Joseph Cough Suppressant syrup OTC *antitussive* [dextromethorphan hydrobromide] 7.5 mg/5 mL

St. Joseph Measured Dose solution (discontinued 1992) OTC *nasal decongestant* [phenylephrine HCl]

ST1-RTA immunotoxin (SR 44163) *(orphan: graft vs. host disease; B-chronic lymphocytic leukemia)*

stable factor [see: factor VII]

Stadol IV or IM injection ℞ *narcotic agonist-antagonist analgesic* [butorphanol tartrate] 1, 2 mg/mL

Stadol NS nasal spray ℞ *narcotic agonist-antagonist analgesic; antimigraine agent* [butorphanol tartrate] 10 mg/mL

Stagesic capsules ℞ *narcotic analgesic* [hydrocodone bitartrate; acetaminophen] 5•500 mg

Stahist sustained-release tablets ℞ *decongestant; antihistamine; anticholinergic* [phenylpropanolamine HCl; phenylephrine HCl; chlorpheniramine maleate; hyoscyamine sulfate; atropine sulfate; scopolamine hydrobromide] 50•25•8•0.19•0.04•0.01 mg

stallimycin INN *antibacterial* [also: stallimycin HCl]

stallimycin HCl USAN *antibacterial* [also: stallimycin]

Stamoist E sustained-release tablets ℞ *decongestant; expectorant* [pseudoephedrine HCl; guaifenesin] 120•500 mg

Stamoist LA sustained-release tablets ℞ *decongestant; expectorant* [phenylpropanolamine HCl; guaifenesin] 75•400 mg

standard VAC *chemotherapy protocol* [see: VAC standard (under VAC)]

Stanford V (mechlorethamine, doxorubicin, vinblastine, vincristine, bleomycin, VePesid, prednisone) *chemotherapy protocol*

stannous chloride USAN *pharmaceutic aid*

stannous fluoride USP *dental caries prophylactic*

stannous pyrophosphate USAN *skeletal imaging aid*

stannous sulfur colloid USAN *bone, liver and spleen imaging aid*

stanolone BAN [also: androstanolone]

stanozolol USAN, USP, INN, BAN *androgen; anabolic steroid*

staphage lysate (SPL) *active bacterin for staphylococcal infections*

Staphcillin powder for IV or IM injection ℞ *bactericidal antibiotic (penicillinase-resistant penicillin)* [methicillin sodium] 1, 4, 6, 10 g

Staphylococcus aureus **vaccine** *investigational anti-infective for renal dialysis patients*

starch NF *dusting powder; pharmaceutic aid*

starch, pregelatinized NF *tablet excipient*

starch, topical USP *dusting powder*

starch carboxymethyl ether, sodium salt [see: sodium starch glycolate]

starch glycerite NF

starch 2-hydroxyethyl ether [see: hetastarch; pentastarch]

Star-Optic eye wash (discontinued 1994) OTC *extraocular irrigating solution* [balanced saline solution]

Star-Otic ear drops OTC *antibacterial/antifungal* [acetic acid; aluminum acetate; boric acid]

Stat-Crit electrode device for professional use *in vitro diagnostic aid for hemoglobin/hematocrit measurement*

Staticin topical solution ℞ *topical antibiotic for acne* [erythromycin] 1.5%

statolon USAN *antiviral* [also: vistatolon]

Stat-One gel OTC *topical antiseptic* [hydrogen peroxide] 3%

Stat-One gel OTC *topical antiseptic* [isopropyl alcohol] 70%

Stat-Pak (trademarked packaging form) *unit-dose package*

Statrol Drop-Tainers (eye drops), ophthalmic ointment (discontinued 1994) ℞ *ophthalmic antibiotic* [polymyxin B sulfate; neomycin sulfate] 16,250 U•3.5 mg per mL; 10,000 U•3.5 mg per g

Statuss Expectorant liquid ℞ *narcotic antitussive; decongestant; expectorant* [codeine phosphate; phenylpropanolamine HCl; guaifenesin; alcohol 5%] 10•12.5•100 mg/5 mL

Statuss Green liquid ℞ *narcotic antitussive; decongestant; antihistamine* [hydrocodone bitartrate; phenylpropanolamine HCl; phenylephrine HCl; pyrilamine maleate; pheniramine maleate; alcohol 5%] 1.67•3.3•5•3.3•3.3 mg/5 mL

stavudine USAN, INN *antiviral for HIV*

Stay Trim gum, mints (discontinued 1995) OTC *diet aid* [phenylpropanolamine HCl] 8.33 mg; 12.5 mg

Stay-Brite solution (discontinued 1993) OTC *cleaning solution for hard contact lenses*

Stay-Wet solution (discontinued 1995) OTC *wetting/rewetting solution for hard contact lenses*

Stay-Wet 3; Stay-Wet 4 solution OTC *disinfecting/wetting/soaking solution for rigid gas permeable contact lenses*

STD (sodium tetradecyl sulfate) [q.v.]

steaglate INN *combining name for radicals or groups*

STEAM (streptonigrin, thioguanine, cyclophosphamide, actinomycin, mitomycin) *chemotherapy protocol*

stearethate 40 [see: polyoxyl 40 stearate]

stearic acid NF *emulsion adjunct; tablet and capsule lubricant*

stearyl alcohol NF *emulsion adjunct*

stearyl dimethyl benzyl ammonium chloride

stearylsulfamide INN

steffimycin USAN, INN *antibacterial; antiviral*

Stelazine film-coated tablets, oral concentrate, IM injection ℞ *antianxiety; antipsychotic* [trifluoperazine HCl] 1, 2, 5, 10 mg; 10 mg/mL; 2 mg/mL

stem cell factor *investigational agent for blood-related disorders*

stenbolone INN *anabolic* [also: stenbolone acetate]

stenbolone acetate USAN *anabolic* [also: stenbolone]

Step 2 creme rinse OTC *for use following a pediculicide shampoo to remove lice eggs from hair*

stepronin INN

Sterapred tablets, Unipak (dispensing pack) (discontinued 1996) ℞ *glucocorticoid* [prednisone] 5 mg

Sterapred DS tablets, Unipak (dispensing pack) ℞ *glucocorticoid* [prednisone] 10 mg

stercuronium iodide INN

Sterecyt ℞ *investigational antineoplastic for leukemia; (orphan: malignant non-Hodgkin's lymphomas)* [prednimustine]

Steri-Dose (trademarked delivery system) *prefilled disposable syringe*

Sterile Lens Lubricant solution (discontinued 1993) OTC *rewetting solution for soft contact lenses*

SteriNail solution OTC *topical antifungal* [undecylenic acid; tolnaftate] 2•2

Steri-Vial (trademarked packaging form) *ampule*

stevaladil INN

stibamine glucoside INN, BAN

stibocaptate BAN [also: sodium stibocaptate]

stibophen NF

stibosamine INN

stilbamidine isethionate [see: stilbamidine isetionate]

stilbamidine isetionate INN

stilbazium iodide USAN, INN *anthelmintic*

stilbestroform [see: diethylstilbestrol]

stilbestrol [see: diethylstilbestrol] ⑨ Stilphostrol

stilbestronate [see: diethylstilbestrol dipropionate]

stilboestroform [see: diethylstilbestrol]

stilboestrol BAN *estrogen* [also: diethylstilbestrol]

stilboestrol DP [see: diethylstilbestrol dipropionate]

Stilnoct; Stilnox (European name for U.S. product Ambien)

stilonium iodide USAN, INN *antispasmodic*

Stilphostrol tablets, IV injection ℞ *antineoplastic for prostatic carcinoma* [diethylstilbestrol diphosphate] 50 mg; 250 mg ⑨ Disophrol; stilbestrol

stilronate [see: diethylstilbestrol dipropionate]

Stimate nasal spray ℞ *pituitary antidiuretic hormone for hemophilia A and von Willebrand's disease (orphan)* [desmopressin acetate] 150 μg/dose

Stimulon QS-21 ℞ *investigational (Phase I/II) immune system stimulant for vaccines*

Stimurub cream (discontinued 1992) OTC *topical anesthetic; counterirritant; anti-inflammatory; vasodilator* [methyl salicylate; menthol; capsicum oleoresin]

Sting-Eze concentrate OTC *topical antihistamine; antipruritic; anesthetic; bacteriostatic* [diphenhydramine HCl; camphor; phenol; benzocaine; eucalyptol]

Stinging Insect Antigen No. 108 subcu or IM injection (discontinued 1993) ℞ *venom sensitivity testing (subcu); venom desensitization therapy (IM)* [bumblebee, honeybee, wasp, hornet, and yellow jacket antigen extracts]

Sting-Kill swabs OTC *topical local anesthetic* [benzocaine; menthol] 20%•1%

stirimazole INN, BAN

stiripentol USAN, INN *anticonvulsant*

stirocainide INN

stirofos USAN *veterinary insecticide*

Stoko Gard cream OTC *topical protection from the effects of poison ivy*

Stop gel ℞ *topical dental caries preventative* [stannous fluoride] 0.4%

storax USP

Storzfen eye drops ℞ *ophthalmic decongestant/vasoconstrictor; mydriatic* [phenylephrine HCl] 2.5%

Storzine 2 eye drops ℞ *antiglaucoma agent; direct-acting miotic* [pilocarpine HCl] 2%

Storz-N-D eye drops ℞ *topical ophthalmic corticosteroidal anti-inflammatory; antibiotic* [dexamethasone sodium phosphate; neomycin sulfate] 0.1%•0.35%

Storz-N-P-D eye drop suspension ℞ *topical ophthalmic corticosteroidal anti-inflammatory; antibiotic* [dexamethasone; neomycin sulfate; polymyxin B sulfate] 0.1%•0.35%•10,000 U/mL

Storzolamide tablets (discontinued 1992) ℞ *anticonvulsant; diuretic* [acetazolamide]

Storz-Sulf eye drops ℞ *ophthalmic bacteriostatic* [sulfacetamide sodium] 10%

Stoxil eye drops, ophthalmic ointment (discontinued 1992) ℞ *ophthalmic antiviral* [idoxuridine]

StrapKap (dosage form) *piggyback vials*

Strep Detect slide tests for professional use *in vitro diagnostic aid for streptococcal antigens in throat swabs*

Streptase powder for IV or intracoronary infusion ℞ *thrombolytic enzyme; lysis of thrombi; catheter clearance* [streptokinase] 38,460, 115,380, 230,770 IU/mL ⓥ Streptonase

streptococcus immune globulin, group B (orphan: *neonatal group B streptococcal infection*)

streptodornase (SD) INN, BAN

streptoduocin USP

streptogramin *investigational treatment for iatrogenic infections*

streptokinase (SK) INN *thrombolytic enzyme* ⓥ Streptonase

streptomycin INN, BAN *aminoglycoside bactericidal antibiotic; primary tuberculostatic* [also: streptomycin sulfate]

streptomycin sulfate USP *aminoglycoside bactericidal antibiotic; primary tuberculostatic* [also: streptomycin] 400 mg/mL injection

Streptonase-B test kit for professional use *in vitro diagnostic test for DNAse-B streptococcal antigens in serum* ⓥ Streptase; streptokinase

streptoniazid INN *antibacterial* [also: streptonicozid]

streptonicozid USAN *antibacterial* [also: streptoniazid]

streptonigrin (SN) USAN *antineoplastic* [also: rufocromomycin]

Strepto-Sec slide test for professional use (discontinued 1991) *in vitro diagnostic test for streptococcal antigens*

streptovarycin INN

streptozocin USAN, INN *antibiotic antineoplastic*

streptozotocin [see: streptozocin]

Streptozyme slide tests for professional use *in vitro diagnostic test for streptococcal extracellular antigens in blood, plasma, and serum*

Stress 600 with Zinc tablets OTC *vitamin/mineral supplement* [multiple vitamins & minerals; folic acid; biotin] ± •400•45 μg

Stress "1000" tablets (discontinued 1993) OTC *vitamin supplement* [multiple vitamins]

Stress B Complex tablets OTC *vitamin/mineral supplement* [multiple vitamins & minerals; folic acid; biotin] ± •400•45 μg

Stress B Complex with Vitamin C timed-release tablets OTC *vitamin/mineral supplement* [multiple B vitamins; vitamin C; zinc] ± •300•15 mg

Stress B with C tablets (discontinued 1995) OTC *vitamin supplement* [multiple B vitamins; vitamin C; folic acid; biotin] ± •250 mg•50 μg•12.5 μg

Stress Formula 500 tablets (discontinued 1993) OTC *vitamin supplement* [multiple vitamins; biotin; folic acid]

Stress Formula 500 Plus Iron tablets (discontinued 1993) OTC *vitamin/iron supplement* [ferrous fumarate; multiple B vitamins; vitamins C and E; folic acid; biotin] 27 mg• ± •500 mg•30 IU•0.4 mg•45 μg

Stress Formula 500 Plus Zinc tablets (discontinued 1993) OTC *vitamin/zinc supplement* [multiple vitamins; zinc; folic acid; biotin]

Stress Formula 600 tablets OTC *vitamin supplement* [multiple vitamins; folic acid; biotin] ± •400•45 μg

Stress Formula 600 plus Iron tablets OTC *antianemic* [ferrous fumarate, dried; vitamins C and E; multiple B vitamins; folic acid]

Stress Formula 600 plus Zinc tablets (discontinued 1993) OTC *vitamin/mineral supplement* [multiple vitamins & minerals; folic acid; biotin]

Stress Formula "605" tablets (discontinued 1995) OTC *vitamin supplement* [multiple vitamins; folic acid; biotin] ± •400•45 μg

Stress Formula "605" with Zinc tablets (discontinued 1995) OTC *vitamin/mineral supplement* [multiple vitamins & minerals; folic acid; biotin] ± •400•45 μg

Stress Formula Vitamins capsules, tablets OTC *vitamin supplement* [multiple vitamins; folic acid; biotin] ± •400•45 μg

Stress Formula with Iron film-coated tablets OTC *vitamin/iron supplement* [multiple B vitamins; vitamins C and E; ferrous fumarate; folic acid; biotin] ± •500 mg•30 IU•27 mg•0.4 mg•45 μg

Stress Formula with Zinc tablets OTC *vitamin/iron supplement* [multiple B vitamins; vitamins C and E; multiple minerals; folic acid; biotin] ± •500 mg•30 IU• ± •0.4 mg•45 μg

Stresscaps capsules (discontinued 1995) OTC *vitamin supplement* [multiple B vitamins; vitamin C] ± •300 mg

StressForm "605" with Iron tablets OTC *vitamin/iron supplement* [multiple B vitamins; vitamins C and E; iron; folic acid; biotin] ± •605 mg•30 IU•27 mg•0.4 mg•45 μg

Stresstabs tablets OTC *vitamin supplement* [multiple vitamins; folic acid; biotin] ± •400•45 μg

Stresstabs 600 with Iron tablets OTC *antianemic* [ferrous fumarate, dried; vitamins E and C; multiple B vitamins; folic acid]

Stresstabs Advanced Formula tablets (name changed to Stresstabs in 1995)

Stresstabs + Iron film-coated tablets OTC *vitamin/iron supplement* [multiple B vitamins; vitamins C and E; ferrous fumarate; folic acid; biotin] ± •500 mg•30 IU•18 mg•0.4 mg•45 μg

Stresstabs + Zinc film-coated tablets OTC *vitamin/mineral supplement* [multiple vitamins & minerals; folic acid; biotin] ± •400•45 μg

Stresstein powder OTC *enteral nutritional therapy for moderate to severe stress or trauma* [branched chain amino acids]

Stri-Dex pads OTC *topical keratolytic cleanser for acne* [salicylic acid; alcohol] 0.5%•28%, 2%•44%, 2%•54%

Stri-Dex Cleansing bar OTC *medicated cleanser for acne* [triclosan] 1%

Stri-Dex Clear gel OTC *topical acne treatment* [salicylic acid; alcohol] 2%•9.3%

Stri-Dex Face Wash solution OTC *antiseptic; disinfectant* [triclosan] 1%

strinoline INN

strong ammonia solution [see: ammonia solution, strong]

Strong Iodine solution, tincture ℞ *thyroid-blocking therapy; topical antimicrobial* [iodine; potassium iodide] 5%•10%; 7%•5%

stronger rose water [see: rose water, stronger]

strontium *element (Sr)*

strontium chloride Sr 85 USAN *radioactive agent*

strontium chloride Sr 89 USAN *radioactive agent; analgesic for metastatic bone pain*

strontium nitrate Sr 85 USAN *radioactive agent*

strontium salicylate NF

strontium Sr 85 USP

Strovite tablets ℞ *vitamin supplement* [multiple B vitamins; vitamin C; folic acid] $\pm$•500•0.5 mg

Strovite Plus caplets ℞ *geriatric vitamin/mineral therapy* [multiple vitamins & minerals; folic acid; biotin] $\pm$•800•150 µg

strychnine NF

strychnine glycerophosphate NF

strychnine nitrate NF

strychnine phosphate NF

strychnine sulfate NF

strychnine valerate NF

Stuart Formula tablets OTC *vitamin/mineral/iron supplement* [multiple vitamins & minerals; iron; folic acid] $\pm$•18•0.1 mg

Stuart Prenatal tablets OTC *vitamin/calcium/iron supplement* [multiple vitamins; calcium; iron; folic acid] $\pm$•200•60•0.8 mg

Stuartinic film-coated tablets (discontinued 1995) OTC *hematinic* [ferrous fumarate; multiple B vitamins; vitamin C] 100•$\pm$•500 mg

Stuartnatal 1 + 1 tablets (name changed to Stuartnatal Plus in 1995)

Stuartnatal Plus tablets ℞ *vitamin/calcium/iron supplement* [multiple vitamins; calcium; iron; folic acid] $\pm$•200•65•1 mg

stugeron [see: cinnarizine]

stutgin [see: cinnarizine]

Stye ophthalmic ointment OTC *emollient* [white petrolatum; mineral oil; boric acid]

Stye ophthalmic ointment (discontinued 1995; replaced by Stye without yellow mercuric oxide) OTC *stye treatment* (*the FDA ruled yellow mercuric oxide "not safe and effective" in 1992*) [yellow mercuric oxide] 1%

Stypto-Caine solution OTC *to stop bleeding of minor cuts* [aluminum chloride; tetracaine HCl; oxyquinoline sulfate] 250•2.5•1 mg/g

styramate INN

styronate resins

subathizone INN

subendazole INN

Sublimaze IV or IM injection ℞ *narcotic analgesic; anesthetic* [fentanyl citrate] 0.05 mg/mL

sublimed sulfur [see: sulfur, sublimed]

Sublingual B Total drops OTC *vitamin supplement* [multiple B vitamins; vitamin C] $\pm$•60 mg/mL

substance F [see: demecolcine]

substance P antagonist *investigational agent for pain, migraine, inflammatory diseases, asthma, and CNS diseases*

Suby's G solution; Suby's solution G (citric acid, magnesium oxide, sodium carbonate) *urologic irrigant to dissolve phosphatic calculi*

succimer USAN, INN, BAN *metal chelating agent; (orphan: lead and mercury poisoning; cysteine kidney stones)*

succinchlorimide NF

succinylcholine chloride USP *neuromuscular blocker; muscle relaxant* [also: suxamethonium chloride]

succinyldapsone [see: succisulfone]

succinylsulfathiazole USP

succisulfone INN

Succus Cineraria Maritima eye drops ℞ *treatment for optic opacity caused by cataract* [aqueous/glycerin solution of senecio compositae, hamamelis water, and boric acid]

suclofenide INN, BAN

Sucostrin IV or IM injection ℞ *neuromuscular blocker* [succinylcholine chloride] 20, 100 mg

sucralfate USAN, INN, BAN *treatment of gastric ulcers; (orphan: oral ulcerations)* 1 g oral

sucralose BAN

sucralox INN, BAN

Sucrasa ℞ *(orphan: congenital sucrase-isomaltase deficiency)* [sucrase]

sucrase *(orphan: congenital sucrase-isomaltase deficiency)*

Sucrets mouthwash/gargle (discontinued 1994) OTC *topical antipruritic/counterirritant; mild local anesthetic* [dyclonine HCl] 0.1%

Sucrets throat spray OTC *topical antipruritic/counterirritant; mild local anesthetic* [dyclonine HCl] 0.1%

Sucrets Children's Sore Throat; Vapor Lemon Sucrets; Sucrets Maximum Strength lozenges OTC *topical antipruritic/counterirritant; mild local anesthetic* [dyclonine HCl] 1.2 mg; 2 mg; 3 mg

Sucrets Cough Control; Sucrets 4-Hour Cough lozenges OTC *antitussive* [dextromethorphan hydrobromide] 5 mg; 15 mg

Sucrets Sore Throat lozenges OTC *oral antiseptic* [hexylresorcinol] 2.4 mg

sucrose NF *flavoring agent; tablet excipient*

sucrose octaacetate NF *alcohol denaturant*

sucrosofate potassium USAN *antiulcerative*

Sudafed tablets OTC *nasal decongestant* [pseudoephedrine HCl] 30, 60 mg

Sudafed, Children's liquid (discontinued 1996) OTC *nasal decongestant* [pseudoephedrine HCl] 30 mg/5 mL

Sudafed 12 Hour Caplets extended-release tablets OTC *nasal decongestant* [pseudoephedrine HCl] 120 mg

Sudafed Cold & Cough liquid caps OTC *antitussive; decongestant; expectorant; analgesic* [dextromethorphan hydrobromide; pseudoephedrine HCl; guaifenesin; acetaminophen] 10•30•100•250 mg

Sudafed Cough syrup (discontinued 1996) OTC *antitussive; decongestant; expectorant* [dextromethorphan hydrobromide; pseudoephedrine HCl; guaifenesin; alcohol 2.4%] 5•15•100 mg/5 mL

Sudafed Plus liquid (discontinued 1996) OTC *decongestant; antihistamine* [pseudoephedrine HCl; chlorpheniramine maleate] 30•2 mg/5 mL

Sudafed Plus tablets OTC *decongestant; antihistamine* [pseudoephedrine HCl; chlorpheniramine maleate] 60•4 mg

Sudafed Severe Cold caplets, tablets OTC *antitussive; decongestant; analgesic* [dextromethorphan hydrobromide; pseudoephedrine HCl; acetaminophen] 15•30•500 mg

Sudafed Sinus tablets, caplets OTC *decongestant; analgesic; antipyretic* [pseudoephedrine HCl; acetaminophen] 30•500 mg

Sudex film-coated sustained-release tablets ℞ *decongestant; expectorant* [pseudoephedrine HCl; guaifenesin] 120•600 mg

Sudex tablets OTC *decongestant* [pseudoephedrine HCl] 30 mg

sudexanox INN

sudismase INN

sudoxicam USAN, INN *anti-inflammatory*

Sudrin tablets (discontinued 1992) OTC *nasal decongestant* [pseudoephedrine HCl]

Sufenta IV injection ℞ *narcotic analgesic; anesthetic* [sufentanil citrate] 50 μg/mL

sufentanil USAN, INN, BAN *analgesic*

sufentanil citrate USAN *narcotic analgesic* 50 μg/mL

sufosfamide INN

sufotidine USAN, INN, BAN *antagonist to histamine H_2 receptors*

sugar, compressible NF *flavoring agent; tablet excipient*

sugar, confectioner's NF *flavoring agent; tablet excipient*

sugar, invert (50% dextrose & 50% fructose) USP *fluid and nutrient replenisher; caloric replacement*

sugar spheres NF *solid carrier vehicle*

Sulamyd [see: Sodium Sulamyd]

Sular extended-release tablets ℞ *calcium channel blocker for hypertension* [nisoldipine] 10, 20, 30, 40 mg

sulazepam USAN, INN *minor tranquilizer*

sulbactam INN, BAN

sulbactam benzathine USAN *β-lactamase inhibitor; penicillin/cephalosporin synergist*

sulbactam pivoxil USAN *β-lactamase inhibitor; penicillin/cephalosporin synergist* [also: pivsulbactam]

sulbactam sodium USAN, USP *β-lactamase inhibitor; penicillin/cephalosporin synergist*

sulbenicillin INN

sulbenox USAN, INN *veterinary growth stimulant*

sulbentine INN

sulbutiamine INN [also: bisibutiamine]

sulclamide INN

sulconazole INN, BAN *antifungal* [also: sulconazole nitrate]

sulconazole nitrate USAN, USP *antifungal* [also: sulconazole]

Suldiazo film-coated tablets (discontinued 1994) ℞ *urinary anti-infective; urinary analgesic* [sulfisoxazole; phenazopyridine HCl] 500•50 mg

sulergine [see: disulergine]

Sulf-10 eye drops ℞ *ophthalmic bacteriostatic* [sulfacetamide sodium] 10% ⓓ Sulten-10

Sulf-15 eye drops (discontinued 1995) ℞ *ophthalmic bacteriostatic* [sulfacetamide sodium] 15%

sulfabenz USAN, INN *antibacterial; coccidiostat for poultry*

sulfabenzamide USAN, USP, INN *bacteriostatic antibiotic*

sulfabromomethazine sodium NF

sulfacarbamide INN [also: sulphaurea]

sulfacecole INN

sulfacetamide USP, INN *bacteriostatic antibiotic*

sulfacetamide sodium USP *bacteriostatic antibiotic* 10%, 30% eye drops

Sulfacet-R lotion ℞ *topical acne treatment* [sulfacetamide sodium; sulfur] 10%•5%

sulfachlorpyridazine INN

sulfachrysoidine INN

sulfacitine INN *antibacterial* [also: sulfacytine]

sulfaclomide INN

sulfaclorazole INN

sulfaclozine INN

sulfacombin [see: sulfadiazine]

sulfacytine USAN *broad-spectrum bacteriostatic* [also: sulfacitine]

sulfadiasulfone sodium INN *antibacterial; leprostatic* [also: acetosulfone sodium]

sulfadiazine USP, INN *broad-spectrum bacteriostatic (orphan: Toxoplasma gondii encephalitis)* 500 mg oral

sulfadiazine silver JAN *broad-spectrum bactericidal; adjunct to burn therapy* [also: silver sulfadiazine]

sulfadiazine sodium USP, INN *antibacterial* [also: sulphadiazine sodium]

sulfadicramide INN

sulfadicrolamide [see: sulfadicramide]

sulfadimethoxine NF [also: sulphadimethoxine]

sulfadimidine INN, BAN *antibacterial* [also: sulfamethazine]

sulfadoxine USAN, USP *bacteriostatic; antimalarial adjunct*

sulfaethidole NF, INN [also: sulphaethidole]

sulfafurazole INN *antibacterial* [also: sulfisoxazole; sulphafurazole]

sulfaguanidine NF, INN

sulfaguanole INN

Sulfa-Gyn vaginal cream (discontinued 1992) ℞ *broad-spectrum bacteriostatic* [sulfathiazole; sulfacetamide; sulfabenzamide; urea]

Sulfair 15 eye drops (discontinued 1992) ℞ *ophthalmic bacteriostatic* [sodium sulfacetamide]

sulfaisodimidine [see: sulfisomidine]

Sulfalax Calcium capsules OTC *stool softener* [docusate calcium] 240 mg

sulfalene USAN, INN *antibacterial* [also: sulfametopyrazine]

sulfaloxic acid INN [also: sulphaloxic acid]

sulfamazone INN
sulfamerazine USP, INN *broad-spectrum bacteriostatic*
sulfamerazine sodium NF, INN
sulfameter USAN *antibacterial* [also: sulfametoxydiazine; sulfamethoxydiazine]
sulfamethazine USP *broad-spectrum bacteriostatic* [also: sulfadimidine]
sulfamethizole USP, INN, JAN *antibacterial* [also: sulphamethizole] ⊘ sulfamethoxazole
Sulfamethoprim IV infusion ℞ *anti-infective; antibacterial* [trimethoprim; sulfamethoxazole] 16•80 mg/mL
sulfamethoxazole (SMX; SMZ) USAN, USP, INN, JAN *broad-spectrum bacteriostatic* [also: sulphamethoxazole; acetylsulfamethoxazole; sulfamethoxazole sodium] 500 mg oral ⊘ sulfamethizole
sulfamethoxazole sodium JAN *broad-spectrum bacteriostatic* [also: sulfamethoxazole; sulphamethoxazole; acetylsulfamethoxazole]
sulfamethoxydiazine BAN *antibacterial* [also: sulfameter; sulfametoxydiazine]
sulfamethoxypyridazine USP, INN [also: sulphamethoxypyridazine]
sulfamethoxypyridazine acetyl
sulfametin [see: sulfameter]
sulfametomidine INN
sulfametopyrazine BAN *antibacterial* [also: sulfalene]
sulfametoxydiazine INN *antibacterial* [also: sulfameter; sulfamethoxydiazine]
sulfametrole INN, BAN
Sulfamide eye drop suspension (discontinued 1993) ℞ *topical ophthalmic corticosteroidal anti-inflammatory; bacteriostatic* [prednisolone acetate; sulfacetamide sodium]
sulfamidothiodiazol [see: glybuzole]
sulfamonomethoxine USAN, INN, BAN *antibacterial*
sulfamoxole USAN, INN *antibacterial* [also: sulphamoxole]
p-**sulfamoylbenzoic acid** [see: carzenide]
4'-sulfamoylsuccinanilic acid [see: sulfasuccinamide]

Sulfamylon cream ℞ *broad-spectrum bacteriostatic* [mafenide acetate] 85 mg/g
Sulfamylon solution ℞ *broad-spectrum bacteriostatic (orphan: meshed autograft loss in burns)* [mafenide acetate]
sulfanilamide NF, INN *bacteriostatic antibiotic* 15% topical
sulfanilanilide [see: sulfabenz]
sulfanilate zinc USAN *antibacterial*
N-sulfanilylacetamide [see: sulfacetamide]
N-sulfanilylacetamide monosodium salt monohydrate [see: sulfacetamide sodium]
N-*p*-sulfanilylphenylglycine sodium [see: acediasulfone sodium]
N-sulfanilylstearamide [see: stearylsulfamide]
4'-sulfanilylsuccinanilic acid [see: succisulfone]
sulfanilylurea [see: sulfacarbamide]
sulfanitran USAN, INN, BAN *antibacterial; coccidiostat for poultry*
sulfaperin INN
sulfaphenazole INN [also: sulphaphenazole]
sulfaphtalythiazol [see: phthalysulfathiazole]
sulfaproxyline INN [also: sulphaproxyline]
sulfapyrazole INN, BAN *antibacterial* [also: sulfazamet]
sulfapyridine USP, INN *dermatitis herpetiformis suppressant (orphan)* [also: sulphapyridine]
sulfapyridine sodium NF
sulfaquinoxaline INN, BAN
sulfarsphenamine NF, INN
sulfasalazine USAN, USP, INN *broad-spectrum bacteriostatic* 500 mg oral
Sulfasim ℞ *investigational (Phase I) immunomodulator for sulfamethoxazole allergy in AIDS patients*
sulfasomizole USAN, INN *antibacterial* [also: sulphasomizole]
sulfastearyl [see: stearylsulfamide]
sulfasuccinamide INN
sulfasymazine INN
sulfated polysaccharide peptidoglycan (SPPG) [see: tecogalan sodium]

sulfathiazole USP, INN *bacteriostatic antibiotic* [also: sulphathiazole] ⑫ sulfisoxazole
sulfathiazole sodium NF
sulfathiocarbamide [see: sulfathiourea]
sulfathiourea INN
sulfatolamide INN
Sulfatrim oral suspension ℞ *anti-infective; antibacterial* [trimethoprim; sulfamethoxazole] 40•200 mg/5 mL ⑫ Sulfa-Trip
Sulfatrim DS tablets ℞ *anti-infective; antibacterial* [sulfamethoxazole; trimethoprim] 160•800 mg
Sulfa-Trip vaginal cream (discontinued 1994) ℞ *broad-spectrum bacteriostatic* [sulfathiazole; sulfacetamide; sulfabenzamide; urea] ⑫ Sulfatrim
sulfatroxazole INN
sulfatrozole INN
sulfazamet USAN *antibacterial* [also: sulfapyrazole]
sulfinalol INN *antihypertensive* [also: sulfinalol HCl]
sulfinalol HCl USAN *antihypertensive* [also: sulfinalol]
sulfinpyrazone USP, INN *uricosuric* [also: sulphinpyrazone] 100, 200 mg oral
sulfiram INN [also: monosulfiram]
sulfisomidine [also: sulphasomidine]
sulfisoxazole USP *broad-spectrum bacteriostatic* [also: sulfafurazole; sulphafurazole] 500 mg oral ⑫ sulfathiazole
sulfisoxazole acetyl USP *broad-spectrum bacteriostatic*
sulfisoxazole diolamine USAN, USP *broad-spectrum bacteriostatic*
Sulfoam shampoo OTC *antiseborrheic; keratolytic* [salicylic acid] 2%
sulfobenzylpenicillin [see: sulbenicillin]
sulfobromophthalein sodium USP *hepatic function test*
sulfobromphthalein sodium [see: sulfobromophthalein sodium]
sulfogaiacol INN *expectorant* [also: potassium guaiacolsulfonate]
Sulfoil liquid OTC *soap-free therapeutic skin cleanser* [sulfonated castor oil]
sulfomyxin USAN, INN *antibacterial* [also: sulphomyxin sodium]
sulfonal [see: sulfonmethane]

sulfonated hydrogenated castor oil [see: hydroxystearin sulfate]
sulfonethylmethane NF
sulfonmethane NF
sulfonterol INN *bronchodilator* [also: sulfonterol HCl]
sulfonterol HCl USAN *bronchodilator* [also: sulfonterol]
Sulforcin lotion OTC *topical acne treatment* [sulfur; resorcinol; alcohol] 5%•2%•11.65%
sulforidazine INN
sulfosalicylic acid
sulfoxone sodium USP *antibacterial; leprostatic* [also: aldesulfone sodium]
Sulfoxyl Regular; Sulfoxyl Strong lotion ℞ *topical keratolytic for acne* [benzoyl peroxide; sulfur] 5%•2%; 10%•5%
sulfur *element (S)* [see: sulfur, precipitated; sulfur, sublimed]
sulfur, precipitated USP *scabicide; topical antibacterial; topical exfoliant*
sulfur, sublimed USP *scabicide; topical antibacterial; topical exfoliant*
sulfur dioxide NF *antioxidant*
Sulfur Soap bar OTC *medicated cleanser for acne* [precipitated sulfur] 10%
sulfurated lime solution [see: lime, sulfurated]
sulfurated potash [see: potash, sulfurated]
sulfuric acid NF *acidifying agent*
sulfuric acid, aluminum ammonium salt, dodecahydrate [see: alum, ammonium]
sulfuric acid, aluminum potassium salt, dodecahydrate [see: alum, potassium]
sulfuric acid, aluminum salt, hydrate [see: aluminum sulfate]
sulfuric acid, barium salt [see: barium sulfate]
sulfuric acid, calcium salt [see: calcium sulfate]
sulfuric acid, copper salt pentahydrate [see: cupric sulfate]
sulfuric acid, disodium salt decahydrate [see: sodium sulfate]
sulfuric acid, magnesium salt [see: magnesium sulfate]

sulfuric acid, manganese salt [see: manganese sulfate]
sulfuric acid, zinc salt hydrate [see: zinc sulfate]
sulfurous acid, monosodium salt [see: sodium bisulfite]
sulglicotide INN [also: sulglycotide]
sulglycotide BAN [also: sulglicotide]
sulicrinat INN
sulindac USAN, USP, INN, BAN *antiarthritic; nonsteroidal anti-inflammatory drug (NSAID); analgesic* 150, 200 mg oral
sulisatin INN
sulisobenzone USAN, INN *ultraviolet screen*
sulmarin USAN, INN *hemostatic*
Sulmasque mask OTC *antibacterial and exfoliant for acne* [sulfur] 6.4%
sulmazole INN
sulmepride INN
sulnidazole USAN, INN *antiprotozoal (Trichomonas)*
sulocarbilate INN
suloctidil USAN, INN, BAN *peripheral vasodilator*
sulodexide INN
sulofenur USAN, INN *antineoplastic*
sulopenem USAN, INN *antibacterial*
sulosemide INN
sulotroban USAN, INN, BAN *treatment for glomerulonephritis*
suloxifen INN *bronchodilator* [also: suloxifen oxalate]
suloxifen oxalate USAN *bronchodilator* [also: suloxifen]
Sulperazon R *investigational antibiotic* [sulbactam; cefoperazone sodium]
sulphabutin [see: busulfan]
sulphadiazine sodium BAN *antibacterial* [also: sulfadiazine sodium]
sulphadimethoxine BAN [also: sulfadimethoxine]
sulphaethidole BAN [also: sulfaethidole]
sulphafurazole BAN *antibacterial* [also: sulfisoxazole; sulfafurazole]
sulphaloxic acid BAN [also: sulfaloxic acid]
sulphamethizole BAN *antibacterial* [also: sulfamethizole]
sulphamethoxazole BAN *broad-spectrum bacteriostatic* [also: sulfamethoxazole; acetylsulfamethoxazole; sulfamethoxazole sodium]
sulphamethoxypyridazine BAN [also: sulfamethoxypyridazine]
sulphamoxole BAN *antibacterial* [also: sulfamoxole]
sulphan blue BAN *lymphangiography aid* [also: isosulfan blue]
sulphaphenazole BAN [also: sulfaphenazole]
sulphaproxyline BAN [also: sulfaproxyline]
sulphapyridine BAN *dermatitis herpetiformis suppressant* [also: sulfapyridine]
sulphasomidine BAN [also: sulfisomidine]
sulphasomizole BAN *antibacterial* [also: sulfasomizole]
sulphathiazole BAN *antibacterial* [also: sulfathiazole]
sulphaurea BAN [also: sulfacarbamide]
sulphinpyrazone BAN *uricosuric* [also: sulfinpyrazone]
sulphocarbolate sodium [see: phenolsulphonate sodium]
Sulpho-Lac cream, soap OTC *antibacterial and exfoliant for acne* [sulfur] 5%
Sulpho-Lac Acne Medication cream OTC *antibacterial; exfoliant* [sulfur; zinc sulfate] 5%•27%
sulphomyxin sodium BAN *antibacterial* [also: sulfomyxin]
sulphonal [see: sulfonmethane]
Sulphrin eye drop suspension (discontinued 1993) R *topical ophthalmic corticosteroidal anti-inflammatory; bacteriostatic* [prednisolone acetate; sulfacetamide sodium] 0.5%•10%
Sulphrin ophthalmic ointment (discontinued 1994) R *topical ophthalmic corticosteroidal anti-inflammatory; bacteriostatic* [prednisolone acetate; sulfacetamide sodium] 0.5%•10%
sulpiride USAN, INN *antidepressant*
Sulpred eye drop suspension R *topical ophthalmic corticosteroidal anti-inflammatory; bacteriostatic* [prednisolone acetate; sodium sulfacetamide]
sulprosal INN
sulprostone USAN, INN *prostaglandin*
Sulster eye drops R *ophthalmic topical corticosteroidal anti-inflammatory; bac-*

teriostatic [prednisolone sodium phosphate; sulfacetamide sodium] 0.25%•1%

sultamicillin USAN, INN, BAN *antibacterial*

Sulten-10 eye drops (discontinued 1992) ℞ *ophthalmic bacteriostatic* [sodium sulfacetamide] ② Sulf-10

sulthiame USAN *anticonvulsant* [also: sultiame]

sultiame INN *anticonvulsant* [also: sulthiame]

sultopride INN

sultosilic acid INN

Sultrin Triple Sulfa vaginal tablets, vaginal cream ℞ *broad-spectrum bacteriostatic* [sulfathiazole; sulfacetamide; sulfabenzamide] 172.5•143.75•184 mg; 3.42%•2.86%•3.7%

sultroponium INN

sulukast USAN, INN *antiasthmatic; leukotriene antagonist*

sulverapride INN

Sumacal powder OTC *carbohydrate caloric supplement* [glucose polymers]

sumacetamol INN, BAN

sumarotene USAN, INN *keratolytic*

sumatriptan INN, BAN *antimigraine; investigational treatment for cluster headache* [also: sumatriptan succinate]

sumatriptan succinate USAN *antimigraine* [also: sumatriptan]

sumetizide INN

Summer's Eve Disposable Douche solution OTC *antifungal; vaginal cleanser and deodorizer; acidity modifier* [sodium benzoate; citric acid]

Summer's Eve Disposable Douche; Summer's Eve Disposable Douche Extra Cleansing solution OTC *vaginal cleanser and deodorizer; acidity modifier* [vinegar (acetic acid)]

Summer's Eve Feminine Bath liquid OTC *for external perivaginal cleansing*

Summer's Eve Feminine Powder OTC *absorbs vaginal moisture* [cornstarch; benzethonium chloride]

Summer's Eve Feminine Wash liquid, wipes OTC *for external perivaginal cleansing*

Summer's Eve Medicated Disposable Douche solution OTC *antiseptic/germicidal; vaginal cleanser and deodorizer* [povidone-iodine] 0.3%

Summer's Eve Post-Menstrual Disposable Douche solution OTC *vaginal cleanser and deodorizer; acidity modifier* [monosodium phosphate; disodium phosphate]

Sumycin syrup ℞ *broad-spectrum antibiotic* [tetracycline HCl] 125 mg/5 mL

Sumycin '250'; Sumycin '500' capsules, tablets ℞ *broad-spectrum antibiotic* [tetracycline HCl] 250 mg; 500 mg

sunagrel INN

suncillin INN *antibacterial* [also: suncillin sodium]

suncillin sodium USAN *antibacterial* [also: suncillin]

SunKist Multivitamins Complete, Children's chewable tablets OTC *vitamin/mineral/iron supplement* [multiple vitamins & minerals; iron; folic acid; biotin] ±•18 mg•400 μg•40 μg

SunKist Multi-Vitamins + Extra C chewable tablets OTC *vitamin supplement* [multiple vitamins; folic acid] ±•0.3 mg

SunKist Multivitamins + Iron, Children's chewable tablets OTC *vitamin/iron supplement* [multiple vitamins; iron; folic acid] ±•15•0.3 mg

SunKist Vitamin C chewable tablets, caplets OTC *vitamin supplement* [ascorbic acid] 60, 250, 500 mg; 500 mg

Sunshine chewable tablets (discontinued 1992) OTC *dietary supplement* [multiple vitamins & minerals; iron; folic acid; biotin]

Supac tablets OTC *analgesic; antipyretic; anti-inflammatory* [acetaminophen; aspirin; caffeine] 160•230•32 mg

Super CalciCaps tablets OTC *dietary supplement* [dibasic calcium phosphate; calcium gluconate; calcium carbonate; vitamin D] 400 mg (Ca)•42 mg (P)•133 IU

Super CalciCaps M-Z tablets OTC *dietary supplement* [vitamins A and D; multiple minerals] 1667 mg•133 IU•±

Super Calcium '1200' softgels OTC *dietary supplement* [calcium; vitamin D] 600 mg•200 IU

Super Citro Cee sustained-release tablets OTC *dietary supplement* [ascorbic acid; lemon & rose hips bioflavonoids; rutin] 500•1000•50 mg

Super Complex C-500 Caplets OTC *dietary supplement* [ascorbic acid; various bioflavonoids; citrus hesperidin; rutin] 500•200•25•50 mg

Super D Perles (capsules) OTC *vitamin supplement* [vitamins A and D] 10,000•400 IU

Super Hi Potency tablets OTC *vitamin/mineral supplement* [multiple vitamins & minerals; folic acid; biotin] ±•0.4 mg•0.075 mg

Super Omega-3 soft capsules OTC *dietary supplement* [eicosapentaenoic acid; docosahexaenoic acid; alpha-linolenic acid]

Super Quints-50 tablets OTC *vitamin supplement* [multiple B vitamins; folic acid; biotin] ±•400•50 µg

Super-1-Daily; Vegetarian Super-1-Daily cellulose-coated caplets OTC *vitamin/mineral supplement* [multiple vitamins & minerals; betaine HCl]

Super-75 cellulose-coated caplets OTC *vitamin/mineral supplement* [multiple vitamins & minerals; bioflavonoids; betaine HCl]

Superdophilus powder OTC *dietary supplement; fever blister treatment; not generally regarded as safe and effective as an antidiarrheal* [Lactobacillus acidophilus] 2 billion U/g

SuperEPA 1200; SuperEPA 2000 softgels OTC *dietary supplement* [omega-3 fatty acids] 1200 mg; 1000 mg

Superfed liquid OTC *decongestant* [pseudoephedrine HCl]

superoxide dismutase (SOD) [see: orgotein]

superoxide dismutase (SOD), recombinant human (*orphan: prevent reperfusion injury to donor organ tissue; neonatal bronchopulmonary dysplasia*)

Superplex-T tablets OTC *vitamin supplement* [multiple B vitamins; vitamin C] ±•500 mg

supidimide INN

Suplena ready-to-use liquid OTC *enteral nutritional therapy for renal failure* [essential amino acids]

Suppap-120; Suppap-650 suppositories OTC *analgesic; antipyretic* [acetaminophen] 120 mg; 650 mg

Suppap-325 suppositories (discontinued 1994) OTC *analgesic; antipyretic* [acetaminophen] 325 mg

Supprelin subcu injection ℞ *gonadotropin-releasing hormone for central precocious puberty (orphan)* [histrelin acetate] 120, 300, 600 µg/0.6 mL

Suppress lozenges OTC *antitussive* [dextromethorphan hydrobromide] 7.5 mg

Supprette (trademarked dosage form) *suppository*

Suprane liquid for vaporization ℞ *inhalation general anesthetic* [desflurane]

Suprax film-coated tablets, powder for oral suspension ℞ *cephalosporin-type antibiotic* [cefixime] 200, 400 mg; 100 mg/5 mL

Suprefact ℞ *investigational antineoplastic for prostatic cancer* [buserelin acetate]

suproclone USAN, INN *sedative*

suprofen USAN, INN, BAN *ocular nonsteroidal anti-inflammatory drug (NSAID); antimiotic*

Supule (trademarked dosage form) *suppository*

suramin sodium USP, BAN *investigational anti-infective for trypanosomiasis & onchocerciasis; investigational antineoplastic*

Surbex Filmtabs (film-coated tablets) OTC *vitamin supplement* [multiple B vitamins] ±

Surbex 750 with Iron Filmtabs (film-coated tablets) OTC *vitamin/iron supplement* [multiple B vitamins; vitamins C and E; ferrous sulfate, dried; folic acid] ±•750 mg•30 IU•27 mg•0.4 mg

Surbex 750 with Zinc Filmtabs (film-coated tablets) OTC *vitamin/zinc supplement* [multiple vitamins; zinc sulfate; folic acid] ±•22.5•0.4 mg

Surbex-T; Surbex with C Filmtabs (film-coated tablets) OTC *vitamin supplement* [multiple B vitamins; vitamin C] ≐•500 mg; ≐•250 mg

Surbu-Gen-T film-coated tablets OTC *vitamin supplement* [multiple B vitamins; vitamin C] ≐•500 mg

Sure Cell Chlamydia Test reagent kit for professional use *in vitro diagnostic aid for Chlamydia trachomatis* [monoclonal antibody-based enzyme-linked immunosorbent assay (ELISA)]

Sure Cell hCG-Urine Test kit (name changed to Sure Cell Pregnancy in 1995)

Sure Cell Herpes (HSV) Test reagent kit for professional use *in vitro diagnostic aid for herpes simplex virus in genital, rectal, oral, or dermal swabs* [monoclonal antibody-based enzyme-linked immunosorbent assay (ELISA)]

Sure Cell Pregnancy test kit for professional use *in vitro diagnostic aid for urine pregnancy test* [monoclonal/polyclonal antibody ELISA test]

Sure Cell Strep A Test kit (name changed to Sure Cell Streptococci in 1995)

Sure Cell Streptococci test kit for professional use *in vitro diagnostic aid for Group A streptococcal antigens in blood and throat swabs* [enzyme-linked immunosorbent assay (ELISA)]

SureLac chewable tablets OTC *digestive aid for lactose intolerance* [lactase enzyme] 3000 U

surface active extract of saline lavage of bovine lungs (*orphan: respiratory failure in premature infants*)

surfactant, human amniotic fluid derived (*orphan status withdrawn 1994*)

surfactant TA [see: beractant]

surfactant TA, modified bovine lung surfactant extract (*orphan: neonatal respiratory distress syndrome*) [see: beractant]

Surfak Liquigels (capsules) OTC *stool softener* [docusate calcium] 50, 240 mg

surfilcon A USAN *hydrophilic contact lens material*

Surfol Post-Immersion Bath Oil OTC *bath emollient*

surfomer USAN, INN *hypolipidemic*

Surgel vaginal gel OTC *lubricant* [propylene glycol; glycerin]

surgibone USAN *internal bone splint*

surgical catgut [see: suture, absorbable surgical]

surgical gut [see: suture, absorbable surgical]

Surgicel strips, Nu-knit pads ℞ *topical local hemostat for surgery* [oxidized cellulose]

suricainide INN *antiarrhythmic* [also: suricainide maleate]

suricainide maleate USAN, INN *antiarrhythmic* [also: suricainide]

suriclone INN, BAN

Surital IV injection (discontinued 1993) ℞ *general anesthetic* [thiamylal sodium] 1, 5, 10 g ⓓ Serentil

suritozole USAN, INN *antidepressant; investigational Alzheimer's treatment*

Surmontil capsules ℞ *tricyclic antidepressant* [trimipramine maleate] 25, 50, 100 mg

suronacrine INN *cholinesterase inhibitor* [also: suronacrine maleate]

suronacrine maleate USAN *cholinesterase inhibitor* [also: suronacrine]

Survanta suspension for intratracheal instillation ℞ *pulmonary surfactant; neonatal respiratory distress syndrome or respiratory failure* (*orphan*) [beractant] 25 mg/mL

Susano elixir ℞ *GI anticholinergic; sedative* [atropine sulfate; scopolamine hydrobromide; hyoscyamine hydrobromide; phenobarbital] 0.0194•0.0065•0.1037•16.2 mg/5 mL

Susano tablets (discontinued 1995) ℞ *GI anticholinergic; sedative* [phenobarbital; atropine sulfate; scopolamine hydrobromide; hyoscyamine hydrobromide] 0.0194•0.0065•0.1037•16.2 mg

Sus-Phrine subcu injection ℞ *bronchodilator for bronchial asthma, bronchospasm and COPD; vasopressor for shock* [epinephrine] 1:200 (5 mg/mL)

Sust-A 10,000; Sust-A 25,000 sustained-release tablets OTC *vitamin supplement* [vitamin A palmitate]

Sustacal powder OTC *enteral nutritional therapy* [milk-based formula]

Sustacal pudding OTC *enteral nutritional therapy* [milk-based formula]

Sustacal ready-to-use liquid OTC *enteral nutritional therapy* [lactose-free formula]

Sustacal Basic; Sustacal Plus ready-to-use liquid OTC *enteral nutritional therapy* [lactose-free formula]

Sustacal HC ready-to-use liquid (discontinued 1994) OTC *high-calorie nutritional supplement* [lactose-free formula] 8 oz.

Sustagen powder OTC *enteral nutritional therapy* [milk-based formula]

Sustaire timed-release tablets ℞ *bronchodilator* [theophylline] 100, 300 mg

sutilains USAN, USP, INN, BAN *topical proteolytic enzymes for necrotic tissue debridement*

sutoprofen [see: suprofen]

suture, absorbable surgical USP *surgical aid*

suture, nonabsorbable surgical USP *surgical aid*

suxamethone [see: succinylcholine chloride]

suxamethonium chloride INN, BAN *neuromuscular blocking agent* [also: succinylcholine chloride]

suxemerid INN *antitussive* [also: suxemerid sulfate]

suxemerid sulfate USAN *antitussive* [also: suxemerid]

suxethonium chloride INN

suxibuzone INN

sweet birch oil [see: methyl salicylate]

sweet orange peel tincture [see: orange peel tincture, sweet]

sweet spirit of nitre [see: ethyl nitrite]

Sweet'n Fresh Clotrimazole-7 cream, vaginal suppositories OTC *antifungal* [clotrimazole] 1%; 100 mg

Swim-Ear ear drops OTC *antiseptic* [isopropyl alcohol] 95%

SWS solution (discontinued 1992) OTC *wetting/soaking solution for hard contact lenses*

Sygen ℞ *investigational treatment for stroke, spinal cord injury, subarachnoid hemorrhage, and parkinsonism* [nerve growth factor GM_1 ganglioside]

Syllact powder OTC *bulk laxative* [psyllium seed husks] 3.3 g/tsp.

Syllamalt powder OTC *laxative* [malt soup extract; psyllium seed husks] 4•3 g/tsp.

Symadine capsules ℞ *antiviral; antiparkinsonian agent* [amantadine HCl] 100 mg

symclosene USAN, INN *topical anti-infective*

Symcor ℞ *investigational treatment for hypertension and congestive heart failure* [tiamenidine]

symetine INN *antiamebic* [also: symetine HCl]

symetine HCl USAN *antiamebic* [also: symetine]

Symmetrel capsules, syrup ℞ *antiviral; antiparkinsonian agent* [amantadine HCl] 100 mg; 50 mg/5 mL

Synacol CF tablets OTC *antitussive; expectorant* [dextromethorphan hydrobromide; guaifenesin] 15•200 mg

Synacort cream ℞ *topical corticosteroid* [hydrocortisone] 1%, 2.5%

Synalar cream, ointment, topical solution ℞ *topical corticosteroid* [fluocinolone acetonide] 0.01, 0.25%; 0.025%; 0.01%

Synalar-HP cream ℞ *topical corticosteroid* [fluocinolone acetonide] 0.2%

Synalgos-DC capsules ℞ *narcotic analgesic* [dihydrocodeine bitartrate; aspirin; caffeine] 16•356.4•30 mg

Synapton SR ℞ *investigational sustained-release cholinesterase inhibitor for Alzheimer's disease* [physostigmine]

Synarel nasal spray ℞ *gonadotropin-releasing hormone for endometriosis; and central precocious puberty (orphan)* [nafarelin acetate] 2 mg/mL (200 μg/spray)

Synemol cream ℞ *topical corticosteroid* [fluocinolone acetonide] 0.025%

Synercid injection ℞ *investigational semi-synthetic antibiotic for iatrogenic infections* [streptogramin]

synestrin [see: diethylstilbestrol]

Synkayvite subcu, IM, or IV injection (discontinued 1992) ℞ *coagulant; for vitamin K deficiency or hypoprothrombinemia* [menadiol sodium diphosphate] 5, 10, 37.5 mg/mL

Synkayvite tablets (discontinued 1992) ℞ *coagulant; for vitamin K deficiency or hypoprothrombinemia* [menadiol sodium diphosphate] 5 mg

synnematin B [see: adicillin]

Synophylate-GG syrup ℞ *antiasthmatic; bronchodilator; expectorant* [theophylline; guaifenesin; alcohol 10%] 150•100 mg/15 mL

Synovir ℞ *investigational treatment for AIDS-related cachexia* [thalidomide]

Syn-Rx controlled-release tablets (14-day treatment regimen) ℞ *decongestant; expectorant* [pseudoephedrine HCl; guaifenesin] 60•600 mg

Synthaloids throat lozenges OTC *oral antiseptic; topical anesthetic* [Calpuridin (q.v.); benzocaine]

synthestrin [see: diethylstilbestrol]

synthetic lung surfactant [see: colfosceril palmitate]

synthetic paraffin [see: paraffin, synthetic]

synthetic spermaceti [now: cetyl esters wax]

synthoestrin [see: diethylstilbestrol]

Synthroid tablets, powder for injection ℞ *thyroid hormone* [levothyroxine sodium] 25, 50, 75, 88, 100, 112, 125, 150, 175, 200, 300 μg; 200, 500 μg ② Euthroid

Syntocinon IV, IM injection ℞ *induction of labor; postpartum bleeding; incomplete abortion* [oxytocin] 10 U/mL

Syntocinon nasal spray ℞ *initial milk let-down* [oxytocin] 40 U/mL

synvinolin [now: simvastatin]

Synvisc ℞ *investigational antiarthritic* [hylan fluid-gel mixture]

Syprine capsules ℞ *chelating agent for copper; for Wilson's disease (orphan)* [trientine HCl] 50 mg

Syracol CF tablets OTC *antitussive; expectorant* [dextromethorphan hydrobromide; guaifenesin] 15•200 mg

syrosingopine NF, INN, BAN

syrup NF *flavoring agent*

syrupus cerasi [see: cherry juice]

Syrvite liquid OTC *vitamin supplement* [multiple vitamins] ±

Sytobex IM or subcu injection (discontinued 1994) ℞ *antianemic; vitamin B_{12} supplement* [cyanocobalamin] 1000 μg/mL

T-2 protocol (dactinomycin, doxorubicin, vincristine, cyclophosphamide, radiation) *chemotherapy protocol*

T_3 (liothyronine sodium) [q.v.]

T_4 (levothyroxine sodium) [q.v.]

T4, recombinant soluble human *investigational (Phase I/II) antiviral for HIV*

T4 endonuclease V, liposome encapsulated *(orphan: prevent cutaneous neoplasms in xeroderma pigmentosum)*

T-10 protocol (methotrexate, doxorubicin, cisplatin, bleomycin, cyclophosphamide, dactinomycin) *chemotherapy protocol*

T-88 *investigational treatment for gram-negative sepsis*

T-3761 *investigational oral fluoroquinolone antibiotic*

T-3762 *investigational injectable fluoroquinolone antibiotic*

T30177 *investigational (Phase I) antiviral oligonucleotide for AIDS*

T4N5 ℞ *(orphan: prevent cutaneous neoplasms in xeroderma pigmentosum)* [T4 endonuclease V, liposome encapsulated]

T-61 ℞ *veterinary anesthesia; veterinary euthanasia* [embutramide]

Tab-A-Vite tablets OTC *vitamin supplement* [multiple vitamins; folic acid] ≟•0.4 mg

Tab-A-Vite + Iron tablets OTC *vitamin/iron supplement* [multiple vitamins; iron; folic acid] ≟•18•0.4 mg

tabilautide INN

Tabloid (trademarked dosage form) *tablet with raised lettering*

Tabron Filmseals (film-coated tablets) (discontinued 1996) ℞ *hematinic* [ferrous fumarate; multiple B vitamins; vitamins C and E; docusate sodium; folic acid] 100 mg•≟•500 mg•30 IU•50 mg•1 mg

Tabules (dosage form) *tablets*

Tac suspension ℞ *topical corticosteroid* [triamcinolone acetonide]

Tac-3 IM, intra-articular, intrabursal, intradermal injection ℞ *glucocorticoids* [triamcinolone acetonide] 3 mg/mL

Tac-40 suspension ℞ *topical corticosteroid* [triamcinolone acetonide] 40 mg/mL

Tacaryl syrup ℞ *antihistamine* [methdilazine HCl] 4 mg/5 mL

Tacaryl tablets, chewable tablets (discontinued 1994) ℞ *antihistamine* [methdilazine HCl] 8 mg; 4 mg

Tace capsules ℞ *hormone for estrogen replacement therapy or inoperable prostatic carcinoma* [chlorotrianisene] 12, 25 mg

taclamine INN *minor tranquilizer* [also: taclamine HCl]

taclamine HCl USAN *minor tranquilizer* [also: taclamine]

tacrine INN, BAN *cognition adjuvant for Alzheimer's dementia* [also: tacrine HCl]

tacrine HCl USAN *cognition adjuvant for Alzheimer's dementia* [also: tacrine]

tacrolimus USAN, INN *immunosuppressant*

TAD (thioguanine, ara-C, daunorubicin) *chemotherapy protocol* [also: DCT; DAT]

Tagamet film-coated tablets ℞ *gastric and duodenal ulcer treatment; for gastric hypersecretory conditions* [cimetidine] 200, 300, 400, 800 mg ② Tegopen

Tagamet liquid, IV or IM injection, premixed injection ℞ *gastric and duodenal ulcer treatment; for gastric hypersecretory conditions* [cimetidine HCl] 300 mg/5 mL; 300 mg/2 mL; 300 mg/vial

Tagamet 100 (British name for U.S. product Tagamet HB)

Tagamet CR ℞ *investigational controlled-release gastric and duodenal ulcer treatment* [cimetidine]

Tagamet HB film-coated tablets OTC H_2 *antagonist for episodic heartburn and acid indigestion* [cimetidine] 100 mg

taglutimide INN

TA-HPV ℞ *(orphan: cervical cancer)* [recombinant vaccinia (human papillomavirus)]

Talacen caplets ℞ *narcotic agonist-antagonist analgesic; antipyretic* [pentazocine HCl; acetaminophen] 25•650 mg

talampicillin INN *antibacterial* [also: talampicillin HCl]

talampicillin HCl USAN *antibacterial* [also: talampicillin]

talastine INN

talbutal USP, INN *sedative; hypnotic*

talc USP *dusting powder; tablet and capsule lubricant*

taleranol USAN, INN *gonadotropin enzyme inhibitor*

talinolol INN

talipexole INN

talisomycin USAN, INN *antineoplastic*

tallimustine INN *investigational antineoplastic for leukemia and solid tumors*

tallysomycin A [now: talisomycin]

talmetacin USAN, INN *analgesic; anti-inflammatory; antipyretic*

talmetoprim INN

talniflumate USAN, INN *anti-inflammatory; analgesic*

Taloin ointment (discontinued 1992) OTC *topical diaper rash treatment* [methylbenzethonium chloride; zinc oxide; calamine; eucalyptol]

talopram INN *catecholamine potentiator* [also: talopram HCl]

talopram HCl USAN *catecholamine potentiator* [also: talopram]

talosalate USAN, INN *analgesic; anti-inflammatory*
Taloxa (foreign name for U.S. product Felbatol)
taloximine INN, BAN
talsaclidine INN
talsaclidine fumarate USAN *muscarinic M₁ agonist for Alzheimer's disease*
talsupram INN
taltibride [see: metibride]
taltrimide INN
taludipine [see: teludipine]
taludipine HCl *(previously used USAN)* [see: teludipine HCl]
Talwin IV, subcu or IM injection ℞ *narcotic agonist-antagonist analgesic* [pentazocine lactate] 30 mg/mL
Talwin Compound caplets ℞ *narcotic agonist-antagonist analgesic; antipyretic* [pentazocine HCl; aspirin] 12.5•325 mg
Talwin NX tablets ℞ *narcotic agonist-antagonist analgesic* [pentazocine HCl; naloxone HCl] 50•0.5 mg
Tambocor tablets ℞ *antiarrhythmic* [flecainide acetate] 50, 100, 150 mg
tameridone USAN, INN, BAN *veterinary sedative*
tameticillin INN
tametraline INN *antidepressant* [also: tametraline HCl]
tametraline HCl USAN *antidepressant* [also: tametraline]
Tamine S.R. sustained-release tablets ℞ *decongestant; antihistamine* [phenylpropanolamine HCl; phenylephrine HCl; brompheniramine maleate] 15•15•12 mg
tamitinol INN
tamoxifen INN, BAN *antiestrogen; antineoplastic* [also: tamoxifen citrate]
tamoxifen citrate USAN, USP, JAN *antiestrogen antineoplastic for breast cancer; investigational for breast cancer prevention* [also: tamoxifen] 10 mg oral
tampramine INN *antidepressant* [also: tampramine fumarate]
tampramine fumarate USAN *antidepressant* [also: tampramine]
Tamp-R-Tel (trademarked packaging form) *tamper-evident cartridge-needle unit*

tamsulosin INN
tamsulosin HCl USAN *alpha₁ antagonist for treatment of BPH*
Tanac gel OTC *topical oral anesthetic; vulnerary* [dyclonine HCl; allantoin] 1%•0.5%
Tanac liquid OTC *topical oral anesthetic; antiseptic* [benzocaine; benzalkonium chloride] 10%•0.12%
Tanac Dual Core stick OTC *topical oral anesthetic; antiseptic; astringent* [benzocaine; benzalkonium chloride; tannic acid] 7.5%•0.12%•6%
Tanac Roll-On liquid (discontinued 1994) OTC *topical oral anesthetic; antiseptic* [benzocaine; benzalkonium chloride] 5%•0.12%
Tanafed oral suspension ℞ *decongestant; antihistamine* [pseudoephedrine tannate; chlorpheniramine tannate] 75•4.5 mg/5 mL
tandamine INN *antidepressant* [also: tandamine HCl]
tandamine HCl USAN *antidepressant* [also: tandamine]
tandospirone INN, BAN *anxiolytic* [also: tandospirone citrate]
tandospirone citrate USAN *anxiolytic* [also: tandospirone]
taniplon INN
tannic acid USP, JAN *astringent; topical mucosal protectant*
tannic acid acetate [see: acetyltannic acid]
tannin [see: tannic acid]
tannyl acetate [see: acetyltannic acid]
Tanoral tablets ℞ *decongestant; antihistamine* [phenylephrine tannate; chlorpheniramine tannate; pyrilamine tannate] 25•8•25 mg
tantalum *element (Ta)*
Tao capsules ℞ *macrolide antibiotic* [troleandomycin] 250 mg
taoryi edisylate [see: caramiphen edisylate]
Tapanol tablets, caplets OTC *analgesic; antipyretic* [acetaminophen] 500 mg
Tapazole tablets ℞ *antithyroid agent* [methimazole] 5, 10 mg
tape, adhesive USP *surgical aid*
taprostene INN
tar [see: coal tar]

Tarabine PFS injection ℞ *antineoplastic* [cytarabine]

Taractan IM injection (discontinued 1994) ℞ *antipsychotic* [clorprothixene HCl] 12.5 mg/mL ⓘ Periactin; Tinactin

Taractan oral concentrate (discontinued 1994) ℞ *antipsychotic* [clorprothixene lactate] 100 mg/5 mL

Taractan tablets (discontinued 1994) ℞ *antipsychotic* [clorprothixene] 10, 25, 50, 100 mg

Taraphilic Ointment OTC *topical antipsoriatic; antiseborrheic* [coal tar] 1%

Targocid (commercially available in 13 foreign countries) ℞ *investigational glycopeptide antibiotic* [teicoplanin]

Targretin oral, topical ℞ *investigational (Phase I/II) antineoplastic for AIDS-related Kaposi sarcoma* [LGD 1069 (code name—generic name not yet approved)] ⓘ Tegopen; Tegrin

Tarlene hair lotion OTC *antiseborrheic; antipsoriatic; keratolytic* [salicylic acid; coal tar] 2.5%•2%

Tarsum shampoo OTC *antipsoriatic; antiseborrheic; keratolytic* [coal tar; salicylic acid] 10%•5%

tartar emetic [see: antimony potassium tartrate]

tartaric acid NF *buffering agent*

Tasmar ℞ *investigational topical treatment for cutaneous actinic damage* [isotretinoin]

tasosartan USAN, INN *antihypertensive*

tasuldine INN

TAT antagonist *investigational (Phase I/II) antiviral for HIV*

T-Athlete cream, powder, aerosol powder, solution OTC *antifungal* [tolnaftate]

Tauricyt ℞ *investigational antineoplastic* [tauromustine]

taurine INN [also: aminoethylsulfonic acid]

taurocholate sodium [see: sodium taurocholate]

taurolidine INN, BAN *investigational antitoxin for the treatment of sepsis*

tauromustine INN *investigational treatment for renal cancer and multiple sclerosis*

tauroselcholic acid INN, BAN

taurultam INN, BAN

Tavist tablets, syrup ℞ *antihistamine* [clemastine fumarate] 2.68 mg; 0.67 mg/5 mL

Tavist-1 tablets OTC *antihistamine* [clemastine fumarate] 1.34 mg

Tavist-D film-coated sustained-release tablets OTC *decongestant; antihistamine* [phenylpropanolamine HCl; clemastine fumarate] 75•1.34 mg

Taxol IV infusion ℞ *antineoplastic for metastatic carcinoma of the ovary and breast and non-small cell lung cancer* [paclitaxel] 30 mg/5 mL

Taxotere IV infusion ℞ *antineoplastic for breast cancer; investigational for ovarian and lung cancers* [docetaxel] 20, 80 mg/vial

tazadolene INN *analgesic* [also: tazadolene succinate]

tazadolene succinate USAN *analgesic* [also: tazadolene]

tazanolast INN

tazarotene USAN *keratolytic*

tazasubrate INN, BAN

tazeprofen INN

Tazicef powder for IV or IM injection ℞ *cephalosporin-type antibiotic* [ceftazidime] 1, 2, 6 g

Tazidime powder for IV or IM injection ℞ *cephalosporin-type antibiotic* [ceftazidime] 0.5, 1, 2, 6 g

tazifylline INN *antihistamine* [also: tazifylline HCl]

tazifylline HCl USAN *antihistamine* [also: tazifylline]

taziprinone INN

tazobactam USAN, INN, BAN *β-lactamase inhibitor*

tazobactam sodium USAN *β-lactamase inhibitor*

Tazocin (European name for U.S. product Zosyn)

tazofelone USAN *treatment for ulcerative colitis and Crohn's disease*

tazolol INN *cardiotonic* [also: tazolol HCl]

tazolol HCl USAN *cardiotonic* [also: tazolol]

TBC-3B *investigational (Phase I) vaccine for AIDS*

TBC-CEA ℞ *investigational cancer vaccine* [vaccinia virus vaccine for carcinoembryonic antigen (CEA)]
TBZ (thiabendazole) [q.v.]
TC (thioguanine, cytarabine) *chemotherapy protocol*
^{99m}**Tc** [see: macrosalb (^{99m}Tc)]
^{99m}**Tc** [see: sodium pertechnetate Tc 99m]
^{99m}**Tc** [see: technetium Tc 99m albumin]
^{99m}**Tc** [see: technetium Tc 99m albumin aggregated]
^{99m}**Tc** [see: technetium Tc 99m albumin colloid]
^{99m}**Tc** [see: technetium Tc 99m albumin microaggregated]
^{99m}**Tc** [see: technetium Tc 99m antimony trisulfide colloid]
^{99m}**Tc** [see: technetium Tc 99m biciromab]
^{99m}**Tc** [see: technetium Tc 99m bicisate]
^{99m}**Tc** [see: technetium Tc 99m disofenin]
^{99m}**Tc** [see: technetium Tc 99m etidronate]
^{99m}**Tc** [see: technetium Tc 99m exametazine]
^{99m}**Tc** [see: technetium Tc 99m ferpentetate]
^{99m}**Tc** [see: technetium Tc 99m furifosmin]
^{99m}**Tc** [see: technetium Tc 99m gluceptate]
^{99m}**Tc** [see: technetium Tc 99m lidofenin]
^{99m}**Tc** [see: technetium Tc 99m mebrofenin]
^{99m}**Tc** [see: technetium Tc 99m medronate]
^{99m}**Tc** [see: technetium Tc 99m medronate disodium]
^{99m}**Tc** [see: technetium Tc 99m mertiatide]
^{99m}**Tc** [see: technetium Tc 99m oxidronate]
^{99m}**Tc** [see: technetium Tc 99m pentetate]
^{99m}**Tc** [see: technetium Tc 99m pentetate calcium trisodium]
^{99m}**Tc** [see: technetium Tc 99m (pyro- & trimeta-) phosphates]
^{99m}**Tc** [see: technetium Tc 99m pyrophosphate]
^{99m}**Tc** [see: technetium Tc 99m red blood cells]
^{99m}**Tc** [see: technetium Tc 99m sestamibi]
^{99m}**Tc** [see: technetium Tc 99m siboroxime]
^{99m}**Tc** [see: technetium Tc 99m succimer]
^{99m}**Tc** [see: technetium Tc 99m sulfur colloid]
^{99m}**Tc** [see: technetium Tc 99m teboroxime]
^{99m}**Tc** [see: technetium Tc 99m tetrofosmin]
^{99m}**Tc** [see: technetium Tc 99m tiatide]
T-Caine lozenges (discontinued 1993) OTC *topical oral anesthetic* [benzocaine] 5 mg
TCC (trichlorocarbanilide) [see: triclocarban]
TC-CYT-380 *investigational imaging aid for breast cancer detection and staging*
TC-CYT-380 fragment *investigational imaging aid for non-small cell lung cancer detection and staging*
TD; Td (tetanus & diphtheria [toxoids]) *the designation TD or DT denotes the pediatric vaccine; Td denotes the adult vaccine* [see: diphtheria & tetanus toxoids, adsorbed]
T-Dry sustained-release capsules (discontinued 1995) OTC *decongestant; antihistamine* [pseudoephedrine HCl; chlorpheniramine maleate] 120•12 mg
T-Dry Jr. sustained-release capsules (discontinued 1992) ℞ *decongestant; antihistamine* [pseudoephedrine HCl; chlorpheniramine maleate]
TEAB (tetraethylammonium bromide) [see: tetrylammonium bromide]
teaberry oil [see: methyl salicylate]
TEAC (tetraethylammonium chloride) [q.v.]
Tear Drop eye drops OTC *ocular moisturizer/lubricant* [polyvinyl alcohol]
TearGard eye drops OTC *ocular moisturizer/lubricant* [hydroxyethylcellulose]
Teargen eye drops OTC *ocular moisturizer/lubricant*

Tearisol eye drops OTC *ocular moisturizer/lubricant* [hydroxypropyl methylcellulose] 0.5%

Tears Naturale; Tears Naturale II; Tears Naturale Free eye drops OTC *ocular moisturizer/lubricant* [hydroxypropyl methylcellulose] 0.3%

Tears Plus eye drops OTC *ocular moisturizer/lubricant* [polyvinyl alcohol] 1.4%

Tears Renewed eye drops OTC *ocular moisturizer/lubricant* [hydroxypropyl methylcellulose] 0.3%

Tears Renewed ophthalmic ointment OTC *ocular moisturizer/lubricant* [white petrolatum; mineral oil]

Tebamide suppositories, pediatric suppositories ℞ *anticholinergic; antiemetic* [trimethobenzamide HCl] 200 mg; 100 mg

tebatizole INN

tebethion [see: thioacetazone; thiacetazone]

tebufelone USAN, INN *analgesic; antiinflammatory*

tebuquine USAN, INN *antimalarial*

tebutate USAN, INN *combining name for radicals or groups*

T.E.C. IV injection (discontinued 1992) ℞ *intravenous nutritional therapy* [multiple trace elements (metals)]

TEC (thiotepa, etoposide, carboplatin) *chemotherapy protocol*

teceleukin USAN, INN, BAN *immunostimulant (orphan: metastatic renal cell cancer; metastatic malignant melanoma)*

TechneScan Q-12 ℞ *investigational radiodiagnostic aid for cardiac disease* [technetium Tc 99m furifosmin]

technetium *element (Tc)*

technetium (^{99m}Tc) dimercaptosuccinic acid JAN *diagnostic aid for renal function testing* [also: technetium Tc 99m succimer]

technetium (^{99m}Tc) human serum albumin JAN *radioactive agent*

technetium (^{99m}Tc) labeled macroaggregated human albumin JAN [also: macrosalb (^{99m}Tc)]

technetium (^{99m}Tc) methylenediphosphonate JAN *radioactive diagnostic aid for skeletal imaging* [also: technetium Tc 99m medronate]

technetium (^{99m}Tc) phytate JAN *radioactive agent*

technetium Tc 99m albumin USP *radioactive agent*

technetium Tc 99m albumin aggregated USAN, USP *radioactive diagnostic aid for lung imaging*

technetium Tc 99m albumin colloid USAN, USP *radioactive agent*

technetium Tc 99m albumin microaggregated USAN *radioactive agent*

technetium Tc 99m antimelanoma murine monoclonal antibody *(orphan: diagnostic imaging agent for metastases of malignant melanoma)*

technetium Tc 99m antimony trisulfide colloid USAN *radioactive agent*

technetium Tc 99m biciromab *radioactive diagnostic aid for deep vein thrombosis* [see: biciromab]

technetium Tc 99m bicisate USAN, INN, BAN *radioactive diagnostic aid for brain imaging*

technetium Tc 99m disofenin USP *radioactive diagnostic aid for hepatobiliary function testing*

technetium Tc 99m DMSA (dimercaptosuccinic acid) [see: technetium Tc 99m succimer]

technetium Tc 99m DTPA (diethylenetriaminepentaacetic acid) [see: technetium Tc 99m pentetate]

technetium Tc 99m etidronate USP *radioactive agent*

technetium Tc 99m exametazine USAN *radioactive agent*

technetium Tc 99m ferpentetate USP *radioactive agent*

technetium Tc 99m furifosmin USAN, INN *radioactive agent; diagnostic aid for cardiac disease*

technetium Tc 99m gluceptate USP *radioactive agent*

technetium Tc 99m HSA (human serum albumin) [see: technetium Tc 99m albumin]

technetium Tc 99m iron ascorbate pentetic acid complex [now: technetium Tc 99m ferpentetate]

technetium Tc 99m lidofenin USAN, USP *radioactive agent*

technetium Tc 99m MAA (microaggregated albumin) [see: technetium Tc 99m albumin aggregated]

technetium Tc 99m MDP (methylenediphosphonate) [see: technetium Tc 99m medronate]

technetium Tc 99m mebrofenin USAN, USP *radioactive agent*

technetium Tc 99m medronate USP *radioactive diagnostic aid for skeletal imaging* [also: technetium (^{99m}Tc) methylenediphosphonate]

technetium Tc 99m medronate disodium USAN *radioactive agent*

technetium Tc 99m mertiatide USAN *radioactive diagnostic aid for renal function testing*

technetium Tc 99m murine monoclonal antibody IgG$_2$a to B cell (*orphan: diagnostic aid for B-cell leukemia and lymphoma*)

technetium Tc 99m murine monoclonal antibody to human alpha-fetoprotein (AFP) (*orphan: diagnostic aid for AFP-producing tumors; hepatoblastoma*)

technetium Tc 99m murine monoclonal antibody to human chorionic gonadotropin (hCG) (*orphan: diagnostic aid for hCG-producing tumors*)

technetium Tc 99m oxidronate USP *radioactive diagnostic aid for skeletal imaging*

technetium Tc 99m pentetate USP *radioactive agent* [also: human serum albumin diethylenetriaminepentaacetic acid technetium (^{99m}Tc)]

technetium Tc 99m pentetate calcium trisodium USAN *radioactive agent*

technetium Tc 99m pentetate sodium [now: technetium Tc 99m pentetate]

technetium Tc 99m (pyro- & trimeta-) phosphates USP *radioactive agent*

technetium Tc 99m pyrophosphate USP, JAN *radioactive agent*

technetium Tc 99m red blood cells USAN *radioactive agent*

technetium Tc 99m sestamibi USAN, INN, BAN *radioactive/radiopaque diagnostic aid for cardiac perfusion imaging*

technetium Tc 99m siboroxime USAN, INN *radioactive diagnostic aid for brain imaging*

technetium Tc 99m sodium gluceptate [now: technetium Tc 99m gluceptate]

technetium Tc 99m succimer USP *diagnostic aid for renal function testing* [also: technetium (^{99m}Tc) dimercaptosuccinic acid]

technetium Tc 99m sulfur colloid (TSC) USAN, USP *radioactive agent*

technetium Tc 99m teboroxime USAN, INN, BAN *radioactive/radiopaque diagnostic aid for cardiac perfusion imaging*

technetium Tc 99m tetrofosmin *radioactive agent for cardiovascular imaging*

technetium Tc 99m tiatide BAN

technetium Tc 99m TSC (technetium sulfur colloid) [see: technetium Tc 99m sulfur colloid]

teclothiazide INN, BAN

teclozan USAN, INN *antiamebic*

Tecnu Poison Oak-N-Ivy liquid OTC *topical poison ivy treatment* [deodorized mineral spirits] 2

tecogalan sodium USAN *antiangiogenic antineoplastic*

tedisamil INN *investigational calcium channel blocker for ischemic heart disease and arrhythmias*

Tedral tablets, suspension (discontinued 1993) OTC *antiasthmatic; bronchodilator; decongestant; sedative* [theophylline; ephedrine HCl; phenobarbital] ☒ Teldrin

Tedral SA sustained-action tablets (discontinued 1993) ℞ *antiasthmatic; bronchodilator; decongestant; sedative* [theophylline; ephedrine HCl; phenobarbital]

Tedrigen tablets OTC *antiasthmatic; bronchodilator; decongestant; sedative* [theophylline; ephedrine HCl; phenobarbital] 120•22.5•7.5 mg

tefazoline INN

tefenperate INN

tefludazine INN
teflurane USAN, INN *inhalation anesthetic*
teflutixol INN
Tega Caine solution (discontinued 1992) OTC *topical local anesthetic* [benzocaine; urea; parachlorometaxylenol]
Tega D & E, SR sustained-release tablets (discontinued 1992) ℞ *decongestant; expectorant* [phenylpropanolamine HCl; guaifenesin]
Tega-Atric; Tega-Atric M elixir (discontinued 1992) OTC *vitamin/mineral supplement* [multiple B vitamins & minerals]
Tega-Cort; Tega-Cort Forte lotion (discontinued 1992) ℞ *topical corticosteroid* [hydrocortisone]
tegafur USAN, INN, BAN *antineoplastic*
Tega-Otic ear drops (discontinued 1992) ℞ *topical corticosteroid; antibacterial/antifungal; anesthetic* [hydrocortisone; pramoxine; chloroxylenol; acetic acid]
Tega-Tussin syrup (discontinued 1992) ℞ *narcotic antitussive; decongestant; antihistamine* [hydrocodone bitartrate; phenylephrine HCl; chlorpheniramine maleate]
Tega-Vert capsules (discontinued 1992) OTC *antinauseant; antiemetic; antivertigo; motion sickness preventative* [dimenhydrinate] 50 mg
Tegison capsules ℞ *systemic antipsoriatic* [etretinate] 10, 25 mg
Tegopen capsules, powder for oral solution ℞ *bactericidal antibiotic (penicillinase-resistant penicillin)* [cloxacillin sodium] 250, 500 mg; 125 mg/5 mL ❷ Tagamet; Tegrin; Targretin
Tegretol chewable tablets, tablets, oral suspension ℞ *anticonvulsant* [carbamazepine] 100 mg; 200 mg; 100 mg/5 mL ❷ Tegrin
Tegretol-XR extended-release tablets ℞ *anticonvulsant* [carbamazepine] 100, 200, 400 mg
Tegrin for Psoriasis cream, lotion, soap OTC *topical antipsoriatic; antiseborrheic; antiseptic* [coal tar solution] 5% ❷ Tegopen; Tegretol; Targretin

Tegrin Medicated cream, lotion (name changed to Tegrin for Psoriasis in 1992)
Tegrin Medicated gel shampoo, lotion shampoo OTC *antiseborrheic; antipsoriatic; antipruritic; antibacterial* [coal tar] 5%
Tegrin Medicated Extra Conditioning; Advanced Formula Tegrin shampoo OTC *antiseborrheic; antipsoriatic; antipruritic; antibacterial* [coal tar] 7%
Tegrin-HC ointment OTC *topical corticosteroid* [hydrocortisone] 1%
Tegrin-LT shampoo/conditioner OTC *pediculicide* [pyrethrins; piperonyl butoxide technical] 0.33%•3.15%
T.E.H. tablets (discontinued 1993) ℞ *antiasthmatic; bronchodilator; decongestant; anxiolytic* [theophylline; ephedrine sulfate; hydroxyzine HCl]
teholamine [see: aminophylline]
TEIB (triethyleneiminobenzoquinone) [see: triaziquone]
teicoplanin USAN, INN, BAN *glycopeptide antibacterial antibiotic*
teicoplanin A_{2-1}, A_{2-2}, A_{2-3}, A_{2-4}, A_{2-5}, and A_{3-1} *components of teicoplanin*
Tekron ℞ *investigational antiglaucoma agent*
Telachlor timed-release capsules ℞ *antihistamine* [chlorpheniramine maleate] 8, 12 mg
Teladar cream ℞ *topical corticosteroid* [betamethasone dipropionate] 0.05%
Teldrin timed-release capsules OTC *antihistamine* [chlorpheniramine maleate] 12 mg ❷ Tedral
Teldrin 12-Hour Allergy Relief sustained-release capsules OTC *decongestant; antihistamine* [phenylpropanolamine HCl; chlorpheniramine maleate] 75•8 mg
Tel-E-Amp (trademarked packaging form) *unit dose ampule*
Tel-E-Dose (trademarked packaging form) *unit dose package*
Tel-E-Ject (trademarked delivery system) *prefilled disposable syringe*
teleleukin (orphan: metastatic renal cell carcinoma)

telenzepine INN
Tel-E-Pack (trademarked packaging form) *packaging system*
Telepaque tablets ℞ *oral cholecystographic radiopaque agent* [iopanoic acid] 500 mg
Tel-E-Vial (trademarked packaging form) *unit dose vial*
telinavir USAN *antiviral; HIV protease inhibitor*
Teline; Teline-500 capsules ℞ *broad-spectrum antibiotic* [tetracycline HCl] 250 mg; 500 mg
tellurium *element (Te)*
teloxantrone INN *antineoplastic* [also: teloxantrone HCl]
teloxantrone HCl USAN *antineoplastic* [also: teloxantrone]
teludipine INN, BAN *antihypertensive; calcium channel antagonist* [also: teludipine HCl]
teludipine HCl USAN *antihypertensive; calcium channel antagonist* [also: teludipine] [USAN previously used: taludipine HCl]
temafloxacin INN, BAN *antibacterial; microbial DNA topoisomerase inhibitor* [also: temafloxacin HCl]
temafloxacin HCl USAN *antibacterial; microbial DNA topoisomerase inhibitor* [also: temafloxacin]
Temaril tablets, syrup, Spansules (sustained-release capsules) (discontinued 1996) ℞ *antihistamine* [trimeprazine tartrate] 2.5 mg; 2.5 mg/5 mL; 5 mg ☑ Demerol; Tepanil
temarotene INN
tematropium methylsulfate USAN *anticholinergic* [also: tematropium metilsulfate]
tematropium metilsulfate INN *anticholinergic* [also: tematropium methylsulfate]
temazepam USAN, INN *minor tranquilizer; hypnotic* 7.5, 15, 30 mg oral
Temazin Cold syrup OTC *decongestant; antihistamine* [phenylpropanolamine HCl; chlorpheniramine maleate] 12.5•2 mg/5 mL
Tembid (trademarked dosage form) *sustained-action capsule*

temefos USAN, INN *veterinary ectoparasiticide*
temelastine USAN, INN, BAN *antihistamine*
Temelin (Japanese name for U.S. product Zanaflex)
Temicef ℞ *investigational cephalosporin antibiotic* [cefodizime]
temocapril HCl USAN *antihypertensive*
temocillin USAN, INN, BAN *antibacterial*
temodox USAN, INN *veterinary growth stimulant*
temoporfin USAN, INN, BAN *photosensitizer for photodynamic cancer therapy*
Temovate ointment, gel, cream, scalp application ℞ *topical corticosteroidal anti-inflammatory* [clobetasol propionate] 0.05%
Temovate Emollient cream ℞ *topical corticosteroidal anti-inflammatory* [clobetasol propionate in an emollient base] 0.05%
temozolomide INN, BAN *investigational cytotoxic alkylating antineoplastic for malignant glioma*
TEMP (tamoxifen, etoposide, mitoxantrone, Platinol) *chemotherapy protocol*
Tempo chewable tablets OTC *antacid; antiflatulent* [aluminum hydroxide; magnesium hydroxide; calcium carbonate; simethicone] 133•81•414•20 mg
Tempra chewable tablets, syrup, drops OTC *analgesic; antipyretic* [acetaminophen] 80 mg; 160 mg/5 mL; 100 mg/mL
Tempule (trademarked dosage form) *timed-release capsule or tablet*
temurtide USAN, INN, BAN *vaccine adjuvant*
10 Benzagel; 5 Benzagel gel ℞ *keratolytic for acne* [benzoyl peroxide] 10%; 5%
10% LMD IV injection ℞ *plasma volume expander for shock due to hemorrhage, burns, or surgery* [dextran 40] 10%
tenamfetamine INN
Tencet capsules ℞ *analgesic; antipyretic; sedative* [acetaminophen; caffeine; butalbital] 325•40•50 mg

Tencon capsules ℞ *analgesic* [acetaminophen; butalbital] 650•50 mg

tendamistat INN

Tenecrin ℞ *investigational agent for cancer chemotherapy, infectious and autoimmune diseases* [tumor necrosis factor]

Tenex tablets ℞ *antihypertensive; antiadrenergic* [guanfacine HCl] 1, 2 mg

tenidap USAN, INN *anti-inflammatory for osteoarthritis and rheumatoid arthritis; cytokine inhibitor*

tenidap sodium USAN *anti-inflammatory for osteoarthritis and rheumatoid arthritis*

tenilapine INN

teniloxazine INN

tenilsetam INN

teniposide USAN, INN, BAN *antineoplastic; for refractory childhood acute lymphocytic leukemia (orphan)*

Ten-K controlled-release tablets ℞ *potassium supplement* [potassium chloride] 750 mg (10 mEq)

tenoate INN *combining name for radicals or groups*

tenocyclidine INN

Tenol-Plus tablets (discontinued 1995) OTC *analgesic; antipyretic; anti-inflammatory* [acetaminophen; aspirin; caffeine] 250•250•65 mg

tenonitrozole INN

Tenoretic 50; Tenoretic 100 tablets ℞ *antihypertensive* [chlorthalidone; atenolol] 25•50 mg; 25•100 mg

Tenormin tablets, IV injection ℞ *antianginal; antihypertensive; β-blocker* [atenolol] 25, 50, 100 mg; 5 mg/10 mL

tenoxicam USAN, INN, BAN *anti-inflammatory*

Tensilon IV or IM injection ℞ *myasthenia gravis treatment; antidote to curare-type overdose* [edrophonium chloride] 10 mg/mL

Ten-Tab (trademarked dosage form) *controlled-release tablet*

Tenuate tablets, Dospan (controlled-release tablets) ℞ *anorexiant* [diethylpropion HCl] 25 mg; 75 mg

tenylidone INN

teoclate INN *combining name for radicals or groups* [also: theoclate]

teopranitol INN

teoprolol INN

T.E.P. tablets OTC *antiasthmatic; bronchodilator; decongestant; sedative* [theophylline; ephedrine HCl; phenobarbital]

Tepanil tablets, Ten-tab (sustained-release tablets) (discontinued 1995) ℞ *anorexiant* [diethylpropion HCl] 25 mg; 75 mg ⓓ Temaril; Tofranil

tepirindole INN

tepoxalin USAN, INN *antipsoriatic; investigational anti-inflammatory for rheumatoid arthritis*

teprenone INN

teprosilate INN *combining name for radicals or groups*

teprotide USAN, INN *angiotensin-converting enzyme (ACE) inhibitor*

Terak ophthalmic ointment ℞ *ophthalmic antibiotic* [oxytetracycline HCl; polymyxin B sulfate] 5 mg•10,000 U per g

Terazol 3 vaginal suppositories, vaginal cream ℞ *antifungal* [terconazole] 80 mg; 0.8%

Terazol 7 vaginal cream ℞ *antifungal* [terconazole] 0.4%

terazosin INN, BAN *antihypertensive; $α_1$-adrenergic blocker* [also: terazosin HCl]

terazosin HCl USAN *antihypertensive; $α_1$-adrenergic blocker* [also: terazosin]

terbinafine USAN, INN, BAN *antifungal*

terbinafine HCl *antifungal*

terbium *element (Tb)*

terbucromil INN

terbufibrol INN

terbuficin INN

terbuprol INN

terbutaline INN, BAN *bronchodilator* [also: terbutaline sulfate]

terbutaline sulfate USAN, USP *bronchodilator* [also: terbutaline]

terciprazine INN

terconazole USAN, INN, BAN *antifungal*

terephthalamidine *investigational antineoplastic*

terfenadine USAN, USP, INN *antihistamine*

terfenadine carboxylate *investigational antihistamine with fewer drug interactions than terfenadine (Seldane)*

terflavoxate INN

terfluranol INN
terguride INN *investigational dopamine agonist for central nervous system disorders*
teriparatide INN *diagnostic aid for hypocalcemia (orphan)* [also: teriparatide acetate]
teriparatide acetate USAN *diagnostic aid for hypocalcemia* [also: teriparatide]
terizidone INN
terlakiren USAN *antihypertensive; renin inhibitor*
terlipressin INN, BAN *(orphan: bleeding esophageal varices)*
ternidazole INN
terodiline INN, BAN, JAN *coronary vasodilator* [also: terodiline HCl]
terodiline HCl USAN *coronary vasodilator; investigational agent for urinary incontinence* [also: terodiline]
terofenamate INN
teroxalene INN *antischistosomal* [also: teroxalene HCl]
teroxalene HCl USAN *antischistosomal* [also: teroxalene]
teroxirone USAN, INN *antineoplastic*
terpin hydrate USP *(disapproved for use as an expectorant in 1991)* 85 mg/5 mL oral
Terpin-Dex elixir (discontinued 1992) OTC *antitussive; expectorant* [dextromethorphan hydrobromide; terpin hydrate]
terpinol [see: terpin hydrate]
Terra-Cortril eye drop suspension ℞ *topical ophthalmic corticosteroidal anti-inflammatory; antibiotic* [hydrocortisone acetate; oxytetracycline HCl] 1.5%•0.5%
terrafungine [see: oxytetracycline]
Terramycin capsules ℞ *tetracycline-type antibiotic* [oxytetracycline HCl] 250 mg ⚕ Garamycin
Terramycin IM injection ℞ *tetracycline-type antibiotic* [oxytetracycline; lidocaine] 50 mg•2%, 125 mg•2% per mL
Terramycin with Polymyxin B ophthalmic ointment ℞ *ophthalmic antibiotic* [oxytetracycline HCl; polymyxin B sulfate] 5 mg•10,000 U per g

Terramycin with Polymyxin B vaginal tablets (discontinued 1992) ℞ *topical antibiotic* [oxytetracycline HCl; polymyxin B sulfate]
Tersaseptic shampoo/cleanser OTC *soap-free therapeutic cleanser*
tertatolol INN, BAN
tertiary amyl alcohol [see: amylene hydrate]
tert-pentyl alcohol [see: amylene hydrate]
Tesamone IM injection ℞ *androgen replacement for delayed puberty or breast cancer* [testosterone] 100 mg/mL
tesicam USAN, INN *anti-inflammatory*
tesimide USAN, INN *anti-inflammatory*
Teslac tablets ℞ *adjunctive hormonal chemotherapy for advanced postmenopausal breast carcinoma* [testolactone] 50 mg
TESPA (triethylenethiophosphoramide) [see: thiotepa]
Tessalon Perles (capsules) ℞ *antitussive* [benzonatate] 100 mg
Test Pack kit for professional use *in vitro diagnostic aid for Group A streptococcal antigens in throat swabs* [enzyme immunoassay]
Testandro IM injection ℞ *androgen replacement for delayed puberty or breast cancer* [testosterone] 100 mg/mL
Tes-Tape reagent strips for home use (discontinued 1996) OTC *in vitro diagnostic aid for urine glucose*
Test-Estro Cypionates IM injection ℞ *estrogen/androgen for menopausal vasomotor symptoms* [estradiol cypionate; testosterone cypionate] 2•50 mg/mL
Testex IM injection (discontinued 1994) ℞ *androgen replacement for delayed puberty or breast cancer* [testosterone propionate] 100 mg/mL
Testoderm transdermal patch (for scrotal area) ℞ *hormone replacement therapy for hypogonadism* [testosterone] 4, 6 mg/day (10, 15 mg)
testolactone USAN, USP, INN *antineoplastic; androgen hormone* ⚕ testosterone
Testone LA 100; Testone LA 200 IM injection (discontinued 1994) ℞ *androgen replacement for delayed puberty or breast cancer* [testosterone ethanate] 100 mg/mL; 200 mg/mL

Testopel pellets for subcu implantation ℞ *hormone replacement therapy for hypogonadism* [testosterone] 75 mg

testosterone USP, INN, BAN *androgen (orphan: sublingual treatment of growth and puberty delay in boys)* ⓢ testolactone

Testosterone Aqueous IM injection ℞ *androgen for hypogonadism, delayed puberty, and androgen-responsive metastatic cancers* [testosterone] 25, 50, 100 mg/mL

testosterone cyclopentanepropionate [see: testosterone cypionate]

testosterone cyclopentylpropionate [see: testosterone cypionate]

testosterone cypionate USP *parenteral androgen* 100, 200 mg/mL

testosterone enanthate USP *parenteral androgen* 100, 200 mg/mL injection

testosterone heptanoate [see: testosterone enanthate]

testosterone ketolaurate USAN, INN *androgen*

testosterone 3-oxododecanoate [see: testosterone ketolaurate]

testosterone phenylacetate USAN *androgen*

testosterone propionate USP *parenteral androgen; (orphan: vulvar dystrophies)* 100 mg/mL injection

TestPack [see: Abbott TestPack]

Testred capsules ℞ *androgen for male hypogonadism, impotence and breast cancer* [methyltestosterone] 10 mg

Testred Cypionate IM injection (discontinued 1994) ℞ *androgen replacement for delayed puberty or breast cancer* [testosterone cypionate] 200 mg/mL

Testrin PA IM injection (discontinued 1994) ℞ *androgen replacement for delayed puberty or breast cancer* [testosterone enanthate] 200 mg/mL

tetanus antitoxin USP *passive immunizing agent*

tetanus & gas gangrene antitoxins NF

tetanus & gas gangrene polyvalent antitoxin [see: tetanus & gas gangrene antitoxins]

tetanus immune globulin USP *passive immunizing agent*

tetanus immune human globulin [now: tetanus immune globulin]

tetanus toxoid USP *active immunizing agent*

tetanus toxoid, adsorbed USP *active immunizing agent*

tetiothalein sodium [see: iodophthalein sodium]

tetnicoran [see: nicofurate]

tetrabarbital INN

tetrabenazine INN, BAN

TetraBriks (trademarked delivery form) *ready-to-use liquid containers*

tetracaine USP, INN *topical local anesthetic* [also: amethocaine]

tetracaine HCl USP, JAN *topical local anesthetic* [also: amethocaine HCl]

Tetracap capsules ℞ *broad-spectrum antibiotic* [tetracycline HCl] 250 mg

tetrachloroethylene USP

tetrachloromethane [see: carbon tetrachloride]

Tetraclear eye drops OTC *topical ocular vasoconstrictor* [tetrahydrozoline HCl; sodium borate; boric acid; sodium chloride]

tetracosactide INN *adrenocorticotropic hormone* [also: cosyntropin; tetracosactrin]

tetracosactrin BAN *adrenocorticotropic hormone* [also: cosyntropin; tetracosactide]

tetracycline USP, INN, BAN *bacteriostatic antibiotic; antirickettsial*

tetracycline HCl USP *bacteriostatic antibiotic; antirickettsial* 100, 250, 500 mg oral; 125 mg/5 mL oral

tetracycline phosphate complex USP, BAN *antibacterial*

Tetracyn; Tetracyn 500 capsules ℞ *antibiotic* [tetracycline HCl]

tetradecanoic acid, methylethyl ester [see: isopropyl myristate]

tetradonium bromide INN

tetraethylammonium bromide (TEAB) [see: tetrylammonium bromide]

tetraethylammonium chloride (TEAC)

tetraethylthiuram disulfide [see: disulfiram]

tetrafilcon A USAN *hydrophilic contact lens material*
tetraglycine hydroperiodide *source of iodine for disinfecting water*
tetrahydroaminoacridine (THA) [see: tacrine HCl]
tetrahydrocannabinol (THC) [see: dronabinol]
tetrahydrolipstatin [see: orlistat]
tetrahydrozoline BAN *vasoconstrictor; nasal decongestant; topical ocular decongestant* [also: tetrhydrozoline HCl; tetryzoline] 0.05% eye drops
tetrahydrozoline HCl USP *vasoconstrictor; nasal decongestant; topical ocular decongestant* [also: tetryzoline; tetrahydrozoline]
tetraiodophenolphthalein sodium [see: iodophthalein sodium]
Tetralan syrup ℞ *broad-spectrum antibiotic* [tetracycline HCl] 125 mg/5 mL
Tetralan "250"; Tetralan-500 capsules ℞ *broad-spectrum antibiotic* [tetracycline HCl] 250 mg; 500 mg
tetrallobarbital [see: butalbital]
Tetram capsules (discontinued 1996) ℞ *broad-spectrum antibiotic* [tetracycline HCl] 250 mg
tetramal [see: tetrabarbital]
tetrameprozine [see: aminopromazine]
tetramethrin INN
tetramethylene dimethanesulfonate [see: busulfan]
tetramisole INN *anthelmintic* [also: tetramisole HCl]
tetramisole HCl USAN *anthelmintic* [also: tetramisole]
Tetramune IM injection ℞ *pediatric vaccine for diphtheria, pertussis, tetanus and Haemophilus influenzae type b* [diphtheria & tetanus toxoids & whole-cell pertussis vaccine; Hemophilus b conjugate vaccine (DTwP-Hib)] 0.5 mL
tetranitrol [see: erythrityl tetranitrate]
tetrantoin
TetraPaks (trademarked delivery form) *ready-to-use open system containers*
Tetrasine; Tetrasine Extra eye drops OTC *topical ocular decongestant/vasoconstrictor* [tetrahydrozoline HCl] 0.05%

tetrasodium ethylenediaminetetraacetate [see: edetate sodium]
tetrasodium pyrophosphate [see: sodium pyrophosphate]
tetrazepam INN
tetrazolast meglumine USAN *antiallergic; antiasthmatic; investigational mediator-release inhibitor*
tetridamine INN *analgesic; anti-inflammatory* [also: tetrydamine]
tetriprofen INN
tetrofosmin USAN, INN, BAN *diagnostic aid*
tetronasin BAN [also: tetronasin 5930]
tetronasin 5930 INN [also: tetronasin]
tetroquinone USAN, INN *systemic keratolytic*
tetroxoprim USAN, INN *antibacterial*
tetrydamine USAN *analgesic; anti-inflammatory* [also: tetridamine]
tetrylammonium bromide INN
tetryzoline INN *vasoconstrictor; nasal decongestant; topical ocular decongestant* [also: tetrahydrozoline HCl; tetrahydrozoline]
tetryzoline HCl [see: tetrahydrozoline HCl]
Texacort solution ℞ *topical corticosteroid* [hydrocortisone] 1%
texacromil INN
6-TG (6-thioguanine) [see: thioguanine]
TG (thyroglobulin) [q.v.]
T/Gel Scalp Solution gel (discontinued 1992) OTC *topical antipsoriatic; antiseborrheic; keratolytic* [coal tar solution; salicylic acid]
T-Gen suppositories, pediatric suppositories ℞ *anticholinergic; antiemetic* [trimethobenzamide HCl] 200 mg; 100 mg
T-Gesic capsules ℞ *narcotic analgesic* [hydrocodone bitartrate; acetaminophen] 5•500 mg
αTGI (α-triglycidyl isocyanurate) [see: teroxirone]
TH (theophylline) [q.v.]
TH (thyroid hormone) [see: levothyroxine sodium]
THA (tetrahydroaminoacridine) [see: tacrine HCl]

thalidomide USAN, INN, BAN *sedative; hypnotic;* (*orphan: bone marrow graft vs. host disease; leprosy; mycobacterial infections*)

Thalitone tablets ℞ *diuretic; antihypertensive* [chlorthalidone] 15, 25 mg

thallium *element (Tl)* ⑨ Valium

thallous chloride Tl 201 USAN, USP *radiopaque medium; radioactive agent*

Tham IV infusion ℞ *corrects systemic acidosis associated with cardiac bypass surgery or cardiac arrest* [tromethamine] 18 g/500 mL (150 mEq/500 mL)

Tham-E powder for IV infusion (discontinued 1992) ℞ *corrects systemic acidosis associated with cardiac bypass surgery or cardiac arrest* [tromethamine]

thaumatin BAN

THC (tetrahydrocannabinol) [see: dronabinol]

THC (thiocarbanidin)

thebacon INN, BAN

Theelin Aqueous IM injection (discontinued 1995) ℞ *estrogen replacement therapy; antineoplastic for prostatic and breast cancer* [estrone] 2 mg/mL

theine [see: caffeine]

thenalidine INN

thenium closilate INN *veterinary anthelmintic* [also: thenium closylate]

thenium closylate USAN *veterinary anthelmintic* [also: thenium closilate]

thenyldiamine INN

thenylpyramine HCl [see: methapyrilene HCl]

Theo-24 timed-release capsules ℞ *bronchodilator* [theophylline] 100, 200, 300 mg

Theobid Duracaps (sustained-release capsules) ℞ *bronchodilator* [theophylline] 260 mg

Theobid Jr. Duracaps (sustained-release capsules) ℞ *bronchodilator* [theophylline] 130 mg

theobromine NF

theobromine calcium salicylate NF

theobromine sodium acetate NF

theobromine sodium salicylate NF

Theochron extended-release tablets ℞ *bronchodilator* [theophylline] 100, 200, 300 mg

theoclate BAN *combining name for radicals or groups* [also: teoclate]

Theoclear L.A. extended-release capsules ℞ *bronchodilator* [theophylline] 130, 260 mg

Theoclear-80 oral solution ℞ *bronchodilator* [theophylline] 80 mg/15 mL ⑨ Theolair

theodrenaline INN, BAN

Theodrine tablets OTC *antiasthmatic; bronchodilator; decongestant* [theophylline; ephedrine HCl] 120•22.5 mg

Theo-Dur extended-release tablets ℞ *bronchodilator* [theophylline] 100, 200, 300, 450 mg

Theo-Dur Sprinkle sustained-release capsules (discontinued 1996) ℞ *bronchodilator* [theophylline] 50, 75, 125, 200 mg

Theofedral tablets (discontinued 1992) ℞ *antiasthmatic* [theophylline; ephedrine HCl]

theofibrate USAN *antihyperlipoproteinemic* [also: etofylline clofibrate]

Theo-G capsules (discontinued 1993) ℞ *antiasthmatic; bronchodilator; expectorant* [theophylline; guaifenesin]

Theolair tablets, liquid ℞ *antiasthmatic* [theophylline] 125, 250 mg; 80 mg/15 mL ⑨ Theoclear; Thyrolar

Theolair-SR sustained-release tablets ℞ *antiasthmatic* [theophylline] 200, 250, 300, 500 mg

Theolate liquid ℞ *antiasthmatic; bronchodilator; expectorant* [theophylline; guaifenesin] 150•90 mg/15 mL

Theomax DF pediatric syrup ℞ *antiasthmatic; bronchodilator; decongestant; anxiolytic* [theophylline; ephedrine sulfate; hydroxyzine HCl; alcohol 5%] 97.5•18.75•7.5 mg/15 mL

Theo-Organidin elixir (discontinued 1995) ℞ *antiasthmatic; bronchodilator; expectorant* [theophylline; iodinated glycerol] 8•2 mg/mL

theophyldine [see: aminophylline]

theophyllamine [see: aminophylline]

Theophyllin KI elixir ℞ *antiasthmatic; bronchodilator; expectorant* [theophylline; potassium iodide] 80•130 mg/15 mL

theophylline (TH) USP, BAN *bronchodilator* 100, 125, 200, 300 mg oral; 80 mg/15 mL oral

theophylline aminoisobutanol [see: ambuphylline]

theophylline calcium salicylate *bronchodilator*

theophylline ethylenediamine [now: aminophylline]

Theophylline Extended-Release tablets ℞ *bronchodilator* [theophylline] 450 mg

theophylline monohydrate [see: theophylline]

theophylline olamine USP

theophylline sodium acetate NF

theophylline sodium glycinate USP *smooth muscle relaxant*

Theo-R-Gen elixir (discontinued 1993) ℞ *antiasthmatic; bronchodilator; expectorant* [theophylline; iodinated glycerol]

Theo-Sav controlled-release tablets ℞ *bronchodilator* [theophylline] 100, 200, 300 mg

Theospan-SR timed-release capsules ℞ *bronchodilator* [theophylline] 130, 260 mg

Theostat 80 syrup ℞ *bronchodilator* [theophylline; alcohol 1%] 80 mg/15 mL

Theotal tablets (discontinued 1993) OTC *antiasthmatic; bronchodilator; decongestant; sedative* [theophylline; ephedrine HCl; phenobarbital]

Theovent timed-release capsules ℞ *bronchodilator* [theophylline] 125, 250 mg

Theo-X controlled-release tablets ℞ *bronchodilator* [theophylline] 100, 200, 300 mg

Theozine tablets ℞ *bronchodilator; antihistamine; decongestant* [theophylline; hydroxyzine HCl; ephedrine sulfate]

Thera Hematinic tablets OTC *hematinic; vitamin supplement* [ferrous fumarate; multiple vitamins; folic acid] 66.7•≛•0.33 mg

Thera Multi-Vitamin liquid OTC *vitamin supplement* [multiple vitamins] ≛

Therabid tablets OTC *vitamin supplement* [multiple vitamins] ≛

Therac lotion OTC *topical acne treatment* [colloidal sulfur] 10%

theraccine *investigational antineoplastic for disseminated melanoma*

Thera-Combex H P Kapseals (capsules) (discontinued 1992) OTC *vitamin supplement* [multiple B vitamins; vitamin C]

TheraCys freeze-dried suspension for intravesical injection ℞ *antineoplastic for urinary bladder cancer* [BCG vaccine, live] 27 mg

TheraDerm-LRS transdermal patch ℞ *investigational hormonal therapy for hypogonadism* [testosterone]

Therafectin ℞ *investigational anti-inflammatory for rheumatoid arthritis* [amiprilose]

TheraFlu Flu, Cold & Cough; NightTime TheraFlu powder for oral solution OTC *antitussive; decongestant; antihistamine; analgesic* [dextromethorphan hydrobromide; pseudoephedrine HCl; chlorpheniramine maleate; acetaminophen] 20•60•4•650 mg/packet; 30•60•4•1000 mg/packet ⊡ Thera-Flur

TheraFlu Flu & Cold Medicine powder for oral solution OTC *decongestant; antihistamine; analgesic* [pseudoephedrine HCl; chlorpheniramine maleate; acetaminophen] 60•4•650 mg/packet

TheraFlu Non-Drowsy powder for oral solution (name changed to TheraFlu Non-Drowsy Flu, Cold & Cough in 1995)

TheraFlu Non-Drowsy Flu, Cold & Cough powder for oral solution OTC *antitussive; decongestant; analgesic* [dextromethorphan hydrobromide; pseudoephedrine HCl; acetaminophen] 30•60•100 mg/packet

TheraFlu Non-Drowsy Formula caplets OTC *antitussive; decongestant; analgesic* [dextromethorphan hydrobromide; pseudoephedrine HCl; acetaminophen] 15•30•500 mg

Thera-Flur; Thera-Flur-N gel drops (for self-application) ℞ *dental caries preventative* [sodium fluoride] 1.1% ⊡ TheraFlu

Theragenerix tablets (name changed to Therapeutic in 1995)

Theragenerix-H tablets (name changed to Therapeutic-H in 1995)

Theragenerix-M tablets (name changed to Therapeutic-M in 1995)

Thera-Gesic cream OTC *counterirritant* [methyl salicylate; menthol] 15%•⚠

Theragran caplets OTC *vitamin supplement* [multiple vitamins; folic acid; biotin] ±•400•30 µg

Theragran liquid OTC *vitamin supplement* [multiple vitamins] ± 🗩 Phenergan

Theragran AntiOxidant softgels OTC *vitamin/mineral supplement* [vitamins A, C, and E; multiple minerals] 5000 IU•250 mg•200 IU•±

Theragran Hematinic tablets ℞ *hematinic; vitamin/mineral supplement* [ferrous fumarate; multiple vitamins and minerals; folic acid] 66.7•±•0.33 mg

Theragran Jr. with Iron chewable tablets (discontinued 1992) OTC *vitamin/iron supplement* [multiple vitamins; iron; folic acid]

Theragran Stress Formula tablets OTC *vitamin/iron supplement* [multiple B vitamins; vitamins C and E; ferrous fumarate; folic acid; biotin] ±•600 mg•30 IU•27 mg•0.4 mg•45 µg

Theragran-M caplets OTC *vitamin/mineral/calcium/iron supplement* [multiple vitamins & minerals; calcium; iron; folic acid; biotin] ±•40•27•0.4•0.03 mg

Thera-Hist powder (discontinued 1993) OTC *decongestant; antihistamine; analgesic* [pseudoephedrine HCl; chlorpheniramine maleate; acetaminophen]

Thera-Hist syrup OTC *decongestant; antihistamine* [phenylpropanolamine HCl; chlorpheniramine maleate] 12.5•2 mg/5 mL

Thera-Ject (trademarked delivery system) *prefilled disposable syringe*

Thera-M tablets OTC *vitamin/mineral/iron supplement* [multiple vitamins & minerals; iron; folic acid; biotin] ±•27 mg•0.4 mg•35 µg

Theramill Forte capsules OTC *vitamin replacement therapy* [multiple vitamins & minerals]

Theramine Expectorant liquid OTC *decongestant; expectorant* [phenylpropanolamine HCl; guaifenesin] 12.5•100 mg/5 mL

Theramycin Z topical solution ℞ *topical antibiotic for acne* [erythromycin] 2%

Therapeutic tablets OTC *vitamin supplement* [multiple vitamins; folic acid; biotin] ±•400•30 µg

Therapeutic B with C capsules OTC *vitamin supplement* [multiple B vitamins; vitamin C] ±•300 mg

Therapeutic Bath lotion, oil OTC *moisturizer; emollient*

Therapeutic Mineral Ice; Therapeutic Mineral Ice Exercise Formula gel OTC *counterirritant* [menthol] 2%; 4%

Therapeutic-H tablets OTC *hematinic; vitamin supplement* [ferrous fumarate; multiple vitamins; folic acid] 66.7•±•0.33 mg

Therapeutic-M tablets OTC *vitamin/mineral/iron supplement* [multiple vitamins & minerals; iron; folic acid; biotin] ±•27 mg•0.4 mg•30 µg

Theraplex T shampoo OTC *antiseborrheic; antipsoriatic; antipruritic; antibacterial* [coal tar] 1%

Theraplex Z shampoo OTC *antiseborrheic; antibacterial; antifungal* [pyrithione zinc] 2%

Theravee tablets OTC *vitamin supplement* [multiple vitamins; folic acid; biotin] ±•400•15 µg

Theravee Hematinic tablets OTC *hematinic; vitamin supplement* [ferrous fumarate; multiple vitamins; folic acid] 66.7•±•0.33 mg

Theravee-M tablets OTC *vitamin/mineral/iron supplement* [multiple vitamins & minerals; iron; folic acid; biotin] ±•27 mg•0.4 mg•15 µg

Theravim tablets OTC *vitamin supplement* [multiple vitamins; folic acid; biotin] ±•400•35 µg

Theravim-M tablets OTC *vitamin/mineral/iron supplement* [multiple vitamins & minerals; iron; folic acid; biotin] ± •27 mg•0.4 mg•30 μg

Theravir ℞ *investigational anti-HIV drug* [monoclonal antibodies]

Theravite liquid OTC *vitamin supplement* [multiple vitamins] ± ② Therevac

Theravit-M tablets OTC *vitamin/mineral supplement* [multiple vitamins & minerals]

Theravits tablets OTC *vitamin supplement* [multiple vitamins]

Therems tablets OTC *vitamin supplement* [multiple vitamins; folic acid; biotin] ± •400•15 μg

Therems-M tablets OTC *vitamin/mineral/iron supplement* [multiple vitamins & minerals; iron; folic acid; biotin] ± •27 mg•0.4 mg•30 μg

Therevac-Plus suppository enema OTC *laxative; stool softener* [docusate sodium; benzocaine] 283•20 mg ② Theravite

Therevac-SB suppository enema OTC *laxative; stool softener* [docusate sodium] 283 mg

Therfectin ℞ *investigational treatment for rheumatoid arthritis* [amiprilose]

Theri bath oil OTC *emollient* [mineral oil; PEG; 4-dilaurate; lanolin oil; benzophenone-3]

Theri-Care lotion OTC *moisturizer; emollient* [mineral oil; propylene glycol; lanolin; trolamine; alcohol]

Thermax gel ℞ *investigational vulnerary for bed sores, chronic skin ulcers, and other wounds*

Thermazene cream ℞ *broad-spectrum bactericidal for adjunctive burn treatment* [silver sulfadiazine] 10 mg/g

ThermoRub ointment, lotion (discontinued 1992) OTC *counterirritant; topical analgesic* [methyl nicotinate; histamine dihydrochloride; salicylamide; dipropylene glycol salicylate; capsicum]

Theroxide lotion (discontinued 1994) ℞ *topical keratolytic for acne* [benzoyl peroxide]

Theroxide wash (discontinued 1994) ℞ *topical keratolytic for acne* [benzoyl peroxide] 10%

ThexForte caplets OTC *vitamin supplement* [multiple B vitamins; vitamin C] ± •500 mg

THF (thymic humoral factor) [q.v.]

thiabendazole (TBZ) USAN, USP *anthelmintic* [also: tiabendazole]

thiabutazide [see: buthiazide]

thiacetarsamide sodium INN

thiacetazone BAN [also: thioacetazone]

Thiacide film-coated tablets (discontinued 1994) ℞ *urinary anti-infective; acidifier* [methenamine mandelate; potassium acid phosphate] 500•250 mg ② Dyazide; thiazides

thialbarbital INN [also: thialbarbitone]

thialbarbitone BAN [also: thialbarbital]

thialisobumal sodium [see: buthalital sodium]

thiamazole INN *thyroid inhibitor* [also: methimazole]

thiambutosine INN, BAN

Thiamilate enteric-coated tablets OTC *vitamin supplement* [thiamine HCl] 20 mg

thiamine INN *vitamin B_1; enzyme cofactor* [also: thiamine HCl]

thiamine HCl USP *vitamin B_1; enzyme cofactor* [also: thiamine] 50, 100, 250, 500 mg oral; 100 mg/mL injection

thiamine mononitrate USP *vitamin B_1; enzyme cofactor*

thiamine propyl disulfide [see: prosultiamine]

thiamiprine USAN *antineoplastic* [also: tiamiprine]

thiamphenicol USAN, INN, BAN *antibacterial*

thiamylal USP *general anesthetic*

thiamylal sodium USP, JAN *general anesthetic*

thiazesim HCl USAN *antidepressant* [also: tiazesim]

thiazinamium chloride USAN *antiallergic*

thiazinamium metilsulfate INN

4-thiazolidinecarboxylic acid [see: timonacic]

thiazolsulfone [see: thiazosulfone]

thiazosulfone INN

thiazothielite [see: antienite]

thiazothienol [see: antazonite]

thiethylperazine USAN, INN *antiemetic; antidopaminergic*
thiethylperazine malate USP *antiemetic; antipsychotic*
thiethylperazine maleate USAN, USP *antiemetic*
thihexinol methylbromide NF, INN
thimerfonate sodium USAN *topical anti-infective* [also: sodium timerfonate]
thimerosal USP *topical anti-infective; preservative (49% mercury)* [also: thiomersal] 1:1000 topical
thioacetazone INN, DCF [also: thiacetazone]
thiocarbanidin (THC)
thiocarlide BAN [also: tiocarlide]
thiocolchicine glycoside [see: thiocolchicoside]
thiocolchicoside INN
thiocyanate sodium NF
thiodiglycol INN
thiodiphenylamine [see: phenothiazine]
thiofuradene INN
thioguanine (6-TG) USAN, USP *antimetabolic antineoplastic* [also: tioguanine] 40 mg oral
thiohexallymal [see: thialbarbital]
thiohexamide INN
Thiola tablets ℞ *prevention of cystine nephrolithiasis in homozygous cystinuria (orphan)* [tiopronin] 100 mg
thiomebumal sodium [see: thiopental sodium]
thiomersal INN, BAN *topical anti-infective; preservative* [also: thimerosal]
thiomesterone BAN [also: tiomesterone]
thiomicid [see: thioacetazone; thiacetazone]
thioparamizone [see: thioacetazone; thiacetazone]
thiopental sodium USP, INN, JAN *general anesthetic; anticonvulsant* [also: thiopentone sodium] 20, 25 mg/mL (2%, 2.5%) injection
thiopentone sodium BAN *general anesthetic; anticonvulsant* [also: thiopental sodium]
thiophanate BAN
thiophosphoramide [see: thiotepa]
Thioplex powder for IV, intracavitary, or intravesical injection ℞ *alkylating antineoplastic for lymphomas and carcinoma of the breast, ovary, or bladder* [thiotepa] 15 mg
thiopropazate INN [also: thiopropazate HCl]
thiopropazate HCl NF [also: thiopropazate]
thioproperazine INN, BAN [also: thioproperazine mesylate]
thioproperazine mesylate [also: thioproperazine]
thioproperazine methanesulfonate [see: thioproperazine mesylate]
thioridazine USAN, USP, INN *antipsychotic; sedative*
thioridazine HCl USP *antipsychotic; sedative* 10, 15, 25, 50, 100, 150, 200 mg oral; 30, 100 mg/mL oral
thiosalan USAN *disinfectant* [also: tiosalan]
Thiosulfil Forte tablets ℞ *broad-spectrum bacteriostatic* [sulfamethizole] 500 mg
thiosulfuric acid, disodium salt pentahydrate [see: sodium thiosulfate]
thiotepa USP, INN *alkylating antineoplastic*
thiotetrabarbital INN
thiothixene USAN, USP, BAN *antipsychotic* [also: tiotixene] 1, 2, 5, 10, 20 mg oral
thiothixene HCl USAN, USP *antipsychotic* 5 mg/mL oral
thiouracil
thiourea *antioxidant*
thioxolone BAN [also: tioxolone]
thiphenamil HCl USAN *smooth muscle relaxant* [also: tifenamil]
thiphencillin potassium USAN *antibacterial* [also: tifencillin]
thiram USAN, INN *antifungal*
Thiuretic tablets (discontinued 1993) ℞ *diuretic; antihypertensive* [hydrochlorothiazide]
Thixo-Flur topical gel (for professional application) ℞ *dental caries preventative* [acidulated phosphate fluoride]
thonzonium bromide USAN, USP *detergent* [also: tonzonium bromide]
thonzylamine HCl USAN, INN
Thorazine tablets, Spansules (capsules), IV or IM injection, syrup,

suppositories, concentrate ℞ *tranquilizer; antiemetic* [chlorpromazine] 10, 25, 50, 100, 200 mg; 30, 75, 150, 200, 300 mg; 25 mg/mL; 10 mg/5 mL; 25, 50 mg; 30, 100 mg/mL

Thorets throat lozenges OTC *topical oral anesthetic* [benzocaine]

thorium *element (Th)*

thozalinone USAN *antidepressant* [also: tozalinone]

THQ (tetrahydroxybenzoquinone) [see: tetroquinone]

THR (trishydroxyethyl rutin) [see: troxerutin]

Threamine DM syrup OTC *antitussive; decongestant; antihistamine* [dextromethorphan hydrobromide; phenylpropanolamine HCl; chlorpheniramine maleate] 10•12.5•2 mg/5 mL

Threamine Expectorant liquid OTC *decongestant; expectorant* [phenylpropanolamine HCl; guaifenesin; alcohol 5%] 12.5•100 mg/5 mL

3 in 1 Toothache Relief gum, liquid, lotion/gel OTC *topical oral anesthetic* [benzocaine]

3118 *investigational antibacterial antibiotic*

311C *investigational antimigraine agent*

348U *investigational antiviral*

3TC [now: lamivudine]

threonine (L-threonine) USAN, USP, INN *essential amino acid; (orphan: spasticity; amyotrophic lateral sclerosis); symbols: Thr, T* 500 mg oral

Threostat ℞ *(orphan: familial spastic paraparesis; amyotrophic lateral sclerosis)* [L-threonine] ② Triostat

Throat Discs lozenges OTC *analgesic; counterirritant* [capsicum; peppermint oil]

Thrombate III ℞ *congenital antithrombin III deficiency (orphan)* [antithrombin III, human]

thrombin USP, INN *topical local hemostatic*

Thrombinar powder ℞ *topical local hemostatic for surgery* [thrombin] 1000, 5000, 50,000 U

Thrombin-JMI powder ℞ *topical local hemostatic for surgery* [thrombin] 10,000, 20,000, 50,000 U

thrombinogen (prothrombin)

Thrombogen powder ℞ *topical local hemostatic for surgery* [thrombin] 1000, 5000, 10,000, 20,000 U

thrombolyse-inj 1500 *investigational tissue-cultured plasminogen activator for acute myocardial infarction*

thromboplastin USP

Thrombostat powder ℞ *topical local hemostatic for surgery* [thrombin] 5000, 10,000, 20,000 U

thromboxane inhibitor *investigational therapy for stroke and heart attack*

thulium *element (Tm)*

Thylline tablets ℞ *bronchodilator* [dyphylline]

Thylline-GG tablets (discontinued 1995) ℞ *antiasthmatic; bronchodilator; expectorant* [dyphylline; guaifenesin] 200•200 mg

thymalfasin USAN *vaccine enhancer for hepatitis, cancer, and infectious diseases*

thymic hormone factor *investigational agent for HIV, genital herpes, and hepatitis*

thymic humoral factor, gamma 2 *investigational (Phase II) immunomodulator for HIV*

thymocartin INN

thymoctonan INN *investigational antiviral for HIV infection, genital herpes, and chronic viral hepatitis*

thymol NF *stabilizer; topical antiseptic*

thymol iodide NF

Thymone ℞ *(orphan: amyotrophic lateral sclerosis)* [protirelin]

thymopentin USAN, INN, BAN *immunoregulator; investigational (Phase III) for HIV*

thymopoietin 32-36 [now: thymopentin]

thymosin alpha-1 [now: thymalfasin]

thymostimulin INN *investigational (Phase III) immunomodulator for AIDS*

thymotrinan INN

thymoxamine BAN [also: moxisylyte]

thymoxamine HCl *(orphan: phenylephrine-induced mydriasis)*

Thypinone IV injection ℞ *in vivo thyroid function test* [protirelin] 500 μg/mL

Thyrar tablets ℞ *thyroid replacement therapy; hypothyroidism; thyroid cancer*

[thyroid (bovine)] 30, 60, 120 mg ⓓ Thyrolar

Thyrel-TRH IV injection ℞ *in vivo thyroid function test* [protirelin] 500 μg/mL

Thyro-Block tablets ℞ *thyroid-blocking therapy* [potassium iodide] 130 mg

thyrocalcitonin [see: calcitonin]

Thyrogen ℞ *investigational thyroid stimulating hormone (orphan: diagnostic aid for thyroid cancer)* [thyrotropin]

thyroglobulin (TG) USAN, USP, INN *thyroid hormone*

thyroid USP *thyroid hormone* 15, 30, 60, 90, 120, 180, 240, 300 mg oral ⓓ euthroid

thyroid hormone (TH) [see: levothyroxine sodium]

thyroid stimulating hormone (TSH) [see: thyrotropin]

Thyroid Strong tablets ℞ *hypothyroidism; thyroid cancer* [thyroid, desiccated] 30, 60, 120, 180 mg

Thyrolar-0.25; -0.5; -1; -2; -3 tablets ℞ *thyroid hormone therapy* [liotrix] 15 mg; 30 mg; 60 mg; 120 mg; 180 mg ⓓ Theolair; Thyrar

thyromedan HCl USAN *thyromimetic* [also: tyromedan]

thyropropic acid INN

thyrotrophic hormone [see: thyrotrophin]

thyrotrophin INN *thyroid stimulating hormone* [also: thyrotropin]

thyrotropin *thyroid stimulating hormone; (orphan: diagnostic aid for thyroid cancer)* [also: thyrotrophin]

thyrotropin-releasing hormone (TRH) [see: protirelin]

thyroxine BAN *thyroid hormone* [also: levothyroxine sodium]

D-thyroxine [see: dextrothyroxine sodium]

L-thyroxine [see: levothyroxine sodium]

thyroxine I 125 USAN *radioactive agent*

thyroxine I 131 USAN *radioactive agent*

Thytropar powder for IM or subcu injection ℞ *thyrotrophic hormone; in vivo thyroid function test* [thyrotropin] 10 IU

TI-23 *investigational (Phase I) antiviral for cytomegalovirus retinitis*

tiabendazole INN *anthelmintic* [also: thiabendazole]

tiacrilast USAN, INN *antiallergic*

tiacrilast sodium USAN *antiallergic*

tiadenol INN

tiafibrate INN

tiagabine INN *investigational anticonvulsant*

tiamenidine USAN, INN *antihypertensive*

tiamenidine HCl USAN *antihypertensive*

tiametonium iodide INN

tiamiprine INN *antineoplastic* [also: thiamiprine]

tiamizide INN *diuretic; antihypertensive* [also: diapamide]

tiamulin USAN, INN *veterinary antibacterial*

tiamulin fumarate USAN *veterinary antibacterial*

tianafac INN

tianeptine INN

tiapamil INN, BAN *antagonist to calcium* [also: tiapamil HCl]

tiapamil HCl USAN *antagonist to calcium* [also: tiapamil]

tiapirinol INN

tiapride INN

tiaprofenic acid INN

tiaprost INN

tiaramide INN, BAN *antiasthmatic* [also: tiaramide HCl]

tiaramide HCl USAN *antiasthmatic* [also: tiaramide]

Tiazac extended-release capsules ℞ *antihypertensive; antianginal; calcium channel blocker* [diltiazem HCl] 120, 180, 240, 300, 360 mg

tiazesim INN *antidepressant* [also: thiazesim HCl]

tiazesim HCl [see: thiazesim HCl]

tiazofurin USAN *antineoplastic* [also: tiazofurine]

tiazofurine INN *antineoplastic* [also: tiazofurin]

Tiazole ℞ *investigational treatment for leukemia* [tiazofurin]

tiazuril USAN, INN *coccidiostat for poultry*

tibalosin INN

tibenelast sodium USAN *antiasthmatic; bronchodilator*

tibenzate INN

tibezonium iodide INN

tibolone USAN, INN, BAN *anabolic*

tibric acid USAN, INN *antihyperlipoproteinemic*

tibrofan USAN, INN *disinfectant*

ticabesone INN *glucocorticoid* [also: ticabesone propionate]

ticabesone propionate USAN *glucocorticoid* [also: ticabesone]

Ticar powder for IV or IM injection ℞ *extended-spectrum penicillin-type antibiotic* [ticarcillin disodium] 1, 3, 6, 20, 30 g ⓓ Tigan

ticarbodine USAN, INN *anthelmintic*

ticarcillin INN *antibacterial* [also: ticarcillin disodium]

ticarcillin cresyl sodium USAN *antibacterial*

ticarcillin disodium USAN, USP *bactericidal antibiotic* [also: ticarcillin]

Tice BCG percutaneous injection for TB, intravesical injection for cancer ℞ *tuberculosis immunizing agent; antineoplastic for bladder cancer* [BCG vaccine, Tice strain] 50 mg

ticlatone USAN, INN *antibacterial; antifungal*

Ticlid film-coated tablets ℞ *platelet aggregation inhibitor for stroke* [ticlopidine HCl] 250 mg

ticlopidine INN, BAN *platelet aggregation inhibitor* [also: ticlopidine HCl]

ticlopidine HCl USAN *platelet aggregation inhibitor* [also: ticlopidine]

Ticon IM injection ℞ *anticholinergic; antiemetic* [trimethobenzamide HCl] 100 mg/mL

ticrynafen USAN *diuretic; uricosuric; antihypertensive* [also: tienilic acid]

tidiacic INN

tiemonium iodide INN, BAN

tienilic acid INN *diuretic; uricosuric; antihypertensive* [also: ticrynafen]

tienocarbine INN

tienopramine INN

tienoxolol INN

tifemoxone INN

tifenamil INN *smooth muscle relaxant* [also: thiphenamil HCl]

tifenamil HCl [see: thiphenamil HCl]

tifencillin INN *antibacterial* [also: thiphencillin potassium]

tifencillin potassium [see: thiphencillin potassium]

tiflamizole INN

tiflorex INN

tifluadom INN

tiflucarbine INN

tiformin INN [also: tyformin]

tifurac INN *analgesic* [also: tifurac sodium]

tifurac sodium USAN *analgesic* [also: tifurac]

Tigan capsules, suppositories, pediatric suppositories, IM injection ℞ *antiemetic* [trimethobenzamide HCl] 100, 250 mg; 200 mg; 100 mg; 100 mg/mL ⓓ Ticar

tigemonam INN *antimicrobial* [also: tigemonam dicholine]

tigemonam dicholine USAN *antimicrobial* [also: tigemonam]

tigestol USAN, INN *progestin*

tigloidine INN, BAN

tiglyl*pseudo*tropine [see: tigloidine]

tiglyltropeine [see: tropigline]

Tiject-20 IM injection (discontinued 1992) ℞ *anticholinergic; antiemetic* [trimethobenzamide HCl] 100 mg/mL

tilactase INN *digestive enzyme*

Tilad (Spanish name for U.S. product Tilade)

Tilade oral inhalation aerosol ℞ *respiratory anti-inflammatory; antiasthmatic; bronchoconstriction inhibitor* [nedocromil sodium] 1.75 mg/dose

Tilarin nasal spray (commercially available in Germany) ℞ *investigational antiasthmatic* [nedocromil sodium]

Tilavist eye drops ℞ *investigational treatment for allergic conjunctivitis* [nedocromil sodium]

tilbroquinol INN

Tilcotil ℞ *investigational analgesic for postoperative and menstrual pain and juvenile arthritis* [tenoxicam]

tiletamine INN *anesthetic; anticonvulsant* [also: tiletamine HCl]

tiletamine HCl USAN *anesthetic; anticonvulsant* [also: tiletamine]

tilidate HCl BAN *analgesic* [also: tilidine HCl; tilidine]

tilidine INN *analgesic* [also: tilidine HCl; tilidate HCl]

tilidine HCl USAN *analgesic* [also: tilidine; tilidate HCl]
tiliquinol INN
tilisolol INN
tilmicosin USAN, INN, BAN *veterinary antibacterial*
tilmicosin phosphate USAN *veterinary antibacterial*
tilomisole USAN, INN *immunoregulator*
tilorone INN *antiviral* [also: tilorone HCl]
tilorone HCl USAN *antiviral* [also: tilorone]
tilozepine INN
tilsuprost INN
Tiltab (trademarked dosage form) *tablet*
tiludronate disodium USAN *bone resorption inhibitor for osteoporosis & Paget's disease*
tiludronic acid INN
Time-B-50 timed-release caplet OTC *vitamin supplement* [multiple B vitamins]
Time-C; Time-C-1500 timed-release capsules OTC *vitamin supplement* [vitamin C]
Timecap (trademarked dosage form) *sustained-release capsule*
Time-C-Bio timed-release caplet OTC *vitamin supplement* [vitamin C; bioflavonoids]
Timecelle (trademarked dosage form) *timed-release capsule*
timefurone USAN, INN *antiatherosclerotic*
timegadine INN
Time-Hist sustained-release capsules ℞ *decongestant; antihistamine* [pseudoephedrine HCl; chlorpheniramine maleate] 120•8 mg
timelotem INN
Timentin powder for IV injection ℞ *extended-spectrum penicillin-type antibiotic* [ticarcillin disodium; clavulanate potassium] 3•0.1 g
timepidium bromide INN
Timespan (trademarked dosage form) *timed-release tablets*
Timesules (dosage form) *sustained-release capsules*
timiperone INN
timobesone INN *topical adrenocortical steroid* [also: timobesone acetate]

timobesone acetate USAN *topical adrenocortical steroid* [also: timobesone]
Timodal eye drops (available only in Canada) ℞ *antiglaucoma agent (β-blocker)* [timolol maleate] 0.25%, 0.5%
timofibrate INN
Timolide 10-25 tablets ℞ *antihypertensive* [timolol maleate; hydrochlorothiazide] 10•25 mg
timolol USAN, INN, BAN *antiadrenergic (β-receptor)* ② atenolol
timolol hemihydrate *topical antiglaucoma agent (β-blocker)*
timolol maleate USAN, USP *antiadrenergic; topical antiglaucoma agent (β-blocker); migraine preventative* 5, 10, 20 mg oral; 0.25%, 0.5% eye drops
timonacic INN
timoprazole INN
Timoptic Ocumeter (eye drops), Ocudose (single-use eye drop dispenser) ℞ *topical antiglaucoma agent (β-blocker)* [timolol maleate] 0.25%, 0.5%
Timoptic-XE ophthalmic gel ℞ *topical once-daily antiglaucoma agent (β-blocker)* [timolol maleate] 0.25%, 0.5%
Timpilo ℞ *investigational treatment for glaucoma* [timolol; pilocarpine]
Timunox ℞ *investigational (Phase III) immunomodulator for asymptomatic HIV infection* [thymopoentin]
tin *element (Sn)*
tin chloride dihydrate [see: stannous chloride]
tin fluoride [see: stannous fluoride]
tinabinol USAN, INN *antihypertensive*
Tinactin cream, powder, spray powder, spray liquid, solution OTC *topical antifungal* [tolnaftate] 1% ② Taractan
Tinactin for Jock Itch cream, spray powder OTC *topical antifungal* [tolnaftate] 1%
tinazoline INN
TinBen tincture OTC *skin protectant* [benzoin; alcohol 75% to 83%]
TinCoBen tincture OTC *skin protectant* [benzoin; aloe; alcohol 77%]
Tincture of Green Soap liquid OTC *antiseptic cleanser* [green soap; alcohol 28-32%]

Tindal sugar-coated tablets (discontinued 1995) ℞ *antipsychotic* [acetophenazine maleate] 20 mg

Tine Test OT [see: Tuberculin Tine Test, Old]

Tine Test PPD single-use intradermal puncture test device ℞ *tuberculosis skin test* [tuberculin purified protein derivative] 5 U

Ting cream, powder, spray powder, spray liquid OTC *topical antifungal* [tolnaftate] 1%

tinidazole USAN, INN *antiprotozoal*

tinisulpride INN

tinofedrine INN

tinoridine INN

Tinver lotion ℞ *topical antifungal; keratolytic; antipruritic; anesthetic* [sodium thiosulfate; salicylic acid; alcohol 10%] 25%•1%

tinzaparin sodium USAN, INN, BAN *anticoagulant; antithrombotic*

T-inzole ℞ *investigational antineoplastic for leukemia* [tizofurin]

tiocarlide INN [also: thiocarlide]

tioclomarol INN

tioconazole USAN, USP, INN, BAN, JAN *antifungal*

tioctilate INN

tiodazosin USAN, INN *antihypertensive*

tiodonium chloride USAN, INN *antibacterial*

tiofacic [see: stepronin]

tioguanine INN *antineoplastic* [also: thioguanine]

tiomergine INN

tiomesterone INN [also: thiomesterone]

tioperidone INN *antipsychotic* [also: tioperidone HCl]

tioperidone HCl USAN *antipsychotic* [also: tioperidone]

tiopinac USAN, INN *anti-inflammatory; analgesic; antipyretic*

tiopronin INN *prevention of cystine nephrolithiasis in homozygous cystinuria* (orphan)

tiopropamine INN

tiosalan INN *disinfectant* [also: thiosalan]

tiosinamine [see: allylthiourea]

tiospirone INN *antipsychotic* [also: tiospirone HCl]

tiospirone HCl USAN *antipsychotic* [also: tiospirone]

tiotidine USAN, INN *antagonist to histamine H_2 receptors*

tiotixene INN *antipsychotic* [also: thiothixene]

tioxacin INN

tioxamast INN

tioxaprofen INN

tioxidazole USAN, INN *anthelmintic*

tioxolone INN [also: thioxolone]

tipentosin INN, BAN *antihypertensive* [also: tipentosin HCl]

tipentosin HCl USAN *antihypertensive* [also: tipentosin]

tipepidine INN

tipetropium bromide INN

tipindole INN

tipredane USAN, INN, BAN *topical adrenocortical steroid*

tiprenolol INN *antiadrenergic (β-receptor)* [also: tiprenolol HCl]

tiprenolol HCl USAN *antiadrenergic (β-receptor)* [also: tiprenolol]

tiprinast INN *antiallergic* [also: tiprinast meglumine]

tiprinast meglumine USAN *antiallergic* [also: tiprinast]

tipropidil INN *vasodilator* [also: tipropidil HCl]

tipropidil HCl USAN *vasodilator* [also: tipropidil]

tiprostanide INN, BAN

tiprotimod INN

tiqueside USAN, INN *antihyperlipidemic*

tiquinamide INN *gastric anticholinergic* [also: tiquinamide HCl]

tiquinamide HCl USAN *gastric anticholinergic* [also: tiquinamide]

tiquizium bromide INN

tirapazamine USAN, INN *antineoplastic*

tiratricol INN (orphan: thyroid cancer)

Tirend tablets OTC *CNS stimulant; analeptic* [caffeine] 100 mg

tirilazad INN, BAN *lipid peroxidation inhibitor; 21-aminosteroid (lazaroid); antioxidant* [also: tirilazad mesylate]

tirilazad mesylate USAN *lipid peroxidation inhibitor; 21-aminosteroid (lazaroid); antioxidant* [also: tirilazad]

tiropramide INN

tisilfocon A USAN *hydrophobic contact lens material*

Tisit liquid, shampoo OTC *pediculicide* [pyrethrins; piperonyl butoxide] 0.3%•2%; 0.3%•3%

Tisit Blue gel OTC *pediculicide* [pyrethrins; piperonyl butoxide; petroleum distillate] 0.3%•3%•1.2%

tisocromide INN

TiSol solution OTC *anesthetic and antimicrobial throat irrigation* [benzyl alcohol; menthol] 1%•0.04%

tisopurine INN

tisoquone INN

tissue factor [see: thromboplastin]

tissue plasminogen activator (tPA; t-PA) [see: alteplase]

Tis-U-Sol solution ℞ *sterile irrigant* [physiologic irrigating solution]

Titan solution OTC *cleaning solution for hard contact lenses*

titanium *element (Ti)*

titanium dioxide USP *topical protectant; astringent*

titanium oxide [see: titanium dioxide]

Titracid chewable tablets (discontinued 1994) OTC *antacid* [calcium carbonate; glycine]

Titradose (trademarked dosage form) *scored tablet*

Titralac chewable tablets OTC *antacid* [calcium carbonate] 420, 750 mg

Titralac Plus chewable tablets, liquid OTC *antacid; antiflatulent* [calcium carbonate; simethicone] 420•21 mg; 500•20 mg/5 mL

tivanidazole INN

tivazine [see: piperazine citrate]

tixadil INN

tixanox USAN *antiallergic* [also: tixanoxum]

tixanoxum INN *antiallergic* [also: tixanox]

tixocortol INN *topical anti-inflammatory* [also: tixocortol pivalate]

tixocortol pivalate USAN *topical anti-inflammatory* [also: tixocortol]

tizabrin INN

tizanidine INN, BAN *antispasmodic* [also: tizanidine HCl]

tizanidine HCl USAN, JAN *antispasmodic for multiple sclerosis and spinal cord injury (orphan); central α_2 agonist* [also: tizanidine]

tizofurin *investigational antineoplastic for leukemia*

tizolemide INN

tizoprolic acid INN

TJ-9 *investigational herbal compound (Sho-Saiko-To) adjunct for HIV*

T-Koff liquid ℞ *narcotic antitussive; decongestant; antihistamine* [codeine phosphate; phenylpropanolamine HCl; phenylephrine HCl; chlorpheniramine maleate] 10•20•20•5 mg/5 mL

^{201}Tl [see: thallous chloride Tl 201]

TLC A-60 *investigational vaccine adjuvant*

TLC ABLC ℞ *investigational systemic antifungal for bone marrow transplants* [amphotericin B lipid complex (ABLC)]

TLC C-53 *investigational cell adhesion antagonist for adult respiratory distress syndrome*

TLC D-99 ℞ *investigational antineoplastic for metastatic breast cancer* [liposome-encapsulated doxorubicin]

TLC D-99 *investigational liposomal form of doxorubicin for Kaposi sarcoma*

T-lymphotrophic virus antigens [see: human T-lymphotropic virus type III (HTLV-III) gp-160 antigens]

TMB (trimedoxime bromide) [q.v.]

T-Medic Cold Syrup OTC *decongestant; antihistamine* [phenylpropanolamine HCl; chlorpheniramine maleate]

T-Medic Expectorant syrup OTC *decongestant; expectorant* [phenylpropanolamine HCl; guaifenesin]

TMP (trimethoprim) [q.v.]

TMP-SMZ (trimethoprim & sulfamethoxazole) [q.v.]

TNF (tumor necrosis factor) [q.v.]

TNP-470 *investigational angiogenesis inhibitor for AIDS-related Kaposi sarcoma*

TOAP (thioguanine, Oncovin, [cytosine] arabinoside, prednisone) *chemotherapy protocol*

TobraDex eye drop suspension ℞ *topical ophthalmic corticosteroidal anti-inflammatory; antibiotic* [dexamethasone; tobramycin] 0.1%•0.3% ② Tobrex

TobraDex ophthalmic ointment ℞ *topical ophthalmic corticosteroidal anti-inflammatory; antibiotic* [dexamethasone; tobramycin; chlorobutanol] 0.1%•0.3%•0.5%

tobramycin USAN, USP, INN, BAN *antibacterial antibiotic (orphan: inhalation therapy for Pseudomonas aeruginosa in cystic fibrosis)* 0.3% eye drops ⊘ Trobicin

tobramycin sulfate USP *aminoglycoside bactericidal antibiotic* 10, 40 mg/mL injection

Tobrex Drop-Tainers (eye drops), ophthalmic ointment ℞ *ophthalmic antibiotic* [tobramycin] 0.3%; 3 mg/g ⊘ TobraDex

tobuterol INN

tocainide USAN, INN, BAN *antiarrhythmic*

tocainide HCl USP *antiarrhythmic*

tocamphyl USAN, INN *choleretic*

tocofenoxate INN

tocofersolan INN *vitamin E supplement* [also: tocophersolan]

tocofibrate INN

tocopherol, *d*-alpha [see: vitamin E]

tocopherol, *dl*-alpha [see: vitamin E]

tocopherols, mixed [see: vitamin E]

tocopherols excipient NF *antioxidant*

tocophersolan USAN *vitamin E supplement; (orphan: cholestatic hepatobiliary disease)* [also: tocofersolan]

tocopheryl acetate, *d*-alpha [see: vitamin E]

tocopheryl acetate, *dl*-alpha [see: vitamin E]

tocopheryl acid succinate, *d*-alpha [see: vitamin E]

tocopheryl acid succinate, *dl*-alpha [see: vitamin E]

tocopheryl polyethylene glycol succinate (TPGS) [see: tocophersolan]

Today vaginal sponge (discontinued 1995) OTC *spermicidal/barrier contraceptive* [nonoxynol 9] 1 g

todralazine INN, BAN

tofenacin INN *anticholinergic* [also: tofenacin HCl]

tofenacin HCl USAN *anticholinergic* [also: tofenacin]

tofesilate INN *combining name for radicals or groups*

tofetridine INN

tofisoline

tofisopam INN

Tofranil film-coated tablets, IM injection ℞ *tricyclic antidepressant; treatment for childhood enuresis* [imipramine HCl] 10, 25, 50 mg; 25 mg/2 mL ⊘ Tepanil

Tofranil-PM capsules ℞ *tricyclic antidepressant; treatment for childhood enuresis* [imipramine pamoate] 75, 100, 125, 150 mg

Tolamide tablets (discontinued 1992) ℞ *antidiabetic* [tolazamide]

tolamolol USAN, INN *vasodilator; antiarrhythmic; antiadrenergic (β-receptor)*

tolazamide USAN, USP, INN, BAN *sulfonylurea-type antidiabetic* 100, 250, 500 mg oral

tolazoline INN *peripheral vasodilator* [also: tolazoline HCl]

tolazoline HCl USP *antihypertensive; peripheral vasodilator* [also: tolazoline]

tolboxane INN

tolbutamide USP, INN, BAN *sulfonylurea-type antidiabetic* 500 mg oral

tolbutamide sodium USP *diagnostic aid for diabetes*

tolcapone USAN, INN *antiparkinsonian*

tolciclate USAN, INN *antifungal*

tolclotide [see: disulfamide]

toldimfos INN, BAN

Tolectin 200; Tolectin 600 tablets ℞ *nonsteroidal anti-inflammatory drug (NSAID); antiarthritic; analgesic* [tolmetin sodium] 200 mg; 600 mg

Tolectin DS capsules ℞ *nonsteroidal anti-inflammatory drug (NSAID); antiarthritic; analgesic* [tolmetin sodium] 400 mg

Tolerex powder OTC *enteral nutritional therapy* [lactose-free formula]

tolfamide USAN, INN *urease enzyme inhibitor*

tolfenamic acid INN, BAN

Tolfrinic film-coated tablets OTC *hematinic* [ferrous fumarate; cyanocobalamin; ascorbic acid] 200 mg•25 μg•100 mg

tolgabide USAN, INN, BAN *anticonvulsant*

tolhexamide [see: glycyclamide]

tolimidone USAN, INN *antiulcerative*

Tolinase tablets ℞ *sulfonylurea-type antidiabetic* [tolazamide] 100, 250, 500 mg ⓘ Orinase

tolindate USAN, INN *antifungal*

toliodium chloride USAN, INN *veterinary food additive*

toliprolol INN

tolmesoxide INN

tolmetin USAN, INN *nonsteroidal anti-inflammatory drug (NSAID); analgesic*

tolmetin sodium USAN, USP *antiarthritic; nonsteroidal anti-inflammatory drug (NSAID); analgesic* 200, 400 mg oral

tolnaftate USAN, USP, INN, BAN *antifungal* 1% topical

tolnapersine INN

tolnidamine INN

toloconium metilsulfate INN

tolofocon A USAN *hydrophobic contact lens material*

tolonidine INN

tolonium chloride INN

toloxatone INN

toloxichloral [see: toloxychlorinol]

toloxychlorinol INN

tolpadol INN

tolpentamide INN, BAN

tolperisone INN, BAN

tolpiprazole INN, BAN

tolpovidone I 131 USAN *hypoalbuminemia test; radioactive agent* [also: radiotolpovidone I 131]

tolpronine INN, BAN

tolpropamine INN, BAN

tolpyrramide USAN, INN *antidiabetic*

tolquinzole INN

tolrestat USAN, INN, BAN *aldose reductase inhibitor*

toltrazuril USAN, INN, BAN *veterinary coccidiostat*

tolu balsam USP *pharmaceutic aid*

***p*-toluenesulfone dichloramine** [see: dichloramine T]

tolufazepam INN

toluidine blue O [see: tolonium chloride]

toluidine blue O chloride [see: tolonium chloride]

Tolu-Sed DM syrup OTC *antitussive; expectorant* [dextromethorphan hydrobromide; guaifenesin; alcohol 10%] 10•100 mg/5 mL

tolycaine INN, BAN

tomelukast USAN, INN *antiasthmatic; leukotriene antagonist*

Tomocat concentrated suspension ℞ *GI contrast radiopaque agent* [barium sulfate] 5%

tomoglumide INN

Tomosar ℞ *investigational antineoplastic for breast, prostatic, and stomach cancers and lymphomas* [menogaril]

tomoxetine INN *antidepressant* [also: tomoxetine HCl]

tomoxetine HCl USAN *antidepressant* [also: tomoxetine]

tomoxiprole INN

Tomudex ℞ *investigational antineoplastic for colorectal cancer*

Tonavite-M liquid (discontinued 1992) OTC *antianemic* [iron ammonium citrate; multiple B vitamins]

tonazocine INN *analgesic* [also: tonazocine mesylate]

tonazocine mesylate USAN *analgesic* [also: tonazocine]

Tonocard film-coated tablets ℞ *antiarrhythmic* [tocainide HCl] 400, 600 mg

Tonopaque powder for suspension ℞ *GI contrast radiopaque agent* [barium sulfate; sorbitol] 95%

tonzonium bromide INN *detergent* [also: thonzonium bromide]

Toothache gel OTC *topical oral anesthetic* [benzocaine] ⓘ

Topamax ℞ *investigational anticonvulsant* [topiramate] 200 mg

Topic gel OTC *antipruritic; counterirritant* [benzyl alcohol; camphor; menthol; alcohol 30%] 5%•ⓘ•ⓘ ⓘ Topicort

topical starch [see: starch, topical]

Topicort ointment, cream, gel ℞ *topical corticosteroidal anti-inflammatory* [desoximetasone] 0.25%; 0.25%; 0.05% ⓘ Topic

Topicort LP cream ℞ *topical corticosteroidal anti-inflammatory* [desoximetasone] 0.05%

Topicycline solution ℞ *topical antibiotic for acne* [tetracycline HCl] 2.2 mg/mL

Topimax ℞ *investigational anticonvulsant; (orphan: Lennox-Gastaut syndrome)* [topiramate]

topiramate USAN, INN, BAN *anticonvulsant (orphan: Lennox-Gastaut syndrome)*

Toposar IV injection ℞ *antineoplastic for testicular and small cell lung cancers* [etoposide; alcohol 30.5%] 20 mg/mL

topotecan INN, BAN *antineoplastic for ovarian cancer; DNA topoisomerase I inhibitor* [also: topotecan HCl]

topotecan HCl USAN *antineoplastic for ovarian cancer; DNA topoisomerase I inhibitor* [also: topotecan]

toprilidine INN

Toprol XL film-coated extended-release tablets ℞ *antihypertensive; long-term antianginal; β-blocker* [metoprolol succinate] 50, 100, 200 mg

topterone USAN, INN *antiandrogen*

TOPV (trivalent oral poliovirus vaccine) [see: poliovirus vaccine, live oral]

toquizine USAN, INN *anticholinergic*

Toradol film-coated tablets, Tubex (cartridge-needle unit) for IM or IV injection ℞ *nonsteroidal anti-inflammatory drug (NSAID); analgesic for acute, moderately severe pain* [ketorolac tromethamine] 10 mg; 15, 30 mg/mL

Toradol gel, transdermal, IV injection ℞ *investigational nonsteroidal anti-inflammatory drug (NSAID)* [ketorolac tromethamine]

torasemide INN, BAN *loop diuretic* [also: torsemide]

torbafylline INN

Torecan tablets, IM injection, suppositories ℞ *antiemetic* [thiethylperazine maleate] 10 mg; 5 mg/mL; 10 mg

toremifene INN, BAN *antiestrogen; antineoplastic (orphan: metastatic carcinoma of the breast; desmoid tumors)* [also: toremifene citrate]

toremifene citrate USAN *antiestrogen; antineoplastic* [also: toremifene]

toripristone INN

Tornalate oral inhalation aerosol, inhalation solution ℞ *bronchodilator* [bitolterol mesylate] 0.8%; 0.2%

torsemide USAN *loop diuretic* [also: torasemide]

tosactide INN [also: octacosactrin]

tosifen USAN, INN *antianginal*

tosilate INN *combining name for radicals or groups* [also: tosylate]

tosufloxacin USAN, INN *antibacterial*

tosulur INN

tosylate USAN, BAN *combining name for radicals or groups* [also: tosilate]

tosylchloramide sodium INN [also: chloramine-T]

Tota Vite tablets OTC *vitamin/mineral supplement* [multiple vitamins & minerals]

Totacillin capsules, powder for oral suspension ℞ *penicillin-type antibiotic* [ampicillin trihydrate] 250, 500 mg; 125, 250 mg/5 mL

Totacillin-N powder for IV or IM injection ℞ *penicillin-type antibiotic* [ampicillin sodium] 0.25, 0.5, 1, 2, 10 g

Total solution OTC *cleaning/soaking/wetting solution for hard contact lenses*

Total Formula; Total Formula-2 tablets OTC *vitamin/mineral/iron supplement* [multiple vitamins & minerals; iron; folic acid; biotin] ±•20•0.4•0.3 mg

Total Formula-3 without Iron tablets OTC *vitamin/mineral supplement* [multiple vitamins & minerals; folic acid; biotin] ±•0.4•0.3 mg

toughened silver nitrate [see: silver nitrate, toughened]

Touro A & H timed-release capsules ℞ *decongestant; antihistamine* [pseudoephedrine HCl; brompheniramine maleate] 60•6 mg

Touro Ex sustained-release caplets ℞ *expectorant* [guaifenesin] 600 mg

Touro LA long-acting caplets ℞ *decongestant; expectorant* [pseudoephedrine HCl; guaifenesin] 120•500 mg

tozalinone INN *antidepressant* [also: thozalinone]

tPA; t-PA (tissue plasminogen activator) [see: alteplase]

T-Panol drops (for infants), oral solution (for children) OTC *analgesic* [acetaminophen]

TPCH (thioguanine, procarbazine, CCNU, hydroxyurea) *chemotherapy protocol*

TPDCV (thioguanine, procarbazine, DCD, CCNU, vincristine) *chemotherapy protocol*

TPGS (tocopheryl polyethylene glycol succinate) [see: tocophersolan]

T-Phyl timed-release tablets ℞ *bronchodilator* [theophylline] 200 mg

TPI tablets (discontinued 1992) OTC *decongestant; antihistamine; antitussive; analgesic* [pseudoephedrine HCl; chlorpheniramine maleate; dextromethorphan hydrobromide; acetaminophen]

TPM Test kit for professional use *in vitro diagnostic aid for Toxoplasma gondii antibodies in serum* [indirect hemagglutination test]

TPN Electrolytes; TPN Electrolytes II; TPN Electrolytes III IV admixture ℞ *intravenous electrolyte therapy* [combined electrolyte solution]

traboxopine INN

Trac Tabs 2X tablets ℞ *urinary anti-infective; analgesic; antispasmodic; acidifier* [methenamine; phenyl salicylate; atropine sulfate; hyoscyamine sulfate; benzoic acid; methylene blue] 120•30•0.06•0.03•7.5•6 mg

tracazolate USAN, INN, BAN *sedative*

Trace Metals Additive in 0.9% NaCl IV injection ℞ *intravenous nutritional therapy* [multiple trace elements (metals)]

Tracelyte; Tracelyte II; Tracelyte with Double Electrolytes; Tracelyte II with Double Electrolytes IV admixture ℞ *intravenous nutritional therapy* [multiple trace elements (metals); electrolytes]

Tracer bG reagent strips for home use (discontinued 1995) OTC *in vitro diagnostic aid for blood glucose*

Tracrium IV infusion ℞ *nondepolarizing neuromuscular blocker; adjunct to anesthesia* [atracurium besylate] 10 mg/mL

tragacanth NF *suspending agent*

tralonide USAN, INN *glucocorticoid*

tramadol INN *central analgesic* [also: tramadol HCl]

tramadol HCl USAN *central analgesic* [also: tramadol]

tramazoline INN *adrenergic* [also: tramazoline HCl]

tramazoline HCl USAN *adrenergic* [also: tramazoline]

Trancopal caplets ℞ *anxiolytic* [chlormezanone] 100, 200 mg

Trandate tablets, IV injection ℞ *antihypertensive; alpha- and beta-adrenergic blocking agent* [labetalol HCl] 100, 200, 300 mg; 5 mg/mL

Trandate HCT tablets (discontinued 1992) ℞ *antihypertensive* [labetalol HCl; hydrochlorothiazide]

trandolapril INN, BAN *antihypertensive; ACE inhibitor*

trandolaprilat INN

tranexamic acid USAN, INN, BAN *systemic hemostatic; (orphan: angioneurotic edema; congenital coagulopathies)*

tranilast USAN, INN *antiasthmatic*

trans AMCHA (*trans*-aminomethyl cyclohexanecarboxylic acid) [see: tranexamic acid]

transcainide USAN, INN *antiarrhythmic*

transclomiphene [now: zuclomiphene]

Transderm Scōp transdermal patch ℞ *motion sickness prevention* [scopolamine hydrobromide] 1.5 mg

Transderm-Nitro transdermal patch ℞ *antianginal* [nitroglycerin] 12.5, 25, 50, 75, 100 mg

transforming growth factor beta *investigational connective tissue growth stimulator (orphan: full-thickness macular holes)*

Trans-Plantar transdermal patch (name changed to Trans-Ver-Sal Plantar-Patch in 1995)

trans- JAN *topical antipruritic; mild local anesthetic; counterirritant* [also: camphor]

***trans*-retinoic acid** [see: tretinoin]

Trans-Ver-Sal Adult-Patch; Trans-Ver-Sal Pedia-Patch; Trans-Ver-Sal Plantar-Patch transdermal patch OTC *topical keratolytic* [salicylic acid] 15%

trantelinium bromide INN

Tranxene T-Tabs ("T"-imprinted tablets) ℞ *anxiolytic; minor tranquilizer;*

anticonvulsant adjunct [clorazepate dipotassium] 3.75, 7.5, 15 mg

Tranxene-SD single-dose tablets ℞ *anxiolytic; minor tranquilizer; anticonvulsant adjunct* [clorazepate dipotassium] 11.25, 22.5 mg

tranylcypromine INN *antidepressant; MAO inhibitor* [also: tranylcypromine sulfate]

tranylcypromine sulfate USP *antidepressant; MAO inhibitor* [also: tranylcypromine]

trapencaine INN

trapidil INN

trapymin [see: trapidil]

Trasylol IV infusion ℞ *systemic hemostatic for coronary artery bypass graft (CABG) surgery (orphan)* [aprotinin] 10,000 KIU/mL (Kallikrein inhibitor units) ② Travasol

TraumaCal ready-to-use liquid OTC *enteral nutritional therapy for moderate to severe stress or trauma* [branched chain amino acids]

Traum-Aid HBC powder (discontinued 1994) OTC *oral nutritional supplement for trauma and sepsis* 125.8 g/packet

Travase ointment (discontinued 1996) ℞ *topical enzyme for biochemical debridement* [sutilains] 82,000 U/g

Travasol 2.75% in 5% (10%, 25%) Dextrose; Travasol 4.25% in 5% (10%, 25%) Dextrose IV infusion ℞ *total parenteral nutrition; peripheral parenteral nutrition* [multiple essential and nonessential amino acids; dextrose] ② Trasylol

Travasol 3.5% (5.5%, 8.5%) with Electrolytes IV infusion ℞ *total parenteral nutrition (all except 3.5%); peripheral parenteral nutrition (all)* [multiple essential and nonessential amino acids & electrolytes] ♀

Travasol 5.5% (8.5%, 10%) IV infusion ℞ *total parenteral nutrition; peripheral parenteral nutrition* [multiple essential and nonessential amino acids] ♀

Travasorb Hepatic Diet powder (discontinued 1996) OTC *enteral nutritional therapy for hepatic failure* [branched chain amino acids] ♀

Travasorb HN; Travasorb MCT; Travasorb STD powder OTC *enteral nutritional therapy* [lactose-free formula]

Travasorb Renal Diet powder OTC *enteral nutritional therapy for acute renal failure* [essential amino acids] ♀

Travert IV infusion ℞ *nonelectrolyte fluid and caloric replacement* [invert sugar (50% dextrose + 50% fructose) in water]

5% Travert and Electrolyte No. 2; 10% Travert and Electrolyte No. 2 IV infusion ℞ *intravenous nutritional/electrolyte therapy* [combined electrolyte solution; invert sugar (50% dextrose + 50% fructose)]

traxanox INN

Traypak (trademarked packaging form) *multivial carton*

trazitiline INN

trazium esilate INN

trazodone INN *antidepressant* [also: trazodone HCl]

trazodone HCl USAN *antidepressant; used for panic disorders and aggressive behavior* [also: trazodone] 50, 100, 150 mg oral

trazolopride INN

trebenzomine INN *antidepressant* [also: trebenzomine HCl]

trebenzomine HCl USAN *antidepressant* [also: trebenzomine]

trecadrine INN

Trecator-SC tablets ℞ *tuberculostatic* [ethionamide] 250 mg

trefentanil HCl USAN *analgesic*

treloxinate USAN, INN *antihyperlipoproteinemic*

trenbolone INN, BAN *veterinary anabolic* [also: trenbolone acetate]

trenbolone acetate USAN *veterinary anabolic* [also: trenbolone]

Trendar tablets (discontinued 1996) OTC *nonsteroidal anti-inflammatory drug (NSAID); antiarthritic; analgesic* [ibuprofen] 200 mg

trengestone INN

trenizine INN

Trental film-coated controlled-release tablets ℞ *hemorheologic agent; to* *improve blood microcirculation* [pentoxifylline] 400 mg

treosulfan INN, BAN *(orphan: ovarian cancer)*

trepibutone INN

trepipam INN *sedative* [also: trepipam maleate]

trepipam maleate USAN *sedative* [also: trepipam]

trepirium iodide INN

treptilamine INN

trequinsin INN

trestolone INN *antineoplastic; androgen* [also: trestolone acetate]

trestolone acetate USAN *antineoplastic; androgen* [also: trestolone]

tretamine INN, BAN [also: triethylenemelamine]

trethinium tosilate INN

trethocanic acid INN

trethocanoic acid [see: trethocanic acid]

tretinoin USAN, USP, INN, BAN *keratolytic; acute promyelocytic leukemia (APL) treatment; (orphan: ophthalmic squamous metaplasia)*

Tretinoin APS (Advanced Polymer System) controlled-release sponge ℞ *investigational keratolytic for acne* [tretinoin]

tretoquinol INN

Trexan tablets (name changed to ReVia in 1995)

TRH (thyrotropin-releasing hormone) [see: protirelin]

Tri Vit drops (discontinued 1992) OTC *vitamin supplement* [vitamins A, C, and D]

Tri Vit with Fluoride drops ℞ *pediatric vitamin supplement and dental caries preventative* [vitamins A, C, and D; fluoride] 1500 IU•35 mg•400 IU•0.25 mg, 1500 IU•35 mg•400 IU•0.5 mg per mL

Triacana ℞ *(orphan: thyroid cancer)* [tiratricol]

Triacet cream ℞ *topical corticosteroid* [triamcinolone acetonide] 0.1%

triacetin USP, INN *antifungal*

triacetyloleandomycin BAN *macrolide bactericidal antibiotic* [also: troleandomycin]

Triacin syrup (discontinued 1992) OTC *decongestant; antihistamine* [pseudoephedrine HCl; triprolidine HCl]

Triacin-C Cough syrup ℞ *narcotic antitussive; decongestant; antihistamine* [codeine phosphate; pseudoephedrine HCl; triprolidine HCl; alcohol] 10•30•1.25 mg/5 mL

triaconazole [now: terconazole]

Triad capsules ℞ *sedative; analgesic* [acetaminophen; caffeine; butalbital] 325•40•50 mg

Triafed syrup (discontinued 1995) OTC *decongestant; antihistamine* [pseudoephedrine HCl; triprolidine HCl] 30•1.25 mg/5 mL ② Trifed

Triafed tablets (discontinued 1994) OTC *decongestant; antihistamine* [pseudoephedrine HCl; triprolidine HCl] 60•2.5 mg

Triafed with Codeine syrup ℞ *narcotic antitussive; decongestant; antihistamine* [codeine phosphate; pseudoephedrine HCl; triprolidine HCl] 10•30•1.25 mg/5 mL

triafungin USAN, INN *antifungal*

Triam Forte IM injection ℞ *glucocorticoids* [triamcinolone diacetate] 40 mg/mL

Triam-A IM, intra-articular, intrabursal, intradermal injection ℞ *glucocorticoids* [triamcinolone acetonide] 40 mg/mL

triamcinolone USP, INN, BAN, JAN *corticosteroid* 4 mg oral ② Triaminicin

triamcinolone acetonide USP, JAN *corticosteroid; inhalant for asthma* 0.025%, 0.1%, 0.5% topical; 40 mg/mL injection

triamcinolone acetonide sodium phosphate USAN *corticosteroid*

triamcinolone benetonide INN

triamcinolone diacetate USP, JAN *corticosteroid* 40 mg/mL injection

triamcinolone furetonide INN

triamcinolone hexacetonide USAN, USP, INN, BAN *corticosteroid*

Triaminic chewable tablets, syrup OTC *pediatric decongestant and antihistamine* [phenylpropanolamine HCl; chlorpheniramine maleate] 6.25•0.5

mg; 6.25•1 mg/5 mL ⓡ Triaminicin; TriHemic

Triaminic oral infant drops ℞ *pediatric decongestant and antihistamine* [phenylpropanolamine HCl; pyrilamine maleate; pheniramine maleate] 20•10•10 mg/mL

Triaminic Allergy; Triaminic Cold tablets OTC *decongestant; antihistamine* [phenylpropanolamine HCl; chlorpheniramine maleate] 25•4 mg; 12.5•2 mg

Triaminic AM Cough & Decongestant Formula liquid OTC *pediatric antitussive and decongestant* [dextromethorphan hydrobromide; pseudoephedrine HCl] 7.5•15 mg/5 mL

Triaminic AM Decongestant Formula syrup OTC *decongestant* [pseudoephedrine HCl] 15 mg/5 mL

Triaminic Decongestant oral infant drops OTC *pediatric decongestant* [pseudoephedrine HCl] 7.5 mg/0.8 mL

Triaminic DM syrup OTC *antitussive; decongestant* [dextromethorphan hydrobromide; phenylpropanolamine HCl] 5•6.25 mg/5 mL

Triaminic DM Day time oral solution (available only in Canada) OTC *pediatric antitussive, decongestant, and expectorant* [dextromethorphan hydrobromide; phenylpropanolamine HCl; guaifenesin] 1.5•1.75•7.5 mg/mL

Triaminic DM Night time for Children syrup (Canadian name for U.S. product Triaminic Nite Light)

Triaminic Expectorant liquid OTC *decongestant; expectorant* [phenylpropanolamine HCl; guaifenesin] 6.25•50 mg/5 mL

Triaminic Expectorant DH liquid ℞ *narcotic antitussive; decongestant; antihistamine; expectorant* [hydrocodone bitartrate; phenylpropanolamine HCl; pyrilamine maleate; pheniramine maleate; guaifenesin; alcohol 5%] 1.67•12.5•6.25•6.25•100 mg/5 mL

Triaminic Expectorant with Codeine liquid ℞ *narcotic antitussive; decongestant; expectorant* [codeine phosphate; phenylpropanolamine HCl; guaifenesin; alcohol 5%] 10•12.5•100 mg/5 mL

Triaminic Nite Light liquid OTC *pediatric antitussive, decongestant, and antihistamine* [dextromethorphan hydrobromide; pseudoephedrine HCl; chlorpheniramine maleate] 7.5•15•1 mg/5 mL

Triaminic Sore Throat Formula liquid OTC *pediatric antitussive, decongestant, and analgesic* [dextromethorphan hydrobromide; pseudoephedrine HCl; acetaminophen] 7.5•15•160 mg/5 mL

Triaminic TR sustained-release tablets (discontinued 1993) ℞ *decongestant; antihistamine* [phenylpropanolamine HCl; pyrilamine maleate; pheniramine maleate]

Triaminic-12 sustained-release tablets OTC *decongestant; antihistamine* [phenylpropanolamine HCl; chlorpheniramine maleate] 75•12 mg

Triaminicin tablets (name changed to Triaminicin Cold, Allergy, Sinus in 1993) ⓡ triamcinolone; Triaminic

Triaminicin Cold, Allergy, Sinus tablets OTC *decongestant; antihistamine; analgesic* [phenylpropanolamine HCl; chlorpheniramine maleate; acetaminophen] 25•4•650 mg ⓡ triamcinolone; Triaminic

Triaminicol Multi-Symptom Cough and Cold tablets OTC *antitussive; decongestant; antihistamine* [dextromethorphan hydrobromide; phenylpropanolamine HCl; chlorpheniramine maleate] 10•12.5•2 mg

Triaminicol Multi-Symptom Relief liquid OTC *antitussive; decongestant; antihistamine* [dextromethorphan hydrobromide; phenylpropanolamine HCl; chlorpheniramine maleate] 10•12.5•2 mg/5 mL

Triaminicol Multi-Symptom Relief Colds with Cough liquid OTC *pediatric antitussive, decongestant, and antihistamine* [dextromethorphan hydrobromide; phenylpropanolamine HCl; chlorpheniramine maleate] 5•6.25•1 mg/5 mL

Triamolone 40 IM injection ℞ *glucocorticoids* [triamcinolone diacetate] 40 mg/mL

Triamonide 40 IM, intra-articular, intrabursal, intradermal injection ℞ *glucocorticoids* [triamcinolone acetonide] 40 mg/mL

triampyzine INN *anticholinergic* [also: triampyzine sulfate]

triampyzine sulfate USAN *anticholinergic* [also: triampyzine]

triamterene USAN, USP, INN *potassium-sparing diuretic* ② trimipramine

trianisestrol [see: chlorotrianisene]

Triaprin capsules ℞ *analgesic; antipyretic; sedative* [acetaminophen; butalbital] 325•50 mg

Tri-Aqua tablets (discontinued 1993) OTC *diuretic* [caffeine; buchu, uva ursi, zea, and triticum extracts]

Triasyn B capsules, tablets (discontinued 1993) OTC *vitamin supplement* [vitamins B_1, B_2, and B_3]

Triavil 2-10; Triavil 2-25; Triavil 4-10; Triavil 4-25; Triavil 4-50 tablets ℞ *antipsychotic; antidepressant* [perphenazine; amitriptyline HCl] 2•10 mg; 2•25 mg; 4•10 mg; 4•25 mg; 4•50 mg

Tri-A-Vite F drops ℞ *pediatric vitamin supplement and dental caries preventative* [vitamins A, C, and D; fluoride] 1500 IU•35 mg•400 IU•0.5 mg per mL

Triaz gel, skin cleanser ℞ *topical keratolytic for acne* [benzoyl peroxide] 6%, 10%; 10%

triaziquone INN, BAN

triazolam USAN, USP, INN *sedative; hypnotic* 0.125, 0.25 mg oral

Triban; Pediatric Triban suppositories ℞ *anticholinergic; antiemetic* [trimethobenzamide HCl; benzocaine] 200 mg•2%; 100 mg•2%

Tri-Barbs capsules (discontinued 1993) ℞ *sedative; hypnotic* [phenobarbital; butabarbital sodium; secobarbital sodium]

tribasic calcium phosphate [see: calcium phosphate, tribasic]

tribavirin BAN *antiviral* [also: ribavirin]

tribendilol INN

tribenoside USAN, INN *sclerosing agent*

Tribiotic Plus ointment OTC *topical antibiotic; anesthetic* [polymyxin B sulfate; bacitracin; neomycin sulfate; lidocaine] 5000 U•500 U•3.5 mg•40 mg per g

tribromoethanol NF

tribromomethane [see: bromoform]

tribromsalan USAN, INN *disinfectant*

Tri-Buffered Aspirin tablets OTC *analgesic; antipyretic; anti-inflammatory* [aspirin; calcium carbonate; magnesium oxide; magnesium carbonate]

tribuzone INN

tricalcium phosphate [see: calcium phosphate, tribasic]

tricarbocyanine dye [see: indocyanine green]

tricetamide USAN *sedative*

Trichinella extract USP

Tri-Chlor liquid ℞ *cauterant; keratolytic* [trichloroacetic acid] 80%

trichlorethoxyphosphamide [see: defosfamide]

Trichlorex tablets (discontinued 1993) ℞ *diuretic; antihypertensive* [trichlormethiazide]

trichlorisobutylalcohol [see: chlorobutanol]

trichlormethiazide USP, INN *diuretic; antihypertensive* 4 mg oral

trichlormethine INN [also: trimustine]

trichloroacetic acid USP *strong keratolytic/cauterant*

trichlorocarbanilide (TCC) [see: triclocarban]

trichloroethylene NF, INN

trichlorofluoromethane [see: trichloromonofluoromethane]

trichlorofon [see: metrifonate]

trichloromonofluoromethane NF *aerosol propellant*

trichlorphon [see: metrifonate]

Trichophyton extract *diagnosis and treatment of Trichophyton-induced skin infections*

trichorad [see: acinitrazole]

trichosanthin *investigational (Phase II) antiviral for AIDS/ARC*

Trichotine Douche powder OTC *antiseptic/germicidal; vaginal cleanser and deodorizer; acidity modifier* [sodium perborate]

Trichotine Douche solution OTC *antiseptic/germicidal; vaginal cleanser and deodorizer; acidity modifier* [sodium borate]

triciribine INN *antineoplastic* [also: triciribine phosphate]

triciribine phosphate USAN *antineoplastic* [also: triciribine]

triclabendazole INN

triclacetamol INN

triclazate INN

triclobisonium chloride NF, INN

triclocarban USAN, INN *disinfectant*

triclodazol INN

triclofenate INN *combining name for radicals or groups*

triclofenol piperazine USAN, INN *anthelmintic*

triclofos INN *hypnotic; sedative* [also: triclofos sodium]

triclofos sodium USAN *hypnotic; sedative* [also: triclofos]

triclofylline INN

triclonide USAN, INN *anti-inflammatory*

triclosan USAN, INN, BAN *disinfectant/antiseptic*

Tricodene Cough and Cold liquid ℞ *narcotic antitussive; antihistamine* [codeine phosphate; pyrilamine maleate] 8.2•12.5 mg/5 mL

Tricodene Forte; Tricodene NN liquid OTC *antitussive; decongestant; antihistamine* [dextromethorphan hydrobromide; phenylpropanolamine HCl; chlorpheniramine maleate] 10•12.5•2 mg/5 mL

Tricodene Pediatric Cough & Cold liquid OTC *pediatric antitussive and decongestant* [dextromethorphan hydrobromide; phenylpropanolamine HCl] 10•12.5 mg/5 mL

Tricodene Sugar Free liquid OTC *antitussive; antihistamine* [dextromethorphan hydrobromide; chlorpheniramine maleate] 10•2 mg/5 mL

Tricom tablets (discontinued 1995) OTC *decongestant; antihistamine; analgesic* [pseudoephedrine HCl; chlorpheniramine maleate; acetaminophen] 60•4•650 mg

Tricomin ℞ *investigational hair growth enhancer* [peptide metal compound]

tricosactide INN

Tricosal film-coated tablets ℞ *analgesic; antipyretic; antirheumatic* [choline magnesium trisalicylate] 500, 750, 1000 mg

tricyclamol chloride INN

Triderm cream ℞ *topical corticosteroid* [triamcinolone acetonide] 0.1%

Tridesilon cream, ointment ℞ *topical corticosteroidal anti-inflammatory* [desonide] 0.05%

Tridesilon Otic [see: Otic Tridesilon]

Tri-Desogen ℞ *investigational triphasic oral contraceptive* [ethinyl estradiol; desogestrel]

tridihexethyl chloride USP *peptic ulcer adjunct*

tridihexethyl iodide INN

Tridil IV infusion ℞ *antianginal; perioperative antihypertensive; for congestive heart failure with myocardial infarction* [nitroglycerin] 0.5, 5 mg/mL

Tridione capsules, Dulcets (chewable tablets) ℞ *anticonvulsant* [trimethadione] 300 mg; 150 mg

Tridione oral solution (discontinued 1995) ℞ *anticonvulsant* [trimethadione] 40 mg/mL

Tridrate Bowel Evacuant Kit oral solution + 3 tablets + 1 suppository OTC *pre-procedure bowel evacuant* [magnesium citrate (solution); bisacodyl (tablets and suppository)] 300 mL; 5 mg; 10 mg

trientine INN *chelating agent* [also: trientine HCl; trientine dihydrochloride]

trientine dihydrochloride BAN *chelating agent* [also: trientine HCl; trientine]

trientine HCl USAN, USP *copper chelating agent for Wilson's disease (orphan)* [also: trientine; trientine dihydrochloride]

triethanolamine [now: trolamine]

triethyl citrate NF *plasticizer*

triethyleneiminobenzoquinone (TEIB) [see: triaziquone]

triethylenemelamine NF [also: tretamine]

triethylenethiophosphoramide (TSPA; TESPA) [see: thiotepa]

Trifed tablets (discontinued 1995) ℞ *decongestant; antihistamine* [pseudoephedrine HCl; triprolidine HCl] 60•2.5 mg ⓓ Triafed

Trifed-C Cough syrup ℞ *narcotic antitussive; decongestant; antihistamine* [codeine phosphate; pseudoephedrine HCl; triprolidine HCl; alcohol 4.4%] 10•30•1.25 mg/5 mL

trifenagrel USAN, INN *antithrombotic*

trifezolac INN

triflocin USAN, INN *diuretic*

Tri-Flor-Vite with Fluoride drops ℞ *pediatric vitamin supplement and dental caries preventative* [vitamins A, C, and D; fluoride] 1500 IU•35 mg•400 IU•0.25 mg per mL

triflubazam USAN, INN *minor tranquilizer*

triflumidate USAN, INN *anti-inflammatory*

trifluomeprazine INN, BAN

trifluoperazine INN *antipsychotic; sedative* [also: trifluoperazine HCl] 1, 2, 5, 10 mg oral; 10 mg/mL oral; 2 mg/mL injection

trifluoperazine HCl USP *antipsychotic; sedative* [also: trifluoperazine]

N-trifluoroacetyladriamicin-14-valerate (orphan: carcinoma in situ of urinary bladder)

trifluorothymidine [see: trifluridine]

trifluperidol USAN, INN *antipsychotic*

triflupromazine USP, INN *antiemetic; antipsychotic; antidopaminergic*

triflupromazine HCl USP *antipsychotic; antiemetic*

trifluridine USAN, INN *ophthalmic antiviral*

triflusal INN

triflutate USAN, INN *combining name for radicals or groups*

Trigesic tablets (discontinued 1995) OTC *analgesic; antipyretic; anti-inflammatory* [acetaminophen; aspirin; caffeine] 125•230•30 mg

trigevolol INN

α-triglycidyl isocyanurate (αTGI) [see: teroxirone]

TriHemic 600 film-coated tablets ℞ *hematinic* [ferrous fumarate; cyanocobalamin; ascorbic acid; vitamin E; intrinsic factor concentrate; docusate sodium; folic acid] 115 mg•25 μg•600 mg•30 IU•75 mg•50 mg•1 mg ⓓ Triaminic

Trihexy-2; Trihexy-5 tablets ℞ *anticholinergic; antiparkinsonian agent* [trihexyphenidyl HCl] 2 mg; 5 mg

trihexyphenidyl INN *anticholinergic; antiparkinsonian* [also: trihexyphenidyl HCl; benzhexol]

trihexyphenidyl HCl USP *anticholinergic; antiparkinsonian* [also: trihexyphenidyl; benzhexol] 2, 5 mg oral

Tri-Hist syrup OTC *decongestant; antihistamine* [phenylpropanolamine HCl; chlorpheniramine maleate]

Tri-Hist Expectorant syrup OTC *decongestant; expectorant* [phenylpropanolamine HCl; guaifenesin]

Tri-Hydroserpine tablets ℞ *antihypertensive* [hydrochlorothiazide; reserpine; hydralazine HCl] 15•0.1•25 mg

Tri-Immunol IM injection ℞ *immunization against diphtheria, tetanus and pertussis* [diphtheria & tetanus toxoids & whole-cell pertussis vaccine, adsorbed (DTwP)] 0.5 mL

triiodothyronine sodium, levo [see: liothyronine sodium]

Tri-K liquid ℞ *potassium supplement* [potassium acetate; potassium bicarbonate; potassium citrate] 45 mEq/15 mL (K)

trikates USP *electrolyte replenisher*

Tri-Kort IM, intra-articular, intrabursal, intradermal injection ℞ *glucocorticoids* [triamcinolone acetonide] 40 mg/mL

Trilafon tablets, oral concentrate, IV or IM injection ℞ *antipsychotic; antidopaminergic; antiemetic* [perphenazine] 2, 4, 8, 16 mg; 16 mg/5 mL; 5 mg/mL

Trileptal (commercially available in Argentina, Finland, and the Netherlands) ℞ *investigational antiepileptic* [oxcarbazepine]

triletide INN

Tri-Levlen tablets ℞ *triphasic oral contraceptive* [levonorgestrel; ethinyl estradiol] Phase 1: 0.05 mg•30 μg; Phase 2: 0.075 mg•40 μg; Phase 3: 0.125 mg•30 μg

Trilisate tablets, liquid ℞ *analgesic; antipyretic; anti-inflammatory; anti-*

rheumatic [choline salicylate; magnesium salicylate] 500, 750, 1000 mg; 500 mg/5 mL

trilithium citrate tetrahydrate [see: lithium citrate]

Trilog IM, intra-articular, intrabursal, intradermal injection ℞ *glucocorticoids* [triamcinolone acetonide] 40 mg/mL

Trilone IM injection ℞ *glucocorticoids* [triamcinolone diacetate] 40 mg/mL

trilostane USAN, INN, BAN *adrenocortical suppressant; antisteroidal antineoplastic*

Trimazide capsules, suppositories, pediatric suppositories ℞ *anticholinergic; antiemetic* [trimethobenzamide HCl] 100 mg; 200 mg; 100 mg

trimazosin INN, BAN *antihypertensive* [also: trimazosin HCl]

trimazosin HCl USAN *antihypertensive* [also: trimazosin]

Trimcaps sustained-release capsules (discontinued 1992) ℞ *anorexiant* [phendimetrazine tartrate] 105 mg

trimebutine INN

trimecaine INN

Trimedine liquid OTC *antitussive; decongestant; antihistamine* [dextromethorphan hydrobromide; phenylephrine HCl; chlorpheniramine maleate]

trimedoxime bromide INN

trimeperidine INN, BAN

trimeprazine BAN *antipruritic; antihistamine* [also: trimeprazine tartrate; alimemazine; alimemazine tratrate] ② trimipramine

trimeprazine tartrate USP *antipruritic; antihistamine* [also: alimemazine; trimeprazine; alimemazine tratrate]

trimeproprimine [see: trimipramine]

trimetamide INN

trimetaphan camsilate INN *antihypertensive* [also: trimethaphan camsylate; trimetaphan camsylate]

trimetaphan camsylate BAN *antihypertensive* [also: trimethaphan camsylate; trimetaphan camsilate]

trimetazidine INN, BAN

trimethadione USP, INN *anticonvulsant* [also: troxidone]

trimethamide [see: trimetamide]

trimethaphan camphorsulfonate [see: trimethaphan camsylate] ② trimethoprim

trimethaphan camsylate USP *emergency antihypertensive* [also: trimetaphan camsilate; trimetaphan camsylate]

trimethidinium methosulfate NF, INN

trimethobenzamide INN *antiemetic; anticholinergic* [also: trimethobenzamide HCl]

trimethobenzamide HCl USP *antiemetic; anticholinergic* [also: trimethobenzamide] 250 mg oral; 100, 200 mg suppositories; 100 mg/mL injection

trimethoprim (TMP) USAN, USP, INN, BAN *antibacterial antibiotic* 100, 200 mg oral ② trimethaphan

trimethoprim sulfate USAN *antibacterial*

trimethoquinol [see: tretoquinol]

trimethylammonium chloride carbamate [see: bethanechol chloride]

trimethylene [see: cyclopropane]

trimethyltetradecylammonium bromide [see: tetradonium bromide]

trimetozine USAN, INN *sedative*

trimetrexate USAN, INN, BAN *antimetabolic antineoplastic; systemic antiprotozoal*

trimetrexate glucuronate USAN *antimetabolic antineoplastic; (orphan: Pneumocystis carinii pneumonia of AIDS; multiple cancers)*

trimexiline INN

Triminol Cough syrup OTC *antitussive; decongestant; antihistamine* [dextromethorphan hydrobromide; phenylpropanolamine HCl; chlorpheniramine maleate] 10•12.5•2 mg/5 mL

Tri-Minulet ℞ *investigational triphasic oral contraceptive* [gestodene]

trimipramine USAN, INN *tricyclic antidepressant* ② imipramine; triamterene; trimeprazine

trimipramine maleate USAN *tricyclic antidepressant*

trimolide [see: trimetozine]

trimopam maleate [now: trepipam maleate]

trimoprostil USAN, INN *gastric antisecretory*

Trimo-San vaginal jelly OTC *antibacterial; astringent; antipruritic* [oxyquinoline sulfate; boric acid; sodium borate] 0.025%•1%•0.7%

Trimox '125'; Trimox '250' powder for oral suspension ℞ *penicillin-type antibiotic* [amoxicillin trihydrate] 125 mg/5 mL; 250 mg/5 mL

Trimox '250'; Trimox '500' capsules ℞ *penicillin-type antibiotic* [amoxicillin trihydrate] 250 mg; 500 mg

trimoxamine INN *antihypertensive* [also: trimoxamine HCl]

trimoxamine HCl USAN *antihypertensive* [also: trimoxamine]

Trimpex tablets ℞ *anti-infective; antibacterial* [trimethoprim] 100 mg

Trimstat tablets (discontinued 1996) ℞ *anorexiant* [phendimetrazine tartrate] 35 mg

Trimtabs tablets (discontinued 1992) ℞ *anorexiant* [phendimetrazine tartrate] 35 mg

trimustine BAN [also: trichlormethine]

Trinalin Repetabs (repeat-action tablets) ℞ *decongestant; antihistamine* [pseudoephedrine sulfate; azatadine maleate] 120•1 mg

Trinasal nasal spray ℞ *investigational treatment for allergic rhinitis*

Trind liquid (discontinued 1995) OTC *decongestant; antihistamine* [phenylpropanolamine HCl; chlorpheniramine maleate; alcohol 5%] 12.5•2 mg/5 mL

Trind-DM liquid (discontinued 1994) OTC *antitussive; decongestant; antihistamine* [dextromethorphan hydrobromide; phenylpropanolamine HCl; chlorpheniramine maleate; alcohol]

Tri-Nefrin tablets OTC *decongestant; antihistamine* [phenylpropanolamine HCl; chlorpheniramine maleate] 25•4 mg

trinitrin [see: nitroglycerin]

trinitrophenol NF

Tri-Norinyl tablets ℞ *triphasic oral contraceptive* [norethindrone; ethinyl estradiol] Phase 1: 0.5 mg•35 μg; Phase 2: 1 mg•35 μg; Phase 3: 0.5 mg•35 μg

Trinsicon capsules ℞ *hematinic* [ferrous fumarate; cyanocobalamin; ascorbic acid; intrinsic factor concentrate; folic acid] 110 mg•15 μg•75 mg•240 mg•0.5 mg

Trinsicon M capsules (discontinued 1992) ℞ *antianemic* [ferrous fumarate; intrinsic factor; vitamins B_{12} and C]

Triofed syrup OTC *decongestant; antihistamine* [pseudoephedrine HCl; triprolidine HCl] 30•1.25 mg/5 mL

triolein I 125 USAN *radioactive agent*

triolein I 131 USAN *radioactive agent*

trional [see: sulfonethylmethane]

Triostat IV injection ℞ *thyroid hormone; treatment of myxedema coma or precoma (orphan)* [liothyronine sodium] 10 μg/mL ② Threostat

Triotann pediatric oral suspension (discontinued 1995) ℞ *decongestant; antihistamine* [phenylephrine tannate; chlorpheniramine tannate; pyrilamine tannate] 5•2•12.5 mg/5 mL

Triotann tablets ℞ *decongestant; antihistamine* [phenylephrine tannate; chlorpheniramine tannate; pyrilamine tannate] 25•8•25 mg

Tri-Otic ear drops ℞ *topical corticosteroid; topical local anesthetic; antiseptic* [hydrocortisone; pramoxine HCl; chloroxylenol] 10•10•1 mg/mL

trioxifene INN *antiestrogen* [also: trioxifene mesylate]

trioxifene mesylate USAN *antiestrogen* [also: trioxifene]

trioxsalen USAN, USP *pigmentation agent for vitiligo; antipsoriatic* [also: trioxysalen]

trioxyethylrutin [see: troxerutin]

trioxymethylene [see: paraformaldehyde]

trioxysalen INN *pigmentation agent* [also: trioxsalen]

Tri-Pain tablets (discontinued 1995) OTC *analgesic; antipyretic; anti-inflammatory* [acetaminophen; aspirin; salicylamide; caffeine] 162•162•162•16.2 mg

Tripalgen Cold syrup (discontinued 1995) OTC *decongestant; antihistamine* [phenylpropanolamine HCl; chlorpheniramine maleate] 12.5•2 mg/5 mL

tripamide USAN, INN *antihypertensive; diuretic*

triparanol INN *(withdrawn from market)*

Tripedia IM injection ℞ *immunization against diphtheria, tetanus and pertussis* [diphtheria & tetanus toxoids & acellular pertussis vaccine (DTaP)] 6.7 LfU•5 LfU• 46.8 μg per 0.5 mL

tripelennamine INN *antihistamine* [also: tripelennamine citrate]

tripelennamine citrate USP *antihistamine* [also: tripelennamine]

tripelennamine HCl USP *antihistamine* 50 mg oral

Triphasil tablets ℞ *triphasic oral contraceptive* [levonorgestrel; ethinyl estradiol] Phase 1: 0.05 mg•30 μg; Phase 2: 0.075 mg•40 μg; Phase 3: 0.125 mg•30 μg

Tri-Phen-Chlor syrup, pediatric syrup, pediatric drops ℞ *decongestant; antihistamine* [phenylpropanolamine HCl; phenylephrine HCl; chlorpheniramine maleate; phenyltoloxamine citrate] 20•5•2.5•7.5 mg/5 mL; 5•1.25•0.5•2 mg/5 mL; 5•1.25•0.5•2 mg/mL

Tri-Phen-Chlor T.R. timed-release tablets ℞ *decongestant; antihistamine* [phenylpropanolamine HCl; phenylephrine HCl; chlorpheniramine maleate; phenyltoloxamine citrate] 40•10•5•15 mg

Tri-Phen-Mine syrup, drops ℞ *pediatric decongestant and antihistamine* [phenylpropanolamine HCl; phenylephrine HCl; chlorpheniramine maleate; phenyltoloxamine citrate] 5•1.25•0.5•2 mg/5 mL; 5•1.25•0.5•2 mg/mL

Tri-Phen-Mine S.R. timed-release tablets ℞ *decongestant; antihistamine* [phenylpropanolamine HCl; phenylephrine HCl; chlorpheniramine maleate; phenyltoloxamine citrate] 40•10•5•15 mg

Triphenyl syrup OTC *decongestant; antihistamine* [phenylpropanolamine HCl; chlorpheniramine maleate] 6.25•1 mg/5 mL

Triphenyl Expectorant liquid OTC *decongestant; expectorant* [phenylpropanolamine HCl; guaifenesin; alcohol 5%] 12.5•100 mg/5 mL

Triphenyl T.D. sustained-release tablets (discontinued 1992) ℞ *decongestant; antihistamine* [phenylpropanolamine HCl; pyrilamine maleate; pheniramine maleate]

Triple Antibiotic ointment OTC *topical antibiotic* [polymyxin B sulfate; neomycin sulfate; bacitracin] 5000 U•3.5 mg•400 U per g

Triple Antibiotic ophthalmic ointment ℞ *ophthalmic antibiotic* [polymyxin B sulfate; neomycin sulfate; bacitracin zinc] 5000 U•3.5 mg•400 U per g

Triple Antibiotic with HC ophthalmic ointment (discontinued 1993) ℞ *topical ophthalmic corticosteroidal anti-inflammatory; antibiotic* [hydrocortisone; neomycin sulfate; bacitracin zinc; polymyxin B sulfate]

Triple Paste ointment (discontinued 1993) OTC *topical diaper rash treatment* [zinc oxide; aluminum acetate]

Triple Sulfa vaginal cream ℞ *broad-spectrum bacteriostatic* [sulfathiazole; sulfacetamide; sulfabenzamide] 3.42%•2.86%•3.7%

triple sulfa (sulfathiazole, sulfacetamide, and sulfabenzamide) [q.v.]

Triple Sulfa No. 2 tablets (discontinued 1995) ℞ *broad-spectrum bacteriostatic* [trisulfapyrimidines] 500 mg

Triple Vita Drops (discontinued 1992) OTC *vitamin supplement* [vitamins A, C, and D]

Triple Vitamin ADC with Fluoride drops ℞ *pediatric vitamin supplement and dental caries preventative* [vitamins A, C, and D; fluoride] 1500 IU•35 mg•400 IU•0.5 mg per mL

Triple Vitamins with Fluoride chewable tablets ℞ *vitamin supplement; dental caries preventative* [vitamins A, C, and D; fluoride]

Triple X Kit liquid + shampoo OTC *pediculicide* [pyrethrins; piperonyl butoxide; petroleum distillate] 0.3%•3%• ?

Triple-Gen eye drop suspension (discontinued 1993) ℞ *topical ophthalmic*

corticosteroidal anti-inflammatory; antibiotic [hydrocortisone; neomycin sulfate; polymyxin B sulfate]

Triple-Vita-Flor drops (discontinued 1993) ℞ *pediatric vitamin supplement and dental caries preventative* [multiple vitamins; fluoride]

Triplevite with Fluoride drops (discontinued 1993) ℞ *pediatric vitamin supplement and dental caries preventative* [multiple vitamins; fluoride]

Tripodrine tablets (discontinued 1992) OTC *decongestant; antihistamine* [pseudoephedrine HCl; triprolidine HCl]

Triposed tablets, syrup OTC *decongestant; antihistamine* [pseudoephedrine HCl; triprolidine HCl] 60•2.5 mg; 30•1.25 mg/5 mL

tripotassium citrate monohydrate [see: potassium citrate]

triprolidine INN *antihistamine* [also: triprolidine HCl]

triprolidine HCl USP *antihistamine* [also: triprolidine] 1.25 mg/5 mL oral

Triptone long-acting caplets OTC *antinauseant; antiemetic; antivertigo; motion sickness preventative* [dimenhydrinate] 50 mg

triptorelin USAN, INN *antineoplastic*

triptorelin pamoate (*orphan: ovarian carcinoma*)

trisaccharides A & B (*orphan: newborn hemolytic disease; ABO blood incompatibility of organ or bone marrow transplants*)

Trisequens ℞ *investigational osteoporosis treatment* [17-beta-estradiol; norethindrone acetate]

trisodium citrate [see: sodium citrate]

trisodium citrate dihydrate [see: sodium citrate]

trisodium hydrogen ethylenediaminetetraacetate [see: edetate trisodium]

Trisoralen tablets ℞ *taken before exposure to sunlight to enhance repigmentation* [trioxsalen] 5 mg

Tri-Statin II cream ℞ *topical corticosteroid; antifungal* [triamcinolone acetonide; nystatin] 0.1%•100,000 U per g

Tristoject IM injection ℞ *glucocorticoids* [triamcinolone diacetate] 40 mg/mL

trisulfapyrimidines (a mixture of sulfadiazine, sulfamerazine, and sulfamethazine) USP *broad-spectrum bacteriostatic*

Tritan tablets ℞ *decongestant; antihistamine* [phenylephrine tannate; chlorpheniramine tannate; pyrilamine tannate] 25•8•25 mg

Tritann Pediatric oral suspension (discontinued 1995) ℞ *pediatric antihistamine and decongestant* [phenylephrine tannate; chlorpheniramine tannate; pyrilamine tannate] 5•2•12.5 mg/5 mL

Tri-Tannate tablets, pediatric oral suspension ℞ *decongestant; antihistamine* [phenylephrine tannate; chlorpheniramine tannate; pyrilamine tannate] 25•8•25 mg; 5•2•12.5 mg/5 mL

Tri-Tannate Plus Pediatric oral suspension ℞ *pediatric antitussive, decongestant, and antihistamine* [carbetapentane tannate; phenylephrine tannate; ephedrine tannate; chlorpheniramine tannate] 30•5•5•4 mg/5 mL

Tritec film-coated tablets ℞ *histamine H_2 antagonist for duodenal ulcers with H. pylori infection* [ranitidine bismuth citrate] 400 mg

Tri-Thalmic ophthalmic ointment, ophthalmic solution ℞ *topical antibiotic* [bacitracin zinc; neomycin sulfate; polymyxin B sulfate]

Tri-Thalmic HC ophthalmic ointment ℞ *topical corticosteroid; antibiotic* [bacitracin zinc; neomycin sulfate; polymyxin B sulfate; hydrocortisone]

tritheon [see: acinitrazole]

tritiated water USAN *radioactive agent*

Tri-Tinic capsules ℞ *antianemic* [ferrous fumarate; intrinsic factor; vitamins B_{12} and C; folic acid]

tritiozine INN

tritoqualine INN

Triva Douche powder OTC *antiseptic/germicidal; vaginal cleanser and deodorizer* [oxyquinoline sulfate] 2%

trivalent oral poliovirus vaccine (TOPV) [see: poliovirus vaccine, live oral]

Tri-Vi-Flor chewable tablets, drops ℞ *pediatric vitamin supplement and dental caries preventative* [vitamins A, C, and D; sodium fluoride] 2500 IU•60 mg•400 IU•1 mg; 1500 IU•35 mg•400 IU•0.25 mg, 1500 IU•35 mg•400 IU•0.5 mg per mL

Tri-Vi-Flor with Iron drops ℞ *pediatric vitamin/iron supplement and dental caries preventative* [vitamins A, C, and D; iron; sodium fluoride] 1500 IU•35 mg•400 IU•0.25 mg per mL

Tri-Vi-Sol drops OTC *pediatric vitamin supplement* [vitamins A, C, and D] 1500 IU•35 mg•400 IU per mL

Tri-Vi-Sol with Iron drops OTC *vitamin/iron supplement* [vitamins A, C, and D; ferrous sulfate] 1500 IU•35 mg•400 IU•10 mg per mL

Trivitamin Fluoride chewable tablets, drops ℞ *pediatric vitamin supplement and dental caries preventative* [vitamins A, C, and D; fluoride] 2500 IU•60 mg•400 IU•1 mg; 1500 IU•35 mg•400 IU•0.25 mg, 1500 IU•35 mg•400 IU•0.5 mg per mL

Tri-Vitamin Infants' Drops OTC *vitamin supplement* [vitamins A, C, and D] 1500 IU•35 mg•400 IU per mL

Tri-Vitamin with Fluoride drops ℞ *pediatric vitamin supplement and dental caries preventative* [vitamins A, C, and D; fluoride] 1500 IU•35 mg•400 IU•0.5 mg per mL

trixolane INN

trizoxime INN

Trizyme (ingredient) OTC *digestive enzymes* [amylolytic, proteolytic and cellulolytic enzymes (amylase; protease; cellulase)]

Trobicin powder for IM injection ℞ *antibiotic* [spectinomycin HCl] 400 mg/mL ② tobramycin

Trocaine lozenges OTC *topical oral anesthetic* [benzocaine] 10 mg

Trocal lozenges OTC *antitussive* [dextromethorphan hydrobromide] 7.5 mg

trocimine INN

troclosene potassium USAN, INN *topical anti-infective*

Trofan; Trofan-DS tablets (discontinued 1993) OTC *dietary amino acid supplement* [L-tryptophan] 500 mg; 1000 mg

trofosfamide INN

troglitazone USAN, INN *antidiabetic; investigational insulin-enhancing agent*

trolamine USAN, NF *alkalizing agent; analgesic*

troleandomycin USAN, USP *macrolide bactericidal antibiotic; (orphan: severe asthma)* [also: triacetyloleandomycin]

trolnitrate INN

trolnitrate phosphate [see: trolnitrate]

tromantadine INN

trometamol INN, BAN *alkalizer for cardiac bypass surgery* [also: tromethamine]

tromethamine USAN, USP *alkalizer for cardiac bypass surgery* [also: trometamol]

Tronolane anorectal cream OTC *topical local anesthetic* [pramoxine HCl] 1% ② Tronothane

Tronolane rectal suppositories OTC *astringent; emollient* [zinc oxide] 11%

Tronothane HCl cream OTC *topical local anesthetic* [pramoxine HCl] 1% ② Tronolane

tropabazate INN

Tropamine + capsules (discontinued 1993) OTC *dietary supplement* [multiple amino acids, vitamins, and minerals]

tropanserin INN, BAN *migraine-specific serotonin receptor antagonist* [also: tropanserin HCl]

tropanserin HCl USAN *migraine-specific serotonin receptor antagonist* [also: tropanserin]

tropapride INN

tropatepine INN

tropenziline bromide INN

TrophAmine 6%; TrophAmine 10% IV infusion ℞ *total parenteral nutrition; peripheral parenteral nutrition* [multiple essential and nonessential amino acids]

Troph-Iron liquid (name changed to Trophite + Iron in 1995)

Trophite liquid (discontinued 1995) OTC *vitamin supplement* [vitamins B_1 and B_{12}] 10 mg•25 μg per 5 mL

Trophite + Iron liquid OTC *hematinic* [ferric pyrophosphate; vitamins B_1 and B_{12}] 60 mg•30 mg•75 µg per 15 mL

trophosphamide [see: trofosfamide]

Tropicacyl eye drops ℞ *cycloplegic; mydriatic* [tropicamide] 0.5%, 1%

tropicamide USAN, USP, INN *ophthalmic anticholinergic; cycloplegic; short-acting mydriatic*

tropigline INN, BAN

tropirine INN

tropisetron INN, BAN *investigational treatment for nausea and vomiting related to chemotherapy*

Tropi-Storz eye drops ℞ *cycloplegic; mydriatic* [tropicamide] 0.5%, 1%

tropodifene INN

troquidazole INN

trospectomycin INN, BAN *broad-spectrum aminocyclitol antibiotic* [also: trospectomycin sulfate]

trospectomycin sulfate USAN *broad-spectrum aminocyclitol antibiotic* [also: trospectomycin]

trospium chloride INN

trovafloxacin mesylate USAN *antibacterial*

troxerutin INN, BAN *vitamin P_4*

troxidone BAN *anticonvulsant* [also: trimethadione]

troxipide INN

troxolamide INN

troxonium tosilate INN [also: troxonium tosylate]

troxonium tosylate BAN [also: troxonium tosilate]

troxundate INN *combining name for radicals or groups*

troxypyrrolium tosilate INN [also: troxypyrrolium tosylate]

troxypyrrolium tosylate BAN [also: troxypyrrolium tosilate]

T.R.U.E. Test patch ℞ *diagnostic aid for contact dermatitis*

Truphylline suppositories ℞ *bronchodilator* [aminophylline] 250, 500 mg

Truquant BR RIA test for professional use *in vitro diagnostic aid for breast cancer recurrence* [radioimmunoassay (RIA) test for CA27.29 antigen]

Trusopt eye drops ℞ *topical carbonic anhydrase inhibitor for glaucoma* [dorzolamide HCl] 2%

Trutol oral liquid ℞ *glucose tolerance test beverage* [glucose]

truxicurium iodide INN

truxipicurium iodide INN

trypaflavine [see: acriflavine HCl]

tryparsamide USP, INN

trypsin, crystallized USP *topical proteolytic enzyme; necrotic tissue debridement*

Tryptacin tablets (discontinued 1993) OTC *dietary amino acid supplement* [L-tryptophan] 500, 1000 mg

tryptizol [see: amitriptyline]

tryptizol HCl [see: amitriptyline HCl]

tryptophan (L-tryptophan) USAN, USP, INN *essential amino acid; serotonin precursor (The FDA has recalled all OTC tryptophan supplements.)*

Trysul vaginal cream ℞ *broad-spectrum bacteriostatic* [sulfathiazole; sulfacetamide; sulfabenzamide] 3.42%•2.86%•3.7%

TSC (technetium sulfur colloid) [see: technetium Tc 99m sulfur colloid]

T/Scalp liquid OTC *topical corticosteroid* [hydrocortisone] 1%

TSH (thyroid stimulating hormone) [see: thyrotropin]

TSPA (triethylenethiophosphoramide) [see: thiotepa]

TST (tuberculin skin test) [see: tuberculin]

T-Stat topical solution, medicated pads ℞ *topical antibiotic for acne* [erythromycin] 2%

T-Tabs (trademarked form) *"T"-imprinted tablets*

T-Tussin CF liquid OTC *expectorant; decongestant; antitussive* [guaifenesin; phenylpropanolamine HCl; dextromethorphan hydrobromide; alcohol]

T-Tussin DM liquid OTC *expectorant; antitussive* [guaifenesin; dextromethorphan hydrobromide; alcohol]

T-Tussin Expectorant liquid OTC *expectorant* [guaifenesin]

T-Tussin PE liquid OTC *expectorant; decongestant* [guaifenesin; pseudoephedrine HCl; alcohol]

tuaminoheptane USP, INN *adrenergic; vasoconstrictor*

tuaminoheptane sulfate USP

tuberculin USP *dermal tuberculosis test*

tuberculin, crude [see: tuberculin]

tuberculin, old (OT) [see: tuberculin]

tuberculin purified protein derivative (PPD) [see: tuberculin]

Tuberculin Tine Test, Old single-use intradermal puncture test device ℞ *tuberculosis skin test* [old tuberculin] 5 U

tuberculosis vaccine [see: BCG vaccine]

Tubersol intradermal injection ℞ *tuberculosis skin test* [tuberculin purified protein derivative] 1, 5, 250 U/0.1 mL

Tubex (trademarked delivery system) *cartridge-needle unit*

tubocurarine chloride USP, INN, BAN *neuromuscular blocker; muscle relaxant* 3 mg (20 U)/mL injection

tubocurarine chloride HCl pentahydrate [see: tubocurarine chloride]

tubulozole INN *antineoplastic; microtubule inhibitor* [also: tubulozole HCl]

tubulozole HCl USAN, INN *antineoplastic; microtubule inhibitor* [also: tubulozole]

tucaresol INN, BAN *investigational (Phase I/II) immunopotentiator for HIV*

Tucks; Tucks Take-Alongs cleansing pads OTC *moisturizer and cleanser for the perineal area; astringent* [witch hazel; glycerin] 50%•10%

Tucks Clear gel OTC *astringent* [hamamelis water; glycerin] 50%•10%

Tucks Hemorrhoidal cream (discontinued 1995) OTC *astringent* [hamamelis water] 50%

tuclazepam INN

Tuinal Pulvules (capsules) ℞ *sedative; hypnotic* [amobarbital sodium; secobarbital sodium] 50•50, 100•100 mg ☒ Luminal; Tylenol

tulobuterol INN, BAN, JAN [also: tulobuterol HCl]

tulobuterol HCl JAN [also: tulobuterol]

tulopafant INN

tumor necrosis factor (TNF) *investigational (Phase I) antiviral for HIV; investigational treatment for septic shock* [also see: anti-TNF]

tumor necrosis factor (TNF)-binding protein I and II (orphan: *symptomatic AIDS patients*)

Tums liquid (discontinued 1994) OTC *antacid* [calcium carbonate] 200 mg/mL

Tums; Tums E-X chewable tablets OTC *antacid* [calcium carbonate] 500 mg; 750 mg

Tums 500; Tums Ultra chewable tablets OTC *antacid* [calcium carbonate] 1.25 g; 1 g

Tums with Simethicone liquid (discontinued 1994) OTC *antacid; antiflatulent* [calcium carbonate; simethicone] 200•6 mg/mL

tungsten *element* (W)

Turbinaire (trademarked delivery system) *nasal inhalation aerosol*

turosteride INN

Tusal IM injection (discontinued 1994) ℞ *analgesic; antipyretic; antiinflammatory; antirheumatic* [sodium thiosalicylate] 50 mg/mL

Tusibron syrup OTC *expectorant* [guaifenesin; alcohol 3.5%] 100 mg/5 mL

Tusibron-DM syrup OTC *antitussive; expectorant* [dextromethorphan hydrobromide; guaifenesin] 15•100 mg/5 mL

Tusquelin syrup ℞ *antitussive; decongestant; antihistamine; analgesic* [dextromethorphan hydrobromide; phenylpropanolamine HCl; phenylephrine HCl; chlorpheniramine maleate; alcohol 5%] 15•5•5•2 mg/5 mL

Tuss-Ade extended-release capsules ℞ *decongestant* [phenylpropanolamine HCl; caramiphen edisylate]

Tussafed syrup, pediatric drops ℞ *antitussive; decongestant; antihistamine* [dextromethorphan hydrobromide; pseudoephedrine HCl; carbinoxamine maleate; menthol] 15•60•4 mg/5 mL; 4•25•2 mg/mL ☒ Tussafin

Tussafin Expectorant liquid ℞ *narcotic antitussive; decongestant; expec-*

torant [hydrocodone bitartrate; pseudoephedrine HCl; guaifenesin; alcohol 12.5%] 5•60•200 mg/5 mL ℞ Tussafed

Tuss-Allergine Modified T.D. capsules ℞ *antitussive; decongestant* [caramiphen edisylate; phenylpropanolamine HCl] 40•75 mg

Tussanil DH syrup ℞ *narcotic antitussive; decongestant; antihistamine* [hydrocodone bitartrate; phenylephrine HCl; chlorpheniramine maleate; alcohol 5%] 2.5•10•4 mg/5 mL

Tussanil DH tablets ℞ *narcotic antitussive; decongestant; expectorant; analgesic* [hydrocodone bitartrate; phenylpropanolamine HCl; guaifenesin; salicylamide] 1.66•25•100•300 mg

Tussanil Plain syrup (discontinued 1995) ℞ *decongestant; antihistamine* [phenylephrine HCl; chlorpheniramine maleate; alcohol 5%] 10•4 mg/5 mL

Tussar DM syrup OTC *antitussive; decongestant; antihistamine* [dextromethorphan hydrobromide; pseudoephedrine HCl; chlorpheniramine maleate] 15•30•2 mg/5 mL

Tussar SF; Tussar-2 liquid ℞ *narcotic antitussive; antihistamine; expectorant* [codeine phosphate; pseudoephedrine HCl; guaifenesin; alcohol 2.5%] 10•30•100 mg/5 mL

Tuss-DA liquid ℞ *decongestant; antitussive* [dextromethorphan; pseudoephedrine HCl]

Tuss-DM tablets OTC *antitussive; expectorant* [dextromethorphan hydrobromide; guaifenesin] 10•200 mg

Tussend syrup ℞ *narcotic antitussive; decongestant; antihistamine* [hydrocodone bitartrate; pseudoephedrine HCl; chlorpheniramine maleate; alcohol 5%] 2.5•30•2 mg/5 mL

Tussex Cough syrup OTC *antitussive; decongestant; expectorant* [dextromethorphan hydrobromide; phenylephrine HCl; guaifenesin] 10•5•100 mg/5 mL ℞ Tussionex; Tussirex

Tussgen liquid (discontinued 1995) ℞ *narcotic antitussive; decongestant* [hydrocodone bitartrate; pseudoephedrine HCl; alcohol 5%] 5•60 mg/5 mL

Tuss-Genade Modified sustained-release capsules (discontinued 1995) ℞ *antitussive; decongestant* [caramiphen edisylate; phenylpropanolamine HCl] 40•75 mg

Tussibron-DM liquid (discontinued 1995) OTC *antitussive; expectorant* [dextromethorphan hydrobromide; guaifenesin] 15•100 mg/5 mL ℞ Tussigon

Tusside liquid (discontinued 1992) ℞ *antitussive; expectorant* [dextromethorphan hydrobromide; iodinated glycerol]

Tussigon tablets ℞ *narcotic antitussive; GI anticholinergic/antispasmodic* [hydrocodone bitartrate; homatropine methylbromide] 5•1.5 mg ℞ Tussibron

Tussionex Pennkinetic extended-release suspension ℞ *narcotic antitussive; antihistamine* [hydrocodone polistirex; chlorpheniramine polistirex] 10•8 mg/5 mL ℞ Tussex; Tussirex

Tussi-Organidin liquid (discontinued 1993; replaced by Tussi-Organidin NR ["Newly Reformulated"] in 1994) ℞ *narcotic antitussive; expectorant* [codeine phosphate; iodinated glycerol] 10•30 mg/5 mL ℞ Tussi-R-Gen

Tussi-Organidin DM liquid (discontinued 1993; replaced by Tussi-Organidin DM NR ["Newly Reformulated"] in 1994) ℞ *antitussive; expectorant* [dextromethorphan hydrobromide; iodinated glycerol] 10•30 mg/5 mL

Tussi-Organidin DM NR liquid ℞ *antitussive; expectorant* [dextromethorphan hydrobromide; guaifenesin] 10•100 mg/5 mL

Tussi-Organidin NR liquid ℞ *narcotic antitussive; expectorant* [codeine phosphate; guaifenesin] 10•100 mg/5 mL

Tussirex syrup, sugar-free liquid ℞ *narcotic antitussive; decongestant; antihistamine; expectorant; analgesic* [codeine phosphate; phenylephrine HCl; pheniramine maleate; sodium citrate; sodium salicylate; caffeine citrate]

10•4.17•13.33•83.3•83.33•25 mg/5 mL ℞ Tussex; Tussionex

Tussi-R-Gen liquid (discontinued 1994) ℞ *narcotic antitussive; expectorant* [codeine phosphate; iodinated glycerol] ℞ Tussi-Organidin

Tussi-R-Gen DM liquid (discontinued 1994) ℞ *antitussive; expectorant* [dextromethorphan hydrobromide; iodinated glycerol]

Tuss-LA sustained-release tablets ℞ *decongestant; expectorant* [pseudoephedrine HCl; guaifenesin] 120•500 mg

Tusso-DM liquid ℞ *antitussive; expectorant* [dextromethorphan hydrobromide; iodinated glycerol] 10•30 mg/5 mL

Tussogest extended-release capsules ℞ *antitussive; decongestant* [caramiphen edisylate; phenylpropanolamine HCl] 40•75 mg

Tuss-Ornade Spansules (sustained-release capsules), liquid ℞ *antitussive; decongestant* [caramiphen edisylate; phenylpropanolamine HCl] 40•75 mg; 6.7•12.5 mg/5 mL

Tusstat syrup ℞ *antihistamine; antitussive* [diphenhydramine HCl; alcohol 5%] 12.5 mg/5 mL

tuvatidine INN

tuvirumab USAN, INN *antiviral monoclonal antibody*

TV-1203 *investigational antiparkinsonism agent*

TVC-2 Dandruff Shampoo OTC *antiseborrheic; antibacterial; antifungal* [pyrithione zinc] 2%

T-Vites tablets OTC *vitamin/mineral supplement* [multiple vitamins & minerals; biotin] ≐•30 μg

12 Hour nasal spray OTC *nasal decongestant* [oxymetazoline HCl] 0.05%

12 Hour Antihistamine Nasal Decongestant sustained-release tablets (discontinued 1995) OTC *decongestant; antihistamine* [pseudoephedrine sulfate; dexbrompheniramine maleate] 120•6 mg

12 Hour Cold sustained-release capsules (discontinued 1995) OTC *decongestant; antihistamine* [phenylpropanolamine HCl; chlorpheniramine maleate] 75•4 mg

12 Hour Cold sustained-release tablets OTC *decongestant; antihistamine* [pseudoephedrine sulfate; dexbrompheniramine maleate] 120•6 mg

Twice-A-Day nasal spray OTC *nasal decongestant* [oxymetazoline HCl] 0.05%

Twilite caplets OTC *antihistaminic sleep aid* [diphenhydramine HCl] 50 mg

Twin-K liquid ℞ *potassium supplement* [potassium gluconate; potassium citrate] 20 mEq/15 mL (K)

TwoCal HN ready-to-use liquid OTC *enteral nutritional therapy* [lactose-free formula]

Two-Dyne capsules ℞ *analgesic; antipyretic; sedative* [acetaminophen; caffeine; butalbital] 325•40•50 mg

tybamate USAN, NF, INN, BAN *minor tranquilizer*

Ty-Cold tablets (discontinued 1995) OTC *antitussive; decongestant; antihistamine; analgesic* [dextromethorphan hydrobromide; pseudoephedrine HCl; chlorpheniramine maleate; acetaminophen] 15•30•2•325 mg

tyformin BAN [also: tiformin]

tylcalsin [see: calcium acetylsalicylate]

tylemalum [see: carbubarb]

Tylenol tablets, caplets, liquid, gelcaps, geltabs OTC *analgesic; antipyretic* [acetaminophen] 160, 325, 500 mg; 325, 500 mg; 500 mg/15 mL; 500 mg; 500 mg ℞ Tuinal

Tylenol, Children's chewable tablets, elixir, oral suspension OTC *analgesic; antipyretic* [acetaminophen] 80 mg; 160 mg/5 mL; 160 mg/5 mL

Tylenol Allergy Sinus caplets, gelcaps OTC *decongestant; antihistamine; analgesic* [pseudoephedrine HCl; chlorpheniramine maleate; acetaminophen] 30•2•500 mg

Tylenol Allergy Sinus NightTime caplets OTC *decongestant; antihistamine; analgesic* [pseudoephedrine HCl; diphenhydramine HCl; acetaminophen] 30•25•500 mg

Tylenol Cold effervescent tablets (discontinued 1995) OTC *deconges-*

tant; antihistamine; analgesic [phenylpropanolamine HCl; chlorpheniramine maleate; acetaminophen] 12.5•2•325 mg

Tylenol Cold, Children's chewable tablets, liquid OTC *pediatric decongestant, antihistamine and analgesic* [pseudoephedrine HCl; chlorpheniramine maleate; acetaminophen] 7.5•0.5•80 mg; 15•1•160 mg/5 mL

Tylenol Cold, Multi-Symptom caplets, tablets OTC *antitussive; decongestant; antihistamine; analgesic* [dextromethorphan hydrobromide; pseudoephedrine HCl; chlorpheniramine maleate; acetaminophen] 10•30•2•325 mg

Tylenol Cold & Flu powder for oral solution (name changed to Tylenol Multi-Symptom Hot Medication in 1995)

Tylenol Cold & Flu No Drowsiness powder for oral solution (discontinued 1995) OTC *antitussive; decongestant; analgesic* [dextromethorphan hydrobromide; pseudoephedrine HCl; acetaminophen] 30•60•650 mg/packet

Tylenol Cold Multi Symptom Plus Cough, Children's liquid OTC *pediatric antitussive, decongestant, antihistamine, and analgesic* [dextromethorphan hydrobromide; pseudoephedrine HCl; chlorpheniramine maleate; acetaminophen] 5•15•1•160 mg/5 mL

Tylenol Cold Night Time liquid (discontinued 1995) OTC *decongestant; antihistamine; analgesic* [pseudoephedrine HCl; diphenhydramine HCl; acetaminophen; alcohol 10%] 2•1.66•21.66 mg

Tylenol Cold No Drowsiness caplets, gelcaps OTC *antitussive; decongestant; analgesic* [dextromethorphan hydrobromide; pseudoephedrine HCl; acetaminophen] 15•30•325 mg

Tylenol Cold Plus Cough, Children's chewable tablets OTC *antitussive; decongestant; antihistamine; analgesic* [dextromethorphan hydrobromide; pseudoephedrine HCl; chlorpheniramine maleate; acetaminophen] 2.5•7.5•0.5•80 mg

Tylenol Cough liquid (name changed to Multi-Sympton Tylenol Cough in 1995)

Tylenol Cough, Multi-Symptom liquid OTC *antitussive; analgesic* [dextromethorphan hydrobromide; acetaminophen; alcohol 5%] 10•216.7 mg/5 mL

Tylenol Cough with Decongestant liquid (name changed to Multi-Symptom Tylenol Cough with Decongestant in 1995)

Tylenol Cough with Decongestant, Multi-Symptom liquid OTC *antitussive; decongestant; analgesic* [dextromethorphan hydrobromide; pseudoephedrine HCl; acetaminophen; alcohol 5%] 10•20•200 mg/5 mL

Tylenol Extended Relief extended-release caplets OTC *analgesic; antipyretic* [acetaminophen] 650 mg

Tylenol Flu gelcaps OTC *antitussive; decongestant; analgesic* [dextromethorphan hydrobromide; pseudoephedrine HCl; acetaminophen] 15•30•500 mg

Tylenol Flu NightTime gelcaps, powder OTC *decongestant; antihistamine; analgesic* [pseudoephedrine HCl; diphenhydramine HCl; acetaminophen] 30•25•500 mg; 60•50•1000 mg/packet

Tylenol Headache Plus caplets OTC *analgesic; antipyretic; antacid* [acetaminophen; calcium carbonate] 500•250 mg

Tylenol Infant's Drops solution, suspension OTC *analgesic; antipyretic* [acetaminophen] 100 mg/mL; 80 mg/0.8 mL

Tylenol Junior Strength chewable tablets OTC *analgesic; antipyretic* [acetaminophen] 160 mg

Tylenol Multisymptom liquid (discontinued 1992) OTC *decongestant; antihistamine; antitussive; analgesic* [pseudoephedrine HCl; chlorpheniramine maleate; dextromethorphan hydrobromide; acetaminophen]

Tylenol Multisymptom tablets, caplets (name changed to Tylenol Cold in 1992)
Tylenol Multi-Symptom Hot Medication powder for oral solution OTC *antitussive; decongestant; antihistamine; analgesic* [dextromethorphan hydrobromide; pseudoephedrine HCl; chlorpheniramine maleate; acetaminophen] 30•60•4•650 mg/packet
Tylenol No. 1, No. 2, No. 3, and No. 4 [see: Tylenol with Codeine]
Tylenol PM tablets, caplets, gelcaps OTC *antihistaminic sleep aid; analgesic* [diphenhydramine HCl; acetaminophen] 25•500 mg
Tylenol Severe Allergy caplets OTC *antihistamine; analgesic* [diphenhydramine HCl; acetaminophen] 12.5•500 mg
Tylenol Sinus tablets, caplets, geltabs, gelcaps OTC *decongestant; analgesic; antipyretic* [pseudoephedrine HCl; acetaminophen] 30•500 mg
Tylenol with Codeine elixir ℞ *narcotic analgesic* [codeine phosphate; acetaminophen] 12•120 mg/5 mL
Tylenol with Codeine No. 1 tablets (discontinued 1994) ℞ *narcotic analgesic* [codeine phosphate; acetaminophen] 7.5•300 mg
Tylenol with Codeine No. 2, No. 3, and No. 4 tablets ℞ *narcotic analgesic* [codeine phosphate; acetaminophen] 15•300 mg; 30•300 mg; 60•300 mg
tylosin INN, BAN
Tylox capsules ℞ *narcotic analgesic* [oxycodone HCl; acetaminophen] 5•500 mg
tyloxapol USAN, USP, INN, BAN *detergent; wetting agent; cleaner/lubricant for artificial eyes*
Tympagesic ear drops ℞ *topical local anesthetic; analgesic; decongestant* [benzocaine; antipyrine; phenylephrine HCl] 5%•5%•0.25%

Typhim Vi IM injection ℞ *typhoid vaccine for adults and children over 2 years* [typhoid Vi capsular polysaccharide vaccine] 25µg/0.5 mL
typhoid vaccine USP *active bacterin for typhoid fever (Salmonella typhi Ty21a, attenuated)*
Typhoid Vaccine (AKD) subcu injection by jet injectors only ℞ *typhoid vaccine for military use only* [typhoid vaccine, acetone-killed and dried] 8 U/mL
Typhoid Vaccine (H-P) subcu injection (incompatible with jet injectors) ℞ *typhoid vaccine for adults and children* [typhoid vaccine, heat- and phenol-inactivated] 8 U/mL
typhoid Vi capsular polysaccharide vaccine *active bacterin for typhoid fever (Salmonella typhi Ty2, inactivated)*
typhus vaccine USP
Tyrex-2 powder OTC *enteral nutritional therapy for tyrosinemia*
Tyrobenz lozenges (discontinued 1992) OTC *topical oral anesthetic* [benzocaine] 10 mg
Tyrodone liquid ℞ *antitussive; decongestant* [hydrodocone bitartrate; pseudoephedrine HCl; alcohol 5%] 5•60 mg/5 mL
tyromedan INN *thyromimetic* [also: thyromedan HCl]
tyromedan HCl [see: thyromedan HCl]
Tyromex-1 powder OTC *formula for infants with tyrosinemia type I*
tyropanoate sodium USAN, USP *cholecystographic radiopaque medium* [also: sodium tyropanoate]
tyrosine (L-tyrosine) USAN, USP, INN *nonessential amino acid; symbols: Tyr, Y*
Tyrosum Cleanser liquid, packets OTC *topical cleanser for acne* [isopropanol; acetone] 50%•10%
tyrothricin USP, INN *antibacterial*
Tyzine nasal spray, nose drops, pediatric drops ℞ *nasal decongestant* [tetrahydrozoline HCl] 0.1%; 0.1%; 0.05%

U89 investigational (Phase I/II) reverse transcriptase inhibitor for AIDS

U-10,483 investigational treatment for diabetes

U-93,385 investigational antidepressant and anxiolytic

U-96,988 investigational protease inhibitor for HIV infections

U-98,079 investigational anxiolytic and antidepressant

U-98,222 investigational treatment for Alzheimer's disease

U-98,950 investigational treatment for Alzheimer's disease

UAA sugar-coated tablets ℞ *urinary anti-infective; analgesic; antispasmodic; acidifier* [methenamine; phenyl salicylate; atropine sulfate; methylene blue; hyoscyamine sulfate; benzoic acid] 40.8•18.1•0.03•5.4•0.03•4.5 mg

UAD cream, lotion ℞ *topical anti-infective; corticosteroid* [clioquinol; hydrocortisone]

UAD Otic ear drop suspension ℞ *topical corticosteroidal anti-inflammatory; antibiotic* [hydrocortisone; neomycin sulfate; polymyxin B sulfate] 1%•5 mg•10,000 U per mL

ubenimex INN

ubidecarenone INN

ubiquinone [see: coenzyme Q10]

ubisindine INN

Ucephan oral solution ℞ *hyperammonemia preventative for urea cycle enzymopathy (orphan)* [sodium benzoate; sodium phenylacetate] 10•10 g/100 mL

UCG Beta Slide Monoclonal II slide tests for professional use *in vitro diagnostic aid for urine pregnancy test*

UCG Slide tests for professional use *in vitro diagnostic aid for urine pregnancy test* [latex agglutination test]

U-Cort cream ℞ *topical corticosteroid* [hydrocortisone acetate] 1%

UDIP (trademarked packaging form) *unit-dose identification package*

Uendex ℞ *investigational (Phase II) antiviral for AIDS/ARC/HIV; (orphan: cystic fibrosis)* [dextran sulfate]

ufenamate INN

ufiprazole INN

U-Ject (trademarked delivery system) *prefilled disposable syringe*

UK-109,496 investigational (Phase II) antifungal for HIV-related candidiasis and aspergillosis

Ulcerease mouth rinse OTC *topical antipruritic/counterirritant; mild local anesthetic* [phenol] 0.6%

uldazepam USAN, INN *sedative*

ulinastatin INN

ulobetasol INN *topical corticosteroidal anti-inflammatory* [also: halobetasol propionate]

ULR-LA long-acting tablets ℞ *decongestant; expectorant* [phenylpropanolamine HCl; guaifenesin] 75•400 mg

Ultane liquid for vaporization ℞ *inhalation general anesthetic* [sevoflurane]

Ultiva IV injection ℞ *narcotic analgesic; adjunct to anesthesia for surgery* [remifentanil HCl] ≟

Ultra B-50 tablets (discontinued 1992) OTC *vitamin supplement* [multiple B vitamins; folic acid; biotin; inositol; choline; lecithin]

Ultra Derm lotion, bath oil OTC *moisturizer; emollient*

Ultra KLB6 tablets OTC *dietary supplement* [vitamin B_6; multiple food supplements] 16.7•≟ mg

Ultra Mide 25 lotion OTC *moisturizer; emollient; keratolytic* [urea] 25%

Ultra Tears eye drops OTC *ocular moisturizer/lubricant* [hydroxypropyl methylcellulose] 1%

Ultra Vent (trademarked delivery system) *jet nebulizer*

Ultra Vita Time tablets OTC *dietary supplement* [multiple vitamins, minerals, and food products; iron; folic acid; biotin] ≟•6•0.4•1 mg

Ultra Vitamin A & D tablets (discontinued 1992) OTC *vitamin supplement* [vitamins A and D]

UltraBrom sustained-release capsules ℞ *decongestant; antihistamine* [pseudoephedrine HCl; brompheniramine maleate] 120•12 mg

UltraBrom PD timed-release capsules ℞ *pediatric decongestant and antihistamine* [pseudoephedrine HCl; brompheniramine maleate] 60•6 mg

Ultracal liquid OTC *enteral nutritional therapy* [lactose-free formula]

Ultra-Care solution + tablets OTC *two-step chemical disinfecting system for soft contact lenses* [hydrogen peroxide-based] 3%

Ultracef capsules, tablets (discontinued 1995) ℞ *cephalosporin-type antibiotic* [cefadroxil monohydrate] 500 mg; 1 g

Ultracef oral suspension (discontinued 1995) ℞ *cephalosporin-type antibiotic* [cefadroxil] 125, 250 mg/5 mL

Ultra-Freeda; Ultra Freeda, Iron Free tablets OTC *geriatric vitamin/mineral supplement* [multiple vitamins & minerals; folic acid; biotin] ±•270•100 μg

Ultraject prefilled syringe ℞ *investigational contrast agent*

Ultralan liquid OTC *enteral nutritional therapy* [lactose-free formula]

Ultralente Iletin I subcu injection (discontinued 1994) OTC *antidiabetic* [insulin zinc (beef-pork)] 100 U/mL

Ultralente Insulin subcu injection (name changed to Ultralente U in 1994)

Ultralente U subcu injection (discontinued 1994) OTC *antidiabetic* [extended insulin zinc (beef)] 100 U/mL

Ultram film-coated tablets ℞ *analgesic* [tramadol HCl] 50 mg

Ultraprin tablets OTC *analgesic; nonsteroidal anti-inflammatory drug (NSAID); antipyretic* [ibuprofen]

Ultrase MT 12; Ultrase MT 20 capsules ℞ *digestive enzymes* [lipase, protease; amylase] 12,000•39,000•39,000 U; 20,000•65,000•65,000 U

Ultrase MT 24 capsules (discontinued 1994) ℞ *digestive enzymes* [lipase, protease; amylase] 24,000•78,000•78,000 U

Ultravate ointment, cream ℞ *topical corticosteroidal anti-inflammatory* [halobetasol propionate] 0.05%

Ultravist IV injection ℞ *radiopaque imaging agent for the head, heart, peripheral vascular system, and genitourinary tract* [iopromide (source of iodine)] 311.7 (150), 498.72 (240), 623.4 (300), 768.86 (370) mg

Ultrazyme Enzymatic Cleaner effervescent tablets OTC *enzymatic cleaner for soft contact lenses* [subtilisin A]

umespirone INN

Unasyn powder for IV or IM injection ℞ *penicillin-type antibiotic* [ampicillin sodium; sulbactam sodium] 1•0.5, 2•1 g

Unavit Therapeutic tablets OTC *vitamin/mineral supplement* [multiple vitamins & minerals]

Unavit-M tablets OTC *vitamin/mineral supplement* [multiple vitamins & minerals]

10-undecenoic acid [see: undecylenic acid]

10-undecenoic acid, calcium salt [see: calcium undecylenate]

undecoylium chloride-iodine

undecylenic acid USP *antifungal*

Unguentine aerosol spray (discontinued 1995) OTC *topical local anesthetic* [benzocaine] 0.99 g/oz.

Unguentine ointment OTC *minor burn treatment* [phenol; zinc oxide; eucalyptus oil] 1%•²•²

Unguentine Plus cream OTC *topical local anesthetic* [lidocaine HCl; phenol] 2%•0.5%

Unguentum Bossi cream ℞ *topical antipsoriatic; anti-infective; bactericidal* [ammoniated mercury; methenamine sulfosalicylate; coal tar] 5%•2%•2%

Uni-Ace infant drops OTC *analgesic; antipyretic* [acetaminophen] 100 mg/mL

Uni-Amp (trademarked packaging form) *single-dose ampule*

Unibase OTC *ointment base*

Uni-Bent Cough syrup OTC *antihistamine; antitussive* [diphenhydramine HCl; alcohol 5%] 12.5 mg/5 mL

Unicap capsules, tablets OTC *vitamin supplement* [multiple vitamins; folic acid] ±•0.4 mg

Unicap Jr. chewable tablets OTC *vitamin supplement* [multiple vitamins; folic acid] ±•0.4 mg

Unicap M; Unicap T tablets OTC *vitamin/mineral/iron supplement* [multiple vitamins & minerals; iron; folic acid] ≜ •18•0.4 mg

Unicap Plus Iron tablets OTC *vitamin/iron supplement* [multiple vitamins; iron; folic acid] ≜ •22.5•0.4 mg

Unicap Sr. tablets OTC *vitamin/mineral/iron supplement* [multiple vitamins & minerals; iron; folic acid] ≜ •10•0.4 mg

Unicard ℞ *investigational antihypertensive and vasodilator* [dilevalol]

Unicomplex T & M tablets OTC *vitamin/mineral/iron supplement* [multiple vitamins & minerals; iron; folic acid] ≜ •18•0.4 mg

Uni-Decon sustained-release tablets ℞ *decongestant; antihistamine* [phenylpropanolamine HCl; phenylephrine HCl; chlorpheniramine maleate; phenyltoloxamine citrate] 40•10•5•15 mg

Uni-Dur extended-release tablets ℞ *once-daily antiasthmatic/bronchodilator* [theophylline] 400, 600 mg

Unifiber powder OTC *bulk laxative* [powdered cellulose]

unifocon A USAN *hydrophobic contact lens material*

Unilax capsules OTC *laxative; stool softener* [phenolphthalein; docusate sodium] 130•230 mg

Unimatic (trademarked delivery system) *prefilled disposable syringe*

Uni-nest (trademarked packaging form) *ampule*

Unipak (packaging form) *dispensing pack*

Unipen film-coated tablets, capsules, powder for IV or IM injection ℞ *bactericidal antibiotic (penicillinase-resistant penicillin)* [nafcillin sodium monohydrate] 500 mg; 250 mg; 0.5, 1, 2, 10 g ▣ Omnipen

Uniphyl timed-release tablets ℞ *bronchodilator* [theophylline] 400, 600 mg

Unipres tablets (discontinued 1996) ℞ *antihypertensive* [hydrochlorothiazide; reserpine; hydralazine HCl] 15•0.1•25 mg

Uniquin (foreign name for U.S. product Maxaquin)

Uni-Rx (trademarked packaging form) *unit-dose containers and packages*

Unisert (trademarked dosage form) *suppository*

Unisol; Unisol 4 solution OTC *rinsing/storage solution for soft contact lenses* [preservative-free saline solution]

Unisol Plus aerosol solution OTC *rinsing/storage solution for soft contact lenses* [preservative-free saline solution]

Unisom Nighttime Sleep-Aid tablets OTC *antihistaminic sleep aid* [doxylamine succinate] 25 mg

Unisom SleepGels (capsules) OTC *antihistaminic sleep aid* [diphenhydramine HCl] 50 mg

Unisom with Pain Relief tablets OTC *antihistaminic sleep aid; analgesic* [diphenhydramine citrate; acetaminophen] 50•650 mg

Unistep hCG test kit for professional use *in vitro diagnostic aid for urine pregnancy test*

Unitrol timed-release capsules OTC *diet aid* [phenylpropanolamine HCl] 75 mg

Unituss HC syrup ℞ *narcotic antitussive; decongestant; antihistamine* [hydrocodone bitartrate; phenylephrine HCl; chlorpheniramine maleate] 2.5•5•2 mg/5 mL

Uni-Tussin syrup OTC *expectorant* [guaifenesin; alcohol 3.5%] 100 mg/5 mL

Uni-Tussin DM syrup OTC *antitussive; expectorant* [dextromethorphan hydrobromide; guaifenesin] 10•100 mg/5 mL

Univasc tablets ℞ *antihypertensive; angiotensin-converting enzyme (ACE) inhibitor* [moexipril HCl] 7.5, 15 mg

Universal Antidote (discontinued 1996) *general-purpose gastric adsorbent/detoxicant* [activated charcoal; magnesium hydroxide; tannic acid] ≜

Univial (trademarked form) *single-dose vials*

Unizime ℞ *investigational cephalosporin antibiotic* [cefodizime]

Unna's boot [see: Dome-Paste bandage]

Urabeth tablets (discontinued 1992) ℞ *postsurgical cholinergic bladder muscle stimulant* [bethanechol chloride]

Uracel 5 enteric-coated tablets (discontinued 1992) OTC *analgesic; antipyretic; anti-inflammatory* [sodium salicylate] ⓘ uracil; Urised

Uracid capsules ℞ *urinary acidifier to control ammonia production* [racemethionine] 200 mg ⓘ uracil; Urised; Urocit

uracil mustard USAN, USP *alkylating antineoplastic* [also: uramustine] 1 mg oral ⓘ Uracel; Uracid

uradal [see: carbromal]

uralenic acid [see: enoxolone]

uramustine INN *antineoplastic* [also: uracil mustard]

Uranap; Uranap 500 capsules (discontinued 1993) OTC *urinary acidifier to control ammonia production; oral amino acid supplement* [racemethionine]

uranin [see: fluorescein sodium]

uranium *element (U)*

urapidil INN, BAN

urea USP *osmotic diuretic; keratolytic; emollient*

urea peroxide [see: carbamide peroxide]

Ureacin-10 lotion OTC *moisturizer; emollient; keratolytic* [urea] 10%

Ureacin-20 cream OTC *moisturizer; emollient; keratolytic* [urea] 20%

Ureacin-40 cream (discontinued 1995) ℞ *for removal of dystrophic nails* [urea] 40%

Ureaphil IV infusion ℞ *osmotic diuretic* [urea] 40 g/150 mL

Urecholine tablets, subcu injection ℞ *postsurgical cholinergic bladder muscle stimulant* [bethanechol chloride] 5, 10, 25, 50 mg; 5 mg/mL

uredepa USAN, INN *antineoplastic*

uredofos USAN, INN *veterinary anthelmintic*

urefibrate INN

p-ureidobenzenearsonic acid [see: carbarsone]

urethan NF [also: urethane]

urethane INN, BAN [also: urethan]

urethane polymers [see: polyurethane foam]

Urethrin injection ℞ *investigational treatment of urinary incontinence*

Urex tablets ℞ *urinary bactericidal* [methenamine hippurate] 1 g ⓘ Eurax; Serax

Uricult culture paddles for professional use *in vitro diagnostic aid for nitrate, uropathogens, or bacteria in the urine*

Uridon Modified sugar-coated tablets ℞ *urinary anti-infective; analgesic; antispasmodic; acidifier* [methenamine; phenyl salicylate; atropine sulfate; methylene blue; hyoscyamine sulfate; benzoic acid] 40.8•18.1•0.03•5.4•0.03•4.5 mg

Urimar-T tablets ℞ *urinary anti-infective; antiseptic; analgesic; antispasmodic* [methenamine; sodium biphosphate; phenyl salicylate; methylene blue; hyoscyamine sulfate] 81.6•40.8•36.2•10.8•0.12 mg

Urimed Modified Formula tablets ℞ *urinary anti-infective; analgesic; antispasmodic; acidifier* [atropine sulfate; hyoscyamine sulfate; methenamine; methylene blue; phenyl salicylate; benzoic acid]

Urinary Antiseptic No. 2 tablets ℞ *urinary anti-infective; analgesic; antispasmodic; acidifier* [methenamine; phenyl salicylate; atropine sulfate; methylene blue; hyoscyamine sulfate; benzoic acid] 40.8•18.1•0.03•5.4•0.03•4.5 mg

Urised sugar-coated tablets ℞ *urinary anti-infective; analgesic; antispasmodic; acidifier* [methenamine; phenyl salicylate; atropine sulfate; methylene blue; hyoscyamine sulfate; benzoic acid] 40.8•18.1•0.03•5.4•0.03•4.5 mg ⓘ Uracel; Uracid; Urispas

Urisedamine tablets ℞ *urinary anti-infective; antispasmodic* [methenamine mandelate; hyoscyamine] 500•0.15 mg

Urispas film-coated tablets ℞ *urinary antispasmodic* [flavoxate HCl] 100 mg ⓘ Urised

Uristat tablets ℞ *urinary analgesic* [phenazopyridine HCl] 95 mg

Uristix; Uristix 4 reagent strips *in vitro diagnostic aid for multiple urine products*

Uritab tablets ℞ *urinary anti-infective; analgesic; antispasmodic; acidifier* [methenamine; phenyl salicylate; atropine sulfate; methylene blue; hyoscyamine; benzoic acid] 40.8•18.1•0.03•5.4•0.03•4.5 mg

Uri-Tet capsules ℞ *antibacterial* [oxytetracycline HCl] 250 mg

Uritin tablets ℞ *urinary anti-infective; analgesic; antispasmodic; acidifier* [methenamine; phenyl salicylate; atropine sulfate; methylene blue; hyoscyamine sulfate; benzoic acid] 40.8•18.1•0.03•5.4•0.03•4.5 mg

Urobak tablets ℞ *broad-spectrum bacteriostatic* [sulfamethoxazole] 500 mg

Urobiotic-250 capsules ℞ *urinary anti-infective* [oxytetracycline HCl; sulfamethizole; phenazopyridine HCl] 250•250•50 mg ② Otobiotic

Urocit-K tablets ℞ *urinary alkalizer; nephrolithiasis and hypocitraturia prevention (orphan)* [potassium citrate] 5, 10 mEq ② Uracid

urodilatin *investigational atrial natriuretic peptide to prevent renal failure after heart transplant*

Urodine tablets ℞ *urinary analgesic* [phenazopyridine HCl] 100, 200 mg

urofollitrophin BAN *follicle-stimulating hormone (FSH)* [also: urofollitropin]

urofollitropin USAN, INN *follicle-stimulating hormone (FSH); ovulation stimulant in polycystic ovarian disease (orphan)* [also: urofollitrophin]

urogastrone *(orphan: corneal transplant surgery)*

Urogesic tablets ℞ *urinary analgesic* [phenazopyridine HCl] 100 mg

Urogesic Blue sugar-coated tablets ℞ *urinary anti-infective; antiseptic; analgesic; antispasmodic* [methenamine; sodium biphosphate; phenyl salicylate; methylene blue; hyoscyamine sulfate] 81.6•40.8•36.2•10.8•0.12 mg

urokinase USAN, INN, BAN *plasminogen activator; thrombolytic enzyme*

Uro-KP-Neutral film-coated tablets ℞ *phosphorus supplement* [disodium phosphate; dipotassium phosphate; monobasic sodium phosphate] 250 mg (P)

Urolene Blue tablets ℞ *urinary anti-infective/antiseptic; antidote to cyanide poisoning* [methylene blue] 65 mg

Uro-Mag capsules OTC *antacid; magnesium supplement* [magnesium oxide] 140 mg

uronal [see: barbital]

Uro-Phosphate film-coated tablets ℞ *urinary anti-infective; acidifier* [methenamine; sodium biphosphate] 300•434.78 mg

Uroplus SS; Uroplus DS tablets (discontinued 1994) ℞ *anti-infective; antibacterial* [trimethoprim; sulfamethoxazole] 80•400 mg; 160•800 mg

Uroqid-Acid sugar-coated tablets (discontinued 1994) ℞ *urinary anti-infective; acidifier* [methenamine mandelate; sodium acid phosphate] 350•200 mg

Uroqid-Acid No. 2 film-coated tablets ℞ *urinary anti-infective; acidifier* [methenamine mandelate; sodium acid phosphate] 500•500 mg

Uro-Ves tablets (discontinued 1994) ℞ *urinary anti-infective; analgesic; antispasmodic; acidifier* [methenamine; phenyl salicylate; atropine sulfate; methylene blue; hyoscyamine; benzoic acid] 40.8•18.1•0.03•5.4•0.03•4.5 mg

Urovist Cysto intracavitary instillation ℞ *urologic radiopaque agent* [diatrizoate meglumine] 30%

Urovist Meglumine DIU/CT injection ℞ *parenteral renal radiopaque agent* [diatrizoate meglumine] 30%

Urovist Sodium 300 injection ℞ *parenteral radiopaque agent* [diatrizoate sodium] 50%

Ursinus Inlay-Tabs (tablets) OTC *decongestant; analgesic; antipyretic* [pseudoephedrine HCl; aspirin] 30•325 mg

ursodeoxycholic acid INN, BAN *anticholelithogenic; (orphan: primary biliary cirrhosis)* [also: ursodiol]

ursodiol USAN *anticholelithogenic; (orphan: primary biliary cirrhosis)* [also: ursodeoxycholic acid]

Ursofalk ℞ *(orphan: primary biliary cirrhosis)* [ursodiol]

ursulcholic acid INN

Uticort cream, lotion, gel (discontinued 1996) ℞ *topical corticosteroid* [betamethasone benzoate] 0.025%

Uvadex ℞ *(orphan: prevent rejection of cardiac allografts; treat diffuse systemic sclerosis)* [methoxsalen]

VA (vincristine, actinomycin D) *chemotherapy protocol*

VAAP (vincristine, asparaginase, Adriamycin, prednisone) *chemotherapy protocol*

VAB; VAB-I (vinblastine, actinomycin D, bleomycin) *chemotherapy protocol*

VAB-II (vinblastine, actinomycin D, bleomycin, cisplatin) *chemotherapy protocol*

VAB-III (vinblastine, actinomycin D, bleomycin, cisplatin, chlorambucil, cyclophosphamide) *chemotherapy protocol*

VAB-V (vinblastine, actinomycin D, bleomycin, cyclophosphamide, cisplatin) *chemotherapy protocol*

VAB-6 (vinblastine, actinomycin D, bleomycin, cyclophosphamide, cisplatin) *chemotherapy protocol*

VABCD (vinblastine, Adriamycin, bleomycin, CCNU, DTIC) *chemotherapy protocol*

VAC (vincristine, Adriamycin, cisplatin) *chemotherapy protocol*

VAC; VAC pulse; VAC standard (vincristine, actinomycin D, cyclophosphamide) *chemotherapy protocol*

VAC; VAC pulse; VAC standard (vincristine, Adriamycin, cyclophosphamide) *chemotherapy protocol* also: CAV

VACA (vincristine, actinomycin D, cyclophosphamide, Adriamycin) *chemotherapy protocol*

VACAD (vincristine, actinomycin D, cyclophosphamide, Adriamycin, dacarbazine) *chemotherapy protocol*

VACAdr-IfoVP (vincristine, actinomycin D, cyclophosphamide, Adriamycin, ifosfamide, VePesid) *chemotherapy protocol*

vaccinia (human papillomavirus) [see: recombinant vaccinia (human papillomavirus)]

vaccinia immune globulin (VIG) USP *passive immunizing agent*

vaccinia immune human globulin [now: vaccinia immune globulin]

VACP (VePesid, Adriamycin, cyclophosphamide, Platinol) *chemotherapy protocol*

VAD (vincristine, Adriamycin, dactinomycin) *chemotherapy protocol*

VAD (vincristine, Adriamycin, dexamethasone) *chemotherapy protocol*

Vademin-Z capsules OTC *vitamin/mineral supplement* [multiple vitamins & minerals] ≚

vadocaine INN

VAdrC (vincristine, Adriamycin, cyclophosphamide) *chemotherapy protocol*

VAD/V (vincristine, Adriamycin, dexamethasone, verapamil) *chemotherapy protocol*

VAFAC (vincristine, amethopterin, fluorouracil, Adriamycin, cyclophosphamide) *chemotherapy protocol*

Vagilia vaginal cream (discontinued 1992) ℞ *bacteriostatic; antiseptic; vulnerary* [sulfisoxazole; aminacrine HCl; allantoin] 10%•0.2%•2%

Vaginex vaginal cream OTC *topical antihistamine* [tripelennamine HCl]

Vagisec Douche solution ℞ *vaginal cleanser and deodorizer*

Vagisec Plus vaginal suppositories ℞ *antiseptic* [aminacrine HCl] 6 mg

Vagisil cream OTC *topical local anesthetic; antipruritic; antifungal* [benzocaine; resorcinol] 5%•2%

Vagisil powder OTC *absorbs vaginal moisture* [cornstarch; aloe]

Vagistat-1 vaginal ointment in pre-filled applicator ℞ *antifungal* [tioconazole] 6.5%

Vagitrol vaginal cream (discontinued 1992) ℞ *broad-spectrum bacteriostatic* [sulfanilamide]

VAI (vincristine, actinomycin D, ifosfamide) *chemotherapy protocol*

valaciclovir INN *antiviral for herpes zoster and herpes simplex* [also: valacyclovir HCl]

valacyclovir HCl USAN *antiviral for herpes zoster and herpes simplex* [also: valaciclovir]

valconazole INN

valdetamide INN

valdipromide INN

valepotriate [see: valtrate]

Valergen 10 IM injection (discontinued 1995) ℞ *estrogen replacement therapy for postmenopausal disorders; antineoplastic for prostatic cancer* [estradiol valerate in oil] 10 mg/mL

Valergen 20; Valergen 40 IM injection ℞ *estrogen replacement therapy for postmenopausal disorders; antineoplastic for prostatic cancer* [estradiol valerate in oil] 20 mg/mL; 40 mg/mL

Valertest No. 1 IM injection ℞ *estrogen/androgen for menopausal vasomotor symptoms* [estradiol valerate; testosterone enanthate] 4•90 mg/mL

valethamate bromide NF

Valihist tablets OTC *antihistamine; decongestant; analgesic; antipyretic* [chlorpheniramine maleate; phenylephrine HCl; acetaminophen; caffeine]

valine (L-valine) USAN, USP, INN, JAN *essential amino acid*; symbols: Val, V

Valisone ointment, cream, lotion ℞ *topical corticosteroid* [betamethasone valerate] 0.1%

Valisone Reduced Strength cream ℞ *topical corticosteroid* [betamethasone valerate] 0.01%

Valium tablets, IV or IM injection, Tel-E-Ject syringes ℞ *sedative; anxiolytic; skeletal muscle relaxant; anticonvulsant adjunct* [diazepam] 2, 5, 10 mg; 5 mg/mL; 10 mg ⑨ thallium; Valpin

valnoctamide USAN, INN *tranquilizer*

valofane INN

Valorin; Valorin Extra tablets OTC *analgesic; antipyretic* [acetaminophen]

Valorin Super tablets OTC *analgesic; antipyretic* [acetaminophen; caffeine]

valperinol INN

Valpin 50 tablets (discontinued 1992) ℞ *anticholinergic; treatment of peptic ulcer; antisecretory* [anisotropine methylbromide] 50 mg ⑨ Valium; Valprin; Velban

Valprin tablets OTC *analgesic; nonsteroidal anti-inflammatory drug (NSAID); antipyretic* [ibuprofen] ⑨ Valpin

valproate pivoxil INN

valproate semisodium INN *anticonvulsant* [also: divalproex sodium; semisodium valproate]

valproate sodium USAN *anticonvulsant* 250 mg/5 mL oral

valproic acid USAN, USP, INN, BAN *anticonvulsant* 250 mg oral

valpromide INN

Valrelease sustained-release capsules (discontinued 1996) ℞ *sedative; anxiolytic; skeletal muscle relaxant; anticonvulsant adjunct* [diazepam] 15 mg

valsartan USAN, INN *antihypertensive; angiotensin II receptor antagonist*

Valsartan ℞ *investigational angiotensin II antagonist for cardiovascular disorders*

valtrate INN

Valtrex film-coated caplets ℞ *antiviral for herpes zoster and herpes simplex* [valacyclovir HCl] 500 mg

VAM (vinblastine, Adriamycin, mitomycin) *chemotherapy protocol*

VAM (VP-16-213, Adriamycin, methotrexate) *chemotherapy protocol*

VAMP (vincristine, actinomycin, methotrexate, prednisone) *chemotherapy protocol*

VAMP (vincristine, Adriamycin, methylprednisolone) *chemotherapy protocol*

VAMP (vincristine, amethopterin, mercaptopurine, prednisone) *chemotherapy protocol*

vanadium *element* (V)

Vancenase Pockethaler (nasal inhalation aerosol) ℞ *intranasal steroidal* *anti-inflammatory* [beclomethasone dipropionate] 42 μg/dose

Vancenase AQ nasal spray ℞ *intranasal steroidal anti-inflammatory* [beclomethasone dipropionate] 0.042%, 0.084%

Vanceril oral inhalation aerosol ℞ *corticosteroid for bronchial asthma* [beclomethasone dipropionate] 42 μg/dose

Vancocin Pulvules (capsules), powder for oral solution, powder for IV or IM injection ℞ *glycopeptide-type antibiotic* [vancomycin HCl] 125, 250 mg; 1, 10 g; 0.5, 1, 10 g

Vancoled powder for IV or IM injection ℞ *glycopeptide-type antibiotic* [vancomycin HCl] 0.5, 1, 5 g

vancomycin INN, BAN *tricyclic glycopeptide bactericidal antibiotic* [also: vancomycin HCl]

vancomycin HCl USP *tricyclic glycopeptide bactericidal antibiotic* [also: vancomycin] 500, 1000 mg/vial injection; 250 mg/mL oral

Vancor Intravenous powder for IV injection (discontinued 1992) ℞ *antibiotic* [vancomycin HCl]

vaneprim INN

Vanex Expectorant liquid ℞ *narcotic antitussive; decongestant; expectorant* [hydrocodone bitartrate; pseudoephedrine HCl; guaifenesin; alcohol 5%] 2.5•30•100 mg/5 mL

Vanex Forte sustained-release caplets ℞ *decongestant; antihistamine* [phenylpropanolamine HCl; phenylephrine HCl; chlorpheniramine maleate; pyrilamine maleate] 50•10•4•25 mg

Vanex-HD liquid ℞ *narcotic antitussive; decongestant; antihistamine* [hydrocodone bitartrate; phenylephrine HCl; chlorpheniramine maleate] 1.67•5•2 mg/5 mL

Vanex-LA long-acting tablets (discontinued 1996) ℞ *decongestant; expectorant* [phenylpropanolamine HCl; guaifenesin] 75•400 mg

Vanicream OTC *cream base*

vanilla NF *flavoring agent*

vanillin NF *flavoring agent*

N-vanillylnonamide [see: nonivamide]

N-vanillyloleamide [see: olvanil]

vanitiolide INN

Vanoxide lotion OTC *topical keratolytic for acne* [benzoyl peroxide] 5%

Vanoxide-HC lotion ℞ *keratolytic for acne; topical corticosteroid* [benzoyl peroxide; hydrocortisone] 5%•0.5%

Vanquish caplets OTC *analgesic; antipyretic; anti-inflammatory* [acetaminophen; aspirin; caffeine] 194•227•33 mg

Vanseb cream, lotion OTC *antiseborrheic; keratolytic* [sulfur; salicylic acid]

Vanseb shampoo (discontinued 1994) OTC *antiseborrheic; keratolytic* [sulfur; salicylic acid] 2%•1%

Vanseb-T cream shampoo, lotion shampoo (discontinued 1994) OTC *antiseborrheic; antipsoriatic; keratolytic* [coal tar; salicylic acid; sulfur] 5%•2%•1%

Vansil capsules ℞ *anthelmintic* [oxamniquine] 250 mg

Vantin film-coated tablets, granules for suspension ℞ *cephalosporin-type antibiotic* [cefpodoxime proxetil] 100, 200 mg; 50, 100 mg/5 mL

Vantol ℞ *investigational beta blocker for hypertension* [bevantolol]

vanyldisulfamide INN

VAP (vinblastine, actinomycin D, Platinol) *chemotherapy protocol*

VAP (vincristine, Adriamycin, prednisone) *chemotherapy protocol*

VAP (vincristine, Adriamycin, procarbazine) *chemotherapy protocol*

VAP (vincristine, asparaginase, prednisone) *chemotherapy protocol*

vapiprost INN, BAN *antagonist to thromboxane* A_2 [also: vapiprost HCl]

vapiprost HCl USAN *antagonist to thromboxane* A_2 [also: vapiprost]

Vaponefrin solution for inhalation OTC *bronchodilator for bronchial asthma* [racepinephrine] 2%

Vaporole (trademarked dosage form) *crushable ampule for inhalation*

vapreotide USAN *antineoplastic*

Vaqta IM injection ℞ *hepatitis A vaccine* [hepatitis A vaccine, inactivated] 25 U/0.5 mL (pediatric), 50 U/mL (adult)

varicella virus vaccine *live, attenuated vaccine for chickenpox*

varicella-zoster immune globulin (VZIG) USP *passive immunizing agent* 10%–18% (125 U/2.5 mL)

Varivax powder for subcu injection ℞ *vaccine for chickenpox* [varicella virus vaccine, live attenuated] 1350 PFU/0.5 mL

Vascor film-coated tablets ℞ *antianginal* [bepridil HCl] 200, 300, 400 mg

Vascoray injection ℞ *parenteral radiopaque agent* [iothalamate meglumine; iothalamate sodium] 52%•26%

Vaseretic 5-12.5; Vaseretic 10-25 tablets ℞ *antihypertensive* [enalapril maleate; hydrochlorothiazide] 5•12.5 mg; 10•25 mg

vasoactive intestinal polypeptide *investigational treatment for male sexual dysfunction (orphan: acute esophageal food impaction)*

Vasocidin eye drops ℞ *ophthalmic topical corticosteroidal anti-inflammatory; bacteriostatic* [prednisolone sodium phosphate; sulfacetamide sodium] 0.25%•10% ⓓ Vasodilan

Vasocidin ophthalmic ointment ℞ *ophthalmic topical corticosteroidal anti-inflammatory; bacteriostatic* [prednisolone acetate; sulfacetamide sodium] 0.5%•10%

VasoClear eye drops OTC *topical ocular decongestant/vasoconstrictor* [naphazoline HCl] 0.02%

VasoClear A eye drops OTC *topical ocular decongestant; astringent* [naphazoline HCl; zinc sulfate] 0.02%•0.25%

Vasocon Regular eye drops ℞ *topical ocular decongestant/vasoconstrictor* [naphazoline HCl] 0.1%

Vasocon-A eye drops ℞ *topical ocular decongestant and antihistamine* [naphazoline HCl; antazoline phosphate] 0.05%•0.5%

Vasoderm; Vasoderm-E cream ℞ *topical corticosteroid* [fluocinonide]

Vasodilan tablets ℞ *peripheral vasodilator* [isoxsuprine HCl] 10, 20 mg ⓓ Vasocidin

vasopressin (VP) USP, INN *posterior pituitary hormone; antidiuretic*

vasopressin tannate USP *posterior pituitary hormone; antidiuretic*

Vasoprost ℞ *investigational prostaglandin; (orphan: severe peripheral arterial occlusive disease)* [prostaglandin E$_1$ alphacyclodextrin]

Vasosulf eye drops ℞ *ophthalmic bacteriostatic and decongestant* [sodium sulfacetamide; phenylephrine HCl] 15%•0.125% ⓓ Velosef

Vasotate HC ear drops ℞ *topical corticosteroidal anti-inflammatory; antibacterial/antifungal* [hydrocortisone; acetic acid] 1%•2%

Vasotec tablets ℞ *antihypertensive; angiotensin-converting enzyme (ACE) inhibitor* [enalapril maleate] 2.5, 5, 10, 20 mg

Vasotec I.V. injection ℞ *antihypertensive; angiotensin-converting enzyme (ACE) inhibitor* [enalaprilat] 1.25 mg/mL

Vasoxyl IV or IM injection ℞ *vasopressor for hypotensive shock during surgery* [methoxamine HCl] 20 mg/mL

VAT (vinblastine, Adriamycin, thiotepa) *chemotherapy protocol*

VATD; VAT-D (vincristine, ara-C, thioguanine, daunorubicin) *chemotherapy protocol*

VATH (vinblastine, Adriamycin, thiotepa, Halotestin) *chemotherapy protocol*

Vatronol [see: Vicks Vatronol]

VAV (VP-16-213, Adriamycin, vincristine) *chemotherapy protocol*

VaxSyn HIV-1 ℞ *investigational antiviral (therapeutic, Phase II) and vaccine (preventative, Phase I) for HIV* [gp160 antigens]

Vazepam tablets, IV or IM injection (discontinued 1992) ℞ *anticonvulsant; anxiolytic; skeletal muscle relaxant* [diazepam]

VB (vinblastine, bleomycin) *chemotherapy protocol*

VBA (vincristine, BCNU, Adriamycin) *chemotherapy protocol*

VBAP (vincristine, BCNU, Adriamycin, prednisone) *chemotherapy protocol*

VBC (VePesid, BCNU, cyclophosphamide) *chemotherapy protocol*

VBC (vinblastine, bleomycin, cisplatin) *chemotherapy protocol*

VBD (vinblastine, bleomycin, DDP) *chemotherapy protocol*

VBM (vincristine, bleomycin, methotrexate) *chemotherapy protocol*

VBMCP (vincristine, BCNU, melphalan, cyclophosphamide, prednisone) *chemotherapy protocol*

VBMF (vincristine, bleomycin, methotrexate, fluorouracil) *chemotherapy protocol*

VBP (vinblastine, bleomycin, Platinol) *chemotherapy protocol*

VC (VePesid, carboplatin) *chemotherapy protocol*

VC (vincristine) [q.v.]

VC (vinorelbine, cisplatin) *chemotherapy protocol*

VCAP (vincristine, cyclophosphamide, Adriamycin, prednisone) *chemotherapy protocol* [see also: V-CAP III]

V-CAP III (VP-16-213, cyclophosphamide, Adriamycin, Platinol) *chemotherapy protocol* [see also: VCAP]

VCF (vaginal contraceptive film) OTC *spermicidal contraceptive* [nonoxynol 9] 28%

VCF (vincristine, cyclophosphamide, fluorouracil) *chemotherapy protocol*

V-Cillin K tablets, powder for oral solution ℞ *bactericidal antibiotic* [penicillin V potassium] 125, 250, 500 mg; 125, 250 mg/5 mL ② Bicillin; Wycillin

VCMP (vincristine, cyclophosphamide, melphalan, prednisone) *chemotherapy protocol*

VCP (vincristine, cyclophosphamide, prednisone) *chemotherapy protocol*

VCP 205 *investigational (Phase I) vaccine for HIV*

VCR (vincristine) [q.v.]

VDA (vincristine, daunorubicin, asparaginase) *chemotherapy protocol*

V-Dec-M sustained-release tablets ℞ *decongestant; expectorant* [pseudoephedrine HCl; guaifenesin] 120•500 mg

VDP (vinblastine, dacarbazine, Platinol) *chemotherapy protocol*

VDP (vincristine, daunorubicin, prednisone) *chemotherapy protocol*

Veasnoid ℞ *keratolytic (orphan: acute promyelocytic leukemia)* [tretinoin]

vecuronium bromide USAN, INN, BAN *nondepolarizing neuromuscular blocker; muscle relaxant; adjunct to anesthesia*

Veetids '125'; Veetids '250' powder for oral solution ℞ *bactericidal antibiotic* [penicillin V potassium] 125 mg/5 mL; 250 mg/5 mL

Veetids '250'; Veetids '500' film-coated tablets ℞ *bactericidal antibiotic* [penicillin V potassium] 250 mg; 500 mg

Vega ℞ *investigational antiasthmatic* [ozagrel]

vegetable oil, hydrogenated NF *tablet and capsule lubricant*

Vehicle/N; Vehicle/N Mild OTC *lotion base*

VeIP (Velban, ifosfamide, Platinol) *chemotherapy protocol*

Velban powder for IV injection ℞ *antineoplastic for lung, breast and testicular cancers, lymphomas, sarcomas, and neuroblastoma* [vinblastine sulfate] 10 mg ② Valpin

Veldona ℞ *investigational (Phase I) cytokine for AIDS*

velnacrine INN, BAN *cholinesterase inhibitor* [also: velnacrine maleate]

velnacrine maleate USAN *cholinesterase inhibitor* [also: velnacrine]

Velosef capsules, oral suspension, powder for IV or IM injection ℞ *cephalosporin-type antibiotic* [cephradine] 250, 500 mg; 125, 250 mg/5 mL; 250, 500, 1000, 2000 mg ② Vasosulf

Velosulin subcu injection (discontinued 1994) OTC *antidiabetic* [insulin (pork)]

Velosulin Human subcu injection OTC *antidiabetic* [human insulin (semisynthetic)] 100 U/mL

Velsar powder for IV injection (discontinued 1992) ℞ *antineoplastic* [vinblastine sulfate] 10 mg

Veltane tablets ℞ *antihistamine* [brompheniramine maleate] 4 mg

Veltap Lanatabs (sustained-release tablets), elixir (discontinued 1993) ℞ *decongestant; antihistamine* [phenylpropanolamine HCl; phenylephrine HCl; brompheniramine maleate]

Velvachol OTC *cream base*

Vendona ℞ *investigational cytokine for AIDS*

venlafaxine INN, BAN *antidepressant* [also: venlafaxine HCl]

venlafaxine HCl USAN *antidepressant* [also: venlafaxine]

Venoglobulin-I powder for IV infusion ℞ *passive immunizing agent; immunomodulator for AIDS/ARC* [immune globulin] 50 mg/mL

Venoglobulin-S IV infusion ℞ *passive immunizing agent; immunomodulator for AIDS/ARC* [immune globulin, solvent/detergent treated] 5%, 10%

Venomil subcu or IM injection ℞ *venom sensitivity testing (subcu); venom desensitization therapy (IM)* [extracts of honeybee, yellow jacket, yellow hornet, white-faced hornet, mixed vespid, and wasp venom]

Ventolin inhalation aerosol ℞ *bronchodilator* [albuterol] 90 μg/dose ② phentolamine

Ventolin Rotacaps (capsules for inhalation), tablets, Nebules (solution for inhalation), syrup ℞ *bronchodilator* [albuterol sulfate] 200 μg; 2, 4 mg; 0.083%; 2 mg/5 mL

VePesid IV injection, capsules ℞ *antineoplastic for testicular and small cell lung cancers* [etoposide] 20 mg/mL; 50 mg

Veracolate tablets OTC *laxative* [phenolphthalein; cascara sagrada extract; capsicum oleoresin] 32.4•75•0.05 mg

veradoline INN *analgesic* [also: veradoline HCl]

veradoline HCl USAN *analgesic* [also: veradoline]

veralipride INN

verapamil USAN, INN, BAN *coronary vasodilator; calcium channel blocker*

verapamil HCl USAN, USP *antianginal; antiarrhythmic; antihypertensive; calcium channel blocker* 40, 80, 120, 180, 240 mg oral; 5 mg/2 mL injection

veratrylidene-isoniazid [see: verazide]

verazide INN, BAN

Verazinc capsules OTC *zinc supplement* [zinc sulfate] 220 mg

Vercyte tablets (discontinued 1994) ℞ *alkylating antineoplastic for polycythemia vera and chronic myelocytic leukemia* [pipobroman] 25 mg

Verelan sustained-release capsules ℞ *antihypertensive; calcium channel blocker* [verapamil HCl] 120, 180, 240, 360 mg

Vergo cream (discontinued 1992) OTC *topical keratolytic* [calcium pantothenate; ascorbic acid; starch]

Vergogel gel (discontinued 1994) OTC *topical keratolytic* [salicylic acid in collodion] 17%

Vergon capsules OTC *anticholinergic; antihistamine; antivertigo agent; motion sickness preventative* [meclizine HCl] 30 mg

verilopam INN *analgesic* [also: verilopam HCl]

verilopam HCl USAN *analgesic* [also: verilopam]

Verin timed-release tablets (discontinued 1992) OTC *analgesic; antipyretic; anti-inflammatory* [aspirin]

verlukast USAN, INN *bronchodilator; antiasthmatic*

Verluma technetium Tc 99 prep kit ℞ *monoclonal antibody imaging agent for small cell lung cancer* [nofetumomab merpentan]

Vermox chewable tablets ℞ *anthelmintic* [mebendazole] 100 mg

verofylline USAN, INN *bronchodilator; antiasthmatic*

veronal [see: barbital]

veronal sodium [see: barbital sodium]

Verr-Canth liquid ℞ *topical keratolytic* [cantharidin] 0.7%

Verrex liquid ℞ *topical keratolytic* [salicylic acid; podophyllum] 30%•10%

Verrusol liquid (discontinued 1996) ℞ *topical keratolytic* [salicylic acid; podophyllum; cantharidin] 30%•5%•1%

Versacaps prolonged-action capsules ℞ *decongestant; expectorant* [pseudoephedrine HCl; guaifenesin] 60•300 mg

Versed IV or IM injection, Tel-E-Ject syringes ℞ *general anesthetic adjunct; preoperative sedative* [midazolam HCl] 1, 5 mg/mL

versetamide USAN *stabilizer; carrier agent for gadoversetamide*

Versiclear lotion ℞ *topical antifungal; keratolytic; antipruritic; anesthetic* [sodium thiosulfate; salicylic acid; alcohol 10%] 25%•1%

Vertab capsules (discontinued 1995) OTC *antinauseant; antiemetic; antivertigo; motion sickness preventative* [dimenhydrinate] 50 mg

verteporfin USAN *antineoplastic (used with phototherapy)*

Verukan solution (discontinued 1994) ℞ *topical keratolytic* [salicylic acid in flexible collodion; lactic acid] 17%•17%

Verukan-20 (discontinued 1992) ℞ *topical keratolytic* [salicylic acid; lactic acid]

Verukan-HP solution (discontinued 1994) ℞ *topical keratolytic* [salicylic acid in flexible collodion] 26%

Vesanoid capsules ℞ *antineoplastic retinoid to induce remission of acute promyelocytic leukemia (APL)* [tretinoin] 10 mg

vesnarinone USAN, INN *cardiotonic; investigational inotropic for congestive heart failure*

vesperal [see: barbital]

Vesprin IV or IM injection ℞ *antipsychotic; antiemetic* [triflupromazine HCl] 10, 20 mg/mL

vetrabutine INN, BAN

Vexol eye drop suspension ℞ *ophthalmic topical corticosteroidal anti-inflammatory* [rimexolone] 1%

V-Gan 25; V-Gan 50 injection (discontinued 1996) ℞ *antihistamine; motion sickness; sleep aid; antiemetic; sedative* [promethazine HCl] 25 mg/mL; 50 mg/mL

Viaflex (trademarked form) *ready-to-use IV*

Vianain *investigational proteolytic enzymes (orphan: enzymatic debridement of severe burns)* [ananain/comosain; bromelains]

vibesate

Vibramycin capsules, powder for IV injection ℞ *tetracycline-type antibiotic* [doxycycline hyclate] 50, 100 mg; 100, 200 mg

Vibramycin powder for oral suspension ℞ *tetracycline-type antibiotic* [doxycycline monohydrate] 25 mg/5 mL

Vibramycin syrup ℞ *tetracycline-type antibiotic* [doxycycline calcium] 50 mg/5 mL

Vibra-Tabs tablets ℞ *tetracycline-type antibiotic* [doxycycline hyclate] 100 mg

VIC (VePesid, ifosfamide [with mesna rescue], carboplatin) *chemotherapy protocol* [also: CVI]

VIC (vinblastine, ifosfamide, CCNU) *chemotherapy protocol*

Vicam injection ℞ *parenteral vitamin therapy* [multiple B vitamins; vitamin C] ≐•50 mg/mL

Vicef capsules OTC *vitamin/iron supplement* [multiple vitamins; iron; folic acid]

Vicks 44 Non-Drowsy Cold & Cough LiquiCaps (capsules) OTC *antitussive; decongestant* [dextromethorphan hydrobromide; pseudoephedrine HCl] 30•60 mg

Vicks 44 Pediatric syrup (name changed to Vicks Pediatric 44d Dry Hacking Cough and Head Congestion in 1994)

Vicks 44D Cough & Head Congestion; Vicks Formula 44D Cough & Decongestant; Vicks Pediatric Formula 44d Cough & Decongestant liquid OTC *antitussive; decongestant* [dextromethorphan hydrobromide; pseudoephedrine HCl] 10•20 mg/5 mL; 10•20 mg/5 mL; 5•10 mg/5 mL

Vicks 44E liquid OTC *antitussive; expectorant* [dextromethorphan hydrobromide; guaifenesin] 6.7•66.7 mg/5 mL

Vicks 44M Cold, Flu & Cough LiquiCaps (capsules) OTC *antitussive; decongestant; antihistamine; anal-*

gesic [dextromethorphan hydrobromide; pseudoephedrine HCl; chlorpheniramine maleate; acetaminophen] 10•30•2•250 mg

Vicks Children's Cough syrup (discontinued 1994) OTC *antitussive; expectorant* [dextromethorphan hydrobromide; guaifenesin]

Vicks Cough Drops; Vicks Menthol Cough Drops OTC *topical antipruritic/counterirritant; mild local anesthetic* [menthol] 10 mg; 8.4 mg

Vicks Cough Silencers lozenges OTC *antitussive; topical oral anesthetic* [dextromethorphan hydrobromide; benzocaine] 2.5•1 mg

Vicks Dry Hacking Cough syrup OTC *antitussive* [dextromethorphan hydrobromide; alcohol 10%] 15 mg/5 mL

Vicks Ice Blue Throat Lozenges (discontinued 1994) OTC *topical antipruritic/counterirritant; mild local anesthetic* [menthol]

Vicks Inhaler OTC *nasal decongestant* [l-desoxyephedrine] 50 mg

Vicks NyQuil products [see: NyQuil]

Vicks Pediatric 44d Dry Hacking Cough and Head Congestion syrup OTC *antitussive* [dextromethorphan hydrobromide] 15 mg/15 mL

Vicks Pediatric Formula 44e liquid OTC *antitussive; expectorant* [dextromethorphan hydrobromide; guaifenesin] 3.3•33.3 mg/5 mL

Vicks Pediatric Formula 44m Multi-Symptom Cough & Cold liquid OTC *pediatric antitussive, decongestant, and antihistamine* [dextromethorphan hydrobromide; pseudoephedrine HCl; chlorpheniramine maleate] 5•10•0.67 mg/5 mL

Vicks Sinex products [see: Sinex]

Vicks Throat lozenges (discontinued 1994) OTC *topical oral anesthetic; antiseptic* [benzocaine; cetylpyridinium chloride] 5•1.66 mg

Vicks VapoRub vaporizing ointment, cream OTC *counterirritant* [camphor; menthol; eucalyptus oil] 4.7%•2.6%•1.2%

Vicks Vatronol nose drops (discontinued 1994) OTC *nasal decongestant* [ephedrine sulfate] 0.5%

Vicks Vitamin C Drops (lozenges) OTC *vitamin supplement* [sodium ascorbate & ascorbic acid] 60 mg

Vicodin; Vicodin ES tablets ℞ *narcotic analgesic* [hydrocodone bitartrate; acetaminophen] 5•500 mg; 7.5•750 mg

Vicodin Tuss syrup ℞ *narcotic antitussive; expectorant* [hydrocodone bitartrate; guaifenesin] 5•100 mg/5 mL ② Hycodan; Hycomine

Vicon Forte capsules ℞ *vitamin/mineral supplement* [multiple vitamins & minerals; folic acid] ±•1 mg

Vicon Plus capsules OTC *vitamin/mineral supplement* [multiple vitamins & minerals] ±

Vicon-C capsules OTC *vitamin/mineral supplement* [multiple B vitamins & minerals; vitamin C] ±•300 mg

vicotrope [see: cosyntropin]

Victors Dual Action Cough Drops; Victors Vapor Cough Lozenges (discontinued 1994) OTC *antipruritic/counterirritant; mild local anesthetic; antiseptic* [menthol; eucalyptus oil]

vidarabine USAN, USP, INN, BAN *antiviral* ② cytarabine

vidarabine monohydrate *antiviral*

vidarabine phosphate USAN *antiviral*

vidarabine sodium phosphate USAN *antiviral*

Vi-Daylin chewable tablets OTC *vitamin supplement* [multiple vitamins; folic acid] ±•0.3 mg

Vi-Daylin ADC drops OTC *vitamin supplement* [vitamins A, C, and D] 1500 IU•35 mg•400 IU per mL

Vi-Daylin ADC Vitamins + Iron drops OTC *vitamin/iron supplement* [vitamins A, C, and D; ferrous gluconate] 1500 IU•35 mg•400 IU•10 mg per mL

Vi-Daylin Multivitamin liquid, drops OTC *vitamin supplement* [multiple vitamins] ±

Vi-Daylin Multivitamin + Iron chewable tablets OTC *vitamin/iron*

supplement [multiple vitamins; iron; folic acid] ≟•12•0.3 mg

Vi-Daylin Multivitamin + Iron liquid, drops OTC *vitamin/iron supplement* [multiple vitamins; ferrous gluconate] ≟•10 mg/5 mL; ≟•10 mg/mL

Vi-Daylin/F ADC drops ℞ *pediatric vitamin supplement and dental caries preventative* [vitamins A, C, and D; sodium fluoride] 1500 IU•35 mg•400 IU•0.25 mg per mL

Vi-Daylin/F ADC + Iron drops ℞ *pediatric vitamin/iron supplement and dental caries preventative* [vitamins A, C, and D; sodium fluoride; ferrous sulfate] 1500 IU•35 mg•400 IU•0.25 mg•10 mg per mL

Vi-Daylin/F Multivitamin chewable tablets ℞ *pediatric vitamin supplement and dental caries preventative* [multiple vitamins; sodium fluoride; folic acid] ≟•1•0.3 mg

Vi-Daylin/F Multivitamin drops ℞ *pediatric vitamin supplement and dental caries preventative* [multiple vitamins; sodium fluoride] ≟•0.25 mg/mL

Vi-Daylin/F Multivitamin + Iron chewable tablets ℞ *pediatric vitamin/iron supplement and dental caries preventative* [multiple vitamins; sodium fluoride; ferrous sulfate; folic acid] ≟•1•12•0.3 mg

Vi-Daylin/F Multivitamin + Iron drops ℞ *pediatric vitamin/iron supplement and dental caries preventative* [multiple vitamins; sodium fluoride; ferrous sulfate] ≟•0.25•10 mg/mL

Videx chewable/dispersible tablets, powder for oral solution, powder for pediatric oral solution ℞ *antiviral for advanced HIV infection and AIDS* [didanosine] 25, 50, 100, 150 mg; 100, 167, 250, 375 mg/packet; 2, 4 g

VIE (vincristine, ifosfamide, etoposide) *chemotherapy protocol*

vifilcon A USAN *hydrophilic contact lens material*

vifilcon B USAN *hydrophilic contact lens material*

Vi-Flor [see: Poly-Vi-Flor; Tri-Vi-Flor]

VIG (vaccinia immune globulin) [q.v.]

vigabatrin USAN, INN, BAN *anticonvulsant for tardive dyskinesia*

Vigomar Forte tablets OTC *vitamin/mineral/iron supplement* [multiple vitamins & minerals; iron] ≟•12 mg

Vigortol liquid OTC *geriatric vitamin/mineral supplement* [multiple B vitamins & minerals; alcohol 18%] ≟

viloxazine INN, BAN *bicyclic antidepressant* [also: viloxazine HCl]

viloxazine HCl USAN *antidepressant; (orphan: cataplexy; narcolepsy)* [also: viloxazine]

Viminate liquid OTC *geriatric vitamin/mineral supplement* [multiple B vitamins & minerals] ≟

viminol INN

VIMRxyn ℞ *investigational (Phase I) antiviral for HIV and AIDS* [hypericin (synthetic)]

vinafocon A USAN *hydrophobic contact lens material*

vinbarbital NF, INN [also: vinbarbitone]

vinbarbital sodium NF

vinbarbitone BAN [also: vinbarbital]

vinblastine INN *antineoplastic* [also: vinblastine sulfate]

vinblastine sulfate USAN, USP *antineoplastic* [also: vinblastine] 10 mg/vial, 1 mg/mL injection

vinburnine INN

vincaleukoblastine sulfate [see: vinblastine sulfate]

vincamine INN, BAN

vincanol INN

vincantenate [see: vinconate]

vincantril INN

Vincasar PFS IV injection ℞ *antineoplastic* [vincristine sulfate] 1 mg/mL

vincofos USAN, INN *anthelmintic*

vinconate INN

vincristine (VC; VCR) INN *antineoplastic* [also: vincristine sulfate]

vincristine sulfate USAN, USP *antineoplastic* [also: vincristine] 1 mg/mL injection

vindeburnol INN

vindesine USAN, INN, BAN *antineoplastic*

vindesine sulfate USAN, JAN *antineoplastic*

vinegar [see: acetic acid]

vinepidine INN *antineoplastic* [also: vinepidine sulfate]
vinepidine sulfate USAN *antineoplastic* [also: vinepidine]
vinformide INN
vinglycinate INN *antineoplastic* [also: vinglycinate sulfate]
vinglycinate sulfate USAN *antineoplastic* [also: vinglycinate]
vinleurosine INN *antineoplastic* [also: vinleurosine sulfate]
vinleurosine sulfate USAN *antineoplastic* [also: vinleurosine]
vinmegallate INN
vinorelbine INN *antineoplastic* [also: vinorelbine tartrate]
vinorelbine tartrate USAN *antineoplastic* [also: vinorelbine]
vinpocetine USAN, INN
vinpoline INN
vinrosidine INN *antineoplastic* [also: vinrosidine sulfate]
vinrosidine sulfate USAN *antineoplastic* [also: vinrosidine]
vintiamol INN
vintoperol INN
vintriptol INN
vinyl alcohol polymer [see: polyvinyl alcohol]
vinyl ether USP
vinyl gamma-aminobutyric acid [see: vigabatrin]
vinylbital INN [also: vinylbitone]
vinylbitone BAN [also: vinylbital]
vinylestrenolone [see: norgesterone]
vinymal [see: vinylbital]
vinyzene [see: bromchlorenone]
vinzolidine INN *antineoplastic* [also: vinzolidine sulfate]
vinzolidine sulfate USAN *antineoplastic* [also: vinzolidine]
Vio-Bec capsules (discontinued 1992) OTC *vitamin supplement* [multiple B vitamins; vitamin C]
Vio-Bec Forte film-coated tablets (discontinued 1993) ℞ *vitamin/mineral therapy* [multiple B vitamins; vitamins C and E; folic acid; multiple minerals]
Vioform cream, ointment OTC *topical antifungal; antibacterial* [clioquinol] 3%

Vioform-Hydrocortisone; Vioform-Hydrocortisone Mild cream, ointment (discontinued 1994) ℞ *topical corticosteroid; antifungal; antibacterial* [hydrocortisone; clioquinol] 1%•3%; 0.5%•3%
Viogen-C capsules OTC *vitamin/mineral supplement* [multiple B vitamins & minerals; vitamin C] $\pm$•300 mg
Viokase tablets, powder ℞ *digestive enzymes* [lipase; protease; amylase] 8000•30,000•30,000 U; 16,800•70,000•70,000 U/0.7 g
viomycin INN [also: viomycin sulfate]
viomycin sulfate USP [also: viomycin]
Viopan-T film-coated tablets (discontinued 1993) OTC *geriatric vitamin/mineral supplement* [multiple vitamins & minerals; folic acid; biotin]
viosterol in oil [see: ergocalciferol]
VIP; VIP-1; VIP-2 (VePesid, ifosfamide [with mesna rescue], Platinol) *chemotherapy protocol*
VIP (vinblastine, ifosfamide [with mesna rescue], Platinol) *chemotherapy protocol*
VIP-B (VP-16, ifosfamide, Platinol, bleomycin) *chemotherapy protocol*
viprostol USAN, INN, BAN *hypotensive; vasodilator*
viprynium embonate BAN *anthelmintic* [also: pyrvinium pamoate]
viqualine INN
viquidil INN
Viquin Forte cream ℞ *hyperpigmentation bleaching agent; sunscreen* [hydroquinone; padimate O; dioxybenzone; oxybenzone] 4%•8%•3%•2%
Vira-A IV infusion (discontinued 1995) ℞ *antiviral for herpes simplex and herpes zoster* [vidarabine monohydrate] 200 mg/mL
Vira-A ophthalmic ointment ℞ *ophthalmic antiviral* [vidarabine monohydrate] 3%
Viracept ℞ *investigational (Phase II) antiviral protease inhibitor for HIV* [nelfinavir]
Viractin cream, gel OTC *topical anesthetic for cold sores and fever blisters* [tetracaine] 2%

Viramune tablets ℞ *antiviral; non-nucleoside reverse transcriptase inhibitor (NNRTI) for HIV-1* [nevirapine] 200 mg

Viranol gel (discontinued 1994) OTC *topical keratolytic* [salicylic acid; lactic acid] 12%• ≟

Viranol Gel Ultra (discontinued 1994) ℞ *topical keratolytic* [salicylic acid in a collodion-like vehicle] 26%

Virazole powder for inhalation aerosol ℞ *antiviral; investigational (Phase II/III) for HIV; (orphan: hemorrhagic fever with renal syndrome)* [ribavirin] 6 g/100 mL (20 mg/mL)

Virend ℞ *investigational (Phase II) antiviral for AIDS-related genital herpes* [SP-303 (code name—generic name not yet assigned)]

virginiamycin USAN, INN *antibacterial; veterinary food additive*

virginiamycin factor M$_1$ [see: virginiamycin]

virginiamycin factor S [see: virginiamycin]

viridofulvin USAN, INN *antifungal*

Virilon capsules ℞ *androgen for male hypogonadism, impotence and breast cancer* [methyltestosterone] 10 mg

Virogen Herpes slide test for professional use *in vitro diagnostic aid for herpes simplex virus antigen in lesions or cell cultures* [latex agglutination test]

Virogen HSV Antibody slide test for professional use (discontinued 1993) *in vitro diagnostic aid for herpes simplex virus antibodies in serum* [latex agglutination test]

Virogen Rotatest slide test for professional use *in vitro diagnostic aid for fecal rotavirus* [latex agglutination test]

Virogen Rubella; Virogen Rubella Microlatex slide test for professional use (discontinued 1995) *in vitro diagnostic aid for rubella virus antibodies in serum* [latex agglutination test]

Viro-Med tablets (discontinued 1995) OTC *antitussive; decongestant; antihistamine; analgesic* [dextromethorphan hydrobromide; pseudoephedrine HCl; chlorpheniramine maleate; acetaminophen] 15•30•2•500 mg

Viroptic Drop-Dose (eye drops) ℞ *ophthalmic antiviral* [trifluridine] 1%

viroxime USAN, INN *antiviral*

viroxime component A [see: zinviroxime]

viroxime component B [see: enviroxime]

Virulizin ℞ *investigational antineoplastic for melanoma*

Visalens Soaking/Cleaning solution (discontinued 1992) OTC *cleaning and soaking solution for hard contact lenses*

Visalens Wetting solution (discontinued 1992) OTC *wetting solution for hard contact lenses*

Viscoat prefilled syringes ℞ *viscoelastic agent for ophthalmic surgery* [hyaluronate sodium; chondroitin sulfate sodium] 30•40 mg/mL

Visine eye drops (discontinued 1996) OTC *topical ocular decongestant/vasoconstrictor* [tetrahydrozoline HCl] 0.05%

Visine A.C. eye drops (name changed to Visine Allergy Relief in 1995)

Visine Allergy Relief eye drops OTC *topical ocular decongestant; astringent* [tetrahydrozoline HCl; zinc sulfate] 0.05%•0.25%

Visine Extra eye drops (name changed to Visine Moisturizing in 1995)

Visine L.R. eye drops OTC *topical ocular decongestant/vasoconstrictor* [oxymetazoline HCl] 0.025%

Visine Moisturizing eye drops OTC *topical ocular decongestant/vasoconstrictor; emollient* [tetrahydrozoline HCl; PEG 400] 0.05%•1%

Vision Care Enzymatic Cleaner tablets OTC *enzymatic cleaner for soft contact lenses* [pork pancreatin]

Visipak (trademarked packaging form) *reverse-numbered package*

Visipaque intra-arterial or IV injection ℞ *nonionic dimeric contrast agent for CECT, CT, x-ray and visceral digital subtraction angiography* [iodixanol] 270, 320 mg iodine/mL

Visken tablets ℞ *antihypertensive; β-blocker* [pindolol] 5, 10 mg

visnadine INN, BAN

visnafylline INN
Vi-Sol [see: Ce-Vi-Sol; Poly-Vi-Sol; Tri-Vi-Sol]
Vistacon IM injection ℞ *anxiolytic* [hydroxyzine HCl] 50 mg/mL
Vistaject-25; Vistaject-50 IM injection (discontinued 1996) ℞ *anxiolytic* [hydroxyzine HCl] 25 mg/mL; 50 mg/mL
Vistaquel 50 IM injection ℞ *anxiolytic* [hydroxyzine HCl] 50 mg/mL
Vistaril capsules, oral suspension ℞ *anxiolytic* [hydroxyzine pamoate] 25, 50, 100 mg; 25 mg/5 mL ⚠ Restoril
Vistaril IM injection ℞ *anxiolytic* [hydroxyzine HCl] 25, 50 mg/mL
vistatolon INN *antiviral* [also: statolon]
Vistazine 50 IM injection ℞ *anxiolytic* [hydroxyzine HCl] 50 mg/mL
Vistide IV infusion ℞ *nucleoside antiviral for AIDS-related cytomegalovirus retinitis and herpes* [cidofovir] 75 mg/mL
Visual-Eyes ophthalmic solution OTC *extraocular irrigating solution* [sterile isotonic solution]
Vita Bee C-800 tablets (discontinued 1995) OTC *vitamin supplement* [multiple B vitamins; vitamins C and E] ± • 800 • 45 mg
Vita-bee with C Captabs (capsule-shaped tablets) OTC *vitamin supplement* [multiple B vitamins; vitamin C] ± • 300 mg
Vita-Bob softgel capsules OTC *vitamin supplement* [multiple vitamins; folic acid] ± • 0.4 mg
Vita-C crystals OTC *vitamin supplement* [ascorbic acid] 4 g/tsp.
VitaCarn oral solution ℞ *carnitine replenisher for deficiency of genetic origin or end-stage renal disease (orphan)* [levocarnitine]
Vit-A-Drops eye drops (discontinued 1995) OTC *ocular moisturizer/lubricant* [vitamin A]
Vita-Feron tablets OTC *hematinic* [iron; folic acid; vitamin B_{12}] 150 • 0.8 • 0.006 mg
Vitafōl film-coated caplets ℞ *hematinic; vitamin supplement* [ferrous fumarate; multiple vitamins; folic acid] 65 mg • ± • 1 mg

Vitafōl syrup ℞ *hematinic* [ferric pyrophosphate; multiple B vitamins; folic acid] 90 • ± • 0.75 mg/15 mL
Vita-Kaps Filmtabs (film-coated tablets) (discontinued 1993) ℞ *vitamin supplement* [multiple vitamins]
VitaKaps-M Filmtabs (film-coated tablets) (discontinued 1993) OTC *vitamin/mineral/iron supplement* [multiple vitamins & minerals; iron]
Vita-Kid chewable wafers OTC *vitamin supplement* [multiple vitamins; folic acid] ± • 0.3 mg
Vital B-50 timed-release tablets OTC *vitamin supplement* [multiple B vitamins; folic acid; biotin] ± • 100 • 50 μg
Vital High Nitrogen powder OTC *enteral nutritional therapy* [lactose-free formula] 79 g
Vitalets chewable tablets OTC *vitamin/mineral/iron supplement* [multiple vitamins & minerals; iron; biotin] ± • 10 mg • 25 μg
VitalEyes capsules (discontinued 1995) OTC *vitamin/mineral supplement* [vitamins A, C, and E; multiple minerals] 10,000 IU • 200 mg • 100 IU • ±
Vitalize SF liquid OTC *hematinic* [ferric pyrophosphate; multiple B vitamins; lysine] 66 • ± • 300 mg/15 mL
vitamin A USP *vitamin; antixerophthalmic; topical emollient* 10,000, 25,000, 50,000 IU oral
vitamin A acid [see: tretinoin]
vitamin A palmitate
vitamin A_1 [see: retinol]
Vitamin B Complex 100 injection ℞ *parenteral vitamin therapy* [multiple B vitamins] ±
vitamin B_1 [see: thiamine HCl]
vitamin B_1 mononitrate [see: thiamine mononitrate]
vitamin B_2 [see: riboflavin]
vitamin B_3 [see: niacin; niacinamide]
vitamin B_5 [see: calcium pantothenate]
vitamin B_6 [see: pyridoxine HCl]
vitamin B_8 [see: adenosine phosphate]
vitamin B_{12} [now: cyanocobalamin; hydroxocobalamin]
vitamin B_c [see: folic acid]
vitamin B_t [see: carnitine]
vitamin C [see: ascorbic acid]

vitamin D (vitamins D$_2$ and/or D$_3$) [see: ergocalciferol (D$_2$); cholecalciferol (D$_3$)]

vitamin D$_1$ [see: dihydrotachysterol]

vitamin D$_2$ [see: ergocalciferol]

vitamin D$_3$ [see: cholecalciferol]

vitamin E USP *vitamin E supplement; topical emollient* 100, 200, 400, 500, 600, 1000 IU oral

vitamin E-TPGS (tocopheryl polyethylene glycol succinate) [see: tocophersolan]

vitamin G [see: riboflavin]

vitamin H [see: biotin]

vitamin K$_1$ [see: phytonadione]

vitamin K$_2$ [see: menaquinone]

vitamin K$_3$ [see: menadione]

vitamin K$_4$ [see: menadiol sodium diphosphate]

vitamin M [see: folic acid]

vitamin P [see: bioflavonoids]

vitamin P$_4$ [see: troxerutin]

Vitamin-Mineral Supplement liquid OTC *vitamin/mineral supplement* [multiple B vitamins & minerals; alcohol 18%] ±

vitamins A & D (topical) *emollient*

Vitaneed liquid OTC *enteral nutritional therapy* [lactose-free formula]

Vita-Plus B-12 injection ℞ *vitamin B$_{12}$ therapy* [cyanocobalamin]

Vita-Plus E softgels OTC *vitamin supplement* [vitamin E] 400 IU

Vita-Plus G softgel capsules OTC *geriatric vitamin/mineral supplement* [multiple vitamins & minerals]

Vita-Plus H softgel capsules OTC *vitamin/mineral/iron supplement* [multiple vitamins & minerals; iron] ± • 13.4 mg

Vita-PMS; Vita-PMS Plus tablets OTC *vitamin/mineral supplement; digestive enzymes* [multiple vitamins & minerals; folic acid; biotin; amylase; protease; lipase; betaine acid HCl] ± • 0.33 mg • 10.4 μg • 2500 U • 2500 U • 200 U • 16.7 mg

Vitarex tablets OTC *vitamin/mineral/iron supplement* [multiple vitamins & minerals; iron] ± • 15 mg

Vitazin capsules (discontinued 1992) OTC *vitamin/mineral supplement* [multiple vitamins & minerals]

Vite E cream OTC *emollient* [vitamin E] 50 mg/g

Vitec cream OTC *emollient* [vitamin E]

Vitrasert intraocular implant ℞ *antiviral for AIDS-associated cytomegalovirus retinitis* [ganciclovir] 4.5 mg

Vitron-C chewable tablets OTC *hematinic* [ferrous fumarate; ascorbic acid] 66 • 125 mg ⑲ Vytone

Vitron-C-Plus tablets OTC *hematinic* [ferrous fumarate; ascorbic acid] 132 • 250 mg

Vivactil film-coated tablets ℞ *tricyclic antidepressant* [protriptyline HCl] 5, 10 mg

Viva-Drops eye drops OTC *ocular moisturizer/lubricant*

Vivalan ℞ *(orphan: cataplexy; narcolepsy)* [viloxazine HCl]

Vivarin tablets OTC *CNS stimulant; analeptic* [caffeine] 200 mg

Vivelle transdermal patch ℞ *estrogen replacement therapy for postmenopausal disorders* [estradiol] 37.5, 50, 75, 100 μg/day

Vivonex T.E.N. powder OTC *enteral nutritional therapy* [lactose-free formula]

Vivotif Berna enteric-coated capsules ℞ *typhoid fever vaccine* [typhoid vaccine] $2–6 \times 10^9$ viable CFU + $5–50 \times 10^9$ nonviable cells

Vi-Zac capsules OTC *vitamin/zinc supplement* [vitamins A, C, and E; zinc] 5000 IU • 500 mg • 50 mg • 18 mg

VLA-4 *investigational anti-inflammatory*

V-Lax powder OTC *bulk laxative* [psyllium hydrophilic mucilloid] 50%

VLP (vincristine, L-asparaginase, prednisone) *chemotherapy protocol*

VM (vinblastine, mitomycin) *chemotherapy protocol*

VM-26 [see: teniposide]

VM-26PP (teniposide, procarbazine, prednisone) *chemotherapy protocol*

VMAD (vincristine, methotrexate, Adriamycin, actinomycin D) *chemotherapy protocol*

VMCP (vincristine, melphalan, cyclophosphamide, prednisone) chemotherapy protocol
VMP (VePesid, mitoxantrone, prednimustine) chemotherapy protocol
VOCAP (VP-16-213, Oncovin, cyclophosphamide, Adriamycin, Platinol) chemotherapy protocol
volazocine USAN, INN analgesic
Volmax extended-release tablets ℞ bronchodilator [albuterol sulfate] 4, 8 mg
Voltaren delayed-release enteric-coated tablets ℞ nonsteroidal anti-inflammatory drug (NSAID); antiarthritic; analgesic [diclofenac sodium] 25, 50, 75 mg
Voltaren eye drops ℞ ocular nonsteroidal anti-inflammatory drug (NSAID) [diclofenac sodium] 0.1%
Voltaren OTC OTC investigational nonsteroidal anti-inflammatory drug (NSAID); antiarthritic; analgesic [diclofenac sodium]
Voltaren Rapide (Canadian name for U.S. product Cataflam)
Voltaren XR extended-release tablets ℞ once-daily antiarthritic for osteoarthritis and rheumatoid arthritis [diclofenac sodium] 100 mg
von Willebrand's factor [see: antihemophilic factor]
Vontrol tablets ℞ antiemetic; antivertigo agent [diphenidol HCl] 25 mg ⓢ Bontril
vorozole USAN, INN, BAN antineoplastic; aromatase inhibitor
vortel [see: clorprenaline HCl]
VōSol HC Otic ear drops ℞ topical corticosteroidal anti-inflammatory; antibacterial/antifungal [hydrocortisone; acetic acid] 1%•2%
VōSol Otic ear drops ℞ antibacterial/antifungal [acetic acid] 2%

votumumab USAN monoclonal antibody for cancer imaging and therapy
voxergolide INN
Voxsuprine tablets ℞ peripheral vasodilator [isoxsuprine HCl] 10, 20 mg
VP (vasopressin) [q.v.]
VP (vincristine, prednisone) chemotherapy protocol
VP + A (vincristine, prednisone, asparaginase) chemotherapy protocol
VPB (vinblastine, Platinol, bleomycin) chemotherapy protocol
VPBCPr (vincristine, prednisone, vinblastine, chlorambucil, procarbazine) chemotherapy protocol
VPCA (vincristine, prednisone, cyclophosphamide, ara-C) chemotherapy protocol
VPCMF (vincristine, prednisone, cyclophosphamide, methotrexate, fluorouracil) chemotherapy protocol
VP-L-asparaginase (vincristine, prednisone, L-asparaginase) chemotherapy protocol
VPP (VePesid, Platinol) chemotherapy protocol
V-TAD (VePesid, thioguanine, ara-C, daunorubicin) chemotherapy protocol
Vumon IV infusion ℞ antineoplastic for acute lymphoblastic leukemia (orphan) and bladder cancer [teniposide] 50 mg (10 mg/mL)
V.V.S. vaginal cream ℞ broad-spectrum bacteriostatic [sulfathiazole; sulfacetamide; sulfabenzamide] 3.42%•2.86%•3.7%
VX-478 investigational (Phase I/II) antiviral protease inhibitor for HIV and AIDS
Vytone cream ℞ topical corticosteroid; antifungal; antibacterial [hydrocortisone; iodoquinol] 1%•1% ⓢ Hytone; Vitron
VZIG (varicella-zoster immune globulin) [q.v.]

Wampole One-Step hCG test kit for professional use (discontinued 1995) *in vitro diagnostic aid for urine/serum pregnancy test*

warfarin INN, BAN *anticoagulant* [also: warfarin potassium]

warfarin potassium USP *anticoagulant* [also: warfarin]

warfarin sodium USP *anticoagulant*

Wart Remover liquid OTC *topical keratolytic* [salicylic acid in flexible collodion] 17%

wart-aid cream (discontinued 1992) OTC *topical keratolytic* [calcium pantothenate; ascorbic acid; starch]

Wart-Off liquid OTC *topical keratolytic* [salicylic acid in flexible collodion] 17%

water, purified USP *solvent*

water, tritiated [see: tritiated water]

water moccasin snake antivenin [see: antivenin (Crotalidae) polyvalent]

water O 15 USAN *radioactive diagnostic aid for vascular disorders*

[^{15}O]water [see: water O 15]

water-d$_2$ [see: deuterium oxide]

wax, carnauba NF *tablet-coating agent*

wax, emulsifying NF *emulsifying and stiffening agent*

wax, microcrystalline NF *stiffening and tablet-coating agent*

wax, white NF *stiffening agent* [also: beeswax, white]

wax, yellow NF *stiffening agent* [also: beeswax, yellow]

Wehdryl injection (discontinued 1996) ℞ *antihistamine; motion sickness preventative; sleep aid; antiparkinsonian* [diphenhydramine HCl] 50 mg/mL

Wehgen IM injection (discontinued 1996) ℞ *estrogen replacement therapy; antineoplastic for prostatic and breast cancer* [estrone] 2 mg/mL

Wehless capsules, Timecelles (sustained-release capsules) (discontinued 1996) ℞ *anorexiant* [phendimetrazine tartrate] 35 mg; 105 mg

Weightrol tablets (discontinued 1996) ℞ *anorexiant* [phendimetrazine tartrate] 35 mg

Wellbutrin tablets ℞ *antidepressant* [bupropion HCl] 75, 100 mg

Wellbutrin SR ℞ *investigational sustained-release formula for smoking cessation and ADD in adults and children* [bupropion HCl]

Wellcovorin powder for IV infusion ℞ *leucovorin "rescue" after methotrexate therapy (orphan)* [leucovorin calcium] 100 mg/vial

Wellcovorin tablets ℞ *leucovorin "rescue" after methotrexate therapy; antidote to folic acid antagonist overdose* [leucovorin calcium] 5, 25 mg

Wellferon ℞ *investigational (Phase III) cytokine for HIV; (orphan: Kaposi sarcoma; human papillomavirus)* [interferon alfa-n1]

Wesprin tablets (discontinued 1994) OTC *analgesic; antipyretic; anti-inflammatory; antirheumatic* [aspirin, buffered with aluminum hydroxide and magnesium hydroxide] 325 mg

Westcort ointment, cream ℞ *topical corticosteroid* [hydrocortisone valerate] 0.2%

Wet-N-Soak solution OTC *rewetting solution for rigid gas permeable contact lenses*

Wet-N-Soak Plus solution OTC *disinfecting/wetting/soaking solution for rigid gas permeable contact lenses* [note: RGP contact indication different from hard contact indication for same product]

Wet-N-Soak Plus solution OTC *wetting/soaking solution for hard contact lenses* [note: hard contact indication different from RGP contact indication for same product]

Wetting solution OTC *wetting solution for hard contact lenses*

Wetting & Soaking solution OTC *disinfecting/wetting/soaking solution for rigid gas permeable contact lenses* [note: one of two different products with the same name]

Wetting & Soaking solution OTC *wetting/soaking solution for hard contact lenses* [note: one of two different products with the same name]

wheat germ oil [see: vitamin E]
white beeswax [see: beeswax, white]
White Cloverine Salve ointment OTC *skin protectant* [white petrolatum] 97%
White Cod Liver Oil Concentrate capsules, chewable tablets OTC *vitamin supplement* [vitamins A, D, and E] 10,000•400•± IU; 4000•200•± IU
White Cod Liver Oil Concentrate with Vitamin C chewable tablets OTC *vitamin supplement* [vitamins A, C, and D] 4000 IU•50 mg•200 IU
white lotion USP *astringent; topical protectant*
white mineral oil [see: petrolatum, white]
white ointment [see: ointment, white]
white petrolatum [see: petrolatum, white]
white phenolphthalein [see: phenolphthalein]
white wax [see: wax, white]
Whitfield's ointment OTC *topical antifungal; keratolytic* [benzoic acid; salicylic acid] 6%•3%
Whitfield's ointment [see: benzoic & salicylic acids]
whole blood [see: blood, whole]
whole root rauwolfia [see: rauwolfia serpentina]
Wibi lotion OTC *moisturizer; emollient*
widow spider species antivenin [now: antivenin (Latrodectus mactans)]
Wigraine suppositories ℞ *migraine-specific vasoconstrictor* [ergotamine tartrate; caffeine; tartaric acid] 2•100•21.5 mg
Wigraine tablets ℞ *migraine-specific vasoconstrictor* [ergotamine tartrate; caffeine] 1•100 mg
wild cherry syrup USP
WIN 59010 *investigational liver imaging aid for MRI*
WinGel chewable tablets, liquid (discontinued 1994) OTC *antacid* [aluminum hydroxide; magnesium hydroxide] 180•180 mg; 36•32 mg/mL
WinRho SD IV or IM injection ℞ *obstetric Rh factor immunity suppressant; treatment for immune thrombocytopenic purpura (orphan)* [Rh$_0$(D) immune globulin] 600, 1500 IU (120, 300 μg)
Winstrol tablets ℞ *anabolic steroid for hereditary angioedema* [stanozolol] 2 mg
wintergreen oil [see: methyl salicylate]
Wintersteiner's compound F [see: hydrocortisone]
witch hazel [see: hamamelis water]
Wolfina tablets (discontinued 1992) ℞ *antihypertensive; antipsychotic* [rauwolfia serpentina (whole root)] 100 mg
Women's Daily Formula capsules OTC *vitamin/calcium/iron supplement* [multiple vitamins; calcium; iron; folic acid] ±•450•25•0.4 mg
Wonder Ice gel OTC *counterirritant* [menthol] 5.25%
Wondra lotion OTC *moisturizer; emollient* [lanolin]
wood creosote [see: creosote carbonate]
Woolley's antiserotonin [see: benanserin HCl]
Wyamine Sulfate IV or IM injection ℞ *vasopressor for hypotensive shock* [mephentermine sulfate] 15, 30 mg/mL
Wyamycin S film-coated tablets (discontinued 1994) ℞ *macrolide antibiotic* [erythromycin stearate] 250, 500 mg
Wyanoids Relief Factor rectal suppositories OTC *emollient* [cocoa butter; shark liver oil] 79%•3%
Wycillin IM injection, Tubex (cartridge-needle units) ℞ *bactericidal antibiotic* [penicillin G procaine] 600,000, 1,200,000, 2,400,000 U ② Bicillin; V-Cillin
Wycillin and Probenecid two prefilled disposable syringes for IM injection + two tablets (discontinued 1992) ℞ *antibiotic for Neisseria gonorrhoeae* [penicillin G procaine (syringes); probenecid (tablets)] 2,400,000 U; 500 mg
Wydase IV or subcu injection, powder for injection ℞ *adjuvant to increase absorption and dispersion of injected drugs* [hyaluronidase] 150 U/mL; 150, 1500 U ② Lidex
Wygesic tablets ℞ *narcotic analgesic* [propoxyphene HCl; acetaminophen] 65•650 mg

Wymox capsules, powder for oral suspension ℞ *penicillin-type antibiotic* [amoxicillin trihydrate] 250, 500 mg; 125, 250 mg/5 mL

Wyseal (trademarked dosage form) *film-coated tablet*
Wytensin tablets ℞ *antihypertensive* [guanabenz acetate] 4, 8 mg

Xact ℞ *investigational treatment for the symptoms of menopause, including osteoporosis* [norethindrone acetate; ethinyl estradiol]
Xalatan eye drops ℞ *prostaglandin agonist for glaucoma and ocular hypertension* [latanoprost] 0.005% (50 μg/mL)
xamoterol USAN, INN, BAN *cardiac stimulant*
xamoterol fumarate USAN *cardiac stimulant*
Xanax tablets ℞ *anxiolytic* [alprazolam] 0.25, 0.5, 1, 2 mg ⚠ Zantac
Xanax SR; Xanax XR ℞ *investigational sustained-release anxiolytic* [alprazolam]
xanomeline USAN *cholinergic agonist for Alzheimer's disease*
xanomeline tartrate USAN *cholinergic agonist for Alzheimer's disease*
xanoxate sodium USAN *bronchodilator*
xanoxic acid INN
xanthan gum NF *suspending agent*
xanthinol niacinate USAN *peripheral vasodilator* [also: xantinol nicotinate]
xanthiol INN
xanthiol HCl [see: xanthiol]
xanthocillin BAN [also: xantocillin]
xanthotoxin [see: methoxsalen]
xantifibrate INN
xantinol nicotinate INN *peripheral vasodilator* [also: xanthinol niacinate]
xantocillin INN [also: xanthocillin]
xantofyl palmitate INN
^{127}Xe [see: xenon Xe 127]
^{133}Xe [see: xenon Xe 133]
xemilofiban HCl USAN *antianginal; prevents reocclusion of coronary arteries after PTCA*
xenalamine [see: xenazoic acid]
xenaldial [see: xenygloxal]
xenalipin USAN, INN *hypolipidemic*

xenazoic acid INN
xenbucin USAN, INN *antihypercholesterolemic*
xenbuficin [see: xenbucin]
Xenical ℞ *investigational adjunct to weight loss* [orlistat]
xenipentone INN
xenon *element (Xe)*
xenon (^{133}Xe) INN *radioactive agent* [also: xenon Xe 133]
xenon Xe 127 USP *diagnostic aid; medicinal gas; radioactive agent*
xenon Xe 133 USAN, USP *radioactive agent* [also: xenon (^{133}Xe)]
xenthiorate INN
xenygloxal INN
xenyhexenic acid INN
xenysalate INN, BAN *topical anesthetic; antibacterial; antifungal* [also: biphenamine HCl]
xenysalate HCl [see: biphenamine HCl]
xenytropium bromide INN
Xerac gel (discontinued 1994) OTC *antibacterial and exfoliant for acne* [microcrystalline sulfur] 4% ⚠ Serax
Xerac AC liquid ℞ *topical cleanser for acne* [aluminum chloride hexahydrate; anhydrous ethyl alcohol] 6.25%•96%
Xerac BP5; Xerac BP10 gel (discontinued 1994) OTC *topical keratolytic for acne* [benzoyl peroxide] 5%; 10%
Xeroderm lotion OTC *moisturizer; emollient*
Xero-Lube oral spray (discontinued 1994) OTC *saliva substitute*
xibenolol INN
xibornol INN, BAN
xilobam USAN, INN *muscle relaxant*
ximoprofen INN

xinafoate USAN, INN, BAN *combining name for radicals or groups*

xinidamine INN

xinomiline INN

xipamide USAN, INN *antihypertensive; diuretic*

xipranolol INN

XomaZyme-791 ℞ *investigational antineoplastic (orphan: metastatic colorectal adenocarcinoma)* [anti-TAP-72 immunotoxin]

XomaZyme-CD5 Plus ℞ *investigational treatment for graft vs. host disease, rheumatoid arthritis, and type I diabetes* [anti-CD5 monoclonal antibodies]

XomaZyme-CD7 Plus ℞ *investigational antineoplastic for T-cell malignancies* [4MRTA (code name—generic name not yet approved)]

XomaZyme-H65 ℞ *(orphan: graft vs. host disease or graft rejection in bone marrow transplants)* [CD5-T lymphocyte immunotoxin]

XomaZyme-Mel ℞ *investigational antineoplastic for melanoma*

Xomen ℞ *investigational treatment for sepsis* [monoclonal antibody E5]

xorphanol INN *analgesic* [also: xorphanol mesylate]

xorphanol mesylate USAN *analgesic* [also: xorphanol]

Xotic ear drops (name changed to Zoto-HC in 1994)

X-Prep liquid OTC *pre-procedure bowel evacuant* [senna extract; alcohol 7%] 74 mL

X-Prep Bowel Evacuant Kit-1 liquid, tablet & suppository in a kit OTC *pre-procedure bowel evacuant* [X-Prep liquid (q.v.); Senokot-S tablets (q.v.); Rectolax suppository (q.v.)]

X-Prep Bowel Evacuant Kit-2 liquid, granules & suppository in a kit OTC *pre-procedure bowel evacuant* [X-Prep liquid (q.v.); Citralax granules (q.v.); Rectolax suppository (q.v.)]

XRT (x-ray therapy) *adjunct to chemotherapy* [not a pharmaceutical agent]

X-Seb shampoo OTC *antiseborrheic; keratolytic* [salicylic acid] 4%

X-Seb Plus shampoo OTC *antiseborrheic; keratolytic; antibacterial; antifungal* [salicylic acid; pyrithione zinc] 2%•1%

X-seb T shampoo OTC *antiseborrheic; antipsoriatic; keratolytic* [coal tar; salicylic acid] 10%•4%

X-seb T Plus shampoo OTC *antiseborrheic; antipsoriatic; keratolytic* [coal tar; salicylic acid; menthol] 10%•3%•1%

xylamidine tosilate INN *serotonin inhibitor* [also: xylamidine tosylate]

xylamidine tosylate USAN *serotonin inhibitor* [also: xylamidine tosilate]

xylazine INN *analgesic; veterinary muscle relaxant* [also: xylazine HCl]

xylazine HCl USAN *analgesic; veterinary muscle relaxant* [also: xylazine]

xylitol NF *sweetened vehicle*

Xylocaine injection ℞ *injectable local anesthetic* [lidocaine HCl] 0.5%, 1%, 2%

Xylocaine liquid, solution, ointment, jelly ℞ *mucous membrane anesthetic* [lidocaine HCl] 5%; 4%; 5%; 2%

Xylocaine ointment OTC *topical local anesthetic* [lidocaine] 2.5%

Xylocaine 10% Oral spray ℞ *mucous membrane anesthetic* [lidocaine HCl] 10%

Xylocaine HCl injection ℞ *injectable local anesthetic* [lidocaine HCl; dextrose] 1.5%•7.5%

Xylocaine HCl injection ℞ *injectable local anesthetic* [lidocaine HCl; epinephrine] 0.5%•1:200,000, 1%•1:100,000, 1%•1:200,000, 2%•1:50,000, 2%•1:100,000, 2%•1:200,000

Xylocaine HCl IV for Cardiac Arrhythmias IV injection, IV admixture ℞ *antiarrhythmic* [lidocaine HCl] 1%, 2%, 4%, 20%

Xylocaine MPF injection ℞ *injectable local anesthetic* [lidocaine HCl] 0.5%, 1%, 1.5%, 2%, 4%

Xylocaine MPF injection ℞ *injectable local anesthetic* [lidocaine HCl; epinephrine] 1%•1:200,000, 1.5%•1:200,000, 2%•1:200,000

Xylocaine MPF injection ℞ *injectable local anesthetic* [lidocaine HCl; glucose] 5%•7.5%

Xylocaine Viscous solution ℞ *mucous membrane anesthetic* [lidocaine HCl] 2%
xylocoumarol INN
xylofilcon A USAN *hydrophilic contact lens material*
xylometazoline INN, BAN *vasoconstrictor; nasal decongestant* [also: xylometazoline HCl]

xylometazoline HCl USP *vasoconstrictor; nasal decongestant* [also: xylometazoline]
Xylo-Pfan tablets OTC *intestinal function test* [xylose] 25 g
xylose (D-xylose) USP *intestinal function test*
xyloxemine INN

yatren [see: chiniofon]
¹⁶⁹**Yb** [see: pentetate calcium trisodium Yb 169]
¹⁶⁹**Yb** [see: ytterbium Yb 169 pentetate]
yeast, dried NF
yeast cell derivative *claimed to promote wound healing*
Yeast-Gard vaginal suppositories OTC *for vaginal irritations, itching, and burning* [pulsatilla 28x]
Yeast-Gard; Yeast-Gard Sensitive Formula vaginal cream OTC *topical local anesthetic; keratolytic; antifungal* [benzocaine; resorcinol] 20%•3%; 5%•2%
Yeast-Gard Medicated Disposable Douche Premix solution OTC *antifungal; vaginal cleanser and deodorizer; acidity modifier* [sodium benzoate; lactic acid]
Yeast-Gard Medicated Douche; Yeast-Gard Medicated Disposable Douche solution OTC *antiseptic/germicidal; vaginal cleanser and deodorizer* [povidone-iodine] 10%; 0.3%
Yeast-X powder OTC *absorbs vaginal moisture; astringent* [cornstarch; zinc oxide]
Yeast-X vaginal suppositories OTC *for vaginal irritations, itching, and burning* [pulsatilla 28x]
Yelets tablets OTC *vitamin/mineral/iron supplement* [multiple vitamins & minerals; ferrous fumarate; folic acid] ≠•20•0.1 mg
yellow beeswax [see: beeswax, yellow]

yellow ferric oxide [see: ferric oxide, yellow]
yellow fever vaccine USP *active immunizing agent for yellow fever*
yellow mercuric oxide [see: mercuric oxide, yellow]
yellow ointment [see: ointment, yellow]
yellow petrolatum JAN *ointment base; emollient/protectant* [also: petrolatum]
yellow phenolphthalein [see: phenolphthalein, yellow]
yellow precipitate [see: mercuric oxide, yellow]
yellow wax [see: wax, yellow]
yerba santa [see: eriodictyon]
YF-Vax subcu injection ℞ *yellow fever vaccine* [yellow fever vaccine] 0.5 mL
Yocon tablets ℞ *no approved uses; sympatholytic; mydriatic; aphrodisiac* [yohimbine HCl] 5.4 mg
Yodoxin tablets, powder ℞ *amebicide* [iodoquinol] 210, 650 mg; 25 g
yohimbic acid INN
yohimbine HCl *alpha₂ adrenergic blocker; claimed to be an aphrodisiac; no FDA-sanctioned uses* 5.4 mg oral
Yohimex tablets ℞ *no approved uses; sympatholytic; mydriatic; aphrodisiac* [yohimbine HCl] 5.4 mg
Your Choice Non-Preserved Saline solution OTC *rinsing/storage solution for soft contact lenses* [preservative-free saline solution]
Your Choice Sterile Preserved Saline solution OTC *rinsing/storage*

solution for soft contact lenses [preserved saline solution]
ytterbium *element (Yb)*
ytterbium Yb 169 pentetate USP *radioactive agent*
yttrium *element (Y)*
Yurelax (Spanish name for U.S. product Flexeril)

Yutopar IV infusion ℞ *uterine relaxant to arrest preterm labor* [ritodrine HCl] 10, 15 mg/mL
Yutopar tablets (discontinued 1995) ℞ *uterine relaxant to arrest preterm labor* [ritodrine HCl] 10 mg

zabicipril INN
zacopride INN *antiemetic; peristaltic stimulant* [also: zacopride HCl]
zacopride HCl USAN, INN *antiemetic; peristaltic stimulant* [also: zacopride]
Zadaxin ℞ *investigational vaccine enhancer for lung cancer and chronic hepatitis B* [thymalfasin]
Zaditen ℞ *investigational antiasthmatic* [ketotifen]
zafirlukast USAN, INN, BAN *antiasthmatic; leukotriene antagonist*
zafuleptine INN
Zagam ℞ *investigational broad-spectrum fluoroquinolone antibiotic* [sparfloxacin]
zalcitabine USAN *antiviral; for AIDS (orphan)*
zaleplon USAN *sedative; hypnotic*
zalospirone INN *anxiolytic* [also: zalospirone HCl]
zalospirone HCl USAN *anxiolytic* [also: zalospirone]
zaltidine INN, BAN *antagonist to histamine H_2 receptors* [also: zaltidine HCl]
zaltidine HCl USAN *antagonist to histamine H_2 receptors* [also: zaltidine]
zamifenacin INN, BAN *investigational treatment for irritable bowel syndrome*
Zanaflex tablets ℞ *investigational antispasmodic for multiple sclerosis and spinal cord injury (orphan)* [tizanidine HCl] 4 mg
zankiren HCl USAN *antihypertensive*
Zanosar powder for IV injection ℞ *antineoplastic for metastatic islet cell carcinoma of pancreas and colon cancer* [streptozocin] 1 g
zanoterone USAN *antiandrogen*

Zantac film-coated tablets, syrup, IV or IM injection ℞ *gastric and duodenal ulcer treatment; histamine H_2 antagonist* [ranitidine HCl] 150, 300 mg; 15 mg/mL; 0.5, 25 mg/mL ⚠ Xanax
Zantac 75 tablets OTC *treatment of episodic heartburn; histamine H_2 antagonist* [ranitidine HCl] 75 mg
Zantac EFFERdose effervescent tablets, effervescent granules ℞ *gastric and duodenal ulcer treatment; histamine H_2 antagonist* [ranitidine HCl] 150 mg; 150 mg/packet
Zantac GELdose capsules ℞ *gastric and duodenal ulcer treatment; histamine H_2 antagonist* [ranitidine HCl] 150, 300 mg
Zantryl capsules ℞ *appetite suppressant* [phentermine HCl] 30 mg
zapizolam INN
zaprinast INN, BAN
zardaverine INN
Zarontin capsules, syrup ℞ *anticonvulsant* [ethosuximide] 250 mg; 250 mg/5 mL ⚠ Zaroxolyn
Zaroxolyn tablets ℞ *diuretic; antihypertensive* [metolazone] 2.5, 5, 10 mg ⚠ Zarontin; Zeroxin
Zartan capsules (discontinued 1995) ℞ *cephalosporin-type antibiotic* [cephalexin monohydrate] 500 mg
zatosetron INN *antimigraine; investigational selective serotonin antagonist for anxiety and schizophrenia* [also: zatosetron maleate]
zatosetron maleate USAN *antimigraine; investigational selective sero-*

tonin antagonist for anxiety and schizophrenia [also: zatosetron]
Zavedos (European name for U.S. product Idamycin)
Z-Bec tablets OTC *vitamin/zinc supplement* [multiple vitamins; zinc sulfate] ≐ • 22.5 mg
ZBT Baby powder OTC *topical diaper rash treatment* [talc]
ZD 0490 *investigational immunotoxin for colorectal cancer*
ZD 0870 *investigational broad-spectrum systemic antifungal*
ZD 1694 *investigational antineoplastic for lung, colorectal, hepatic, breast, and ovarian cancer*
ZD 2079 *investigational treatment for diabetes and obesity*
ZD 2138 *investigational 5-lipoxygenase inhibitor for rheumatoid arthritis and asthma*
ZD 3523 *investigational leukotriene receptor antagonist for asthma*
ZD 7288 *investigational sinoatrial node modulator for angina*
ZE Caps soft capsules OTC *dietary supplement* [vitamin E; zinc gluconate] 200 • 9.6 mg
Zeasorb powder OTC *absorbent* [microporous cellulose; talc]
Zeasorb-AF powder OTC *topical antifungal* [miconazole nitrate] 2%
Zebeta film-coated tablets ℞ *antihypertensive; β-blocker* [bisoprolol fumarate] 5, 10 mg
Zecnil (discontinued 1996) ℞ *(orphan: secreting cutaneous gastrointestinal fistulas)* [somatostatin]
Zefazone powder for IV injection ℞ *cephalosporin-type antibiotic* [cefmetazole sodium] 1, 2 g
zein NF *coating agent*
Zeisin Autohaler (metered-dose inhaler) ℞ *investigational antiasthmatic*
Zemuron IV injection ℞ *neuromuscular blocking agent for anesthesia* [rocuronium bromide] 10 mg/mL
Zenate, Advanced Formula film-coated tablets ℞ *vitamin/iron supplement* [multiple vitamins; iron; folic acid] ≐ • 65 • 1 mg

Zenate Prenatal film-coated tablets (name changed to Advanced Formula Zenate in 1994)
zenazocine mesylate USAN *analgesic*
Zeneca 182,780 *investigational steroidal antiestrogen for breast cancer*
Zeneca 200,880 *investigational treatment for adult respiratory distress syndrome*
zepastine INN
Zephiran Chloride tincture, tincture spray, aqueous solution, towelettes, disinfectant concentrate OTC *topical antiseptic* [benzalkonium chloride] 1:750; 1:750; 1:750; 1:750; 17%
zephirol [see: benzalkonium chloride]
Zephrex film-coated tablets ℞ *decongestant; expectorant* [pseudoephedrine HCl; guaifenesin] 60 • 400 mg
Zephrex LA timed-release tablets ℞ *decongestant; expectorant* [pseudoephedrine HCl; guaifenesin] 120 • 600 mg
zeranol USAN, INN *anabolic*
Zerit capsules ℞ *antiviral for HIV infection* [stavudine] 15, 20, 30, 40 mg
Zeroxin-5; Zeroxin-10 gel (discontinued 1994) ℞ *topical keratolytic for acne* [benzoyl peroxide] 5%; 10% ⓘ Zaroxolyn
Zestoretic tablets ℞ *antihypertensive* [hydrochlorothiazide; lisinopril] 12.5 • 10, 25 • 20 mg
Zestril tablets ℞ *antihypertensive; angiotensin-converting enzyme (ACE) inhibitor for CHF and acute MI* [lisinopril] 2.5, 5, 10, 20, 40 mg
Zetar shampoo OTC *antiseborrheic; antipsoriatic; antipruritic; antibacterial* [coal tar] 1%
Zetar Emulsion bath oil ℞ *antipsoriatic; antiseborrheic; antipruritic; emollient* [coal tar] 30%
zetidoline INN, BAN
Zetran IV or IM injection (discontinued 1996) ℞ *sedative; anxiolytic; skeletal muscle relaxant; anticonvulsant adjunct* [diazepam] 5 mg/mL
Z-gen tablets OTC *vitamin/zinc supplement* [multiple vitamins; zinc] ≐ • 22.5 mg
Ziac tablets ℞ *antihypertensive* [hydrochlorothiazide; bisoprolol fumarate] 6.25 • 2.5, 6.25 • 5, 6.25 • 10 mg

zidapamide INN
zidometacin USAN, INN *anti-inflammatory*
zidovudine USAN, INN, BAN *antiviral for AIDS and AIDS-related complex (orphan)*
zifrosilone USAN *acetylcholinesterase inhibitor for Alzheimer's disease*
Zilactin Medicated gel OTC *astringent for oral canker and herpes lesions* [tannic acid; alcohol 80%] 7%
Zilactin-B Medicated gel OTC *topical oral anesthetic* [benzocaine; alcohol 76%] 10%
Zilactin-L liquid OTC *topical local anesthetic* [lidocaine] 2.5%
Zilactol Medicated liquid (discontinued 1993) OTC *astringent for pre-emergent oral herpes lesions* [tannic acid]
ZilaDent gel (discontinued 1995) OTC *topical oral anesthetic* [benzocaine; alcohol 74.9%] 6%
zilantel USAN, INN *anthelmintic*
zileuton USAN, INN, BAN *5-lipoxygenase inhibitor; investigational anti-inflammatory for asthma, arthritis, and lupus*
zilpaterol INN
zimeldine INN, BAN *antidepressant* [also: zimeldine HCl]
zimeldine HCl USAN *antidepressant* [also: zimeldine]
zimelidine HCl [now: zimeldine HCl]
zimidoben INN
Zinacef powder for IV or IM injection ℞ *cephalosporin-type antibiotic* [cefuroxime sodium] 0.75, 1.5, 7.5 g
zinc *element* (Zn)
Zinc 15 tablets OTC *zinc supplement* [zinc sulfate] 66 mg
zinc acetate USP (*orphan: Wilson's disease*)
zinc acetate, basic INN
zinc acetate dihydrate [see: zinc acetate]
zinc bacitracin [see: bacitracin zinc]
zinc caprylate *antifungal*
zinc carbonate USAN *zinc supplement*
zinc chloride USP *astringent; dentin desensitizer; dietary zinc supplement*
zinc chloride Zn 65 USAN *radioactive agent*

zinc complex bacitracins [see: bacitracin zinc]
zinc gelatin USP
zinc gluconate USP *dietary zinc supplement* 10, 15, 50, 78 mg oral
zinc mesoporphyrin [see: hemin and zinc mesoporphyrin]
zinc oleate NF
zinc oxide USP, JAN *astringent; topical protectant; emollient; antiseptic* 20% topical
zinc peroxide, medicinal USP
zinc phenolsulfonate NF *not generally regarded as safe and effective as an antidiarrheal*
zinc propionate *antifungal*
zinc pyrithione [see: pyrithione zinc]
zinc stearate USP *dusting powder; tablet and capsule lubricant; antifungal*
zinc sulfate USP, JAN *ophthalmic astringent; dietary zinc supplement* 200, 250 mg oral; 1, 5 mg/mL injection
zinc sulfate heptahydrate [see: zinc sulfate]
zinc sulfate monohydrate [see: zinc sulfate]
Zinc Sulfide Compound Lotion, Improved (discontinued 1992) OTC *topical acne treatment* [zinc sulfide; sulfur]
zinc sulfocarbolate [see: zinc phenolsulfonate]
Zinc Trace Metal Additive IV injection (discontinued 1992) ℞ *intravenous nutritional therapy* [zinc sulfate]
zinc undecylenate USP *antifungal*
zinc valerate USP
Zinc-220 capsules OTC *zinc supplement* [zinc sulfate] 220 mg
Zinca-Pak IV injection ℞ *intravenous nutritional therapy* [zinc sulfate] 1, 5 mg/mL
Zincate capsules ℞ *zinc supplement* [zinc sulfate] 220 mg
zinc-eugenol USP
Zincfrin Drop-Tainers (eye drops) OTC *topical ocular decongestant; astringent* [phenylephrine HCl; zinc sulfate] 0.12%•0.25%
Zincon shampoo OTC *antiseborrheic; antibacterial; antifungal* [pyrithione zinc] 1%

Zincvit capsules ℞ *vitamin/mineral supplement* [multiple vitamins and minerals; folic acid] ≐•1 mg

zindotrine USAN, INN *bronchodilator*

Zinecard powder for IV drip or push ℞ *cardioprotectant for doxorubicin-induced cardiomyopathy (orphan)* [dexrazoxane] 250, 500 mg/vial

Zinkaps-220 capsules (discontinued 1992) OTC *zinc supplement* [zinc sulfate]

zinoconazole INN *antifungal* [also: zinoconazole HCl]

zinoconazole HCl USAN *antifungal* [also: zinoconazole]

zinostatin USAN, INN *antineoplastic*

zinterol INN *bronchodilator* [also: zinterol HCl]

zinterol HCl USAN *bronchodilator* [also: zinterol]

zinviroxime USAN, INN *antiviral*

zipeprol INN

ziprasidone *investigational antipsychotic for schizophrenia*

ziprasidone HCl *antipsychotic*

Ziradryl lotion OTC *topical antihistamine; astringent; antiseptic* [diphenhydramine HCl; zinc oxide; alcohol 2%] 1%•2%

zirconium *element (Zr)*

zirconium oxide *astringent*

Zithromax capsules, tablets ℞ *macrolide antibiotic* [azithromycin dihydrate] 250 mg

Zithromax oral suspension ℞ *pediatric macrolide antibiotic* [azithromycin dihydrate] 100, 200 mg/5 mL

Zixoryn ℞ *(orphan: neonatal hyperbilirubinemia)* [flumecinol]

^{65}Zn [see: zinc chloride Zn 65]

ZNP cleansing bar OTC *antiseborrheic; antibacterial; antifungal* [pyrithione zinc] 2%

zocainone INN

Zocor tablets ℞ *cholesterol-lowering antihyperlipidemic* [simvastatin] 5, 10, 20, 40 mg

Zodeac-100 tablets ℞ *hematinic; vitamin/mineral supplement* [ferrous fumarate; multiple vitamins & minerals; folic acid; biotin] 60 mg•≐•1 mg•300 μg

zofenopril INN, BAN *angiotensin-converting enzyme (ACE) inhibitor* [also: zofenopril calcium]

zofenopril calcium USAN *angiotensin-converting enzyme (ACE) inhibitor* [also: zofenopril]

zofenoprilat INN *antihypertensive* [also: zofenoprilat arginine]

zofenoprilat arginine USAN *antihypertensive* [also: zofenoprilat]

zoficonazole INN

Zofran tablets, IV infusion ℞ *antiemetic for chemotherapy and radiotherapy; investigational anxiolytic and Alzeimer treatment* [ondansetron HCl] 4, 8 mg; 2 mg/mL, 32 mg/50 mL

Zoladex subcu implant in preloaded syringe ℞ *palliative hormonal chemotherapy for prostatic carcinoma, breast cancer, and endometriosis* [goserelin acetate] 3.6 mg (1-month implant), 10.8 mg (3-month implant)

zolamine INN *antihistamine; topical anesthetic* [also: zolamine HCl]

zolamine HCl USAN *antihistamine; topical anesthetic* [also: zolamine]

zolazepam INN, BAN *sedative* [also: zolazepam HCl]

zolazepam HCl USAN *sedative* [also: zolazepam]

zolenzepine INN

zolertine INN *antiadrenergic; vasodilator* [also: zolertine HCl]

zolertine HCl USAN *antiadrenergic; vasodilator* [also: zolertine]

Zolicef powder for IV or IM injection ℞ *cephalosporin-type antibiotic* [cefazolin sodium] 0.5, 1 g

zolimidine INN

zolimomab aritox USAN *anti-T lymphocyte monoclonal antibody*

zoliprofen INN

zoliridine [see: zolimidine]

Zoloft film-coated tablets ℞ *antidepressant; selective serotonin reuptake inhibitor* [sertraline HCl] 50, 100 mg

zoloperone INN

zolpidem INN, BAN *imidazopyridine-type sedative/hypnotic* [also: zolpidem tartrate]

zolpidem tartrate USAN *imidazopyridine-type sedative/hypnotic* [also: zolpidem]

Zolyse ophthalmic solution (discontinued 1993) ℞ *enzymatic zonulolytic for intracapsular lens extraction* [chymotrypsin] 750 U

zomebazam INN

zomepirac INN, BAN *analgesic; anti-inflammatory* [also: zomepirac sodium]

zomepirac sodium USAN, USP *analgesic; anti-inflammatory* [also: zomepirac]

zometapine USAN *antidepressant*

Zonalon cream ℞ *topical antihistamine/antipruritic* [doxepin HCl] 5%

Zonavir ℞ *investigational treatment for varicella zoster virus* [5-propynylarabinofuranosyluracil]

Zone-A lotion, cream (discontinued 1993) ℞ *topical corticosteroid; anesthetic* [hydrocortisone acetate; pramoxine]

Zone-A Forte lotion ℞ *topical corticosteroid; local anesthetic* [hydrocortisone acetate; pramoxine] 2.5%•1%

zoniclezole INN *anticonvulsant* [also: zoniclezole HCl]

zoniclezole HCl USAN *anticonvulsant* [also: zoniclezole]

zonisamide USAN, INN, BAN *anticonvulsant*

Zonite Douche solution concentrate OTC *antiseptic; antipruritic/counterirritant; vaginal cleanser and deodorizer* [benzalkonium chloride; menthol; thymol]

Zophren (European name for U.S. product Zofran)

zopiclone INN, BAN, JAN *sedative; hypnotic*

zopolrestat USAN *antidiabetic; aldose reductase inhibitor*

zorbamycin USAN *antibacterial*

ZORprin Zero Order Release tablets ℞ *analgesic; antipyretic; anti-inflammatory; antirheumatic* [aspirin] 800 mg

zorubicin INN *antineoplastic* [also: zorubicin HCl]

zorubicin HCl USAN *antineoplastic* [also: zorubicin]

Zostrix; Zostrix-HP cream OTC *topical analgesic* [capsaicin] 0.025%; 0.075%

Zosyn powder for IV injection ℞ *extended-spectrum penicillin-type antibiotic* [piperacillin sodium; tazobactam sodium] 2•0.25, 3•0.375, 4•0.5 g

zotepine INN *investigational antipsychotic*

Zoto-HC ear drops ℞ *topical corticosteroidal anti-inflammatory; antibacterial; local anesthetic* [hydrocortisone; chloroxylenol; pramoxine HCl] 10•1•10 mg/mL

Zovia tablets ℞ *monophasic oral contraceptive* [ethynodiol diacetate; ethinyl estradiol] 1 mg•35 µg; 1 mg•50 µg

Zovirax powder for IV infusion ℞ *antiviral for herpes infections* [acyclovir sodium] 500, 1000 mg

Zovirax tablets, capsules, oral suspension, ointment ℞ *antiviral for herpes simplex, herpes zoster, and adult-onset chickenpox; investigational for AIDS* [acyclovir] 400, 800 mg; 200 mg; 200 mg/5 mL; 5%

Zovirax OTC *investigational (awaiting approval) OTC formulation for recurrent genital herpes* [acyclovir]

zoxazolamine NF, INN

zucapsaicin USAN *topical analgesic*

zuclomifene INN

zuclomiphene USAN

zuclopenthixol INN, BAN

Zumenon; Zumeston ℞ *investigational treatment of postmenopausal symptoms* [estrogen; progestogen]

Zurinol tablets ℞ *uricosuric for gout* [allopurinol]

Zydone capsules ℞ *narcotic analgesic* [hydrocodone bitartrate; acetaminophen] 5•500 mg

zylofuramine INN

Zyloprim injection ℞ *investigational antineoplastic (orphan: leukemia, lymphoma, and solid tumor malignancies)* [allopurinol sodium]

Zyloprim tablets ℞ *xanthine oxidase inhibitor for gout* [allopurinol] 100, 300 mg

Zymacap capsules OTC *vitamin supplement* [multiple vitamins; folic acid] ±•0.4 mg

Zymase capsules containing enteric-coated spheres ℞ *digestive enzymes* [lipase; protease; amylase] 12,000•24,000•24,000 U

Zyrtec film-coated tablets ℞ *once-daily antihistamine* [cetirizine HCl] 5, 10 mg

APPENDIX A
Sound-Alikes

Listed below are 961 pairs of drugs that sound alike or sufficiently alike that they may be confused in transcription. The list is not all-inclusive, and we would appreciate hearing of any additions the reader might suggest. These sound-alikes have also been included in the main section of the book where appropriate. Look for the "ear" icon (👂).

A-Caine	Anocaine
Accurbron	Accutane
Accutane	Accurbron
Achromycin	actinomycin
Achromycin	Aureomycin
Actidil	Actifed
Actifed	Actidil
actinomycin	Achromycin
actinomycin	Aureomycin
Adapin	Atabrine
Adapin	Ativan
Adapin	Betapen
adrenaline	adrenalone
adrenalone	adrenaline
Advil	Avail
Aerolone	Aralen
Aerolone	Arlidin
Afrin	Afrinol
Afrin	aspirin
Afrinol	Afrin
Agoral	Argyrol
Ak-Mycin	Akne-Mycin
Akne-Mycin	Ak-Mycin
Alamag	Alma-Mag
Aldactazide	Aldactone
Aldactone	Aldactazide
Aldomet	Aldoril
Aldoril	Aldomet
Aldoril	Elavil
Allergan	allergen
Allergan	Auralgan
allergen	Allergan
allergen	Auralgan
Alma-Mag	Alamag
ALOMAD	Alomide
Alomide	ALOMAD
Ambenyl	Aventyl
Amicar	Amikin

Appendix A: Sound-Alikes

Amikin	Amicar
amitriptyline	nortriptyline
amoxapine	amoxicillin
amoxapine	Amoxil
amoxicillin	amoxapine
Amoxil	amoxapine
Anafranil	enalapril
Analbalm	Analpram
Analpram	Analbalm
Ancobon	Oncovin
Anocaine	A-Caine
Anturane	Artane
Anusol	Aplisol
APAC	APAP
APAP	APAC
Aplisol	Anusol
Aplisol	Apresoline
Appedrine	aprindine
Appedrine	ephedrine
Apresoline	Aplisol
Apresoline	Priscoline
aprindine	Appedrine
aprindine	ephedrine
ara-C	ERYC
Aralen	Aerolone
Aralen	Arlidin
Argyrol	Agoral
Arlidin	Aerolone
Arlidin	Aralen
Artane	Anturane
aspirin	Afrin
Atabrine	Adapin
Atarax	Marax
atenolol	timolol
Ativan	Adapin
Ativan	Avitene
Auralgan	Allergan
Auralgan	allergen
Aureomycin	Achromycin
Aureomycin	actinomycin
Avail	Advil
Aventyl	Ambenyl
Aventyl	Bentyl
Avitene	Ativan
Azlin	Mezlin
azolimine	Azulfidine
Azulfidine	azolimine
Bacid	Banacid
bacitracin	Bacitrin
bacitracin	Bactrim
Bacitrin	bacitracin
Bactocill	Pathocil

Bactrim	bacitracin
Banacid	Bacid
Banophen	Barophen
Banthine	Brethine
Barophen	Banophen
Belladenal	belladonna
Belladenal	Benadryl
belladonna	Belladenal
Beminal	Benemid
Benadryl	Belladenal
Benadryl	Bentyl
Benadryl	Benylin
Benadryl	Caladryl
Benemid	Beminal
Benoxyl	PanOxyl
Bentyl	Aventyl
Bentyl	Benadryl
Bentyl	Bontril
Benylin	Benadryl
Benylin	Betalin
Betagan	Betagen
Betagen	Betagan
Betalin	Benylin
Betapen	Adapin
Betapen	Phenaphen
Bichloracetic acid	dichloroacetic acid
Bicillin	V-Cillin
Bicillin	Wycillin
bleomycin	Cleocin
boil	Boyol
Bonain	Bonine
Bonine	Bonain
Bontril	Bentyl
Bontril	Vontrol
Boyol	boil
Brethine	Banthine
Bretylol	Brevital
Brevital	Bretylol
Bromfed	Bromphen
Bromophen	Bromphen
Bromphen	Bromfed
Bromphen	Bromophen
Broncholate	Brondelate
Brondecon	Bronitin
Brondelate	Broncholate
Bronitin	Brondecon
butabarbital	butalbital
butalbital	butabarbital
butalbital	Butibel
Butazolidin	Butisol
Butibel	butalbital
Butisol	Butazolidin

Appendix A: Sound-Alikes 563

564 Appendix A: Sound-Alikes

Byclomine	Hycomine
Bydramine	Hydramine
Caladryl	Benadryl
Calamox	Camalox
calcitonin	calcitriol
calcitriol	calcitonin
Camalox	Calamox
Capastat	Cepastat
Capitrol	captopril
captopril	Capitrol
Catapres	Catarase
Catapres	Combipres
Catapres	Ser-Ap-Es
Catarase	Catapres
cefazolin	cephalexin
cefazolin	cephalothin
cefotaxime	cefoxitin
cefoxitin	cefotaxime
ceftizoxime	cefuroxime
cefuroxime	ceftizoxime
Cefzil	Kefzol
Cepastat	Capastat
cephalexin	cefazolin
cephalexin	cephalothin
cephalothin	cefazolin
cephalothin	cephalexin
cephapirin	cephradine
cephradine	cephapirin
chlorpheniramine	chlorphentermine
chlorphentermine	chlorpheniramine
cimetidine	dimethicone
claretin	Claritin
claretin	Clarityne
Claritin	claretin
Claritin	Clarityne
Clarityne	claretin
Clarityne	Claritin
Cleocin	bleomycin
Cleocin	Lincocin
Clinoxide	clioxanide
Clinoxide	Clipoxide
clioxanide	Clinoxide
Clipoxide	Clinoxide
clomiphene	clonidine
clonidine	clomiphene
clonidine	Klonopin
clonidine	quinidine
clotrimazole	co-trimoxazole
co-trimoxazole	clotrimazole
Codafed	Codaphen
Codaphen	Codafed
Codegest	Codehist

Codehist	Codegest
codeine	Kaodene
Colestid	colistin
colestipol	colistin
colistin	Colestid
colistin	colestipol
Combipres	Catapres
Cort-Dome	Cortone
Cortenema	quart enema
Cortin	Cotrim
cortisone	Cortizone
Cortizone	cortisone
Cortone	Cort-Dome
Cotrim	Cortin
Coumadin	Kemadrin
cytarabine	vidarabine
dacarbazine	Dicarbosil
dacarbazine	procarbazine
dactinomycin	daunorubicin
Dalmane	Dialume
danthron	Dantrium
Dantrium	danthron
Daranide	Daraprim
Daraprim	Daranide
Daricon	Darvon
Darvocet-N	Darvon-N
Darvon	Daricon
Darvon-N	Darvocet-N
daunorubicin	dactinomycin
daunorubicin	doxorubicin
Decaderm	Decadron
Decadron	Decaderm
Decadron	Percodan
Deconal	Deconsal
Deconsal	Deconal
Delacort	Delcort
Delcort	Delacort
Demerol	Demulen
Demerol	dicumarol
Demerol	Dymelor
Demerol	Temaril
Demolin	Demulen
Demulen	Demerol
Demulen	Demolin
Dermacort	DermiCort
DermiCort	Dermacort
deserpidine	desipramine
Desferal	Disophrol
desipramine	deserpidine
desoximethasone	dexamethasone
Desoxyn	digitoxin
Desoxyn	digoxin

Appendix A: Sound-Alikes 565

Appendix A: Sound-Alikes

dexamethasone	desoximethasone
Dexedrine	dextran
dextran	Dexedrine
dextran	dextrin
dextrin	dextran
Dialume	Dalmane
Dicarbosil	dacarbazine
dichloroacetic acid	Bichloracetic acid
dicumarol	Demerol
digitoxin	Desoxyn
digitoxin	digoxin
digoxin	Desoxyn
digoxin	digitoxin
Dilantin	Dilaudid
Dilaudid	Dilantin
Dimacol	dimercaprol
dimenhydrinate	diphenhydramine
dimercaprol	Dimacol
Dimetabs	Dimetane
Dimetabs	Dimetapp
Dimetane	Dimetabs
Dimetapp	Dimetabs
dimethicone	cimetidine
diphenhydramine	dimenhydrinate
Diphenylin	Dyphenylan
Disophrol	Desferal
Disophrol	disoprofol
Disophrol	Stilphostrol
disoprofol	Disophrol
Ditropan	Intropin
Diutensen	Salutensin
dobutamine	dopamine
Dommanate	Dramanate
Donnagel	Donnatal
Donnatal	Donnagel
Donnazyme	Entozyme
dopamine	dobutamine
dopamine	Dopram
Dopar	Dopram
Dopram	dopamine
Dopram	Dopar
doxepin	Doxidan
Doxidan	doxepin
doxorubicin	daunorubicin
Dramanate	Dommanate
Dyazide	Thiacide
Dyazide	thiazides
Dymelor	Demerol
Dymelor	Pamelor
Dyphenylan	Diphenylin
Dyrenium	Pyridium
Ecotrin	Edecrin

Edecrin	Ecotrin
Edecrin	Ethaquin
Elavil	Aldoril
Elavil	Enovil
Elavil	Equanil
Elavil	Mellaril
emetine	Emetrol
Emetrol	emetine
Endal	Intal
Enduron	Imuran
Enduron	Inderal
Enduronyl	Inderal
Enovil	Elavil
Entozyme	Donnazyme
ephedrine	Appedrine
ephedrine	aprindine
Epifrin	epinephrine
Epifrin	EpiPen
Epinal	Epitol
epinephrine	Epifrin
EpiPen	Epifrin
Epitol	Epinal
Equanil	Elavil
erythromycin	clarithromycin
ERYC	ara-C
Esidrix	Lasix
Esimil	Estinyl
Esimil	Isomil
Estinyl	Esimil
Estraderm	Estradurin
Estradurin	Estraderm
Estratab	Ethatab
ethacridine	ethacrynic
ethacrynic	ethacridine
Ethaquin	Edecrin
Ethatab	Estratab
ethinamate	ethionamide
ethionamide	ethinamate
Eurax	Serax
Eurax	Urex
Euthroid	Synthroid
Euthroid	thyroid
Eutonyl	Eutron
Eutron	Eutonyl
Evac-Q-Kit	Evac-Q-Kwik
Evac-Q-Kwik	Evac-Q-Kit
Feosol	Feostat
Feosol	Fer-in-Sol
Feosol	Festal
Feostat	Feosol
Fer-in-Sol	Feosol
Festal	Feosol

Festal	Festalan
Festalan	Festal
Feverall	Fiberall
Fiberall	Feverall
Fioricet	Lorcet
Fiorinal	Florinef
Flaxedil	Flexeril
Flexeril	Flaxedil
Florinef	Fiorinal
fluocinolone	fluocinonide
fluocinonide	fluocinolone
folacin	Fulvicin
Fostex	pHisoHex
Fulvicin	folacin
Fulvicin	Furacin
Furacin	Fulvicin
Gamastan	Garamycin
Gantanol	Gantrisin
Gantrisin	Gantanol
Garamycin	Gamastan
Garamycin	kanamycin
Garamycin	Terramycin
Gelfoam	Ger-O-Foam
Genapap	Genatap
Genatap	Genapap
gentamicin	Jenamicin
gentamicin	kanamycin
Ger-O-Foam	Gelfoam
glucose	Glutose
Glutose	glucose
Glycotuss	Glytuss
Glytuss	Glycotuss
Gonak	Gonic
Gonic	Gonak
guaifenesin	guanfacine
guanethidine	guanidine
guanfacine	guaifenesin
guanidine	guanethidine
Guiatuss	Guiatussin
Guiatussin	Guiatuss
Haldol	Halenol
Haldol	Halog
Halenol	Haldol
Halog	Haldol
Halotestin	Halotex
Halotestin	Halotussin
Halotex	Halotestin
Halotussin	Halotestin
Hespan	Histastan
Hexadrol	Hexalol
Hexalen	Hexalol
Hexalol	Hexadrol

Hexalol	Hexalen
Hiprex	Hispril
Hispril	Hiprex
Histastan	Hespan
Histastan	Histatime
Histatime	Histastan
Hycodan	Hycomine
Hycodan	Vicodin
Hycomine	Byclomine
Hycomine	Hycodan
Hycomine	Vicodin
Hydergine	Hydramine
Hydramine	Bydramine
Hydramine	Hydergine
Hydramine	Hydramyn
Hydramine	Hytramyn
Hydramyn	Hydramine
Hydropane	Hydropine
Hydrophen	Hydropine
Hydropine	Hydropane
Hydropine	Hydrophen
Hygroton	Regroton
Hyper-Tet	HyperHep
Hyper-Tet	Hyperstat
HyperHep	Hyper-Tet
HyperHep	Hyperstat
Hyperstat	Hyper-Tet
Hyperstat	HyperHep
Hyperstat	Nitrostat
Hytone	Vytone
Hytramyn	Hydramine
Ilosone	inosine
Imferon	imipramine
Imferon	Imuran
imipramine	Imferon
imipramine	Norpramin
imipramine	trimipramine
Imuran	Enduron
Imuran	Imferon
Inderal	Enduron
Inderal	Enduronyl
Inderal	Inderide
Inderide	Inderal
Indocin	Lincocin
Indocin	Minocin
inosine	Ilosone
insulin	inulin
Intal	Endal
Intropin	Ditropan
Intropin	Isoptin
inulin	insulin
Ismelin	Ritalin

Appendix A: Sound-Alikes

Isomil	Esimil
Isoptin	Intropin
Isopto Carpine	Isopto Eserine
Isopto Eserine	Isopto Carpine
Isordil	Isuprel
Isuprel	Isordil
K-LOR	Kaochlor
K-LOR	Klor
kanamycin	Garamycin
kanamycin	gentamicin
Kaochlor	K-LOR
Kaodene	codeine
kaolin	Kaon
Kaon	kaolin
Kaopectate	Kapectalin
Kapectalin	Kaopectate
Kay Ciel	KCl
KCl	Kay Ciel
Keflet	Keflex
Keflet	Keflin
Keflex	Keflet
Keflex	Keflin
Keflin	Keflet
Keflin	Keflex
Kefzol	Cefzil
Kemadrin	Coumadin
Kenalog	Ketalar
Ketalar	Kenalog
Klonopin	clonidine
Klor	K-LOR
Klotrix	Liotrix
Komex	Koromex
Koromex	Komex
lanolin	Lanoline
Lanoline	lanolin
Lanoxin	Levoxine
Lasix	Esidrix
Lasix	Lidex
levallorphan	levorphanol
levodopa	methyldopa
levorphanol	levallorphan
levothyroxine	liothyronine
Levoxine	Lanoxin
Lidex	Lasix
Lidex	Lidox
Lidex	Wydase
Lidox	Lidex
Lincocin	Cleocin
Lincocin	Indocin
liothyronine	levothyroxine
Liotrix	Klotrix
Loniten	clonidine

Lorcet	Fioricet
Lotrimin	Otrivin
Luminal	Tuinal
LuVax	Luvox
Luvox	LuVax
Maalox	Marax
Mandol	nadolol
Marax	Atarax
Marax	Maalox
Marcaine	Narcan
mazindol	mebendazole
Mebaral	Medrol
Mebaral	Mellaril
mebendazole	mazindol
Meclan	Meclomen
Meclan	Mezlin
Meclomen	Meclan
Medrol	Mebaral
Mellaril	Elavil
Mellaril	Mebaral
Mellaril	Moderil
meperidine	meprobamate
mephenytoin	Mephyton
mephenytoin	Mesantoin
Mephyton	mephenytoin
Mephyton	methadone
meprobamate	meperidine
Meprospan	Naprosyn
Mesantoin	mephenytoin
Mesantoin	Mestinon
Mesantoin	Metatensin
Mestinon	Mesantoin
Mestinon	Metatensin
Metahydrin	Metandren
Metandren	Metahydrin
metaproterenol	metoprolol
Metatensin	Mesantoin
Metatensin	Mestinon
metaxalone	metolazone
methadone	Mephyton
methenamine	methionine
methionine	methenamine
methixene	methoxsalen
methoxsalen	methixene
methyldopa	levodopa
metolazone	metaxalone
Metopirone	metyrapone
metoprolol	metaproterenol
metyrapone	Metopirone
metyrapone	metyrosine
metyrosine	metyrapone
Mezlin	Azlin

Mezlin	Meclan
MICRhoGAM	microgram
microgram	MICRhoGAM
Midrin	Mydfrin
Milontin	Miltown
Milontin	Mylanta
Miltown	Milontin
Minocin	Indocin
Minocin	Mithracin
Minocin	niacin
Mithracin	Minocin
mithramycin	mitomycin
mitomycin	mithramycin
mitomycin	Mity-Mycin
mitomycin	Mutamycin
Mity-Mycin	mitomycin
Moban	Mobidin
Moban	Modane
Mobidin	Moban
Modane	Moban
Modane	Mudrane
Moderil	Mellaril
Modicon	Mylicon
Moi-Stir	moisture
moisture	Moi-Stir
Monocete	Monoket
Mono-Chlor	Monocor
Monocor	Mono-Chlor
Monoket	Monocete
Mudrane	Modane
Mutamycin	mitomycin
Myambutol	Nembutal
Mydfrin	Midrin
Mydfrin	Myfedrine
Myfedrine	Mydfrin
Mylanta	Milontin
Myleran	Mylicon
Mylicon	Modicon
Mylicon	Myleran
nadolol	Mandol
Naldecon	Nalfon
Nalfon	Naldecon
Naprosyn	Meprospan
Naprosyn	naproxen
Naprosyn	Natacyn
naproxen	Naprosyn
Narcan	Marcaine
Nardil	Norinyl
Natacyn	Naprosyn
Nembutal	Myambutol
Neomixin	neomycin
neomycin	Neomixin

Appendix A: Sound-Alikes 573

niacin	Minocin
Nicobid	Nitro-Bid
Nilstat	Nitrostat
Nilstat	nystatin
Nitro-Bid	Nicobid
nitroglycerin	Nitroglyn
Nitroglyn	nitroglycerin
Nitrostat	Hyperstat
Nitrostat	Nilstat
Nitrostat	nystatin
Norinyl	Nardil
Norlutate	Norlutin
Norlutin	Norlutate
Norpramin	imipramine
nortriptyline	amitriptyline
nystatin	Nilstat
nystatin	Nitrostat
Omnipen	Unipen
Oncovin	Ancobon
Ophthochlor	Ophthocort
Ophthocort	Ophthochlor
Orabase	Orinase
Oracin	orarsan
Oracin	Orasone
orarsan	Oracin
orarsan	Orasone
Orasone	Oracin
Orasone	orarsan
Oretic	Oreton
Oreton	Oretic
Orex	Ornex
Orinase	Orabase
Orinase	Ornade
Orinase	Ornex
Orinase	Tolinase
Ornade	Orinase
Ornade	Ornex
Ornex	Orex
Ornex	Orinase
Ornex	Ornade
Ortho-Creme	Orthoclone
Orthoclone	Ortho-Creme
Otobiotic	Urobiotic
Otrivin	Lotrimin
oxymetazoline	oxymetholone
oxymetholone	oxymetazoline
oxymetholone	oxymorphone
oxymorphone	oxymetholone
Pamelor	Dymelor
Panarex	Panorex
Panasol	Panscol
Panorex	Panarex

PanOxyl	Benoxyl
Panscol	Panasol
Pantopon	Parafon
Parafon	Pantopon
paramethadione	paramethasone
paramethasone	paramethadione
Pathilon	Pathocil
Pathocil	Bactocill
Pathocil	Pathilon
Pathocil	Placidyl
Pavabid	Pavased
Pavased	Pavabid
Pavatine	Pavatym
Pavatym	Pavatine
Paverolan	Pavulon
Pavulon	Paverolan
penicillamine	penicillin
penicillin	penicillamine
penicillin	Polycillin
Pentazine	Phenazine
pentobarbital	phenobarbital
Pentothal	pentrinitrol
pentrinitrol	Pentothal
Percodan	Decadron
Perdiem	Pyridium
Periactin	Taractan
Persantine	Pertofrane
Pertofrane	Persantine
Phazyme	Pherazine
phenacetin	phenazocine
Phenaphen	Betapen
Phenaphen	Phenergan
Phenazine	Pentazine
Phenazine	phenelzine
Phenazine	Phenoxine
Phenazine	Pherazine
phenazocine	phenacetin
phenelzine	Phenazine
phenelzine	Phenylzin
Phenergan	Phenaphen
Phenergan	Theragran
phenobarbital	pentobarbital
Phenoxine	Phenazine
phentermine	phentolamine
phentolamine	phentermine
phentolamine	Ventolin
Phenylzin	phenelzine
Pherazine	Phazyme
Pherazine	Phenazine
pHisoHex	Fostex
physostigmine	pyridostigmine
physostigmine	Prostigmin

Appendix A: Sound-Alikes 575

piperacetazine	piperazine
piperazine	piperacetazine
piracetam	piroxicam
piroxicam	piracetam
Pitocin	Pitressin
Pitressin	Pitocin
Placidyl	Pathocil
Pod-Ben	Podoben
Podoben	Pod-Ben
Podoben	Podofin
Podofin	Podoben
Podofin	podophyllin
podophyllin	Podofin
Polycillin	penicillin
Ponstel	Pronestyl
pralidoxime	pramoxine
pralidoxime	pyridoxine
Pramosone	pramoxine
pramoxine	pralidoxime
pramoxine	Pramosone
prazepam	prazepine
prazepam	Prazosin
prazepine	prazepam
Prazosin	prazepam
prednisolone	prednisone
prednisone	prednisolone
Priscoline	Apresoline
procaine	Procan
Procan	procaine
procarbazine	dacarbazine
Prolene	proline
proline	Prolene
promazine	Promethazine
Promethazine	promazine
Pronestyl	Ponstel
Prostigmin	physostigmine
Protamine	Protopam
Protopam	Protamine
Psorex	Serax
Pyridium	Dyrenium
Pyridium	pyridoxine
Pyridium	pyrithione
Pyridium	pyritidium
pyridostigmine	physostigmine
pyridoxine	pralidoxime
pyridoxine	Pyridium
pyrithione	Pyridium
pyritidium	Pyridium
quart enema	Cortenema
Quarzan	Questran
Questran	Quarzan
quinacrine	quinidine

Quinatime	quinidine
quinidine	clonidine
quinidine	quinacrine
quinidine	Quinatime
quinidine	quinine
quinine	quinidine
Regain	Rogaine
Reglan	Regonol
Regonol	Reglan
Regroton	Hygroton
Repan	Riopan
Resperol	Risperdal
Resperol	Restoril
Restoril	Resperol
Restoril	Vistaril
Rheumatex	Rheumatrex
Rheumatrex	Rheumatex
Rifadin	rifampin
Rifadin	Ritalin
rifampin	Rifadin
Riopan	Repan
Risperdal	Resperol
Ritalin	Ismelin
Ritalin	Rifadin
Robaxacet	Robaxisal
Robaxisal	Robaxacet
Rogaine	Regain
Salutensin	Diutensen
Sepo	Septa
Septa	Sepo
Septa	Septra
Septra	Septa
Ser-Ap-Es	Catapres
Serax	Eurax
Serax	Psorex
Serax	Urex
Serax	Xerac
Serentil	Surital
Simplet	Singlet
Singlet	Simplet
Soprodol	Sopronol
Sopronol	Soprodol
stilbestrol	Stilphostrol
Stilphostrol	Disophrol
Stilphostrol	stilbestrol
Streptase	Streptonase
streptokinase	Streptonase
Streptonase	Streptase
Streptonase	streptokinase
Sulf-10	Sulten-10
Sulfa-Trip	Sulfatrim
sulfamethizole	sulfamethoxazole

sulfamethoxazole	sulfamethizole
sulfathiazole	sulfisoxazole
Sulfatrim	Sulfa-Trip
sulfisoxazole	sulfathiazole
Sulten-10	Sulf-10
Surital	Serentil
Synthroid	Euthroid
Tagamet	Tegopen
Taractan	Periactin
Taractan	Tinactin
Tedral	Teldrin
Tegopen	Tagamet
Tegopen	Tegrin
Tegretol	Tegrin
Tegrin	Tegopen
Tegrin	Tegretol
Teldrin	Tedral
Temaril	Demerol
Temaril	Tepanil
Tepanil	Temaril
Tepanil	Tofranil
Terramycin	Garamycin
testolactone	testosterone
testosterone	testolactone
thallium	Valium
Theoclear	Theolair
Theocolate	Theolate
Theolair	Theoclear
Theolair	Thyrolar
Theolate	Theocolate
Thera-Flur	TheraFlu
TheraFlu	Thera-Flur
Theragran	Phenergan
Theravite	Therevac
Therevac	Theravite
Thiacide	Dyazide
Thiacide	thiazides
thiazides	Dyazide
thiazides	Thiacide
Threostat	Triostat
Thyrar	Thyrolar
thyroid	Euthroid
Thyrolar	Theolair
Thyrolar	Thyrar
Ticar	Tigan
Tigan	Ticar
timolol	atenolol
Tinactin	Taractan
TobraDex	Tobrex
tobramycin	Trobicin
Tobrex	TobraDex
Tofranil	Tepanil

Tolinase	Orinase
Topic	Topicort
Topicort	Topic
Trasylol	Travasol
Travasol	Trasylol
Triafed	Trifed
triamcinolone	Triaminicin
Triaminic	Triaminicin
Triaminic	TriHemic
Triaminicin	triamcinolone
Triaminicin	Triaminic
triamterene	trimipramine
Trifed	Triafed
TriHemic	Triaminic
trimeprazine	trimipramine
trimethaphan	trimethoprim
trimethoprim	trimethaphan
trimipramine	imipramine
trimipramine	triamterene
trimipramine	trimeprazine
Triostat	Threostat
Trobicin	tobramycin
Tronolane	Tronothane
Tronothane	Tronolane
Tuinal	Luminal
Tuinal	Tylenol
Tussafed	Tussafin
Tussafin	Tussafed
Tussex	Tussionex
Tussex	Tussirex
Tussi-Organidin	Tussi-R-Gen
Tussi-R-Gen	Tussi-Organidin
Tussionex	Tussex
Tussionex	Tussirex
Tussirex	Tussex
Tussirex	Tussionex
Tylenol	Tuinal
Unipen	Omnipen
Uracel	uracil
Uracel	Urised
Uracid	uracil
Uracid	Urised
Uracid	Urocit
uracil	Uracel
uracil	Uracid
Urex	Eurax
Urex	Serax
Urised	Uracel
Urised	Uracid
Urised	Urispas
Urispas	Urised
Urobiotic	Otobiotic

Appendix A: Sound-Alikes

Urocit	Uracid
V-Cillin	Bicillin
V-Cillin	Wycillin
Valium	thallium
Valium	Valpin
Valmid	Valpin
Valpin	Valium
Valpin	Valmid
Valpin	Valprin
Valpin	Velban
Valprin	Valpin
Vasocidin	Vasodilan
Vasodilan	Vasocidin
Vasosulf	Velosef
Velban	Valpin
Velosef	Vasosulf
Ventolin	phentolamine
Vicodin	Hycodan
Vicodin	Hycomine
vidarabine	cytarabine
Vigran	Wigraine
Vistaril	Restoril
Vitron	Vytone
Vontrol	Bontril
Vytone	Hytone
Vytone	Vitron
Wigraine	Vigran
Wycillin	Bicillin
Wycillin	V-Cillin
Wydase	Lidex
Xanax	Zantac
Xerac	Serax
Zantac	Xanax
Zarontin	Zaroxolyn
Zarontin	Zentron
Zaroxolyn	Zarontin
Zaroxolyn	Zeroxin
Zentron	Zarontin
Zeroxin	Zaroxolyn

APPENDIX B
Investigational Code Names

A code name is a temporary identification assigned to a product by the manufacturer. The number or letter-number combination is used while the substance is undergoing testing, before a generic name is given. Below are 3665 code names and their subsequently assigned generic names.

10275-S	epitiostanol
106223	cefamandole nafate
1069C	generic not yet assigned—see main list
10-EDAM	edatrexate
110264	cefaparole
125 I NM-113	iomethin I 125
129Y83	colfosceril palmitate
12C	velaresol
1314 TH	ethionamide
131 I NM-113	iomethin I 131
1370U	generic not yet assigned—see main list
1380U	baquiloprim
142780	generic not yet assigned—see main list
1589 RB	pefloxacin
1592U89	generic not yet assigned—see main list
16726	symetine HCl
16842	bitoscanate
1709 CERM	niaprazine
177 J.D.	aminocaproic acid
1875 CERM	fepromide
18894	nifungin
194-B	zolamine HCl
20025	clorprenaline HCl
205 E	calcium dobesilate
21401-Ba	tribenoside
21679-CH	malethamer
22-708	endralazine mesylate
24281	mitocarcin
249-16	deditonium bromide
2-5410-3A	iodixanol
256U87 HCl	valacyclovir HCl
26383	thiphencillin potassium
26P	aliflurane
27165	temefos
27-400	cyclosporine
28002	epipropidine
29060-LE	vinblastine sulfate
2936	proscillaridin
29866	levopropoxyphene napsylate

30038CB	minaprine HCl
3-01003	guanoxan sulfate
3-01029	guanoclor sulfate
30109	noracymethadol HCl
30639	polyethadene
3118	generic not yet assigned—see main list
311C	generic not yet assigned—see main list
3123L	puromycin
31518	pyrroliphene HCl
31595C	mitosper
31814	heteronium bromide
32-046	edetate dipotassium
32379	dromostanolone propionate
32645	vinleurosine sulfate
33006	acetohexamide
33355	mestranol
33379	flurandrenolide
33876	anthelmycin
348U	generic not yet assigned—see main list
34977	capreomycin sulfate
349 C59	moxipraquine
35483	cyclothiazide
36781	vinrosidine sulfate
36-801	etifoxine
37 162 R.P.	suproclone
37231	vincristine sulfate
38000	clometherone
38253	cephalothin sodium
38389	levopropylcillin potassium
38489	nortriptyline HCl
38851	bolmantalate
39435	cephaloglycin
3 MS	hydroxytoluic acid
3TC	lamivudine
40 045	articaine
40045	trimetazidine
403U	generic not yet assigned—see main list
40602	cephaloridine
4091 C.B.	benfurodil hemisuccinate
41071	cefalonium
41-123	clazolam
4197X-RA	generic not yet assigned—see main list
41 982 RP	pefloxacin mesylate
42-348	lifibrate
42406	metoquizine
42-548	mazindol
4306 CB	clorazepate dipotassium
4311 CB	clorazepate monopotassium
43-663	guanoxabenz
43-715	proquazone
43853	clobenoside
44089	valproic acid

44106	toquizine
44328	dexproxibutene
447C	generic not yet assigned—see main list
46083	cefazolin sodium
46236	dobutamine HCl
46-790	fluproquazone
46 R.P.	benzylsulfamide
47-210 (as sodium)	tetriprofen
47599	pyrazofurin
47657	apramycin
47663	tobramycin
48-674	furacrinic acid
49040	vinglycinate sulfate
4909 RP	chlorproethazine HCl
49825	nylestriol
4A65	imidocarb HCl
4-C-32	ticlopidine HCl
4MRTA	generic not yet assigned—see main list
5048	dimethisterone
5052	acetylcysteine
5054	prodilidine HCl
5058	oxybutynin chloride
5071	megestrol acetate
5107	chloral betaine
516 MD	cinnarizine
5190	amidephrine mesylate
51W89	cisatracurium besylate
520C9x22	generic not yet assigned—see main list
52230	pyrrolnitrin
53183	aranotin
53-32C	ticlopidine HCl
5373	melengestrol acetate
53858	fenoprofen
566C	atovaquone
566C80	atovaquone
57C65	cloguanamil
589C	tucaresol
59156	enpromate
5A8	generic not yet assigned—see main list
5IUDR	idoxuridine
60284	cyclophenazine HCl
611 C 65	thenium closylate
619C	generic not yet assigned—see main list
640/1	cefuracetime
640/359	cefuroxime
64716	cinoxacin
65-318	bidimazium iodide
66-269	pretamazium iodide
66873	cephalexin
673-082	nexeridine HCl
67314	monensin
68618	mycophenolic acid

69323	fenoprofen calcium
711 SE	pipratecol
7162 RP	trimipramine
7432-S	ceftibuten
786-723	anilopam HCl
79907	lergotrile
79 T61	lucanthone HCl
7-OMEN	menogaril
7U85	generic not yet assigned—see main list
80066	bufilcon A
8088 C.B.	benfotiamine
8102 CB	bamifylline HCl
83636	lergotrile mesylate
8599 R.P. mesylate	fonazine mesylate
882	generic not yet assigned—see main list
882C	generic not yet assigned—see main list
88BV59	votumumab
935U	generic not yet assigned—see main list
A-118	sultroponium
A-12253A	nebramycin
A-16612	teroxalene HCl
A-16686	ramoplanin
A-17624	ditolamide
A-19120	paragyline HCl
A-19757	encyprate
A-1981-12	prodilidine HCl
A-20968	piposulfan
A-2205	profadol HCl
A-2371	plicamycin
A-2655	dioxamate
A-27053	chromonar HCl
A-272	rutamycin
A-3217	ocfentanil HCl
A-32686	proscillaridin
A-3331	brifentanil HCl
A-33547	remoxipride
A-33547.HCl.H$_2$O	remoxipride HCl
A-3508.HCl	mirfentanil HCl
A-35957	altrenogest
A-3665.HCl	trefentanil HCl
A-4020 Linz	midodrine HCl
A 40664 (as tartrate)	raclopride
A-41-304	desoximetasone
A-4180	isometamidium chloride
A-4492	pentamorphone
A 46 745	gestrinone
A-4696	actaplanin
A-4828	trofosfamide
A-53986	fostedil
A-5610	azelastine HCl
A 5MP	adenosine phosphate
A-60386X	beractant

A-61589	docebenone
A-65006	lansoprazole
A-7283	guanoctine HCl
A-73001	seratrodast
A-77000	pazinaclone
A-8103	pipobroman
A-82	nitroxoline
A-8999	aspartocin
AA-2414	seratrodast
AA-673	amlexanox
AA-861	docebenone
AAFC	flurocitabine
AB08	doxycycline fosfatex
AB-100	uredepa
AB-103	benzodepa
AB-132	meturedepa
AB-A 663	cimaterol
Abbott-16900	teflurane
Abbott-19957	lorbamate
Abbott-22370	trimetozine
Abbott-24091	berythromycin
Abbott-34842	butamben picrate
Abbott-35616	clorazepate dipotassium
Abbott-36581	butamirate citrate
Abbott-38579	protirelin
Abbott-38642	fosfonet sodium
Abbott-39083	clorazepate monopotassium
Abbott-40728	cetocycline HCl
Abbott-41070	gonadorelin acetate
Abbott-43326	carteolol HCl
Abbott-43818	leuprolide acetate
Abbott 44090	valproate sodium
Abbott-44747	astromicin sulfate
Abbott-45975	terazosin HCl
Abbott-46811	cefsulodin sodium
Abbott-47631	estazolam
Abbott-48999	cefotiam HCl
Abbott-50192 (HCl)	cefmenoxime HCl
Abbott-50711	divalproex sodium
Abbott-56268	clarithromycin
Abbott-56619	difloxacin HCl
Abbott-56620	sarafloxacin HCl
Abbott-57135 (sarafloxacin)	sarafloxacin HCl
Abbott-61827	tosufloxacin
Abbott-62254	temafloxacin HCl
Abbott-64077	zileuton
Abbott-64662	enalkiren
Abbott-72517	zankiren HCl
Abbott-73001	seratrodast
Abbott-76745	fenleuton
Abbott-84538	ritonavir
ABC 12/3	doxofylline

Appendix B: Investigational Code Names

Code	Generic
ABOB	moroxydine
ABT-001	seratrodast
ABT-538	ritonavir
AC 1198	dimethadione
AC 137	generic not yet assigned—see main list
AC 1370	cefpimizole
AC 263,780	cimaterol
AC 3810	bamifylline HCl
AC4464	torsemide
AC-528	dioxation
AC-601	buramate
AC625	generic not yet assigned—see main list
ACA-147	generic not yet assigned—see main list
ACC-9089	flestolol sulfate
ACC-9653-010	fosphenytoin sodium
AD 106	cicrotoic acid
AD-439	generic not yet assigned—see main list
AD-519	generic not yet assigned—see main list
AD-810	zonisamide
ADD-3878	ciglitazone
ADR-033	tripamide
ADR-529	dexrazoxane
AE-0047	generic not yet assigned—see main list
AE-705W	neutramycin
AE-9	feclobuzone
AF102B	generic not yet assigned—see main list
AF-1161	trazodone HCl
AF 1934 (lysine)	bendazac
AF-2139	dapiprazole HCl
AF 2838	bindarit
AF-438 (as citrate)	oxolamine
AF-634	proxazole citrate
AF-864	benzydamine HCl
AG-1343	nelfinavir
AG-1749	lansoprazole
AG-3	chromonar HCl
AG-337	generic not yet assigned—see main list
AG 58107	ioxitalamic acid
Agent M-01	sucrosofate potassium
AGN 190168	tazarotene
AGN 190342-LF	brimonidine tartrate
AGN 20	metamfazone
AGN 511 (as HCl)	prazitone
AGN 616	fantridone HCl
AGR-1240	minaprine
AH 19065	ranitidine HCl
AH 22216	lamtidine
AH 23844A	lavoltidine succinate
AH 23844 (lavoltidine)	lavoltidine succinate
AH 25352X	sufotidine
AH 3923	salmefamol
AH 5158A	labetalol HCl

AH 8165D	fazadinium bromide
AHR-10282B	bromfenac sodium
AHR-10718	suricainide maleate
AHR-1118	pridefine HCl
AHR-11190-B	zacopride HCl
AHR-11325-D	rocastine HCl
AHR-11748	dezinamide
AHR-1680	fenpipalone
AHR-224	pyroxamine maleate
AHR-2277 (as HCl)	lenperone
AHR-2438B	polignate sodium
AHR-3000	butaperazine
AHR-3002	fenfluramine HCl
AHR-3015	cintazone
AHR-3018	apazone
AHR-3053	carbocysteine
AHR-3070-C	metoclopramide HCl
AHR-438	metaxalone
AHR-4698	isosorbide mononitrat
AHR-504	glycopyrrolate
AHR-5531C	dazopride fumarate
AHR-5850D	amfenac sodium
AHR-6134	cloroperone HCl
AHR-619	doxapram HCl
AHR 6646	duoperone fumarate
AHR-8559	fluzinamide
AHR-857	sulfameter
AHR-9377	tampramine fumarate
AI204	generic not yet assigned—see main list
AI-27,303	cetamolol HCl
AICA	orazamide
A IX	demecycline
AJ-2615	monatepil maleate
AL02145	apraclonidine HCl
AL02725	pyrithione sodium
Al-0361	hydroxyphenamate
AL 0559	fenamole
AL-1021	carperone
AL1577A	levobetaxolol HCl
AL 20 (as HCl)	clemizole
AL-721	generic not yet assigned—see main list
AL 842	deterenol HCl
ALCA	alcloxa
ALDA	aldioxa
Allergan 211	idoxuridine
ALO 1401-02	betaxolol HCl
ALO 2184	resocortol butyrate
ALO4943A	olopatadine HCl
ALRT 1057	9-cis-retinoic acid
AL-T150	oxyfilcon A
AL-T30	vinafocon A
ALVAC-120TMG	generic not yet assigned—see main list

ALVAC-HIV 1	generic not yet assigned—see main list
AM-684-Beta	relomycin
AMA 1080(2Na)	carumonam sodium
AMI-121	ferumoxsil
AMI-227	generic not yet assigned—see main list
AMI-25	ferumoxides
AMR-69	pirfenidone
AN021	tizanidine HCl
AN-051	dezinamide
AN 1317	perimetazine
AN 1324	glybuzole
ANA-756	generic not yet assigned—see main list
anesthetic compound no. 347	enflurane
ANP 246	clofexamide
ANP 3260	clofezone
antibiotic 241a	biniramycin
antibiotic $273a_1$	paldimycin
antibiotic A-5283	natamycin
antifoam A	simethicone
antifoam AF	simethicone
AO-407	hydrofilcon A
AOMA	surfomer
AO-PLUTO	mesifilcon A
AP 67	chlorthenoxazine
APM	aspartame
APSAC	anistreplase
AQ-110	tretoquinol
AR 12008	trapidil
AR-121	generic not yet assigned—see main list
AR-177	generic not yet assigned—see main list
AR-623	generic not yet assigned—see main list
ARC I-K-1	methopholine
ARDF 26	gliquidone
ARI-509	generic not yet assigned—see main list
AS-013	generic not yet assigned—see main list
AS 101	arsanilic acid
AS-17665	nifurthiazole
ASA 158/5 (as phosphate)	benproperine
ASL-279	dopamine HCl
ASL-601	acecainide HCl
ASL-603	bretylium tosylate
ASL-607	pentastarch
ASL-8052	esmolol HCl
Asta 3746	ciclonium bromide
Astra 1512	prilocaine HCl
Astra 1572	iron sorbitex
AT-101	isosorbide
AT-125	acivicin
AT-2266	enoxacin
AT 327	tipepidine
AT-4140	sparfloxacin
AW 10	sitogluside

AW 105-843	naftifine HCl
AW 14'2333	perlapine
AW-14'2446	clodazon HCl
AY-11,440	clogestone acetate
AY-11,483	estrofurate
AY-15,613	citenamide
AY-20,385	nequinate
AY-20,694	dexpropranolol HCl
AY-21,011	practolol
AY-21,367	furobufen
AY-21,554	talopram HCl
AY-22,124	intriptyline HCl
AY-22,214	taclamine HCl
AY-22,241	actodigin
AY-22,284A	alrestatin sodium
AY-22,469	deprostil
AY-22989	sirolimus
AY-23,028	butaclamol HCl
AY-23,289	prodolic acid
AY-23,713	pirandamine HCl
AY-23,946	tandamine HCl
AY-24,031	gonadorelin HCl
AY-24,169	dexclamol HCl
AY-24,236	etodolac
AY-24,269	proroxan HCl
AY-24,559	doxaprost
AY-24,856	pareptide sulfate
AY-25,329	azaclorzine HCl
AY-25,712	acifran
AY-27,110	ciladopa HCl
AY-27,255	vinpocetine
AY-27,773	tolrestat
AY-28,228	atiprosin maleate
AY-28,768	pelrinone HCl
AY-30,715	pemedolac
AY-5312	chlorhexidine HCl
AY-5710	magaldrate
AY-6108	ampicillin
AY-61122	methallibure
AY-61123	clofibrate
AY-62014	butriptyline HCl
AY-62021	clopenthixol
AY-62022	medrogestone
AY 6204 (as HCl)	pronetalol
AY-64043	propranolol HCl
AY-6608	pentagastrin
AY-8682	cyheptamide
AZQ	diaziquone
AZT-P-ddI	zidovudine + didanosine
B 10610	iodoxamic acid
B 11420	iopronic acid
B 1312 (as HCl)	bupranolol

B 1464	guanacline sulfate
B1 61.012	sargramostim
B19036/7	gagobenate dimeglumine
B1Q 16	hedaquinium chloride
B-2311	morinamide
B-35251	mitocromin
B-360	paroxypropione
B-4130	iodamide
B-436	prenylamine
Ba 13155 (as tartrate)	meladrazine
Ba-20684	etonitazene
Ba-29038	boldenone undecylenate
Ba-29837	deferoxamine HCl
Ba-30803	benzoctamine HCl
BA 32644	niridazole
Ba-32968	delfantrine
Ba-33112	deferoxamine mesylate
Ba-34,276 (as HCl)	maprotiline
Ba-34,647	baclofen
BA 36278A	cephacetrile sodium
Ba-39,089	oxprenolol HCl
Ba-40088	proxibutene
Ba 41166/E	rifampin
BA 4164-8	diflumidone sodium
Ba-41795	codactide
BA 4197	flucrylate
BA 4223	triflumidate
BA 7602-06	talniflumate
BA 7604-02	talosalate
BA 7605-06	talmetacin
BAQD 10	dequalinium chloride
BASF 43915	pelretin
BASF 47011	doretinel
BASF 52404	linarotene
BAX 1400Z	dimethadione
BAX 1515	sutilains
BAX 1526	chymopapain
BAX 2739Z	bamifylline HCl
BAX 422Z	albutoin
BAY 1500	mefruside
BAY 1521	noxiptiline
BAY 2353	niclosamide
BAY 4059 Va	brotianide
BAY 4503	propiram fumarate
BAY 5097	clotrimazole
BAY 9002	naftalofos
Bay a 1040	nifedipine
BAY B 4231	glisoxepide
Bay d 1107	etofenamate
BAY d 8815 (HCl)	amidantel
Bay e 5009	nitrendipine
BAY e 9736	nimodipine

Appendix B: Investigational Code Names 591

Bayer 1362	butaperazine
Bayer 1420	propanidid
Bayer 205	suramin sodium
Bayer 21199	coumaphos
Bayer 2502	nifurtimox
Bayer 3231	triaziquone
Bayer 5360	metronidazole
Bayer 9015	niclofolan
Bayer 9037	quintiofos
Bayer 9053	phoxim
Bayer A 128	aprotinin
Bayer L 1359	metrifonate
BAY g 2821	muzolimine
Bay g 5421	acarbose
Bay g 6575	nafazatrom
BAY h 2049	daniquidone
Bay h 4502	bifonazole
Bay h 5757	febantel
BAY i 3930	isomalt
BAY i 7433	copovithane
Bay k 5552	nisoldipine
BAY m 1099	miglitol
BAYNAC	fenfluthrin
BAY o 1248	emiglitate
Bay o 9867 monohydrate	ciprofloxacin HCl
Bay q 3939	ciprofloxacin
Bay q 4218	butaprost
BAY q 7821	ipsapirone HCl
BAY V1 4718	etisomicin
BAY V1 6045	flumethrin
BAY Va 1470	xylazine HCl
Bay VA 9387	etisazole
BAY Va 9391	olaquindox
BAY Vh 5757	febantel
Bay Vi 9142	toltrazuril
BAY Vk 4999	fuzlocillin
Bay Vl 1704	cyfluthrin
Bay Vn 6528	fenfluthrin
Bay Vp 2674	enrofloxacin
BAY w 6240	factor VIII (rDNA)
BAY y 7432	ecadotril
BB-882	lexipafant
BB-94	batimastat
BB-K8	amikacin sulfate
BBM-2478A	elsamitrucin
BC-105	pizotyline
BCM	mannomustine
BCX 2600	stiripentol
BCX-34	generic not yet assigned—see main list
BDH 1298	megestrol acetate
BDH 1921	melengestrol acetate
Be-100	ibuprofen piconol

Be-1293	xipamide
BE 419	ioglycamic acid
BG 8301	teceleukin
BG8967	bivalirudin
BIIP 20 XX	apaxifylline
BI-L-239	enofelast
BILA 2011 BS	palinavir
BIM-23014C	lanreotide acetate
BIRG 0587	nevirapine
BIRM-270	ontazolast
BI-RR-0001	enlimomab
BL 191	pentoxifylline
BL-3912A	dimoxamine HCl
BL-4162a	anagrelide HCl
BL-5111	tiodazosin
BL-5572M	proxorphan tartrate
BL-5641A	etintidine HCl
BL-P 1322	cephapirin sodium
BL-P 1462	suncillin sodium
BL-P 1761	sarpicillin
BL-P 1780	sarmoxicillin
BL-P 804	hetacillin
BL-R 743	intrazole
BL-S578	cefadroxil
BL-S640	cefatrizine
BL-S786	ceforanide
BM01.004	metipranolol
BM02.015	torsemide
BM 06.019	epoetin beta
BM 13.177	sulotroban
BM 13.505	daltroban
BM 14.190	carvedilol
BM 14802	generic not yet assigned—see main list
BM 15.075	bezafibrate
BM 22.145	isosorbide mononitrate
BM 41.332	ciamexon
BM 41.440	ilmofosine
BM 51052	carazolol
BMS 180048	generic not yet assigned—see main list
BMS-180194	lobucavir
BMS-180291	ifetroban
BMS-180291-02	ifetroban sodium
BMS 181101	generic not yet assigned—see main list
BMS-181173	gusperimus trihydrochloride
BMS-181339-01	paclitaxel
BMS-186091	ammonium lactate
BMY-05763-1-D	dexsotalol HCl
BMY 13754	nefazodone HCl
BMY 13805-1	gepirone HCl
BMY 13859-1	tiospirone HCl
BMY 14802	generic not yet assigned—see main list
BMY-21891	belfosdil

BMY-25182	cefbuperazone
BMY-25801-01	batanopride HCl
BMY-26517	pemirolast potassium
BMY-27857	stavudine
BMY-28090	elsamitrucin
BMY-28100-03-800	cefprozil
BMY-28142	cefepime
BMY-28142 2HCl H$_2$O	cefepime HCl
BMY-30056	halobetasol propionate
BMY-30120	chlorhexidine phosphanilate
BMY-40327	modecainide
BMY 40481	etoposide phosphate
BMY-40900	didanosine
BMY-41606	vapreotide
BMY-42215-1	gusperimus trihydrochloride
BMY-45622	generic not yet assigned—see main list
BN-1270	cicletanine
BP 1.02; S.049	ecadotril
BP-1184	guanoctine HCl
BP 400	pimethixene
BRL-1241	methicillin sodium
BRL 12594	ticarcillin cresyl sodium
BRL-1288	benapryzine HCl
BRL-1341	ampicillin
BRL 13856	clopirac
BRL 14151	clavulanic acid
BRL 14151K	clavulanate potassium
BRL 14777	nabumetone
BRL-1621	cloxacillin sodium
BRL-1702	dicloxacillin
BRL 17421 (as sodium)	temocillin
BRL-2039	floxacillin
BRL-2064	carbenicillin disodium
BRL 2288	ticarcillin disodium
BRL 2333	amoxicillin
BRL 2534	azidocillin
BRL 26921	anistreplase
BRL-284	levopropylcillin potassium
BRL 29060	paroxetine
BRL 30892	denbufylline
BRL-3475	carbenicillin phenyl sodium
BRL 34915	cromakalim
BRL-38227	levcromakalim
BRL 38705	epsiprantel
BRL-39123	penciclovir
BRL 40015	diproteverine
BRL-42810	famciclovir
BRL 43694	granisetron
BRL 43694A	granisetron HCl
BRL 46470	generic not yet assigned—see main list
BRL 4664	nonabine
BRL 4910A	mupirocin

BRL 4910F	mupirocin calcium
BRL55834	generic not yet assigned—see main list
BRL 61063	cipamfylline
BRL-804	hetacillin
BRL 8988 HCl	talampicillin HCl
BS 100-141	guanfacine HCl
B.S. 6534	bufenadrine
BS 6748	xyloxemine
BS 6987	deptropine citrate
BS 7161D (as HCl)	pytamine
B.S. 7173-D	xylocoumarol
BS 749	metacetamol
B.S. 7561 (as HCl)	tixadil
B.S. 7573-a	acridorex
BS 7723 (as maleate)	tropirine
BS 7977 D (as dihydrochloride)	xipranolol
BSH	borocaptate sodium B 10
BSSG	sitogluside
BT 621 (as HCl)	todralazine
BTPABA, PFT	bentiromide
BTS 13622	hexaprofen
BTS 17345	fluprofen
BTS 18,322	flurbiprofen
BTS 24332	esflurbiprofen
BTS 49 465	flosequinan
BTS 54524	sibutramine HCl
BTS67,583	generic not yet assigned—see main list
BTS 7706	debropol
BU-2231A	talisomycin
BW 12C	generic not yet assigned—see main list
BW 207U	xenalipin
BW 234U dihydrochloride	rimcazole HCl
BW 248U sodium	acyclovir sodium
BW256U	valacyclovir
BW 301U isethionate	piritrexim isethionate
BW 325U	trifenagrel
BW 33A	atracurium besylate
BW 33-T-57	methisazone
BW 356-C-61	gloxazone
BW 430C	lamotrigine
BW-467-C-60	bethanidine sulfate
BW 49-210	diaveridine
BW 532U	cinflumide
BW 56-158	allopurinol
BW 56-72	trimethoprim
BW-57-322	azathioprine
BW 57-323	thiamiprine
BW 58-271	rolodine
BW-61-32	stilbazium iodide
BW 63-90	butacetin
BW 647U HCl	bipenamol HCl
BW 64-9	butoxamine HCl

Appendix B: Investigational Code Names 595

BW 72U	trimethoprim sulfate
BW 759U	ganciclovir
BW 825C	acrivastine
BW A256C	palatrigine
BW A509U	zidovudine
BW A515U	desciclovir
BW A770U mesylate	crisnatol mesylate
BW A938U dichloride	doxacurium chloride
BW B109OU	mivacurium chloride
Bx 311	cinoxolone
BX 341	bifluranol
BX 363A (as disodium salt)	cicloxolone
BX 591	acefluranol
BX 650A	ipsalazide
BX 661A	balsalazide; balsalazide disodium
BY 1023	pantoprazole
BZ 55	carbutamide
C-11925	phanquone
C-12669	demecolcine
C-1428	cyclarbamate
C 1656	clometacin
C-238	pridinol
C-3	capobenate sodium
C-3	capobenic acid
C-4	imciromab pentetate
C-434	trimedoxime bromide
C-49802B-Ba	oxaprotiline HCl
c7E3	abciximab
Ca 1022	carbutamide
CA-7	brinolase
CAM-807	bialamicol HCl
CARN 750	acemannan
CAS 276	molsidomine
CAS 936	pirsidomine
CB 1048	chlornaphazine
CB 10615	nifurmazole
CB 11380	nifurizone
CB 11 (as HCl)	phenadoxone
CB 12592	subendazole
CB-154	bromocriptine
CB-154 mesylate	bromocriptine mesylate
CB 1664	aceprometazine
CB 1678	propiomazine
CB 2201	amfepentorex
CB-30038	minaprine
CB 302	ferric fructose
CB 3025	melphalan
CB 304	azaribine
CB 309	fenabutene
CB-311	somatropin
CB 313	mitotane
CB-337	meglutol

CB 3697	racefemine
CB 4260	nortetrazepam
CB 4261	tetrazepam
CB 4857	menitrazepam
CB 4985	acequinoline
CB 7432	idoxifene
CB 804	bucloxic acid
CCA	lobenzarit sodium
CCD 1042	generic not yet assigned—see main list
C.C.I. 12923	minaxolone
CCI 15641	cefuroxime axetil
CCI 18773	cloticasone propionate
CCI 18781	fluticasone propionate
CCI 23628	cefuroxime pivoxetil
CCI 4725	clobetasol propionate
CCI 5537	clobetasone butyrate
CD 271	adapalene
CDDD 1815	alprenoxime HCl
CDDD 2803	adaprolol maleate
CDDD 3602	tematropium methylsulfate
CDDD 5604	loteprednol etabonate
CEP 1538	modafinil
CEPH (as HCl)	todralazine
CERM 1978	bepridil HCl
CERM 730	amoproxan
CG 201	bevonium metilsulfate
CG-315E	tramadol HCl
GCA 18809	azamethiphos
CGA-23654	nitroscanate
CGA 72662	cyromazine
CGP-14221/E	cefotiam HCl
CGP 14,458	halobetasol propionate
CGP 21690E	oxiracetam
CGP 2175C	metoprolol fumarate
CGP-2175E	metoprolol tartrate
CGP 23339AE	pamidronate disodium
CGP 25827A	formoterol
CGP 30694	edatrexate
CGP 32349	formestane
CGP 39393	desirudin
CGP 45840B	diclofenac potassium
CGP 48933	valsartan
CGP 57701	generic not yet assigned—see main list
CGP-7174/E	cefsulodin sodium
CGP 7760B	prenalterol HCl
CGP 9000	cefroxadine
CGS 10078B	bendacalol mesylate
CGS 10746B	pentiapine maleate
CGS 10787D	prinomide tromethamine
CGS 13080	pirmagrel
CGS 13429A	batelapine maleate
CGS 13945	pentopril

CGS 14824A HCl	benazepril HCl
CGS 14831	benazeprilat
CGS 15040A	serazapine HCl
CGS 16617	libenzapril
CGS 16949A	fadrozole HCl
CGS 18416A	zoniclezole HCl
CGS 19755	selfotel
CGS 20267	letrozole
CGS 5391B (anhydrous)	enolicam sodium
CGS 7135A	azaloxan fumarate
CGS 7525A	aptazapine maleate
CH 3565	triclosan
CHX-100	masoprocol
CHX-3673	amlexanox
CI-100	acetosulfone sodium
CI-107	argipressin tannate
CI-301	bialamicol HCl
CI-336	carbocloral
CI-366	ethosuximide
CI-379	benzilonium bromide
CI-395	phencyclidine HCl
CI 403A	pararosaniline pamoate
CI-406	oxymetholone
CI-416	triclofenol piperazine
CI-419	fenimide
CI 427	prodilidine HCl
CI-433	clamoxyquin HCl
CI 440	flufenamic acid
CI-456	diapamide
CI-473	mefenamic acid
CI-501	cycloguanil pamoate
CI-515	guanoxyfen sulfate
CI-546	alipamide
CI 556	acedapsone
CI-572	profadol HCl
CI-581	ketamine HCl
CI-583	meclofenamic acid
CI-633	clioxanide
CI-634	tiletamine HCl
CI-636	sulfacytine
CI-642	butirosin sulfate
CI 673	vidarabine
CI-686 HCl	trebenzomine HCl
CI-705	methaqualone
CI-716	zolazepam HCl
CI-718	bentazepam
CI-719	gemfibrozil
CI-720	gemcadiol
CI-781	zometapine
CI 787	tioperidone HCl
CI-825	pentostatin
CI-874	indeloxazine HCl

CI-879	pramiracetam HCl
CI-879 (sulfate)	pramiracetam sulfate
CI-880	amsacrine
CI-881	ametantrone acetate
CI-882	sparfosate sodium
CI-888	procaterol HCl
CI-897	tebuquine
CI-898	trimetrexate
CI-904	diaziquone
CI-906	quinapril HCl
CI-907	indolapril HCl
CI-908	dezaguanine
CI-908 mesylate	dezaguanine mesylate
CI-909	tiazofurin
CI-911	rolziracetam
CI-912	zonisamide
CI-914	imazodan HCl
CI-9148	cysteamine HCl
CI-919	enoxacin
CI-920	fostriecin sodium
CI 925	moexipril HCl
CI-928	quinaprilat
CI-942	piroxantrone HCl
CI-945	gabapentin
CI-946	ralitoline
CI-960 HCl	clinafloxacin HCl
CI-970	tacrine HCl
CI-977	enadoline HCl
CI-978	sparfloxacin
CI-979	generic not yet assigned—see main list
CI-980	generic not yet assigned—see main list
CI-981	atorvastatin calcium
CI-982	fosphenytion sodium
CI-983	cefdinir
CI-988	generic not yet assigned—see main list
CI-991	troglitazone
CIBA 1906	thiambutosine
CJ 91B	olsalazine sodium
CK-0383	verofylline
CK-0569 (as the base)	ipexidine mesylate
CK-1752A	sematilide HCl
CL09	icomethasone enbutate
CL 10304	aminocaproic acid
CL 106359	triamcinolone acetonide sodium phosphate
CL 108,756	brocresine
CL 112,302	buprenorphine HCl
CL 115,347	viprostol
CL 118,532	triptorelin
CL 12,625	natamycin
CL-1388R	guanadrel sulfate
CL 13,900	puromycin

Appendix B: Investigational Code Names

CL 14377	methotrexate
CL 16,536	puromycin HCl
CL 184,116	porfimer sodium
CL 184,824	alovudine
CL-1848C	etoxadrol HCl
CL 186,815	biapenem
CL 203,821	cetaben sodium
CL 205925	iprocinodine HCl
CL 206,214	butamisole HCl
CL 206,576	sulbenox
CL 206,797	cypothrin
CL 216,942	bisantrene HCl
CL 217,658	imcarbofos
CL 220,075	bicifadine HCl
CL 22415	demecycline
CL 227,193	piperacillin sodium
CL 232,315	mitoxantrone HCl
CL 2422	guancydine
CL 25477	azetepa
CL 26193	simtrazene
CL 27,071	descinolone acetonide
CL 273,547	ocinaplon
CL 273,703	maduramicin
CL 274,471	colestolone
CL 284,635	cefixime
CL 284,846	zaleplon
CL 286,558	zeniplatin
CL 287,088	nemadectin
CL 287,110	enloplatin
CL 287,389	nilvadipine
CL 291,894	somagrebove
CL 297,939	bisoprolol
CL 297,939	bisoprolol fumarate
CL 298,741	tazobactam
CL 301,423	moxidectin
CL 307,579	tazobactam sodium
CL 307,782	levoleucovorin calcium
CL 318,952	verteporfin
Cl 337	azaserine
CL 34433	triamcinolone hexacetonide
CL 34699	amcinonide
CL 36467	methotrimeprazine
CL 369	ketamine HCl
CL 39743	methotrimeprazine
CL 39808	thozalinone
CL 399	tiletamine HCl
CL 40881	ethambutol HCl
CL 48156	imidoline HCl
CL 5,279	nithiamide
CL 53415	cyproximide
CL 54131	piperamide maleate
CL 54998	brocresine

Cl-583.Na salt	meclofenamate sodium
CL 59112	roletamide
CL 61965	triamcinolone acetonide sodium phosphate
CL 62,362	loxapine
CL-639C	dioxadrol HCl
Cl-64,976	zilantel
CL 65205	boxidine
CL 65336	tranexamic acid
CL 65,562	triflocin
Cl-661	oxiramide
CL 67,772	amoxapine
Cl-683	ripazepam
CL 71563	loxapine succinate
Cl-775	bevantolol HCl
Cl-808	vidarabine phosphate
Cl-808 sodium	vidarabine sodium phosphate
CL 81,587	avoparcin
CL 82,204	fenbufen
CL 83,544	felbinac
Cl-845	pirmenol HCl
CL 84,633	nimidane
CL-867	piridicillin sodium
Cl-871	piracetam
CL 88,893	clazolimine
CL 90,748	azolimine
CL-911C	dexoxadrol HCl
CL-912C	levoxadrol HCl
CL 98984	cinodine HCl
CLY-503	simfibrate
CM 31-916	ceftiofur sodium
CN-10,395	ethosuximide
CN-14,329-23A	cycloguanil pamoate
CN-15,573-23A	pararosaniline pamoate
CN-15,757	azaserine
CN-16146	carbocloral
CN-17,900-2B	clamoxyquin HCl
CN-1883	acedapsone
CN-20,172-3	benzilonium bromide
CN-25,253-2	phencyclidine HCl
CN-27,554	flufenamic acid
CN-34,799-5A	guanoxyfen sulfate
CN-35355	mefenamic acid
CN-36,337	diapamide
CN-38,474	alipamide
CN 38703	methaqualone
CN-52,372-2	ketamine HCl
CN-54521-2	tiletamine HCl
CN-5834-5931B	triclofenol piperazine
CN 59,567	clioxanide
CNS 1102	generic not yet assigned—see main list
CO 405	butidrine

Appendix B: Investigational Code Names 601

compound 109168	nifluridide
compound 112531	vindesine
compound 113878	ciprefadol succinate
compound 113935	pentomone
compound 122587	drobuline
compound 133314	trioxifene mesylate
compound 24266	pentetate calcium trisodium Yb 169
compound 42339	acronine
compound 469	isoflurane
compound 497	dieldrin
compound 53616	frentizole
compound 56063	melizame
compound 57926	sinefungin
compound 68-198	diamfenetide
compound 79891	narasin
compound 81929	dobutamine
compound 83405	cefamandole
compound 83846	aprindine HCl
compound 85287	nibroxane
compound 89218	nisoxetine
compound 904	alexidine
compound 90459	benoxaprofen
compound 90606	isamoxole
compound 93819	fluretofen
compound 99170	aprindine
compound 99638	cefaclor
compound LY 131126	butopamine
compound S	zidovudine
CP-10,188	fenclonine
CP-10,303-8	quinterenol sulfate
CP-10,423-16	pyrantel pamoate
CP-10,423-18	pyrantel tartrate
CP 1044 J3	bufexamac
CP-11,332-1	quinazosin HCl
CP-12,009-18	morantel tartrate
CP-12,252-1	thiothixene HCl
CP-12,299-1	prazosin HCl
CP-12,521-1	piquizil HCl
CP-12,574	tinidazole
CP-13,608	tesicam
CP-14,185-1	hoquizil HCl
CP-14,368-1	lometraline HCl
CP-14,445-16	oxantel pamoate
CP-15,464-2	carbenicillin indanyl sodium
CP-15,467-61	lithium carbonate
CP 1552 S	milacemide HCl
CP-15-639-2	carbenicillin disodium
CP-15,973	sudoxicam
CP-16,171	piroxicam
CP-16,171-85	piroxicam olamine
CP-16,533-1	verapamil
CP 172 AP	clopirac

CP-18,524	tibric acid
CP-19,106-1	trimazosin HCl
CP-20,961	avridine
CP-22,341	temodox
CP-22,665	flumizole
CP-24,314-1	pirbuterol HCl
CP-24,314-14	pirbuterol acetate
CP-24,441-1	tametraline HCl
CP-24,877	drinidene
CP-25,673	tiazuril
CP-26,154	tolimidone
CP-27,634	gliamilide
CP-28,720	glipizide
CP-31,081	polydextrose
CP-32,387	pirolate
CP-33,994-2	pirbenicillin sodium
CP-34,089	sulprostone
CP-36,584	flutroline
CP-38,754	plauracin
CP-44,001-1	nantradol HCl
CP-45,634	sorbinil
CP-45,899-2	sulbactam sodium
CP-45,899-99	sulbactam benzathine
CP-47,904	sulbactam pivoxil
CP-48,810-27	fanetizole mesylate
CP-48,867-9	ristianol phosphate
CP-49,952	sultamicillin
CP-50,556-1	levonantradol HCl
Cp-51,974-1	sertraline HCl
CP-52,640-2	cefoperazone sodium
CP-54,802	alitame
CP-556S	suloctidil
CP-57,361-01	zaltidine HCl
CP-62,993	azithromycin
CP-65703	ampiroxicam
CP-66,248	tenidap
CP-66,248-2	tenidap sodium
CP-70,429	sulopenem
CP-70,490-09	enazadrem phosphate
CP-72,133	ilonidap
CP-72,467-2	englitazone sodium
CP-73,049	binfloxacin
CP-73,850	zopolrestat
CP-76,136-27	danofloxacin mesylate
CP-80,794	terlakiren
CP-86,325-2	darglitazone sodium
CP-88,059	ziprasidone
CP-88,059-1	ziprasidone HCl
CP-88,818	tiqueside
CP-99,219-27	trovafloxacin mesylate
Cpd 109514	nabilone
Cpd. 5411	iopentol

CPT-11	irinotecan
CR/662	tipepidine
CRL 40476	modafinil
CS-045	troglitazone
CS-151	crofilcon A
CS-514	pravastatin sodium
CS-622	temocapril HCl
CS-807	cefpodoxime proxetil
CSAG-144	mebeverine HCl
CT 1501R	lisofylline
CTR 6110	nitrodan
CTX	lornoxicam
CV 57533	xenyhexenic acid
CV 58903	xenazoic acid
CY-116	aminocaproic acid
CY-1503	generic not yet assigned—see main list
CY 153	acexamic acid
CY-1787	generic not yet assigned—see main list
CY-1899	generic not yet assigned—see main list
CY 216	nadroparin calcium
CY 39	psilocybine
CYT-103 ^{111}In	indium In 111 satumomab pendetide
CYT-103-Y-90	generic not yet assigned—see main list
CYT-356	capromab pendetide
CYT-356-In-111	generic not yet assigned—see main list
CYT-356-Y-90	generic not yet assigned—see main list
CYT-372-In-111	generic not yet assigned—see main list
CYT-424	samarium Sm 153 lexidronam pentasodium
D 00079	anoxomer
D-1262	cloxypendyl
D-1593	diapamide
D-1721	alipamide
D-1959 HCl	reproterol HCl
D2083	desonide
D 237	cloforex
D-254	pipazethate
D-365	verapamil
D 4028	enprofylline
D 47	sulbentine
d4T	stavudine
D 7093	mesna
D-775	homofenazine
D-9998	flupirtine maleate
DA 1773	sodium picosulfate
DA 2370	feprazone
DA-398	epirizole
DA 688	gefarnate
DA-708	teflurane
DA-808	nafcaproic acid
DA-893	roflurane
DA-914	nafiverine

DA-992	naftypramide
DAC	decitabine
D.A.T.	acetiamine
DATC	tiocarlide
DBV	buformin
DCH 21 (as sodium salt)	exiproben
DETF	trichlorfon
DF 118	dihydrocodeine bitartrate
DH-524	fenmetozole HCl
DH-581	probucol
DIM-SA	succimer
DL 152	bietaserpine
DL-164	tiodonium chloride
DL-588	napactadine HCl
DL-8280	ofloxacin
dl HM-PAO	exametazime
dl HM-PAO	hexametazime
DMI	desipramine HCl
DMP 266	generic not yet assigned—see main list
DMP 728	generic not yet assigned—see main list
DMP 840	bisnafide dimesylate
DMSC	doxycycline fosfatex
DN-2327	pazinaclone
DO6	lexipafant
DS 103-282	tizanidine HCl
DS-4152	tecogalan sodium
DT-3	detrothyronine
DT-327	clopamide
DTC 101	generic not yet assigned—see main list
DTPA-SMS	pentetreotide
D-Trp LHRH-PEA	deslorelin
DU-21220	ritodrine
DU-21445	tiprenolol HCl
DU 22550 (as sulfate)	caproxamine
DU23000	fluvoxamine maleate
DU-23187	quincarbate
DuP 128	lecimibide
DuP 753	losartan potassium
Dup 785	brequinar sodium
DuP 921	sibopirdine
DUP 937	teloxantrone HCl
DUP 941	losoxantrone
DuP 996	linopirdine
DV-1006	cetraxate HCl
DW-61	flavoxate HCl
DW-62	dimefline HCl
DW 75	norleusactide
DyDTPA-BMA	sprodiamide
E-0659	azelastine HCl
E-106-E (as cyclamate)	furfenorex
E 141	ethamsylate
E-2020	generic not yet assigned—see main list

Appendix B: Investigational Code Names

E-2663	bentiromide
E-3810	rabeprazole sodium
E 39	inproquone
E-52	pentafilcon A
E-614	tripamide
E 9002	naftalofos
EA-166	guanoxyfen sulfate
EDU	edoxudine
EE$_3$ME	mestranol
EF9	temoporfin
EGTA	egtazic acid
EGYT 201	bencyclane fumarate
EHB 776	foscarnet sodium
EL10	dehydroepiandrosterone
EL349	somidobove
EL737	ractopamine HCl
EL-857	apramycin
EL870	tilmicosin
EL-970	fampridine
EL-974	ticarbodine
ELD 950	eledoisin
EMBAY 8440	praziquantel
EMD 15 700	nitrefazole
EMD 19698 (as hydrogen maleate)	peratizole
EMD 33 512	bisoprolol
EMD 9806	pramiverine
EN-1010	pyrrocaine
EN-141	josamycin
EN-15304	naloxone HCl
EN-1620A	nalmexone HCl
EN-1639A (as HCl)	naltrexone
EN-1661L	bisobrin lactate
EN-1733A	molindone HCl
EN-2234A	nalbuphine HCl
EN-313	moricizine
EN-970	fluquazone
ENT-20852	butonate
ENT-23969	carbaril
ENT-25567	naftalofos
ENT 29,106	nimidane
EPOCH	epoetin beta
ES 304	nicofuranose
ET-394	tribromsalan
ET-495	piribedil
ETTN	propatyl nitrate
EU-1063	proquinolate
EU-1085	leniquinsin
EU-1093	buquinolate
EU-1806	nafronyl oxalate
EU-2826	benurestat
EU-2972	nolinium bromide
EU-3120	acodazole HCl

EU-3325	triafungin
EU-3421	oxifungin HCl
EU-4093	azumolene sodium
EU-4200	piribedil
EU-4534	flurofamide
EU-4584	tolfamide
EU-4891	diacetolol HCl
EU-4906	sitogluside
EU-5306	pefloxacin
EUDR	edoxudine
EV2-7	sevirumab
EX 10-029-C	elantrine
EX 10-781	metizoline HCl
EX 12-095	eterobarb
EX 4355	desipramine HCl
EX 4810	ambuside
Ex 4883	rolicyprine
EXP-105-1	amantadine HCl
EXP 126	rimantadine HCl
EXP 338	midaflur
EXP 999	metopimazine
F 1500	succisulfone
F 1983	pyrovalerone HCl
F28249α	nemadectin
F-368	dantrolene
F-413	clodanolene
F-440	dantrolene sodium
F-605 (as the sodium)	clodanolene
F 6066	cyclofenil
F-691	furodazole
F-776	orpanoxin
F-853	nitrafudam HCl
Fa 402	fentonium bromide
FBA 1420	propanidid
FBA 4059	brotianide
FBB 4231	glisoxepide
FBB 6896	clenpirin
FC-1157a	toremifene citrate
FCE 21336	cabergoline
FCF 89	roquinimex
FER-1443	ticlatone
FG-10571	panadiplon
FG 5111	melperone
FGN-1	generic not yet assigned—see main list
FI 5852	oxabolone cipionate
F.I. 6146	buzepide metiodide
FI 6337	metergoline
FI 6339 (as the base)	daunorubicin HCl
F.I. 6426	stallimycin HCl
F.I. 6654	caroxazone
F.I. 6820	brofoxine
FK 027	cefixime

FK-037	generic not yet assigned—see main list
FK-1052	generic not yet assigned—see main list
FK-143	generic not yet assigned—see main list
FK-176	generic not yet assigned—see main list
FK-201	quinotolast
FK-224	generic not yet assigned—see main list
FK 235	nilvadipine
FK-3311	generic not yet assigned—see main list
FK-366	generic not yet assigned—see main list
FK-409	generic not yet assigned—see main list
FK-453	generic not yet assigned—see main list
FK-480	generic not yet assigned—see main list
FK 482	cefdinir
FK-506	tacrolimus
FK-508	generic not yet assigned—see main list
FK-565	generic not yet assigned—see main list
FK-613	generic not yet assigned—see main list
FK-739	generic not yet assigned—see main list
FK 749	ceftizoxime sodium
FK-780	generic not yet assigned—see main list
FK-906	generic not yet assigned—see main list
FLA 731	remoxipride
FLA 731(−)	remoxipride HCl
FPL 12924AA	remacemide HCl
FPL 58668KC	probicromil calcium
FPL 59002	nedocromil
FPL 59002KC	nedocromil calcium
FPL 59002KP	nedocromil sodium
FPL 59360	minocromil
FPL 60278	dopexamine
FPL 60278AR	dopexamine HCl
FPL64170	generic not yet assigned—see main list
FPL.670	cromolyn sodium
FPL67085	generic not yet assigned—see main list
FR 13749	ceftizoxime sodium
FR 17027	cefixime
FU-02	fumoxicillin
FUT-175	nafamostat mesylate
FWH 399	troxonium tosilate
G-101	erythromycin salnacedin
G-201	salnacedin
G-203	fluocinonide
G-24480	dimpylate
G-25178	prodeconium bromide
G-25766	clorindione
G 26,872	phenbutazone sodium glycerate
G 30320	clofazimine
G-32883	carbamazepine
G-33040	opipramol HCl
G-33182	chlorthalidone
G 34586	clomipramine HCl
G-35020	desipramine HCl

G 35259	ketipramine fumarate
G-4	dichlorophen
G-704,650	alendronate sodium
GEA 654	alaproclate
GEM 91	generic not yet assigned—see main list
GER-11	pimagedine HCl
GI 87084B	remifentanil HCl
GLQ 223	trichosanthin
GM 6001	generic not yet assigned—see main list
GMC 89-107	regramostim
Go 1213	atolide
Go 1733	suloxifen oxalate
Go 2782	iproxamine HCl
Go 3026A	ciclafrine HCl
Go-560	febarbamate
Go 919	piprozolin
GOE 3450	gabapentin
Goedecke 3282	ozolinone
GP-1-110	acadesine
gp120	generic not yet assigned—see main list
GP-121	phencyclidine HCl
gp 160	generic not yet assigned—see main list
GP-2-121-3	arbutamine HCl
GP 31406	depramine
GP 45840	diclofenac sodium
GP 51084	glibutimine
GPA-878	metazamide
GR109714X	lamivudine
GR 114297A	picumeterol fumarate
GR 114297X (picumeterol)	picumeterol fumarate
GR 122311X	ranitidine bismuth citrate
GR 138950C	saprisartan potassium
GR 20263	ceftazidime
GR 2/1214	clobetasone butyrate
GR 2/1574	alfadolone
GR 2/234	alfaxalone
GR 2/443 (as propionate)	doxibetasol
GR 2/925	clobetasol propionate
Gr 30921	mitoquidone
GR 32191B	vapiprost HCl
GR 32191 (vapiprost)	vapiprost HCl
GR 33207	ovandrotone albumin
GR 33343 G	salmeterol xinafoate
GR 33343 X	salmeterol
GR 38032F	ondansetron HCl
GR 412	dodeclonium bromide
GR 43175C	sumatriptan succinate
GR 43659X	lacidipine
GR50360A	fluparoxan HCl
GR 50692	cefempidone
GR 53992B (GX 1296B)	teludipine HCl
GR 63178K	fosquidone

GR 68755C	alosetron HCl
GR 81225C	galdansetron HCl
GR 85478	generic not yet assigned—see main list
GR 85548A	naratriptan HCl
GR 87442 N	luroseron mesylate
GR92132	troglitazone
GR 69153X	cefetecol
GS-0504	cidofovir
GS-1339	dymanthine HCl
GS 2147	sancycline
GS-2876	methacycline
GS-2989	meclocycline
GS-3065	doxycycline
GS-3159	carbenicillin potassium
GS 393	generic not yet assigned—see main list
GS 504	generic not yet assigned—see main list
GS-6244	carbadox
GS-6742	sulfomyxin
GS-7443	mequidox
GS 840	generic not yet assigned—see main list
GS-95	thiethylperazine maleate
GV 104326B	sanfetrinem sodium
GV 118819X	sanfetrinem cilexetil
GW-80126	seprilose
H 102/09 HCl	zimeldine HCl
H 104/08	pamatolol sulfate
H 133/22	prenalterol HCl
H 154/82	felodipine
H 168/68	omeprazole
H 168/68 sodium	omeprazole sodium
H 365	paroxypropione
H 3774	alibendol
H 4132	dotefonium bromide
H 4170	tolpiprazole
H 4723	clobazam
H 56/28	alprenolol HCl
H65-RTA	zolimomab aritox
H 93/26 succinate	metoprolol succinate
HA-1A	nebacumab
HB 115	nifurprazine
HB 419	glyburide
H.B.F. 386	cactinomycin
HBY097	generic not yet assigned—see main list
HC 1528	decoquinate
HC 20,511 fumarate	ketotifen fumarate
HF 1854	clozapine
HF 1927	dibenzepin HCl
HF-2159	clothiapine
HF 241	bufeniode
HGP-1	loteprednol etabonate
HGP-2	adaprolol maleate
HGP-30	generic not yet assigned—see main list

HGP-5	alprenoxime HCl
HGP-6	tematropium methylsulfate
HH105	butetamate
HH 197	butamirate citrate
HL 267	dipenine bromide
HL 362	colforsin
HL 523 (as HCl)	tiformin
HMD	oxymetholone
Hoe 045	articaine
HOE 062 (roxatidine)	roxatidine acetate HCl
HOE 077	lufironil
Hoe 105	citenazone
HOE 118	piretanide
HOE 140	icatibant acetate
HOE 18 680	embutramide
HOE 216V	luxabendazole
HOE 280	ofloxacin
HOE 296	ciclopirox olamine
HOE 296b	ciclopirox
Hoe 296 V	resorantel
HOE 304	desoximetasone
HOE 36801	etifoxine
HOE 39-893d	penbutolol sulfate
HOE 42-440	tiamenidine HCl
HOE440	tiamenidine
Hoe 473	aclantate
HOE 490	glimepiride
HOE 498	ramipril
HOE 760	roxatidine acetate HCl
HOE 766	buserelin acetate
HOE 777	prednicarbate
Hoe 881V	fenbendazole
HOE 893d	penbutolol sulfate
HOE 984	nomifensine maleate
Hoechst 10495	norpipanone
Hoechst 10582	normethadone
HP 029	velnacrine maleate
HP 128	suronacrine maleate
HP 1598	guanoxyfen sulfate
HP 3522	brocrinat
HP 494	fluradoline HCl
HP 522	brocrinat
HP 549	isoxepac
HP 749	besipirdine HCl
HP 873	iloperidone
HPA-23	generic not yet assigned—see main list
HPEK-1	tetroquinone
hPTH 1-34 (acetate salt)	teriparatide acetate
HR111V-sulfate	cefquinome sulfate
HR 221 (as sodium)	cefodizime
HR 376	clobazam
HR 756	cefotaxime sodium

HR 810 sulfate	cefpirome sulfate
HR 930	fosazepam
HRP 543	dazepinil HCl
HRP 913	neflumozide HCl
HS-592	clemastine
HSP 2986	pramiverine
HT-11	cloperastine
HTO	tritiated water
HU-211	generic not yet assigned—see main list
HUF-2446	clodazon HCl
HWA 285	propentofylline
HY-185	carbocloral
Hyal-ct 1101	generic not yet assigned—see main list
^{123}I labeled IMP	iofetamine HCl I 123
^{123}I-M123	iofetamine HCl I 123
I-653	desflurane
IA-307	acetosulfone sodium
ICI 118,587	xamoterol
ICI 118,630	goserelin
ICI 125,211	tiotidine
ICI 128,436	ponalrestat
ICI 136,753	tracazolate
ICI 139603	tetronasin
ICI 141,292	epanolol
ICI 156,834	cefotetan
ICI 176,334	bicalutamide
ICI 194,660	meropenem
ICI 204,219	zafirlukast
ICI 28257	clofibrate
ICI 29661	pyrimitate
ICI 32865	etoglucid
ICI-33,828	methallibure
ICI 35,868	propofol
ICI 38174 (as HCl)	pronetalol
ICI 45520	propranolol HCl
ICI 45763 (as HCl)	toliprolol
ICI 46,474	tamoxifen citrate
ICI 46683	oxyclozanide
I.C.I. 47,319	dexpropranolol HCl
ICI 48213	cyclofenil
ICI 50,123	pentagastrin
I.C.I. 50,172	practolol
I.C.I. 54,450	fenclozic acid
ICI 54,594 (as sodium salt)	brofezil
ICI 55,052	nequinate
ICI 55,897	clobuzarit
ICI 58,834	viloxazine HCl
ICI 59118	razoxane
ICI 66,082	atenolol
ICI 80,008 (as sodium salt)	fluprostenol sodium
ICI 80,996	cloprostenol sodium
ICI 81,008	fluprostenol sodium

ICI 8173	quindoxin
ICI D1033	anastrozole
ICI-U.S. 457	octazamide
ICN-542	ribaminol
ICRF 159	razoxane
ICRF-187	dexrazoxane
IL-17803A (as HCl)	acebutolol
IL-19552	pipotiazine palmitate
IL 22811 HCl	meptazinol HCl
IL 5902	spiramycin
IL 6001	trimipramine
IL-6302 mesylate	fonazine mesylate
IMI-28	epirubicin HCl
IMI 30	idarubicin HCl
IMI 58	esorubicin HCl
IN 1060	cyprolidol HCl
IN 29-5931B	triclofenol piperazine
IN 379	pimetine HCl
IN 461	benzindopyrine HCl
IN 511	phenyramidol HCl
IN 836	fenyripol HCl
INF-1837	flufenamic acid
INF-3355	mefenamic acid
INF 4668	meclofenamic acid
IP 302 sodium	citicoline sodium
IP 456	pagoclone
IPA	riboprine
IS 2596	domoxin
I.S. 499	poldine methylsulfate
ISIS 2105	generic not yet assigned—see main list
ISIS 2922	generic not yet assigned—see main list
isomer A	zuclomiphene
isomer B	enclomiphene
Janssen R 4929	benzetimide HCl
JAV 852	benfosformin
JB-8181	desipramine HCl
JD-96	vinylbital
JF-1	nalmefene
JL-1078	dihexyverine HCl
JL 512	fenadiazole
JM-8	carboplatin
JM-9	iproplatin
K 11941	alfaprostol
K 12148	lifibrol
K-17	thalidomide
K-1900	nimorazole
K-38	glycyclamide
K-386	glycyclamide
K 4024	glipizide
K 4277	indoprofen
K 9147	tolciclate
Kabi 2234	generic not yet assigned—see main list

KABI 925	emylcamate
KAT 256 (as HCl)	clobutinol
KB-944	fostedil
KB 95	benzpiperylon
K-F 224	naftoxate
KL-255 (as HCl)	bupranolol
KNI-272	generic not yet assigned—see main list
Ko 1173 Cl	mexiletine HCl
KO 1366	bunitrolol
Ko 592 (as HCl)	toliprolol
KS 33	oxyridazine
KW-110	aceglutamide aluminum
KW4679	olopatadine HCl
KWD 2019	terbutaline sulfate
L1	deferiprone
L-1573	cysteamine
L-1633	sodium dibunate
L-1718	osalmid
L-1777	medazomide
L 2197	benzarone
L-2214	benzbromarone
L 2329	benziodarone
L 2642	etabenzarone
L-3428	amiodarone
L-364,718	devazepide
L-4269	pyridarone
L-5103 Lepetit	rifampin
L-5418	diftalone
L 542	mercurobutol
L-554	tritoqualine
L 566	dibemethine
L 5818 (as HCl)	coumazoline
L-6257	oxetorone fumarate
L-627	biapenem
L-637,510	nelezaprine maleate
L-6400	fluazacort
L-647,339	naxagolide HCl
L-668,019	verlukast
L-669,455	dexibuprofen lysine
L-67	prilocaine HCl
L-696,229	generic not yet assigned—see main list
L-697,661	generic not yet assigned—see main list
L-735,524	indinavir sulfate
L-749	salacetamide
L 75 1362B	colforsin
L-8	lypressin
L 8027	nictindole
L-9394	butoprozine HCl
LA-012 (as HCl)	quatacaine
LA 1221 (as HCl)	butalamine
LA III	diazepam
LA 391	sodium picosulfate

La 6023	metformin
LAC-43	bupivacaine HCl
LAS 30451	pancopride
LAS 3876	almagate
LAS 9273	clebopride
LAS W-090	ebastine
LB 125	cyprodenate
LB-46	pindolol
LB-502	furosemide
LC 44	flupentixol
LD 2351 (as hydrobromide)	butopiprine
LD 2480	piprocurarium iodide
LD 2630	difencloxazine HCl
LD 2988	folescutol
LD 3055	oxypyrronium bromide
LD 335	propyromazine bromide
LD 3394	fenozolone
LD 3612	paraflutizide
LD 4644	pipebuzone
LD 935	dipiproverine HCl
Leo 1031	prednimustine
Leo 114	polyestradiol phosphate
levo-BC-2605	oxilorphan
levo-BC-2627	butorphanol
levo-BC-2627 tartrate	butorphanol tartrate
levo-BL-4566	moxazocine
LFA3TIP	generic not yet assigned—see main list
LGD 1069	generic not yet assigned—see main list
LJ 206	carbocysteine
LJC 10,141	felbinac
LJ C10,627	biapenem
LL 1530	nadoxolol
LL-705W	neutramycin
LM-1404	lortalamine
LM 176	cobamamide
LM 192	viquidil
LM 2717	clobazam
LM-427	rifabutin
LM-94	hymecromone
L.N. 107	broparestrol
LS-121	nafronyl oxalate
LS 2616	roquinimex
LS 519 C12	pirenzepine HCl
Lu 23-174	sertindole
LU3-010	talopram HCl
LVD	dextran 40
LY031537	ractopamine HCl
LY 048 740	avilamycin
LY061188	cephalexin HCl
LY097964	cefetamet
LY099094	vindesine sulfate
LY104208	vinzolidine sulfate

Appendix B: Investigational Code Names

LY 108380	doxpicomine HCl
LY110140	fluoxetine HCl
LY 119863	vinepidine sulfate
LY120363	flumezapine
LY121019	cilofungin
LY 122512	anitrazafen
LY 12271-72	viroxime
LY 122772	enviroxime
LY 123508	lorzafone
LY 127123	enviradene
LY 127623	metkephamid acetate
LY 127809	pergolide mesylate
LY 127935	moxalactam disodium
LY 135837	indecainide HCl
LY137998	somatropin
LY 139037	nizatidine
LY 139381	ceftazidime
LY 139603	tomoxetine HCl
LY 141894	amflutizole
LY 146032	daptomycin
LY 150378	clofilium phosphate
LY 150720	picenadol HCl
LY156758	raloxifene HCl
LY163502	quinelorane HCl
LY163892 monohydrate	loracarbef
LY167005	proinsulin human
LY170053	olanzapine
LY170680	sulukast
LY171555	quinpirole HCl
LY171883	tomelukast
LY 174008	dobutamine tartrate
LY 175326	isomazole HCl
LY177370	tilmicosin
LY177370 phosphate	tilmicosin phosphate
LY177837	somidobove
LY186641	sulofenur
LY 186655	tibenelast sodium
LY188011	gemcitabine
LY188011 HCl	gemcitabine HCl
LY 195115	indolidan
LY 201116	ameltolide
LY206243 lactobionate	levdobutamine lactobionate
LY207506	dobutamine lactobionate
LY 210448 HCl	dapoxetine HCl
LY 213829	tazofelone
LY215229 HCl	seproxetine HCl
LY 237216	dirithromycin
LY237733	amesergide
LY246708	xanomeline
LY246708 tartrate	xanomeline tartrate
LY248686 HCl	duloxetine HCl
LY253351	tamsulosin HCl

LY264618	lometrexol sodium
LY275585	insulin lyspro
LY277359	zatosetron maleate
LY281067	sergolexole maleate
LY 293111	generic not yet assigned—see main list
LY293404	rismorelin porcine
LY294468 sulfate	efegatran sulfate
LY295337	basifungin
LY307640 sodium	rabeprazole sodium
LYO31537	ractopamine HCl
M-1028 (Meiji)	haloprogin
M-14	rifamycin
M-141	spectinomycin HCl
M 285	cyprenorphine HCl
M. 5050	diprenorphine
M-811	salverine
M. 99 (as HCl)	etorphine
MA 1277	zolertine HCl
MA 1291	quipazine maleate
MA 1337	cloperidone HCl
MA-1443	letimide HCl
MA-540	quinuclium bromide
MA-593	salethamide maleate
MAB35	indium In 111 altumomab pentetate
MAK 195 F	generic not yet assigned—see main list
MAS-1	polyglyconate
Material A	pentetate calcium trisodium Yb 169
M&B 15497	decoquinate
M&B 16942A	diacetolol HCl
M&B 17803A (as HCl)	acebutolol
M&B 22948	zaprinast
M&B 33153	oxoprostol
M&B 39831	temozolomide
M&B 5062 A	amicarbalide
M&B 782 (as isethionate)	propamidine
MB 800 (as isethionate)	pentamidine
M&B 9302	clorgiline
MBR-4164-8	diflumidone sodium
MBR-4197	flucrylate
MBR 4223	triflumidate
MC 903	calcipotriene
MCE	metergoline
McN-1075	fenmetramide
McN-1107	clominorex
McN-1210	pyrinoline
McN-1231	fluminorex
McN-1546	flumetramide
McN-1589	mixidine
McN-2378	mefenidil
McN-2378-46	mefenidil fumarate
McN-2453	azepindole
McN-2559	tolmetin

McN-2559-21-98	tolmetin sodium
McN-2783-21-98	zomepirac sodium
McN-3113	xilobam
McN-3377-98	fenobam
McN-3495	pirogliride tartrate
McN-3716	methyl palmoxirate
McN-3802-21-98	palmoxirate sodium
McN-3802 (anhydrous free acid)	palmoxirate sodium
McN 3935	linogliride
McN-3935	linogliride fumarate
McN-4097-12-98	fenoctimine sulfate
McN-4853	topiramate
McN-742	aminorex
McN-A-2673-11	etoperidone HCl
McN-A-2833	perindopril
McN-A-2833-109	perindopril erbumine
McN-JR-13,558-11	fetoxylate HCl
McN-JR-15,403-11	difenoxin
McN-JR-1625	haloperidol
McN-JR-16,341	penfluridol
McN-JR-2498	trifluperidol
McN-JR-4263-49	fentanyl citrate
McN-JR-4584	benperidol
McN-JR-4749	droperidol
McN-JR-4929-11	benzetimide HCl
McN-JR-6218	fluspirilene
McN-JR-6238	pimozide
McN-JR-7242-11	difluanine HCl
McN-JR-7904	lidoflazine
McN-JR-8299-11	tetramisole HCl
McN-R-1162-22	potassium glucaldrate
McN-R-1967	fenretinide
McN-R-726-47	poldine methylsulfate
McN-R-73-Z	rotoxamine
McN-X-181	valnoctamide
McN-X-94	capuride
MD 141	ethamsylate
MD 2028	fluanisone
MD 67350 (as maleate)	cinepazide
MDL 100,240	generic not yet assigned—see main list
MDL 11,939	glemanserin
MDL 14,042	lofexidine HCl
MDL 16,455A	fexofenadine HCl
MDL 17,043	enoximone
MDL 18,962	plomestane
MDL 19,205	piroximone
MDL 19,744	tipentosin HCl
MDL-201129	beraprost sodium
MDL-201229	beraprost
MDL 201,404	generic not yet assigned—see main list
MDL 257	zindotrine
MDL 26,024G0	tetrazolast meglumine

MDL 26,479	suritozole
MDL 27,192	generic not yet assigned—see main list
MDL 28,314	generic not yet assigned—see main list
MDL 28,574	generic not yet assigned—see main list
MDL 458	deflazacort
MDL 473	rifapentine
MDL 507	teicoplanin
MDL 62,198	ramoplanin
MDL 62,769	rifamexil
MDL 71,754	vigabatrin
MDL 71,782 A	eflornithine HCl
MDL 72,222	bemesetron
MDL 72,422	tropanserin HCl
MDL 72,974A	mofegiline HCl
MDL 73,005EF	binospirone mesylate
MDL 73,147EF	dolasetron mesylate
MDL 73,745	zifrosilone
MDL 73,945	camiglibose
MEDR-640	generic not yet assigned—see main list
MER-29	triparanol
MER-41	clomiphene citrate
MF 934	rufloxacin
M.G. 13054	fenquizone
M.G. 13608	domiodol
M.G. 143	sulmarin
M.G. 1559	xenbucin
Mg 4833	fencibutirol
M.G. 5454	guaiapate
MG 559	metamfepramone
M.G. 5771	butixirate
M.G. 624	stilonium iodide
M.G. 652	oxamarin HCl
M.G. 8823	exaprolol HCl
M.G. 8926 (as HCl)	droprenilamine
MH-532	phenprobamate
MI-216	iothalamic acid
Mi-85	apazone
MJ 10061	benzbromarone
MJ 12,175-170	tiprinast meglumine
MJ 12,880-1	tipropidil HCl
MJ 13,105-1	bucindolol HCl
MJ 13401-1-3	fenprinast HCl
MJ 13,754-1	nefazodone HCl
MJ 1986	indriline HCl
MJ 1987	mesuprine HCl
MJ 1988	quazodine
MJ 1992	soterenol HCl
MJ 1998	metalol HCl
MJ 1999	sotalol HCl
MJ 4309-1	oxybutynin chloride
MJ 505	phenyramidol HCl
MJ 9022-1	buspirone HCl

MJ 9067-1	encainide HCl
MJ 9184-1	zinterol HCl
MJF 10,938	xipamide
MJF 11567-3	cefadroxil
MJF-12264	tegafur
MJF 12637	suloctidil
MJF 9325	ifosfamide
MK-0681	trientine HCl
MK-0787	imipenem
MK-0936	abamectin
MK-130 (as the base)	cyclobenzaprine HCl
MK-188	zeranol
MK-196	indacrinone
MK-208	famotidine
MK-217	alendronate sodium
MK-233	dexibuprofen lysine
MK-240	protriptyline HCl
MK-250	emylcamate
MK-329	devazepide
MK-341	tranilast
MK-351	methyldopa
MK-360	thiabendazole
MK-366	norfloxacin
MK-383	generic not yet assigned—see main list
MK-397	eprinomectin
MK-401	clorsulon
MK-417	sezolamide HCl
MK-422	enalaprilat
MK-458	naxagolide HCl
MK-462	generic not yet assigned—see main list
MK-476	montelukast sodium
MK-499	generic not yet assigned—see main list
MK-507	dorzolamide HCl
MK-521	lisinopril
MK 57	methyldesorphine
MK-591	quiflapon sodium
MK-595	ethacrynic acid
MK-621	efrotomycin
MK-639	indinavir sulfate
MK-678	seglitide acetate
MK-733	simvastatin
MK790	levomethadyl acetate HCl
MK-791	cilastatin sodium
MK-793	diltiazem maleate
MK-801	dizocilpine maleate
MK-803	lovastatin
MK-906	finasteride
ML-1024	theofibrate
ML 1034	celucloral
ML-1129	beraprost sodium
ML-1229	beraprost
MO-1255	encyprate

MO-911	pargyline HCl
MP-10013	iogulamide
MP-1051	silodrate
MP-1177	gadoversetamide
MP-1196	versetamide
MP-1554	technetium Tc 99m furifosmin
MP-1727	indium In 111 pentetreotide
MP 2032	iocarmic acid
MP 2032-meglumine	iocarmate meglumine
MP-271	iosefamic acid
MP 302 (with ioxaglate sodium)	ioxaglate meglumine
MP 328	ioversol
MP 4006	albumin, aggregated
MP 4018	stannous pyrophosphate
MP-537	iomethin I 125
MP-537	iomethin I 131
MP-600	betiatide
MP-6026	ioglucol
MP-620	iocetamic acid
MP 7010	stannous sulfur colloid
MP-8000	ioglucomide
MPV-1248	atipamezole
MPV-1440	dexmedetomidine
MPV-253 AII	detomidine HCl
MPV-785	medetomidine HCl
MR6S4	sevoflurane
MRL 38	hexadiline
MRL-41	clomiphene citrate
MRP-10	pentetate calcium trisodium Yb 169
MSI-78	generic not yet assigned—see main list
MSL-109	sevirumab
MTS 263	tropenziline bromide
MY-25 (as bitartrate)	metergotamine
MY-33-7 (as HCl)	lotucaine
MY-5116	repirinast
MYC 8003	mocimycin
MZ-144	rimazolium metilsulfate
N-0252	laurocapram
N-137	carbetimer
N-3	methetoin
N-399	xenytropium bromide
N-553 (as HCl)	tolperisone
N-7009	flupentixol
N-7020	meprotixol
N-714	chlorprothixene
N-746	clopenthixol
NA-119	bromamid
NA 274	bromhexine HCl
NA-66	pimeclone
NAB 365	clenbuterol
NASH	borocaptate sodium B 10
NAT-327	trimoxamine HCl

NAT-333	fenspiride HCl
NB 68	dacuronium bromide
NC-123	mesoridazine
NC 1264	thonzonium bromide
NC 150	phenazopyridine HCl
NC-1968	fungimycin
NC-7197	esproquin HCl
NCNU	pentamustine
ND 50	octopamine
NDC 0082-4155	daunorubicin HCl
NDR 263	propenzolate HCl
NDR 304	ethyl dibunate
NDR-5061A	aletamine HCl
NDR-5523A	trimoxamine HCl
NDR-5998A	fenspiride HCl
NE-10064	azimilide dihydrochloride
NE 11740	tebufelone
NE-19550	olvanil
NE-58095	risedronate sodium
NE 97221	piridronate sodium
NF-1010	nifurdazil
NF-1088	nifurquinazol
NF-1120	nifurimide
NF-1425	furazolium tartrate
NF-161	nifursemizone
NF-246	nifuradene
NF-602	levofuraltadone
NF-71	nifurmerone
NF-84	nifuraldezone
NF-902 (as HCl)	levofuraltadone
NF-963	furazolium chloride
NG-29	generic not yet assigned—see main list
NGD 91-1	generic not yet assigned—see main list
NIB	nabitan HCl
NIH 2933	dimepheptanol
NIH 7574	benzethidine
NIH 7607	etonitazene
NIH 7667	noracymethadol HCl
NIH 7672	methopholine
NIH 8805	buprenorphine HCl
NK 1006	bekanamycin
NK 204	basifungin
NK-631	peplomycin sulfate
NKK-105	malotilate
NKT-01	gusperimus trihydrochloride
NPAP	prajmalium bitartrate
NPT 15392	nosantine
NSD 1055	brocresine
Nu-1779	betaprodine
Nu-1932	betameprodine
NU-2121	nicotinyl alcohol
NU-445	sulfisoxazole diolamine

NY-198	lomefloxacin HCl
ODA 914	demoxytocin
OK-B7	generic not yet assigned—see main list
OLX-102	generic not yet assigned—see main list
OM 401	generic not yet assigned—see main list
OM-977	etaminile
OMDS	dipyrithione
OMS No 1825	azamethiphos
ONO-1078	generic not yet assigned—see main list
OP 21-23	parnaparin sodium
OPC-1085	carteolol HCl
OPC-14117	generic not yet assigned—see main list
OPC-17116	grepafloxacin HCl
OPC-8212	vesnarinone
ORF 10131	norgestimate
ORF 11676	nalmefene
ORF 15244	thymopentin
ORF 15817	edoxudine
ORF 15927	rioprostil
ORF 16600	bemarinone HCl
ORF 17070	histrelin
ORF 18704	pelretin
ORF 20257	doretinel
ORF 20485	tepoxalin
ORF 22164	atosiban
ORF 22867	bemoradan
ORF-8063	triflubazam
ORF 9326	nisterime acetate
ORG 10172	danaparoid sodium
ORG 2969	desogestrel
ORG 3236	etonogestrel
Org 32489	generic not yet assigned—see main list
ORG 3770	mirtazapine
Org 6216	rimexolone
ORG7417	resocortol butyrate
Org 817	epimestrol
ORG 9426	rocuronium bromide
Org GB 94	mianserin HCl
Org NA 97	pancuronium bromide
ORG NC 45	vecuronium bromide
Org OD 14	tibolone
P 071	cetirizine HCl
P-1011	dicloxacillin sodium
P-113	saralasin acetate
P-12	oxacillin sodium
P-1306	glyparamide
P-1496	zeranol
P-1560	taleranol
P-165	azaserine
P-1742	fluperolone acetate
P-1779	althiazide
P-1888	isosulfan blue

P-2105	epithiazide
P-248	levopropylcillin potassium
P-25	cloxacillin sodium
P-2525	polythiazide
P-2530	methalthiazide
P-2647	benzquinamide
P-286	ioxaglic acid
P-301	hydroxyphenamate
P-3232	somfasepor
P-3693A	doxepin HCl
P-3895	somfasepor
P-3896	guanisoquin sulfate
P-4125	isosulfan blue
P-4385B	clothixamide maleate
P-4599	cidoxepin HCl
P-463	fenamole
P-4657 B	thiothixene
P-50	ampicillin
P-5227	pinoxepin HCl
P53	tetrofosmin
P-5604	loteprednol etabonate
P-638	puromycin
P 7	lauroguadine
P-71	lycetamine
P 71-0129	fendosal
P-7138	nifurpirinol
P 720549	isoxepac
P 76 2494A	fluradoline HCl
P 76 2543	dazepinil HCl
P 78 3522	brocrinat
P79 3913	neflumozide HCl
P83 6029A	velnacrine maleate
PA-144	plicamycin
PAA-3854	clamoxyquin HCl
PAA-701	bialamicol HCl
PAM-MR-1165	acedapsone
PAM-MR-807-23a	cycloguanil pamoate
PAMN (as methonitrate)	prampine
PASIT	glyprothiazol
PAT	fenamole
PB 89 (as HCl)	fominoben
p-BIDA	butilfenin
PC1020 acetate	prezatide copper acetate
PC-1421	piperacetazine
PC-603	iproclozide
PD 107779	enoxacin
PD-110843	zonisamide
PD 81565	pentostatin
PD 90,695-73	dezaguanine mesylate
PD-93	piromidic acid
PDA-641	generic not yet assigned—see main list
PDB	prifinium bromide

PE1-1	tuvirumab
PEM-420	generic not yet assigned—see main list
pentapeptide DSDPR	pentigetide
PF-26	mepramidil
PFA-186	salicylate meglumine
PG 430	febuverine
PG-501	mazaticol
PH 218	edogestrone
pierrel-TQ 86	azipramine HCl
PIXY321	generic not yet assigned—see main list
PK 10169	enoxaparin
PM 1807	fenimide
PM-185184	secnidazole
PM-1952	fenacetinol
PM-3944	flucetorex
PM-671	ethosuximide
PMD-387	crilvastatin
PN 200-110	isradipine
POLI 67	tetrydamine
POR 8	ornipressin
PP 563	cyhalothrin
PPI-002	generic not yet assigned—see main list
PR-0818-156A	verilopam HCl
PR-122	redox phenytoin
PR-225	redox acyclovir
PR-239	redox penicillin G
PR-320	molecusol & carbamazepine
PR-3847	teroxalene HCl
PR-741-976A	somantadine HCl
PR-870-714A	veradoline HCl
PR-877-530L	flavodilol maleate
PR 879-317A	oxamisole HCl
PR 934-423A	remacemide HCl
PR-G 138-CL (as HCl)	ciclosidomine
protease 1	brinolase
PS-1286	pararosaniline pamoate
PS 2383	trimetozine
PSC-833	generic not yet assigned—see main list
PT-9	betahistine HCl
PU-239	benzilonium bromide
PY 108-068	darodipine
PZ 1511	carpipramine dihydrochloride
PZ68	pentosan polysulfate sodium
Q-12	technetium Tc 99m furifosmin
QB-1	cloquinozine
QZ-2	methaqualone
R 10.100	ethonam nitrate
R106-1	basifungin
R 10,948	diamocaine cyclamate
R 11,333	bromperidol
R 12,563 (as HCl)	dexamisole
R 12,564	levamisole HCl

Appendix B: Investigational Code Names

R 1303	carbofenotion
R-13423	dicloxacillin
R 13,558	fetoxylate HCl
R-13,672	haloperidol decanoate
R 1406	phenoperidine
R-148	methaqualone
R 14,827	econazole nitrate
R 14,889	miconazole nitrate
R 14,950	flunarizine HCl
R 15,403 (as HCl)	difenoxin
R-15,454 (as nitrate salt)	isoconazole
R 15,556	orconazole nitrate
R 1575	cinnarizine
R 15,889	lorcainide HCl
R-1625	haloperidol
R 16,341	penfluridol
R 16,470 (as HCl)	dexetimide
R 1658	moperone
R 1707	glafenine
R 17,147	cyclobendazole
R 17,635	mebendazole
R 17,889	flubendazole
R 17,934	nocodazole
R 18,553	loperamide HCl
R 1881	metribolone
R 18,910	fluperamide
R 1929	azaperone
R 19,317	rodocaine
R 2028	fluanisone
R 2113	desoximetasone
R 2159	anisopirol
R 2167	fluanisone
R 22,700 (as HCl)	rodocaine
R 23,050	salantel
R 2323	gestrinone
R 23,633	fludazonium chloride
R 23,979	enilconazole
R 2453	demegestone
R-2498	trifluperidol
R-25,061	suprofen
R-25,160	cliprofen
R 25,540	imafen HCl
R 25,831 (as the free base)	carnidazole
R 26,412	sulnidazole
R 27,500	sepazonium chloride
R 28,096 (as HCl)	carnidazole
R 2858	moxestrol
R-28,644	azaconazole
R 28,930	fluspiperone
R 2962	amiperone
R 29,764	clopimozide
R 29,860	nitramisole HCl

R 30,730	sufentanil
R 31,520	closantel
R 3248	aceperone
R 33,204	declenperone
R 3345	pipamperone
R 3365	piritramide
R 33,799	carfentanil citrate
R 33800	sufentanil citrate
R 33,812	domperidone
R 34,000	doconazole
R 34,009	milenperone
R 34,301	halopemide
R-34,803	etibendazole
R 34,995	lofentanil oxalate
R 35,443	oxatomide
R 38,198	buterizine
R 39,209	alfentanil HCl
R 39,500	parconazole HCl
R 3959	clometacin
R 4082	propyperone
R 41,400	ketoconazole
R-41,468	ketanserin
R-42,470	terconazole
R-4263	fentanyl citrate
R 4318	floctafenine
R 43,512	astemizole
R 4444	duometacin
R-45,486	flumeridone
R-4584	benperidol
R-46,541	bromperidol decanoate
R 46,846	tubulozole HCl
R 4714	oxiperomide
R-47,465	pirenperone
R-4749	droperidol
R 48	chlornaphazine
R 4845	bezitramide
R 5046	cinperene
R 50,547	levocabastine HCl
R 50 970	metrenperone
R 51 163	tameridone
R 51,211	itraconazole
R-51,469	mioflazine HCl
R 5147	spiperone
R 516	cinnarizine
R-51,619	cisapride
R 5188	spiroxatrine
R-52	mannosulfan
R 52,245	setoperone
R-53,200	altanserin tartrate
R 5385	acoxatrine
R 54,718	transcainide
R-548	tricetamide

R 55104	erbulozole
R 55,667	ritanserin
R 5808	spiramide
R58425	loperamide oxide
R 58735	sabeluzole
R 60844	irtemazole
R 610	racemoramide
R 6109	spirilene
R 6218	fluspirilene
R 6238	pimozide
R62,690	clazuril
R 62 818	lorcinadol
R 6438	antazonite
R64,433	diclazuril
R 64 766	risperidone
R 64947	noberastine
R65,824	nebivolol
R 661	buzepide metiodide
R 66905	saperconazole
R 67408	fenclofenac
R 68070	ridogrel
R 72063	loreclezole
R 7242	difluanine HCl
R 7464	propoxate
R 75231	draflazine
R 75251	liarozole HCl
R 77975	pirodavir
R 7904	lidoflazine
R 79598	ocaperidone
R 798	rimiterol hydrobromide
R 8025	antienite
R-803	furaprofen
R 805	nimesulide
R 8141	antienite
R-8193	antafenite
R 8284	proclonol
R 8299	tetramisole HCl
R-830	prifelone
R-830T	prifelone
R-835	ibafloxacin
R-837	imiquimod
R 83842	vorozole
R 85246	liarozole fumarate
R 87 926	generic not yet assigned—see main list
R 89 439	generic not yet assigned—see main list
R 91,274	generic not yet assigned—see main list
R 9298	seperidol HCl
R 93,777	generic not yet assigned—see main list
R 93,877	generic not yet assigned—see main list
RA-8	dipyridamole
RA-C-384	iodocetylic acid I 123
RBC-CD4	generic not yet assigned—see main list

Code	Generic
RC-160	vapreotide
RC-167	niceverine
RC-172	aldioxa
RC-173	alcloxa
RC-27109	nifuroxazide
RC 61-91	ifenprodil
RCH 314	benhepazone
RCM 258	fepentolic acid
RD 11654	ibufenac
RD 17345	fluprofen
RD 2801	pyritidium bromide
Rd 292	fenpentadiol
RD 328	pasiniazid
RD 406	cyprodenate
RD 9338 (as HCl)	norbudrine
Rec 15 0122	nifurpipone
Rec 15/1476	fenticonazole nitrate
Rec 7/0267	dimefline HCl
REV 3659-(S)	pivopril
REV 6000A	delapril HCl
RG 12525	generic not yet assigned—see main list
RG 12561	dalvastatin
RG-12915	generic not yet assigned—see main list
RG 12986	generic not yet assigned—see main list
RG 201	generic not yet assigned—see main list
RG 270	iomeglamic acid
RG 83606	diltiazem HCl
RG 83894	generic not yet assigned—see main list
RGH 1106	pipecuronium bromide
rgp160	generic not yet assigned—see main list
rgp160 MN	generic not yet assigned—see main list
RGW-2938	prinoxodan
RH-32,565	uredofos
RH-565	uredofos
RHC 2871	eclazolast
RHC 2906	flordipine
RHC 3659-(S)	pivopril
RHC 3988	quazolast
RI-64	pifexole
Riker 52G	aprotinin
Riker 594	sulthiame
Riker 595	butaperazine
Riker 601	triaziquone
RIT 1140	apicycline
RJW 60235	becaplermin
r-metHuG-CSF	filgrastim
RMI 10,482A	metizoline HCl
RMI 16,238	eterobarb
RMI 16,289	enclomiphene
RMI 16,312	zuclomiphene
RMI 80,029	elantrine
RMI 8090DJ	quindecamine acetate

RMI 81,182EF	cilobamine mesylate
RMI 81,968	medroxalol
RMI 81,968 A	medroxalol HCl
RMI 83,027	rolicyprine
RMI 83,047	ambuside
RMI 9,384A	desipramine HCl
RMI 9918	terfenadine
RMP-7	generic not yet assigned—see main list
Ro 01-6794/706	dextrorphan HCl
Ro 03-7355/000	avizafone
Ro 03-8799	pimonidazole
Ro 09-1978/000	capecitabine
Ro 10-1670/000	acitretin
Ro 10-6338	bumetanide
Ro 10-9070	amdinocillin
Ro 10-9071	amdinocillin pivoxil
Ro 10-9359	etretinate
Ro 11-1163/000	moclobemide
Ro 11-1430	motretinide
Ro 11-1781/023	tiapamil HCl
Ro 12-0068/000	tenoxicam
Ro 13-5057	aniracetam
Ro 13-6438/006	quazinone
RO 13-8996	oxiconazole nitrate
Ro-13-9297	lornoxicam
Ro 13-9904	ceftriaxone sodium
Ro 14-4767/000	amorolfine
Ro 14-9706/000	sumarotene
RO 1-5155	nicotinyl alcohol
Ro 15-1570/000	etarotene
Ro 15-1788/000	flumazenil
Ro 16-6028/000	bretazenil
Ro 1-6794	dextrorphan
Ro 17-2301/006	carumonam sodium
Ro 18-0647/002	orlistat
Ro 1-9334/19	dehydroemetine
Ro 1-9569	tetrabenazine
Ro 19-6327/000	lazabemide
Ro 20-5720/000	carprofen
Ro 21-0702	flurocitabine
Ro 21-3981/001	midazolam maleate
Ro 21-3981/003	midazolam HCl
Ro 21-5535	calcitriol
Ro 21-5998	mefloquine
Ro 21-5998/001	mefloquine HCl
Ro 21-6937/000	trimoprostil
Ro 21-8837/001	estramustine phosphate sodium
Ro 22-1319/003	piquindone HCl
Ro 22-2296/000	estramustine
Ro 22-3747/000	tiacrilast
Ro 22-3747/007	tiacrilast sodium
Ro 22-7796	cifenline

Code	Generic
Ro 22-7796/001	cifenline succinate
Ro 22-8181	interferon alfa-2a
Ro 22-9000	alfaprostol
Ro 2-2985	lasalocid
Ro 23-0731/000	sedecamycin
Ro 23-3544/000	ablukast
Ro 23-3544/001	ablukast sodium
Ro 23-6019	teceleukin
Ro 23-6240/000	fleroxacin
Ro 2-3773	clidinium bromide
Ro 24-2027/000	zalcitabine
Ro 24-5913	cinalukast
Ro 24-7375	dacliximab
Ro 24-7429	generic not yet assigned—see main list
Ro 2-9757	fluorouracil
Ro 2-9915	flucytosine
Ro-31-2848/006	cilazapril
Ro 31-3113	cilazaprilat
Ro-31-3948/000	romazarit
Ro 31-8959	saquinavir
Ro 31-8959/003	saquinavir mesylate
Ro 4-0403	chlorprothixene
Ro 40-5967/001	mibefradil dihydrochloride
Ro 40-7592	tolcapone
Ro 4-1544-6	sodium stibocaptate
Ro 4-1778/1	methopholine
Ro 4-2130	sulfamethoxazole
Ro 42-1611	arteflene
Ro 4-3780	isotretinoin
RO 4-3816	alcuronium chloride
Ro 4-4393	sulfadoxine
Ro 4-4602	benserazide
Ro 44-9883/000	lamifiban
Ro 4-5282	mefenorex HCl
Ro 4-5360	nitrazepam
Ro 4-6467/1	procarbazine HCl
Ro 46-6240/000	napsagatran
Ro 47-0203/029	bosentan
Ro 48347	trengestone
Ro 5-0690	chlordiazepoxide HCl
Ro 5-2092	demoxepam
Ro 5-2807	diazepam
Ro 5-3059	nitrazepam
RO 5-3307/1	debrisoquin sulfate
Ro 5-3350	bromazepam
Ro 5-4023	clonazepam
Ro 5-4200	flunitrazepam
Ro 5-4556	medazepam HCl
Ro 5-4645/010	coumermycin sodium
Ro 5-6901	flurazepam HCl
Ro 5-9110/1	dorastine HCl
Ro 5-9754	ormetoprim

Ro 6-4563	glibornuride
Ro 7-0207	ornidazole
Ro 7-0582	misonidazole
Ro 7-1554	ipronidazole
Ro 7-4488/1	cuprimyxin
RP 12222	penmesterol
RP 13057 (as the base)	daunorubicin HCl
RP 13607	clotioxone
RP 14539	secnidazole
RP 16091	metiazinic acid
RP 19552	pipotiazine palmitate
R.P. 19,583	ketoprofen
R.P. 20 578	bamnidazole
RP 22,050 HCl	zorubicin HCl
RP 22410	glisoxepide
RP 2254	glyprothiazol
RP 2259	glybuthiazol
rp24	generic not yet assigned—see main list
RP 2512 (as isethionate)	pentamidine
RP 27267	zopiclone
RP 2921	aminothiazole
RP 2987	diethazine HCl
RP 31264	suriclone
RP 3854	melarsoprol
RP 4763 (as sodium salt)	difetarsone
RP 5171	proadifen HCl
RP 5337	spiramycin
RP 54274	rulizole
RP 54476	dalfopristin
RP 54563	enoxaparin sodium
RP 56976	docetaxel
RP 57669	quinupristin
RP 60180	generic not yet assigned—see main list
RP 60475	intoplicine
RP 62955	pagoclone
RP 64305	ebastine
RP 64477	generic not yet assigned—see main list
RP 6484	etymemazine HCl
RP 6847	oxomemazine
RP 6870	inproquone
RP 7044	methotrimeprazine
RP 7204	cyamemazine
RP 7293	pristinamycin
RP 73401	generic not yet assigned—see main list
RP 7891	glybuzole
RP 8595	dimetridazole
RP 8823	metronidazole
RP 8909	periciazine
RP 9159	perimetazine
RP 9671	nosiheptide
RP 9778	protionamide
RP 9921	aprotinin

RP 9955	melarsonyl potassium
RR No. 32705	rutamycin
RS-10085-197	moexipril HCl
RS-11988	laidlomycin propionate potassium
RS-1301	delmadinone acetate
RS-1320	flunisolide acetate
RS 15385	generic not yet assigned—see main list
RS-15385-197	delequamine HCl
RS-21361	imiloxan HCl
RS-21592	ganciclovir
RS-21592 sodium	ganciclovir sodium
RS-21607-197	azalanstat dihydrochloride
R&S 218-M	alletorphine
RS-2208	amadinone acetate
RS-2252	flucloronide
RS-2362	procinonide
RS-2386	ciprocinonide
RS 25259	generic not yet assigned—see main list
RS-26306	ganirelix acetate
RS-3268R	nandrolone cyclotate
RS-3540	naproxen
RS-35887	butoconazole nitrate
RS-35887-00-10-3	butoconazole nitrate
RS-35909-00-00-0	ticabesone propionate
RS-3650	naproxen sodium
RS-3694R	cormethasone acetate
RS-37326	anirolac
RS-37449	temurtide
RS-3999	flunisolide
RS-4034	naproxol
RS-40584	flumoxonide
RS-40974-00-00-0	tiopinac
RS-43179	lonapalene
RS-43285	ranolazine HCl
RS-4464	triclonide
RS-44872	sulconazole nitrate
RS-44872-00-10-3	sulconazole nitrate
RS-4691	cloprednol
RS-49014	tazifylline HCl
R&S 5205-M	homprenorphine
RS-61443	mycophenolate mofetil
RS-6245	tazolol HCl
RS 66271	generic not yet assigned—see main list
RS-6818	xanoxate sodium
RS-68439	detirelix acetate
RS-69216	nicardipine HCl
RS-69216-XX-07-0	nicardipine HCl
RS-7337	tixanox
RS-82856	lixazinone sulfate
RS-82917-030	tifurac sodium
RS-84043	fenprostalene
RS-84135	enprostil

RS-85446-007	timobesone acetate
RS-87476-000	lifarizine
RS-8858	oxfendazole
RS-9390	prostalene
RS-94991-298	nafarelin acetate
RU 15060	tiaprofenic acid
Ru 15750	floctafenine
RU-1697	trenbolon acetate
RU-19110	halofuginone hydrobromide
RU-2267	altrenogest
RU 2323	gestrinone
RU 23908	nilutamide
RU 24756	cefotaxime sodium
RU 28965	roxithromycin
RU 38486	mifepristone
RU 38882	inocoterone acetate
RU 44570	trandolapril
RU 486	mifepristone
RU 882	inocoterone acetate
RU 965	roxithromycin
RWJ 10131	norgestimate
RWJ 15817	edoxudine
RWJ 15927	rioprostil
RWJ 16600	bemarinone HCl
RWJ-17021	topiramate
RWJ 17070	histrelin
RWJ 18704	pelretin
RWJ 20257	doretinel
RWJ 20485	tepoxalin
RWJ 21757	loroxibine
RWJ 22164	atosiban
RWJ 23989	generic not yet assigned—see main list
RWJ 24517	carsatrin succinate
RWJ 24834	linarotene
RWJ 29091	generic not yet assigned—see main list
RWJ 26127	generic not yet assigned—see main list
RWJ 26251	cladribine
RWJ 37796	mazapertine succinate
RX 6029-M HCl	buprenorphine HCl
Rx 67408	fenclofenac
RX77989	pentamorphone
R-(−)-YM-12617	tamsulosin HCl
S-041	gadodiamide
S-043	sprodiamide
S 10036	fotemustine
S-1210	bietaserpine
S-1320	budesonide
S 1530	nimetazepam
S-16820	prifelone
S-210	morsuximide
S-222	ditazole
S-2395	tertatolol

S-2539F	phenothrin
S-25930	ibafloxacin
S26308	imiquimod
S 314	fusafungine
S 4105	medibazine
S 5614 HCl	dexfenfluramine HCl
S-62	chlorphentermine HCl
S 7	fenticlor
S 73 4118	piretanide
S 77 0777	prednicarbate
S-940	naftalofos
S-9490	perindopril
S-9490-3	perindopril erbumine
S-9780	perindoprilat
SA-267	dipenine bromide
SB 7505	ibopamine
SBW-22	ketorfanol
SC 10363	megestrol acetate
SC 11585	oxandrolone
SC 11800	ethynodiol diacetate
SC-12350	nitralamine HCl
SC-12937	azacosterol HCl
SC-13504	ropizine
SC-13957	disopyramide phosphate
SC-14207	metogest
SC-14266	canrenoate potassium
SC-16148	silandrone
SC 1749 (as sodium salt)	menbutone
SC-18862	aspartame
SC-19198	methynodiol diacetate
SC-21009	norgestomet
SC-23992	prorenoate potassium
SC-25469	pinadoline
SC-26100	difenoximide HCl
SC-26304	dicirenone
SC-26438	pirolazamide
SC-26714	mexrenoate potassium
SC-27123	octriptyline phosphate
SC-27166	nufenoxole
SC-27761	pranolium chloride
SC-29333	misoprostol
SC-31828	disobutamide
SC-32642	metronidazole HCl
SC-32840	oxagrelate
SC-33643	bemitradine
SC-33963	reclazepam
SC-34301	enisoprost
SC-35135	edifolone acetate
SC-36602	actisomide
SC-37681	gemeprost
SC-38390	zinoconazole HCl
SC-39026	lodelaben

SC-40230	bidisomide
SC-4642	norethynodrel
SC-47111	lomefloxacin HCl
SC-47111A	lomefloxacin
SC-47111B	lomefloxacin mesylate
SC-48834	remiprostol
SC-49483	generic not yet assigned—see main list
SC-52151	telinavir
SC-52458	forasartan
SC-54684A	xemilofiban HCl
SC-55389A	droxinavir HCl
SC-7031	disopyramide
SC-7294	propetandrol
SC-7525	bolandiol dipropionate
SC-9376	canrenone
SC-9880	flurogestone acetate
SCE-1365 (Takeda) (base)	cefmenoxime HCl
Sch 1000-Br-monohydrate	ipratropium bromide
Sch 10144	tolnaftate
Sch 10159	triclofos sodium
Sch 10304	clonixin
Sch 10595	bupicomide
Sch 10649	azatadine maleate
Sch 11460	betamethasone dipropionate
Sch 11572	meclorisone dibutyrate
Sch 11973	tosifen
Sch 12041	halazepam
Sch 12149	pazoxide
Sch 12169	closiramine aceturate
Sch 12650	dazadrol maleate
Sch 12679	trepipam maleate
Sch 12707	clonixeril
Sch 13166 D fumarate	domazoline fumarate
Sch 13430.2KH$_2$PO$_4$	megalomicin potassium phosphate
Sch 13475 sulfate	sisomicin sulfate
Sch 13521	flutamide
Sch 13949W Sulfate	albuterol sulfate
Sch 14342	betamicin sulfate
Sch 14714	flunixin
Sch 14714 meglumine	flunixin meglumine
Sch 14947	rosaramicin
Sch 14947.NaH$_2$PO$_4$	rosaramicin sodium phosphate
Sch 14947 stearate	rosaramicin stearate
Sch 15280	azanator maleate
Sch 15427	carmantadine
Sch 15507	dopamantine
Sch 15698	fletazepam
Sch 15719W	labetalol HCl
Sch 16134	quazepam
Sch 16524	repromicin
Sch 17894	rosaramicin propionate
Sch 18020W	beclomethasone dipropionate

Sch 18667	rosaramicin butyrate
Sch 19741	picotrin diolamine
Sch 19927	dilevalol HCl
Sch 20569	netilmicin sulfate
Sch 21420	isepamicin
Sch 21480	tioxidazole
Sch 22219	alclometasone dipropionate
Sch 22591	pentisomicin
Sch 25298	florfenicol
Sch 2544	cycliramine maleate
Sch 28316Z	indenolol
Sch 29851	loratadine
Sch 30500	interferon alfa-2b
Sch 31353	dexamethasone acefurate
Sch 32088	mometasone furoate
Sch 32481	netobimin
Sch 33844	spirapril HCl
Sch 33861	spiraprilat
Sch 3444	parapenzolate bromide
Sch 35852	cisconazole
Sch 39300	molgramostim
Sch 39720	ceftibuten
SCH 40054 HCl	nemazoline HCl
Sch 4358	meprednisone
Sch 4831	betamethasone
Sch 4855	pseudoephedrine sulfate
Sch 6620	prednazate
Sch 6673	acetophenazine maleate
Sch 6783	diazoxide
Sch 7056	acrisorcin
Sch 9384	oxymetazoline HCl
Sch 9724	gentamicin sulfate
Scha-306	cintazone
SCL-70	alofilcon A
SCT 1	salcatonin
SCTZ (as edisylate)	clomethiazole
SCY-Er	erythromycin salnacedin
SD 1223-01	trazitiline
SD 1248-17 (as HCl)	tropatepine
SD 14112	sulclamide
SD 149-01	feneritrol
SD 15803	vincofos
SD 17102	meticrane
SD 1750	dichlorvos
SD 2102-18	acrocinonide
SD 2124-01	procinolol
SD 25	dicarfen
SD 270-07 (as succinate)	oxaprazine
SD 270-31 (as disuccinate)	oxaflumazine
SD 271-12	clobenzorex
SD 27115 (as cyclamate)	furfenorex
SD 286-03	cimemoxin

SD 7859	clofenvinfos
SDZ 215-811	pentetreotide
SDZ 215-811s	pentetreotide
SDZ MSL 109	sevirumab
SDZ OST 577	tuvirumab
SE 1702	gliclazide
SEB-324	generic not yet assigned—see main list
SEC-579	generic not yet assigned—see main list
SeHCAT	tauroselcholic acid
SF 86-327	terbinafine
SF-R11	bovactant
SG-75	nicorandil
SGD 301-76	oxiconazole nitrate
SGP 3	unifocon A
SH 100	oxapium iodide
SH 1040	gestaclone
SH 1051	glicetanile sodium
SH 2.1139/H 248 AB	ioxotrizoic acid
SH 213 AB	iotroxic acid
SH 240	moxnidazole
SH 263	droxacin sodium
SH 3.1168	gliflumide
SH 567	methenolone acetate
SH 570	generic not yet assigned—see main list
SH 582	gestonorone caproate
SH 601	methenolone enanthate
SH 714	cyproterone acetate
SH 717	glymidine sodium
SH 723	mesterolone
SH 741	clomegestone acetate
SH 742	fluocortolone
SH 770	fluocortolone caproate
SH 818	clocortolone acetate
SH 863	clocortolone pivalate
SH 926	iodamide
SH 968	diflucortolone pivalate
SH B 331	gestodene
SH E 199	etoformin HCl
SH G 318 AB	sermetacin
SH H 200 AB	ioglicic acid
SH H 239 AB	ioseric acid
SH K 203	fluocortin butyl
SH L 451 A	gadopentetate dimeglumine
SJ 1977	methixene HCl
SK&F 101468-A	ropinirole HCl
SK&F 102,362	nilvadipine
SK&F 104353-Q	pobilukast edamine
SKF 105657	epristeride
SK&F 10623	generic not yet assigned—see main list
SK&F 108566	eprosartan
SK&F 108566-J	eprosartan mesylate
SK&F 110679	generic not yet assigned—see main list

SK&F 12866	clorethate
SKF 13338	ampyrimine
SK&F 13364-A	thyromedan HCl
SK&F 1340	dimefadane
SK&F 14287	idoxuridine
SK&F 14336	clomacran phosphate
SK&F 15601A	toliodium chloride
SKF 16046	anisacril
SK&F 18,667	poloxalene
SK&F 1995	dicloralurea
SKF 20716	periciazine
SK&F 2208	hetaflur
SK&F 24529	lobendazole
SKF 2599	doxenitoin
SK&F 28175	fluotracen HCl
SK&F 29044	parbendazole
SK&F 30310	oxibendazole
SK&F 3050	cortodoxone
SKF 33134-A	amiodarone
SK&F 38094	dectaflur
SK&F 38095	olaflur
SK&F 39162	auranofin
SK&F 39186	amicloral
SK&F 40383	carbuterol HCl
SK&F 41558	cefazolin sodium
SK&F 478	diphenidol
SK&F 478-A	diphenidol HCl
SK&F 478-J	diphenidol pamoate
SK&F 51	octodrine
SK&F 5116	methotrimeprazine
SK&F 525-A	proadifen HCl
SK&F 53705-A	sulfonterol HCl
SK&F 59962	cefazaflur sodium
SK&F 61636	bromoxanide
SK&F 62698	ticrynafen
SK&F 62979	albendazole
SK&F 63797	dribendazole
SK&F 6539	flurothyl
SK&F 69634	clopipazan mesylate
SK&F 70230-A	pipazethate
SK&F 72517	elfazepam
SK&F 7690	benorterone
SK&F 7988	virginiamycin
SK&F 82526-J	fenoldopam mesylate
SKF-8318	xenazoic acid
SK&F 8542	triamterene
SK&F 88373-Z	ceftizoxime sodium
SKF 8898-A	moroxydine
SK&F 92058	metiamide
SK&F 92657-A_2	prizidilol HCl
SK&F 92676-A_3	impromidine HCl
SK&F 92994-A_2	oxmetidine HCl

SK&F 92994-J$_2$	oxmetidine mesylate
SK&F 93319	icotidine
SK&F 93479	lupitidine HCl
SK&F 93574	donetidine
SK&F 93944	temelastine
SK&F 94836	siguazodan
SK&F 95587	sulotroban
SK&F 96022	pantoprazole
SK&F 96148	daltroban
SK&F 97426	generic not yet assigned—see main list
SKF 9976 (as citrate)	oxolamine
SK&F D-39304	cephradine
SK&F D-75073-Z	cefonicid monosodium
SK&F D-75073-Z$_2$	cefonicid sodium
SK&F S-104846-A	topotecan HCl
SL 501	chlophedianol HCl
SL 75 177-10	cicloprolol HCl
SL 75.212-10	betaxolol HCl
SL 76 002	progabide
SL 77 499-10	alfuzosin HCl
SL 79.229-00	fengabine
SL 80.0342-00	alpidem
SL 80.0750-23N	zolpidem tartrate
SL 81.0142-00	tolgabide
SM-1213 (free base)	amiprilose HCl
SM-3997	tandospirone citrate
SM-7338	meropenem
SMP 68-40	pyrabrom
SMP-78 Acid S	ambruticin
SMS-201-995	octreotide
SMS-201-995 ac	octreotide acetate
Sms2PA	strontium chloride Sr 89
SN-166 (as the sodium salt)	glucosulfone
SN-263	sodium amylosulfate
S.N. 44	insulin, dalanated
SN 654	mepartricin
SNR 1804	clamidoxic acid
SNX-111	generic not yet assigned—see main list
SP-106	nabitan HCl
SP-119	tinabinol
SP-175	nabazenil
SP-204	menabitan HCl
SP-303	generic not yet assigned—see main list
SP-304	pirnabine
SP-325	naboctate HCl
SP54	pentosan polysulfate sodium
SP63	otilonium bromide
SPA-S-132	partricin
SPA-S-160	mepartricin
SPA-S-510	piroxicam cinnamate
SPA-S-565	rifametane
SPC-100270	safingol

SPC-100271	safingol HCl
SPC-101210	cedefingol
SPC 297 D	azidocillin
SPI-77	mitopodozide
SPM 925	moexipril HCl
SQ 10,269	carbiphene HCl
SQ 10,496	thiazesim HCl
SQ 10,643	cinanserin HCl
SQ 1089	hydroxyurea
SQ 11,302	epicillin
SQ 11436	cephradine
SQ 11725	nadolol
SQ 13050	econazole nitrate
SQ 13,396	iopamidol
SQ 13847	pirquinozol
SQ 14055	tiamulin
SQ 14,225	captopril
SQ 1489	thiram
SQ 15,101	algestone acetophenide
SQ 15,102	amcinafal
SQ 15,112	amcinafide
SQ 15,659	rolitetracycline
SQ 15,860	glyhexamide
SQ 15,874	pipazethate
SQ 16,123	methicillin sodium
SQ 16,150	estradiol enanthate
SQ 16360	fusidate sodium
SQ 16374	methenolone enanthate
SQ 16,401	halquinols
SQ 16,423	oxacillin sodium
SQ 16496	methenolone acetate
SQ 16,603	fusidic acid
SQ 18566	halcinonide
SQ 19844	sincalide
SQ 20009	etazolate HCl
SQ 20824	cicloprofen
SQ 20881	teprotide
SQ 2128	ethoxazene HCl
SQ 21982	iodoxamic acid
SQ 21983	iopronic acid
SQ 22022 (dihydrate)	cephradine
SQ 22947	tiamulin fumarate
SQ 26490	naflocort
SQ 26,703	zofenoprilat arginine
SQ 26776	aztreonam
SQ 26962	mebrofenin
SQ 26991	zofenopril calcium
SQ 27,239	tipredane
SQ 27,519	fosinoprilat
SQ 28555	fosinopril sodium
SQ 29,852	ceronapril
SQ 30217	technetium Tc 99m teboroxime

SQ 30836	tigemonam dicholine
SQ-31,000	pravastatin sodium
SQ 32,097	technetium Tc 99m siboroxime
SQ 32,692	gadoteridol
SQ 32,756	sorivudine
SQ 33,248	calteridol calcium
SQ 34,514	lobucavir
SQ 65396	cartazolate
SQ 82291	oximonam
SQ 82531	gloximonam
SQ 82629	oximonam sodium
SQ 83360	pirazmonam sodium
SQ 9343	phytate sodium
SQ 9453	dimethyl sulfoxide
SQ 9538	testolactone
SQ 9993	estradiol undecylate
SR-202	mifobate
SR 2508	etanidazole
SR 25990 C	clopidogrel
SR 33557	fantofarone
SR 41319B	tiludronate disodium
SR-7037	belfosdil
SR 720-22	metolazone
SR 96225	adenosine
SRG 95213	diazoxide
St 1085 (as the base)	midodrine HCl
ST12	dexamethasone dipropionate
St 1411	dimepregnen
ST1512/SO4	hexoprenaline sulfate
ST-155	clonidine HCl
ST-155-BS	clonidine
ST 375	tolonidine
St 567-BR (as hydrobromide)	alinidine
ST 600	flutonidine
ST-813	oxiconazole nitrate
ST 9067	azintamide
STA-307	tiomesterone
St. Peter 224	midodrine HCl
Su-10568	clortermine HCl
Su-13437	nafenopin
Su-18137	cyproquinate
Su 21524	pirprofen
Su-4885	metyrapone tartrate
Su-5864	guanethidine sulfate
Su-6518	dimethindene maleate
Su-8341	cyclopenthiazide
Su-9064	metoserpate HCl
SUD919CL2Y	pramipexole
SUM 3170	loxapine
SUR 2647	sumacetamol
SYD-230	clioxanide
synthetic TRH	protirelin

T-1220	piperacillin sodium
T-1551	cefoperazone sodium
T-1982	cefbuperazone
T-2636	sedecamycin
T-2636A	sedecamycin
T2G1s	biciromab
T30177	generic not yet assigned—see main list
T-3761	generic not yet assigned—see main list
T-3762	generic not yet assigned—see main list
T-88	generic not yet assigned—see main list
TA-3090	clentiazem maleate
TA 5901	cefempidone
TAP031 (as the base)	fertirelin acetate
TAP-144	leuprolide acetate
TAT-3	picoperine
TATBA	triamcinolone hexacetonide
TBC-3B	generic not yet assigned—see main list
Tc 924 (DPD)	butedronate tetrasodium
Tc99m-MP 4006	technetium Tc 99m albumin aggregated
Tc99m RP-30A	technetium Tc 99m sestamibi
TC-CYT-380	generic not yet assigned—see main list
TC-CYT-380 fragment	generic not yet assigned—see main list
Tc-MAG$_3$	technetium Tc 99m mertiatide
TE-031	clarithromycin
TE 114	tiemonium iodide
tenite butyrate formula 264 H4	cabufocon B
TH 1165a (as hydrobromide salt)	fenoterol
TH-1321	protionamide
Th-152	metaproterenol sulfate
TH-2151	hydracarbazine
TH-2180	propanidid
Th 322	metrifudil
THFES (HM)	zeranol
THR 221 (as sodium)	cefodizime
TI-23	generic not yet assigned—see main list
TJ-9	generic not yet assigned—see main list
TLC A-60	generic not yet assigned—see main list
TLC ABLC	generic not yet assigned—see main list
TLC C-53	generic not yet assigned—see main list
TLC D-99	generic not yet assigned—see main list
TMB-4	trimedoxime bromide
TNO-6	spiroplatin
TNP-470	generic not yet assigned—see main list
TP-1	thymostimulin
TP-21	thioridazine
TP-5	thymopentin
TPN-12	sulforidazine
TPS-23	mesoridazine
TR-2378	broperamole
TR-2515	pelanserin HCl
TR-2855	cromitrile sodium

TR-2985	ropitoin HCl
TR-3369	indorenate HCl
TR-4698	rioprostil
TR-495	methaqualone
TR-4979	butaprost
TR-5109	conorphone HCl
TR-5379M	xorphanol mesylate
TS 408	hydrocortisone buteprate
TSAA-291	oxendolone
TTFD	fursultiamine
TV-1203	generic not yet assigned—see main list
TVP-1012	rasagiline mesylate
TVX485	etofenamate
TWSB; TWSb	sodium stibocaptate
U-10,136	alprostadil
U-101.440E	irinotecan HCl
U-10,149	lincomycin
U-10,483	generic not yet assigned—see main list
U-10,858	minoxidil
U-10,974	flumethasone
U-10,997	mibolerone
U-11100A	nafoxidine HCl
U-12,019E	methylprednisolone sodium phosphate
U-12,062	dinoprostone
U-12,241	cirolemycin
U-12898	bluensomycin
U-13,933	asperlin
U-14,583	dinoprost
U-14,583E	dinoprost tromethamine
U-14,743	porfiromycin
U-15167	nogalamycin
U-15,614	trestolone acetate
U-15,965	lydimycin
U-17312E	etryptamine acetate
U-17,323	fluorometholone acetate
U-17835	tolazamide
U-18,409AE	spectinomycin HCl
U-18,496	azacitidine
U-18,573	ibuprofen
U-18,573G	ibuprofen aluminum
U-19183	sparsomycin
U-19,646	chlorphenesin carbamate
U-19,718	kalafungin
U-19763	bolasterone
U-19,920	cytarabine
U-19920A	cytarabine HCl
U-2032	kethoxal
U-20,661	steffimycin
U-21,251	clindamycin
U-22020	indoxole
U-22,550	calusterone
U-22,559A	dexoxadrol HCl

U-24,729A	mirincamycin HCl
U-24,792	lomofungin
U-24,973A	melitracen HCl
U-25,179 E	clindamycin palmitate HCl
U-25,873	ranimycin
U-26,225A	tramadol HCl
U-26,452	glyburide
U-27,182	flurbiprofen
U-28,009	denofungin
U-28,288D	guanadrel sulfate
U-28,508	clindamycin phosphate
U-28,774	ketazolam
U-29,479	scopafungin
U-30,604	zorbamycin
U-31,889	alprazolam
U-31,920	uldazepam
U-32,070E	calcifediol
U-32,921	carboprost
U-32,921E	carboprost tromethamine
U-33,030	triazolam
U-34,865	diflorasone diacetate
U-36,059	amitraz
U-36,384	carboprost methyl
U-41,123	adinazolam
U-41,123F	adinazolam mesylate
U-42,126	acivicin
U-42,585E	lodoxamide tromethamine
U-42,718	lodoxamide ethyl
U-42,842	arbaprostil
U-43,120	paulomycin
U-4527	cycloheximide
U-46,785	meteneprost
U-47,931E	bromadoline maleate
U-48,753E	eclanamine maleate
U-52,047	menogaril
U-53,059	itazigrel
U-53,217	epoprostenol
U-53,217A	epoprostenol sodium
U-53,996H	tazadolene succinate
U-54,461	bropirimine
U-54,555	metronidazole phosphate
U-54,669F	losulazine HCl
U-56,321	timefurone
U-57,930E	pirlimycin HCl
U-5956	filipin
U-6013	isoflupredone acetate
U-60,257	piriprost
U-60,257B	piriprost potassium
U-61,431F	ciprostene calcium
U-62066E	spiradoline mesylate
U-63,196	cefpimizole
U-63,196E	cefpimizole sodium

U-63287	ciglitazone
U-63,366F	trospectomycin sulfate
U-63,557A	furegrelate sodium
U-64279A	ceftiofur HCl
U-64279E	ceftiofur sodium
U-66858	bunaprolast
U-67,590A	methylprednisolone
U-67,590A	methylprednisolone suleptanate
U-69689E	fertirelin acetate
U-6987	carbutamide
U-70138	paldimycin
U-70226E	ibutilide fumarate
U-71038	ditekiren
U-72107A	pioglitazone HCl
U-72791	cefmetazole
U-72791A	cefmetazole sodium
U-73,975	adozelesin
U-74006F	tirilazad mesylate
U-75630	ibuprofen piconol
U-76252	cefpodoxime proxetil
U-77,233	ormaplatin
U-7743	mercufenol chloride
U-7750	streptovaricin
U-77779	bizelesin
U-7800	fluprednisolone
U-78875	panadiplon
U-78,938	dexormaplatin
U-80244	carzelesin
U-8344	uracil mustard
U-8471	medrysone
U-85,855	alvircept sudotox
U-87201E	atevirdine mesylate
U-88943E	artilide fumarate
U89	generic not yet assigned—see main list
U-90152S	delavirdine mesylate
U-93,385	generic not yet assigned—see main list
U-935	amiquinsin HCl
U-95376	premafloxacin
U-96988	generic not yet assigned—see main list
U-98079	generic not yet assigned—see main list
U-98222	generic not yet assigned—see main list
U-98528E	pramipexole
U-9889	streptozocin
U-98950	generic not yet assigned—see main list
UCB 1402	decloxizine
UCB 1474	chlorbenzoxamine HCl
UCB 1549	minepentate
UCB 1967	dropropizine
UCB 2073	etoxeridine
UCB 3928	fedrilate
UCB 4445	buclizine HCl
UDCG-115	pimobendan

UK-109,496	generic not yet assigned—see main list
UK-11,443	primidolol
UK-14304-18	brimonidine tartrate
UK-18,892	butikacin
UK-20,349	tioconazole
UK-2054	famotine HCl
UK-2371	memotine HCl
UK-25,842	oxfenicine
UK-31,214	propikacin
UK-31,557	carbazeran
UK-33,274-27	doxazosin mesylate
UK-3540-1	amedalin HCl
UK-3557-15	daledalin tosylate
UK-37,248-01	dazoxiben HCl
UK-38,485	dazmegrel
UK-4271	oxamniquine
UK-48,340-11	amlodipine maleate
UK-48,340-26	amlodipine besylate
UK-49,858	fluconazole
UK-61260-27	nanterinone
UK-61,689	semduramicin
UK-61,689-2	semduramicin sodium
UK-67,994	doramectin
UK-68,798	dofetilide
UK-738	ethybenztropine
UK-73,967	candoxatrilat
UK-76654-2 (as fumarate)	zamifenacin
UK-79,300	candoxatril
UK-80067	modipafant
UK-88060	espatropate
UM 952	buprenorphine HCl
UP 106	propizepine
UP 107	bepiastine
UP 164	morniflumate
UP 74	nixylic acid
UP 83	niflumic acid
USV 3659-(S)	pivopril
V-C 13	dichlofenthion
VCP 205	generic not yet assigned—see main list
VK-57	glyprothiazol
VLA-4	generic not yet assigned—see main list
VM-26	teniposide
VP-16-213	etoposide
VUAB6453 (SPOFA)	metipranolol
VX-478	generic not yet assigned—see main list
W-1015	nisobamate
W 10168	vifilcon A
W-1372	beloxamide
W 1655	phenazopyridine HCl
W 1760A	namoxyrate
W-19053 (as HCl)	etidocaine
W 1929	colistimethate sodium

W 2180	suxemerid sulfate
W 2197	pentrinitrol
W 2291A	mimbane HCl
W-2354	seclazone
W 2394A	pemerid nitrate
W-2395	meseclazone
W 2426	chlorphentermine HCl
W 2900A	etozolin
W-2946M	reproterol HCl
W-2964M	flupirtine maleate
W 2965 A	acetryptine
W-2979M	azelastine HCl
W 3207B	modaline sulfate
W 3366A	quindonium bromide
W 3395	algestone acetonide
W 3399	quingestrone
W 3566	quinestrol
W 3580B	ampyzine sulfate
W-36095	tocainide
W 3623	cyprazepam
W 3676	sulazepam
W 3699	piprozolin
W 37	buformin
W 3746	cetophenicol
W 3976B	triampyzine sulfate
W 4020	prazepam
W 42782	iproxamine HCl
W 43026A	ciclafrine HCl
W 4425	almadrate sulfate
W 4454A	estrazinol hydrobromide
W 4540	quingestanol acetate
W 4565	oxolinic acid
W 4600	algeldrate
W 4701	hexedine
W 4744	mecloqualone
W 4869	prednival
W-5219	proglumide
W 5494A	naranol HCl
W-554	felbamate
W 5733	atolide
W 5759A	tilidine HCl
W-583	mebutamate
W 5975	betamethasone benzoate
W 6309	difluprednate
W 6412A	bunolol HCl
W 6439A	suloxifen oxalate
W 6495	oxisuran
W 7000A	levobunolol HCl
W 713	tybamate
W 7320	alclofenac
W 7783	ambruticin
W 8495	isoxicam

WA 184	sitogluside
W-A 335	danitracen
WAL 2014 FU	talsaclidine fumarate
WAY-ANA-756	tasosartan
WAY-PEM-420	dexpemedolac
WAY-SEC-579	mirisetron maleate
WE352	triflubazam
We 941	brotizolam
We 973-BS	ciclotizolam
WG-253	rimiterol hydrobromide
WG 537 (as acetate)	flumedroxone
WH 5668	propanidid
WHR-1051B	biclodil HCl
WHR-1142A	lidamidine HCl
WHR-2908A	lofepramine HCl
WHR-5020	etofenamate
WHR-539	fenclorac
Win 11,318	bupivacaine HCl
Win 11450	benorilate
Win 11,464	fludorex
Win 11,530	menoctone
Win 11831	lorajmine HCl
Win 13,146	teclozan
Win 1344	gamfexine
Win 13820	becanthone HCl
Win 14833	stanozolol
Win 17625	azastene
Win 17665	topterone
Win 17,757	danazol
Win 1783	isomethadone
Win 18,320	nalidixic acid
Win 18,320-3	nalidixate sodium
Win 18,413-2	solypertine tartrate
Win 18,501-2	oxypertine
Win 18,935	milipertine
Win 19356	clorindanic acid
Win 20,228	pentazocine
Win 20,740	cyclazocine
Win 21,904	alexidine
WIN 22118	pegorgotein
Win 23,200	volazocine
Win 24,540	trilostane
Win 24,933	hycanthone
Win 25,347	nimazone
Win 25,978	amfonelic acid
Win 27147-2	cyclindole
Win 27,914	nivazol
Win 29194-6	carbantel lauryl sulfate
Win 31,665	alpertine
Win 32,729	epostane
Win 32,784	bitolterol mesylate
Win 3406	isoetharine

Appendix B: Investigational Code Names 649

Win 34,276	ketazocine
Win 34284	oxarbazole
Win 34886	nisbuterol mesylate
Win 35150	flucindole
Win 35,213	rosoxacin
Win 35833	ciprofibrate
Win 38020	arildone
Win 38770	azarole
Win 39103	metrizamide
Win 39424	iohexol
Win 40014	quinfamide
Win 40350	durapatite
Win 40680	amrinone
Win 40808-7	sulfinalol HCl
Win 41464-2	octenidine HCl
Win 41,464-6	octenidine saccharin
Win 41528-2	fezolamine fumarate
Win 42156-2	tonazocine mesylate
Win 42,202	fosarilate
Win 42964-4	zenazocine mesylate
Win 44,441-3	quadazocine mesylate
Win 47,203-2	milrinone
Win 48,049	ofornine
Win 48,098-6	pravadoline maleate
Win 49,016	medorinone
Win 49,375	amifloxacin
Win 49,375-3	amifloxacin mesylate
Win 49,596	zanoterone
Win 5063	racephenicol
Win 5063-2	thiamphenicol
Win 51,181-2	napamezole HCl
Win 51,711	disoxaril
Win 54,177-4	ipazilide fumarate
Win 5563-3	colterol mesylate
WIN 59010	generic not yet assigned—see main list
Win 59075	tirapazamine
Win 771	hydroxypethidine
Win 8851-2	tyropanoate sodium
Win 90,000	cicletanine
Win 9154	inositol niacinate
Win 9317	propatyl nitrate
Wl 140	calcium polycarbophil
Wl 287	euprocin HCl
Wl 291	zolamine HCl
WP-973	chlorhexidine phosphanilate
WR 142,490	mefloquine
WR-171669	halofantrine HCl
WR 180,409	enpiroline phosphate
WR-228,258	tebuquine
WR-2721	amifostine
WV 569 (as HCl)	norfenefrine
WX 14812	alofilcon A

WX 14822	hydrofilcon A
WX 2412	fungimycin
Wy-1359	propiomazine
WY-15,705	ciramadol
WY-15,705 HCl	ciramadol HCl
WY-16,225	dezocine
WY-18,251	tilomisole
Wy-2039	etoxeridine
WY-20,788	penamecillin
WY-21,743	oxaprozin
WY-21,894	fentiazac
Wy 21901	indoramin
WY-21,901 HCl	indoramin HCl
WY-22811 HCl	meptazinol HCl
WY-23,409	ciclazindol
WY-24,081 HCl	tiquinamide HCl
WY-24,377	isotiquimide
Wy-2445	carphenazine maleate
WY-25,021	rolgamidine
Wy-2837	potassium aspartate & magnesium aspartate
Wy-2838	potassium aspartate & magnesium aspartate
Wy-3263	iprindole
Wy-3277	nafcillin sodium
Wy-3467	diazepam
Wy-3475	norbolethone
Wy-3478	sodium oxybate
Wy-3498	oxazepam
Wy-3707	norgestrel
Wy-3917	temazepam
Wy-4036	lorazepam
WY-4082	lormetazepam
WY-40,972	lutrelin acetate
WY-42,362 HCl	recainam HCl
WY-42,362 tosylate	recainam tosylate
WY-44,417 sodium	apalcillin sodium
WY-44,635	cefpiramide
WY-44,635 sodium	cefpiramide sodium
WY-45,030	venlafaxine HCl
Wy-4508	cyclacillin
WY-460E	thiazinamium chloride
WY-47384	gevotroline HCl
WY-47,663 acetate	anaritide acetate
WY-47791 HCl	carvotroline HCl
WY-47846 HCl	zalospirone HCl
WY-48252	ritolukast
WY-48314	lexithromycin
WY-48624	enciprazine HCl
WY-48986	risotilide HCl
WY-50324 HCl	adatanserin HCl
WY-5104	levonorgestrel

Wy-806	oxethazaine
Wy-8138	bisoxatin acetate
Wy-8678	guanabenz
WY-8678 acetate	guanabenz acetate
WY-90493 RD	ardeparin sodium
X-1497	methicillin sodium
XLG	polyglactin 910
XM-72	polybutester
XU 62-320	fluvastatin sodium
XZ-450	azithromycin
Y 3642	tinoridine
Y 4153 (as HCl)	clocapramine
Y 6124 (as HCl)	bufetolol
YC-93	nicardipine HCl
YM-09330	cefotetan disodium
YM-12617-1	tamsulosin HCl
YM617	tamsulosin HCl
YN-72	sorivudine
YTR-830H	tazobactam
Z 1282	fosfomycin tromethamine
Z 326	fentonium bromide
Z 424	viminol
Z-4828	trofosfamide
Z4942	ifosfamide
Z 6000	troxerutin
ZCE025	indium In 111 altumomab
ZD 0490	generic not yet assigned—see main list
ZD 0870	generic not yet assigned—see main list
ZD1033	anastrozole
ZD 1694	generic not yet assigned—see main list
ZD2079	generic not yet assigned—see main list
ZD 2138	generic not yet assigned—see main list
ZD 3523	generic not yet assigned—see main list
ZD 7288	generic not yet assigned—see main list
Zeneca 182,780	generic not yet assigned—see main list
Zeneca 200,880	generic not yet assigned—see main list
ZK 10 720	ioprocemic acid
ZK 35760	iopromide
ZK 39 482	iotrolan
ZK 57 671	sulprostone
ZK 62 711	rolipram
ZK 71 630	iotetric acid
ZK 76 604	pirazolac
ZK 79 112	iotasul

APPENDIX C
Abbreviations Used with Medications and Dosages

Abbreviation	Literally	Meaning
a.c.	ante cibum	before meals or food
ad	ad	to, up to
A.D., AD	auris dextra	right ear
ad lib.	ad libitum	at pleasure
A.L.	auris laeva	left ear
a.m., A.M.	ante meridiem	morning
Aq.	aqua	water
A.S., AS	auris sinistra	left ear
A.U., AU*	auris uterque	each ear
b.i.d.	bis in die	twice daily
b.m.	bowel movement	
cc, cm³	cubic centimeter	
d.	die	day
et	et	and
g	gram(s)	
gt. (plural gtt.)	gutta (plural guttae)	a drop (drops)
h.	hora	hour
h.s.	hora somni	at bedtime
IM†	intramuscular	
IV†	intravenous	
mcg, μg	microgram(s)	
mg	milligram(s)	
mEq	milliequivalent(s)	
mL, ml	milliliter(s)	
O.D.	oculus dexter	right eye
O.L.	oculus laevus	left eye
O.S.	oculus sinister	left eye
O.U.§	oculus uterque	each eye
p.c.	post cibum	after meals
p.m., P.M.	post meridiem	afternoon or evening
p.o.	per os	by mouth
p.r.n.	pro re nata	as needed
q.a.d.	quaque alterni die	every other day
q.d.	quaque die	every day
q.h.	quaque hora	every hour
q.i.d.	quater in die	four times a day
q.o.d.		every other day
q.s.	quantum satis	sufficient quantity
q.s. ad	quantum satis ad	a sufficient quantity to make
℞, Rx	recipe	take; a recipe

Abbreviation	Literally	Meaning
Sig.	signetur	label
s.o.s.	si opus sit	if there is need
stat	statim	at once, immediately
t.i.d.	ter in die	three times a day
tsp.	teaspoonful	
μg, mcg	microgram(s)	

---

* Although some references have aures unitas (Latin, both ears), this cannot be justified by classical Latin.

† Some references suggest that IM and IV be typed with periods to distinguish from Roman numerals, but we believe context is sufficient to make this distinction.

§ Although some references have oculi unitas (Latin, both eyes), this cannot be justified by classical Latin.

APPENDIX D
Therapeutic Drug Levels

Drug	Class	Serum Levels metric units (SI units)
amantadine	antiviral	300 ng/mL
amikacin	aminoglycoside	16-32 μg/mL
amiodarone	antiarrhythmic	0.5-2.5 μg/mL
amitriptyline	antidepressant	110-250 ng/mL
amoxapine	antidepressant	200-500 ng/mL
amrinone	cardiotonic	3.7 μg/mL
bretylium	antiarrhythmic	0.5-1.5 μg/mL
bupropion	antidepressant	25-100 ng/mL
carbamazepine	anticonvulsant	4-12 μg/mL (17-51 μmol/L)
chloramphenicol	antibiotic	10-20 μg/mL (31-62 μmol/L)
chlorpromazine	antipsychotic	30-500 ng/mL
clomipramine	antidepressant	80-100 ng/mL
cyclosporine	immunosuppressive	250-800 ng/mL (whole blood, RIA*)
trough values:		50-300 ng/mL (plasma, RIA*)
desipramine	antidepressant	125-300 ng/mL
digitoxin	antiarrhythmic	9-25 μg/L (11.8-32.8 nmol/L)
digoxin	antiarrhythmic	0.5-2.2 ng/mL (0.6-2.8 nmol/L)
disopyramide	antiarrhythmic	2-8 μg/mL (6-18 μmol/L)
doxepin	antidepressant	100-200 ng/mL
flecainide	antiarrhythmic	0.2-1 μg/mL
fluphenazine	antipsychotic	0.13-2.8 ng/mL
gentamicin	aminoglycoside	4-8 μg/mL
haloperidol	antipsychotic	5-20 ng/mL
hydralazine	antihypertensive	100 ng/mL
imipramine	antidepressant	200-350 ng/mL
kanamycin	aminoglycoside	15-40 μg/mL
lidocaine	antiarrhythmic	1.5-6 μg/mL (4.5-21.5 μmol/L)
lithium	antipsychotic	0.5-1.5 mEq/L (0.5-1.5 mmol/L)
maprotiline	antidepressant	200-300 ng/mL
mexiletine	antiarrhythmic	0.5-2 μg/mL
netilmicin	aminoglycoside	6-10 μg/mL
nortriptyline	antidepressant	50-150 ng/mL
perphenazine	antipsychotic	0.8-1.2 ng/mL

Drug	Class	Serum Levels metric units (SI units)
phenobarbital	anticonvulsant	15-40 µg/mL (65-172 µmol/L)
phenytoin	anticonvulsant	10-20 µg/mL (40-80 µmol/L)
primidone	anticonvulsant	5-12 µg/mL (25-46 µmol/L)
procainamide	antiarrhythmic	4-8 µg/mL (17-34 µmol/L)
propranolol	antiarrhythmic	50-200 ng/mL (190-770 nmol/L)
protriptyline	antidepressant	100-200 ng/mL
quinidine	antiarrhythmic	2-6 µg/mL (4.6-9.2 µmol/L)
salicylate	analgesic	100-200 mg/L (725 1448 µmol/L)
streptomycin	aminoglycoside	20-30 µg/mL
sulfonamide	antibiotic	5-15 mg/dL
terbutaline	bronchodilator	0.5-4.1 ng/mL
theophylline	bronchodilator	10-20 µg/mL (55-110 µmol/L)
thiothixene	antipsychotic	2-57 ng/mL
tobramycin	aminoglycoside	4-8 µg/mL
tocainide	antiarrhythmic	4-10 µg/mL
trazodone	antidepressant	800-1600 ng/mL
valproic acid	anticonvulsant	50-100 µg/mL (350-700 µmol/L)
vancomycin	antibiotic	30-40 ng/mL (peak)
verapamil	antiarrhythmic	0.08-0.3 µg/mL

* radioimmunoassay

APPENDIX E
The Most Prescribed Drugs

Drug	Class/Indications
Accupril (quinapril HCl)	antihypertensive, ACE inhibitor
acetaminophen with codeine	analgesic, anti-inflammatory
Adalat CC (nifedipine)	antianginal, antihypertensive
Advil, Children's (ibuprofen)	NSAID, antiarthritic, analgesic
albuterol sulfate	bronchodilator
alprazolam	anxiolytic, sedative
Altace (ramipril)	antihypertensive, ACE inhibitor
Ambien (zolpidem tartrate)	sedative, hypnotic
amitriptyline HCl	antidepressant
amoxicillin trihydrate	antibiotic
Amoxil (amoxicillin trihydrate)	antibiotic
atenolol	antiadrenergic
Atrovent (ipratropium bromide)	bronchodilator
Augmentin (amoxicillin trihydrate, clavulanate potassium)	antibiotic
Axid (nizatidine)	H_2 antagonist, antiulcer
Azmacort (triamcinolone acetonide)	corticosteroid for asthma
Bactroban (mupirocin)	topical antibiotic
Beconase AQ (beclomethasone dipropionate)	steroidal anti-inflammatory
Biaxin (clarithromycin)	antibiotic
BuSpar (buspirone HCl)	anxiolytic
Calan SR (verapamil HCl)	antianginal, antiarrhythmic, antihypertensive
Capoten (captopril)	antihypertensive, ACE inhibitor
Carafate (sucralfate)	antiulcer
Cardizem (diltiazem HCl)	antiarrhythmic, antihypertensive, antianginal
Cardura (doxazosin mesylate)	antihypertensive, antiadrenergic
carisoprodol	skeletal muscle relaxant
Ceclor (cefaclor)	antibiotic
cefaclor	antibiotic
Ceftin (cefuroxime axetil)	antibiotic
Cefzil (cefprozil)	antibiotic
cephalexin	antibiotic
cimetidine	antiulcer
Cipro (ciprofloxacin)	antibiotic
Claritin (loratadine)	antihistamine
Claritin-D (loratadine, pseudoephedrine sulfate)	antihistamine, decongestant
Compazine (prochlorperazine maleate)	antiemetic, tranquilizer
Cotrim DS (sulfamethoxazole, trimethoprim)	anti-infective, antibacterial

Coumadin (warfarin sodium)	anticoagulant
cyclobenzaprine HCl	skeletal muscle relaxant
Cycrin (medroxyprogesterone acetate)	progestin
Darvocet-N (propoxyphene napsylate, acetaminophen)	narcotic analgesic
Daypro (oxaprozin)	NSAID
Deltasone (prednisone)	glucocorticoid
Demulen (ethynodiol diacetate, ethinyl estradiol)	oral contraceptive
Depakote (divalproex sodium)	anticonvulsant
Desogen (ethinyl estradiol, desogestrel)	oral contraceptive
DiaBeta (glyburide)	antidiabetic
diazepam	anxiolytic, skeletal muscle relaxant
dicyclomine HCl	antispasmodic, anticholinergic
Diflucan (fluconazole)	systemic antifungal
Dilacor XR (diltiazem HCl)	antihypertensive
Dilantin (phenytoin sodium)	anticonvulsant
doxycycline hyclate	antibacterial
Duricef (cefadroxil monohydrate)	antibiotic
Dyazide (hydrochlorothiazide, triamterene)	diuretic, antihypertensive
E.E.S. (erythromycin ethylsuccinate)	antibiotic
Effexor (venlafaxine)	antidepressant
Elocon (mometasone furoate)	topical corticosteroid
Ery-Tab (erythromycin)	antibiotic
Erythrocin Stearate (erythromycin stearate)	antibiotic
erythromycin base	antibiotic
Estrace (estradiol)	topical estrogen
Estraderm (estradiol)	estrogen replacement
Fiorinal with Codeine (codeine phosphate, acetaminophen, caffeine, butalbital)	narcotic analgesic, sedative
Flonase (fluticasone propionate)	steroidal anti-inflammatory
Floxin (ofloxacin)	antibiotic
furosemide	diuretic, antihypertensive
gemfibrozil	antihyperlipoproteinemic
glipizide	antidiabetic
Glucotrol (glipizide)	antidiabetic
glyburide	antidiabetic
Glynase (glyburide)	antidiabetic
guaifenesin with phenylpropanolamine	expectorant, decongestant
Hismanal (astemizole)	antihistamine
Humulin (human insulin)	antidiabetic
hydrochlorothiazide	diuretic, antihypertensive
hydrocodone with acetaminophen	antitussive, analgesic
Hytrin (terazosin HCl)	antihypertensive
Imitrex (sumatriptan succinate)	antimigraine
K-Dur (potassium chloride)	potassium supplement
Klonopin (clonazepam)	anticonvulsant
Klor-Con (potassium chloride)	potassium supplement
Lanoxin (digoxin)	antiarrhythmic
Lasix (furosemide)	diuretic

Appendix E: The Most Prescribed Drugs

Lescol (fluvastatin sodium)	antihyperlipidemic
Levoxyl (levothyroxine sodium)	thyroid hormone
Lodine (etodolac)	NSAID, analgesic, antiarthritic
Loestrin Fe (norethindrone acetate, ethinyl estradiol, ferrous fumarate)	oral contraceptive with iron
Lo/Ovral (ethinyl estradiol, norgestrel)	oral contraceptive
Lopressor (metoprolol tartrate)	antianginal, antihypertensive, beta blocker
Lorabid (loracarbef)	antibiotic
lorazepam	anxiolytic, tranquilizer
Lorcet (hydrocodone bitartrate, acetaminophen)	narcotic analgesic
Lorcet Plus (hydrocodone bitartrate, acetaminophen)	narcotic analgesic
Lotensin (benazepril HCl)	antihypertensive, ACE inhibitor
Lotrisone (betamethasone dipropionate, clotrimazole)	topical corticosteroid, antifungal
Lozol (indapamide)	antihypertensive, diuretic
Macrobid (nitrofurantoin macrocrystals, nitrofurantoin monohydrate)	urinary antibacterial
medroxyprogesterone	progestin
methylphenidate HCl	CNS stimulant for ADHD
methylprednisolone	corticosteroidal anti-inflammatory
metoprolol tartrate	antiadrenergic
Mevacor (lovastatin)	antihyperlipidemic
Micronase (glyburide)	antidiabetic
Monopril (fosinopril sodium)	antihypertensive, ACE inhibitor
Motrin (ibuprofen)	NSAID, antiarthritic, analgesic
Motrin, Childen's (ibuprofen)	NSAID, antiarthritic, analgesic
naproxen sodium	NSAID, antiarthritic, analgesic
Nasacort (triamcinolone acetonide)	corticosteroidal anti-inflammatory
neomycin/polymyxin/hydrocortisone	antibiotic, steroidal anti-inflammatory
Nitro-Dur (nitroglycerin)	antianginal
Nitrostat (nitroglycerin)	antianginal
Nizoral (ketoconazole)	systemic antifungal
nortriptyline HCl	tricyclic antidepressant
Norvasc (amlodipine)	antianginal, antihypertensive
Ortho-Cept (ethinyl estradiol, desogestrel)	oral contraceptive
Ortho-Novum 1/35 (norethindrone, ethinyl estradiol)	oral contraceptive
Ortho-Novum 7/7/7 (norethindrone, ethinyl estradiol)	oral contraceptive
Oruvail (ketoprofen)	NSAID, antiarthritic, analgesic
Paxil (paroxetine HCl)	antidepressant
PCE [polymer-coated erythromycin]	antibiotic
Penicillin-VK (penicillin V potassium)	antibiotic
Pepcid (famotidine)	antiulcer
Phenergan (promethazine HCl)	antihistamine, antiemetic, sedative
potassium chloride	potassium supplement
Pravachol (pravastatin sodium)	antihyperlipidemic
prednisone	corticosteroidal anti-inflammatory

Premarin (conjugated estrogen)	estrogen replacement
Prilosec (omeprazole)	antiulcer
Principen (ampicillin trihydrate)	antibiotic
Prinivil (lisinopril)	antihypertensive, ACE inhibitor
Procardia XL (nifedipine)	antianginal, antihypertensive
promethazine with codeine	narcotic antitussive, antihistamine
Propacet (propoxyphene napsylate, acetaminophen)	narcotic analgesic
propoxyphene napsylate with acetaminophen	narcotic analgesic
Propulsid (cisapride)	gastroesophageal reflux
Proventil aerosol (albuterol)	bronchodilator
Provera (medroxyprogesterone acetate)	progestin
Prozac (fluoxetine HCl)	antidepressant
Relafen (namubetone)	NSAID, antiarthritic
Retin-A (tretinoin)	topical keratolytic
Ritalin (methylphenidate HCl)	CNS stimulant for ADHD
Roxicet (oxycodone HCl, acetaminophen)	narcotic analgesic
Seldane (terfenadine)	antihistamine
Seldane-D (terfenadine, pseudoephedrine HCl)	antihistamine, decongestant
Serevent (salmeterol xinafoate)	antiasthmatic, bronchodilator
sulfamethasoxazole with trimethoprim	anti-infective, antibacterial
Sumycin (tetracycline HCl)	antibiotic
Suprax (cefixime)	antibiotic
Synthroid (levothyroxine sodium)	thyroid replacement
Tegretol (carbamazepine)	anticonvulsant
temazepam	tranquilizer, hypnotic
Tenormin (atenolol)	antianginal, antihypertensive, beta blocker
Terazol (terconazole)	antifungal
Theo-Dur (theophylline)	bronchodilator
Timoptic (timolol maleate)	antiglaucoma
Toprol XL (metoprolol succinate)	antihypertensive, antianginal
Toradol (ketorolac tromethamine)	NSAID
Trental (pentoxifylline)	hemorrheologic agent, improve circulation
triamterene with hydrochlorothiazide	diuretic, antihypertensive
Tri-Levlen (levonorgestrel, ethinyl estradiol)	oral contraceptive
trimethoprim with sulfamethoxazole	anti-infective, antibacterial
Trimox (amoxicillin trihydrate)	antibiotic
Triphasil (levonorgestrel, ethinyl estradiol)	oral contraceptive
Tylenol with Codeine (acetaminophen, codeine phosphate)	analgesic
Ultram (tramadol HCl)	analgesic
Valium (diazepam)	sedative, skeletal muscle relaxant, anticonvulsant adjunct
Vancenase AQ (beclomethasone dipropionate)	steroidal anti-inflammatory

Appendix E: The Most Prescribed Drugs

Vanceril (beclomethasone dipropionate)	corticosteroid for bronchial asthma
Vasotec (enalaprilat maleate)	antihypertensive, ACE inhibitor
Veetids (penicillin V potassium)	antibiotic
Ventolin (albuterol sulfate)	bronchodilator
verapamil HCl	antianginal, antiarrhythmic, calcium channel blocker
Verelan (verapamil HCl)	antianginal, antiarrhythmic, calcium channel blocker
Vicodin (hydrocodone bitartrate, acetaminophen)	narcotic analgesic
Voltaren (diclofenac sodium)	NSAID, antiarthritic, analgesic
Xanax (alprazolam)	anxiolytic
Zantac (ranitidine HCl)	antiulcer
Zestril (lisinopril)	antihypertensive
Zithromax (azithromycin dihydrate)	antibiotic
Zocor (simvastatin)	antihyperlipidemic
Zoloft (sertraline)	antidepressant
Zovirax (acyclovir)	antiviral

Dropped from the previous list:

Ansaid (flurbiprofen)	NSAID
Ativan (lorazepam)	anxiolytic
Bumex (bumetanide)	diuretic
doxepin HCl	tricyclic antidepressant, anxiolytic
DynaCirc (isradipine)	antihypertensive
E-Mycin (erythromycin)	antibiotic
Entex LA (phenylpropanolamine HCl, guaifenesin)	decongestant, expectorant
Inderal (propranolol HCl)	antianginal, antihypertensive
Intal (cromolyn sodium)	bronchodilator, antiasthmatic
isosorbide dinitrate	coronary vasodilator, antianginal
Levoxine (levothyroxine sodium)	thyroid replacement
Lopid (gemfibrozil)	antihyperlipoproteinemic
Lortab (hydrocodone bitartrate, acetaminophen)	narcotic analgesic
Maxzide (triamterene, hydrochlorothiazide)	diuretic, antihypertensive
Micro-K (potassium chloride)	potassium supplement
Naprosyn (naproxen)	NSAID, antiarthritic, analgesic
Nolvadex (tamoxifen citrate)	hormonal therapy for breast cancer
Ogen (estropipate sulfate)	estrogen replacement therapy
Orasone (prednisone)	glucocorticoid
Ovcon (norethindrone, ethinyl estradiol)	oral contraceptive
penicillin V	antibiotic
Peridex (chlorhexidine gluconate)	antimicrobial
Proventil Repetabs (albuterol sulfate)	bronchodilator
Sinemet (carbidopa, levodopa)	antiparkinsonian
Slo-bid (theophylline)	antiasthmatic, bronchodilator
Tagamet (cimetidine)	antiulcer
thyroid	thyroid hormone replacement